Quick Reference

Chapter	Title[a]	Procedures[b]	Case Studies[c]
1	Foundations of Immunology	• Identification of Leukocytes Related to Immune Function • Screening Test for Phagocytic Engulfment	**CASE 1.1** A 1-month-old female infant born 6 weeks prematurely was admitted to the hospital because she had a high fever and was crying all of the time.
2	Soluble Mediators of the Immune System	• C-Reactive Protein Rapid Latex Agglutination Test	**CASE 2.1** A 39-year-old woman was admitted for a cholecystectomy. The patient became febrile 1 day after surgery.
3	Antigens and Antibodies	• ABO Blood Grouping (Forward Antigen Typing)	**CASE 3.1** A 38-year-old White woman presented to the emergency department of her local hospital with increased difficulty in breathing and chronic diarrhea.
4	Cellular Activities and Clinical Disorders of Innate and Adaptive Immunity	• Screening Test for Phagocytic Engulfment • Assessment of Cellular Immune Status	**CASE 4.1** A family had a son who died age 2 weeks because of overwhelming bacterial infection. When their newborn daughter began developing recurrent infections, she was immediately taken to a pediatrician. **CASE 4.2** A 6-year-old White male patient was taken to a pediatrician because of recurring abscesses since the age of 1 month. **CASE 4.3** A 33-year-old man, the child of unrelated parents of Mexican descent, was examined because of a history of frequent sore throats and sinus headaches.
5	Safety in the Immunology-Serology Laboratory	• Test Your Safety Knowledge	**CASE 5.1** When a new employee in a rural laboratory started to work, she wiped down the work bench with 5% bleach and donned latex gloves that she had rinsed off the night before.
6	Quality Control and Quality Assurance Practices	• Validation of a New Procedure Write-Up	**CASE 6.1** A new employee was asked to examine a CLISI procedural protocol worksheet and rate the write-up.
7	Serologic Laboratory: Techniques and Clinical Applications	• Card Pregnancy Testing	**CASE 7.1** A 9-year-old boy was taken to the emergency department with a sore throat. **CASE 7.2** A 28-year-old woman has been trying to get pregnant for the past 6 months. Although she has no health problems, conceiving a child is proving to be difficult.
8	Precipitation and Particle Agglutination Methods	• ABO Blood Grouping (Reverse Grouping)	**CASE 8.1** An 85-year-old man had a discrepancy between his forward grouping (ABO antigens) and reverse grouping (ABO antibodies).
9	Electrophoresis Techniques and Chromatography	• Immunofixation Electrophoresis	**CASE 9.1** A 40-year-old woman with a long-term history of alcohol abuse comes to the emergency department complaining of difficulty breathing.
10	Labeling Techniques in Immunoassay	• Pregnancy Testing • Direct Fluorescent Antibody Test for *Neisseria gonorrhoeae*	**CASE 10.1** A 25-year-old woman had a missed menstrual period 3 weeks earlier.
11	Flow Cytometry	• Laboratory Activities	**CASE 11.1** The parents of a 6-year-old boy brought him to the hospital complaining of back pain and refusal to walk since falling a week earlier.
12	Molecular Laboratory Techniques	• Molecular testing—Group A *Streptococcus* Direct Test	**CASE 12.1** A 38-year-old man drove himself to the emergency department because of a worsening condition of shortness of breath. He had a sore throat, felt tired, and had a fever, unproductive cough, and mild chest pain.
13	Infectious Diseases: Overview and TORCH Diseases	• Rapid TORCH Testing • Passive Latex Rubella Agglutination Test • Passive Latex Agglutination for Detection of Antibodies to Cytomegalovirus • Quantitative Determination of Antibodies to Cytomegalovirus	**CASE 13.1** A 34-year-old Black male was a local delivery truck driver until 2 weeks ago when he was laid off because of the SARS-CoV-2 pandemic. He has been an organist at his local church for the past 5 years. Two weeks ago, he began to feel very tired but had no other medical complaints. **CASE 13.2** A 24-year-old woman with a history of acquired immunodeficiency syndrome (AIDS) comes to the clinic for evaluation of left-sided weakness. She has been experiencing headaches and seizures, and others had observed an alteration in her mental status. **CASE 13.3** A 20-year-old college junior comes to the student health office because she had been exposed to rubella during a recent outbreak at the college. She had been immunized as a child. **CASE 13.4** A 35-year-old man recently received a kidney transplant. He had been feeling well until 2 weeks before, when he experienced a sore throat, fever, chills, profound malaise, and myalgia.

(Continued)

Quick Reference—cont'd

Chapter	Title[a]	Procedures[b]	Case Studies[c]
14	Streptococcal Infections	• Antistreptolysin O Latex Test Kit • OSOM Ultra Streptococcus A Test • Group A Streptococcus Direct Test • Antistreptolysin O Classic Procedure	**CASE 14.1** A 19-year-old woman visited the emergency department (ED) with swelling and redness of her right leg.
15	Syphilis	• Classic Venereal Disease Research Laboratory Test—Venereal Disease Research Laboratory Qualitative Slide Test • Rapid Plasma Reagin Card Test • Fluorescent Treponemal Antibody Absorption Test	**CASE 15.1** A 25-year-old woman comes to an ambulatory center with pain in the right side of her pelvis and a slightly elevated temperature.
16	Vector-Borne Diseases	Rapid *Borrelia burgdorferi* Antibody Detection Assay	**CASE 16.1** A 42-year-old executive lives in New York City. Her company annually sponsors a Memorial Day weekend golf outing at a Long Island club. In early June, she noticed a solid bright red spot on her left thigh. **CASE 16.2** A 25-year-old graduate student visits his local family physician because of episodic arthromyalgia, sporadic global headaches, fatigue, irritability, and depression. Over the last several months, he has become seriously dysfunctional at work and home. **CASE 16.3** A 45-year-old man from upstate New York visits his physician because of a worsening headache, myalgia, arthralgia, and generalized weakness. He had been in good health until about 1 week before the appointment. **CASE 16.4** A 73-year-old previously healthy man had spent the previous summer on Martha's Vineyard. On returning to his home in Boston after Labor Day, he began to feel unusually tired and had difficulty breathing. **CASE 16.5** A 35-year-old field biologist from central Missouri was positive for human immunodeficiency virus (HIV). Her work required that she spend a great deal of time in the woods in the surrounding areas. Although she was in good health despite the HIV positivity, she began having back pain, fever, chills, sweats, productive cough, and extreme tiredness before her visit to the emergency department.
17	Infectious Mononucleosis	• Paul-Bunnell Screening Test • Davidsohn Differential Test • MonoSlide Test	**CASE 17.1** A female college freshman visits the infirmary complaining of extreme fatigue, frequent headaches, and a sore throat.
18	Viral Hepatitis	• Rapid Hepatitis C Virus Testing	**CASE 18.1** Several workers at a local fast food restaurant called in sick and reported to the local ambulatory clinic for treatment. All of them complain of extreme fatigue. In addition, another 26-year-old food handler, who returned from visiting his relatives in Costa Rica a month ago, is sick. **CASE 18.2** A 30-year-old phlebotomist presents with fever, persistent fatigue, and joint pain. She reports that a needle in a plastic garbage bag nicked her finger about 2 months ago. **CASE 18.3** A 75-year-old woman had an 18-month history of right-sided abdominal pain and progressive fatigue. Her other medical problems include insulin-dependent diabetes mellitus and hypertension. **CASE 18.4** A 45-year-old previously healthy medical technologist visits her primary care physician because of increasing fatigue and loss of appetite.
19	Primary and Acquired Immunodeficiency Syndromes	• Rapid HIV Antibody Test • GS HIV Combo Ag/Ab EIA • Simulation of HIV-1 Detection	**CASE 19.1** Mary is a freshman in college. She began to feel ill with diarrhea and a cough. She tried to ignore the symptoms but woke up the next morning with a severe headache and a painful stiff neck. **CASE 19.2** Mr. J.J. Smith, aged 68 years, had retired to Florida and was meeting with his new primary care provider for the first time. His medical history indicated that he had suffered from recurrent upper and lower respiratory and gastrointestinal infections throughout his life. **CASE 19.3** A 40-year-old man with a history of IV drug use came to the emergency department because of a rash and fever. In addition, the patient complained of a several-day history of malaise, fatigue, fever, headache, and sore throat.

Quick Reference—cont'd

Chapter	Title[a]	Procedures[b]	Case Studies[c]
20	Hypersensitivity Reactions	• Rapid Test for Food Allergy • Direct Antiglobulin Test	CASE 20.1 A 60-year-old man was stung by a bee while gardening. CASE 20.2 A 35-year-old gravida 4 para 1 + 2 was seen by her gynecologist when she was 8 weeks pregnant. Her first pregnancy 4 years ago was unremarkable. The patient reported that her second and third pregnancies had resulted in a stillbirth at 36 weeks and a spontaneous abortion at 10 weeks of gestation. CASE 20.3 A patient had a medical history that included frequent sore throats as a child. He had been treated with antibiotics, particularly penicillin. Eventually, he developed a rash. He was told that he had developed an allergy to penicillin and should not have it again. CASE 20.4 A 19-year-old college student went to the Student Health Services because she had a slowly developing rash on both earlobes, her hands and her wrists, and around her neck. CASE 20.5 A 35-year-old woman reported that she had experienced three bouts of urticaria of unknown origin about 10 years ago.
21	Plasma Cell Neoplasms and Other Diseases with Paraproteins	• Bence Jones Protein Screening Procedure	CASE 21.1 A 58-year-old nuclear power plant worker saw his family physician because of increasing fatigue and weakness.
22	Tolerance, Autoimmunity, and Autoimmune Disorders	• Rapid Slide Test for Antinucleoprotein	CASE 22.1 A 50-year-old White woman visited her primary care provider because of extreme fatigue. She also reported experiencing mild pain in her abdominal region. CASE 22.2 A right-handed 25-year-old woman had no significant medical history. She came to the emergency department because of a sudden onset of slurred speech.
23	Systemic Lupus Erythematosus	• Antinuclear Antibody Visible Method • Rapid Slide Test for Antinucleoprotein • Autoimmune Enzyme Immunoassay ANA Screening Test	CASE 23.1 A 39-year-old Black woman with SLE was diagnosed with the illness 20 years ago. CASE 23.2 A 27-year-old White woman sought medical attention because of persisting pain in her wrists and ankles and an unexplained skin irritation on her face.
24	Rheumatoid Arthritis	• Rapid Agglutination	CASE 24.1 A 62-year-old woman experienced pain in her left knee unrelated to trauma. The pain occurred primarily with weight bearing. She is currently being treated for hypertension but is otherwise healthy. CASE 24.2 A 31-year-old patient was referred to a rheumatologist because of pain and stiffness in her fingers and wrists. Before her last pregnancy 3 years earlier, she had experienced similar symptoms, but these had gone away.
25	Transplantation: Human Leukocyte Antigens, Solid Organ, and Hematopoietic Stem Cells	• Longitudinal Assessment of Posttransplant Immune Status	CASE 25.1 A 40-year-old was seen by her family physician after several episodes of painless hematuria. On direct questioning, she complained of worsening malaise and swelling of her legs and hands over the previous 2 weeks.
26	Tumor Immunology and Applications of Massive Parallel Sequencing/Next-Generation Sequencing	• Prostate-Specific Antigen Rapid Test of Seminal Fluid (Seratec)	CASE 26.1 A 59-year-old White man visited his primary care provider because of his need to urinate frequently and urgently. Over the past several years, his urine output had been in small volumes, with a decreasing flow rate. CASE 26.2 A 65-year-old Black woman visited her primary care provider for an annual examination, including a routine pelvic examination. Although she had gained some weight since her last examination, she reported that her general health was good, but that she had been experiencing some gastrointestinal problems over the last 6 weeks.
27	Vaccines-Development and Applications	• Tetanus Antibodies (IgG)	CASE 27.1 A 25-year-old female medical student came to the emergency department because of a fever, cough, and shortness of breath.

[a]Digital enrichment files for animated content, virtual labs, web-based videos, and additional chapter-specific outline web resources are available on the Elsevier Evolve website for approved textbook adopters (instructors).
[b]The principles and clinical applications of these procedures are explained in the textbook. Procedural protocols and other technical details are posted and explained on the Elsevier Evolve website for approved textbook adopters (instructors).
[c]Fully developed case studies and associated questions are published in associated chapters. A full, narrative discussion of the questions for each case study is posted on the Elsevier Evolve website for approved textbook adopters (instructors).

EIGHTH EDITION
Immunology & Serology
in Laboratory Medicine

Mary Louise Turgeon
EdD, MLS(ASCP)CM

Clinical Laboratory Education Consultant,
Mary L. Turgeon and Associates
Boston, Massachusetts;
St. Petersburg, Florida

Associate Professor
Chair, Department of Medical Laboratory Science (previous)
Northeastern University
Bouve College of Health Professions
Boston, Massachusetts

Professor
Program Director (previous)
Medical Laboratory Technology
Corning Community College
Corning, New York

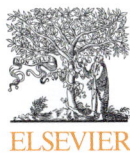
ELSEVIER

Elsevier
3251 Riverport Lane
St. Louis, Missouri 63043

IMMUNOLOGY & SEROLOGY IN LABORATORY MEDICINE, EIGHTH EDITION ISBN: 978-0-443-12298-9
Copyright © 2026 by Elsevier Inc. All rights are reserved, including those for text and data mining, AI training, and similar technologies.

For accessibility purposes, images in electronic versions of this book are accompanied by alt text descriptions provided by Elsevier. For more information, see https://www.elsevier.com/about/accessibility.

Publisher's note: Elsevier takes a neutral position with respect to territorial disputes or jurisdictional claims in its published content, including in maps and institutional affiliations.

No part of this publication may be reproduced or transmitted in any form or by any means, electronic or mechanical, including photocopying, recording, or any information storage and retrieval system, without permission in writing from the publisher. Details on how to seek permission, further information about the Publisher's permissions policies and our arrangements with organizations such as the Copyright Clearance Center and the Copyright Licensing Agency, can be found at our website: www.elsevier.com/permissions.

This book and the individual contributions contained in it are protected under copyright by the Publisher (other than as may be noted herein).

Notice

Practitioners and researchers must always rely on their own experience and knowledge in evaluating and using any information, methods, compounds or experiments described herein. Because of rapid advances in the medical sciences, in particular, independent verification of diagnoses and drug dosages should be made. To the fullest extent of the law, no responsibility is assumed by Elsevier, authors, editors or contributors for any injury and/or damage to persons or property as a matter of products liability, negligence or otherwise, or from any use or operation of any methods, products, instructions, or ideas contained in the material herein.

Previous editions copyrighted © 2022, 2018, 2014, 2009, 2003, 1996, 1990.

Content Strategist: Melissa J. Rawe
Senior Content Development Specialist: Shilpa Kumar
Publishing Services Manager: Deepthi Unni
Project Manager: Manchu Mohan
Senior Design Direction: Amy Buxton

Printed in India

Last digit is the print number: 9 8 7 6 5 4 3 2 1

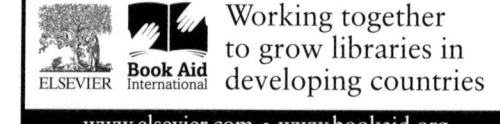

To the continuing support and learning adventures shared with Dick.

REVIEWERS

Denise Pacovsky, MS, MLS (ASCP)^{CM}
MLT Program Director, Faculty, Clinical Coordinator
Flathead Valley Community College
Kalispell, MT

Stephen M. Johnson, MLS (ASCP), MS
Program Director
Saint Vincent Hospital
Iowa City, IA

Cynthia Funne Doby, EdD, MAED, MS, BS, MT (AMT), CPT(NPA)
Assistant Professor
City Colleges of Chicago
Chicago, IL

Michele G. Harms, MS, MLS (ASCP)
Program Director
UPMC Chautauqua Medical Laboratory Science Program-
Jamestown, NY

Deborah Josko, PhD, MLT (ASCP)M, SM
Associate Professor
Rutgers, The State University of New Jersey – School of Health Professions
Newark, NJ

PREFACE

The overall goal of the 8th edition of *Immunology & Serology in Laboratory Medicine* is to facilitate mastery of the knowledge required by medical laboratory technician (MLT) and medical laboratory science (MLS) students to achieve excellent scores on national board certification or licensure examinations upon graduation and to display entry-level professional competencies for career success.

Immunology & Serology in Laboratory Medicine was the first textbook in this discipline to be designed and written specifically for MLT and MLS students and faculty. Every edition of this book is classroom and laboratory "field tested" by MLT and MLS students and instructors including the book's author. Consequently, instructor and student feedback is a voice in recognizing the newest professional curriculum instructor and student needs and state-of-the-art educational content.

The presentation of content in *Immunology & Serology in Laboratory Medicine* strives to convey relevant content in sufficient detail for MLT and MLS students. The style of presentation in the book underscores the importance of clarity, conciseness, and continuity of information for medical laboratory science students. Sole authorship of this textbook ensures a smooth transition from chapter to chapter without unnecessary redundancy, content gaps, or a change in writing style.

Sharp focusing on the most important principles and laboratory practices at the undergraduate level contributes to the popularity and continuing success of each edition of this book. Every chapter of the 8th edition of *Immunology & Serology in Laboratory Medicine* reflects the most recent concepts and practices related to the study of immunology and serology as it applies to the clinical laboratory. Each revision of the book clearly addresses the changes in content and the challenges for students to learn more and for instructors to teach more in a fixed time frame. Each chapter in a current edition capitalizes on the strengths of previous editions based on up-to-date information presented at annual meetings and conferences, publications in professional literature, web-based research, and comments received from students, faculty, prepublication faculty book reviewers, and comments from professionals working around the globe.

Immunology & Serology in Laboratory Medicine continues to be a distinctly unique textbook because of the recognition of the importance of the professional knowledge and practice guidelines in the current American Society for Clinical Laboratory Science (ASCLS) documents including the ASCLS Professional Body of Knowledge in immunology and applicable molecular science diagnostic applications. In addition, the latest ASCP Board of Certification Examination Content Outline for the Medical Laboratory Technician, MLT(ASCP), and Medical Laboratory Scientist, MLS(ASCP), categories of certification are used as reference guidelines.

DISTINCTIVE FEATURES OF *IMMUNOLOGY & SEROLOGY IN LABORATORY MEDICINE* 8TH EDITION

The 8th edition of *Immunology & Serology in Laboratory Medicine* continues to use an original platform to present and integrate new content and practices. This edition of the book continues to strengthen the robust pedagogy that was established in the first edition and continues to be enriched as a quality benchmark.

Immunology & Serology in Laboratory Medicine continues to recognize critical thinking as an essential component of learning. To promote critical thinking, a total of 50 clinical cases are fully developed and presented in the 8th edition. These cases have extensively developed content, case-related multiple-choice questions, and open-ended critical analysis group discussion questions. These cases promote critical thinking and stimulate an overall interest in medicine, including highlighting the essential role of the laboratory in patient diagnosis and treatment.

Students in the digital age are visual learners. To accommodate this learning style, many colorful and highly acclaimed illustrations, tables, and boxes are incorporated throughout the book. Many algorithms are featured in *Immunology & Serology in Laboratory Medicine* because of the value of high-impact visuals that accommodate learning preferences of today's students.

The organization of the book allows for tremendous flexibility in instructional design and delivery. The book is well suited for traditional on-campus instruction, hybrid, or blended modes of teaching, and online delivery of courses. The 8th edition provides students with a basic foundation in the theory and practice of clinical immunology and practical serology in a one- or two-term course at MLT or MLS levels of instruction.

To enhance learning, there are a total of 650 end-of-chapter multiple-choice review questions. Some traditional content has been retained in the book or transferred to the web-based Evolve platform, because some questions related to classic content may appear on certification or licensure examinations, and under-resourced locations in the United States and worldwide may use classic manual techniques.

The procedural protocol, including specimen collection, the required materials, actual procedure, and expected reference results, is published on the Evolve websites for students and instructors who wish to select a particular laboratory exercise in their curriculum. Instructors can easily select procedures and create a customized laboratory manual that students can print, as needed. This reduces the risk of soiling or contaminating their textbook in a wet laboratory. By reducing the number of pages devoted to laboratory procedures in the text, which may not be desired in a course, the planet gets a little greener in addition to the associated savings in the production cost.

Content correlation between lecture and reading, procedures, and case studies is featured in the inside cover of the book for easy reference. Suggestions for web-based videos and virtual laboratories have been compiled by chapter and are presented on the Evolve site.

HIGHLIGHTS OF SIGNIFICANT CONTENT REVISIONS OR ADDITIONS

The content in *Immunology & Serology in Laboratory Medicine* 8th edition is organized into six parts. All of the content has been reviewed and refreshed as needed. Statistical reports of clinical diseases or disorders is carefully monitored with the most recent available data included in relevant chapters. In addition, key concepts are interwoven throughout each chapter in order to highlight important facts. Use of these key concepts enables more focused learning of the content narrative as it unfolds in a chapter. End-of-chapter review questions have been reviewed and revised as needed.

Part I—Basic Immunologic Mechanisms (Chapters 1–4)

In this section, content is arranged into Chapters 1 to 4. The arrangement focuses on examining the immune system in a holistic manner rather than as independent entities.

Chapter 1, Foundations of Immunology, begins with the history of immunology by presenting a classic timeline of discoveries and Black scientists. However, a unique addition to this topic is the inclusion of diverse women and Black scientists who contributed significant milestones in the history of immunology.

This chapter organizes the cells and tissues of innate and adaptive immune systems to enable students to relate new immunology content to various blood cells that may have been studied in previous courses. A comparison of the three lines of immunologic defense introduces student to normal immunologic body defense activities.

In **Chapter 2, Soluble Mediators of the Immune System** are introduced early in the book. The early introduction of information related to soluble mediator substances, e.g., complement and cytokines, allows students to link the activities of these constituents to innate body defenses discussed in Chapter 1.

To assist with the understanding of the importance of testing complement, current testing algorithms and tables summarizing complement testing are included in Chapter 2.

In addition to a discussion of complement disorders, a new disorder, Complement Deficiency Disorder-Hereditary Angioedema, has been added with a detailed narrative of the disorder.

Chapter 3, **Antigens and Antibodies**, the hallmarks of immunologic activities, has been placed in this position in the flow of information to facilitate association of content with the previous chapters.

Chapter 4, Cellular Activities and Clinical Disorders of Innate and Adaptive Immunity, integrates the content from the first three chapters of the book into the functional characteristics of body defenses and associated clinical disorders. Content related to Chédiak-Higashi Syndrome has been expanded in the Innate (Congenital) Neutrophil Abnormalities section of this chapter.

Part II—The Theory of Immunologic and Serologic Procedures (Chapters 5–12)

Chapter 5, Safety in the Immunology-Serology Laboratory, continues to include all of the traditional safety practices. However, additional new topics include risk and risk management, reducing risk of surface-based infection, and the laboratory safety team

Chapter 6, Serologic Laboratory: Techniques & Clinical Applications, now features integrated laboratory techniques supported by examples of noninstrument, rapid testing techniques, including syphilis, malaria, HIV, and pregnancy testing.

Chapter 12, Molecular Laboratory Techniques, has been revised to keep up with the latest innovations in testing. The chapter begins with genetic information that bridges classic information with exciting state-of-the-art molecular techniques and applications. Molecular diagnostic testing and treatment strategies have assumed a more visible presence in the clinical laboratory. The content of this chapter as well as throughout the book reflects the importance of molecular diagnostics in today's medical laboratories.

Single nucleotide polymorphisms (SNPs) content is introduced early in the chapter because they are the most abundant source of genetic variation in the human genome. This chapter has expanded content on molecular amplification methods and the molecular analysis of amplification products.

Alternatives to electrophoresis-based techniques of pyrosequencing, mass spectrophotometry, and high-performance liquid chromatography continue to be important topics in this chapter. Other important and expanding topics are microarrays and Next-Generation Sequencing Technology/Massively Parallel Sequencing.

Part III—Immunologic Manifestations of Infectious Diseases (Chapters 13–18)

Statistics for Chapters 13 to 18 have been reviewed and updated. The numerous testing algorithms have been reviewed and updated with most recent published data.

Chapter 13, Infectious Diseases: Overview & TORCH Diseases, continues to present a traditional overview of laboratory testing in infectious diseases. However, in this edition, TORCH (Toxoplasmosis, Other Viruses, Rubella, and Cytomegalovirus) infectious diseases are combined into a single chapter to emphasize their similarities. The use of infectious diseases immunohistochemistry (IHC), advantages of polymer-based immunohistochemistry methods, and newer molecular testing approaches are carried over into the new chapter.

Chapter 15, Syphilis, has increased in incidence in the United States. In addition to classic diagnostic test methods, point-of-care rapid testing is available in the United States.

Chapter 16, Vector-Borne Diseases, can be bacterial, parasitic, viral diseases transmitted by mosquitoes, ticks, or fleas. These diseases include some of the world's most destructive diseases, many of which are increasing threats to human health as environment climate changes and globalization increases.

After being absent since 2003, malaria made a reappearance in 2023 in Florida and Texas as domestically-acquired rather than travel-related infections. The presence of malarial parasites can be detected by microscopy which continues to be the gold standard. Three main groups of antigens detected by commercially available rapid diagnostic test RDTS are histidine-rich protein II (HPR-II), which is specific to *P. falciparum* antigen, parasite-specific plasmodium lactate dehydrogenase (pLDH), and aldolase. Prevention strategies include several drugs and a newly approved vaccine for children in Africa.

Another vector-borne disease discussed in this chapter is Lyme disease. Lyme disease has become the most commonly reported (95%) vector-borne illness in the United States. It has demonstrated a significant increase in the number of infected patients. The disease is concentrated heavily in the northeast and upper Midwest, but the geographic distribution of high-incidence states of patients with Lyme disease appears to be increasing.

Dengue fever and West Nile virus are being carefully observed for an increased incidence.

Part IV—Immune Disorders (Chapters 19–24)

Chapter 19, Primary and Acquired (Secondary) Immunodeficiencies, has been expanded to include additional content related to innate immunity with two newly associated clinical case studies. Laboratory testing algorithms are emphasized in order to simplify the diagnostic process. Therapeutic drugs in an extensive number of viral mechanistic categories for the treatment of human immunodeficiency virus are described in terms of viral impact.

Chapter 21, Plasma Cell Neoplasms and Other Diseases with Paraproteins, such as (Multiple Myeloma and monoclonal gammopathies were reorganized in 2022 by the World Health Organization (WHO) into various disease with paraproteins. Representative examples of these neoplasms include multiple myeloma (MM) and Waldenström primary macroglobulinemia (WM) are presented in this chapter. Expanded discussion of etiology, pathophysiology, and new diagnostic criteria is presented in the chapter.

Monoclonal gammopathy of renal significance and cold agglutinin disease are two new entities that fall under the umbrella of plasma cell neoplasms/other diseases with paraproteins.

Part V—Transplantation and Tumor Immunology (Chapters 25 and 26)

Chapter 26, *Tumor Immunology and Applications of Next-Generation Sequencing/Massive Parallel Sequencing*, has an extensively updated table of diagnostic tumor markers currently in common use. Tumor markers have traditionally been proteins or other substances that can be made by both normal and cancer cells but at higher amounts in cancer or certain benign conditions. Markers can be found in blood, urine, stool, tumors, or other tissues or bodily fluids. A tumor marker provides information that can be used to determine aggressiveness of the cancer, stage of cancer, potential for types of treatment, and responsiveness to treatment or prognosis based on detection of minimal residual disease.

Content on Next-Generation Sequencing, now called Massive Parallel Sequencing, is re-introduced as an important aspect of tumor immunology. In addition, continuous field-flow–assisted dielectrophoresis, a new method to isolate and characterize rare circulating tumor cells (CTCs) is presented in this chapter. In addition, examples of currently approved monoclonal antibodies and mechanisms of action have been updated.

Part VI—Vaccines (Chapter 27)

Chapter 27, Vaccines: Development and Applications. Knowledge of vaccines has never been more important to healthcare professionals. The SARS-CoV-2 (COVID-19) pandemic vaccine development directed at prevention of COVID-19 has raised awareness of the importance of vaccines. Continuing research on human immunodeficiency virus (HIV), malaria, and cancer vaccines is discussed in this chapter. Immunization schedules have been reviewed and updated as needed.

OVERALL IN-TEXT FEATURES

- **Basic and Advanced Learning Outcomes** clarify what MLT and MLS students need to know upon successful completion of each chapter.
- **Key Terms (Italicized in Text and Defined in Glossary)** help students master the vocabulary of immunology and serology.
- **Key Concepts** interwoven in every chapter assist students to focus on important topics as narrative content unfolds in each chapter.
- **Numerous Case Studies** with etiology, pathophysiology, laboratory findings, multiple-choice questions, and critical thinking group discussion questions linked to key concepts and procedures with a disorder, disease, or condition.
- **More Visual Learning Content** to meet the needs of today's students and to promote effective learning of concepts and procedures.
- **End-of-Chapter Certification-Style Review Questions (total of more than 650 questions)** assist students in self-evaluation of content upon successful completion of each chapter.
- **Applicable Procedures** help students solidify concepts and gain practical skills.

ANCILLARIES

Immunology & Serology in Laboratory Medicine includes additional resources for both instructors and students that are available on the book's companion website, Evolve.

For the Instructor
Evolve

The companion Evolve website offers several features to aid instructors:

- **Critical Analysis Group Discussion Questions:** Complete explanations are on the instructor's side of Evolve for the open-ended, case-related discussion questions.
- **Test Bank:** This test bank of more than 990 multiple-choice questions features answers, explanations, and cognitive levels. The test bank can be used for review in class or for test development. More than 330 of the questions in the instructor test bank are available for student use.
- **PowerPoint Presentations:** One PowerPoint presentation is given per chapter; this feature can be used as is or as a template to prepare lectures.
- **Image Collection:** All the images from the book can be downloaded into PowerPoint presentations. The figures can be used during lectures to illustrate important concepts.
- **Procedures:** This feature presents the principles and application of procedures in every chapter.
- **Sample Syllabi for MLT and MLS Students:** One- and two-semester courses are available.
- **Answers to Additional Review Questions:** Students have access to more than 330 questions that test their knowledge on the concepts presented in the text. The questions and answers are available to instructors.
- **Chapter-Linked Digital Enrichment References:** References to videos, animations, and virtual laboratories are available.

For the Student
Evolve

The student resources on Evolve include the following:

- **Additional Review Questions:** A set of more than 330 multiple-choice questions provides extra review and practice.
- **Case Studies:** Case studies provide additional opportunities for student application of chapter content in real-life scenarios.

ACKNOWLEDGMENTS

My objective in writing *Immunology & Serology in Laboratory Medicine*, 8th edition, continues to be to share basic scientific concepts, procedural theory, and clinical applications with colleagues and students. Because the knowledge base and technology in immunology and serology continue to expand, writing and revising a book that addresses the needs of teachers and students continue to be a challenge. In addition, this book continues to provide me with the opportunity to learn and share my laboratory and teaching experience, and insight as an educator, with others.

Thank you to Ellen Wurm-Cutter, my original editor, and Kelly Skelton and Melissa Rawe, Senior Content Strategists for guiding this project. Also, thank you to the faculty reviewers and students for their valuable feedback. The contributions of Shilpa Kumar, Senior Content Development Specialist, and Manchu Mohan, Book Specialist, are greatly appreciated.

Comments from instructors and students are always welcome at Turgeonbooks@gmail.com.

Mary L. Turgeon
St. Petersburg, Florida

ABOUT THE AUTHOR

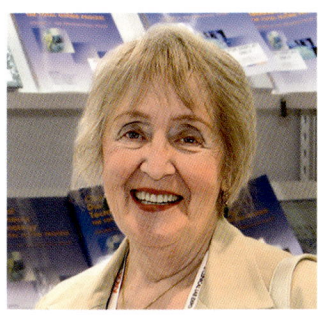

Mary Louise Turgeon, EdD, MLS(ASCP)^{CM}, is an educator, author, and consultant in medical laboratory science education. Her career as an educator includes 15 years as a community college professor and Medical Laboratory Technology (MLT) program director and 14 years as an undergraduate (MLS) and graduate university professor, Medical Laboratory Science program director, and departmental chairperson. Other university teaching has included teaching graduate Physician Assistant students at South University, Tampa, Florida and Northeastern University, Boston, Massachusetts. Most recently, Dr. Turgeon taught a graduate immunology course to students in the Doctorate in Clinical Laboratory Science program at the University of Texas Medical Branch, Galveston, Texas.

Dr. Turgeon is currently an ad hoc educational content specialist for the College of Professional Studies, Northeastern University, Boston, and maintains an active clinical laboratory science consulting practice. Mary L. Turgeon and Associates focuses on new undergraduate and post-graduate program development, curriculum revisions, and increasing teaching effectiveness through the use of technology and interactive teaching strategies.

The presentation of numerous professional workshops and lectures complements Dr. Turgeon's extensive teaching and writing activities. Her career in medical laboratory science has spanned the globe with active participation in a wide variety of professional meetings and workshops. Enthusiastic professional involvement has offered her the opportunity to share leading-edge knowledge with students and to meet and collaborate with medical laboratory science colleagues in the United States and worldwide, including China, Italy, Japan, Qatar, Saudi Arabia, and the United Arab Emirates.

Professional volunteer activities with the American Society of Clinical Pathologists, ASCP, include numerous regional workshops focusing on Increasing Teaching Effectiveness and Curriculum Development. In addition as an ASCP volunteer, she has traveled to distant locations such as Cambodia and Lesotho, Africa.

Dr. Turgeon is a longstanding member of the American Society for Clinical Laboratory Science (ASCLS), and an active volunteer on various organizational committees, e.g. Clinical Laboratory Educators Steering Committee for the CLEC-23 and CLEC-24. In addition, she is a member of the American Association of Immunology (AAI) and the American Association of Clinical Chemistry (AACC) renamed in 2023 to the Association for Diagnostics and Laboratory Medicine (ADLM).

Dr. Turgeon's most significant professional career accomplishment is authoring multiple editions of undergraduate medical laboratory science textbooks (sold in more than 45 countries):

- *Immunology & Serology in Laboratory Medicine,* 7th edition (2022), Elsevier
- *Clinical Laboratory Science,* 9th edition (2021) formerly *Linné & Ringsrud's Clinical Laboratory Science,* 8th edition (2020), Elsevier
- *Clinical Hematology,* 7th edition (2026), Jones & Bartlett

Immunology & Serology in Laboratory Medicine has been translated into Italian and Chinese. *Clinical Hematology* has been translated into Spanish.

CONTENTS

PART I Basic Immunologic Mechanisms

1. Foundations of Innate and Adaptive Immune Systems, 2
2. Soluble Mediators of the Immune System, 28
3. Antigens and Antibodies, 47
4. Cellular Activities and Clinical Disorders of Innate and Adaptive Immunity, 67

PART II The Theory of Immunologic and Serologic Procedures

5. Basic Safety in the Immunology-Serology Laboratory, 98
6. Basic Quality Control and Quality Assurance Practices, 107
7. Basic Serologic Laboratory: Techniques and Clinical Applications, 117
8. Precipitation and Particle Agglutination Methods, 128
9. Electrophoresis Techniques and Chromatography, 143
10. Labeling Techniques in Immunoassay, 150
11. Flow Cytometry, 159
12. Molecular Laboratory Techniques, 168

PART III Immunologic Manifestations of Infectious Diseases

13. Infectious Diseases: Overview and TORCH Diseases, 190
14. Streptococcal Infections, 221
15. Syphilis, 228
16. Vector-Borne Diseases, 240
17. Infectious Mononucleosis, 267
18. Viral Hepatitis, 273

PART IV Immune Disorders

19. Primary and Acquired Immunodeficiency Syndromes, 300
20. Hypersensitivity Reactions, 337
21. Plasma Cell Neoplasms and Other Diseases With Paraproteins, 353
22. Tolerance, Autoimmunity, and Autoimmune Disorders, 369
23. Systemic Lupus Erythematosus, 396
24. Rheumatoid Arthritis, 414

PART V Transplantation and Tumor Immunology

25. Transplantation: Human Leukocyte Antigens, Solid Organ, Tissues, and Hematopoietic Stem Cells, 428
26. Tumor Immunology and Applications of Massive Parallel Sequencing/Next-Generation Sequencing, 454

PART VI Vaccines

27. Vaccines: Development and Applications, 478

Appendix A: Answers to Case Study Multiple-Choice Questions, 500
Appendix B: Answers to Review Questions, 503
Appendix C: Origin and Immunoregulatory Activity of Cytokines, 510
Appendix D: Coronavirus Disease 2019 (COVID-19), 514
Appendix E: Vaccines Licensed for Use in the United States by the Federal Drug Administration, 516
Bibliography, 518
Glossary, 528
Index, 550

PART I

Basic Immunologic Mechanisms

Chapter 1: Foundations of Innate and Adaptive Immune Systems, 2

Chapter 2: Soluble Mediators of the Immune System, 28

Chapter 3: Antigens and Antibodies, 47

Chapter 4: Cellular Activities and Clinical Disorders of Innate and Adaptive Immunity, 67

1

Foundations of Innate and Adaptive Immune Systems

LEARNING OUTCOMES

- Describe the classic milestones in immunology.
- Compare examples of diversity in immunology.
- Explain the functions of the immune system.
- Describe the characteristics of five mature leukocytes and their immune function.
- Describe the general functions of granulocytes, monocytes-macrophages, lymphocytes, and plasma cells as components of the immune system.
- Differentiate and compare the functions of primary and secondary lymphoid tissues.
- Describe the structure and function of a lymph node.
- Explain the role of the thymus in T lymphocyte maturation.
- Describe the maturation of a B lymphocyte from origination to plasma cell development.
- Describe the first, second, and third lines of body defense against microbial diseases.
- Compare innate immunity and adaptive immunity.
- Differentiate and compare the functions of primary and secondary lymphoid tissues.
- Analyze a case study related to immunity.
- Correctly answer case study–related multiple-choice questions.
- Participate in a discussion of critical-thinking questions.
- Correctly answer 80% of the end-of-chapter review questions.

OUTLINE

Milestones in Immunology, 3
Diversity in Immunology, 3
    Black Male Scientists, 3
        William Augustus Hinton, 3
        Julian H. Lewis, 3
    Black Non-Scientific Contributors to Immunology, 4
        Onesimus, 4
        Henrietta Lacks, 4
    Pioneer Women in Immunology, 4
        Olga Raissa Povitzky, M.D., 4
        Elise L'Esperance, M.D., 4
        Winifred Ashby, Ph.D., 4
        Rebecca Craighill Lancefield, 4
        Kizzmekia S. Corbett, Ph.D., 4
        Katalin Karikó, Ph.D., 5
What is Immunology?, 5
Cells of the Innate and Adaptive Immune Systems, 6
Origin and Development of Blood Cells, 6
Blood and Tissue Cells Associated With Innate and Adaptive Immune Systems, 8
Granulocytes, 8
    Neutrophils, 8
    Eosinophils, 9
    Basophils, 9
    Tissue Basophils (Mast Cells), 10
Mononuclear Phagocyte System, 10
Monocytes, 10
    Macrophages, 10
    Dendritic Cells, 11
Lymphocyte Variations, 13
    Lymphocyte Development, 13
        T Cells, 14
        B Cells, 14
        Plasma Cells, 14
        Natural Killer Lymphocytes, 15
Innate Lymphoid Cells, 16
    Primary Lymphoid Organs, 16
        Bone Marrow, 16
        Thymus, 16
    Secondary Lymphoid Organs, 17
        Lymph Nodes, 17
        Spleen, 19
        Gut-Associated Lymphoid Tissue, 19
        Thoracic Duct, 19
        Bronchus-Associated Lymphoid Tissue, 19
        Skin-Associated Lymphoid Tissue, 19
        Blood, 19
    Circulation of Lymphocytes, 19
Comparison of Innate and Adaptive Immunity, 19
    Role of Microbiota, 19
    Innate Immunity: The Early Defense, 20
    First Line of Defense, 20
    Second Line of Defense: Innate (Natural) Immunity, 20
    Pathogen-Associated Molecular Patterns and Pattern Recognition Receptors, 22
        Pattern Recognition Receptors, 22
    Third Line of Defense: Adaptive Immunity, 22
        Humoral-Mediated Immunity, 23
        Cell-Mediated Immunity, 25
Case Study 1.1, 25
Procedure: Identification of Leukocytes Related to Immune Function, 27.e1
Procedure: Screening Test for Phagocytic Engulfment, 27.e1

CHAPTER 1 Foundations of Innate and Adaptive Immune Systems

KEY TERMS

- acquired immunity
- active immunity
- adaptive immune system
- adaptive immunity
- allografts
- antibodies
- antigen
- autoimmune disorder
- basophils
- biological aging
- B lymphocytes
- cell-mediated immunity
- chemokines
- clonal selection
- cluster of differentiation (CD)
- complement
- cytokines
- endotoxin
- endogenous
- eosinophils
- exogenous
- exudate (pus)
- genome
- gut-associated lymphoid tissue (GALT)
- hematopoiesis
- humoral-mediated immunity
- immune senescence
- immunity
- immunocompetent
- immunogenic
- immunosuppression
- inflammation
- innate immune system
- interleukins (ILs)
- lymphocyte recirculation
- macrophages
- major histocompatibility complex (MHC)
- microbiome
- microbiota
- monoclonal antibodies (MAbs)
- monoclonal gammopathies
- mononuclear phagocyte system
- negative selection
- neutrophils
- passive immunity
- pathogen-associated molecular patterns (PAMPs)
- pattern recognition receptors (PRRs)
- phagocytosis
- plasma cells
- positive selection
- T lymphocytes
- vaccination

MILESTONES IN IMMUNOLOGY

Louis Pasteur is generally considered to be the "father of immunology." Some historic benchmarks in immunology dominated by White European and American males are listed in Table 1.1. Owing to the exclusion of people of color and women, recognition of examples of diversity is important in order to complete the profile of significant benchmark events in the history of immunology.

DIVERSITY IN IMMUNOLOGY

Black Male Scientists

Black scientists are underrepresented in scientific fields, including immunology. Although their numbers are small, their contributions to the field are significant. Outstanding early examples of the accomplishments of Black Americans include William A. Hinton, M.D. and Julian H. Lewis, M.D.

William Augustus Hinton (1883–1959)

William Augustus Hinton's achievements were remarkable and changed the course of medicine. In 1912, Dr. Hinton worked at the Wassermann Laboratory at the Massachusetts State Laboratory for communicable diseases at Harvard Medical School. He became an expert on syphilis and created a new serological blood test for diagnosing syphilis, the Hinton test, which became the standard of the day for laboratory testing. Subsequently, this testing method was adopted by the US Public Health Service. In addition, Dr. Hinton was the first Black person to write a medical textbook in the United States: *Syphilis and its treatment*, published in 1936.

Julian H. Lewis (1891–1989)

Julian H. Lewis, a Black pathologist, is considered to be the "Father of Anthropathology." Anthropathology is the study of racial differences in the expression of disease. Dr. Lewis's primary area of research was the evolution of human blood types, with a particular emphasis on how the blood types of Black people had been shaped by interactions with other groups, including White people. His research challenged

TABLE 1.1 Classic Timeline of Milestones in Immunology

Date	Scientist(s)	Discovery
1798	Jenner	Smallpox vaccination
1862	Haeckel	Phagocytosis
1880–1881	Pasteur	Live attenuated chicken cholera and anthrax vaccines
1883–1905	Metchnikoff	Cellular theory of immunity through phagocytosis
1885	Pasteur	Therapeutic vaccination
		First report of live "attenuated" vaccine for rabies
1890	Von Behring, Kitasatoa	Humoral theory of immunity proposed
1891	Koch	Demonstration of cutaneous (delayed-type) hypersensitivity
1900	Ehrlich	Antibody formation theory
1902	Portier, Richet	Immediate hypersensitivity anaphylaxis
1903	Arthus	Arthus reaction of intermediate hypersensitivity
1938	Marrack	Hypothesis of antigen–antibody binding
1944		Hypothesis of allograft rejection
1949	Salk, Sabin	Development of polio vaccine
1951	Reed	Vaccine against yellow fever
1953		Graft-versus-host reaction
1957	Burnet	Clonal selection theory
1957		Interferon
1958–1962		Human leukocyte antigens
1964–1968		T-cell and B-cell cooperation in immune response
1972		Identification of antibody molecule
1975	Köhler	First monoclonal antibodies
1985–1987		Identification of genes for T-cell receptor
1986		Monoclonal hepatitis B vaccine
1986	Mosmann	Th1 versus Th2 model of helper T-cell function
1996–1998		Identification of Toll-like receptors
2001		*FOXP3*, the gene directing regulatory T-cell development
2005	Frazer	Development of human papillomavirus vaccine

the idea of race and its perceived permanence as a biological and/or social category.

Examples of People of Color as Contributors to Immunology

Black Non-Scientific Contributors to Immunology
Onesimus
An enslaved Black African, Onesimus helped to save hundreds of Bostonians from smallpox in 1721. His owner, Cotton Mather, gave him the name Onesimus, after an enslaved man in the Bible whose name meant "useful." When Boston experienced a smallpox epidemic, Mather promoted inoculation and cited Onesimus and African folk medicine as a protective practice used in Africa and Asia.

Dr. Zabdiel Boylston carried out the method described by Onesimus that involved sticking a needle into a pustule on the skin of an infected person and scraping the infected needle across the skin of a healthy person. Dr. Boylston initially inoculated his 6-year-old son and two of his slaves. Subsequently, 280 people were inoculated in Boston during the 1721–1722 smallpox epidemic. There were only six smallpox deaths among the treated people (approximately 2.2%) compared with the approximately 14.3% death rate of untreated people. To memorialize this event, an inscription on Dr. Boylston's grave headstone identifies him as the "first" to have introduced the practice of inoculation in America.

Inoculation (variolation) was a common practice long before vaccines were established in 1796 and were replaced by Edward Jenner's development of vaccination for smallpox and cowpox. Subsequently, vaccination became compulsory in Wales and England and inoculation was banned.

Henrietta Lacks
Henrietta Lacks was the donor of the incredible malignant cells—nicknamed "HeLa" cells, from the first two letters of her first and last names. She was a poor, Black woman who died of cervical cancer at the age of 31 years in 1951. Doctors at Johns Hopkins Hospital (Baltimore, MD) gave a biopsy of Henrietta's cancerous cells to Dr. George Otto Gey, a cell biologist based at the hospital's medical school. As a result, these extraordinary cells are used today throughout the world for research without experimenting on humans. HeLa cells are uniquely aggressive—they double in volume every 20 to 24 hours compared with other cultures that would normally die out. If HeLa cells are fed the right mixture of nutrients to allow them to grow, the cells are effectively immortal.

HeLa cells are the most widely used human cell line in biological research, and for almost 70 years they have played a central role in many of mankind's most significant biomedical breakthroughs. For example, these cells were used in 1954 to develop the polio vaccine, in the 1980s to identify and understand HIV, and even in research for vaccines against coronavirus disease 2019 (COVID-19) (Box 1.1). HeLa cells have formed the foundation of clinical trials to treat and cure cancer, contributed to space travel research, and allowed researchers to identify the number of human chromosomes. They have helped to develop treatments for Parkinson disease and hemophilia, establish methods of freezing cells for storage, and discover the telomerase enzyme that contributes to aging and death.

Pioneer Women in Immunology
Olga Raissa Povitzky, M.D. (1877–1948)
Dr. Povitzky published in *The Journal of Immunology* and other journals throughout the 1920s and 1930s. Her focus was primarily on developments that refined production techniques for diphtheria toxoid and antitoxin, and pertussis. In the 1930s, Dr. Povitzky designed a rectangular 2-L Pyrex culture bottle for diphtheria antitoxin production that was later adopted in a larger 5-L size as the standard vessel for the Salk polio vaccine. The durable "Povitsky bottle" proved ideal for culturing poliovirus in a custom-made rocking rack.

Elise L'Esperance, M.D. (1878–1959)
Dr. L'Esperance became the first woman to be a lead author on an article published in *The Journal of Immunology*: L'Esperance ES, Coca EF: Further experiences with the isolated organ lipoids as 'antigen' in the Wassermann test, J Immunol 1(2):129–158, 1916. This article examined sources of error in the Wassermann reaction—the newly developed test for syphilis.

In 1937, Dr. L'Esperance was the founding pioneer of the Kate Depew Strang Tumor Clinic, devoted to the early diagnosis of cancer in women. As the result of her focus on cancer, she authored L'Esperance ES: The early diagnosis of cancer. Bull New York Acad Med 23(7):394–409, 1947.

Winifred Ashby, Ph.D. (1879–1975)
Dr. Ashby made her imprint on immunology as the result of developing the first technique to determine red blood cell lifespan in human beings. The Ashby technique of differential agglutination employs the principles of antigen-antibody agglutination.

This technique was based on the fact that type AB, A, or B blood cells (group I, II, and III in her terminology) will agglutinate when treated with serum from a person of another blood type, while type O blood cells (group IV) lacking ABO antigens will not agglutinate.

Rebecca Craighill Lancefield (1895–1981)
Dr. Lancefield is best known as a world-renowned authority on streptococcal bacteria. She developed the classification system of *Streptococcus* bearing her name that is still in use today.

Lancefield's identification of streptococcal types proved essential to revealing the complexities of the immune response to the bacteria and elucidating streptococci as the primary infectious agent for many diseases—understandings that enabled improved methods for identifying and controlling streptococcal infections. Lancefield assisted Oswald Theodore Avery and Alphonse Raymond Dochez in the laboratory, and they cited Lancefield as a coauthor in the article Studies on the Biology of *Streptococcus*: I. Antigenic Relationships Between Strains of Streptococcus hemolyticus."

Dr. Lancefield also identified two new surface proteins on group A streptococci: T-antigen (she later determined, in 1957, that it did not contribute to virulence) and R-antigen in 1940. Lancefield's attention later turned to group B streptococci—bacteria once thought to infect only bovine but soon discovered to be responsible for neonatal pneumonia and meningitis. Lancefield found that streptococci of this group did not contain the M-protein; instead, it was found that their virulence was determined by surface polysaccharides. This research was an important first step in preventing the life-threatening diseases in newborns caused by group B streptococci.

Kizzmekia S. Corbett, Ph.D. (1986–)
Kizzmekia S. Corbett, a Black scientist, will go down in history as one of the key players in developing the vaccine concept that would end the COVID-19 pandemic. She was a research fellow and the scientific lead for the Coronavirus Vaccines & Immunopathogenesis Team at the National Institutes of Health (Bethesda, MD). In that position, Dr. Corbett was an expert on the front lines of the global race for a severe acute respiratory syndrome coronavirus 2 (SARS-CoV-2) vaccine, and she used her viral immunology expertise to propel a novel vaccine development concept for a vaccine against SARS-CoV-2.

CHAPTER 1 Foundations of Innate and Adaptive Immune Systems

> ### BOX 1.1 Timeline of Representative Achievements with HeLa cells
>
> **1956: Developing Cancer Research Methods**
> HeLa cells are used by scientists to develop a cancer research method that tests whether a cell line is cancerous or not. This method proves so reliable that scientists use it to this day.
>
> **1985: Slowing Cancer Growth**
> Scientists discover that when HeLa cells are treated with a drug called campothecin, cancer cell growth slows. These findings support future studies that verify that camptothecin can limit uncontrollable cell growth in cancer cells beyond HeLa cells. Camptothecin was later approved by the United States Food and Drug Administration (FDA) as a treatment for certain types of ovarian, lung, and cervical cancers.
>
> **1988: Advancing Understanding of HIV Infection**
> In the early days of the HIV-AIDS epidemic, scientists discover that HeLa cells are not easily infected by HIV. Using this information, researchers gain important basic understanding of how HIV infection works. This knowledge later facilitates drug development aimed at limiting the spread of HIV.
>
> **1989: Learning How Cells Age**
> Research involving HeLa cells shows that the telomerase enzyme produces "caps" on the ends of DNA chromosomes that prevent them from degrading over time. This is important for understanding the underlying biology of aging as well as diseases that cause premature aging.
>   The impact of this work later leads to a 2009 Nobel Prize for Dr. Elizabeth Blackburn, Dr. Carol Greider, and Dr. Jack Szostak.
>
> **1993: Exploring How Tuberculosis Makes People Sick**
> Scientists use HeLa cells to see for the first time, at the molecular level, how tuberculosis makes people sick. Tuberculosis has caused disease since ancient times and is thought to infect 25% of the world's population. The discovery of how this disease works provides vital information for the potential development of treatments and more effective vaccines.
>
> **2001: Understanding the Infectivity of Ebola and HIV**
> Scientists uncover that HIV and Ebola share a similar process to enter cells and cause disease. This finding, based on previous HIV research results, provides vital information on the quest to develop a more effective Ebola vaccine.
>
> **2001: Innovating Single-Cell Imaging**
> Scientists use HeLa cells to develop a new and innovative single-cell microscopic imaging method. This method allows scientists to see the mechanism by which viruses enter cells and allows for the clearest view of the inner workings of a living cell. This groundbreaking approach leads to a 2014 Nobel Prize for Dr. Eric Betzig, Dr. Stefan W. Hell, and Dr. William E. Moerner.
>
> **2010: Repurposing Thalidomide to Fight Cancer**
> Researchers use HeLa cells to describe how birth defects were caused by the anti-morning sickness drug, thalidomide. Scientists were able to take this information about how thalidomide works and apply it to halt the progress of certain cancers such as multiple myeloma.
>
> **Cancer Research and Basic Research Methodology**
>
> **2013: Allowing Research to Continue to Advance Science While Protecting Privacy**
> The National Institutes of Health (NIH) reaches an agreement with the descendants of Henrietta Lacks to allow biomedical researchers controlled access to the whole-genome data of HeLa cells. Access to the whole-genome data of these cells will be a valuable reference tool for researchers to study the cause and effect of many diseases with the goal of developing treatments. This landmark agreement exemplifies NIH's continued commitment to seeing research participants as partners in the research enterprise.
>
> **2019–**
> Because of prior experience with HIV and Ebola vaccine development, research scientists had a knowledge base related to the use of HeLa cells. This prior experience provided a quicker and experienced research foundation for the development of the mRNA COVID-19 vaccine.
>   Data Source: National Institutes of Health (NIH). https://nih.gov. Accessed June 28, 2023.

This was the vaccine concept incorporated into mRNA from a viral sequence and rapidly deployed to industry partner, Moderna, Inc.

Katalin Karikó, Ph.D. (January 17, 1955–)

Katalin Karikó, a Hungarian-American biochemist, and her co-collaborator, Drew Weissman, M.D., Ph.D., were awarded the 2023 Nobel Prize in Medicine and Physiology for their vaccine research that was critical for developing effective mRNA vaccines against COVID-19 during the pandemic that began in 2020. Their groundbreaking findings fundamentally changed the scientific understanding of how mRNA can be processed and delivered to our immune system. This knowledge contributed to the unprecedented rate of vaccine development during one of the greatest infectious disease threats to human health in modern times.

Dr. Karikó grew up in a small village in Hungary, where from an early age she expressed an interest in nature and excelled academically in science. Dr. Karikó received her bachelor's degree in biology in 1978 and a doctorate in biochemistry in 1982 from the University of Szeged in her native Hungary. Before immigrating to the United States in 1985, Dr. Karikó conducted vaccine research in Hungary.

WHAT IS IMMUNOLOGY?

> **KEY CONCEPTS: An Overview of Immunology**
>
> The term **immunity** has historically referred to resistance to pathogens based on the ability of the immune system to recognize and dispose of foreign (nonself) material. Today it is recognized that the immune system plays a critical role in both health and disease (Table 1.2). Desirable consequences of immunity include natural resistance, recovery, and acquired resistance to infectious diseases. Another advantage is the scientific ability to manipulate the immune system to protect against or treat a wide variety of clinical conditions. A deficiency or dysfunction of the immune system can cause various disorders. Undesirable consequences of immunity include allergy, rejection of a transplanted organ, or an **autoimmune disorder**, in which the body's own tissues are attacked as if they were foreign.
>
> The immune system is usually conceptualized as having two divisions: the **innate immune system** (also called *natural immunity* or *native immunity*), the immediate protection component, and the **adaptive immune system**, the slower but more focused defense component (Fig. 1.1).

TABLE 1.2 Importance of the Immune System in Health and Disease

Role of Immune System	Health Implications
Defense against infections	Deficient immunity results in increased susceptibility to infections
	Vaccination boosts immune defenses and protects against infections
Defense against tumors	Potential for immunotherapy to treat malignancies
Control of tissue regeneration and scarring	Repair of damaged tissues
Injury to cells and induction of pathologic inflammation	Immune responses cause allergic, autoimmune, and other inflammatory diseases
Recognition and response to tissue grafts and newly introduced proteins	Immune responses are barriers to transplantation and gene therapy

Adapted from Abbas AK, Lichtman AH, Pillae S: *Basic immunology: functions and disorders of the immune system,* Philadelphia, 2020, Elsevier.

> **KEY CONCEPTS: Characteristics of the Immune System**
> - The function of the immune system is to recognize self from nonself and to defend the body against nonself.
> - An effective immune response requires cooperative interaction between specific cells of the immune system's cellular elements, cell products, and nonlymphoid elements for optimal functioning.
> - Desirable consequences of immunity include natural resistance, recovery, and acquired resistance to infectious diseases.
> - Undesirable consequences of immunity include allergy, rejection of a transplanted organ, or an autoimmune disorder, in which the body's own tissues are attacked as nonself.
> - The immune system is usually conceptualized as having two divisions: the innate immune system, the immediate protection component, and the adaptive immune system, the slower but more focused defense component.

Innate immunity reflects a person's ability to resist infections with first and second lines of defense that are nonspecifically directed at all pathogens or foreign particles without memory of prior exposure. Cells in the innate division have receptors to recognize microbial products. The innate division can respond rapidly, but rather indiscriminately, to a danger signal.

In contrast, adaptive immunity is specific and exhibits memory of prior exposure to individual pathogens or foreign particles. Antibody formation is a significant characteristic of adaptive immunity. In addition, the adaptive division can rearrange genes, such as antibody or antigen receptors, and achieve a highly targeted, precise response. This process takes time, but it is much more selective than innate immunity.

Various specific cells and nonspecific constituents of the immune system, including soluble mediators (e.g., complement, the proteins that are the major [fluid] component of natural immunity; see Chapter 2, Soluble Mediators), in addition to antibodies, participate in body defenses. The entire leukocytic cell system is designed to defend the body against disease. Each cell type has a unique function and behaves independently, or, in many cases, in cooperation with other cell types.

This chapter presents the general features of cornerstone concepts that support modern immunology. These themes are woven into subsequent chapters throughout this book.

> **KEY CONCEPTS: Overview of Cells of the Innate and Adaptive Immune Systems**
> - The major blood and tissue cell components of the innate immune system include surface epithelial barriers.
> - Tissue sentinel cells include macrophages, dendritic cells (DCs), and mast cells.
> - Leukocytes associated with the innate immune system include neutrophils, eosinophils, and basophils, monocytes and macrophages derived from monocytes, natural killer (NK) cells, and innate lymphoid cells (ILCs).
> - Lymphocytes are the key mediators of the adaptive immune system.
> - Tissue-resident cells (DCs, macrophages, and mast cells) act as sentinels to detect the presence of microbes in tissues and initiate immune responses.

CELLS OF THE INNATE AND ADAPTIVE IMMUNE SYSTEMS

The cells of the immune system are located in the peripheral blood and different tissues. These cells function differently in host defense. Most of the cells derived from bone marrow precursors circulating in the peripheral blood are leukocytic white blood cells. Other immunologically active cells reside in tissues. Some cells function mainly in innate immunity, others in adaptive immunity, and some in both innate and adaptive immune responses.

Leukocytes can be functionally divided into the general categories of granulocyte, monocyte-macrophage, lymphocyte, or plasma cell. The primary phagocytic cells are the polymorphonuclear neutrophil (PMN) leukocytes and the mononuclear monocytes-macrophages. The response of the body to pathogens involves cross-talk among many immune cells, including macrophages, DCs, and T lymphocytes.

The role of the innate system in tissue injury, particularly neutrophils and macrophages, is that these types of cells are recruited to sites of ischemic injury. Macrophages have a complex program in which they first release proinflammatory mediators to fight pathogens but may then initiate programs to help in the clearance of dead tissue and tissue repair. Although the latter response is beneficial if short-lived, continued activation of the repair program may be detrimental if it becomes chronic.

In contrast, lymphocytes participate in adaptive body defenses primarily through the recognition of foreign antigens and production of antibodies. Plasma cells are antibody-synthesizing cells.

ORIGIN AND DEVELOPMENT OF BLOOD CELLS

Blood cell production, or hematopoiesis, begins in embryonic development. Embryonic blood cells, excluding the lymphocyte type of white blood cell (WBC), originate from the mesenchymal tissue that arises from the embryonic germ layer, the mesoderm (Fig. 1.2). The sites of hematopoiesis follow a definite sequence in the embryo and fetus:

1. In the embryo, self-renewing hematopoietic stem cells develop initially in the primitive yolk sac. The first blood cells are primitive red blood cells (RBCs or erythroblasts), which are formed in the islets of the yolk sac during the first 2 to 8 weeks of life. Advances in molecular genetics have concluded that a large proportion of tissue-resident macrophage populations, including those in the pancreas, liver, brain, and skin, are derived from embryonic yolk sac progenitors.

2. Gradually the liver and spleen replace the yolk sac as the sites of blood cell development. By the second month of gestation, the liver becomes the major site of hematopoiesis. Beginning in the fetal liver

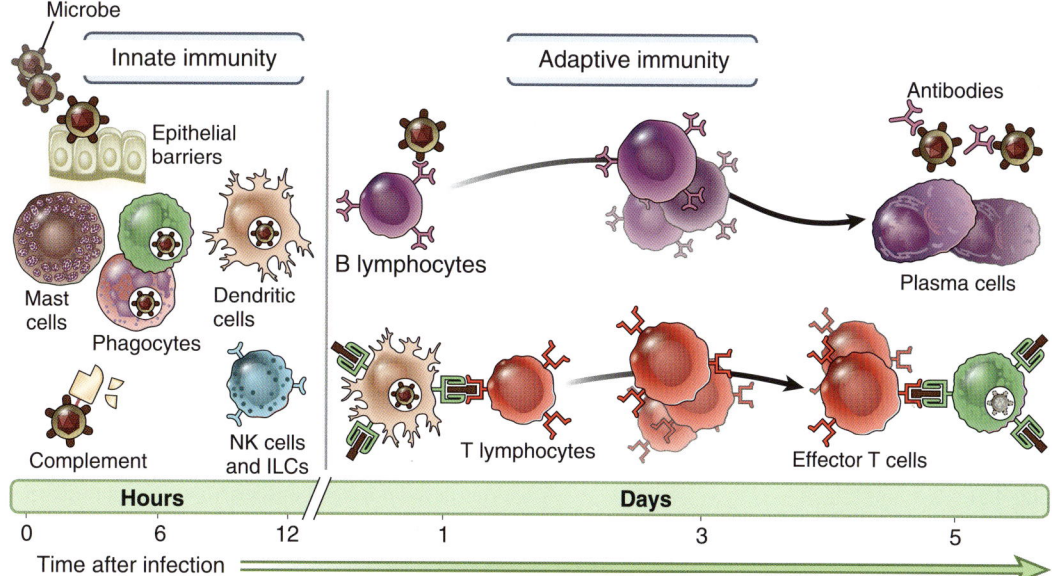

Fig. 1.1 Principal Mechanisms of Innate and Adaptive Immunity. The mechanisms of innate immunity provide the initial defense against infections. Some mechanisms (e.g., epithelial barriers) prevent infections, and other mechanisms (e.g., phagocytes, natural killer [NK] cells, and other innate lymphoid cells [ILCs] and the complement system) eliminate microbes. Adaptive immune responses develop later and are mediated by lymphocytes and their products. Antibodies block infections and eliminate microbes, and T lymphocytes eradicate intracellular microbes. The kinetics of the innate and adaptive immune responses are approximations and may vary in different infections. (From Abbas AK, Lichtman, AH, Pillai S: *Basic immunology: functions and disorders of the immune system,* ed 5, Philadelphia, 2016, Elsevier.)

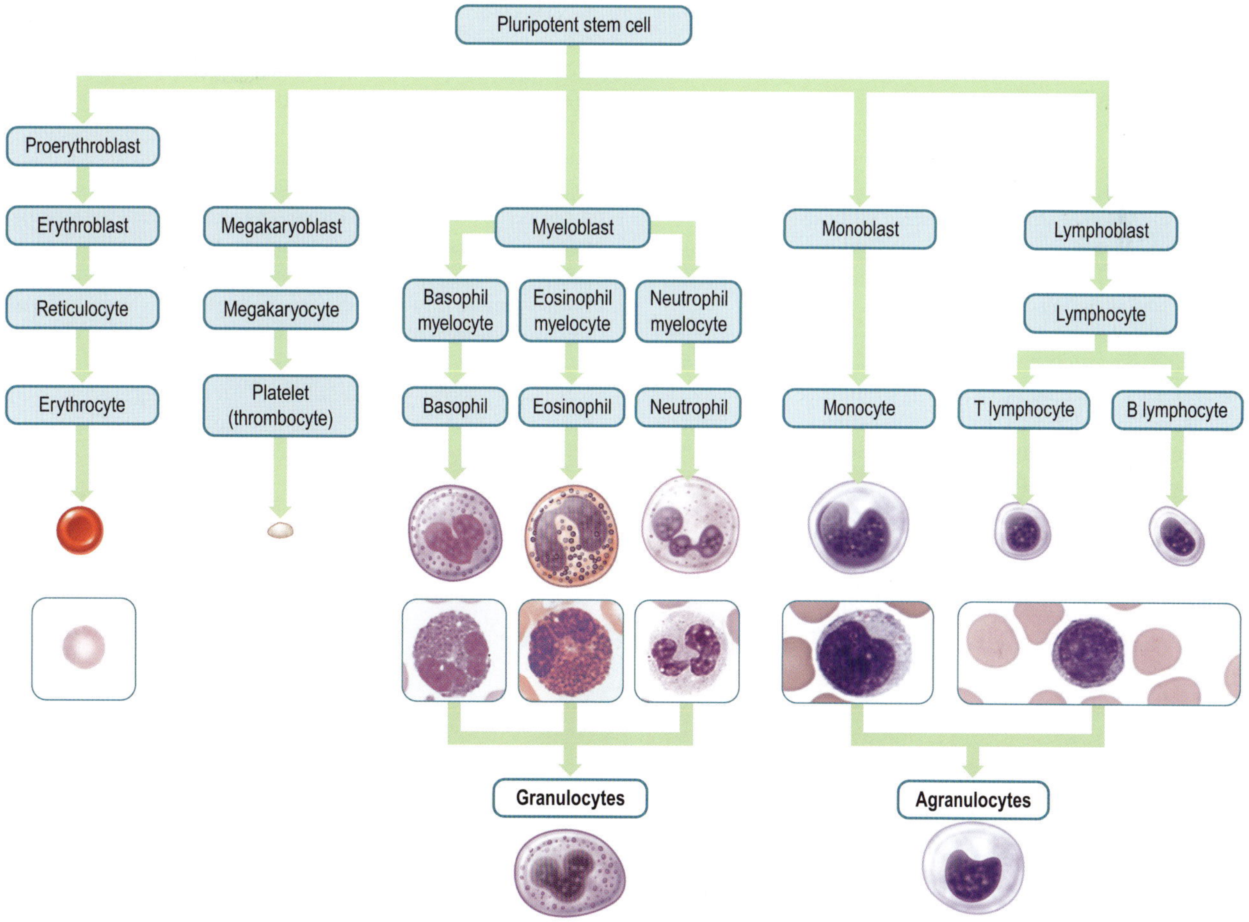

Fig. 1.2 Diagram of Hematopoiesis. Diagram shows derivation of cells from the pluripotential stem cell. (From Waugh A, Grant A: *Ross and Wilson anatomy and physiology in health and illness,* ed 13, Philadelphia, 2018, Elsevier. Photographic inserts from Telser AG, Young JK, Baldwin KM: *Elsevier's integrated histology,* Edinburgh, 2007, Mosby; and Young B, Lowe JS, Stevens A, et al: *Wheater's functional histology: a text and colour atlas,* Edinburgh, 2006, Churchill Livingstone. Reproduced with permission.)

and later in bone marrow, hematopoietic stem cells give rise to the earliest myeloid and lymphoid progenitors. Pancreatic Langerhans cells in the epidermis were discovered to originate from embryonic tissue, predominantly from the fetal liver. The liver and spleen predominate from about 2 to 5 months of fetal life.

3. In the fourth month of gestation, bone marrow begins to produce blood cells. After the fifth fetal month, bone marrow begins to assume its ultimate role as the primary site of hematopoiesis.

The cellular elements of the blood are produced from a common CD34+ multipotential hematopoietic cell, the stem cell. *Cluster of differentiation (CD)* nomenclature for cell surface markers is a common system. The CD system can identify and discriminate between, or "mark," different cell populations, or it can differentiate maturational stages of various leukocytes, particularly lymphocytes (Table 1.3; also see Fig. 4.5 and Table 4.3).

After stem cell differentiation, blast cells arise for each of the major categories of cell types. Subsequent maturation of these blast cells produces the major cellular elements of the circulating blood, the erythrocytes (RBCs), thrombocytes (platelets), and specific types of leukocytes (WBCs). In normal peripheral or circulating blood, the following types of leukocytes can be found, in order of frequency: neutrophils, lymphocytes, monocytes, eosinophils, and basophils.

BLOOD AND TISSUE CELLS ASSOCIATED WITH INNATE AND ADAPTIVE IMMUNE SYSTEMS

Cooperation is required for optimal function of the immune system. This cooperative interaction involves specific cells of the immune system, cell products, and soluble mediators. Cells of the immune system consist of specialized cells that capture and display microbial antigens, effector cells that eliminate microbes, and various subsets of lymphocytes.

The principal functions of the major cell types involved in the immune response are:
1. Specific recognition of antigens or foreign particles
2. Capture and processing of antigens or foreign particles for display to lymphocytes
3. Elimination of offending antigens or foreign particles

The major blood and tissue cell components of the innate immune system are surface epithelial barriers; tissue sentinel cells, including macrophages, DCs, and mast cells; leukocytes, including granulocytes (neutrophils, eosinophils, and basophils), monocytes and macrophages derived from monocytes, and NK cells; and ILCs. Lymphocytes are the key mediators of the adaptive immune system. Some cells, such as tissue-resident cells (DCs, macrophages, and mast cells), act as sentinels to detect the presence of microbes in tissues and initiate immune responses. Formed elements of the circulating blood go through a series of developmental stages. Normally only mature cells are seen in the peripheral blood circulation, but immature cells may appear in the peripheral blood in certain disease states. Each mature cell type has an identifiable appearance, a unique function, independent behavior, or cooperative interaction with other cell types. Each cell type has a normal life span and function.

GRANULOCYTES

Granulocytic leukocytes can be further subdivided on the basis of morphology into neutrophils, eosinophils, and basophils. Granulocytes develop in the bone marrow. The maturation stages are similar for all granulocytes; each begins as a multipotential stem cell in the bone marrow.

Neutrophils

The most numerous of the granulocytes are PMN leukocytes, or segmented neutrophil leukocytes. *Neutrophils* make up about 59% of the leukocytes in the peripheral blood of adults, with a range of 35% to 71%. Infants and children have fewer neutrophils and more lymphocytes.

Cells of the neutrophil series are generally round with smooth margins or edges. As the cells mature, they become progressively smaller. Most immature cells have cytoplasm that stains dark blue and becomes light pink as the cells mature. As the cells mature, nonspecific granules that stain blue to reddish purple appear in the cytoplasm. Eventually, these nonspecific granules are replaced by specific neutrophilic granules.

Nuclear changes also occur as the cells mature. As the cell matures, the nucleus decreases in relative size and begins to contort or form lobes. At the same time the nuclear chromatin changes from a fine, delicate pattern to the more clumped pattern characteristic of the mature cell. The staining of the nucleus also changes from reddish purple to bluish purple as the cell matures. Nucleoli may be apparent in the early forms but gradually disappear as the chromatin thickens and the cell matures.

Neutrophils (Fig. 1.3) are recognized as an essential part of the innate immune response. Previously neutrophils were believed to be directly eliminated in the marrow, liver, and spleen after circulating for

TABLE 1.3 Examples of Cluster of Differentiation (CD) Molecules	
CD Number	**Main Cellular Expression**
CD2	T lymphocytes, NK cells
CD4	Class II MHC–restricted T lymphocytes, some macrophages
CD8b	Class I MHC–restricted T lymphocytes
CD16b	Neutrophils
CD20	Most B lymphocytes
CD36	Platelets, monocytes, macrophages, endothelial cells
CD80	Dendritic cells, activated B lymphocytes, macrophages

MHC, Major histocompatibility complex; *NK,* natural killer.
Adapted from Abbas AK, Lichtman AH, Pillae S: *Basic immunology: functions and disorders of the immune system,* ed 6, St. Louis, 2020, Elsevier.

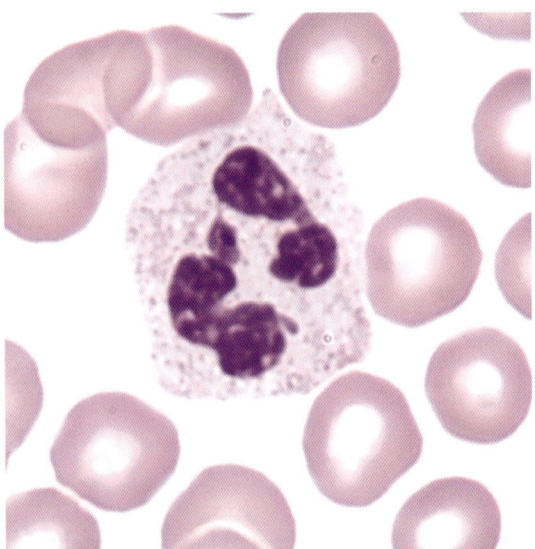

Fig. 1.3 Segmented Neutrophil. (From Rodak BF, Carr JH: *Clinical hematology atlas,* ed 4, St. Louis, 2013, Elsevier.)

less than 1 day. It has now been established that neutrophils redistribute into multiple tissues. Neutrophils exist in the peripheral blood for about 10 hours after they are released from the marrow. During this time they move back and forth between the general blood circulation and the walls of the blood vessels, where they accumulate. They also leave the blood and enter the tissues, where they carry out their primary functions. In the tissues, neutrophils fight bacterial infections and are then destroyed or eliminated from the body by the excretory system (intestinal tract, urine, lungs, or saliva).

Neutrophilic leukocytes, particularly the PMN type, provide an effective host defense against bacterial and fungal infections. The antimicrobial function of PMNs is essential in the innate immune response. Although other granulocytes are also phagocytic cells, the PMNs and macrophages are the principal cells associated with **phagocytosis** (i.e., the capture and destruction of invading microorganisms; see Chapter 4) and a localized inflammatory response. Inflammatory **exudate (pus)**, which develops rapidly in an inflammatory response, is composed primarily of neutrophils and monocytes.

PMNs can prolong **inflammation** by the release of soluble substances, such as **cytokines** and chemokines. The role of neutrophils in influencing the adaptive immune response is believed to include shuttling pathogens to draining lymph nodes, antigen presentation, and modulation of T-lymphocyte responses.

Mature neutrophils are found in two evenly divided pools: the circulating and the marginating pools. The marginating granulocytes adhere to the vascular endothelium. In the peripheral blood, these cells are only in transit to their potential sites of action in the tissues. Movement of granulocytes from the circulating pool to the peripheral tissues occurs by movement through the vessel wall. Once in the peripheral tissues, the neutrophils are able to carry out their function of capture and destruction of invading pathogens or foreign particles.

Eosinophils

Although capable of participating in phagocytosis, eosinophils and basophils have less phagocytic activity. The ineffectiveness of these cells results from the small number of cells in the circulating blood and a lack of powerful digestive enzymes. However, both eosinophils and basophils are functionally important in the body's defense.

Eosinophils (Fig. 1.4) are granulocytes and generally make up about 3% of the circulating leukocytes. They are slightly larger than neutrophils. The nucleus occupies a relatively small part of the cell. The nucleus is usually bilobed, and occasionally three lobes are seen. The nuclear structure is similar to that of the neutrophil, but the lobes are plumper and the chromatin often stains lighter purple than in the neutrophil. The nuclear membrane is distinct, and no nucleoli are visible. The cytoplasm is usually colorless, but it may be faintly basophilic. It is crowded with spheric acidophilic granules, which stain red-orange with eosin and are larger and more distinct than neutrophilic granules. The granules are evenly distributed throughout the cytoplasm but are rarely seen overlying the nucleus. A second population of eosinophilic granules is highly refractive, a feature that is often a valuable distinguishing characteristic.

The eosinophil is considered to be a regulator of inflammation. Functionally this means that the eosinophil attempts to suppress an inflammatory reaction to prevent the excessive spread of the inflammation. The eosinophil may also play a role in the host defense mechanism because of its ability to kill certain parasites. Although capable of participating in phagocytosis, eosinophils and basophils are less effective in phagocytosis than neutrophils. Eosinophils exist in the peripheral blood for less than 8 hours after release from the marrow and have a short survival time in the tissues.

An increase in eosinophils is associated with a wide variety of conditions, but especially with allergic reactions, drug reactions, certain skin disorders, parasitic infestations, collagen vascular diseases, Hodgkin disease, and myeloproliferative diseases.

Basophils

Basophils (Fig. 1.5) are granulocytes that normally constitute an average of 0.6% of the total circulating leukocytes. They are about the same size as neutrophils, but their nuclei usually occupy a relatively greater portion of the cell. The nucleus is often extremely irregular in shape, varying from a lobular form to a form showing indentations that are not deep enough to divide it into definite lobes. The nuclear pattern is indistinct and stains purple or blue. The nuclear membrane is fairly distinct, and no nucleoli are visible. The cytoplasm is usually colorless; it contains a variable number of deeply stained, coarse, round, or angular basophilic granules. The granules (metachromatic) stain deep purple or black;

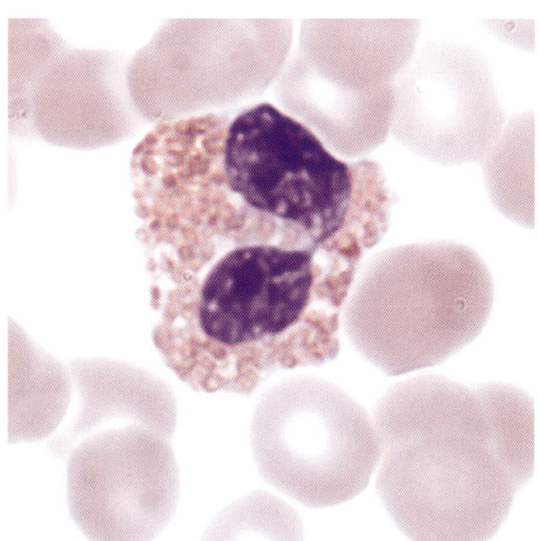

Fig. 1.4 Eosinophil. (From Rodak BF, Carr JH: *Clinical hematology atlas*, ed 4, St. Louis, 2013, Elsevier.)

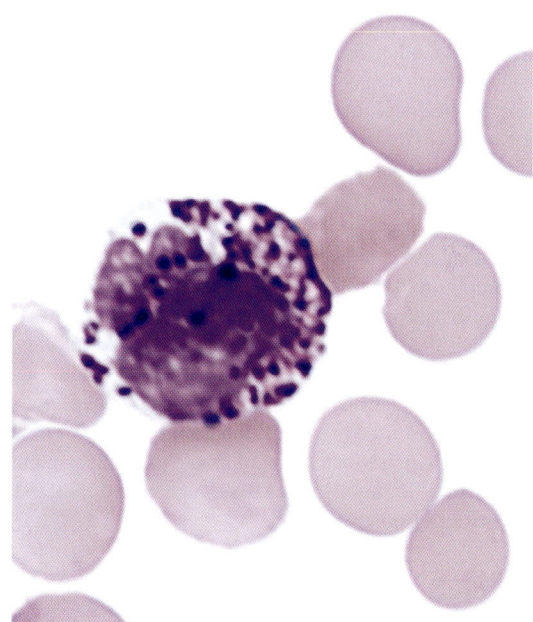

Fig. 1.5 Basophil. (From Rodak BF, Carr JH: *Clinical hematology atlas*, ed 4, St. Louis, 2013, Elsevier.)

occasionally a few smaller, brownish granules may be present. They may overlie and obscure the nucleus. Because the granules are soluble in water, occasionally a few or even most of them may be dissolved during the staining procedure. When this occurs, the cell contains vacuoles in place of granules, and the cytoplasm may appear grayish or brownish in their vicinity. The cytoplasm of a mature basophil is colorless.

Basophils have high concentrations of heparin and histamine in their granules. If events are triggered by antigens from pollen, food, drugs, or insect venom, the result is an immediate hypersensitivity reaction.

Tissue Basophils (Mast Cells)

Tissue basophils are also called *mast cells*. Mast cells are bone marrow–derived cells found in the skin and mucosal barriers. These cells resemble basophils with abundant basophilic, cytoplasmic granules.

Tissue basophils are activated by microbial binding and complement components as part of innate immunity or by an antibody-dependent mechanism of adaptive immunity. Degranulation occurs when an antigen such as pollen binds to two adjacent immunoglobulin E (IgE) antibody molecules located on the surface of mast cells. The events resulting from the release of the contents of these basophilic granules include increased vascular permeability, smooth muscle spasm, and vasodilation. If severe, this reaction can result in anaphylactic shock (see Chapter 20).

Tissue basophils are an important defense against parasitic helminths and other pathogens, in addition to snake and insect venom. Some subsets of basophils are involved in normal tissue homeostasis (e.g., neurogenic and endocrine responses).

MONONUCLEAR PHAGOCYTE SYSTEM

In the past the mononuclear phagocyte system (MPS) was known only as a scavenger cell system. Recently the role of the MPS as a complex component of the immune system in the host defense against infection has been recognized. The MPS is considered a cellular system because of the common origin, similar morphology, and shared functions, including rapid phagocytosis, mediated by receptors and a major fragment of complement (C1).

Cells of the MPS system originate in the bone marrow from the multipotential stem cell. This common committed progenitor cell can differentiate into the granulocyte or monocyte-macrophage pathway, depending on the microenvironment and chemical regulators. Maturation and differentiation of these cells may occur in various directions. Circulating monocytes may continue to be multipotential and give rise to different types of macrophages.

The MPS consists of monocytes, DCs, and macrophages. The system, comprised of promonocytes and their precursors in the bone marrow, monocytes in circulation, and terminally differentiated macrophages at peripheral tissue sites, represents a continuum that is dynamically controlled through proliferation, differentiation, maturation, and precise movement of cells (trafficking). Macrophages and monocytes resident in the tissues of the body are already strategically placed to recognize and deal with an intruding agent. They migrate freely into the tissues from the blood to replenish and reinforce the macrophage population.

The MPS contributes to various functions that are essential for maintaining homeostasis, activation of innate immunity, and bridging it with the adaptive immunity. The MPS is highly significant in bolstering immunity against pathogens.

MONOCYTES

Monocytes (Fig. 1.6), as with granulocytes, are produced mainly in the bone marrow. Monocytes, like granulocytes, are derived from the

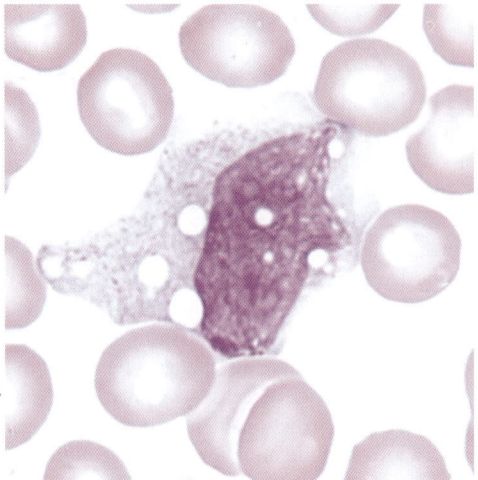

Fig. 1.6 Monocyte. (From Rodak BF, Carr JH: *Clinical hematology atlas*, ed 4, St. Louis, 2013, Elsevier.)

myeloid cell line. They make up about 4% to 6% of normal circulating leukocytes, ranging from 2% to 10%, depending on the laboratory or author. Monocytes are the largest of the normal leukocytes.

The nucleus is fairly large; it may be round, oval, indented, lobular, notched, or rarely even segmented, but most frequently it is indented or horseshoe shaped. The nuclear chromatin stains light purple and is delicate or lacy. Chromatin and parachromatin are sharply segregated, and the chromatin is distributed in a linear arrangement of delicate strands, which gives the nucleus a stringy appearance. The nuclear membrane is delicate but not distinct, and nucleoli usually are not seen.

The cytoplasm is abundant and stains gray or gray-blue. It may contain numerous small, poorly defined granules, resulting in a "ground-glass" appearance, and is often vacuolated. Extremely fine and abundant azurophilic granules are present; this granulation is called *azure dust* and is seen only in monocytes. The granules vary in color from light pink to bright purplish red. In addition, phagocytized particles may be seen in the cytoplasm.

Macrophages

The macrophage (Fig. 1.7) and its precursors are widely distributed throughout the body. Macrophages have long been viewed as major components of the innate immune system as a result of their ability to coordinate directional movement with the detection and elimination of foreign entities. Macrophages also facilitate tissue repair and remodeling, resolution of inflammation, maintenance of homeostasis, and disease progression.

Although distinct macrophage subsets populate the developing embryo and fetus in three distinct waves, little is known about the functional differences between in utero macrophage populations and how they might contribute to fetal and neonatal immunity. Macrophage populations may share common functional properties in the moments after their differentiation from myeloid progenitors during fetal hematopoiesis. Upon trafficking to the circulation and into various tissues, the local microenvironment then shapes macrophage biology and promotes specialized, tissue-specific functions.

An initial concept was that tissue macrophages were derived from multiple organs in early-stage monocyte differentiation, the kinetics of tissue macrophage repopulation by circulating monocytes, and macrophage proliferation in tissues. Now it is recognized that a steady-state maintenance of tissue macrophage populations is not the result of the recruitment of circulating macrophages, but rather of proliferation of tissue-resident cells. There is a fundamental distinction in macrophage

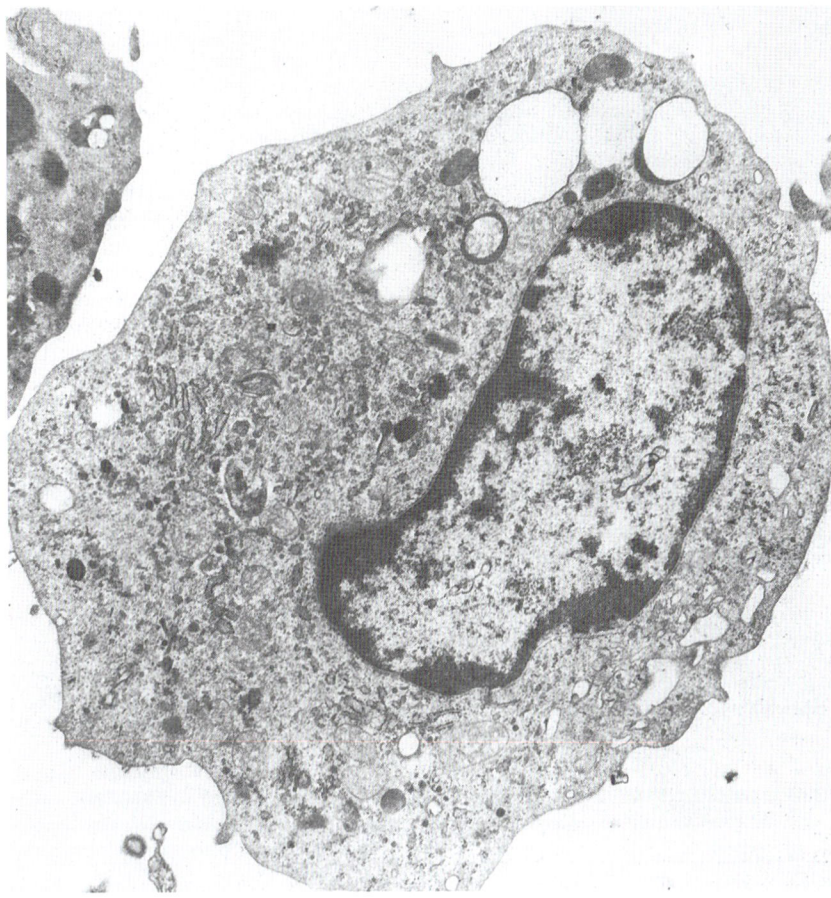

Fig. 1.7 Electron Micrograph of a Macrophage. (From Barrett JT: *Textbook of immunology*, ed 5, St. Louis, 1988, Mosby.)

populations and function. Tissue homeostasis is maintained by resident macrophages established during development; macrophages generated from adult hematopoiesis participate predominantly in response to tissue insult and disease resolution. Resident macrophages can be distinguished from macrophages that enter tissues from the circulation because they tend to express higher levels of the G-protein–coupled receptor F4/80.

Specialized macrophages, such as pulmonary alveolar macrophages, are the so-called dust phagocytes of the lung that function as the first line of defense against inhaled foreign particles and bacteria. Macrophages line the endothelium of capillaries and the sinuses of organs such as the bone marrow, spleen, and lymph nodes. Kupffer cells, also known as *stellate macrophages*, are specialized macrophages located in the liver, lining the walls of the sinusoids that form part of the MPS (Fig. 1.8).

Functionally the most important step in the maturation of macrophages is the mediator (cytokine)–driven conversion of the normal resting macrophage to the activated macrophage. Macrophages can be activated during infection by the release of macrophage-activating cytokines, such as interferon-γ (IFN-γ) and granulocyte colony-stimulating factor (G-CSF), from T lymphocytes specifically sensitized to antigens from the infecting microorganisms. This interaction constitutes the basis of cell-mediated immunity. In addition, macrophages exposed to an **endotoxin** release a hormone, tumor necrosis factor α (TNF-α), or cachectin, which can activate macrophages itself under certain in vitro conditions.

The terminal stage of development in the mononuclear phagocyte cell line is the multinucleated giant cell, which characterizes granulomatous inflammatory diseases, such as tuberculosis. Both monocytes and macrophages can be shown in the lesions in these diseases before the formation of giant cells, thought to be precursors of the multinucleated cells.

Macrophages and neutrophils have different characteristics, but they are the most effective phagocytic cells (Table 1.4).

Dendritic Cells

DCs (also known as *accessory cells*) resemble the microscopic appearance of nerve cells (i.e., dendrites) with long, string-like extensions. DCs act as sentinels in tissues that respond to microbes by producing soluble substances, cytokines. They act as messengers between the innate and the adaptive immune systems.

The common portals of entry for microbes are the skin and the gastrointestinal, respiratory, and urogenital tracts. These tissue locations contain the classic, or conventional, DCs (Table 1.5). DCs or macrophages residing in tissues capture microbes or antigens and present processed antigens to lymphocytes; these are the first steps in the development of an adaptive immune response.

The main function of tissue DCs is to process antigens and present them on the cell surface to the T lymphocytes of the immune system. Other antigen-presenting cells (APCs; macrophages and B lymphocytes) present antigens to differentiated effector T lymphocytes in various immune responses.

Follicular dendritic cells (FDCs) reside in the germinal centers (GCs) of lymphoid follicles in peripheral lymphoid organs and display antigens that stimulate the differentiation of B lymphocytes in the follicles.

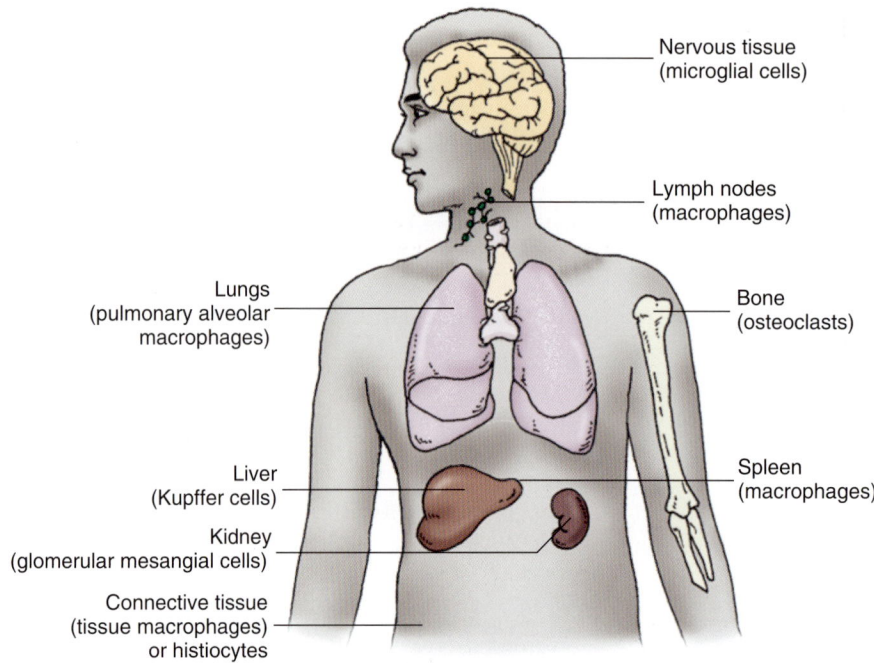

Fig. 1.8 Mononuclear Phagocyte System. (Adapted from Roitt IM: *Essential immunology,* ed 5, Oxford, 1984, Blackwell Scientific.)

TABLE 1.4	Comparison of Characteristics of Neutrophils and Macrophages	
Characteristic	**Neutrophils**	**Monocytes-Macrophages**
Life cycle	Highly variable concentration in peripheral circulating blood, but react with increased concentration in infection	Consistent concentration produced at a steady state
	Only migrate to inflamed tissue injury	Migrate into tissues without the presence of inflammation
	Die a few hours after migrating into tissue and encountering pathogen	Can survive for many years after encountering pathogens
Killing of pathogens	Phagocytosis	Phagocytosis
	Kill pathogens by release of toxic molecules and enzymes	Kill pathogens by release of toxic molecules and enzymes
	Produce neutrophil cellular traps[a]	
Interaction with other immune components	Short-lived secretion of soluble mediators, chemokines, that recruits more neutrophils to the site of inflammation/infection	Recruit neutrophils to site of inflammation/infection by secreting soluble mediators, cytokines
	Respond to soluble mediator interleukin (IL-17) from the adaptive immune system	Respond to soluble mediator, interferon, from adaptive immune system
	Do not provide many signals to interact with adaptive immune system	Stimulate adaptive immune system by presenting processed antigen and secreting soluble mediators, cytokines

[a]Neutrophil extracellular traps (NETs) are networks of extracellular fibers, primarily composed of DNA from neutrophils, which bind pathogens. NETs are a first line of defense against infection because NETs kill invading pathogens by engulfing microbes and secreting antimicrobial mediators.
Adapted from Helbert M: *Immunology for medical students,* ed 3, St. Louis, 2017, Elsevier.

TABLE 1.5	Classic Human Dendritic Cell Subsets		
	Major	**Crosspresenting[a]**	**Plasmacytoid Dendritic Cells[b]**
Major proposed functions	Innate immunity: Source of inflammatory cytokines		Antiviral immunity: Early innate response; priming of antiviral T lymphocytes
	Adaptive immunity: Capture and presentation of antigens mostly to CD4+ T lymphocytes	Adaptive immunity: Capture and crosspresentation of antigens to CD8+ T lymphocytes	

[a]Presentation of exogenous antigens on major histocompatibility complex class I molecules, which is essential for the initiation of CD8+ T-cell responses.
[b]A rare type of immune cell that circulates in the blood and is found in peripheral lymphoid organs. These cells secrete large quantities of type 1 interferon in response to a viral infection.
Adapted from Abbas AK, Lichtman AH, Pillai S: *Cellular and molecular immunology,* ed 9, Philadelphia, 2018, Elsevier.

LYMPHOCYTE VARIATIONS

The adaptive immune system is composed of the cellular and humoral systems. Each of the two arms of the adaptive immune system has fundamental mechanisms allowing the body to attack an invading pathogen. The immunologically specific cellular component of the immune system is organized around two classes of specialized cells, T lymphocytes and B lymphocytes. Lymphocytes recognize foreign antigens, directly destroy some cells, or produce antibodies as plasma cells.

Virgin, or naïve, lymphocytes (Fig. 1.9) are mature T or B lymphocytes that have not encountered or been stimulated by a foreign antigen. Naïve and memory lymphocytes are both called *resting lymphocytes* because they are not actively dividing or performing immune functions.

A newly discovered lymphocyte, the ILC, straddles the innate and adaptive immune systems. Unlike lymphocytes associated with the adaptive immune system, ILCs cannot perform gene rearrangement of their antigen receptors. Although conventional classes of lymphocytes greatly outnumber ILCs, innate cells have been implicated in a variety of diseases, especially ones associated with mucosal surfaces such as the skin, lung, and gut.

> **KEY CONCEPTS: Facts About Lymphocyte Development**
> - In mammalian immunologic development the precursors of lymphocytes arise from progenitor cells of the yolk sac and liver in the embryo.
> - Later in fetal development and throughout the life cycle, the bone marrow becomes the sole provider of undifferentiated progenitor cells, which can further develop into lymphoblasts.
> - Continued cellular development and proliferation of lymphoid precursors occur as the cells travel to the primary and secondary lymphoid tissues.
> - Mature lymphocytes differentiate into the main categories of T lymphocytes or B lymphocytes and include different subsets of highly specialized lymphocytes.
> - T cells arise in the thymus from fetal liver or bone marrow precursors that seed the thymus during embryonic development.
> - B lymphocytes most likely mature in the bone marrow and function primarily in antibody production or the formation of antibodies.
> - Plasma cells arise as the end stage of B-cell differentiation into a large, activated plasma cell.
> - An increase in the number of lymphocytes is associated with viral infections.
> - NK lymphocytes are very important in host defense and are recognized as a unique and important part of the immune system with roles in both infectious disease defense and tumor surveillance.
> - A newly discovered type of lymphocyte, the ILC, straddles the innate and adaptive immune systems.

Lymphocyte Development

In mammalian immunologic development the precursors of lymphocytes arise from progenitor cells of the yolk sac and liver in the embryo (Fig. 1.10). Later in fetal development and throughout the life cycle the bone marrow becomes the sole provider of undifferentiated progenitor cells, which can further develop into lymphoblasts. Continued cellular development and proliferation of lymphoid precursors occur as the cells travel to the primary and secondary lymphoid tissues. Mature lymphocytes differentiate into the main categories of T lymphocytes or B lymphocytes (Table 1.6) and include different subsets of highly specialized lymphocytes (discussed in Chapter 4).

Naïve lymphocytes must see proteins displayed by DCs to initiate clonal expansion and differentiation of T lymphocytes into effector and memory cells. Naïve lymphocytes produce cytokines similar to helper T cells but do not express T-cell antigen receptors.

Lymphocytes make up about 34% of the leukocytes in the normal adult. Infants and children normally have more lymphocytes and fewer neutrophils than adults, a reversed differential. Lymphocytes fall into two general groups, small and large. Most normal lymphocytes are small.

When observed microscopically, lymphocytes are described based on their size and cytoplasmic granularity. Small lymphocytes are found in the greatest numbers. The small lymphocyte is composed chiefly of nucleus and is the type of lymphocyte predominating in normal adult blood. It is about the same size as a normocytic (nucleated) RBC and is a useful size marker during examination of the peripheral blood film, especially in cases of megaloblastic anemia, in which all cell forms other than lymphocytes are increased in diameter.

The nucleus is round or slightly notched, and the nuclear chromatin is in the form of coarse, dense, deeply staining blocks. There is relatively little parachromatin, and it is not very distinct. Almost the entire nucleus stains deep purple. The nuclear membrane is heavy and distinct, and nucleoli are not usually seen. The cytoplasm appears in the form of a narrow band that stains pale blue with few, if any, red (azure) granules.

The large lymphocyte shows a further increase in the size of the nucleus and an increase in the relative amount of cytoplasm. The nucleus contains more parachromatin and thus stains more lightly than the nuclei of the smaller forms. The chromatin is still present in clumps, without distinct outlines because of the blending of chromatin and parachromatin. The nuclear membrane is distinct, and nucleoli usually are not seen. The cytoplasm in this form can be abundant, and azure granules are frequently seen. The cytoplasm color varies from colorless to a clear light or medium blue. The cytoplasm of the large granular lymphocyte (LGL) can be deeply basophilic. Morphologically T and B lymphocytes appear identical on a Wright-stained blood film, but their appearance is very different with scanning electron microscopy (Fig. 1.11)

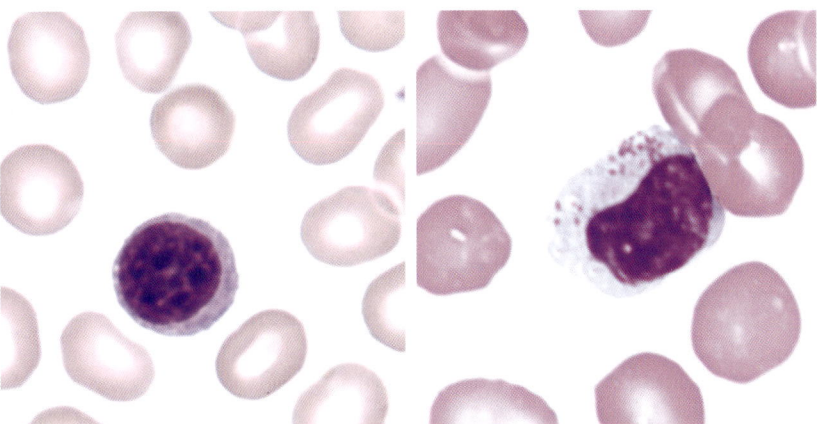

Fig. 1.9 Lymphocytes. (From Rodak BF, Carr JH: *Clinical hematology atlas*, ed 4, St. Louis, 2013, Elsevier.)

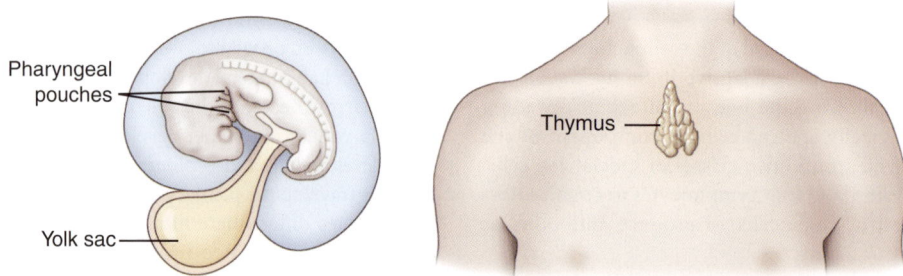

Fig. 1.10 Development of Immunologic Organs. The anatomy of the human fetus illustrates the development of the mammalian immune system. Cells of the pharyngeal pouches migrate into the chest and form the thymus. Precursors of lymphocytes originate early in embryonic life in the yolk sac and eventually migrate to the bone marrow via the spleen and liver.

TABLE 1.6 Stages of Maturation of T and B Lymphocytes			
Stages of Maturation	Stem Cell	Immature Cell	Mature Cell
T Lymphocyte			
Anatomic location	Bone marrow	Thymus	Peripheral blood
Response to antigen	None	Positive and negative selection	Activation (and differentiation)
B Lymphocyte			
Anatomic location	Bone marrow	Bone marrow/ peripheral blood	Peripheral blood
Response to antigen	None	Negative selection (deletion), receptor editing	Activation (proliferation and differentiation)

Adapted from Turgeon ML: *Clinical hematology*, ed 6, Philadelphia, 2018, Lippincott.

After antigenic stimulation, small lymphocytes can undergo transformation. These transformed cells appear large on Wright-stained films, with a relatively large amount of deep blue cytoplasm, and are called *large granular lymphocytes*. The large nucleus has a reticular appearance, with uniform chromatin and prominent nucleoli. Such cells have various names, including *reactive*, *atypical*, *variant*, and *reticular lymphocytes*.

Nucleoli can be observed in reactive or neoplastic lymphocyte nucleoli but are not routinely observed in normal resting lymphocytes.

An increase in the number of lymphocytes is associated with viral infections. It is characteristic of certain acute infections, such as infectious mononucleosis; pertussis, mumps, and rubella; and German measles, and of chronic infections, such as tuberculosis, brucellosis, and infectious hepatitis. The changes seen in these diseases have been referred to as *reactive* or *atypical changes* and are particularly associated with infectious mononucleosis. The cells are called *reactive lymphocytes* because the increased amount and apparent activity of the cytoplasm indicate that it may be reacting to some sort of stimulus. These cells can be referred to as *variant forms*.

Lymphocytes act to direct the immune response system of the body. Maturation of lymphocytes in the bone marrow or thymus results in cells that are immunocompetent. The cells are able to respond to antigenic challenges by directing the immune responses of the host defense. They migrate to various sites in the body to await antigenic stimulus and activation. Only when immunologic studies are performed can these cells be identified as belonging to specific subsets of lymphocytes. As lymphocytes mature, their identity and function are specified by the antigenic structures on their external membrane surface.

T Cells

T cells arise in the thymus from fetal liver or bone marrow precursors that seed the thymus during embryonic development. These CD34+ progenitor cells develop in the thymic cortex. B lymphocytes are derived from hematopoietic stem cells by a complex series of differentiation events. T lymphocytes mature in the thymus and function in cell-mediated immune responses, such as delayed hypersensitivity, graft-versus-host reactions, and allograft rejection. T cells make up the majority of the lymphocytes circulating in the peripheral blood. In the periphery of the thymus they further differentiate into multiple different T-cell subpopulations with different functions, including cytotoxicity and the secretion of soluble factors (cytokines). Many different cytokines have been identified, including 25 interleukin molecules and more than 40 chemokines; their functions include growth promotion, differentiation, chemotaxis, and cell stimulation.

B Cells

B lymphocytes most likely mature in the bone marrow and function primarily in antibody production or the formation of immunoglobulins. B cells constitute about 10% to 30% of the blood lymphocytes. Some activated B cells differentiate into memory B cells, long-lived cells that circulate in the blood. Memory B cells may live for years, but mature B cells that are not activated live only for days. B lymphocytes undergo blast transformation into plasma cells with appropriate antigen stimulation.

Mammalian B-cell development encompasses a continuum of stages that begins in primary lymphoid tissue, such as human fetal liver and fetal or adult marrow, with subsequent functional maturation in secondary lymphoid tissue, such as human lymph nodes and spleen. The functional or protective endpoint is antibody production by terminally differentiated plasma cells. At least 10 distinct transcription factors regulate the early stages of B-cell development.

B cells are derived from progenitor cells through an antigen-independent maturation process occurring in the bone marrow and **gut-associated lymphoid tissue (GALT)**. Plasma cells or antibody-forming cells are terminally differentiated B cells. These cells are entirely devoted to antibody production, a primary host defense against microorganisms.

Plasma Cells

Plasma cells (Fig. 1.12) are not normally found in the circulating blood but are found in the bone marrow in concentrations that do not normally exceed 2%. A greater concentration of plasma cells can be seen in the bone marrow.

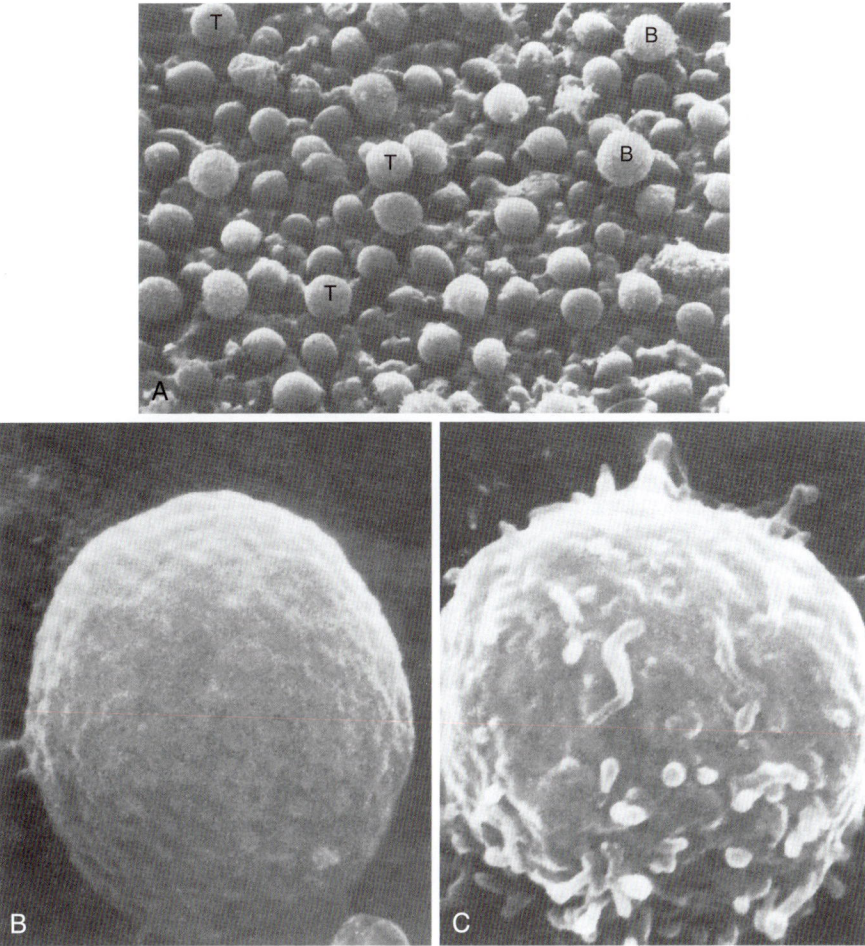

Fig. 1.11 Scanning Electron Photomicrographs of Lymphocyte Cell Surface Membranes. (A) T and B lymphocytes. (B) T lymphocyte. (C) B lymphocyte. (From Polliack A, Lampen N, Clarkson BD, et al: Identification of human B and T lymphocytes by scanning electron microscopy, *J Exp Med* 138:607–624, 1973.)

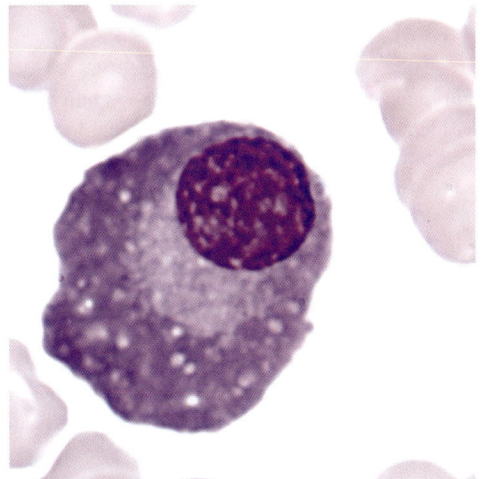

Fig. 1.12 Plasma Cell. (From Rodak BF, Carr JH: *Clinical hematology atlas*, ed 4, St. Louis, 2013, Elsevier.)

After binding and cooperative interaction with T cells, B cells undergo transformation into plasma cells. B-lymphocyte differentiation is complex and proceeds through both an antigen-independent and an antigen-dependent state, culminating in the generation of mature, end-stage, plasma cells.

Plasma cells are large with a round or an oval nucleus that is usually in an eccentric position. The chromatin consists of deeply stained, heavy masses that may be arranged in a radial pattern. The cytoplasm is strongly basophilic. There may be a pale, clear zone in the cytoplasm to one side of the nucleus, referred to as a *hof*. Immature forms may occasionally be seen.

Plasma cells function in the synthesis of immunoglobulins. They may be seen in the peripheral blood of patients with measles, chickenpox, or scarlet fever, and in the malignant conditions of multiple myeloma and plasmacytic leukemia.

Natural Killer Lymphocytes

The third major population of lymphocytes, NK lymphocytes, uses different strategies to discriminate self from nonself. These cells are very important in host defense and are recognized as a unique and important part of the immune system, with roles in both infectious disease defense and tumor surveillance. Originally described in terms of natural killing of tumors, NK lymphocytes have a major role in controlling pathogens, especially viruses. Clonal expansion of NK cells occurs after viral exposure. Human patients with selective NK cell deficiencies have recurrent, severe viral infections.

NK cells vary morphologically from typical lymphocytes and appear as large lymphocytes with characteristic azurophilic granules in the cytoplasm. There are two phenotypically distinct subsets of NK cells. A total of 70% to 80% of NK cells have the appearance of LGLs. Up to about 75% of LGLs function as NK cells, and LGLs appear to account fully for the NK activity in mixed cell populations.

The NK subpopulation is approximately 10% of circulating lymphocytes. NK lymphocytes lack conventional antigen receptors of T or B cells. Monoclonal antibodies (MAbs) demonstrate that NK cells express a variety of surface membrane markers (see Table 4.3). NK cells synthesize a number of cytokines involved in the modulation of hematopoiesis and immune responses and in the regulation of their own activities.

NK cells destroy target cells through an extracellular, nonphagocytic mechanism referred to as a *cytotoxic reaction*. Target cells include tumor cells, some cells of the embryo, cells of the normal bone marrow and thymus, and microbial agents. A considerable number of NK cells may be present in other tissues, particularly in the lungs and liver, where they may play important roles in inflammatory reactions and in host defense, including defense against certain viruses (e.g., cytomegalovirus, hepatitis). NK cells actively kill virally infected target cells, and if this activity is completed before the virus has time to replicate, a viral infection may be stopped.

INNATE LYMPHOID CELLS

As mentioned previously, ILCs straddle the innate and adaptive immune systems. ILCs are lymphocyte-like cells that produce cytokines and perform similar functions to CD4+ and CD8+ effector cells; however, they do not express T-cell receptors (TCRs). ILCs include several developmentally related subsets of bone marrow–derived cells with lymphoid morphology and effector functions similar to those of T cells, but lacking T-cell antigen receptors.

Unlike lymphocytes associated with the adaptive immune system, ILCs cannot perform gene rearrangement of their antigen receptors. Although conventional classes of lymphocytes greatly outnumber ILCs, innate cells have been implicated in a variety of diseases, especially ones associated with mucosal surfaces such as the skin, lung, and gut.

> **KEY CONCEPTS: Primary and Secondary Lymphoid Organs**
> - In mammals, both the bone marrow (and/or fetal liver) and thymus are classified as primary or central lymphoid organs.
> - The bone marrow is the source of progenitor stem cells.
> - In mammals the bone marrow also supports eventual differentiation of mature T and B lymphocytes, probably from a common lymphoid cell progenitor.
> - Bone marrow and GALT may also play a role in the differentiation of progenitor cells into B lymphocytes.
> - The secondary lymphoid tissues include lymph nodes, spleen, GALT, thoracic duct, bronchus-associated lymphoid tissue (BALT), skin-associated lymphoid tissue, and blood.
> - Lymphocytes move freely between the blood and lymphoid tissues. This lymphocyte recirculation enables lymphocytes to come into contact with processed foreign antigens and disseminate antigen-sensitized memory cells throughout the lymphoid system

Primary Lymphoid Organs

In mammals both the bone marrow (and/or fetal liver) and thymus are classified as primary or central lymphoid organs (Fig. 1.13).

Bone Marrow

The bone marrow is the source of progenitor stem cells. Less than 1% of the marrow consists of stem cells. They have the ability to repopulate the bone marrow after injury or lethal radiation, which is the basis of bone marrow transplantation. These cells can differentiate into lymphocytes and other hematopoietic cells (e.g., granulocytes, erythrocytes, and megakaryocyte populations). In mammals the bone marrow also supports eventual differentiation of mature T and B lymphocytes,

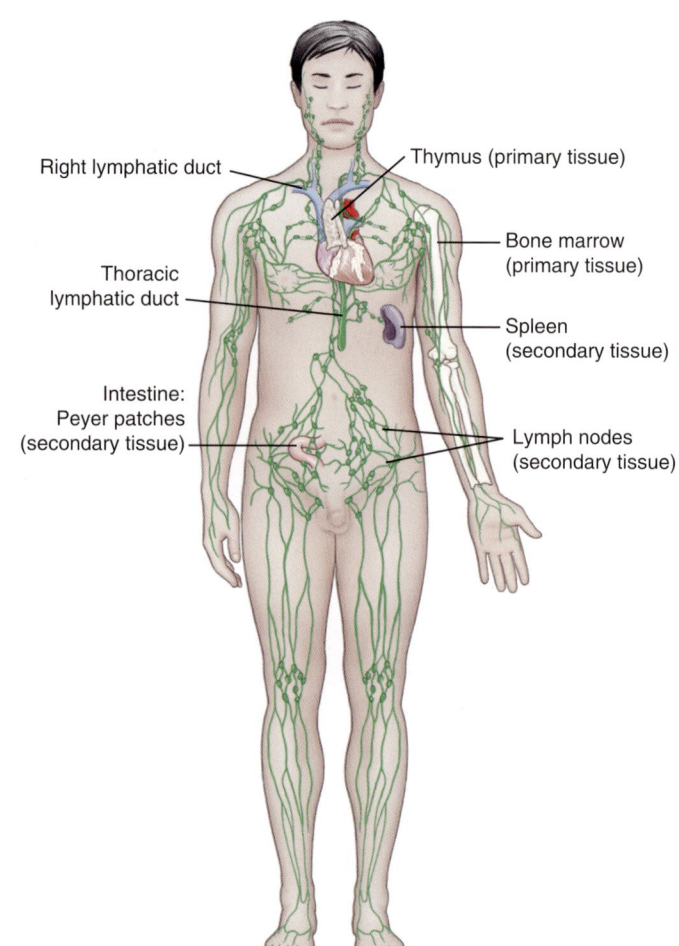

Fig. 1.13 Human Primary and Secondary Tissues.

probably from a common lymphoid cell progenitor. It is believed that the bone marrow and GALT may also play a role in the differentiation of progenitor cells into B lymphocytes.

Thymus

Early in embryonic development, the stroma and nonlymphoid epithelium of the thymus are derived from the third and fourth pharyngeal pouches. The characteristics of the thymus gland change with aging. Older persons are immunologically challenged because aging causes a reduction in the production of naïve T cells by the thymus. Intrinsic defects in mature T-cell function and alterations in the life span of naïve T cells and in naïve or memory T-cell ratios in the peripheral lymphoid tissues occur as the result of the decline of the T-cell response in older persons.

The thymus, located in the mediastinum, exercises control over the entire immune system. It is believed that the development of diversity occurs mainly in the thymus and bone marrow, although clonal expansion can occur anywhere in the peripheral lymphoid tissue.

Progenitor cells that migrate to the thymus proliferate and differentiate under the influence of the humoral factor thymosin. These lymphocyte precursors with acquired surface membrane antigens are referred to as *thymocytes*.

The reticular structure of the thymus allows a significant number of lymphocytes to pass through it to become fully immunocompetent (able to function in the immune response) thymus-derived T cells. The thymus also regulates immune function by the secretion of multiple soluble hormones.

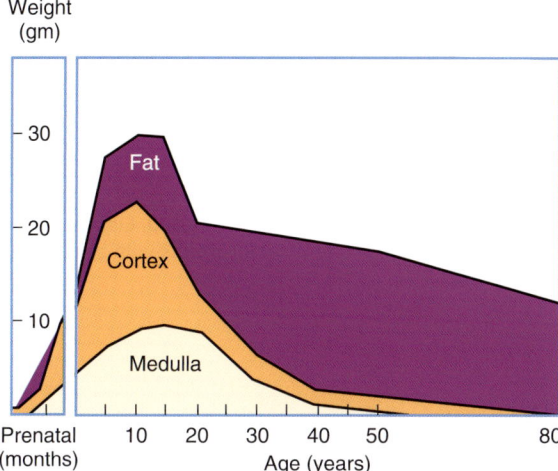

Fig. 1.14 Thymic Development. The histology of the thymus changes with age. The main feature of these changes is a loss of cellularity with advancing age.

TABLE 1.7 Approximate Concentrations of Lymphocytes of the Adaptive Immune System[a]	
Site	Number of Lymphocytes
Spleen	70×10^9/L
Lymph nodes	190×10^9/L
Bone marrow	50×10^9/L
Blood	10×10^9/L
Skin	20×10^9/L
Intestines	50×10^9/L
Liver	10×10^9/L
Lungs	30×10^9/L

[a]Concentrations are approximations based on data from human peripheral blood and mouse lymphoid organs. Not included are natural killer cells and other innate lymphoid cells.
Adapted from Abbas AK, Lichtman AH, Pillai S: *Basic immunology: functions and disorders of the immune system,* ed 6, Elsevier, 2020; Figs. 1.9 and 1.13. Valiathan R, Deeb K, Diamante M, et al: Reference ranges of lymphocyte subsets in healthy adults and adolescents with special mention of T cell maturation subsets in adults of South Florida, *Immunobiology* 219(7):487–496, 2014.

Many cells die in the thymus and apparently are phagocytized, a mechanism to eliminate lymphocyte clones reactive against self. It is estimated that approximately 97% of the cortical cells die in the thymus before becoming mature T cells. Viable cells migrate to the secondary tissues. The absence or abnormal development of the thymus results in a T-lymphocyte deficiency.

Involution of the thymus is the first age-related change occurring in the human immune system. In postnatal life, the thymus is the primary organ that produces naïve T cells for the peripheral T-cell pool, but production of cells declines as early as 3 months of age. The thymus gradually loses up to 95% of its mass during the first 50 years of life (Fig. 1.14). The accompanying functional changes of decreased synthesis of thymic hormones and the loss of ability to differentiate immature lymphocytes are reflected in an increased number of immature lymphocytes within the thymus and as circulating peripheral blood T cells. Most changes in immune function, such as dysfunction of T and B lymphocytes, elevated levels of circulating immune complexes, increases in autoantibodies, and monoclonal gammopathies (see Chapter 21), are correlated with involution of the thymus. Immune senescence, or biological aging, may account for the increased susceptibility of older adults to infections, autoimmune diseases, and neoplasms.

Secondary Lymphoid Organs

Secondary lymphoid organs provide a unique microenvironment for the initiation and development of immune responses. The secondary lymphoid tissues include lymph nodes, spleen, GALT, thoracic duct, BALT, skin-associated lymphoid tissue, and blood.

Mature lymphocytes and accessory cells (e.g., APCs) are found throughout the body, although the relative percentages of T and B cells vary in different locations (Tables 1.7 and 1.8).

The majority of mature B cells outside of the GALT reside within lymphoid follicles of the spleen and lymph nodes, where they encounter and respond to T-cell–dependent foreign antigens bound to FDCs, proliferate, and either differentiate into plasma cells or enter GC reactions. Antigen-induced B-cell activation and differentiation in secondary lymphoid tissues are mediated by dynamic changes in gene expression that give rise to the GC reaction.

GCs containing rapidly proliferating cells were first described in 1884 but were not identified as the main site for high-affinity antibody-secreting plasma cell and memory B–cell generation until a century later.

It is within GCs that purifying selection produces the higher affinity B-cell clones that form the memory component of humoral immunity. The dynamics of lymphocyte entry into follicles and their selection for migration into and within GCs represent a complex set of molecular interactions orchestrated by chemotactic gradients.

The highly sophisticated structure of secondary lymphoid organs allows migration and interactions between APCs, T and B lymphocytes, and FDCs and other stromal cells. The cooperative activities of lymphoid cells within secondary organs dramatically increase the probability of interactions of rare B cells, T cells, and APCs that result in effective generation of humoral immune responses.

Tumor necrosis factor (TNF) and lymphotoxin are essential to the formation and maintenance of secondary organs. These cytokines are produced by B and T lymphocytes. Proliferation of the T and B lymphocytes in the secondary or peripheral lymphoid tissues (Fig. 1.15) is primarily dependent on antigenic stimulation.

The T lymphocytes or T cells populate the following:
1. Perifollicular and paracortical regions of the lymph nodes
2. Medullary cords of the lymph nodes
3. Periarteriolar regions of the spleen
4. Thoracic duct of the circulatory system

The B lymphocytes or B cells multiply and populate the following:
1. Follicular and medullary regions (GCs) of the lymph nodes
2. Primary follicles and red pulp of the spleen
3. Follicular regions of the GALT
4. Medullary cords of the lymph nodes

Lymph Nodes

Lymph fluid is constantly drained from tissue through lymphatics into lymph nodes and eventually into the blood. Microbial antigens are carried in soluble form and within DCs in the lymph to lymph nodes, where they are recognized by lymphocytes.

Lymph nodes act as lymphoid filters in the lymphatic system. Lymph nodes respond to antigens introduced distally and routed to them by afferent lymphatics (Fig 1.16).

No membrane separates T and B lymphocytes in a lymph node. Chemokines, a family of cytokines that function in the regulation of the immune system, enhance immunity by guiding naïve CD8+ T cells

TABLE 1.8 Distribution of Lymphocytes in Lymphoid Organs and Other Tissues[a]

Site	CD4+ T Lymphocytes (%)	CD8+ T Lymphocytes (%)	T (T$_{reg}$) Lymphocytes (%)	B Lymphocytes (%)
Blood	35–60	15–40	0.5–2	5–20
Lymph nodes	50–60	15–20	5–10	20–25
Spleen	50–60	10–15	5–10	40–45

[a]Approximate numbers of lymphocytes in different organs of healthy adults.
Adapted from Abbas AK, Lichtman AH, Pillai S: *Basic immunology: functions and disorders of the immune system,* ed 6, 2020, Elsevier; Figs. 1.9 and 1.13 Valiathan R, Deeb K, Diamante M, et al: Reference ranges of lymphocyte subsets in healthy adults and adolescents with special mention of T cell maturation subsets in adults of South Florida, *Immunobiology* 219(7):487–496, 2014.

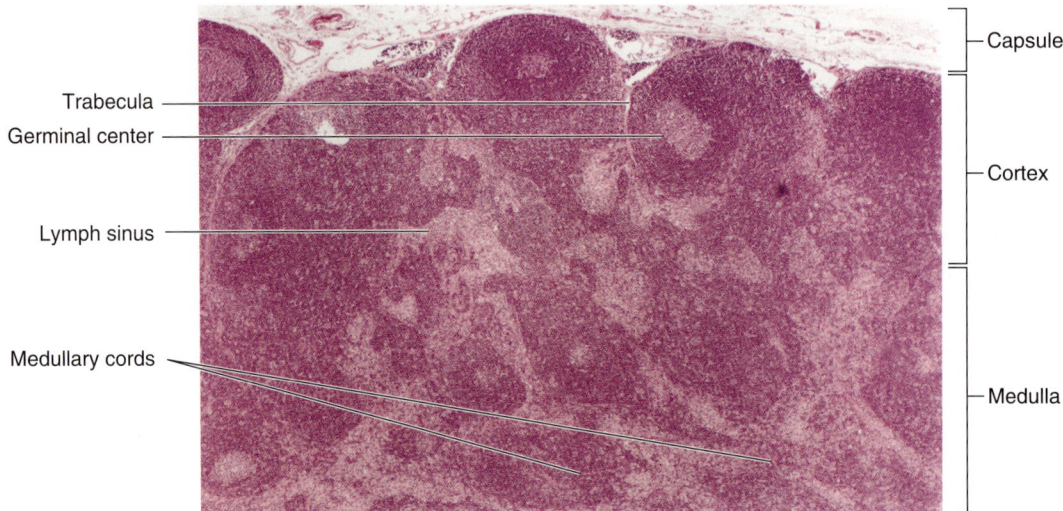

Fig. 1.15 Internal Structure of a Lymph Node. Photomicrography shows a portion of the cortex and medulla. (From Patton KT, Thibodeau GA: *Anthony's textbook of anatomy and physiology,* ed 20, St. Louis, 2013, Elsevier.)

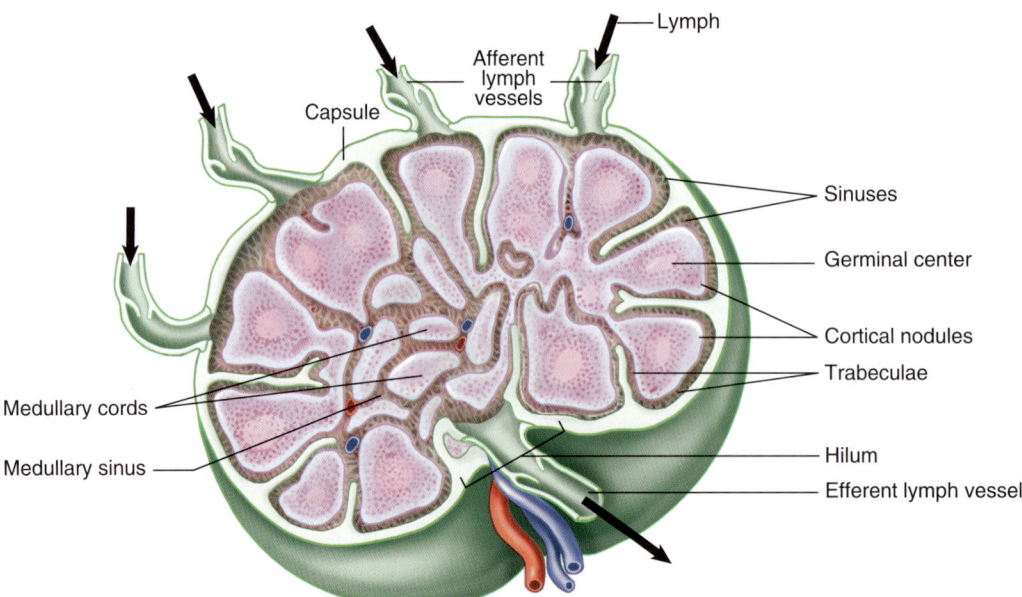

Fig. 1.16 Structure of a Lymph Node. Several afferent valved lymphatics bring lymph to the node. In this example, a single efferent lymphatic leaves the node at a concave area called the *hilum.* Note that the artery and vein enter and leave at the hilum. (From Patton KT, Thibodeau GA: *Anthony's textbook of anatomy and physiology,* ed 20, St. Louis, 2013, Elsevier.)

to sites of CD4+ T-cell–DC interaction. Antigen-activated T and B cells migrate to the T-B border by reversing resting chemokine receptor expression patterns.

Generalized lymph node reactivity can occur after systemic antigen challenge (e.g., serum sickness). During antibody responses, B cells undergo a series of migratory events that guide them to the appropriate microenvironments for activation and differentiation.

Spleen
The spleen acts as a lymphatic filter within the blood vascular tree. It is an important site of antibody production in response to IV particulate antigens (e.g., bacteria). The spleen is also a major organ for the clearance of particles.

Gut-Associated Lymphoid Tissue
GALT includes lymphoid tissue in the intestines (Peyer patches) and the liver. GALT features immunoglobulin A (IgA) production and involves a unique pattern of lymphocyte recirculation. Pre–B cells develop in Peyer patches and, after meeting antigen from the gut, many enter the general circulation and then return to the gut. GALT is also important for the development of tolerance to ingested antigens.

Thoracic Duct
The thoracic duct lymph is a rich source of mature T cells. Chronic thoracic duct drainage can cause T-cell depletion and has been used as a method of immunosuppression.

Bronchus-Associated Lymphoid Tissue
BALT includes lymphoid tissue in the lower respiratory tract and hilar lymph nodes. It is mainly associated with IgA production in response to inhaled antigens.

Skin-Associated Lymphoid Tissue
Antigens introduced through the skin are presented by epidermal Langerhans cells, which are bone marrow–derived accessory cells. These epidermal cells then interact with lymphocytes in the skin and in draining lymph nodes.

Blood
The blood is an important lymphoid organ and immunologic effector tissue. Circulating blood has enough mature T cells to produce a graft-versus-host reaction. In addition, blood transfusions have been responsible for inducing acquired immunologic tolerance in kidney transplant patients (see Chapter 25).

Blood is the most frequently sampled lymphoid organ. It is assumed that what is found in blood samples represents what is present in other lymphoid tissues. Although this may be a true representation, it is not always accurate.

Circulation of Lymphocytes
Mature T lymphocytes survive for several months or years, whereas the average life span of B lymphocytes is only a few days. Lymphocytes move freely between the blood and lymphoid tissues. This activity, termed *lymphocyte recirculation*, enables lymphocytes to come into contact with processed foreign antigens and disseminate antigen-sensitized memory cells throughout the lymphoid system. Clonal expansion may occur regionally, as when lymph nodes drain a contact allergic reaction. The whole body then becomes susceptible to rechallenge because T cells recirculate but generally are excluded from returning to the thymus. Research has shown that a pool of T-cell clonal elements is developed by a combination of positive selection of clones able to recognize and react to foreign antigens and negative selection (purging) of clones able to interact with self-antigens in a damaging way.

Recirculation of lymphocytes back to the blood is through the major lymphatic ducts. Lymphocytes enter the lymph node from the blood circulation via arterioles and capillaries to reach the specialized postcapillary venules. From the venule, the lymphocytes enter the node and either remain in the node or pass through the node and return to the circulating blood. Lymphatic fluid, lymphocytes, and antigens from certain body sites enter the lymph node through the afferent lymphatic duct and exit the lymph node through the efferent lymphatic duct.

> **KEY CONCEPTS: Major Characteristics of Innate and Adaptive Immunity**
> - The innate immune system is composed of DCs, monocytes, macrophages, granulocytic cell lines, NK lymphocytes, and ILCs.
> - The innate immune system and the alternative complement pathways are activated immediately after infection and quickly begin to control multiplication of infecting microorganisms.
> - The adaptive immune system is organized around two classes of cells, T and B lymphocytes. If a microorganism overwhelms the body's natural, innate resistance, the third line of defense, adaptive immunity, steps in.

COMPARISON OF INNATE AND ADAPTIVE IMMUNITY

The innate immune system and the adaptive immune system both defend the body, but they differ in many characteristics (Table 1.9). The innate immune system, an ancient form of host defense, appeared before the adaptive immune system. It is composed of a diverse array of evolutionarily ancient hematopoietic cell types, including DCs, monocytes, macrophages, granulocytic cell lines, and NK lymphocytes. ILCs are the most recently identified cells of the innate immune system. These cells have an emerging role in controlling tissue homeostasis in situations of infection, chronic inflammation, metabolic disease, and cancer. The innate immune system and the alternative complement pathways are activated immediately after infection and quickly begin to control multiplication of infecting microorganisms. Some form of innate immunity probably exists in all multicellular organisms. Innate immune recognition is mediated by germline-encoded receptors, which means that the specificity of each receptor is genetically predetermined. Germline-encoded receptors evolved by natural selection to have defined specificities for infectious microorganisms. The problem is that every organism has a limit as to the number of genes it can encode in its genome.

In contrast, the adaptive immune system is organized around two classes of cells, T and B lymphocytes. When an individual lymphocyte encounters an antigen that binds to its unique antigen receptor site, activation and proliferation of that lymphocyte occur. This is called clonal selection and is responsible for the basic properties of the adaptive immune system.

Random generation of a highly diverse database of antigen receptors allows the adaptive immune system to recognize virtually any antigen. The downside to this recognition is the inability to distinguish foreign antigens from self-antigens. Activation of the adaptive immune response can be harmful to the host when the antigens are self or environmental antigens. They can mimic other antigens and trigger an autoimmune condition.

Role of Microbiota
Bacteria, fungi, protozoa, and viruses colonize our skin, eyes, ears, nose, mouth, anus, vagina, and gastrointestinal tract. The term microbiome

TABLE 1.9 Comparison of Timeframe of Innate Immunity and Adaptive Immunity

Action	Innate Immediate Immunity (0–4 hours)	Innate Induced Immunity (4–96 hours)	Adaptive Immunity (3–5 days)
Initial phase	Exposure to pathogen	Exposure to pathogen	Exposure to pathogen
	Pathogen recognition by preformed nonspecific effectors	Pathogen recognized by receptors encoded in the germline	Pathogen recognized by receptors generated randomly
Second phase	Removal of infectious agent	Receptors have broad specificity (i.e., they recognize many related molecular structures [PAMPs])	Receptors have very narrow specificity (i.e., they recognize a specific epitope)
		Inflammatory response—recruitment and activation of effector cells	Recognition by naïve: T and B lymphocytes
Action		Removal of infectious agent	Clonal expansion and differentiation to effector cells
			Memory of antigenic exposure
			Removal of infectious agent

PAMP, Pathogen-associated molecular pattern.

refers to all of the microbes that inhabit these locations of our bodies. This relatively new field of science has discovered that there is a unique and different mix of microbes for everyone. Most related studies investigate the relationship of the microbiome with health and diseases.

The mammalian gut harbors trillions of microorganisms known as the microbiota. Recent evidence suggests that host microbiota and the immune system interact to maintain tissue homeostasis in healthy individuals. Among the numerous microorganisms in the gut, some bacteria are known to provide health benefits to the host when acquired in adequate amounts; these are labeled "probiotics." Probiotics and other beneficial bacteria provide colonization resistance to pathogens. Beneficial microbes can also indirectly diminish pathogen colonization by stimulating the development of the innate and adaptive immune systems, in addition to the function of the mucosal barrier.

Microbiota regulate development and differentiation of local and systemic immune and nonimmune components by:
- Regulation of innate immune functions and homeostasis
- Regulation of adaptive immune functions in intestines
- Regulation of systemic innate and adaptive immune functions

Disruption of the host microbiota, especially in the gut, has been shown to be associated with many autoimmune diseases (see Chapter 22).

Innate Immunity: The Early Defense

The innate immune system responds almost immediately to microbes or injured cells. Repeated exposures invoke virtually identical innate immune responses to groups of related microbes. Three lines of defense exist in the human body (Fig. 1.17). The first two of these three lines of defense form the principal components of innate immunity. If a microorganism overwhelms the body's natural resistance, a third line of defensive resistance, acquired (or adaptive) immunity, allows the body to recognize, remember, and respond to a specific stimulus, an antigen.

> **KEY CONCEPTS: Lines of Defense**
> - The first line of defense against infection is unbroken skin, mucosal membrane surfaces, and secretions.
> - Natural immunity, consisting of cellular and humoral defense mechanisms, forms the second line of body defenses.
> - The innate immune response may not be able to recognize every possible antigen but may focus on a few large groups of microorganisms, called *pathogen-associated molecular patterns (PAMPs)*.
> - The receptors of the innate immune system that recognize these PAMPs are called *pattern recognition receptors (PRRs)* (e.g., Toll-like receptors [TLRs]).

First Line of Defense

Before a pathogen can invade the human body, it must overcome the resistance provided by the body's first line of defense. The first barrier to infection is unbroken skin and mucosal membrane surfaces. These surfaces are essential in forming a physical barrier to many microorganisms because this is where foreign materials usually first contact the host.

Keratinization of the upper layer of the skin and the constant renewal of the skin's epithelial cells, which repairs breaks in the skin, assist in the protective function of skin and mucosal membranes. In addition to the normal microbiota, microorganisms normally inhabiting the skin and membranes deter penetration or facilitate elimination of foreign microorganisms from the body (Fig. 1.18).

In addition to the physical ability to wash away potential pathogens, tears and saliva have chemical properties that defend the body. The enzyme lysozyme, which is found in tears and saliva, attacks and destroys the cell walls of susceptible bacteria, particularly certain Gram-positive bacteria. IgA antibody, which is formed by the adaptive immune response, is an important protective substance in tears and saliva.

Secretions are also an important component in the first line of defense against microbial invasion. Mucus adhering to the membranes and the wet mucosal surfaces of the nose and nasopharynx trap microorganisms (Fig. 1.19), which can be expelled by coughing or sneezing. Sebum (oil) produced by the sebaceous glands of the skin and lactic acid in sweat both have antimicrobial properties. The production of earwax (cerumen) protects the auditory canals from infectious disease. Secretions produced in the elimination of liquid and solid wastes (e.g., urinary and gastrointestinal processes) are important in physically removing potential pathogens from the body. The acidity and alkalinity of the fluids of the stomach and intestinal tract, in addition to the acidity of the vagina, can destroy many potentially infectious microorganisms. Additional protection is provided to the respiratory tract by the constant motion of the cilia of the tubules.

In viral infections, the host innate immune system is designed to act as a first-line defense to prevent viral invasion or replication before more specific protection by the adaptive immune system kicks in. Since the appearance of COVID-19, there has been an increased interest in this virus that causes SARS-CoV-2.

Second Line of Defense: Innate (Natural) Immunity

Innate, or natural, immunity is one of the ways the body resists infection after microorganisms have penetrated the first line of defense. Acquired resistance, which specifically recognizes and selectively

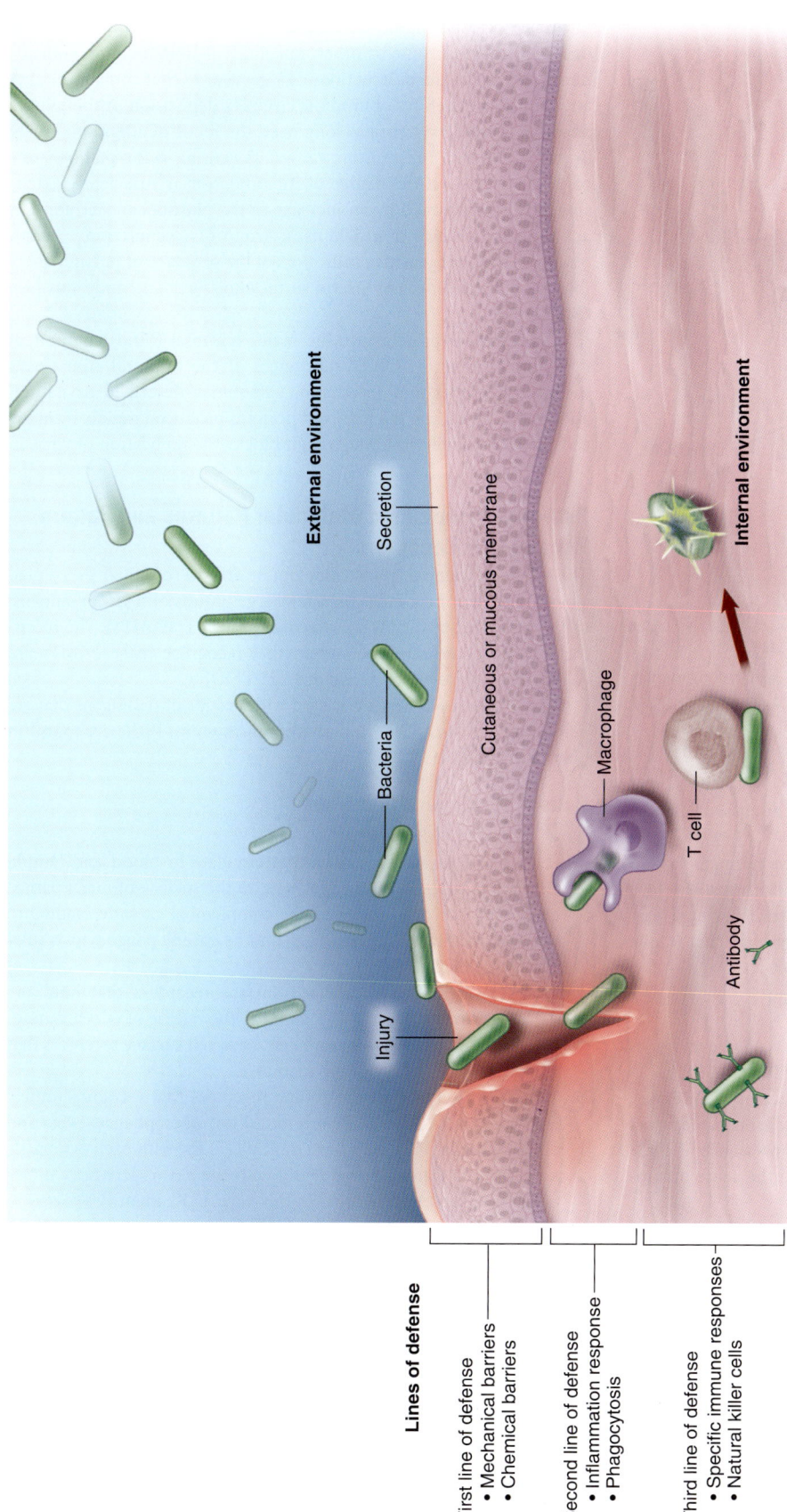

Fig. 1.17 Lines of Defense. Immune function—that is, defense of the internal environment against foreign cells, proteins, and viruses—includes three layers of protection. The first line of defense is a set of barriers between the internal and external environments; the second line involves the innate inflammatory response (including phagocytosis); and the third line includes the adaptive immune responses and the innate defense offered by natural killer cells. Of course, tumor cells that arise within the body are not affected by the first two lines of defense and must be attacked by the third line of defense. This diagram is a simplification of the complex function of the immune system; in reality, a great deal of crossover of mechanisms occurs between these lines of defense. (From Patton KT, Thibodeau GA: *Anthony's textbook of anatomy and physiology*, ed 20, St. Louis, 2013, Elsevier.)

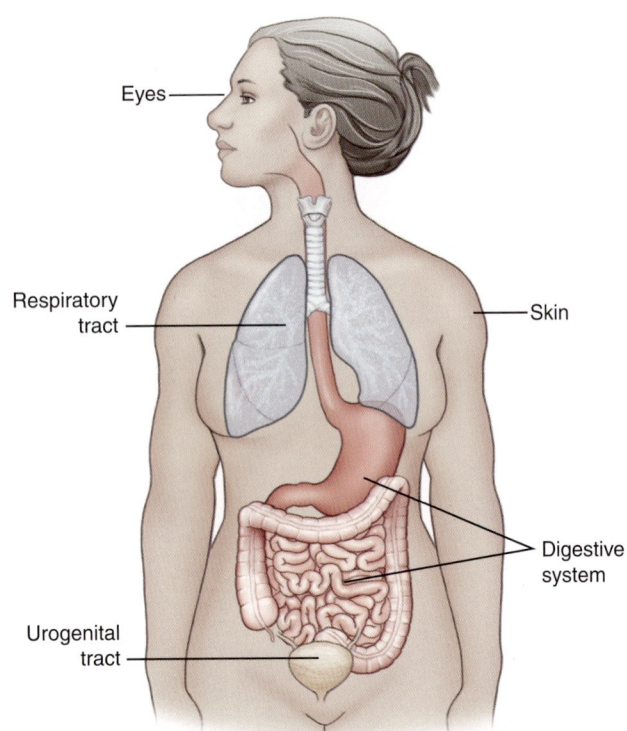

Fig. 1.18 First Line of Defense, Nonspecific. Body fluids, specialized cells, and resident bacteria (normal biota) allow the respiratory, digestive, urogenital, integumentary, and other systems to defend the body against microbial infection.

eliminates *exogenous* or *endogenous* agents, is discussed later in adaptive immunity.

The innate immune system predates the adaptive immune system and is common to all living organisms. All multicellular organisms face the same challenges, such as bacteria, viruses, parasites, and fungi. Natural immunity is characterized as a nonspecific mechanism. Unique characteristics of innate immunity include:
- Rapid recognition of microbes
- No prior exposure required
- Use of widely expressed nonvariant receptors to recognize microbes
- Receptors to distinguish between nonself and self

If a microorganism penetrates the skin or mucosal membranes, a second line of cellular and humoral defense mechanisms becomes operational (Box 1.2). The elements of natural resistance include phagocytic cells, complement (see Chapter 2), and the acute inflammatory reaction.

Detection of microbial pathogens is carried out by sentinel cells of the innate immune system located in tissues (macrophages and DCs) in close contact with the host's natural environment or that are rapidly reunited to the site of infection (neutrophils). There are common molecular signatures (patterns) that define kinds of bacteria, such as bacterial cell wall components.

Patterns that define classes of viruses include double-strand RNA, unmethylated CpG DNA, and uncapped RNA. *Pattern recognition receptors (PRRs)* determine which molecules are *immunogenic*. Recently innate immune receptors and their unique downstream pathways have been identified. In the innate immune response, PRRs are engaged to detect specific viral components or viral intermediate products and to induce proinflammatory cytokine (see Chapter 2, Soluble Mediators) responses in infected cells and other immune cells.

Tissue damage produced by infectious or other agents results in inflammation, a series of biochemical and cellular changes that facilitate phagocytosis (engulfment and destruction) of microorganisms or damaged cells. Chronic or other, intermittent inflammation contributes over time to the destruction of target organs that contain inciting antigens or are the sites of immune complex deposition. Although the adaptive immune system has long been the focus of attention, innate immune mechanisms are now viewed as central to the pathogenesis of these diseases. If the degree of inflammation is sufficiently extensive, it is accompanied by an increase in the plasma concentration of acute-phase proteins or reactants, a group of glycoproteins. Acute-phase proteins are sensitive indicators of the presence of inflammatory disease and are especially useful in monitoring such conditions (see Chapter 2).

Complement proteins are the major humoral (fluid) component of natural immunity. Other substances of the humoral component include lysozymes and interferon, sometimes described as natural antibiotics. Interferon is a family of proteins produced rapidly by many cells in response to viral infection; it blocks the replication of virus in other cells.

Pathogen-Associated Molecular Patterns and Pattern Recognition Receptors

The innate immune response may not be able to recognize every possible antigen but may focus on a few large groups of microorganisms, called *pathogen-associated molecular patterns (PAMPs)*. The receptors of the innate immune system that recognize these PAMPs are called *pattern recognition receptors* (e.g., TLRs).

PAMPs are molecules associated with groups of pathogens that are recognized by cells of the innate immune system. PRRs are found in plants and animals.

Pattern Recognition Receptors

Three groups of PRRs exist:
1. Secreted PRRs are molecules that circulate in blood and lymph; circulating proteins bind to PAMPs on the surface of many pathogens. This interaction triggers the complement cascade, leading to the opsonization of the pathogen and its speedy phagocytosis (discussed in Chapter 4).
2. Phagocytosis receptors are cell surface receptors that bind the pathogen, initiating a signal leading to the release of effector molecules (e.g., cytokines). Macrophages have cell surface receptors that recognize PAMPs containing mannose.
3. TLRs are a set of transmembrane receptors that recognize different types of PAMPs. TLRs are found on macrophages, DCs, and epithelial cells. Mammals have multiple TLRs, with each exhibiting a specialized function, frequently with the aid of accessory molecules, in a subset of PAMPs. In this way, TLRs identify the nature of the pathogen and turn on an effector response appropriate for counteracting it. These signaling cascades lead to the expression of various cytokine genes. Examples include TLR-1, which binds to the peptidoglycan of Gram-positive bacteria, and TLR-2, which binds lipoproteins of Gram-negative bacteria.

In all these cases, binding of the pathogen to the TLR initiates a signaling pathway, leading to the activation of nuclear factor κB (NF-κB, light-chain enhancer of activated B cells). This transcription factor turns on many cytokine genes, such as TNF-α, interleukin-1 (IL-1), and chemokines. All these effector molecules lead to the inflammation site.

Third Line of Defense: Adaptive Immunity

If a microorganism overwhelms the body's natural, innate resistance, a third line of defensive *adaptive immunity* comes into play (Table 1.10).

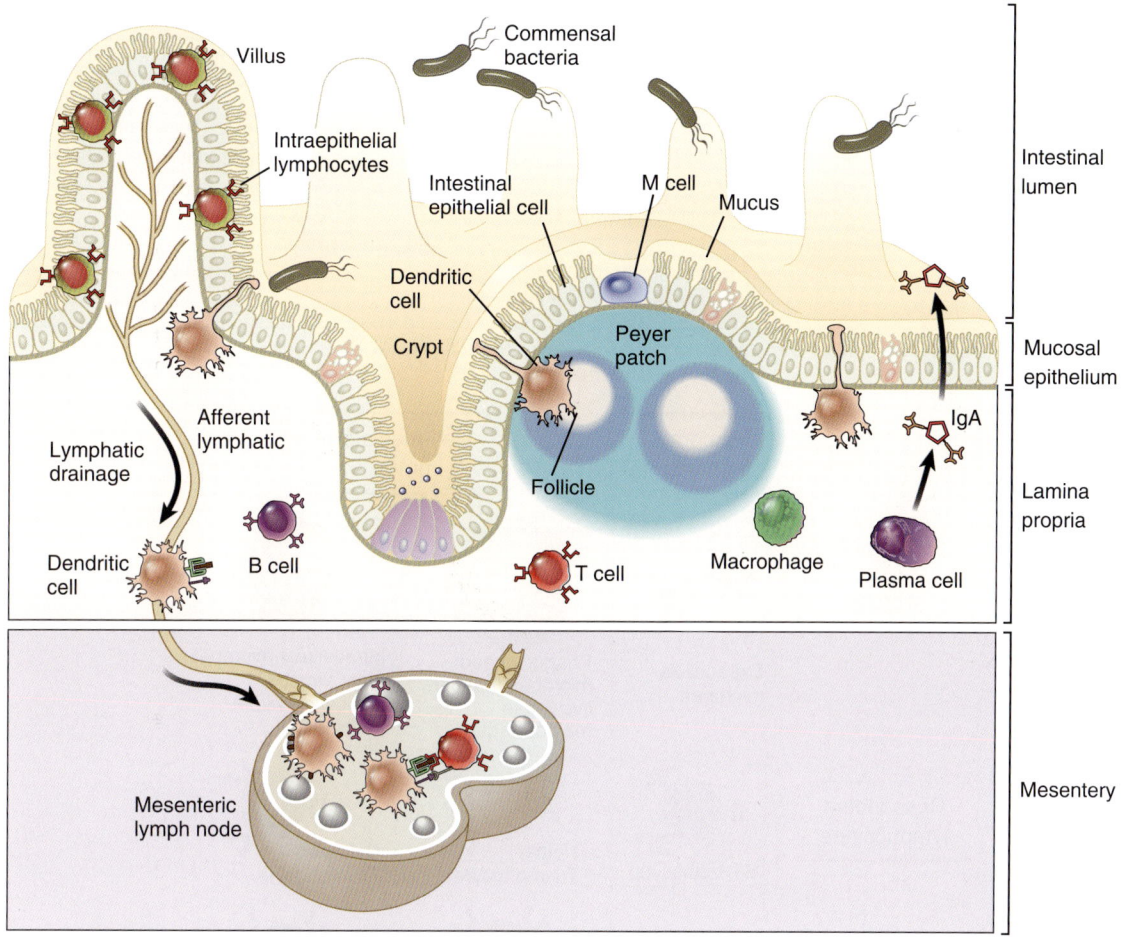

Fig. 1.19 Mucosal Immune System. This schematic diagram of the mucosal immune system uses the small bowel as an example. Many commensal bacteria are present in the lumen. The mucus-secreting epithelium provides an innate barrier to microbial invasion. Specialized epithelial cells, such as M cells, promote the transport of antigens from the lumen into underlying tissues. Cells in the lamina propria, including DCs, T lymphocytes, and macrophages, provide innate and adaptive immune defense against invading microbes; some of these cells are organized into specialized structures, such as Peyer patches in the small intestine. Immunoglobulin A (IgA) is a type of antibody abundantly produced in mucosal tissues that is transported into the lumen, where it binds and neutralizes microbes. (From Abbas AK, Lichtman AH, Pillai S: *Basic immunology: functions and disorders of the immune system*, ed 5, Philadelphia, 2016, Elsevier.)

BOX 1.2 Components of the Natural Immune System: the Second Line of Defense

Cellular
1. Mast cells
2. Neutrophils
3. Macrophages

Humoral
1. Complement
2. Lysozyme
3. Interferon

Acquired, or adaptive, immunity is a more recently evolved mechanism that allows the body to recognize, remember, and respond to a specific stimulus, an **antigen**. Adaptive immunity can result in the elimination of microorganisms and recovery from disease, and the host often acquires a specific immunologic memory. This condition of memory or recall (acquired resistance) allows the host to respond more effectively if reinfection with the same microorganism occurs.

Adaptive immunity is composed of cellular and humoral components (Fig. 1.20 and Box 1.3). The major cellular component of **acquired immunity** is the lymphocyte (see Chapter 4); the major humoral component is the antibody.

Lymphocytes selectively respond to nonself materials (antigens), which leads to immune memory and a permanently altered pattern of response or adaptation to the environment. Most actions in the two categories of the adaptive response, **humoral-mediated immunity** and cell-mediated immunity, are exerted by the interaction of antibody with complement and the phagocytic cells (natural immunity), and of T cells with macrophages.

Humoral-Mediated Immunity

If specific **antibodies** have been formed in response to antigenic stimulation, they are available to protect the body against foreign substances. The recognition of foreign substances and subsequent production of antibodies to these substances define immunity. Antibody-mediated

TABLE 1.10	Features of Innate Immunity and Adaptive Immunity	
Major Characteristics	**Innate Immunity**	**Adaptive Immunity**
Memory lymphocytes	None or limited	Yes
Physical barriers	Skin, mucosal epithelia	Lymphocytes in epithelia
Chemical barriers	Antimicrobial chemicals	Antibodies secreted at epithelial surfaces
Blood proteins	Complement	Antibodies
Blood cells	Macrophages, neutrophils, natural killer cells	Lymphocytes
Nonreactivity to self	Yes	Yes
Specificity	For molecules shared by groups of related microbes and molecules produced by damaged host cells	For microbial and nonmicrobial antigens

Adapted from Abbas AK, Lichtman AH: *Cellular & molecular immunology,* ed 9, Philadelphia, 2018, Elsevier.

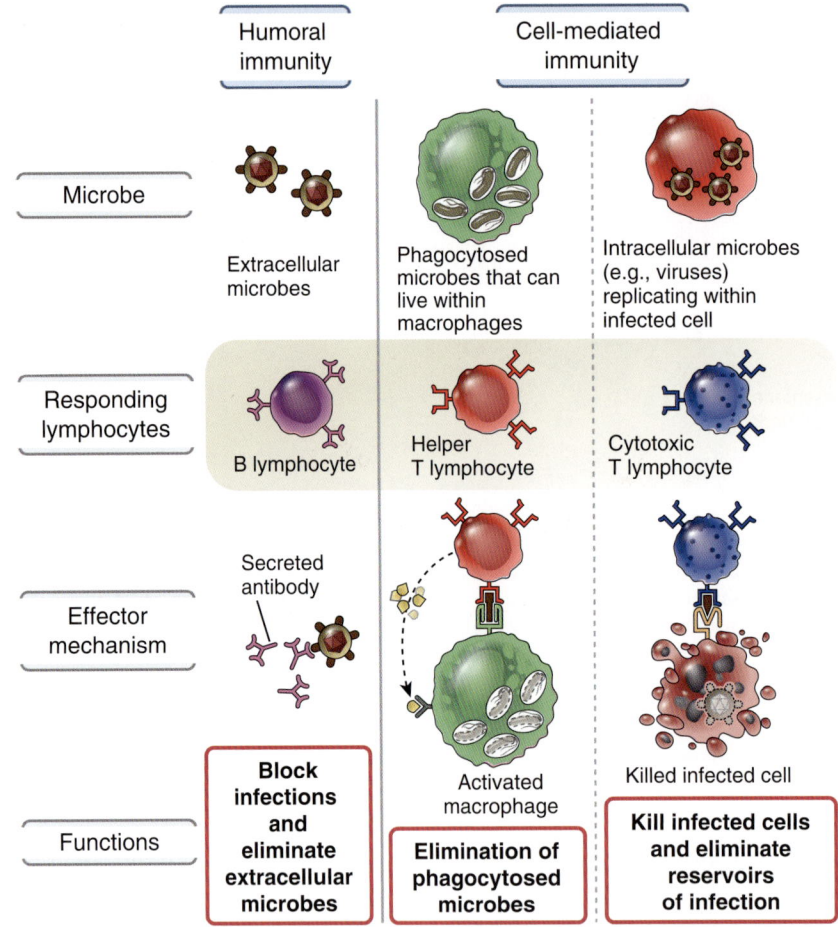

Fig. 1.20 Types of Adaptive Immunity. In humoral immunity, B lymphocytes secrete antibodies that eliminate extracellular microbes. In cell-mediated immunity, different types of T lymphocytes recruit and activate phagocytes to destroy ingested microbes and kill infected cells. (From Abbas AK, Lichtman AH, Pillai S: *Basic immunology: functions and disorders of the immune system,* ed 5, Philadelphia, 2016, Elsevier.)

BOX 1.3 Components of the Adaptive Immune System

Cellular
1. T lymphocytes
2. B lymphocytes
3. Plasma cells

Humoral
1. Antibodies
2. Cytokines

---

immunity to infection can be acquired if the antibodies are formed by the host or if they are received from another source; these two types of acquired immunity are called *active immunity* and *passive immunity*, respectively (Table 1.11).

Active immunity can be acquired by natural exposure in response to an infection or a natural series of infections or through intentional injection of an antigen. The latter, *vaccination* (see Chapter 27), is an effective method of stimulating antibody production and memory (acquired resistance) without contracting the disease. Suspensions of antigenic materials used for immunization may be of animal or plant origin. These products may consist of living suspensions of weak or

TABLE 1.11	Comparison of Active Immunity and Passive Immunity			
	Type	Mode of Acquisition	Antibody Produced by Host	Duration of Immune Response
Active	Natural	Infection	Yes	Long[a,b]
	Artificial	Vaccination	Yes	Long [a,b]
Passive	Natural	Transfer in vivo or colostrum	No	Short
	Artificial	Infusion of serum/plasma	No	Short

[a]Immunocompetent host.
[b]IgG immune antibody half-life is 23 days. Lifespan of memory cells (memory lymphocytes) can be decades or years.

TABLE 1.12	Adaptive Immunity: Classes of Lymphocytes	
	Humoral-Mediated Immunity	Cell-Mediated Immunity
Mechanism	Antibody mediated	Cell mediated
Cell type	B lymphocytes	T lymphocytes
Mode of action	Antibodies in serum	Direct cell-to-cell contact or soluble products secreted by cells
Purpose	Primary defense against bacterial infection	Defense against viral and fungal infections, intracellular organisms, tumor antigens, and graft rejection

attenuated cells or viruses, killed cells or viruses, or extracted bacterial products (e.g., altered and no longer poisonous toxins used to immunize against diphtheria and tetanus). The selected agents should stimulate the production of antibodies without clinical signs and symptoms of disease in an **immunocompetent** host (a host able to recognize a foreign antigen and build specific antigen-directed antibodies) and result in permanent antigenic memory. Booster vaccinations may be needed in some cases to expand the pool of memory cells. The mechanisms of antigen recognition and antibody production are discussed in Chapter 3.

Artificial **passive immunity** is achieved by the infusion of serum or plasma containing high concentrations of antibody or lymphocytes from an actively immunized individual. Passive immunity via preformed antibodies in serum provides immediate, temporary antibody protection against microorganisms (e.g., hepatitis A) through the administration of preformed antibodies. The recipient will benefit only temporarily from passive immunity for as long as the antibodies persist in the circulation. Immune antibodies are usually of the IgG type, with a half-life of 23 days. Antibody half-life is a measure of the mean survival time of antibody molecules after their formation. It is usually expressed as the time required to eliminate 50% of a known quantity of immunoglobulin from the body. Half-life varies from one immunoglobulin class to another.

The main strategies for cancer immunotherapy aim to provide antitumor effectors (T lymphocytes and antibodies) to patients. The purpose is to immunize patients actively against their own tumors and to stimulate the patient's own antitumor immune responses.

In addition, passive immunity can be acquired naturally by the fetus through the transfer of antibodies by the maternal placental circulation in utero during the last 3 months of pregnancy. Maternal antibodies are also transferred to the newborn after birth by breast milk, especially the first breast milk, colostrum. The amount and specificity of maternal antibodies depend on the mother's immune status to infectious diseases that she has experienced.

Passively acquired immunity in newborns is only temporary because it starts to decrease after the first several weeks or months after birth. Breast milk, especially the thick yellowish milk (colostrum) produced for a few days after the birth of a baby, is very rich in antibodies. However, for a newborn to have lasting protection, active immunity must occur.

Cell-Mediated Immunity

In contrast to humoral-mediated immunity, **cell-mediated immunity** consists of immune activities that differ from antibody-mediated immunity (Table 1.12). Lymphocytes are the unique bearers of immunologic specificity, which depends on their antigen receptors. The full development and expression of immune responses, however, require that nonlymphoid cells and molecules primarily act as amplifiers and modifiers.

Cell-mediated immunity is moderated by the link between T lymphocytes and phagocytic cells (i.e., monocytes-macrophages). A B lymphocyte can probably respond to a native antigenic determinant of the appropriate fit. A T lymphocyte responds to antigens presented by other cells in the context of **major histocompatibility complex (MHC)** proteins (i.e., a group of genes that code for proteins found on cellular surfaces that assist the immune system in recognizing foreign substances). In human beings, the complex is also called the human leukocyte antigen (HLA) system. The T lymphocyte does not directly recognize the antigens of microorganisms or other living cells, such as **allografts** (tissue from a genetically different member of the same species, such as a human kidney), but it recognizes when the antigen is present on the surface of an APC (see Chapter 4), the macrophage. APCs were first thought to be limited to cells of the **mononuclear phagocyte system**. Recently other types of cells (e.g., endothelial, glial) have been shown to possess the ability to present antigens.

Lymphocytes are immunologically active through various types of direct cell-to-cell contact and by the production of soluble factors. Nonspecific soluble factors are made by or act on various elements of the immune system. These molecules are collectively called *cytokines* (see Chapter 2). Some of these mediators that act between leukocytes are called **interleukins (ILs)**.

Under some conditions, the activities of cell-mediated immunity may not be beneficial. Suppression of the normal adaptive immune response by drugs or other means is necessary in conditions or procedures such as organ transplantation, hypersensitivity, and autoimmune disorders.

CASE STUDY 1.1

A 1-month-old infant female neonate born 6 weeks premature was admitted for surgery to her foot. Several days after hospital discharge, her parents brought her back to the emergency department because she had a high fever and was crying all of the time. Physical examination revealed increased body temperature, increased respiration rate, and increased heart rate. She also had redness around the site of an inserted percutaneous central line related to her surgery.

Continued

CASE STUDY 1.1—CONT'D

Her blood count was normal except for a decreased concentration of blood platelets. A smear and a culture were taken from the inflamed area. The direct smears revealed the presence of yeast. Pending results of the culture, the patient was started on antifungal therapeutics. She was admitted to the hospital, where her condition improved within the first 24 hours.

Subsequently, the culture demonstrated *Candida albicans*.

Questions
1. A risk factor for the development of a fungal infection in this child is:
   a. Sex
   b. Body weight
   c. Premature birth
   d. Decreased blood platelet count
2. The child's immune problem is related to:
   a. A lack of immune antibodies to yeast
   b. A defect in her cellular immune response
   c. Lack of sunshine and vitamins
   d. Acquiring the infection from her mother

See Appendix A for the answers to these questions.

Critical Thinking Group Discussion Questions
1. Why is the child at risk for developing an infection of this type?
2. Why did this child acquire an infection?

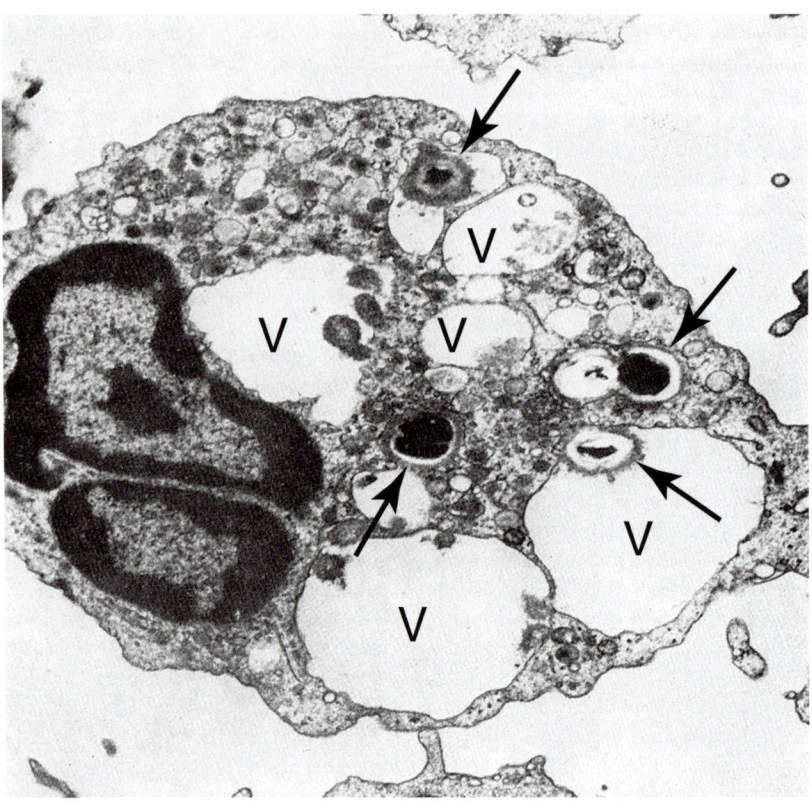

Fig. 1.21 Electron Photomicrograph of Polymorphonuclear Leukocyte from Normal Control Patient Incubated with Staphylococci for 30 Minutes. Many bacteria *(arrows)* in various stages of destruction are evident within the cell. Note the cytoplasmic vacuoles *(V)* around and adjacent to degenerating bacteria. (From Bauer JD: *Clinical laboratory methods*, ed 9, St. Louis, 1982, Mosby.)

REVIEW QUESTIONS

1. The type of blood cell that participates in regulation of inflammation is a:
   a. Polymorphonuclear neutrophil (PMN)
   b. Eosinophil
   c. Basophil
   d. B lymphocyte
2. A component of the *first line* of body defense against infections includes:
   a. Microbiota
   b. Unbroken skin
   c. Antibody production
   d. Both a and b
3. Which components characterized the *second line* of body defense against microbial pathogens?
   a. Unbroken skin and antibodies
   b. Tears, saliva, and antibodies
   c. Phagocytic neutrophils
   d. Unbroken mucous membranes
4. A component of the *second line* of innate body defense against infection is:
   a. Complement
   b. Antibodies
   c. Cytokines
   d. Both a and b

5. Cellular components of the *third line* of body defense are:
   a. T and B Lymphocytes
   b. Neutrophils
   c. Eosinophils
   d. Basophils
6. A secondary lymphoid tissue in mammals is:
   a. Thymus
   b. Lymph nodes
   c. Bone marrow
   d. Macrophage
7. In mammalian immunologic development, the precursors of neutrophils arise from progenitor cells of the:
   a. Thymus
   b. Lymph nodes
   c. Spleen
   d. Bone marrow
8. The thymus is embryologically derived from the:
   a. Yolk sac
   b. Pharyngeal pouches
   c. Lymphoblasts
   d. Bone marrow
9. A primary function of the eosinophil is:
   a. Phagocytosis
   b. Suppression of the inflammatory response
   c. Response in acute, systemic hypersensitivity reactions
   d. Antigen recognition
10. The cells of the mononuclear phagocyte system include:
    a. Monocytes and promonocytes
    b. Monocytes and macrophages
    c. Lymphocytes and monocytes
    d. Both a and b
11. Another term for adaptive immunity is:
    a. Antigenic immunity
    b. Acquired immunity
    c. Lymphocyte-reactive immunity
    d. Phagocytosis
12. Humoral components of the adaptive immune system include:
    a. T lymphocytes
    b. B lymphocytes
    c. Antibodies
    d. Saliva
13. In adaptive immunity, the mode of acquisition of active natural immunity is:
    a. Infusion of serum or plasma
    b. Transfer in vivo or by colostrum
    c. Vaccination
    d. Infection
14. In adaptive immunity, the mode of acquisition of passive natural immunity is:
    a. Infusion of serum or plasma
    b. Transfer in vivo or by colostrum
    c. Vaccination
    d. Infection
15. In adaptive immunity, the mode of acquisition of artificial passive immunity is:
    a. Infusion of serum or plasma
    b. Transfer in vivo or by colostrum
    c. Vaccination
    d. Infection
16. In adaptive immunity acquired by active natural immunity, the duration of the presence of circulating antibody is _____ some other types of responses.
    a. Shorter than
    b. Longer than
    c. Equivalent to
    d. Not measurable
17. In adaptive immunity acquired by artificial active immunity, the duration of the presence of circulating antibody is _____ some other types of responses.
    a. Shorter than
    b. Longer than
    c. Equivalent to
    d. Not measurable
18. In adaptive immunity acquired by passive natural immunity, the duration of the presence of circulating antibody is _____ some other types of responses.
    a. Shorter than
    b. Longer than
    c. Equivalent to
    d. Not measurable
19. In adaptive immunity acquired by artificial passive immunity, the duration of the presence of circulating antibody is _____ some other type of responses.
    a. Shorter than
    b. Longer than
    c. Equivalent to
    d. Not measurable

2

Soluble Mediators of the Immune System

LEARNING OUTCOMES

- Name and compare the three complement activation pathways.
- Describe the central role played by C3 for all pathways.
- Describe the mechanisms and consequences of complement activation.
- Name three reasons for measuring complement.
- Explain the biological functions of the complement system.
- Name and describe alterations in complement levels.
- Interpret the results of the assessment of complement levels.
- Describe the characteristics of hereditary angioedema.
- Compare other types of nonspecific mediators of the immune system, including cytokines, interleukins, tumor necrosis factor, hematopoietic growth factors, and chemokines.
- Discuss the clinical applications of C-reactive protein.
- Compare acute-phase reactant methods.
- Analyze a patient history, clinical signs and symptoms, and laboratory data; answer the related multiple choice and critical thinking questions and conclude the most likely diagnosis.
- Describe the principle, reporting results, sources of error, limitations, and clinical applications of the C-reactive protein procedure.
- Correctly answer 80% of end-of-chapter review questions.

OUTLINE

Complement System, 29
  Activation of Complement, 29
  Enzyme Activation, 29
  Complement Receptors, 29
Classic Pathway, 30
  Recognition, 31
  Amplification of the Proteolytic Complement Cascade, 31
  Membrane Attack Complex, 31
Alternative Pathway, 32
Mannose-Binding Lectin Pathway, 33
Biological Functions of Complement Proteins, 33
  Biological Effects of Complement Activation, 33
Alterations in Complement Levels, 34
  Elevated Complement Levels, 34
  Decreased Complement Levels, 34
Diagnostic Evaluation, 36
  Hemolytic Method, 38
  Enzyme Immunoassay, 38
  Liposome Assay, 38
Complement Deficiency Testing, 38
Complement Deficiency Disorder: Hereditary Angioedema, 38
  Etiology, 38
  Epidemiology, 38
  Pathophysiology, 38
  Signs and Symptoms, 38

Laboratory Assays, 38
  Interpretation of Laboratory Results, 38
Prevention and Treatment, 39
  Other Soluble Immune Response Mediators, 39
  Biological Response Modifiers, 39
  Cytokines, 39
Cytokines, 40
  A Cytokine Storm, 40
  Interleukins, 40
  Interferons, 40
  Tumor Necrosis Factor, 41
Hematopoietic Stimulators, 41
  Stem Cell Factor (c-kit Ligand), 41
  Colony-Stimulating Factors, 41
  Transforming Growth Factors, 41
  Chemokines, 41
Acute-Phase Proteins, 41
  Overview, 41
  Synthesis and Catabolism, 42
  C-Reactive Protein, 42
  Other Acute-Phase Reactants, 43
  Laboratory Assessment Methods, 43
Case Study 2.1, 43
Procedure: C-Reactive Protein Rapid Latex Agglutination Test, 46.e1

KEY TERMS

acute-phase proteins (acute-phase reactants)
agglutination
α$_1$-antitrypsin
angioedema

antineoplastic agents
ceruloplasmin
colony-stimulating factors (CSFs)
complement cascade
convertase

cytokine storm
effector cells
factor H
febrile
haptoglobin

hemolysis
hydrophilic
hydrophobic
immunomodulators
integrins
ligands
lipemic
lysis
malignant neoplasia
membrane attack complex (MAC)
natural immune system
nephelometry
osmotic cytolytic reaction
peptide
polymerize
procalcitonin (PCT)
properdin
proteinases
proteolytic
pyogenic
tumor necrosis factor (TNF)
zymosan

The immune system is composed of the phylogenetically oldest, highly diversified innate immune system and the adaptive immune system. Some components of the innate immune system, or natural immune system (e.g., phagocytosis), are discussed in Chapter 1. As part of the innate immunity, the complement system is one of the first lines of defense against gram-negative pathogens. Besides its direct bactericidal activity, activation of the complement system stimulates phagocytosis and triggers proinflammatory signaling. The principal functions of complement are:
- chemotaxis,
- opsonization and cellular activation,
- lysis of target cells, and
- priming of the adaptive immune response.

This chapter discusses other components of the innate immune system: the complement system and other circulating effector proteins of innate immunity, including cytokines and acute-phase reactants.

Regulatory mechanisms of complement are finely balanced. The activation of complement is focused on the surface of invading microorganisms, with limited complement deposited on normal cells and tissues. If the mechanisms that regulate this delicate balance malfunction, the complement system may cause injury to cells, tissues, and organs, such as destruction of the kidneys in systemic lupus erythematosus (SLE) or hemolytic anemias.

> **KEY CONCEPTS: Facts About Complement**
> - The complement system is a heat-labile series of 18 plasma proteins, many of which are enzymes or proteinases.
> - Normally complement components are present in the circulation in an inactive form.
> - Complement is composed of three interrelated enzyme cascades: the classic, alternative, and mannose-binding lectin pathways.

COMPLEMENT SYSTEM

Complement is a heat-labile series of 18 plasma proteins, many of which are enzymes or proteinases. Collectively, these proteins are a major fraction of the β-1 and β-2 globulins.

The classic complement system proteins are named with a capital C followed by a number. A small letter after the number indicates that the protein is a smaller protein resulting from the cleavage of a larger precursor by a protease. Several complement proteins are cleaved during activation of the complement system; the fragments are designated with lowercase suffixes, such as C3a and C3b. Usually the larger fragment is designated as "b" and the smaller fragment as "a." The exception is the designation of the C2 fragments; the larger fragment is designated C2a and the smaller fragment is C2b.

Proteins of the alternative activation pathway are called *factors* and are symbolized by letters, such as B. Control proteins include the inhibitor of C1 (C1 INH), factor I, and factor H.

The complement system as a component of the natural immune system is crucial for host defense from microbial infections, an interface between innate and adaptive immunity, including enhancement of immunologic memory, and for clearance of immune complexes from tissues and apoptotic or injured cells.

These activities are initiated in various ways through the following three pathways:
1. Classic pathway (coevolved with active immunity)
2. Alternative pathway (oldest pathway in evolution)
3. Mannose-binding lectin pathway (associated with pathogen recognition receptors)

The three pathways (Fig. 2.1) converge at the point of cleavage of C3 to C3b, the central event of the common final pathway, which in turn leads to activation of the lytic complement sequence, C5 through C9, and cell destruction.

Activation of Complement

Normally complement components are present in the circulation in an inactive form. In addition, the control proteins C1 INH, factor I, factor H, and C4-binding protein (C4-bp) are normally present to inhibit uncontrolled complement activation. Under normal physiologic conditions, activation (Table 2.1) of one pathway probably also leads to the activation of another pathway, as follows:
- The classic pathway is initiated by the bonding of the C1 complex, consisting of C1q, C1r, and C1s, to antibodies bound to an antigen on the surface of a bacterial cell.
- The alternative pathway is initiated by contact with a foreign surface, such as the polysaccharide coating of a microorganism and the covalent binding of a small amount of C3b to hydroxyl groups on cell surface carbohydrates and proteins. The pathway is activated by low-grade cleavage of C3 in plasma.
- The mannose-binding lectin pathway is initiated by binding of the complex of mannose-binding lectin and associated serine proteases (MASP1 and MASP2) to arrays of mannose groups on the surface of a bacterial cell.

Enzyme Activation

After complement is initially activated, each enzyme precursor is activated by the previous complement component or complex, which is a highly specialized proteinase. This converts the enzyme precursor to its catalytically active form by limited proteolysis.

The pathways leading to the cleavage of C3 are triggered by enzyme cascades. During this activation process a small peptide fragment is cleaved, a membrane-binding site is exposed, and the major fragment binds. As a consequence, the next active enzyme of the sequence is formed. Because each enzyme can activate many enzyme precursors, each step is amplified until the C3 stage; therefore the whole system forms an amplifying cascade.

Complement Receptors

Various cell types express surface membrane glycoproteins that react with one or more of the fragments of C3 produced during complement

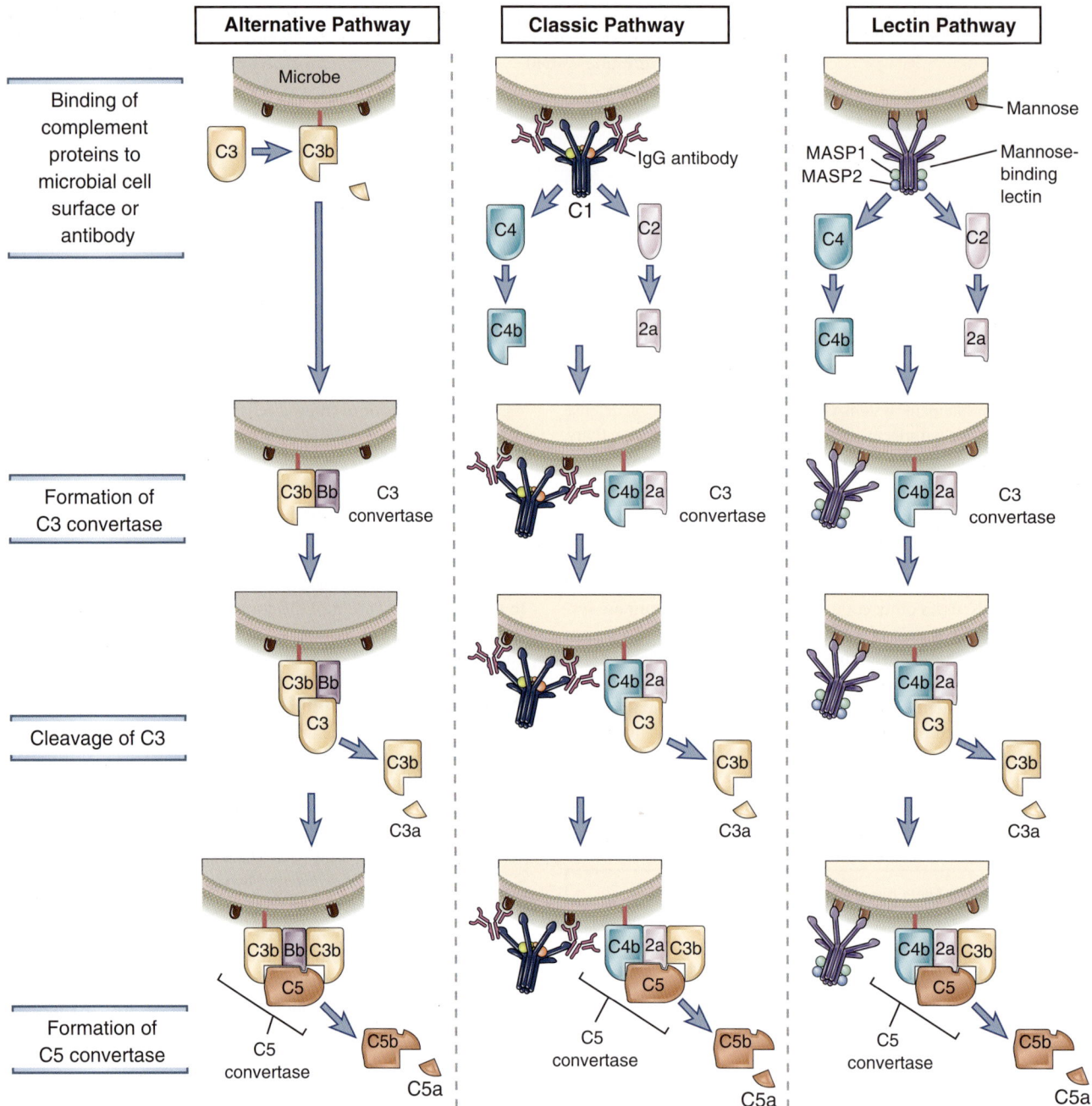

Fig. 2.1 **The Early Stages of Complement Activation.** The alternative pathway is activated by C3b binding to various activating surfaces, such as microbial cell walls; the classic pathway is initiated by C1 binding to antigen–antibody complexes; and the lectin pathway is activated by binding of a plasma lectin to microbes. The C3b that is generated by the action of the C3 convertase binds to the microbial cell surface or the antibody and becomes a component of the enzyme that cleaves C5 (C5 convertase) and initiates the late steps of complement activation. The late steps of all three pathways are the same (not shown), and complement activated by all three pathways serves the same function. (From Abbas AK, Lichtman AH, Pillai S: *Cellular and molecular immunology*, ed 8, Philadelphia, 2015, Saunders.)

activation and degradation. The functions of these receptors depend on the type of cell and often are incompletely understood. Complement receptor 1 (CR1) is important in enhancing phagocytosis and CR3b is also important in these host defense mechanisms.

For example, *Plasmodium falciparum* adhesin PfRh4 binds to CR1 on human erythrocytes. CR1 is a complement regulator and an immune adherence receptor on erythrocytes required for shuttling C3bC4b-opsonized particles to the liver and spleen for phagocytosis.

CLASSIC PATHWAY

The classic complement pathway is one of the major effector mechanisms of antibody-mediated immunity. The principal components of

CHAPTER 2 Soluble Mediators of the Immune System

TABLE 2.1 Activators of the Classic, Alternative, and Lectin Pathways

	Immunoglobulin	Microorganisms	Other Activators
Classic	Immune complexes with IgM, IgG1, IgG2, or IgG3	Viruses HIV and other retroviruses Vesicular stomatitis virus Other *Mycoplasma* sp.	Heparin Dextran sulfate
Alternative	Immune complexes with IgG, IgA, or IgE[a]	Viruses Some virus-infected cells, e.g., Epstein-Barr virus Bacteria Many gram-positive and gram-negative microorganisms Other Trypanosomes, e.g., *Leishmania* sp. Many types of fungi	Dextran sulfate Heterologous (mixed population) of red blood cells Complex carbohydrates, e.g., zymosan
Lectin		Viruses HIV and other retroviruses Bacteria Many gram-positive and gram-negative microorganisms	Arrays of terminal mannose groups acetylated sugars

[a]Less efficient than classic pathway.
Modified from Male D, Peebles RS, Male V. Immunology ed.9, Table 4.1 Summary of the Activators of the Classical, Lectin and Alternative Pathways. Elsevier, 2021, p.63.

the classic pathway are C1 through C9. The sequence of component activation—C1, -4, -2, -3, -5, -6, -7, -8, and -9—does not follow the expected numerical order.

C3 is present in the plasma in the largest quantities; fixation of C3 is the major quantitative reaction of the complement cascade. Although the principal source of synthesis of complement in vivo is debatable, the majority of the plasma complement components are made in hepatic parenchymal cells, except for C1 (a calcium-dependent complex of the three glycoproteins C1q, C1r, and C1s), which is primarily synthesized in the epithelium of the gastrointestinal and urogenital tracts.

The classic pathway has three major stages:
1. Recognition
2. Amplification of proteolytic complement cascade
3. Membrane attack complex

Recognition
The recognition unit of the classic complement system is the C1 complex: C1q, C1r, and C1s, an interlocking enzyme system. In the classic pathway, the first step is initiation of the pathway, triggered by recognition by complement factor C1 of antigen–antibody complexes on the cell surface. When the C1 complex interacts with aggregates of immunoglobulin G (IgG) with antigen on a cell's surface, two C1-associated proteases, C1r and C1s, are activated. A single IgM molecule is potentially able to fix C1, but at least two IgG molecules are required for this purpose. The amount of C1 fixed is directly proportional to the concentration of IgM antibodies, although this is not true of IgG molecules. C1s is weakly proteolytic for free intact C2 but is highly active against C2 that has complexed with C4b molecules in the presence of magnesium (Mg^{2+}) ions. This reaction occurs only if the C4bC2 complex forms close to the C1s.

The resultant C2a fragment joins with C4b to form the new C4bC2a enzyme, or classic pathway C3 **convertase**. The catalytic site of the C4bC2a complex is probably in the C2a **peptide**. A smaller C2b fragment from the C2 component is lost to the surrounding environment.

Amplification of the Proteolytic Complement Cascade
Once C1s is activated, the **proteolytic** complement cascade is amplified on the cell membrane through sequential cleavage of complement factors and recruitment of new factors until a cell surface complex containing C5b, C6, C7, and C8 is formed.

The complement cascade reaches its full amplitude at the C3 stage, which represents the heart of the system. The C4bC2a complex, the classic pathway C3 convertase, activates C3 molecules by splitting the peptide, C3 anaphylatoxin, from the N-terminal end of the peptide of C3. This exposes a reactive binding site on the larger fragment, C3b. Consequently, clusters of C3b molecules are activated and bound near the C4bC2a complex. Each catalytic site can bind several hundred C3b molecules, even though the reaction is very efficient because C3 is present in high concentration. Only one C3b molecule combines with C4bC2a to form the final proteolytic complex of the complement cascade.

Membrane Attack Complex
The **membrane attack complex (MAC)** is a unique system that builds up a lipophilic complex in cell membranes from several plasma proteins. To initiate C5b fixation and the MAC, C3b splits C5a from the alpha chain of C2. No further proteinases are generated in the classic complement sequence. Other bound C3b molecules not involved in the C4b2a3b complex form an opsonic macromolecular coat on the erythrocyte or other target, which renders it susceptible to immune adherence by C3b receptors on phagocytic cells.

When fully assembled in the correct proportions, C7, C6, C5b, and C8 form the MAC (Fig. 2.2). The C5bC6 complex is **hydrophilic** but, with the addition of C7, it also has additional detergent and phospholipid-binding properties. The presence of **hydrophobic** and hydrophilic groups within the same complex may account for its tendency to **polymerize** and form small protein micelles (a packet of chain molecules in parallel arrangement). It can attach to any lipid bilayer within its effective diffusion radius, which produces the phenomenon of reactive lysis on innocent so-called *bystander cells*. Once membrane bound, C5bC6C7 is relatively stable and can interact with C8 and C9.

The C5bC6C7C8 complex polymerizes C9 to form a tubule (pore), which spans the membrane of the cell being attacked, allowing ions to flow freely between the cellular interior and exterior. Complexing with C9 accelerates the **osmotic cytolytic reaction**. This tubule is a hollow cylinder with one end inserted into the lipid bilayer and the

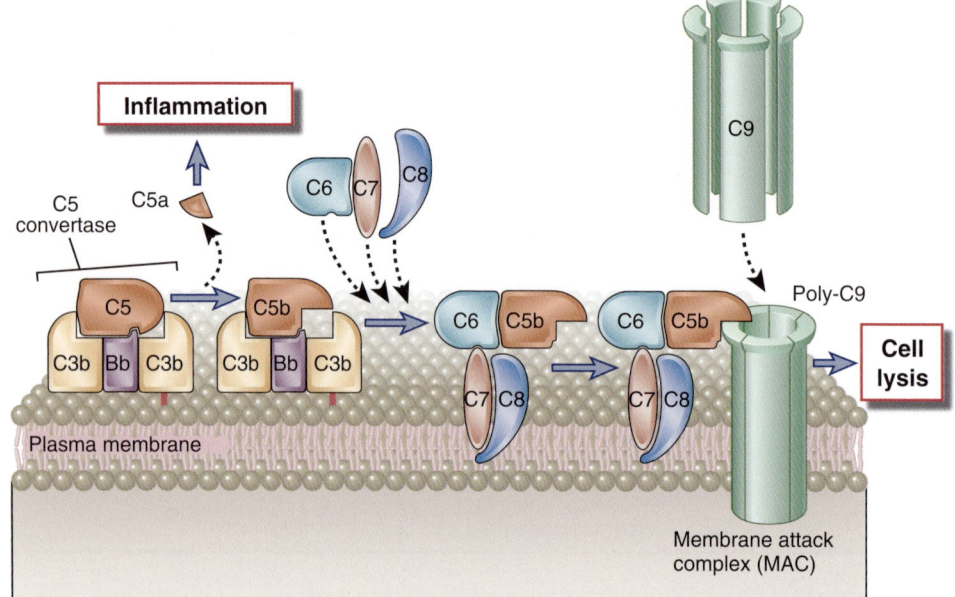

Fig. 2.2 Late Steps of Complement Activation and Formation of the Membrane Attack Complex (MAC). Cell-associated C5 convertase cleaves C5 and generates C5b, which becomes bound to the convertase. C6 and C7 bind sequentially, and the C5b,6,7 complex inserts into the plasma membrane, followed by insertion of C8. Up to 15 C9 molecules may then polymerize around the complex to form the MAC, which creates pores in the membrane and induces cell lysis. C5a, released on proteolysis of C5, stimulates inflammation. (From Abbas AK, Lichtman AH, Pillai S: *Cellular and molecular immunology*, ed 8, Philadelphia, 2015, Saunders.)

other projecting from the membrane. A structure of this form can be assumed to disturb the lipid bilayer sufficiently to allow the free exchange of ions and water (H_2O) molecules across the membrane. Ions flow out, but large molecules stay in, causing H_2O to flood into the cell. The consequence in a living cell is that the influx of sodium (Na^+) ions and H_2O leads to disruption of the osmotic balance, which produces cell lysis.

ALTERNATIVE PATHWAY

The alternative pathway shows points of similarity with the classic sequence. Both pathways generate a C3 convertase that activates C3 to provide the pivotal event in the final common pathway of both systems. However, in contrast to the classic pathway, which is initiated by the formation of antigen–antibody reactions, the alternative complement pathway is predominantly a non–antibody-initiated pathway.

Microbial and mammalian cell surfaces can activate the alternative pathway in the absence of specific antigen–antibody complexes. Factors capable of activating the alternative pathway include inulin; **zymosan** (a polysaccharide complex from the surface of yeast cells); bacterial polysaccharides and endotoxins; and the aggregated IgG2, IgA, and IgE. In paroxysmal nocturnal hemoglobinuria (PNH) the patient's erythrocytes act as an activator, which results in excessive **lysis** of these erythrocytes. This nonspecific activation is a major physiologic advantage because host protection can be generated before the induction of a humoral immune response.

A key feature of the alternative pathway is that the first three proteins of the classic activation pathway—C1, C4, and C2—do not participate in the cascade sequence. The C3a component is considered to be the counterpart of C2a in the classic pathway. C2 of the classic pathway structurally resembles factor B of the alternative pathway. The omission of C1, C4, and C2 is possible because activators of the alternative pathway catalyze the conversion of another series of normal serum proteins, which leads to the activation of C3. It was previously believed that **properdin**, a normal protein of human serum, was the first protein to function in the alternative pathway; thus the pathway was originally named after this protein.

The uptake of factor B onto C3b occurs when C3b is bound to an activator surface. However, C3b in the fluid phase or attached to a nonactivator surface preferentially binds to and therefore prevents C3b,B formation. C3b and factor B combine to form C3b,B, which is converted into an active C3 convertase, C3b,Bb. This results from the loss of a small fragment, Ba (glycine-rich α_2-globulin, believed to be physiologically inert), through the action of the enzyme, factor D. The C3b,Bb complex is able to convert more C3 to C3b, which binds more factor B, and the feedback cycle continues.

The major controlling event of the alternative pathway is **factor H**, which prevents the association between C3b and factor B. Factor H blocks the formation of C3b,Bb, the catalytically active C3 convertase of the feedback loop. Factor H (formerly β_1-H) competes with factor B for its combining site on C3b, eventually leading to C3 inactivation. Factors B and H apparently occupy a common site on C3b. The factor that is preferentially bound to C3b depends on the nature of the surface to which C3b is attached. Polysaccharides are called *activator surfaces* and favor the uptake of factor B on the chain of C3b, with the corresponding displacement of factor H. In this situation, binding of factor H is inhibited, and consequently factor B replaces factor H at the common binding site. When factor H is excluded, C3b is thought to be formed continuously in small amounts. Another controlling point in the amplification loop depends on the stability of the C3b,Bb convertase. Ordinarily C3b,Bb decays because of the loss of Bb, with a half-life of approximately 5 minutes. However, if properdin (P) binds to C3b,Bb, forming C3b,BbP, the half-life is extended to 30 minutes.

The association of numerous C3b units, factor Bb, and properdin on the surface of an aggregate of protein or the surface of a microorganism has potent activity as a C5 convertase. With the cleavage of C5, the remainder of the complement cascade continues as in the classic pathway.

MANNOSE-BINDING LECTIN PATHWAY

Mannose-binding lectin is a member of a family of calcium-dependent lectins, the collectins (collagenous lectins), and is homologous in structure to C1q. Mannose-binding lectin, a pattern recognition molecule of the innate immune system, binds to arrays of terminal mannose groups on a variety of bacteria.

A deficiency of mannose-binding lectin is caused by one of three point mutations in its gene, each of which reduces levels of the lectin. After the discovery that the binding of mannose-binding lectin to mannose residues can initiate complement activation, the mannose-binding lectin–associated serine protease (MASP) enzymes were discovered. MASP activates complement by interacting with two serine proteases, MASP1 and MASP2. These components make up the mannose-binding lectin pathway.

BIOLOGICAL FUNCTIONS OF COMPLEMENT PROTEINS

> **KEY CONCEPTS: Impact of Complement**
> - Three reasons for measuring complement are to detect an absence of a specific protein or a protein that is nonfunctional; to assess consumption of complement; and to monitor patients on immunosuppressive drugs.
> - Complement levels may be abnormal in certain disease states.
> - Increased complement levels are often associated with inflammatory conditions, trauma, and acute illness. Separate complement components (e.g., C3) are acute-phase proteins.
> - The biological functions of the complement system fall into two general categories: cell lysis by the membrane attack complex and biological effects of proteolytic fragments of complement.

Biological Effects of Complement Activation

The three reasons for measuring complement are:
- To detect an absence of a specific protein or a protein that is nonfunctional
- To assess consumption of complement
- To monitor patients on immunosuppressive drugs

The activation of complement and the products formed during the complement cascade have a variety of physiologic and cellular consequences (Box 2.1). The effects of complement in immunity and inflammation that are mediated by the proteolytic fragments generated during complement activation, such as opsonization in phagocytosis and anaphylatoxins, are an important consequence of complement activation. These fragments may remain bound to the same cell surfaces at which complement has been activated or may be released into the blood or extracellular fluid. In either situation, active fragments mediate their effects by binding to specific receptors expressed on various types of cells, including phagocytic leukocytes and the endothelium (Table 2.2).

In addition to the function of complement as a major effector of antigen–antibody interaction, physiologic concentrations of complement have been found to induce profound alterations in the molecular weight, composition, and solubility of immune complexes (Fig. 2.3). The activation of complement may also play a role in mediating hypersensitivity reactions. This process may occur from direct alternative pathway activation by IgE–antigen complexes or through a sequence initiated by the activated Hageman coagulation factor that causes the

> **BOX 2.1 Biological Results of Complement Activation**
> - Coating of pathogens (opsonization) to enhance phagocytosis
> - Recruitment of phagocytes (e.g., neutrophils)
> - Cell activation (e.g., basophils and mast cells)
> - Immune complex removal
> - Cell lysis

TABLE 2.2 Selected Complement Components and Functions

Complement Component(s)	Function
Classic complement pathway	Immune complex removal
	B lymphocyte activation
C3 to C3b	Opsonization in phagocytosis
C5A >C3A >>C4A	Anaphylatoxins C3a and C5a/inflammation (vascular responses)
	C5a and C3a both act on mast cells (basophils) to cause degranulation and the release of vasoactive amines, including histamine and 5-hydroxytryptamine that enhances vascular permeability and local blood flow
C5A	Polymorphonuclear leukocyte activation
C5–C9	Lysis of cells

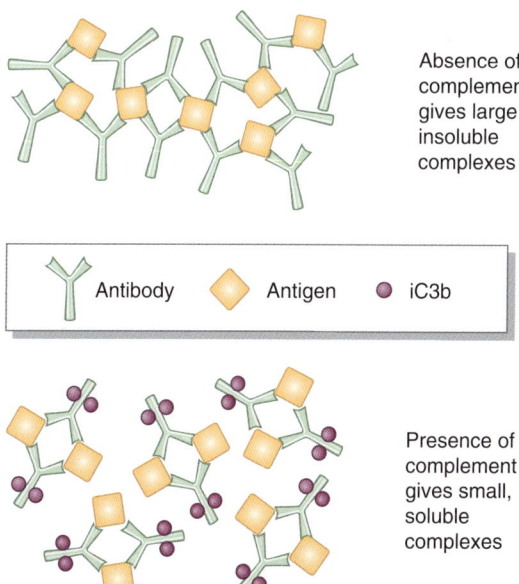

Fig. 2.3 Lattice Formation and the Role of Complement in Immune Complex Solubilization. Because antibodies are divalent (two antigen-binding arms), large antigen–antibody complexes form. C3b binds antibody and forms a complex that stoichiometrically inhibits other antibodies from binding. Soluble complexes can be transported to the spleen and liver for clearance by red blood cells bearing C3b receptors. (From Peakman M, Vergani D: *Basic and clinical immunology*, ed 2, London, 2009, Churchill Livingstone.)

generation of plasmin, which subsequently activates the classic pathway. In either case, activation of complement components from C3 onward leads to the generation of anaphylatoxins in an immediate hypersensitivity reaction.

ALTERATIONS IN COMPLEMENT LEVELS

The complement system can cause significant tissue damage in response to abnormal stimuli. Biological effects of complement activation can occur as a reaction to persistent infection or an autoantibody response to self-antigens. In these infectious or autoimmune conditions, the inflammatory or lytic effects of complement may contribute significantly to the pathology of the disease.

Complement activation is also associated with intravascular thrombosis, which leads to ischemic injury to tissues. Complement levels may be abnormal in certain disease states, such as rheumatoid arthritis (RA) and SLE, and in some genetic disorders.

Elevated Complement Levels

The complement level can be elevated in many inflammatory conditions. Increased complement levels are often associated with inflammatory conditions, trauma, or acute illness (e.g., myocardial infarction [MI]) because separate complement components (e.g., C3) are acute-phase proteins. However, these elevations are common and nonspecific. Therefore increased levels are of limited clinical significance.

Decreased Complement Levels

In contrast, the absence of an integral component of the classic, alternative, or terminal lytic pathways can lead to decreased complement activation and a lack of complement-mediated biological functions.

Low levels of complement suggest one of the following biological effects:

- Complement has been excessively activated recently.
- Complement is currently being consumed.
- A single complement component is absent because of a genetic defect.

Specific component deficiencies are associated with a variety of disorders (Table 2.3). Deficiencies of complement account for a small percentage of primary immunodeficiencies (<2%), but depression of complement levels frequently coexists with SLE and other disorders associated with an immunopathologic process (Box 2.2).

Deficiencies in any of the protein components of complement are usually caused by a genetic defect that leads to abnormal

TABLE 2.3 Complement Deficiency in Human Beings

Classic Pathway Deficiency	Level	Clinical Notes: Associated Diseases or Conditions
C1q, C1r, C1s	Decreased	Infections: encapsulated bacteria (septicemia, meningitis)
		Immune complex disease: SLE-like syndrome; decreased secondary to a gammaglobulinemia
Anti-C1q antibodies		High values of C1q antibodies are associated with the presence of circulating immune complexes. Assess risk for lupus nephritis and global SLE disease activity.
		This assay can be useful as a prognostic tool at diagnosis and during remission of acute myelogenous leukemia.
C1 INH	Increased	HAE, lupus nephritis
		HAE is caused by a low level or improper function of C1, a genetic deficiency. Infections are not usually a significant problem. HAE is autosomal dominant, unlike other complement deficiencies. Two types exist: type 1 (low antigen level and low functional protein) and type 2 (normal antigen level with low function).
	Nonfunctional	Acquired angioedema
C2	Decreased	Infections: recurrent pyogenic infections, septicemia.
		Immune complex disease: SLE, SLE-like syndrome, discoid lupus, membranoproliferative glomerulonephritis, dermatomyositis, synovitis, purpura, Henoch-Schönlein purpura, hypertension, Hodgkin disease, chronic lymphocytic leukemia, dermatitis herpetiformis, polymyositis, cardiovascular disease.
		C2 is the most common complement deficiency. It is an autosomal-recessive disorder; the C2 gene is on chromosome 6 in the MHC. The incidence is 1:28,000–1:40,000; the carrier state is 1.2% in the general population.
		Half of patients with homozygous C2 deficiency have no symptoms; those with symptoms have infections with *Streptococcus pneumoniae, Neisseria meningitidis,* and *Haemophilus influenzae.* Of symptomatic patients, 50% exhibit a lupus-like disorder with photosensitivity and rash.
C3	Decreased with normal C4 level	Decreased levels of C3 with a normal level of C4 indicate complement activation via the alternative pathway.
		Activation of the classic pathway (and sometimes with accompanying alternative pathway activation) is associated with disorders such as immune complex diseases, various forms of vasculitis, and acute glomerulonephritis.
		Activation of the alternative pathway is associated with many disorders, including chronic hypocomplementemic glomerulonephritis, DIC, septicemia, subacute bacterial endocarditis, PNH, and sickle cell anemia.
		In SLE, both the classic and alternative pathways are activated.
C3	Decreased with decreased C4	Decreased levels of C3 and C4 demonstrate activation of the classic pathway.
		The C3b component of complement causes low complement C3 levels.
		Extremely decreased levels are seen in patients with poststreptococcal glomerulonephritis and in those with inherited (C3) complement deficiency. This component is also decreased in cases of severe liver disease and in SLE patients with renal disease.

TABLE 2.3 Complement Deficiency in Human Beings—cont'd

Classic Pathway Deficiency	Level	Clinical Notes: Associated Diseases or Conditions
C3	Increased	Also an acute-phase protein, elevated C3 levels can indicate an acute inflammatory disease. Although C3 lies at the junction of the two pathways, it is much more severely depressed when activation occurs via the alternative pathway. Acute inflammation, malignancy.
C4	Decreased with normal C3 level	Infections: encapsulated bacteria (*Streptococcus pneumoniae*), immune complex disease: cryoglobulinemic vasculitis and HAE The C4 level often provides the most sensitive indicator of disease activity. C4 is also an acute-phase reactant. Elevated C4 levels can indicate an acute inflammatory reaction or a malignant condition. Measurement of C4 may demonstrate inflammation or infection long before it is clinically evident by standard assessment methods (e.g., total WBC and leukocyte differential, febrile response, or elevated ESR). C4 is destroyed only when the classic pathway is activated. A decreased C4 level with elevated anti-nDNA and ANA titers confirm the diagnosis of SLE in a patient. In these cases of SLE, the periodic assessment of C4 can monitor the progress of the disorder. Patients with extremely low C4 levels in the presence of normal levels of the C3 component may be demonstrating the effects of a genetic deficiency of C1 inhibitor or C4. Reduction of C3 and C4 components implies that activation of the classic pathway has been initiated. C4 allotypes: The antigenically distinct forms of C4A and C4B are located on chromosome 6 in the MHC. C4 allotypes in conjunction with specific HLAs are markers for disease susceptibility.
C4	Decreased with increased C3 level	Infections: pyogenic (*S. pneumoniae*), endocarditis. Immune complex diseases: SLE with glomerulonephritis, serum sickness, chronic hepatitis (most commonly with HBV, HCV).
Terminal Pathway		
C5–C9	Decreased	Infections: pyogenic (*Neisseria meningitidis* and *Neisseria gonorrhoeae*). Immune complex disease: SLE (much less frequent than with C1–C4 deficiencies).
C5	Decreased	A genetic deficiency of the C5 component is associated with increased susceptibility to bacterial infection and is expressed as an autoimmune disorder (e.g., SLE). Patients with dysfunction of C5 (Leiner disease) are predisposed to infections of the skin and bowel, characterized by eczema. Their C5 level is normal, but the C5 component fails to promote phagocytosis.
C6	Decreased	A decreased quantity of C6 predisposes an individual to significant neisserial (bacterial) infections.
C7	Decreased	A decreased level of C7 is associated with Raynaud phenomenon, sclerodactyly, telangiectasia, and severe bacterial infections caused by *Neisseria* spp.
C8	Decreased	A decreased quantity of C8 is associated with SLE. A C8 deficiency makes patients highly susceptible to *Neisseria* infections.
Factor H	Decreased	Infections: pyogenic Immune complex disease: membranoproliferative glomerulonephritis, HUS Preeclampsia
Factor I	Decreased	Infections: pyogenic Immune complex disease: membranoproliferative glomerulonephritis Atypical HUS Preeclampsia
Alternative Pathway		
Properdin	Decreased	Properdin acts to stabilize the alternative pathway C3 convertase (C3bBb). A deficiency leads to bacterial infections, often meningococcemia. This disorder is an X-linked–recessive trait. Infections: pyogenic (*Neisseria* spp. and *S. pneumoniae*).
Factor B	Decreased	The factor B component is consumed by activation of the alternative complement pathway. Associated diseases are hemolytic uremic anemia, atypical HUS.
Lectin Pathway		
Mannose-binding lectin	Decreased	Associated infections: pyogenic, fungal (yeasts, molds), recurrent respiratory infections in infants. Immune complex disease: SLE.

ANA, Antinuclear antibody; *DIC*, disseminated intravascular coagulation; *ESR*, erythrocyte sedimentation rate; *HAE*, hereditary angioedema; *HLA*, human leukocyte antigens; *HUS*, hemolytic uremic syndrome; *MHC*, major histocompatibility complex; *PNH*, paroxysmal nocturnal hemoglobinuria; *SLE*, systemic lupus erythematosus; *WBC*, white blood cell.

ARUP Laboratories Consult: Complement deficiency. https://www.arupconsult.com. Revised August 19, 2013; Colten HR, Rosen FS: Complement deficiencies, *Ann Rev Immunol* 10:809–834, 1992; Delgado J, Hill H: ARUP Laboratories: Complement deficiency, https://www.arupconsult.com; and Nusinow SR, Zuraw BL, Curd JG: The hereditary and acquired deficiencies of complement, *Med Clin North Am* 69:487–504, 1985.

patterns of complement activation. If regulatory components are absent, excess activation may occur at the wrong time or at the wrong site. The potential consequences of increased activation are excess inflammation and cell lysis, and consumption of complement components.

Hypocomplementemia can result from the complexing of IgG or IgM antibodies capable of activating complement. Depressed values of complement are associated with diseases that give rise to circulating immune complexes. Because of the rapid normal turnover of the complement proteins (i.e., within 1 or 2 days of the cessation of complement activation by immune complexes), complement levels return to normal rapidly.

Three types of complement deficiency can cause increased susceptibility to pyogenic infections:
- Deficiency of the opsonic activities of complement
- Any deficiency that compromises the lytic activity of complement
- Deficient functioning of the mannose-binding lectin pathway

Increased susceptibility to pyogenic bacteria (e.g., *Haemophilus influenzae*, and *Streptococcus pneumoniae*) occurs in patients with defects of antibody production, complement proteins of the classic pathway, or phagocyte function. The sole clinical association between an inherited deficiency of MAC components and infection is with neisserial infection, particularly *Neisseria meningitidis*. Low levels of mannose-binding lectin in young children with recurrent infections suggest that the mannose-binding lectin pathway is important during the interval between the loss of passively acquired maternal antibody and the acquisition of a mature immunologic repertoire of antigen exposure.

DIAGNOSTIC EVALUATION

During immune complex reactions, certain complement proteins become physically bound to the tissue in which the immunologic reaction is occurring. These proteins can be demonstrated in tissue by appropriate immunopathologic stains.

Indications for testing include:
- Recurrent pyogenic infections, especially meningococcal meningitis, and *Streptococcus pneumoniae* and *Neisseria* species
- Angioedema without urticaria
- Autoimmune disorders

The most frequent evaluation of complement is by fresh serum or plasma assay. Initial testing for suspected complement deficiency includes testing for both the classic (CH50) and alternative (AH50) pathways. Initial testing may also include mannose-binding lectin testing, depending on the clinical circumstance. Further testing follows an algorithm (Fig. 2.4 and Table 2.4).

Measurement of CH50 is the most common method for detecting a deficiency of the classic or terminal complement pathways. The three methods for testing CH50 are:
- Hemolytic method
- Enzyme immunoassay (EIA)
- Liposome assay

> **BOX 2.2 Diseases Associated With Hypocomplementemia**
>
> **Rheumatic Diseases With Immune Complexes**
> - Systemic lupus erythematosus
> - Rheumatoid arthritis (with extraarticular disease)
> - Systemic vasculitis
> - Essential mixed cryoglobulinemia
> - Glomerulonephritis
> - Poststreptococcal type
> - Membranoproliferative type
>
> **Infectious *Diseases***
> - Subacute bacterial endocarditis
> - Infected atrioventricular shunts
> - Pneumococcal sepsis
> - Gram-negative sepsis
> - Viremias (e.g., hepatitis B surface antigenemia, measles)
> - Parasitic infections (e.g., malaria)
>
> **Deficiency of Control Proteins**
> - C1 inhibitor deficiency: hereditary angioedema
> - Factor I deficiency
> - Factor H deficiency

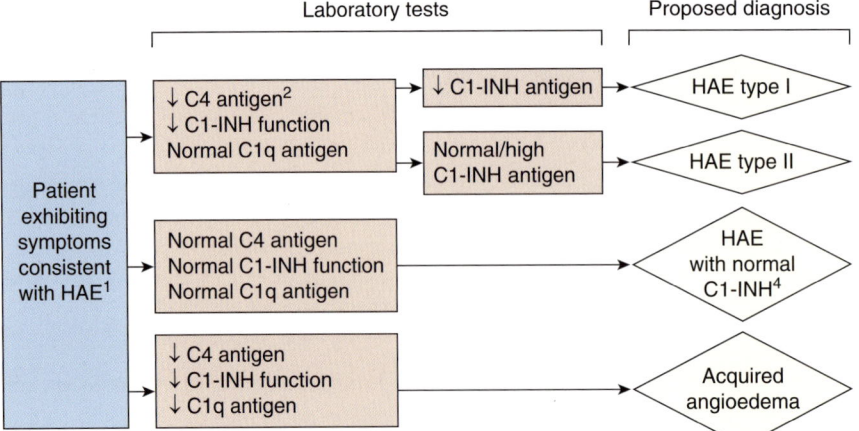

Fig. 2.4 Laboratory Tests Results and Proposed Diagnosis of HAE. *Notes:* (1) Key clinical symptoms include episodic attacks of subcutaneous and/or submucosal swellings without urticaria and/or recurrent abdominal pain. (2) C4 may still be low in some patients with HAE. Scenarios not represented in the figure include (3) pharmacologically induced angioedema and (4) the finding of low C4 and normal C1-INH function. In the latter case, other causes of C4 consumption should be considered, such as cryoglobulins, HCV infection, B-cell dyscrasia, and paraproteins. (Frazer-Abel A, Sepiashvili L, Mbughuni MM, Willrich MAV: Chapter one—Overview of laboratory testing and clinical presentations of complement deficiencies and dysregulation, *Adv Clin Chem* 77:1–75, 2016.)

TABLE 2.4 Summary of Complement Assays

Basic Assays	Methodology
Complement activity enzyme immunoassay, total (CH50) Initial screening for suspected deficiency in the classic complement pathway	Semiquantitative enzyme-linked immunosorbent assay
Complement activity, alternative pathway (AH50) Initial screening for suspected deficiency in the alternative complement pathway	Semiquantitative radial immunodiffusion
Mannose-binding lectin Initial screening for suspected deficiency in the lectin complement pathway	Quantitative enzyme-linked immunosorbent assay
Follow-Up Assays	
Complement factor B When CH50 is normal and AH50 is low	Quantitative radial immunodiffusion
Complement factor I When both CH50 and AH50 are low or absent	Quantitative radial immunodiffusion
Complement factor H (B1H) When both CH50 and AH50 are low or absent	Quantitative radial immunodiffusion
Complement component 1Q level	Radial immunodiffusion
Anti-C1q antibody, IgG	Semiquantitative enzyme-linked immunosorbent assay
Complement component 2 When CH50 is low or absent and AH50 is normal and high suspicion remains for complement deficiency	Quantitative radial immunodiffusion
Complement components 3 and 4 Secondary testing based on initial screening (CH50, AH50) and clinical presentation	Quantitative immunoturbidimetry
Complement component 3 Secondary testing based on initial screening (CH50, AH50) and clinical presentation	Quantitative radial immunodiffusion
Complement component 3A When CH50 and AH50 are low or absent and high suspicion remains for complement deficiency	Radioimmunoassay
Complement C3 nephritic factor	Qualitative immunofixation electrophoresis
Complement component 4 Secondary testing based on initial screening (CH50, AH50) and clinical presentation	Quantitative immunoturbidimetry
Complement component 4A When CH50 is low or absent and AH50 is normal and high suspicion remains for complement deficiency	Radioimmunoassay
Complement component 5 When CH50 and AH50 are low or absent and high suspicion remains for complement deficiency	Quantitative radial immunodiffusion
Complement component 6 When CH50 and AH50 are low or absent and high suspicion remains for complement deficiency	Quantitative radial immunodiffusion
Complement component 7 When CH50 and AH50 are low or absent and high suspicion remains for complement deficiency	Quantitative radial immunodiffusion
Complement component 8 When CH50 and AH50 are low or absent and high suspicion remains for complement deficiency	Quantitative radial immunodiffusion
Complement component 9 When CH50 and AH50 are low or absent and high suspicion remains for complement deficiency	Quantitative radial immunodiffusion
Complement component 1, functional When CH50 is low or absent and AH50 is normal and high suspicion remains for complement deficiency	Quantitative hemolytic assay
Complement component 9, functional When CH50 and AH50 are low or absent and high suspicion remains for complement deficiency	Quantitative hemolytic assay
Complement component 7, functional When CH50 and AH50 are low or absent and high suspicion remains for complement deficiency	Quantitative hemolytic assay
Complement component 6, functional	Quantitative hemolytic assay
Complement component 8, functional	Quantitative hemolytic assay
C1-esterase inhibitor	Quantitative nephelometry
C1-esterase inhibitor Functional	Semiquantitative enzyme-linked immunosorbent assay
C1q-binding assay Assessment of circulating complement	Semiquantitative enzyme-linked immunosorbent assay

From ARUP Laboratories. An ARUP Laboratories test selection tool for healthcare professionals: complement deficiency. http://www.arupconsult.com. All rights reserved. Reviewed May 15, 2023.

Hemolytic Method

The hemolytic method result is associated with hemolytic activity of the classic complement pathway and the C1–C9 components of the MAC. It is measured as hemolysis of sheep erythrocytes sensitized by specific antibodies. Each complement component is required to be activated to obtain a normal value if the immune system is effectively eliminating pathogens or damaged cells. The MAC causes a pore on the surface of a cellular membrane that ultimately results in destruction of a cell membrane, or lysis. The degree of cell lysis is proportional to the total classic complement activity present in the serum. Interpretation of CH50 units is as follows: <100, low; 100 to 300, normal; and >300, high.

Enzyme Immunoassay

The EIA combines the principles of the hemolytic assay with the use of a monoclonal antibody specific for neoantigen (C5b-9 complex [MAC]) produced as a result of complement activation. The amount of the final, polymerized C5b-9 product is proportional to the functional activity of C1 through C9. The interpretation of EIA units is as follows: <60, low; 60 to 140, normal; and >140, high.

Liposome Assay

One version of an automated liposome assay uses dinitrophenyl (DNP)-coated liposomes that contain the enzyme glucose-6-phosphate dehydrogenase. When serum is mixed with the liposomes and a substrate containing anti-DNP antibody, glucose-6-phosphate, and nicotinamide adenine dinucleotide, activated liposomes lyse and an enzymatic colorimetric reaction occurs that is proportional to total classic complement activity. Interpretation of LIA units is as follows: <23, low; 23 to 60, normal and >60, high.

AH50 is an analogous test to measure the alternative pathway. This test is available only in specialized laboratories.

Low levels of CH50 or AH50 require further evaluation. A low CH50 level suggests deficiency of a classic or terminal C component. In a C1–C8 deficiency the CH50 value is about 0. In a C9 deficiency, the CH50 value is approximately one-half of the normal value. A low AH50 level suggests a deficiency in factor B, factor D, or properdin. A low level of both CH50 and AH50 suggests a deficiency of one of the components shared by both pathways (i.e., C3–C9).

COMPLEMENT DEFICIENCY TESTING

Complement deficiency is a category of primary immunodeficiency diseases. A deficiency of any of the proteins in the three complement cascade pathways may lead to recurrent infections such as infections from *Neisseria* sp. Or an inflammatory response. A deficiency can involve complement proteins and regulators such as C3 and factors such as factor B.

Laboratory testing for complement deficiency (Algorithm Fig. 2.4) includes primary testing to determine which pathway is affected, followed by secondary testing to identify the deficient complement protein and/or its regulators to reach a definitive diagnosis. An initial complement deficiency workup includes testing total complement activity (CH50) and alternative complement activity (AH50).

Laboratory testing may also be used to monitor complement blockage in patients treated with anticomplement therapeutics.

COMPLEMENT DEFICIENCY DISORDER: HEREDITARY ANGIOEDEMA

Etiology

Hereditary angioedema (HAE) disease disorder can be either acquired or hereditary. Type I and II HAE are autosomal dominant inherited disorders caused by a qualitative or quantitative deficiency of the serine protease inhibitor, C1 esterase inhibitor (C1-INH). In contrast to acquired angioedema, which is a secondary process, HAE is associated with genetic variation. There is a specific variation in the *SERPING1* gene.

C1-INH plays important roles in the regulation of both vascular permeability and the suppression of inflammation.

Epidemiology

Prevalence estimates for HAE are difficult to determine due to low awareness of the condition and the resemblance of symptoms to other disorders resulting in delayed or incorrect diagnoses.

It is estimated that HAE occurs in 1 in 10,000 to 1 in 50,000 individuals with no known predominance for specific ethnic groups.

Factors associated with the onset of HAE episodes include emotional stress, infections, minor trauma, and minor surgical procedures. Certain medications, such as angiotensin-converting enzyme (ACE) inhibitors and exogenous estrogens, are known to increase risk of HAE. HAE is believed to be associated with increased risk of autoimmune disorders, particularly glomerulonephritis.

Pathophysiology

C1-INH regulates the protein, C1. It is an important multifunctional plasma glycoprotein that is uniquely involved in the regulatory network of the complement cascade, the contact system of the intrinsic coagulation pathway, and the fibrinolytic system. Reduced levels of C1-INH and dysfunctional C1-INH prevent autoactivation of the C1 complement system and impair production of coagulation factors XIIa, XIIf, and XIa. CI-INH is a direct inhibitor of activated kallikrein.

Activation of each of the regulatory network results in the release of vasoactive peptides, such as bradykinin. Subsequently, this release of bradykinin increases the permeability of vascular tissue, resulting in angioedema.

Signs and Symptoms

The initial symptoms of HAE usually present in childhood with exacerbations associated with the onset of puberty.

Acute respiratory attacks and abdominal distress are the most serious, life-threatening symptoms and leading causes of HAE-related morbidity and mortality. HAE typically manifests as acute attacks with edema, with the most frequently affected areas including anatomical sites such as the arms, legs, hands, feet, face, tongue, and larynx. Swelling gradually increases over the first 24 hours, then gradually subsides over the next 48 to 72 hours.

Laboratory Assays

Specific signs and symptoms are indications for testing. In addition, a family history of angioedema would be a reason for laboratory testing.

Initial laboratory assessment is a complement 1 esterase inhibitor (C1-INH) panel—C4. The ARUP Laboratories panel involves testing for:

- C-1-esterase inhibitor
- C-1-esterase inhibitor functional and
- Complement component 4

After primary testing determines the affected complement pathway, it is followed by secondary testing to identify the deficient complement protein and/or its regulators to reach a definitive diagnosis.

Interpretation of Laboratory Results

According to ARUP testing results, the HAE types are identified as follows:

Type 1—low complement 1 esterase inhibitor (C1-INH) level and low function (85%).

    If C1q is also low, suspect acquired angioedema

Type 2—normal C1-INH level but low function (15%)

Type 3 (familial angioedema) —normal C1-INH and normal function (rare)

PREVENTION AND TREATMENT
Other Soluble Immune Response Mediators

> **KEY CONCEPTS: Other Soluble Immune Mediators**
> - Cytokines are a family of proteins that are synthesized and secreted by the cells associated with innate and adaptive immunity in response to microbial and other antigen exposure.
> - Cytokines also participate in host defense. In innate immunity, cytokines mediate early inflammatory reactions to microbial organisms and stimulate adaptive immune responses. In contrast, in adaptive immunity, cytokines stimulate proliferation and differentiation of antigen-stimulated lymphocytes and activate specialized effector cells (e.g., macrophages).
> - The interferons (IFNs) are a group of cytokines discovered in virally infected cultured cells. IFNs are one of the body's natural defensive responses to foreign components (e.g., microbes, tumors, and antigens).
> - Tumor necrosis factor (TNF) is the principal mediator of the acute inflammatory response to gram-negative bacteria and other infectious microbes. TNF is responsible for many of the systemic complications of severe infections.
> - Hematopoietic stimulators include stem cell factor, a cytokine that acts on immature stem cells.
> - Chemokines are a large family of structurally homologous cytokines that stimulate transendothelial leukocyte movement from the blood to the tissue site of infection and regulate the migration of polymorphonuclear neutrophil leukocytes (PMNs) and mononuclear leukocytes within tissues. Chemokines appear to control the phased arrival of different cell populations at sites of inflammation.

Biological Response Modifiers

Biological response modifiers (BRMs) modulate an individual's own immune response. The four main sources of major BRMs secreted by mononuclear leukocytes are:
1. B lymphocytes that secrete specific antibodies.
2. T lymphocytes that secrete soluble mediators, such as interleukin-2 (IL-2) and other ILs, granulocyte–monocyte colony-stimulating factor (GM-CSF), IFN-γ, and TNF-β.

   In addition to activated type 1 helper T (Th1) lymphocytes, cytotoxic T cells and natural killer (NK) cells are a source of IFN-γ. IFN-γ is associated with innate and adaptive immunity. It is a major macrophage-activating cytokine that serves a critical function in innate and cell-mediated immunity. Other functional characteristics of IFN-γ are the induction of major histocompatibility complex (MHC) class II molecules on various cells and the ability to synergize with TNF.

   IL-5 and IL-13 are examples of cytokines secreted by type 2 helper T (Th2) CD4 lymphocytes. IFN-γ is a potent effector cytokine that is secreted by activated CD8 cytotoxic T lymphocytes. In addition, activated Th1 CD4 T lymphocytes can also produce IFN-γ.
3. NK lymphocytes that secrete IFN-α. IFN-γ is an antagonist to IL-4.
4. Monocytes and macrophages that secrete IFN-α, IL-1, and other ILs; TNF-α; and GM-CSF and monocyte colony-stimulating factor (M-CSF).

BRMs can be used therapeutically. The classes of immunotherapy are as follows:
- Active—Use of microbial or chemical immunomodulators (adjuvants) in a specific or nonspecific form
- Adoptive—Use of soluble mediators, such as ILs, to regulate components of the immune system
- Passive—Transfer of preformed antibodies to tumorous recipients, such as monoclonal antibodies
- Restorative—Application of soluble substances, such as IFNs, for a wide range of diseases

TABLE 2.5 Examples of Cytokines of Innate and Adaptive Immunity

Innate Immunity	Adaptive Immunity
Chemokines	IFN-γ
IFN type 1 (IFN-α, IFN-β)	IL-2
IL-1	IL-4
IL-6	IL-5
IL-10	IL-13
IL-12	Lt
IL-15	TGF-β
IL-18	
TNF	

IFN, Interferon; *IL*, interleukin; *Lt*, lymphotoxin; *TGF*, transforming growth factor; *TNF*, tumor necrosis factor.

Cytokines

T cells mediate their responses through the release of soluble proteins called **cytokines**. Migratory inhibitory factor (MIF) was the first cytokine activity to be described. MIF performs a T-cell–derived activity that immobilizes macrophage migration, which may cause retention and accumulation of phagocytes at sites of inflammation.

Cytokines are synthesized and secreted by the cells associated with innate and adaptive immunity in response to microbial and other antigen exposures (Tables 2.5 and 2.6).

The generic term *cytokines* has become the preferred name for this class of mediators. *Lymphokines* is another term used to describe cytokines produced by activated lymphocytes. Cytokines produced by leukocytes that act on other leukocytes are also referred to by the imperfect but descriptive term *interleukins* (ILs). As cytokines are discovered and characterized, they are assigned a number using a standard nomenclature (e.g., IL-1).

Cytokines are polypeptide products of activated cells that control a variety of cellular responses and thereby regulate the immune response. Many cytokines are released in response to specific antigens; however, cytokines are nonspecific in that their chemical structure is not determined by the stimulating antigen. Most cytokines have multiple activities and act on numerous cell types. Hematopoietic and lymphoid cell compartments are regulated by a complex network of interacting cytokines. The colony-stimulating factors (CSFs) and ILs have been shown to play important roles in normal proliferation, differentiation, and activation of several hematopoietic and lymphoid lineages (see Appendix C).

Cytokines have a variety of roles in host defense. In innate immunity, cytokines mediate early inflammatory reactions to microbial organisms and stimulate adaptive immune responses. In contrast, in adaptive immunity, cytokines stimulate proliferation and differentiation of antigen-stimulated lymphocytes and activate specialized effector cells (e.g., macrophages).

Cytokines are very potent, even in minute concentrations. Their action is usually limited to affecting cells in the local area of their production, but they can also have systemic effects. As a group, cytokines differ in molecular structure but share the following actions:
- Secrete cytokines in rapid bursts, synthesized in response to cellular activation
- Bind to specific membrane receptors on target cells
- Regulate receptor expression in T and B cells, which drives positive amplification or negative feedback
- Act on different cell types
- Excite the same functional effects with multiple cytokines (redundancy)

TABLE 2.6 Comparative Features of Innate and Adaptive Immunity

	TYPE OF IMMUNITY	
	Innate	Adaptive
Examples	TNF-α, IFN-β, IL-1, IL-12	IFN-γ, IL-2, IL-4, IL-5
Major cell source	Macrophages, NK cells	T lymphocytes
Major physiologic function	Mediators of innate immunity and inflammation (local and systemic)	Regulation of lymphocyte growth and differentiation
		Activation of effector cells (macrophages, eosinophils, mast cells)
Stimuli	LPS (endotoxin), bacterial peptidoglycans, viral RNA, T-cell–derived cytokines (e.g., IFN-β)	Protein antigens
Quantity produced	Possibly high, detectable in serum	Usually low, usually undetectable in serum
Effects on body	Local and systemic	Usually local
Roles in disease	Systemic diseases	Local tissue injury
Inhibitors	Corticosteroids	Cyclosporine, FK-506

IFN, Interferon; *IL*, interleukin; *LPS*, lipopolysaccharide; *NK*, natural killer; *RNA*, ribonucleic acid; *TNF*, tumor necrosis factor.
Adapted from Abbas AK, Lichtman AH, Pober JS: *Cellular and molecular immunology*, ed 4, Philadelphia, 2000, Saunders.

- Act close to the site of synthesis on the same cell or on a nearby cell
- Influence the synthesis and actions of other cytokines

Cytokines act on other cells by bonding to cytokine receptors on the surface of cells. Individual cytokines have characteristic functions and differ in how they transduce signals as a result of binding. All cytokine receptors consist of one or more transmembrane proteins whose extracellular portions are responsible for cytokine binding and whose cytoplasmic portions are responsible for initiating the intracellular signaling pathways. These six pathways are as follows:

1. Janus kinase (JAK/STAT) pathway
2. TNF receptor signaling by tumor necrosis receptor–associated factors (TRAFs)
3. TNF receptor signaling by death domains
4. Toll receptor signaling
5. Receptor-associated tyrosine kinases
6. G-protein signaling

CYTOKINES

A Cytokine Storm

Cytokines play an important role in the normal immune response but an overwhelming release of high concentrations of cytokines can be very harmful and create a cytokine storm. A simple definition of a cytokine storm is that it is a severe immune reaction characterized by the rapid release of a high concentration of cytokines into the peripheral blood circulation. The term *cytokine storm* was initially used in the H5N1 influenza virus "bird flu" infection in 2005 and is now associated with the severe increase of cytokines seen in coronavirus disease 2019 (COVID-19) caused by severe acute respiratory syndrome coronavirus 2 (SARS-CoV-2). Although the concept of a cytokine storm and the biological consequences of cytokine overproduction are not yet completely understood, one important molecular factor associated with overproduction is the kinetics of cytokine and chemokine gene expression.

Various cytokines from the major classes of IFNs, ILs, chemokines, CSFs, and TNFs are at the heart of the cytokine storm. The IFNs are a family of cytokines that play a central role in innate immunity to viruses and other microbial pathogens. Higher levels of the cytokine IL-6 have been specifically linked to the risk of death in SARS-CoV-2 infection. The release of proinflammatory chemokines produces the recruitment of immune system cells (neutrophils, monocytes/macrophages, and lymphocytes) to the site of infection. SARS is an example of a chemokine response that leads to a strong proinflammatory response in the lungs with the development of pulmonary fibrosis. CSFs may be part of a dependent proinflammatory cytokine network that includes IL-1 and TNF and may be part of an amplification cascade that perpetuates inflammatory reactions. TNF is now considered to be a central cytokine in acute viral diseases.

If a cytokine storm occurs, severe damage can occur because the body begins to attack its own cells and tissues rather than just fighting off the virus. Cytokine storms can occur in a variety of infectious and noninfectious diseases (e.g., autoimmune diseases, juvenile arthritis, some cancer immunotherapies, graft-versus-host disease, and various viral infections). SARS-CoV-2 virus acts differently from other viruses. The cytokine response to SARS-CoV-2 infection is about 50 times higher than seen in response to Zika or West Nile virus infections. Type II pneumocytes in the alveolar walls of the lungs lead to respiratory failure, sepsis, and a cytokine storm. The intensity of the inflammatory response in the lungs reflects a balance between proinflammatory cytokines (e.g., TNF and IL-1β) and their soluble receptors or inhibitors. Acute lung injury is a common consequence of a cytokine storm in the lung alveolar environment and systemic circulation.

Interleukins

Many different individual families and superfamilies of ILs have been identified. A characteristic of ILs is that secreted peptides and proteins mediate local interactions between leukocytes but do not bind antigens. ILs include molecules that are made by and act on lymphocytes.

Interleukins have widely overlapping functions. These molecules modulate inflammation and immunity by regulating growth, mobility, and differentiation of lymphoid cells. Each of the ILs has been shown to be a distinct molecule by gene cloning and sequencing.

Interferons

The IFNs are a group of cytokines discovered in virally infected cultured cells. This interference with viral replication in the cells by another virus led to the term *interferon*.

The IFNs are one of the body's natural defensive responses to foreign components (e.g., microbes, tumors, and antigens). IFNs are among the most broadly active physiologic regulators, enhancing the expression of specific genes, inhibiting cell proliferation, and augmenting immune effector cells. IFNs have been demonstrated to act as antiviral agents, immunomodulators, and antineoplastic agents.

Type I IFNs mediate the early innate immune response to viral infections. They consist of two distinct groups of proteins, IFN-α and IFN-β, that are structurally different but bind to the same cell surface receptor and induce similar biological responses.

IFN-γ is the principal macrophage-activating cytokine and serves a critical function in innate immunity and in specific cell-mediated immunity. It stimulates expression of MHC class I and II molecules and costimulates antigen-presenting cells (APCs), promotes the differentiation of naïve CD4+ T cells to the Th1 subset, and inhibits the proliferation of Th2 cells. In addition, IFN-γ acts on B cells to promote switching to certain IgG subclasses, activates neutrophils, and stimulates the cytolytic activity of NK cells. It is also antagonistic to IL-2. IFN-γ is the subject of much immunologic interest owing to its diverse effects on the immune response. Its ability to augment the activity of many cytokines has resulted in clinical trials in a number of different diseases.

Tumor Necrosis Factor

TNF is the principal mediator of the acute inflammatory response to gram-negative bacteria and other infectious microbes. TNF is responsible for many of the systemic complications of severe infections. The TNF receptor family stimulates gene transcription or induces apoptosis in a variety of cells. The gene encoding TNF-α is located in the human leukocyte antigen (HLA) region between the HLA-DR and HLA-B loci.

TNF-α and TNF-β share similar activities. The principal physiologic functions of TNF are (1) to stimulate the recruitment of neutrophils and monocytes to sites of infection and (2) to activate these cells to eradicate microbes.

In low concentrations, TNF acts on leukocytes and the endothelium to induce acute inflammation. At moderate concentrations, TNF mediates the systemic effects of inflammation. In severe infections, TNF is produced in large amounts and causes clinical and pathologic abnormalities (e.g., septic shock). When TNFs gain access to the circulation during infection, they mediate a series of reactions that induce shock and can result in death. The syndrome known as *septic shock* is a complication of severe gram-negative bacterial sepsis.

HEMATOPOIETIC STIMULATORS

Stem Cell Factor (c-kit Ligand)

Stem cell factor is a cytokine that interacts with a tyrosine kinase membrane receptor, the protein product of the cellular oncogene *c-kit*. The cytokine that interacts with this receptor is called *c-kit ligand*, or *stem cell factor*, because it acts on immature stem cells.

Stem cell factor is needed to make bone marrow stem cells responsive to other CSFs, but it does not cause colony formation itself. Stem cell factor may also play a role in sustaining the viability and proliferative capacity of immature T cells in the thymus and mast cells in mucosal tissues.

Colony-Stimulating Factors

A variety of CSFs, such as granulocyte CSF (G-CSF) and GM-CSF, are also made by T cells. These pathways provide a link between the lymphoid and hematopoietic systems. For example, G-CSF and GM-CSF regulate the production of granulocytes and monocytes, thus enabling the T-cell system to promote the inflammatory response.

The biological activity of CSF is measured by its ability to stimulate hematopoietic progenitor cells to form colonies in semisolid medium. These proteins are necessary for the survival, proliferation, and differentiation of precursor cells of the immune system.

CSFs are potentially important in the treatment of human disease. GM-CSF has been used in a number of clinical trials to increase circulating leukocytes in patients who have acquired immunodeficiency syndrome (AIDS), other immunocompromised patients (e.g., those recovering from chemotherapy), and bone marrow transplant recipients.

Transforming Growth Factors

As with the IFNs, transforming growth factors (TGFs) were identified as products of virally transformed cells. These factors were found to induce phenotypic transformation in nonneoplastic cells and subsequently were termed *transforming growth factors*. TGF-β is a group of five cytokines released by many cell types, including macrophages and platelets. TGF-β is known to be a potent inhibitor of IL-1–induced T-cell proliferation.

The principal action of TGF-β in the immune system is to inhibit the proliferation and activation of lymphocytes and other leukocytes. It inhibits the proliferation and differentiation of T cells and the activation of macrophages.

Chemokines

Chemokines are a large family of structurally homologous cytokines that stimulate transendothelial leukocyte movement from the blood to the tissue site of infection and regulate the migration of PMNs and mononuclear leukocytes within tissues (see Chapter 4). The largest family consists of CC chemokines that attract mononuclear cells to sites of chronic inflammation, such as monocyte chemoattractant protein 1 (MCP-1). A second family of chemokines consists of CXC chemokines, of which IL-8 (CXCL8) is the prototype. CXCL8 attracts PMNs to sites of acute inflammation, activates monocytes, and may direct the recruitment of these cells to vascular lesions. The third family, CX3, forms a cell adhesion receptor capable of arresting cells under physiologic flow conditions. TNF-α–converting enzyme can cleave CX3CL1 from the cell membrane.

Other functions of various chemokines include:

- Increasing the affinity of leukocyte integrins for their ligands on endothelium (e.g., intercellular adhesion molecule-1 [ICAM-1], ICAM-2, and vascular cell adhesion molecule-1 [VCAM-1])
- Regulating the traffic of lymphocytes and other leukocytes through peripheral lymphoid tissues
- Maintaining normal migration of immune cells into lymphoid organs or other specialized cells to particular sites

ACUTE-PHASE PROTEINS

> **KEY CONCEPTS: Acute-Phase Reactants**
> - The acute-phase response is an innate body defense. This response is a nonspecific indicator of an inflammatory process. C-reactive protein (CRP) binds to the membrane of certain microorganisms and activates the complement system.
> - CRP is used clinically for monitoring infection, autoimmune disorders, and, more recently, healing after an MI. CRP levels parallel the course of the inflammatory response and return to lower undetectable levels as the inflammation subsides.

Overview

A group of glycoproteins associated with the acute-phase response are collectively called acute-phase proteins or acute-phase reactants. The various acute-phase proteins rise at different rates and in varying levels in response to tissue injury (e.g., inflammation, infection, malignant neoplasia, various diseases or disorders, trauma, surgical procedures, and drug response). The increased synthesis of these proteins takes place shortly after a trauma and is initiated and sustained by proinflammatory cytokines.

The main biological sign of inflammation is an increase in the erythrocyte sedimentation rate (ESR). In addition to the ESR, measurement of the plasma concentration of acute-phase reactants is usually a good indicator of local inflammatory activity and tissue damage. More than 20 acute-phase proteins have a definable role in inflammation (Box 2.3). These reactants constitute most of the serum glycoproteins (Table 2.7).

An acute-phase protein that binds to the membrane of certain microorganisms and activates complement is CRP. In addition to CRP, other acute inflammatory reactants include inflammatory mediators (e.g., complement components C3 and C4), fibrinogen, transport proteins (e.g., haptoglobin), inhibitors (e.g., α_1-antitrypsin), and α_1-acid glycoprotein. Profiles of inflammatory changes yield detailed information but rarely provide major evidence for diagnosis or treatment.

Produced by the liver under the control of IL-6, CRP is a parameter of inflammatory activity. Serum concentrations can increase 1000-fold with an acute inflammatory reaction. Persistent increases in CRP can also occur in chronic inflammatory disorders (e.g., autoimmune disease and malignancy).

CRP is prominent among the acute-phase proteins because its changes show great sensitivity. Changes in CRP are independent of those of ESR and parallel the inflammatory process. CRP is a direct and quantitative measure of the acute-phase reaction and, as a result of its fast kinetics, provides adequate information about the actual clinical situation (discussed later in the chapter). In contrast, ESR is an indirect measure of the acute-phase reaction. It reacts much slower to changes of inflammatory activity and is influenced by other factors. ESR can be falsely normal in conditions such as polyglobulinemia, cryoglobulinemia, and hemoglobinopathy. ESR may also be spuriously high in the absence of inflammation in patients with anemia or hypergammaglobulinemia.

Synthesis and Catabolism

All the acute-phase proteins are synthesized rapidly in response to tissue injury. The elevation is twofold to fivefold in certain disease states. In addition, strenuous exercise triggers an inflammatory response similar to that in sepsis. Indices of the inflammatory response, especially to exercise, include leukocytosis, release of inflammatory mediators and acute-phase reactants, tissue damage, priming of various white blood cell lines, production of free radicals, and activation of complement, coagulation, and fibrinolytic cascades.

Acute-phase proteins have different kinetics and various degrees of increase. Some of the negative acute-phase proteins, actually decrease,

BOX 2.3 Major Applications of Acute-Phase Protein Measurements

- Monitoring the progress of diagnosed disease activity
- Assessing response to therapy in inflammatory diseases (e.g., rheumatoid arthritis, juvenile chronic arthritis, ankylosing spondylitis, Reiter syndrome, psoriatic arthropathy, vasculitis, and rheumatic fever)
- Detection of complications of a known disease (e.g., immune complex deposition, and postsurgical infection)

possibly resulting from a loss of protein from the vascular space. In addition, acute-phase proteins can be modified by causes other than inflammation; for example, by a low fibrinogen level in disseminated intravascular coagulation (DIC), a very low haptoglobin level in hemolysis, an elevated α_1-acid glycoprotein (orosomucoid) in renal insufficiency, and an elevated transferrin level in iron deficiency. Liver insufficiency or leakage through the kidney or gut lesions can also lower these reactants.

The rate of change and peak concentration of separate acute-phase reactants vary with the component and the clinical situation. In acute inflammation, CRP and α_1-antichymotrypsin levels become elevated within the first 12 hours. CRP has the fastest rate of change of any of the acute-phase proteins. The levels of complement components C3 and C4 and of ceruloplasmin do not rise for several days.

Acute-phase proteins do not always change in parallel. This mismatch in acute-phase protein levels is most often the result of increased catabolism and elimination from the circulation of certain proteins. Differences may also be caused by discrepancies in rates of synthesis. Most acute-phase proteins have half-lives of 2 to 4 days, but CRP has a half-life of 5 to 7 hours. Thus the CRP level falls much more rapidly than that of the other acute-phase proteins when the patient recovers.

C-Reactive Protein

Traditionally CRP has been used clinically for monitoring infection, autoimmune disorders, and, more recently, healing after an MI. Levels of CRP parallel the course of the inflammatory response and return to lower, undetectable levels as the inflammation subsides. CRP demonstrates a large incremental change, with as much as a 100-fold increase in concentration in acute inflammation, and is the fastest responding and most sensitive indicator of acute inflammation. CRP increases faster than ESR in responding to inflammation, whereas the leukocyte count may remain within normal limits despite infection. An elevated CRP level can signal infection many hours before it can be confirmed by culture results; therefore treatment can be prompt. Because of these characteristics, CRP is the method of choice for screening for inflammatory and malignant organic diseases and monitoring therapy in inflammatory diseases.

Elevations of the CRP level occur in about 70 disease states, including septicemia and meningitis in neonates, infections in immunosuppressed patients, burns complicated by infection, serious postoperative infections, MI, malignant tumors, and rheumatic disease. Measurement of CRP may add to the diagnostic procedure in select cases (e.g., differentiation between a bacterial and a viral infection). An extremely elevated CRP level suggests a possible bacterial infection (see the procedure C-Reactive Protein Rapid Latex Agglutination Test later in the chapter). In general, CRP is advocated as an indicator of bacterial infection in at-risk patients in whom the clinical assessment of infection is difficult to make, but a lack of specificity rules out CRP as a definitive diagnostic tool.

Levels of CRP rise after tissue injury or surgery. In uncomplicated cases the CRP level peaks about 2 days after surgery and gradually returns to normal levels within 7 to 10 days. If the CRP level is

TABLE 2.7 Examples of Clinically Useful Acute-Phase Proteins

Protein	Normal Concentration (g/L)	Concentration in Acute Inflammation (g/L)	Response Time (Hours)
C-reactive protein	0.0008–0.004	0.4	6–10
α_1-Antichymotrypsin	0.3–0.6	3.0	10
α_1-Antitrypsin	2.0–4.0	7.0	24
Orosomucoid	0.5–1.4	3.0	24
Haptoglobin	1.0–3.0	6.0	24
Fibrinogen	2.0–4.5	10.0	24
C3	0.55–1.2	3.0	48–72
C4	0.2–0.5	1.0	48–72
Ceruloplasmin	0.15–0.6	2.0	48–72

persistently elevated or returns to an increased level, it may indicate underlying sepsis preceding clinical signs and symptoms and should alert the clinician to postoperative complications.

In clinical practice, CRP is particularly useful when serial measurements are performed. The course of the CRP level may be useful for monitoring the effect of treatment and for early detection of postoperative complications or intercurrent infections. In RA, the CRP level reflects short-term and long-term disease activity. Monitoring of CRP levels allows for early prediction of response to a particular drug, often months before clinical and radiologic confirmation is possible. In disorders such as RA, CRP can be used to assess the effect of antiinflammatory drugs (e.g., aspirin) and the nature of their action. Aspirin-like drugs do not suppress acute-phase proteins in inflammation, allowing optimal therapy in the shortest time and minimizing ongoing inflammation and joint damage. Assessment of CRP is also valuable in monitoring therapy and disease activity in other arthritides. Rheumatic fever and Crohn's disease can also be monitored by CRP. In addition, CRP level assessment has been found to enhance the value of traditional enzyme measurements in MI.

In a number of chronic inflammatory diseases, however, CRP is an unreliable indicator. CRP values may be normal when other acute-phase proteins are altered in disorders such as SLE, dermatomyositis, and ulcerative colitis. SLE shows little or no CRP response despite apparently active inflammation.

Both CRP and low-density lipoprotein (LDL) cholesterol levels are known to be elevated in persons at risk for cardiovascular disease. The CRP level may be a stronger predictor of cardiovascular events than the LDL cholesterol level, an established benchmark of cardiovascular risk.

Other Acute-Phase Reactants

Procalcitonin (PCT) is a biomarker that exhibits greater specificity than other proinflammatory markers (e.g., cytokines) in identifying patients with sepsis and can be used in the diagnosis of bacterial infections. Several clinical laboratory tests have been applied to the diagnosis of sepsis. Microbial culture is the gold standard for the diagnosis of bacterial infection, but a definitive result can take 24 hours or more before a conclusive diagnosis. A number of the inflammatory markers, such as leukocyte cell count, CRP, and cytokines (TNF-α, IL-1β, or IL-6), have been applied in the diagnosis of inflammation and infection, but their lack of specificity has led to the development of more specific clinical laboratory tests. Currently, available methods include a rapid immunochromatographic test and automated assays using various methods, including lateral flow immunoassay and time-resolved amplified cryptate emission (TRACE) technology.

α_1-**Antitrypsin** is an acute-phase protein that increases in acute inflammatory reactions. Generalized vasculitis, such as in immune complex disease, may result in inappropriately low levels of α_1-antitrypsin, probably resulting from increased elimination of complexes with leukocyte lysosomal enzymes.

Defects in the complement components C3a and C5a and the opsonin C3b result in serious infections. In addition, immune complex disease and gram-negative bacteremia result in low levels of complement components, particularly C3 and C4, because the components are consumed during complement activation. Acute inflammation leads to normal or slightly elevated levels. If both disorders are present, complement consumption may be masked, making it deceptive to use complement measurement as the only index of immune complex deposition in disease. The detection of complement breakdown products is more useful than the measurement of total complement component concentrations. It is more desirable to measure C3 breakdown products than total C3 in conditions such as peritonitis or pancreatitis.

Ceruloplasmin, often measured as serum copper, is used to monitor Hodgkin's disease; increases are considered specific indicators of relapse. Although not definitely established, ceruloplasmin monitoring may provide similar information in non-Hodgkin lymphoma.

Laboratory Assessment Methods

Inflammation almost always follows acute tissue damage. Diagnostic categories of acute inflammation can include bacterial causes and nonbacterial causes such as trauma, chronic inflammation, and viral disease. Many laboratory tests have been advocated for the early diagnosis of acute inflammation: total white blood cell (WBC) count (including the absolute count and percentage of band and segmented neutrophils, as determined by a 100-cell differential count on a peripheral blood smear), acute-phase proteins, and the ESR.

The ESR ("sed rate") is a nonspecific indicator of disease, with increased sedimentation of erythrocytes seen in acute and chronic inflammation and malignancies. Although nonspecific, the ESR is one of the most frequently performed laboratory tests.

In addition to these hematologic tests, several tests are of direct value in immunologic testing. These procedures include specific biomarker assessment for inflammation and the determination of CRP (discussed earlier).

CASE STUDY 2.1

A 39-year-old woman was admitted for a cholecystectomy. She had a history of chronic cholecystitis; recent x-ray studies revealed stones in the gallbladder and a large stone in the biliary duct (Fig. 2.5). During surgery, a large stone was removed from the duct, and a cholangiogram showed no further obstructions of the hepatic or common bile ducts.

The patient became febrile 1 day after surgery. A 48-hour postoperative complete blood count (CBC) and CRP were ordered (Fig. 2.6). On the seventh postoperative day, she had abdominal pain and began vomiting. A CBC, ESR, CRP, and blood culture were ordered at that time. Immediately after drawing the blood work, the patient was started on a broad-spectrum antibiotic and discharged on hospital day 12.

Laboratory Data

At 48 hours after surgery, the CBC was within normal limits and the CRP was 7.5 g/L.

Results after the episode of abdominal pain showed a CRP of 8.4 g/L and subsequently positive blood culture for *Pseudomonas* spp.

Review Questions

1. The patient's CRP was elevated at 7 days postoperatively because:
   a. It reflects the leukocyte (WBC) response
   b. It is a sensitive indicator of inflammation
   c. It is diagnostic of sepsis
   d. It is normal to manifest an extremely elevated CRP 7 days after surgery
2. In an uncomplicated cholecystectomy:
   a. The highest level of CRP is at 48 hours postoperatively
   b. The highest level of CRP is at 72 hours postoperatively
   c. The lowest level of CRP is at 5 days postoperatively
   d. The lowest level of CRP is at 7 days postoperatively

See Appendix A for the answers to these questions.

Critical Thinking Group Discussion Questions

1. Which test was the most rapid and sensitive indicator of infection?
2. Is the CRP diagnostic?
3. Why was the CRP level elevated immediately after surgery?

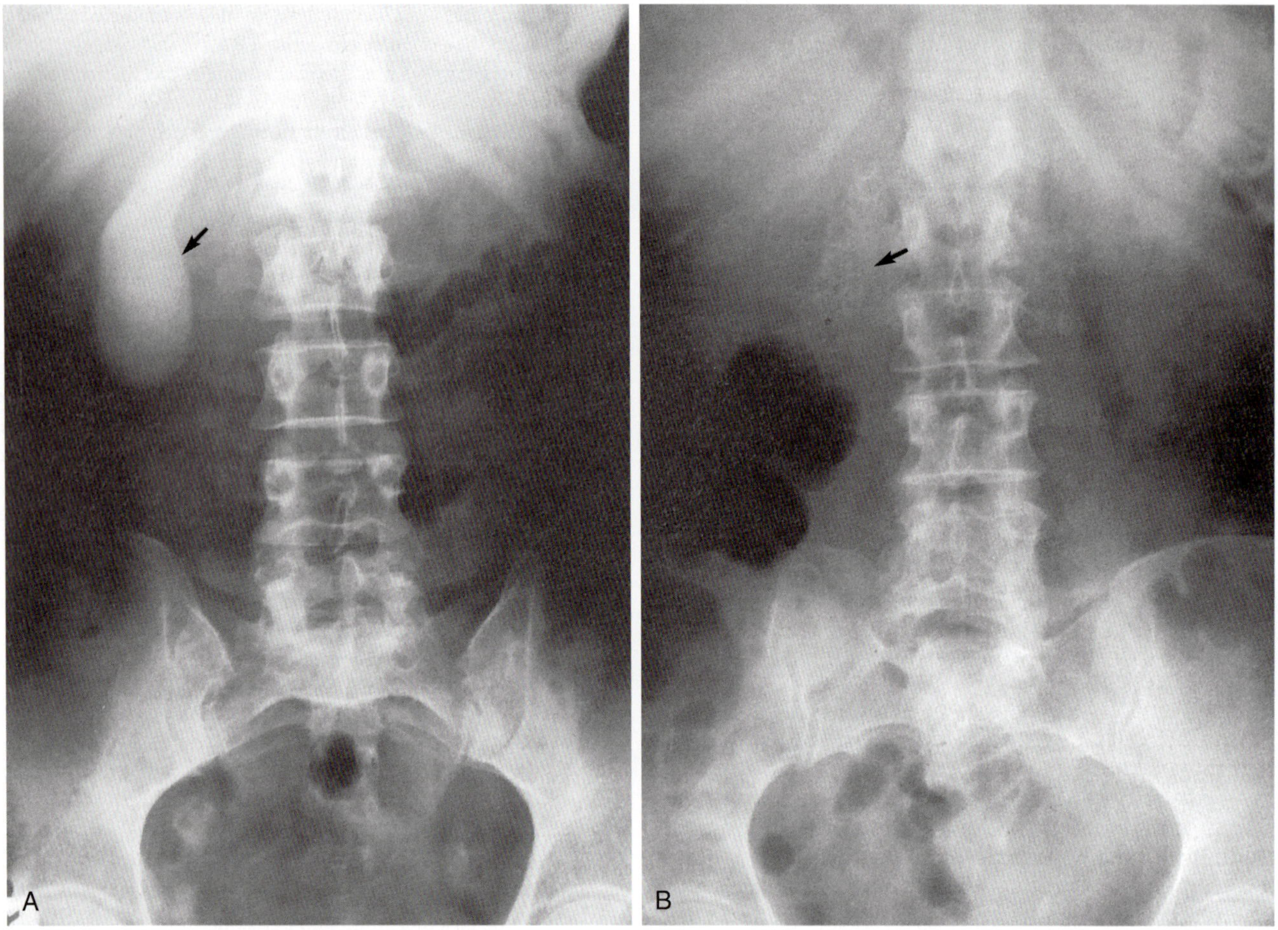

PART I Basic Immunologic Mechanisms

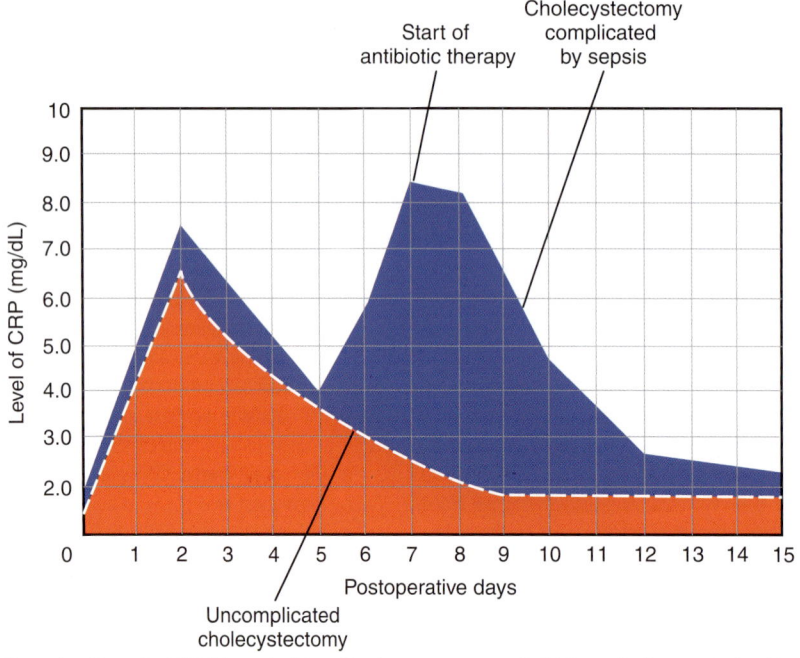

Fig. 2.5 Radiographs of Gallbladder (Contrast Dye). A, Normal gallbladder *(arrow)*. B, Gallbladder filled with stones *(arrow)*.

Fig. 2.6 C-Reactive Protein (CRP) Levels After Cholecystectomy. *Solid lines*, Patients; *dashed line*, example.

REVIEW QUESTIONS

1. A characteristic of the complement system includes all of the following except:
   a. A heat-labile series of plasma proteins
   b. Composed of many proteinases
   c. Composed of two interrelated pathways
   d. Composed of three interrelated pathways
2. Which complement component is found in both the classical and alternative pathways?
   a. C1
   b. C4
   c. Factor B
   d. C3
3. The complement cascade reaches full amplitude at the ____ component level.
   a. C3
   b. C5
   c. C7
   d. C8
4. Which complement pathway and a related initiator can activate complement?
   a. Classic pathway; antigen–IgG antibody complexes
   b. Classic pathway; tumor cells
   c. Alternative pathway; certain viruses and gram-negative bacteria
   d. Mannose–lectin pathway; apoptotic cells
5. Which complement component is present in the greatest quantity in plasma?
   a. C2
   b. C3
   c. C4
   d. C8
6. The first of the stages of the classic complement pathway is:
   a. Enzymatic activation
   b. Membrane attack complex
   c. Recognition
7. The second of the three stages of the classic complement pathway is:
   a. Amplification of the proteolytic complement cascade
   b. Membrane attack complex
   c. Recognition
8. The last of the three stages of the classic complement pathway is:
   a. Enzymatic activation
   b. Membrane attack complex
   c. Recognition
9. Which of the following is a component of the recognition unit in the classic complement pathway?
   a. C1q
   b. C3
   c. C5
   d. C9
10. The complement component, C3b, is:
    a. A T lymphocyte multiplication agent
    b. A powerful opsonin
    c. An antibody production stimulant
    d. A blocker of anaphylaxis
11. The complement component associated with only the alternative pathway of complement activation is:
    a. C1q
    b. Properdin factor B
    c. C3b
    d. C3a
12. The complement component that stimulates the release of histamine and other soluble mediators from basophilic granulocytes is:
    a. C3a
    b. C3b
    c. C5
    d. C9
13. Fixation of the C1 complement component is related to each of the following factors *except*:
    a. Molecular weight of the antibody
    b. The presence of IgM antibody
    c. The presence of most IgG subclasses
    d. Spatial constraints
14. The final steps of complement activation lead to:
    a. Cell lysis
    b. Phagocytosis
    c. Immune opsonin adherence
    d. Virus neutralization
15. Which complement component is associated with the "recognition unit" in the classic complement pathway?
    a. C1q
    b. C3a
    c. C7
    d. C9
16. The alternative complement pathway is (can be):
    a. Initiated by the formation of antigen–antibody reactions
    b. Considered to be a predominantly, non–antibody-initiated pathway
    c. Activated by factors such as endotoxins
    d. Both b and c
17. A complement deficiency state associated with a deficiency of C2 is:
    a. Xeroderma pigmentosa
    b. Leiner disease
    c. Raynaud phenomenon
    d. Recurrent pyogenic infections
18. A complement deficiency state associated with C5 dysfunction is:
    a. Xeroderma pigmentosa
    b. Leiner disease
    c. Raynaud phenomenon
    d. Recurrent pyogenic infections
19. A complement deficiency state associated with a deficiency of C3 and C4 related to disease activity is:
    a. Systemic lupus erythematosus
    b. Leiner disease
    c. Raynaud phenomenon
    d. Recurrent pyogenic infections
20. A complement deficiency associated with a deficiency of C8 that makes a patient highly susceptible to *Neisseria* infections is:
    a. Xeroderma pigmentosa
    b. Leiner disease
    c. Raynaud phenomenon
    d. Recurrent pyogenic infections
21. A (the) nonspecific component(s) of the immune system is (are):
    a. Complement
    b. T cells
    c. B cells
    d. Both a and b
22. What is the purpose of the CH_{50} assay?
    a. Measures classical or terminal complement pathway deficiency
    b. Detects a deficiency in factor B, factor D, or properdin
    c. Detects a lectin pathway component deficiency
    d. Measures the alternative complement pathway

23. Which activity is associated with interferon?
    a. Enhances phagocytosis
    b. Retards the expression of specific genes
    c. Promotes complement-mediated cytolysis
    d. Interferes with viral replication
24. In severe infections, tumor necrosis factor (TNF):
    a. Blocks recruitment of neutrophils
    b. Blocks recruitment of monocytes
    c. Induces acute inflammation
    d. Causes septic shock
25. A characteristic associated with tumor necrosis factor-gamma (TNF-α) is:
    a. Stimulates hematopoietic growth factor
    b. Encoding a gene located in the HLA region between the HLA-DR and HLA-B loci
    c. Induces phenotype transformation in nonneoplastic cells
    d. Also known as IL-2
26. The characteristic associated with colony-stimulating factor is:
    a. Stimulates hematopoietic progenitor cells
    b. Encoding a gene located in the HLA region between the HLA-DR and HLA-B loci
    c. Induces phenotype transformation in nonneoplastic cells
    d. Also known as IL-2
27. The characteristic associated with transforming growth factor (TGF) is:
    a. Stimulates hematopoietic growth factor
    b. Encoding a gene located in the HLA region between the HLA-DR and HLA-B loci
    c. Induces phenotype transformation in nonneoplastic cells
    d. Also known as IL-2
28. A major macrophage cytokine is:
    a. Interferon gamma (IFN-γ)
    b. Interleukin 3 (IL-3)
    c. Interleukin 4 (IL-4)
    d. Interleukin 5 (IL-5)
29. Examples of cytokines originating from activated T cells include:
    a. IL-3, IL-8
    b. IL-18, IL-19
    c. IL-1 superfamily, IL-2
    d. IL-2, IL-3
30. A characteristic of an acute-phase protein includes the following *except*:
    a. An acute-phase protein response is a nonspecific indicator of an inflammatory response.
    b. Acute-phase proteins are slowly synthesized in response to tissue injury.
    c. C-reactive protein is an acute-phase protein.
    d. Laboratory measurement of an acute phase can monitor the progress of tissue healing.

3

Antigens and Antibodies

LEARNING OUTCOMES

- Define the terms *antigen* and *antibody*.
- Compare the characteristics of major histocompatibility complex (MHC) classes I and II.
- Differentiate the characteristics of each of the five immunoglobulin classes.
- Draw and describe a typical immunoglobulin G (IgG) molecular structure.
- Compare the differences between isotype, idiotype, and allotype.
- Name the four phases of an antibody response.
- Describe the characteristics of a primary and secondary (anamnestic) response.
- Compare the terms antibody *avidity* and antibody *affinity*.
- Describe the method of production of a monoclonal antibody.
- Correctly answer case study–related multiple-choice questions.
- Analyze a patient history, clinical signs and symptoms, and laboratory data; answer the related multiple-choice and critical-thinking questions; and conclude the most likely diagnosis.
- Describe the principal and agglutination reactions in ABO blood grouping.
- Correctly answer 80% of the end-of-chapter review questions.

OUTLINE

Antigen Characteristics, 48
    General Characteristics of Immunogens and Antigens, 48
    Histocompatibility Antigens, 48
        Major Histocompatibility Complex Regions, 49
        Classes of Human Leukocyte Antigen Molecules, 49
    Autoantigens, 50
    Blood Group Antigens, 50
Chemical Nature of Antigens, 51
    Adjuvant, 51
Physical Nature of Antigens, 51
    Foreignness, 51
    Degradability, 51
    Molecular Weight, 51
    Structural Stability, 51
    Complexity, 51
General Characteristics of Antibodies, 51
Immunoglobulin Classes, 51
    Immunoglobulin M, 52
    Immunoglobulin G, 53
    Immunoglobulin A, 53
    Immunoglobulin D, 53
    Immunoglobulin E, 53
Antibody Structure, 53
    Typical Immunoglobulin Molecule, 54
        Heavy Chains, 54
        Light Chains, 54
    Specific Immunoglobulin Characteristics, 55
        Immunoglobulin M, 56
        Immunoglobulin A, 56
        Immunoglobulin D, 56
        Immunoglobulin E, 56
Immunoglobulin Variants, 56
    Isotype Determinants, 56
    Allotype Determinants, 56
    Idiotype Determinants, 56
Antibody Synthesis, 56
    Primary Antibody Response, 57
    Secondary (Anamnestic) Response, 57
Functions of Antibodies, 58
Antigen–Antibody Interaction: Specificity and Crossreactivity, 58
    Antibody Affinity, 58
    Antibody Avidity, 59
    Immune Complexes, 59
Molecular Basis of Antigen–Antibody Reactions, 59
    Types of Bonding, 59
        Hydrophobic Bonds, 59
        Hydrogen Bonds, 60
        Van der Waals Forces, 60
        Electrostatic Forces, 60
    Goodness of Fit, 60
    Detection of Antigen–Antibody Reactions, 60
    Influence of Antibody Types on Agglutination, 60
Neutralizing Antibodies, 61
Monoclonal Antibodies, 61
    Discovery of the Technique, 61
    Monoclonal Antibody Production, 61
    Uses of Monoclonal Antibodies, 62
Case Study 3.1   History and Physical Examination, 63
Procedure: ABO Blood Grouping (Forward Antigen Typing), 66.e1

KEY TERMS

- adjuvant
- affinity
- alloantibodies
- anamnestic response
- antibodies
- antigen
- autoantigens
- avidity
- clonal selection
- epitope
- haptens
- human leukocyte antigen (HLA)
- hybridoma
- idiotypes
- immune complex
- immunogens
- major histocompatibility complex (MHC)
- monoclonal antibodies (MAbs)
- neonatal Fc receptor (FcRn)
- opsonin effect
- precipitating
- soluble
- zeta potential

ANTIGEN CHARACTERISTICS

General Characteristics of Immunogens and Antigens

An immune response is triggered by **immunogens**, macromolecules capable of triggering an adaptive immune response by inducing the formation of **antibodies** or sensitized T cells in an immunocompetent host (a host capable of recognizing and responding to a foreign **antigen**). Immunogens can specifically react with corresponding antibodies or sensitized T lymphocytes.

> **KEY CONCEPTS: Characteristics of Antigens**
> - Foreign substances can be immunogenic if their membrane or molecular components contain structures (antigenic determinants or epitopes) recognized as foreign by the immune system.
> - The normal immune system responds to foreignness by producing antibodies.
> - Cellular antigens of importance to immunologists include the major histocompatibility complex (MHC) groups and human leukocyte antigens (HLAs), autoantigens, and blood group antigens. Some of these MHC antigens are more potent than others in provoking an immune response.

In contrast, an antigen is any substance that may be specifically bound by an antibody molecule or T-lymphocyte receptor. Although all antigens are recognized by specific lymphocytes or by antibodies, only some antigens are capable of activating antibody formation. Some may not be able to evoke an immune response initially. For example, lower molecular–weight particles, haptens, can bind to an antibody but must be attached to a macromolecule as a carrier to stimulate a specific immune response. In reality, all immunogens are antigens, but not all antigens are immunogens.

The two terms *immunogens* and *antigens* are frequently used interchangeably without making a distinction between the two. Foreign substances can be immunogenic or antigenic (capable of provoking a humoral and/or cell-mediated immune response) if their membrane or molecular components contain structures recognized as foreign by the immune system. Internal antigens can also be immunogenic if they are processed by phagocytic cells and expressed properly or are produced within a cell, such as a viral protein from an infected cell. An **epitope**, as part of an antigen, reacts specifically with an antibody or T-lymphocyte receptor.

Not all surfaces act as antigenic determinants. Only prominent determinants on the surface of a protein are normally recognized by the immune system, and some of these are much more immunogenic than others. An immune response is directed against specific determinants, and resultant antibodies will bind to them, with much of the remaining molecule being immunogenic.

The cellular membrane of mammalian cells consists chemically of proteins, phospholipids, cholesterol, and traces of polysaccharides. Polysaccharides (carbohydrates) in the form of glycoproteins or glycolipids can be found attached to the lipid and protein molecules of the membrane. When antigen-bearing cells, such as red blood cells (RBCs), from one person, a donor, are transfused into another person, a recipient, they can be immunogenic. Outer surfaces of bacteria, such as the capsule or the cell wall, in addition to the surface structures of other microorganisms, can also be immunogenic.

Cellular antigens of importance to immunologists include histocompatibility antigens, **autoantigens**, and blood group antigens (see Procedure: ABO Blood Grouping [Forward Antigen Typing]). The normal immune system responds to foreignness by producing antibodies. For this reason, microbial antigens are also important to immunologists in the study of the immunologic manifestations of infectious diseases.

Histocompatibility Antigens

Nucleated cells such as leukocytes and tissues have many cell surface–protein antigens that readily provoke an immune response if transferred into a genetically different (allogenic) individual of the same species. Some of these antigens, which constitute the **major histocompatibility complex (MHC)**, are more potent than others in provoking an immune response. The MHC is referred to as the **human leukocyte antigen (HLA)** system in humans because its gene products were originally identified on white blood cells (WBCs, leukocytes). The HLA system is of primary importance in hematopoietic stem cell transplants (see Chapter 25 for a discussion of the importance of MHC/HLA in transplantation). These antigens are second only to the ABO antigens in influencing the survival or graft rejection of transplanted organs. There is a strong association between individual HLAs and immunologic disorders (Box 3.1).

HLA-matched platelets are useful for patients who are refractory to treatment with random donor platelets.

In paternity testing, HLA typing is used, along with the determination of ABO; Rh; MNS; and Kell, Duffy, and Kidd erythrocyte antigens. In the past, most laboratories involved in testing individuals in disputed parentage cases used only the ABO, Rh, and MNS systems. The chances of identifying a falsely accused man with these tests were 58%. Additional testing for Kell, Duffy, and Kidd erythrocyte antigens and for HLA typing has an exclusion rate estimated at 92%.

HLA typing is also useful in forensic medicine, anthropology, and basic research in immunology. In studies of racial ancestry and migration, some antigens are almost excluded or confined to a race (e.g., A1 and B8 are rarely detected in peoples indigenous to central and eastern Asia, and Bw57 is uncommon in White and African American individuals). These distinctions allow for precise conclusions to be drawn regarding origin and ancestry.

HLA testing has increasingly been used as a diagnostic and genetic counseling tool. Knowledge of HLA antigens and their linkage has become important because of the recognized association of certain antigens with distinct immunologic-mediated reactions, autoimmune diseases, some neoplasms, and other disorders; these disorders, although nonimmunologic, are influenced by non-HLA genes also located within the major MHC region.

BOX 3.1 Relationship of Certain Human Leukocyte Antigens and Diseases

B27
Ankylosing spondylitis[a]
Reiter syndrome
Anterior uveitis
Arthritic infection with *Yersinia* or *Salmonella* sp.
Psoriatic arthritis with spinal involvement
Spondylitis associated with inflammatory bowel disease
Juvenile chronic arthritis with spinal involvement

B8
Celiac disease
Addison disease
Myasthenia gravis
Dermatitis herpetiformis
Chronic active hepatitis
Sjögren syndrome
Diabetes mellitus (insulin dependent)
Thyrotoxicosis

B5
Behçet syndrome

BW38
Psoriatic arthritis

BW15
Diabetes mellitus (insulin dependent)

Cw6
Psoriasis vulgaris

DR2
Goodpasture syndrome
Multiple sclerosis

DR3
Gluten-sensitive enteropathy
Dermatitis herpetiformis
Subacute cutaneous lupus erythematosus
Addison's disease
Sjögren syndrome (primary)

DR4
Pemphigus[b]
Giant-cell arthritis
Rheumatoid arthritis
Juvenile (insulin dependent) diabetes mellitus

DR5
Pauciarticular juvenile arthritis
Scleroderma
Hashimoto thyroiditis

[a]If HLA-B27 is present, there is an overall greater increased risk in the general population for developing the disease over a lifetime. Varies with ethnic groups (e.g., three-times greater risk for Pima Indians to 300 times greater risk for Japanese).
[b]Increased incidence in patients of Ashkenazi Jewish descent and patients of Mediterranean origin.

The estimated relative risks or chances of developing a disease if a given antigen is present may be elevated in individuals bearing certain HLA antigens compared with individuals who lack the antigen. The HLA-B27 antigen is the only HLA antigen with a disease association strong enough to be useful in differential diagnosis. Although the degree of association between HLA antigens and other diseases may be statistically significant, it is not strong enough to be of diagnostic or prognostic value.

Although only 8% of White individuals carry the HLA-B27 antigen; 90% of patients with ankylosing spondylitis (AS) or spondylitis in association with Reiter syndrome (see Chapter 24) are positive for the antigen. An elevated percentage of HLA-B27–positive patients is also observed in juvenile chronic arthritis with spinal involvement. Therefore the major indication for screening for HLA-B27 is to rule out AS when back pain develops in relatives of patients with the disease and to help distinguish incomplete Reiter syndrome from gonococcal arthritis, or chronic or atypical Reiter syndrome from rheumatoid arthritis. A negative test result for HLA-B27, however, does not exclude the diagnosis of AS or Reiter syndrome.

Major Histocompatibility Complex Regions

The MHC is divided into four major regions (Fig. 3.1): D, B, C, and A. The A, B, and C regions are the classic or class Ia genes that code for class I molecules. The D region codes for class II molecules. Class I includes HLA-A, HLA-B, and HLA-C. The three principal loci (A, B, and C) and their respective antigens are numbered; for example, 1, 2, and 3. The class II gene region antigens are encoded in the HLA-D region and can be subdivided into three families: HLA-DR, HLA-DC (DQ), and HLA-SB (DP).

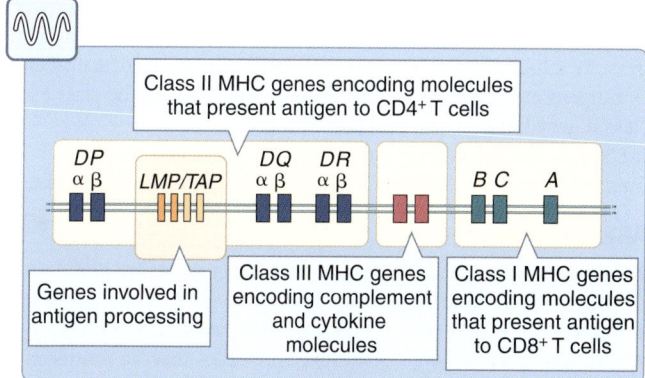

Fig. 3.1 Genetic Organization of MHC (HLA) Antigen. *HLA,* Human leukocyte antigen; *LMP,* large multifunctional protease; *MHC,* major histocompatibility complex; *TAP,* transporter associated with antigen presentation. (From Nairn R, Helbert M: *Immunology for medical students,* ed 2, St. Louis, 2007, Elsevier.)

Classes of Human Leukocyte Antigen Molecules

Structurally there are two classes of HLA molecules, class I (Fig. 3.2) and class II (Fig. 3.3) (Table 3.1). Both class I and class II antigens function as targets of T lymphocytes (see Chapter 4 for a further discussion of lymphocytes) that regulate the immune response. Class I molecules

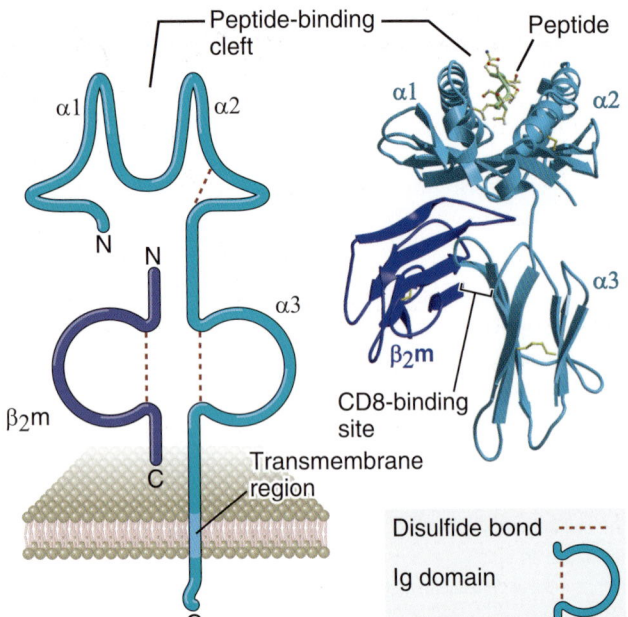

Fig. 3.2 Structure of Class I MHC Molecule. The schematic diagram *(left)* illustrates the different regions of the MHC molecule (not drawn to scale). Class I molecules are composed of a polymorphic α chain noncovalently attached to the nonpolymorphic $β_2$-microglobulin, $β_2m$. The α chain is glycosylated; carbohydrate residues are not shown. The ribbon diagram *(right)* shows the structure of the extracellular portion of the HLA-B27 molecule with a bound peptide, resolved by x-ray crystallography. *Ig,* Immunoglobulin; *MHC,* major histocompatibility complex. (From Abbas AK, Lichtman AH: *Cellular and molecular immunology,* ed 8, Philadelphia, 2015, Elsevier. Courtesy Dr. P. Bjorkman, California Institute of Technology, Pasadena, CA.)

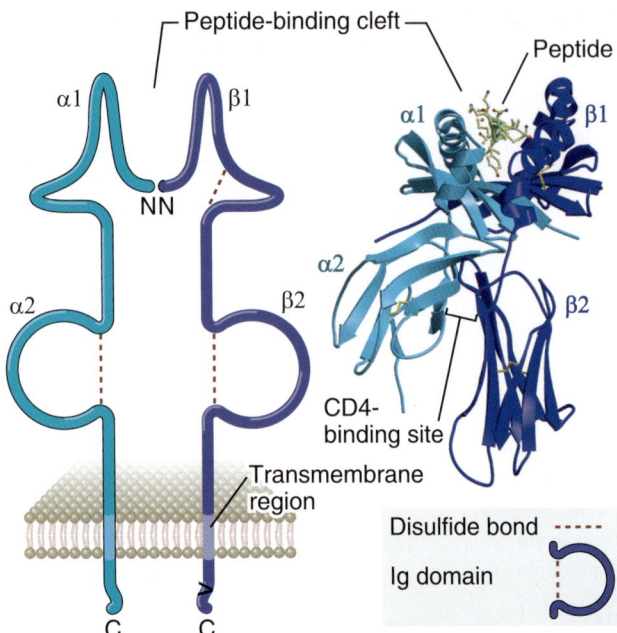

Fig. 3.3 Structure of Class II MHC Molecule. The schematic diagram *(left)* illustrates the different regions of the MHC molecule (not drawn to scale). Class II molecules are composed of a polymorphic α chain noncovalently attached to a polymorphic β chain. Glycosylated; carbohydrate residues are not shown. The ribbon diagram *(right)* shows the structure of the extracellular portion of the HLA-DR1 molecule with a bound peptide, resolved by x-ray crystallography. *Ig,* Immunoglobulin; *MHC,* major histocompatibility complex. (From Abbas AK, Lichtman AH: *Cellular and molecular immunology,* ed 8, Philadelphia, 2015, Elsevier. Courtesy Dr. P. Bjorkman, California Institute of Technology, Pasadena, CA.)

regulate the interaction between cytolytic T cells and target cells, and class II molecules restrict the activity of regulatory T cells. Thus class II molecules regulate the interaction between helper T cells and antigen-presenting cells (APCs). Cytotoxic T cells directed against class I antigens are inhibited by CD8 cells; cytotoxic T cells directed against class II antigens are inhibited by CD4 cells. Many genes in the class I and class II gene families have no known function.

Note: Additional HLA information is presented in Chapter 25, Transplantation: HLA, Solid Organ, and Hematopoietic Stem Cells.

Autoantigens

The evolution of a recognition system that can recognize and destroy nonself material must also have safeguards to prevent damage to self-antigens. The body's immune system usually exercises tolerance to self-antigens, but in some situations, antibodies may be produced in response to normal self-antigens. This failure to recognize self-antigens can result in autoantibodies directed at hormones, such as thyroglobulin (see Chapter 22).

Blood Group Antigens

Blood group substances are widely distributed throughout the tissues, blood cells, and body fluids. When foreign RBC antigens are introduced to a host, a transfusion reaction or hemolytic disease of the fetus and newborn can result (see Chapter 20). In addition certain antigens, especially those of the Rh system, are integral structural components of the erythrocyte (RBC) membrane. If these antigens are missing, the erythrocyte membrane is defective and results in hemolytic anemia. When antigens do not form part of the essential membrane structure (e.g., A, B, and H antigens), the absence of antigen has no effect on membrane integrity.

TABLE 3.1	Comparison of Major Histocompatibility Complex Class I and Class II	
	Class I	**Class II**
Loci	HLA-A, -B, and -C	HLA-DN, -DO, -DP, -DQ, and -DR
Distribution	Most nucleated cells	B lymphocytes, macrophages, other antigen-presenting cells, activated T lymphocytes
Function	To present endogenous antigen to cytotoxic T lymphocytes	To present endogenous antigen to helper T lymphocytes

HLA, Human leukocyte antigen; *MHC,* major histocompatibility complex.

> **KEY CONCEPTS: Chemical Composition of Antigens and Antibodies**
> - Antigens are usually large organic molecules that are proteins or polysaccharides.
> - Large foreign molecules are better antigens, but haptens can bind to larger carrier molecules and behave like antigens.
> - Antibodies that are specific proteins are known as *immunoglobulins* (Igs).
> - Many antibodies can be isolated in the gamma globulin fraction of protein by electrophoretic separation.
> - The primary function of an antibody in body defenses is to combine with antigen.
> - If soluble antigen is added to antibody, the antigen–antibody reaction is precipitation (see Chapter 8).

CHEMICAL NATURE OF ANTIGENS

Antigens, or immunogens, are usually large organic molecules that are proteins or large polysaccharides and, less commonly, lipids. Antigens, especially cell surface or membrane-bound antigens, can be composed of combinations of biochemical classes (e.g., glycoproteins, glycolipids). For example, histocompatibility HLAs are glycoproteins in nature and are found on the surface membranes of nucleated body cells composed of solid tissue and most circulating blood cells (e.g., granulocytes, lymphocytes, and thrombocytes).

Proteins are excellent antigens because of their high molecular weight (MW) and structural complexity. Lipids are considered less antigenic because of their relative simplicity and lack of structural stability. When lipids are linked to proteins or polysaccharides, they may function as antigens. Nucleic acids are less antigenic because of their relative simplicity, molecular flexibility, and rapid degradation. Antinucleic acid antibodies can be produced by artificially stabilizing them and linking them to an immunogenic carrier. Carbohydrates (polysaccharides) by themselves are considered too small to function as antigens. In the case of erythrocyte blood group antigens, protein or lipid carriers may contribute to the necessary size, and the polysaccharides present in the form of side chains confer immunologic specificity.

Adjuvant

The response to immunization can be enhanced by a number of agents, collectively called *adjuvants*. An adjuvant is a substance, distinct from antigen, that enhances T-cell activation by promoting the accumulation of APCs at a site of antigen exposure and by enhancing the expression of costimulators and cytokines by the APCs. An adjuvant in humans with vaccines is alum.

PHYSICAL NATURE OF ANTIGENS

Important factors in the effective functioning of antigens include foreignness, degradability, MW, structural stability, and complexity.

Foreignness

Foreignness is the degree to which antigenic determinants are recognized as nonself by an individual's immune system. The immunogenicity of a molecule depends to a great extent on its degree of foreignness. In addition, the dose of foreign exposure, the route of antigen exposure, and the timing of exposure to foreign antigens all influence immunogenicity.

For example, if a transplant recipient receives a donor organ with several major HLA differences, the organ is perceived as foreign and is subsequently rejected by the recipient. Normally, an individual's immune system does not respond to self-antigens.

Degradability

For an antigen to be recognized as foreign by an individual's immune system, sufficient antigens to stimulate an immune response must be present. In the case of vaccination, an adequate dose of vaccine at appropriate intervals must be administered for an immune response to be stimulated.

Molecular Weight

The higher the MW, the better the molecule will function as an antigen. The number of antigenic determinants on a molecule is directly related to its size. For example, proteins are effective antigens because they have a large MW.

Although large foreign molecules (MW 10,000 daltons [Da]) are better antigens, haptens, which are tiny molecules, can bind to a larger carrier molecule and behave as antigens. If a hapten is chemically linked to a large molecule, a new surface structure is formed on the large molecule, which may function as an antigenic determinant.

Structural Stability

If a molecule is an effective antigen, structural stability is mandatory. If a structure is unstable (e.g., gelatin), the molecule will be a poor antigen. Similarly, totally inert molecules are poor antigens. The structural stability of an antigen is important when the goal is to elicit a patient antibody response when administering a vaccine.

Complexity

The more complex an antigen, the greater its effectiveness. Complex proteins are better antigens than large repeating polymers, such as lipids, carbohydrates, and nucleic acids, which are relatively poor antigens.

GENERAL CHARACTERISTICS OF ANTIBODIES

Antibodies are specific proteins referred to as *immunoglobulins*. Many antibodies can be isolated in the gamma globulin fraction of protein by electrophoresis separation. The term *immunoglobulin* (Ig) has replaced gamma globulin because not all antibodies have gamma electrophoretic mobility. Antibodies can be found in blood plasma and in many body fluids (e.g., tears, saliva, and colostrum).

The primary function of an antibody in body defenses is to combine with antigens, which may be enough to neutralize bacterial toxins or some viruses. A secondary interaction of an antibody molecule with another effector agent (e.g., complement) is usually required to dispose of larger antigens (e.g., bacteria).

Determining Ig concentration can be of diagnostic significance in infectious and autoimmune diseases. Test methods to detect the presence and concentration of Igs are discussed in Part II of this textbook and in chapters relating to specific diseases.

> **KEY CONCEPTS: Immunoglobulin Classes and Variants**
> - Five distinct classes of Ig molecules are recognized: IgM, IgG, IgA, IgD, and IgE.
> - Antibodies exhibit diversity among the different classes, suggesting different functions in addition to their primary function of antigen binding.
> - A typical monomeric IgG molecule consists of three globular regions (two Fab regions and an Fc portion) linked by a flexible hinge region.
> - An antigenic determinant is the specific chemical determinant group or molecular configuration against which the immune response is directed.
> - Immunoglobulins are proteins that can function as effective antigens when used to immunize mammals of a different species. The resulting anti-Igs or antiglobulins can be in three principal categories of antigenic determinants: isotype, allotype, and idiotype.

IMMUNOGLOBULIN CLASSES

Five distinct classes of Ig molecules are recognized in most higher mammals: IgM, IgG, IgA, IgD, and IgE. These Ig classes differ from each other in characteristics such as MW and serum concentrations (Table 3.2), and functions (Table 3.3).

The serum levels of Igs (IgM, IgG, and IgA) vary by demographic factors (e.g., age and gender), common habits (e.g., alcohol consumption and smoking), and metabolic abnormalities (e.g., abdominal obesity and hypertriglyceridemia). Values may be reported in mg/dL or international units (IU/mL).

TABLE 3.2	Characteristics of Immunoglobulin Classes				
	IgM	IgG	IgA	IgE	IgD
Molecular weight (daltons [Da])	900,000 serum pentamer 180,000 B-cell surface monomer	150,000	320,000 (secretory)	200,000	180,000
Subclasses	—	IgG$_{1-4}$	α_1, α_2	2	—
Serum half-life[a] (days)	10 days	IgG$_1$ – 21 days, IgG$_2$ – 20 days, IgG$_3$ – 7 days, IgG$_4$ – 21 days	6 days IgA$_1$ and IgA$_2$ Secretory IgA –unknown	2 days, except: cell-bound IgE associated with high-affinity receptor on mast cells has a very long half-life (90 days)	3 days

[a]Half-life (days); the half-life of circulating antibodies is a measure of how long those antibodies remain in the blood after secretion from B cells or after injection in the case of an injected antibody, or the amount of time to reach one-half activity concentration. Serum values are average concentrations in normal, healthy individuals.
Adapted from Peakman M, Vergani D: *Basic and clinical immunology*, St. Louis, 2009, Elsevier. Male, D, Brostoff J, Roth, DB, Roitt I. *Immunology* 8th ed., St. Louis, 2013, Elsevier. Fig. 3.3 Physicochemical properties of human immunoglobulin classes. p.53.

TABLE 3.3	Immunoglobulin Functional Characteristics
Immunoglobulin Class	Characteristics
IgM	First antibody produced in an immune response
	First effective defense against bacteremia
	Multiple binding sites enable higher avidity
	Activation of the classic complement pathway
	Antigen receptor of naïve B lymphocytes, mediated by membrane-bound and not secreted antibodies
IgG	Predominant (highest concentration) antibody class in plasma or serum
	Opsonization of antigens for phagocytosis by macrophages and neutrophils
	Combats microorganisms and their toxins in extravascular fluid
	Activation of the classic complement pathway
	Antibody-dependent, cell-mediated cytotoxicity mediated by natural killer cells
	Neonatal immunity by transfer of maternal antibody across the placenta and gut, except IgG$_2$, which is variable (+/–)
	Feedback inhibition of B-lymphocyte activation
IgA	Mucosal immunity
	Defends external body surfaces
	Secretion of IgA into the lumens of the gastrointestinal and respiratory tracts
	Dimers held together by J chain
	Because secretory chain is wrapped around the Fc regions, IgA is less susceptible to proteolytic cleavage
IgE	Mast cell degranulation (immediate hypersensitivity reaction)
	Immediate hypersensitivity reaction provides protection against parasitic helminthic infections by promoting IgE- and eosinophil-mediated, antibody-dependent, cell-mediated cytotoxicity, and gut peristalsis
IgD	Present on lymphocyte surface of immunocompetent cells, important for B-cell activation and/or immunoregulation
	Naïve B-cell antigen receptor

Immunoglobulin M

IgM accounts for about 10% of the Ig pool and is largely confined to the intravascular pool because of its large size. This antibody is produced early in an immune response and is largely confined to the blood. IgM is highly effective (the most effective antibody class) in agglutination and cytolytic reactions. In humans, IgM is found in smaller concentrations than IgG or IgA. The molecule has five individual heavy chains, with an MW of 65,000 Da; the whole molecule has an MW of 900,000 Da.

Normal values of IgM are approximately 60 to 250 mg/dL (70–290 IU/mL) for males and approximately 70 to 280 mg/dL (80–320 IU/mL) for females. At 4 months of age, 50% of the adult level is present; adult levels are reached by 8 to 15 years. Cord blood contains more than 20 mg/dL. IgM is usually undetectable in cerebrospinal fluid (CSF).

IgM is decreased in primary (genetically determined) Ig disorders and in secondary Ig deficiencies (acquired disorders associated with certain diseases). IgM can be increased in the following conditions:

- Infectious diseases, such as subacute bacterial endocarditis, infectious mononucleosis, leprosy, trypanosomiasis, malaria, and actinomycosis
- Collagen disorders, such as scleroderma
- Hematologic disorders, such as polyclonal gammopathies, monocytic leukemia, and monoclonal gammopathies (e.g., Waldenström macroglobulinemia)

IgM and IgD are commonly found Igs on circulating B lymphocytes. The antigen receptors of these naïve B lymphocytes and helper T lymphocytes are membrane-bound IgM and IgD. Naïve B lymphocytes are mature B lymphocytes that lack previous exposure to an antigen. After exposure to an antigen, an antigen-specific B lymphocyte clone may expand and differentiate into offspring that secrete antibodies. Some of the descendants of the IgM- and IgD-expressing B lymphocytes may secrete IgM. However, after antigenic stimulation of descendant cells from the same B lymphocytes, these cells may secrete antibodies of other heavy-chain classes.

Immunoglobulin G

The Ig with the highest concentration in normal serum is IgG. It diffuses more readily than other Igs into the extravascular spaces and neutralizes toxins or binds to microorganisms in extravascular spaces. IgG can cross the placenta. In addition, when IgG complexes are formed, complement can be activated. IgG accounts for 70% to 75% of the total Ig pool. It has an MW of approximately 150,000 Da. One of the subclasses, IgG3, is slightly larger (170,000 Da) than the other subclasses.

Normal human adult serum values of IgG are approximately 800 to 1800 mg/dL (90–210 IU/mL). In infants aged 3 to 4 months, the IgG level is approximately 350 to 400 mg/dL (40–45 IU/mL); it gradually increases to approximately 700 to 800 mg/dL (80–90 IU/mL) by the end of the first year of life (Fig. 3.4). The average adult level is achieved before age 16 years. Other body fluids containing IgG include cord blood (800–1800 mg/dL) and CSF (2–4 mg/dL).

IgG has a long half-life (refer back to Table 3.2), which is attributed to its ability to bind to a specific Fc receptor (FcR) called the **neonatal Fc receptor (FcRn)**. This receptor is involved in the transport of IgG from the maternal circulation across the placental barrier and the transfer of maternal IgG across the intestine in neonates. FcRn structurally resembles MHC class I molecules. In the placenta and neonatal intestine, FcRn transports IgG molecules across cells without targeting them to lysosomes. FcRn recycles to the cell surface and releases IgG to the circulation. Intracellular sequestration of IgG away from lysosomes prevents it from being degraded as rapidly as most other serum proteins. IgG is the first isotype of Ig made by a fetus that may increase in concentration during an "in utero" infection.

Decreased levels of IgG can be manifested in primary (genetic) or secondary (acquired) Ig deficiencies. Significant increases in IgG are seen in the following conditions:

- Infectious diseases, such as hepatitis, rubella, and infectious mononucleosis
- Collagen disorders, such as rheumatoid arthritis and systemic lupus erythematosus
- Hematologic disorders, such as polyclonal gammopathies, monoclonal gammopathies, monocytic leukemia, and Hodgkin disease

Immunoglobulin A

Immunoglobulin A represents 15% to 20% of the total circulatory Ig pool. It is the predominant Ig in secretions such as tears, saliva, colostrum, milk, and intestinal fluids. IgA is synthesized largely by plasma cells located on body surfaces. If produced by cells in the intestinal wall, IgA may pass directly into the intestinal lumen or diffuse into the blood circulation. As IgA is transported through intestinal epithelial cells or hepatocytes it binds to a glycoprotein called the *secretory component*. The secretory piece protects IgA from digestion by gastrointestinal proteolytic enzymes. It forms a complex molecule termed *secretory IgA*, which is critical in protecting body surfaces against invading microorganisms because of its presence in seromucous secretions (e.g., tears, saliva, nasal fluids, and colostrum).

IgA monomer is present in relatively high concentrations in human serum; it has a concentration of 90 to 450 mg/dL (55–270 IU/mL) in normal adult humans. At the end of the first year of life 25% of the adult IgA level is reached, and 50% at 3.5 years of age. The average adult level is attained by age 16 years. IgA concentration in cord blood is greater than 1 mg/dL; CSF contains 0.1 to 0.6 mg/dL of IgA.

IgA is decreased in primary or secondary Ig deficiencies. Significant increases in the serum IgA concentration are associated with the following:

- Infectious diseases, such as tuberculosis and actinomycosis
- Collagen disorders, such as rheumatoid arthritis

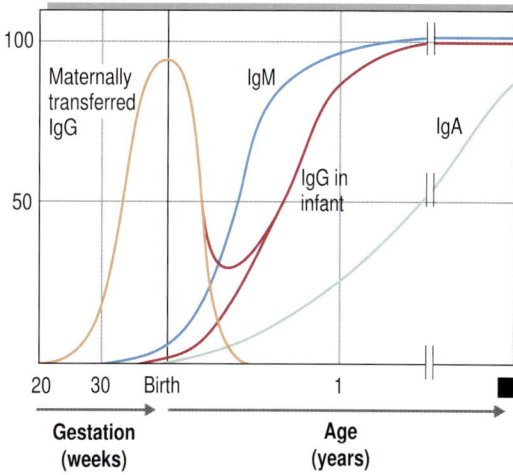

Fig. 3.4 Serum Immunoglobulin Levels in the Fetus During the Last Trimester and in the Newborn Period. (From Peakman M, Vergani D: *Basic and clinical immunology*, ed 2, London, 2009, Churchill Livingstone.)

- Hematologic disorders, such as polyclonal gammopathies, monocytic leukemia, and monoclonal gammopathy (e.g., IgA myeloma)
- Liver diseases, such as Laënnec cirrhosis and chronic active hepatitis

Immunoglobulin D

IgD is found in very low concentrations in plasma, accounting for less than 1% of the total Ig pool. IgD is extremely susceptible to proteolysis and is primarily a cell membrane Ig found on the surface of B lymphocytes in association with IgM.

Immunoglobulin E

IgE is a trace plasma protein found in the blood plasma of unparasitized individuals (MW, 188,000 Da). IgE is crucial because it mediates some types of hypersensitivity (allergic) reactions and anaphylaxis and it is generally responsible for an individual's immunity to invading parasites. The IgE molecule is unique in that it binds strongly to a receptor on mast cells and basophils and, together with antigen, mediates the release of histamines and heparin from these cells.

ANTIBODY STRUCTURE

Antibodies exhibit diversity among the different classes, which suggests that they perform different functions in addition to their primary function of antigen binding. Essentially, each Ig molecule is bifunctional; one region of the molecule involves binding to antigen, and a different region mediates binding of the Ig to host tissues, including cells of the immune system and the first component (C1q) of the classic complement system.

The primary core of an antibody consists of the sequence of amino acid residues linked by the peptide bond. All antibodies have a common, basic polypeptide structure with a three-dimensional configuration. The polypeptide chains are linked by covalent and noncovalent bonds, which produce a unit composed of a four-chain structure based on pairs of identical heavy (H) and light (L) chains. IgG, IgD, and IgE occur only as monomers of the four-chain unit; IgA occurs in both monomeric and polymeric forms; and IgM occurs as a pentamer with five four-chain subunits linked together.

Typical Immunoglobulin Molecule

A general feature of the Ig chains is their amino acid sequence. The first 110 to 120 amino acids of both light and heavy chains have a variable sequence and form the V region.

The basic unit of an antibody structure is the domain unit. An antibody molecule is composed of four polypeptide chains: two identical heavy (H) chains and two identical light (L) chains. Each chain contains a variable region and a constant region. The two identical heavy chains and two identical light chains are linked through cysteine residues by disulfide bonds so that the domains lie in pairs.

The antigen-binding portion of the molecule (N-terminal end) shows such heterogeneity that it is known as the *variable (V) region*; the remainder is composed of relatively constant amino acid sequences, the *constant (C) region*. Short segments of about 10 amino acid residues within the variable regions of antibodies (or T-cell receptor [TCR] proteins) form loop structures called **complementary-determining regions (CDRs)**. Three hypervariable loops, also called CDRs, are present in each antibody H-chain and L-chain. Most of the variability among different antibodies or TCRs is located within these loops.

The IgG molecule provides a classic model of antibody structure, appearing Y-shaped under electron microscopy (Fig. 3.5). If the molecule is studied by chemical treatment and the interchain disulfide bonds are broken, the molecule separates into four polypeptide chains.

Heavy Chains

Large H chains (50,000–77,000 Da) extend the full length of the antibody molecule. There are five types of heavy chains (μ, δ, γ, ε, and α) and two of the α chains (α_1 and α_2). Antibodies that contain different heavy chains belong to different classes or isotypes and are named according to their heavy chains (IgM, IgG, IgA, IgE, and IgD). The class and subclass of an Ig molecule are determined by its constant-region H-chain type.

Each isotype has distinct physical and biological properties as well as effector functions. The IgG subtypes differ from one another in functional characteristics but the IgA subtypes do not.

Light Chains

Light chains are small chains (25,000 Da) common to all Ig classes. The light chains are of two subtypes: kappa (κ) and lambda (λ), which

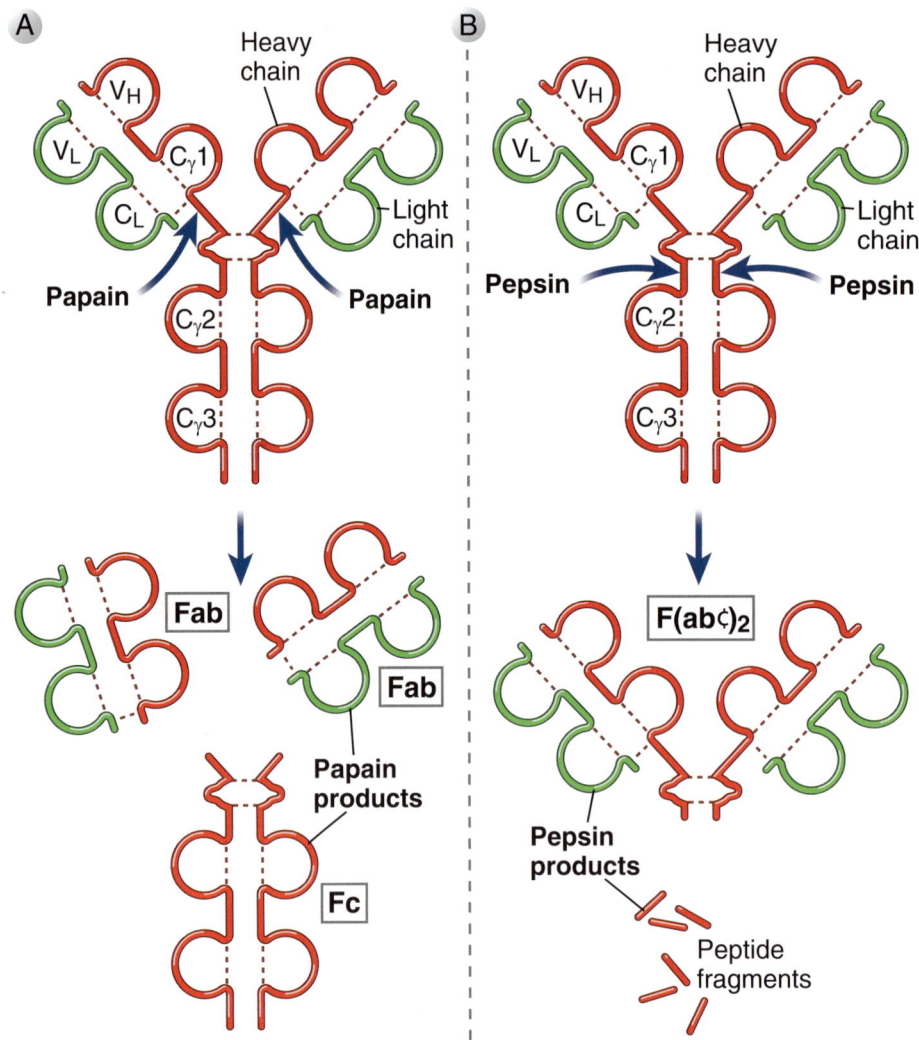

Fig. 3.5 Proteolytic Fragments of an Immunoglobulin G (IgG) Molecule. IgG molecules are cleaved by the enzymes (A) papain and (B) pepsin at the sites indicated by arrows. Papain digestion allows separation of two antigen-binding regions (the Fab fragments) from the portion of the IgG molecule that binds to complement and Fc receptors (the Fc fragment). Pepsin generates a single bivalent antigen-binding fragment, F(ab')2. (From Abbas AK, Lichtman AH, Pillai S: *Cellular and molecular immunology,* ed 9, Philadelphia, 2018, Elsevier.)

have different amino acid sequences and are antigenically different. In humans, about 65% of Ig molecules have κ chains and 35% have λ chains (ratio of 2:1).

Each type of light chain can join with any type of heavy chain in an antibody molecule. The function of light chains is to form the antigen-binding surface of antibodies, along with the heavy chains. All of the antibodies made by any B lymphocytes have the same type of light chain. The light-chain class remains fixed for the life of each B-cell clone. Light chains do not participate in effector functions, except binding and neutralizing toxins or microorganisms.

Specific Immunoglobulin Characteristics

Each specific Ig class has associated characteristics, such as plasma concentration, plasma half-life in days, secreted form, and functions (Fig. 3.6). Immunoglobulin subclasses have different biological functions that reflect the differences between each other in the Fc region of the molecule. The diversity—idiotypic differences—of the variable region of an Ig provides for many different antigens to bind with an antibody. This diversity is best described by the theory of germline recombination that impacts the recombinant events of the heavy chain and different recombinant events for the light chain.

Isotype of antibody	Subtypes (H chain)	Plasma concentration (mg/mL)	Plasma half-life (days)	Secreted form	Functions
IgA	IgA1,2 (α1 or α2)	3.5	6	Mainly dimer, also monomer, trimer 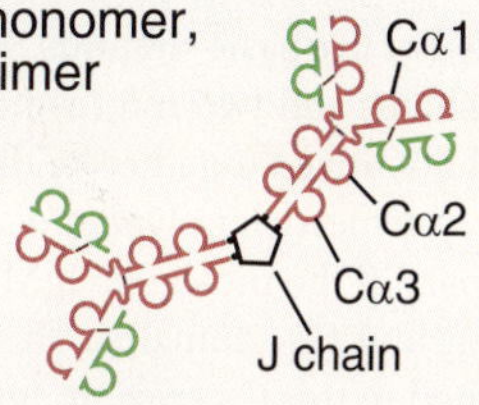	Mucosal immunity
IgD	None (δ)	Trace	3	Monomer	Naïve B cell antigen receptor
IgE	None (ε)	0.05	2	Monomer 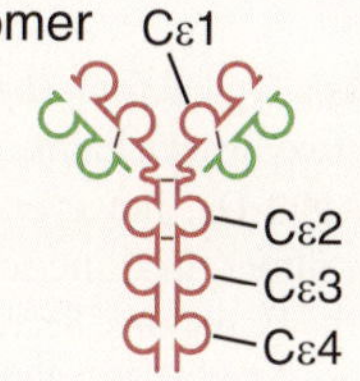	Defense against helminthic parasites, immediate hypersensitivity
IgG	IgG1–4 (γ1, γ2, γ3 or γ4)	13.5	23	Monomer 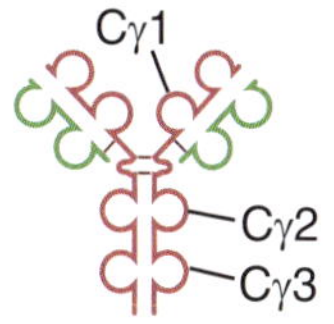	Opsonization, complement activation, antibody-dependent cell-mediated cytotoxicity, neonatal immunity, feedback inhibition of B cells
IgM	None (μ)	1.5	5	Pentamer 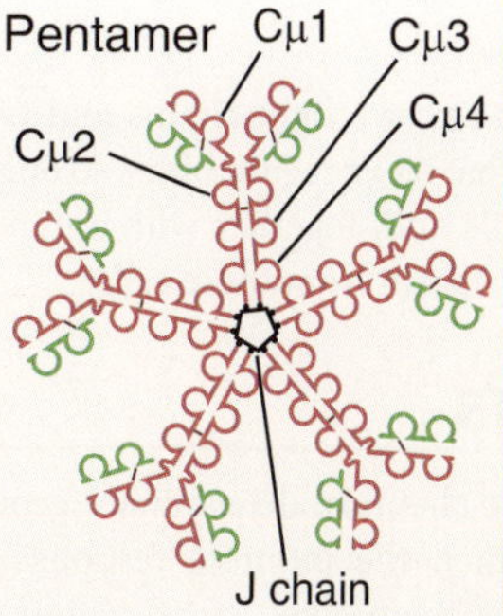	Naïve B cell antigen receptor (monomeric form), complement activation

Fig. 3.6 Features of the Major Isotypes (Classes) of Antibodies. This figure summarizes some important features of the major antibody isotypes of humans. Isotypes are classified on the basis of their heavy (H) chains; each isotype may contain either kappa or lambda light chains. The schematic diagrams illustrate the distinct shapes of the secreted forms of these antibodies. Note that immunoglobulin A (IgA) consists of two subclasses, called *IgA1* and *IgA2*, and IgG consists of four classes, called *IgG1, IgG2, IgG3,* and *IgG4*. Most of the opsonizing and complement fixation functions of IgG are attributable to IgG1 and IgG3. The domains of the heavy chains in each isotype are labeled. The plasma concentrations and half-lives are average values in normal individuals. (From Abbas AK, Lichtman AH, Pillae S: *Basic immunology: functions and disorders of the immune system,* ed 6, Philadelphia, 2020, Elsevier.)

TABLE 3.4 Immunoglobulin Variants

Variant	Distribution	Location	Examples
Isotype	All variants in normal persons	C_H	IgM, IgE
		C_H	IgA1, IgA2
		C_L	Kappa subtype
		C_L	Lambda subtype
Allotype	Genetically controlled alternative forms; not present in all individuals	Mainly C_H/C_L, sometimes V_H/V_2	Gm groups in humans
Idiotype	Individually specific to each immunoglobulin molecule	Variable regions	Probably one or more hypervariable regions forming the antigen-combining site

C, Constant region; *Gm*, marker on IgG; *H*, heavy chain; *L*, light chain; *V*, variable region.

Immunoglobulin M

The IgM molecule is structurally composed of five basic subunits. Each subunit consists of two κ or two λ light chains and two mu (μ) heavy chains. The individual monomers of IgM are linked together by disulfide bonds in a circular fashion. A small, cysteine-rich polypeptide, the J chain, must be considered an integral part of the molecule. IgM has carbohydrate residues attached to the C_{H3} and C_{H4} domains. The site for complement activation by IgM is located in this C_{H4} region. IgM is more efficient than IgG in activities such as complement cascade activation and agglutination.

Immunoglobulin A

In humans, more than 80% of IgA occurs as a typical four-chain structure consisting of paired κ or λ chains and two heavy chains. The basic four-chain monomer has an MW of 160,000 Da; however, in most mammals, plasma IgA occurs mainly as a dimer. In dimeric IgA, the molecules are joined by a J chain linked to the Fc regions. Secretory IgA exists mainly in the dimeric form and has an MW of 385,000 Da. This form of IgA is present in fluids and is stabilized against proteolysis when combined with another protein, the secretory component. In humans, variations in the heavy chains account for the subclasses IgA1 and IgA3.

Immunoglobulin D

The IgD molecule has an MW of 184,000 Da and consists of two κ or λ light chains and two delta (δ) heavy chains. It has no interchain disulfide bonds between its heavy chains and an exposed hinge region.

Immunoglobulin E

The IgE molecule is composed of paired κ or λ light chains and two epsilon (ε) heavy chains. It is unique in that its Fc region binds strongly to a receptor on mast cells and basophils and, together with antigen, mediates the release of histamines and heparin from these cells.

IMMUNOGLOBULIN VARIANTS

An antigenic determinant is the specific chemical determinant group or molecular configuration against which the immune response is directed. Because they are proteins, Igs themselves can function as effective antigens when used to immunize mammals of a different species. When the resulting anti-Igs or antiglobulins are analyzed, three principal categories of antigenic determinants can be recognized: isotype, allotype, and idiotype (Table 3.4).

Isotype Determinants

The isotypic class of antigenic determinants is the dominant type found on the Igs of all animals of a species. The heavy-chain, constant-region structures associated with the different classes and subclasses are termed *isotypic variants*. Genes for isotypic variants are present in all healthy members of a species. Determinants in this category include those specific for each Ig class, such as gamma (γ) for IgG, mu (μ) for IgM, and alpha (α) for IgA, in addition to the subclass-specific determinants κ and λ.

Allotype Determinants

The second principal group of determinants is found on the Igs of some, but not all, animals of a species. Antibodies to these allotypes (**alloantibodies**) may be produced by injecting the Igs of one animal into another member of the same species. The allotypic determinants are genetically determined variations representing the presence of allelic genes at a single locus within a species. Typical allotypes in humans are the Gm specificities on IgG (Gm is a marker on IgG). In humans, five sets of allotypic markers have been found: Gm, Km, Mm, Am, and Hv.

Idiotype Determinants

As a result of the unique structures on light and heavy chains, individual determinants characteristic of each antibody are called **idiotypes**. The idiotypic determinants are located in the variable part of the antibody associated with the hypervariable regions that form the antigen-combining site.

> **KEY CONCEPTS: Antibody Synthesis Facts**
> - Production of antibodies is induced when the host's immune system comes into contact with a foreign antigenic substance and reacts to this antigenic stimulation.
> - When an antigen is encountered initially, the cells of the immune system recognize the antigen as nonself and either elicit an immune response or become tolerant of it.

ANTIBODY SYNTHESIS

When an antigen is initially encountered, the cells of the immune system recognize the antigen as nonself and either elicit an immune response or become tolerant of it, depending on the circumstances. An immune reaction can take the form of cell-mediated immunity (immunity dependent on T cells and macrophages) or may involve the production of antibodies (B lymphocytes and plasma cells) directed against the antigen.

Production of antibodies is induced when the host's lymphocytes come into contact with a foreign antigenic substance that binds to its receptor. This triggers activation and proliferation, or **clonal selection**. Clonal expansion of lymphocytes in response to infection is necessary for an effective immune response (Fig. 3.7). However it requires 3 to 5 days for a sufficient number

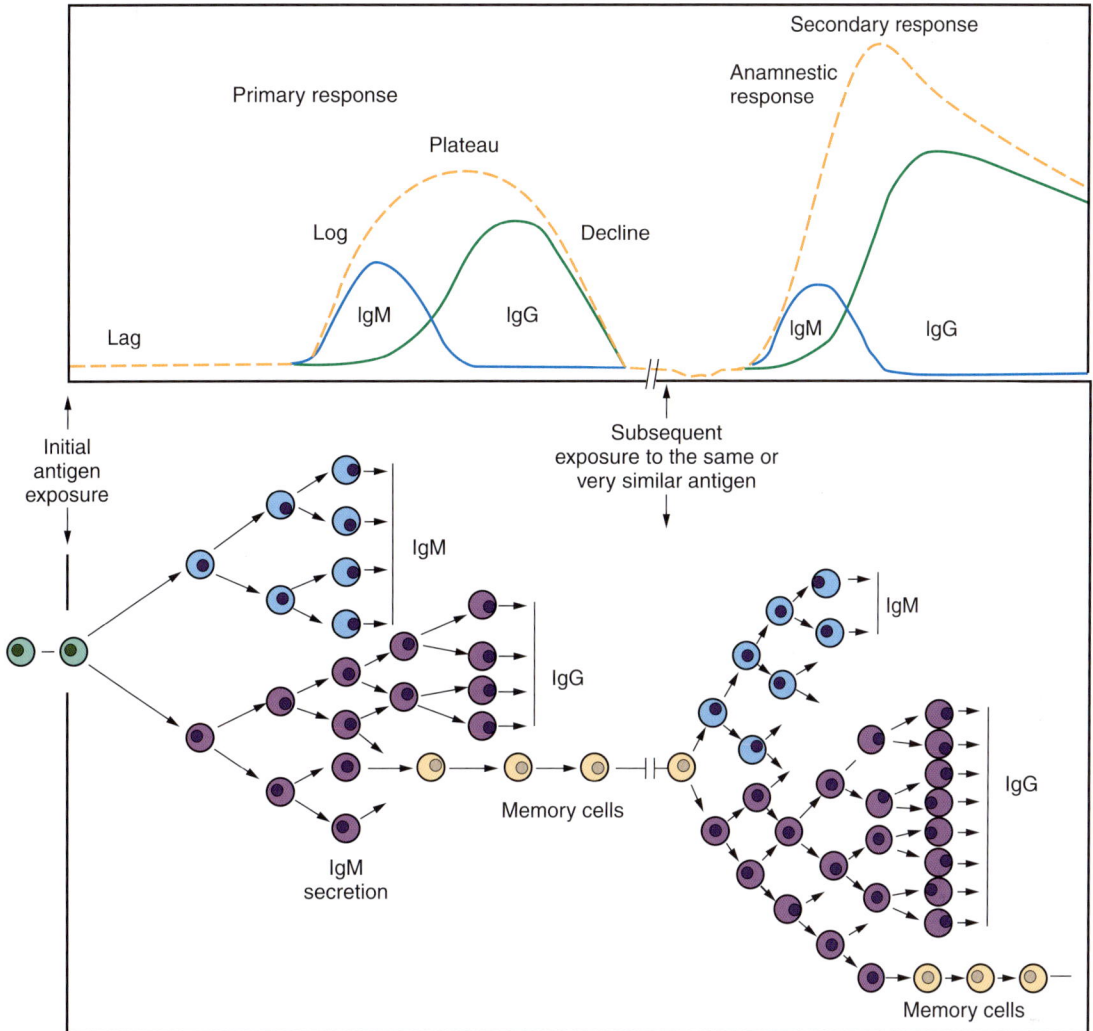

Fig. 3.7 Primary and Secondary Antibody Response. (Adapted from Turgeon ML: *Fundamentals of immunohematology*, ed 2, Baltimore, 1995, Williams & Wilkins.)

of clones to be produced and to differentiate into antibody-producing cells. This allows time for most pathogens to damage host tissues and cells.

Whether a cell-mediated response or an antibody response takes place depends on how the antigen is presented to the lymphocytes; many immune reactions display both types of responses. The antigenicity of a foreign substance is also related to the route of entry. Intravenous and intraperitoneal routes are stronger stimuli than subcutaneous and intramuscular routes.

Subsequent exposure to the same antigen produces a memory response, or **anamnestic response**, and reflects the outcome of the initial challenge. In the case of antibody production, the quantity of IgM-IgG varies.

> **KEY CONCEPTS: Types of Antibody Responses**
> - An immune reaction can be cell-mediated immunity (dependent on T cells and macrophages) or may involve the production of antibodies directed against the antigen.
> - After a foreign antigen challenge, a primary IgM antibody response proceeds in four phases: lag, log, plateau, and decline.
> - Subsequent exposure to the same antigenic stimulus produces an anamnestic (secondary) response, which exhibits the same four phases as a primary response but differs from a primary response in terms of time, type of antibody produced, and antibody titer.

Primary Antibody Response

Although the duration and levels of antibody (titer) depend on the characteristics of the antigen and the individual, an IgM antibody response proceeds in the following four phases after a foreign antigen challenge:
1. Lag phase—no antibody is detectable
2. Log phase—the antibody titer increases logarithmically
3. Plateau phase—the antibody titer stabilizes
4. Decline phase—the antibody is catabolized

Secondary (Anamnestic) Response

Subsequent exposure to the same antigenic stimulus produces an antibody response that exhibits the same four phases as the primary response. Repeated exposure to an antigen can occur many years after the initial exposure, but clones of memory cells will be stimulated to proliferate, with subsequent production of antibodies by the individual. An anamnestic response differs from a primary response as follows:
1. *Time.* A secondary response has a shorter lag phase, longer plateau, and more gradual decline.
2. *Type of antibody.* IgM-type antibodies are the principal class formed in the primary response. Although some IgM antibody is formed in a secondary response, the IgG class is the predominant type formed.

3. *Antibody titer.* In a secondary response, antibody levels attain a higher titer. The plateau levels in a secondary response are typically tenfold or greater than the plateau levels in the primary response.

An example of an anamnestic response can be observed in hemolytic disease, when an Rh-negative mother is pregnant with an Rh-positive baby (see Chapter 20). During the mother's first exposure, the Rh-positive RBCs of the fetus leak into the maternal circulation and elicit a primary response. Subsequent pregnancies with an Rh-positive fetus will elicit a secondary (anamnestic) response.

Vaccination is the application of primary and secondary responses. Humans can become immune to microbial antigens through artificial and natural exposure. A vaccine is designed to provide artificially acquired active immunity to a specific disease (e.g., hepatitis B). Booster vaccine (repeated antigen exposure) allows for an anamnestic response, with an increase in antibody titer and clones of memory cells (see Chapter 27).

FUNCTIONS OF ANTIBODIES

The principal function of an antibody is to bind antigens, but antibodies may also exhibit secondary effector functions and behave as antigens. The significant secondary effector functions of antibodies are complement fixation and placental transfer (Table 3.5). The activation of complement is one of the most important effector mechanisms of IgG1 and IgG3 molecules (see Chapter 2). IgG2 seems to be less effective in activating complement; IgG4, IgA, IgD, and IgE are ineffective in terms of complement activation. IgG4-related disease is a newly recognized inflammatory condition characterized by often, but not always, elevated serum IgG4 concentrations.

In humans most IgG subclass molecules are capable of crossing the placental barrier; no consensus exists on whether IgG2 crosses the placenta. Passage of antibodies across the placental barrier is important in the etiology of hemolytic disease of the fetus and newborn and in conferring passive immunity to the newborn during the first few months of life.

> **KEY CONCEPTS: Antigen–Antibody Reactions**
> - Specificity is the ability of a particular antibody to combine with one antigen instead of another.
> - Affinity is the bonding strength between an antigenic determinant and antibody-combining site.
> - Avidity is the strength with which a multivalent antibody binds a multivalent antigen.
> - Agglutination and other tests (e.g., precipitation reactions, hemolysis testing, enzyme-linked immunosorbent assay [ELISA]) are widely used in immunology to detect and measure the consequences of antigen–antibody interaction.

ANTIGEN–ANTIBODY INTERACTION: SPECIFICITY AND CROSSREACTIVITY

The ability of a particular antibody to combine with a particular antigen is referred to as its *specificity*. This property resides in the portion of the Fab molecule called the *combining site*, a cleft formed largely by the hypervariable regions of heavy and light chains. Evidence indicates that an antigen may bind to larger, or even separate, parts of the variable region. The closer the fit between this site and the antigen determinant, the stronger are the noncovalent forces (e.g., hydrophobic or electrostatic bonds) between them, and the higher is the affinity between the antigen and antibody. Binding depends on a close three-dimensional fit, allowing weak intermolecular forces to overcome the normal repulsion between molecules. When more than one combining site interacts with the same antigen, the bond has greatly increased strength.

Antigen–antibody reactions can show a high level of specificity. Specificity exists when the binding sites of antibodies directed against determinants of one antigen are not complementary to determinants of another, dissimilar antigen. When some of the determinants of an antigen are shared by similar antigenic determinants on the surface of apparently unrelated molecules, a proportion of the antibodies directed against one type of antigen will also react with the other type of antigen; this is called *crossreactivity*. Antibodies directed against a protein in one species may also react in a detectable manner with the homologous protein in another species.

Crossreactivity occurs between bacteria that have the same cell wall polysaccharides as mammalian erythrocytes. Intestinal bacteria, in addition to other substances found in the environment, have A-like or B-like antigens similar to the A and B erythrocyte antigens. If A or B antigens are foreign to an individual, production of anti-A or anti-B occurs, despite lack of previous exposure to these erythrocyte antigens.

Antibody Affinity

Affinity (Fig. 3.8) is the initial force of attraction that exists between a single Fab site on an antibody molecule and a single epitope or determinant site on the corresponding antigen. The antigen is univalent and is usually a hapten. Several types of noncovalent bonds hold an epitope and binding site close together (see the section Types of Bonding later in the chapter).

The strength of the sum total of noncovalent interactions between a single antigen-binding site on an antibody and a single epitope is the affinity of the antibody for that epitope. Low-affinity antibodies bind antigens weakly and tend to dissociate readily. High-affinity antibodies bind antigens more tightly and tend to remain bound longer. The term *association constant*, K, is a measure of affinity.

TABLE 3.5 Comparison of Properties of Immunoglobulins

	IgM	IgG	IgA	IgD	IgE
Classic pathway Complement fixation (binding)	4+	Variable[a]	**No** Classic pathway **Yes** Alternative pathway	No	No
Placental transfer	No	Variable[b]	No	No	No
Opsonin effect[c]	Yes	Yes	Yes	No	No
Agglutination/precipitation	Yes	Yes	Yes	No	No

[a]IgG1+, IgG2+/−, IgG3+, IgG4−.
[b]IgG1+, IgG2+/−, IgG3+, IgG4+.
[c]Opsonin effect means relating to or influenced by an opsonin (various proteins [e.g., antibodies or complement] that bind to foreign particles and cells [e.g., bacteria], making them more susceptible to phagocytosis [engulfment by various types of leukocytes]).

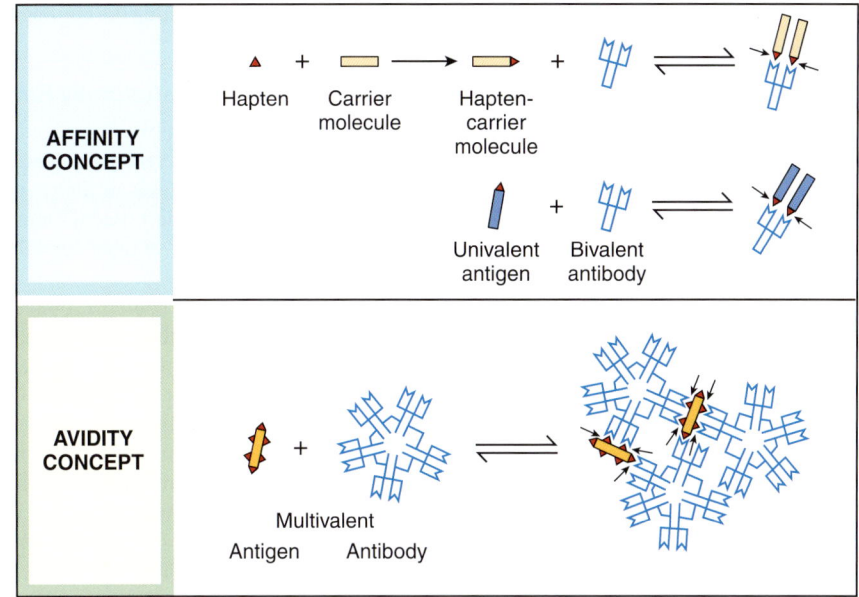

Fig. 3.8 Affinity Versus Avidity. (From Zane HD: *Immunology: theoretical and practical concepts in laboratory medicine*, Philadelphia, 2001, Elsevier.)

Antibodies produced in the late primary response exhibit higher affinity for antigens than antibodies produced in the early primary response.

Antibody Avidity

Based on the heavy-chain isotype, antibodies can have 2 to 10 antigen-binding sites. The total functional strength of all interactions between an antibody and its antigen is called **avidity** (see Fig. 3.8). When a multivalent antigen combines with more than one of an antibody's combining sites, the strength of the bonding is significantly increased. For the antigen and antibody to dissociate, all the antigen–antibody bonds must be broken simultaneously.

Decreased avidity can result when an antigen (e.g., hapten) has only one antigenic determinant (monovalent).

Immune Complexes

The noncovalent combination of antigen with its respective specific antibody is called an **immune complex**. An immune complex may be of the small (**soluble**) or large (**precipitating**) type, depending on the nature and proportion of antigen and antibody. Under conditions of antigen or antibody excess, soluble complexes tend to predominate. If equivalent amounts of antigen and antibody are present, a precipitate may form. However, all antigen–antibody complexes will not precipitate, even at equivalence.

Antibody can react with antigen that is fixed or localized in tissues or that is released or present in the circulation. Once formed in the circulation, the immune complex is usually removed by phagocytic cells through the interaction of the Fc portion of the antibody with complement and cell surface receptors.

Under normal circumstances this process does not lead to pathologic consequences, and it may be viewed as a major host defense against the invasion of foreign antigens. It is only in unusual circumstances that the immune complex persists as a soluble complex in the circulation, escapes phagocytosis, and is deposited in endothelial or vascular structures—where it causes inflammatory damage, the principal characteristic of immune complex disease—or in organs (e.g., kidney), or inhibits useful immunity (e.g., tumors and parasites). The level of circulating immune complex is determined by the rate of formation, rate of clearance, and, most importantly, nature of the complex formed. Detection of immune complexes and identification of the associated antigens are important to the clinical diagnosis of immune complex disorders.

MOLECULAR BASIS OF ANTIGEN–ANTIBODY REACTIONS

The basic Y-shaped Ig molecule is a bifunctional structure. The V regions are primarily concerned with antigen binding. When an antigenic determinant and its specific antibody combine, they interact through the chemical groups found on the surface of the antigenic determinant and on the surface of the hypervariable regions of the Ig molecule. Although the C regions do not form antigen-binding sites, the arrangement of the C regions and hinge region gives the molecule segmental flexibility, which allows it to combine with separated antigenic determinants.

Types of Bonding

Bonding of an antigen to an antibody results from the formation of multiple, reversible, intermolecular attractions between an antigen and amino acids of the binding site. These forces require proximity of the interacting groups. The optimum distance separating the interacting groups varies for different types of bonds; however, all these bonds act only across a very short distance and weaken rapidly as that distance increases.

The bonding of antigen to antibody is exclusively noncovalent. The attractive force of noncovalent bonds is weak compared with that of covalent bonds, but the formation of multiple noncovalent bonds produces considerable total binding energy. The strength of a single antigen–antibody bond (antibody affinity) is produced by the summation of the attractive and repulsive forces. The four types of noncovalent bonds involved in antigen–antibody reactions are hydrophobic bonds, hydrogen bonds, van der Waals forces, and electrostatic forces.

Hydrophobic Bonds

The major bonds formed between antigens and antibodies are hydrophobic. Many of the nonpolar side chains of proteins are hydrophobic.

When antigen and antibody molecules come together, these side chains interact and exclude water molecules from the area of the interaction. The exclusion of water frees some of the constraints imposed by the proteins, which results in a gain in energy and forms an energetically stable complex.

Hydrogen Bonds

Hydrogen bonding results from the formation of hydrogen bridges between appropriate atoms. Major hydrogen bonds in antigen–antibody interactions are O–H–O, N–H–N, and O–H–N.

Van der Waals Forces

Van der Waals forces are nonspecific attractive forces generated by the interaction between electron clouds and hydrophobic bonds. These bonds result from minor asymmetry in the charge of an atom caused by the position of its electrons. They rely on the association of nonpolar hydrophobic groups so that contact with water molecules is minimized. Although extremely weak, van der Waals forces may become collectively important in an antigen–antibody reaction.

Electrostatic Forces

Electrostatic forces result from the attraction of oppositely charged amino acids located on the side chains of two amino acid residues. The relative importance of electrostatic bonds is unclear.

Goodness of Fit

The strongest bonding develops when antigens and antibodies are close to each other and when the shapes of the antigenic determinants and the antigen-binding site conform to each other. This complementary matching of determinants and binding sites is referred to as *goodness of fit* (Fig. 3.9).

A good fit will create ample opportunities for the simultaneous formation of several noncovalent bonds and few opportunities for disruption of the bond. If a poor fit exists, repulsive forces can overpower any small forces of attraction. Variations from the ideal complementary shape will produce a decrease in the total binding energy because of increased repulsive forces and decreased attractive forces. Goodness of fit is important in determining the binding of an antibody molecule for a particular antigen.

Detection of Antigen–Antibody Reactions

In vitro tests detect the combination of antigens and antibodies. Agglutination is the process whereby particulate antigens (e.g., cells) aggregate to form larger complexes in the presence of a specific antibody. Agglutination tests are widely used in immunology to detect and measure the consequences of antigen–antibody interaction. Other tests include the following:

- Precipitation reactions combine soluble antigens with soluble antibody to produce insoluble complexes that are visible.
- Hemolysis testing involves the reaction of antigen and antibody with a cellular indicator (e.g., lysed RBCs).
- ELISA measures immune complexes formed in an in vitro system. This method is the most sensitive for antigen detection.

The theories of immunologic methods are discussed in Part II Chapters 8 to 12 of this text. Detection and quantitation of Igs are important in the laboratory investigation of infectious diseases and immunologic disorders (Table 3.6).

Influence of Antibody Types on Agglutination

Immunoglobulins are relatively positively charged and, after sensitization or coating of particles, they reduce the zeta potential, which is the difference in electrostatic potential between the net charge at the cell membrane and the charge at the surface of shear. Antibodies can bridge charged particles by extending beyond the effective range of the zeta potential, which results in the erythrocytes closely approaching each other, binding, and agglutinating.

Antibodies differ in their ability to agglutinate. IgM-type antibodies, sometimes referred to as *complete antibodies*, are more efficient than IgG or IgA antibodies in exhibiting in vitro agglutination when the antigen-bearing erythrocytes are suspended in physiologic saline (0.9% sodium chloride solution). Antibodies that do not exhibit visible agglutination of saline-suspended erythrocytes, even when bound to the cell's surface membrane, are considered to be nonagglutinating antibodies and have been called *incomplete antibodies*. Incomplete antibodies may fail to exhibit agglutination because the antigenic

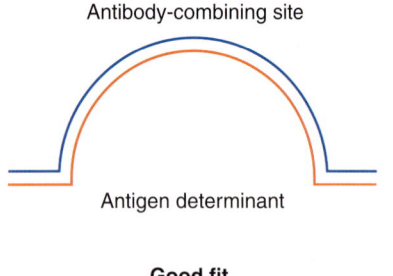
Good fit

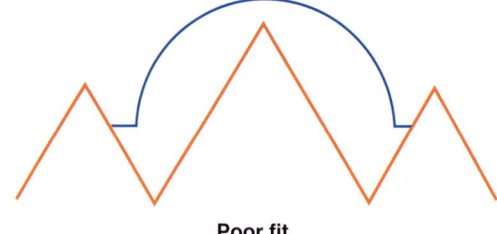
Poor fit

Fig. 3.9 Goodness of Fit.

TABLE 3.6 Role of Specific Immunoglobulins in Diagnostic Tests

	IgG	IgM	IgA
Agglutination	+/−	4+	2+
Complement fixation Classic pathway	1+	4+	Negative
Time of appearance after exposure to antigen (days)	3–7	3.5	3–7
Time to reach peak titer (days)	7–21	5–14	7–21

determinants are located deep within the surface membrane or may show restricted movement in their hinge region, causing them to be functionally monovalent.

NEUTRALIZING ANTIBODIES

> **KEY CONCEPTS: Neutralizing Antibodies**
> - Neutralizing antibodies (NAbs) are a subset of antibodies that are an important specific defense against viral invaders.
> - Neutralizing antibodies bind to a virus and bind in a way that blocks infection.
> - During viral infections, the human immune system develops NAbs, broadly neutralizing antibodies (bNAbs), and nonneutralizing antibodies (n-NAbs).

Neutralizing antibodies are a subset of antibodies that are an important specific defense against viral invaders. Neutralizing antibodies bind to a virus and bind in a way that blocks infection. During viral infections, the human immune system develops NAbs, bNAbs, and n-NAbs. NAbs are a hallmark of infections associated with various viruses (e.g., SARS-CoV-2 coronavirus, influenza viruses). In contrast, only 10% to 30% of infected individuals develop bNAbs that show broad neutralization activity. These bNAbs are found after 2 to 4 years of infection. Identification of bNAbs has opened up ways to explore their use as potential vaccine targets. n-NAbs show antiviral activity against conserved regions of the envelope glycoprotein (Env).

The NAbs are an essential part of the human immune response with a complicated relationship between the innate and adaptive immune systems to prevent viral infection. Identification of the main target for NAbs on coronaviruses is the spike (S) protein, a glycoprotein that is anchored in the viral membrane. The S protein of SARS-CoV-2 bears considerable structural similarity to SARS-CoV, with the S protein consisting of two subdomains: the N-terminal S1 domain and the receptor-binding domain (RBD) for the host cell receptor angiotensin-converting enzyme-2 (ACE2), and the S2 domain, which contains the fusion peptide. The surface of the SARS-CoV-2 virus is coated with a spike glycoprotein, which binds to receptor proteins on the surface of healthy cells, leading to viral entry and infection throughout the body. Following infection, most individuals will develop an immune response to the virus, including the production of NAbs against the SARS-CoV-2 spike glycoprotein. These antibodies can prevent future infection by blocking the binding activity of the spike glycoprotein. At this time, the length of the antibody response following infection is unknown and the level of NAbs needed to confer protective immunity is unknown. Some convalescent COVID-19 patients show strong anti-SARS-CoV-2 S protein-specific B-cell responses and developed memory and antibody-producing B cells that may have participated in the control of infection and the establishment of humoral immunity. Structural identification of these potent NAbs can guide vaccine design.

The level of NAbs against SARS-CoV-2 can be determined in the clinical laboratory. But a Nab test is not a replacement for existing serology testing for COVID-19, which detects antibodies that recognize the virus and serves as an indicator of current or prior infection but does not directly assess the virus-neutralizing capacity of those antibodies. The IMMUNO-COV™ neutralizing antibody test (Vyriad, Rochester, MN.) adds that next level of detail for an accurate estimate of SARS-CoV-2 neutralizing activity. The IMMUNO-COV antibody test uses a mimic virus, a noninfectious virus that has been engineered to display the SARS-CoV-2 spike glycoprotein on its surface. This procedure analyzes human blood serum to detect only the antibodies capable of blocking or neutralizing the action of this spike glycoprotein, which prevents the mimic virus from infecting new cells.

MONOCLONAL ANTIBODIES

> **KEY CONCEPTS: Characteristics of Monoclonal Antibodies**
> - Monoclonal antibodies (MAbs) are purified antibodies cloned from a single cell, called a *hybridoma*.
> - MAbs bound to cell surface antigens now provide a method for classifying and identifying specific cellular membrane characteristics and leukocyte antigens.
> - Identification and follow-up therapy in leukemias and lymphomas can be performed with MAbs.
> - MAbs allow for the diagnosis of many infectious and systemic diseases.
> - MAbs can be used to identify tumor antigens and autoantibodies and also to identify and quantify hormones.
> - Immunohistochemistry uses MAbs to determine the tissue source of tumors.
> - MAbs can be used to deliver immunotherapy.

Discovery of the Technique

In 1975 Köhler, Milstein, and Jerne discovered how to fuse lymphocytes to produce a cell line that was both immortal and a producer of specific antibodies. These scientists were awarded the Nobel Prize in Physiology or Medicine in 1984 for developing this **hybridoma** (cell hybrid) from different lines of cultured myeloma cells (plasma cells derived from malignant tumor strains). To induce the cells to fuse, they used Sendai virus, an influenza virus that characteristically causes cell fusion. Initially, the scientists immunized donors with sheep erythrocytes to provide a marker for the normal cells. The hybrids were tested to determine whether they still produced antibodies against the sheep erythrocytes. Köhler discovered that some of the hybrids were manufacturing large quantities of specific antisheep erythrocyte antibodies.

Hybrid cells secrete the antibody that is characteristic of the parent cell (e.g., antisheep erythrocyte antibodies). The multiplying hybrid cell culture is a hybridoma. Hybridoma cells can be cloned. The Igs derived from a single clone of cells are termed **monoclonal antibodies (MAbs)**.

Monoclonal Antibody Production

Modern methods for producing MAbs are refinements of the original technique. Basically, the hybridoma technique enables scientists to inoculate crude antigen mixtures into animals such as rabbits that are used more commonly today and then select clones producing specific antibodies against a single cell surface antigen (Fig. 3.10). The process of producing MAbs takes 3 to 6 months.

Animals are immunized with a specific antigen; several doses are given to ensure a vigorous immune response. After 2 to 4 days spleen cells are mixed with cultured mouse myeloma cells. Polyethylene glycol (PEG) rather than Sendai virus is added to the cell mixture to promote cell membrane fusion. Only 1 in 200,000 spleen cells actually forms a viable hybrid with a myeloma cell. The fused cell mixture is placed in a medium containing hypoxanthine, aminopterin, and thymidine (HAT medium). Aminopterin is a drug that prevents myeloma cells from making their own purines and pyrimidines; they cannot use hypoxanthine from the medium, so they die.

Hybrids resulting from the fusion of spleen cells and myeloma cells contain transferase provided by the normal spleen cells. Consequently, the hybridoma cells are able to use the hypoxanthine and thymidine in the culture medium and survive. They divide rapidly in the HAT medium,

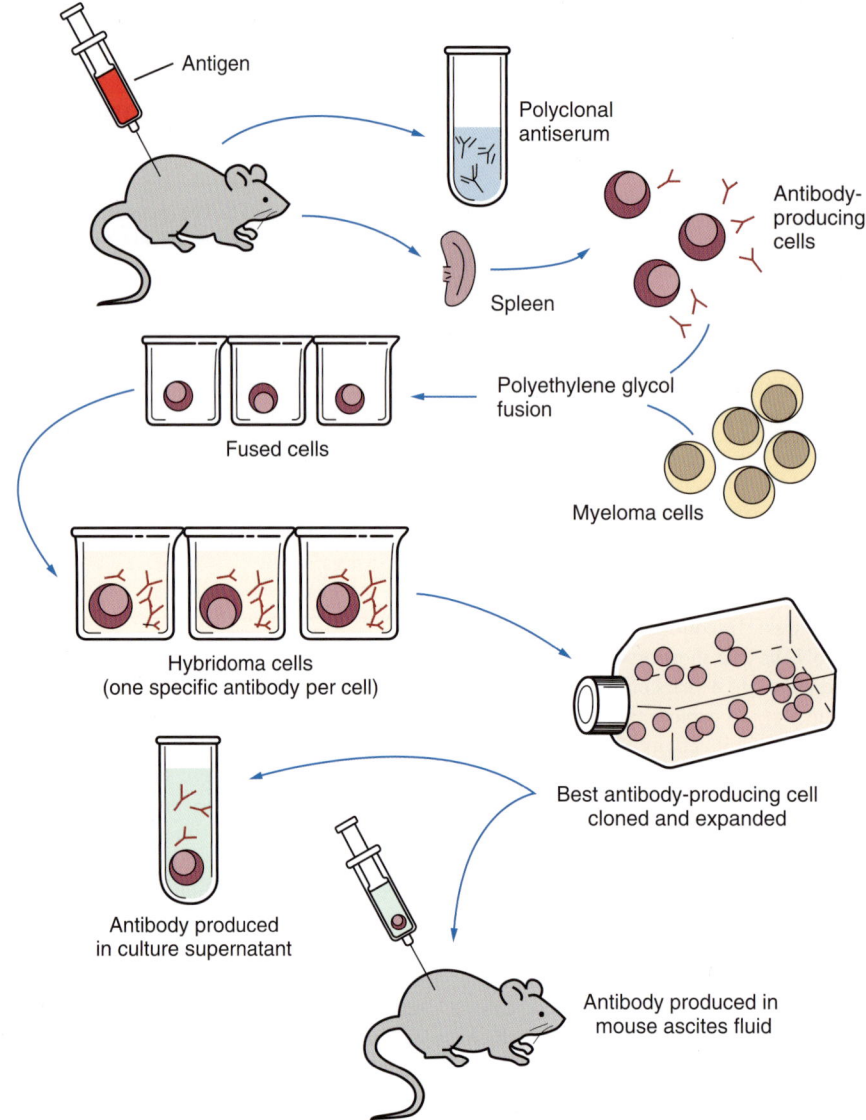

Fig. 3.10 Production of Monoclonal Antibodies (MAbs). (Adapted from Forbes BA, Sahm DF, Weissfeld AS: *Bailey & Scott's diagnostic microbiology,* ed 12, St. Louis, 2007, Elsevier.)

doubling in number every 24 to 48 hours. About 300 to 500 hybrids can be generated from the cells of a single mouse spleen, although not all will be making the desired antibodies. After the hybridomas have been growing for 2 to 4 weeks, the supernatant is tested for specific antibodies using methods such as ELISA. Clones that produce the desired antibody are grown in mass culture and recloned to eliminate non–antibody-producing cells.

Antibody-producing clones lose their ability to synthesize or secrete antibodies after being cultured for several months. Hybridoma cells are usually frozen and stored in small aliquots. The cells may then be grown in mass culture or injected intraperitoneally into mice. Because hybridomas are tumor cells, they grow rapidly and induce the effusion of large quantities of fluid into the peritoneal cavity. This ascites fluid is rich in MAbs and can be easily harvested.

Uses of Monoclonal Antibodies

The greatest impact of MAbs in immunology has been on the analysis of cell membrane antigens and antibody-based treatment strategies. Another example of the use of MAbs is in blood bank laboratory reagents for RBC typing.

Because they have a single specificity rather than the range of antibody molecules present in the serum, MAbs have multiple clinical and research applications, including the following:

- Identifying clusters of differentiation for the classification of leukemias and lymphomas and follow-up therapy. Identification of phenotypic markers unique to particular cell types through the use of MAbs is the basis for automated classification of lymphocytes (see Chapter 11).
- Immunoassay development. MAbs allow for the diagnosis of many infectious and systemic diseases.
- Identification of tumor antigens and autoantibodies, in addition to identification and quantification of hormones.
- Immunohistochemistry uses MAbs to determine the tissue source of tumors.
- Delivering immunotherapy.

CASE STUDY 3.1 History and Physical Examination

A 38-year-old White woman presented to the emergency department of her local hospital with increasing difficulty in breathing. She also reported that she had experienced chronic diarrhea for the past 18 months.

Her physical examination revealed a cachectic woman with bilateral rales and splenomegaly. After a chest x-ray film confirmed the presence of pneumonia and bronchiectasis, the patient was admitted to the hospital.

The patient's condition worsened. Her respiratory insufficiency increased, and she developed renal failure and disseminated intravascular coagulation (DIC). She was subsequently transferred to a tertiary care medical center.

Medical History
The patient had a childhood history of multiple episodes of bronchitis and middle-ear infections (otitis media). In her late 20s, she developed sinusitis, frequent diarrhea, and a chronic productive cough. She had two bouts of pneumonia, one of which required hospitalization. One year before the current episode, the patient developed extreme difficulty in breathing when exercising. During the past year, she lost almost 30 pounds and became so weak that she could no longer lead a normal life.

Family History
She had no family history of frequent infections, immunodeficiency, or autoimmune disorders.

Laboratory Data
On admission to the tertiary medical center, a blood count, serum protein, serum protein electrophoresis, immunoglobulin electrophoresis, stool culture, and ova and parasite examination were performed.

Assay	Patient's Results	Reference Range
Complete Blood Count		
Hemoglobin	9.8 g/dL	11.5–13.5 g/dL
Hematocrit	24%	34–42%
Total leukocyte count	9.0×10^9/L	$4.5–9.0 \times 10^9$/L
Polymorphonuclear leukocytes	87%	40%–60%
Lymphocytes	13%	20%–40%
Absolute lymphocytes	1.17×10^9/L	$>1.1 \times 10^9$/L
Other Tests		
Stool culture	Normal biota (flora)	Normal biota (flora)
Ova and parasite examination	*Giardia lamblia*	Negative for all ova and parasites
Serum total protein	5.5 g/dL	
Immunoelectrophoresis		
IgM	0.7 g/L	0.6–3.5 g/L
IgG	3.2 g/L	6.8–15.5 g/L
IgA	Undetectable	0.7–3.0 g/L
Follow-Up		
CD4+	20%	35%–55%
CD8+	26%	18%–32%
Absolute CD4+ count	0.26×10^9/L	$>0.43 \times 10^9$/L

The patient was found to be anergic. Tetanus, rubella, and diphtheria titers were nonprotective, despite previous immunizations.

The patient was diagnosed with common variable immunodeficiency (CVID). She was treated with IV immunoglobulin monthly. She also received metronidazole for *Giardia lamblia* intestinal infection. After 1 year of Ig therapy, the patient gained weight and returned to a normal lifestyle.

Questions
1. An immunodeficiency disorder may be suggested by:
   a. Presence of anemia
   b. History of repeated childhood infections
   c. Presence of anergy
   d. Elevated total leukocyte count
2. The most significant laboratory finding contributing to a diagnosis is:
   a. Absolute lymphocyte count
   b. Decreased CD4+ cell count
   c. Decreased immunoglobulin levels
   d. Both b and c

See Appendix A for the answers to these questions.

Critical-Thinking Group Discussion Questions
1. Does the patient's medical history suggest an immunodeficiency?
2. Which laboratory findings are significant?
3. What are possible diagnoses for this patient?

REVIEW QUESTIONS

1. A synonym for an antigenic determinant is:
   a. Immunogen
   b. Epitope
   c. Binding site
   d. Polysaccharide
2. Genetically different individuals of the same species are referred to as:
   a. Allogenic
   b. Heterogenic
   c. Autogenic
   d. Isogenic
3. Class III MHC genes encode _____ molecules.
   a. Antigens
   b. Antibodies
   c. Lymphocytes
   d. Complement and cytokine
4. Class I MHC genes _____ encode heavy or alpha chains of molecules.
   a. Complement
   b. Cytokines
   c. HLA-A, HLA-B, HLA-C
   d. HLA-DP, HLA-DP, HLA-DR
5. Class I MHC genes encode for molecules that present:
   a. Antigen to CD8+ T cells
   b. Complement and cytokine to cells
   c. Antigen to CD4+ T cells
   d. Genes involved in antigen processing
6. A characteristic of class I HLA molecules is:
   a. Regulation of interactive behavior between cytolytic T cells and target cells
   b. Restriction of activity of regulatory T cells
   c. Regulation of the interaction between helper T cells and antigen-presenting cells
   d. Inhibition of B lymphocytes by T lymphocytes

7. A specific disease associated with B27 antigen is:
   a. Ankylosing spondylitis
   b. Celiac disease
   c. Multiple sclerosis
   d. Rheumatoid arthritis
8. Which of the following substances cannot stimulate an immune response unless attached to a bigger molecule?
   a. Large polysaccharides
   b. Proteins
   c. Glycoproteins
   d. Hapten
9. Which of the following characteristics of an antigen is the least important?
   a. Foreignness
   b. Degradability
   c. Molecular weight
   d. Presence of large repeating polymers
10. The chemical composition of an antibody is:
    a. Protein
    b. Lipid
    c. Carbohydrate
    d. Any of the above
11. The IgM antibody class:
    a. Has the highest plasma or serum concentration in normal individuals
    b. Has the shortest half-life
    c. Has the highest molecular weight
    d. Can exist as a dimer
12. The IgG antibody class:
    a. Has the highest plasma or serum concentration in normal individuals
    b. Has the shortest half-life
    c. Has the highest molecular weight
    d. Can exist as a dimer
13. The IgA antibody class:
    a. Has the highest plasma or serum concentration in normal individuals
    b. Has the shortest half-life
    c. Has the highest molecular weight
    d. Can exist as a dimer
14. The IgE antibody class:
    a. Has the highest plasma or serum concentration in normal individuals
    b. Associated with mast cell degranulation
    c. Can exist as a dimer
    d. Can be used for diagnostic allergy testing
15. The IgD antibody class:
    a. Has the highest plasma or serum concentration in normal individuals
    b. Has the shortest half-life
    c. Can exist as a dimer
    d. Has no known subclasses
16. The characteristic associated with IgG is:
    a. Predominant immunoglobulin in secretions
    b. Ability to cross the placental barrier
    c. Mediates some types of hypersensitivity reactions
    d. Produced earliest in the immune response
17. The characteristic associated with IgG is:
    a. Predominant immunoglobulin in secretions
    b. Increased in collagen disorders and hematologic disorders
    c. Mediates some types of hypersensitivity reactions
    d. Can activate the classic pathway that concludes with cellular hemolysis
18. The characteristic associated with IgA is:
    a. Predominant immunoglobulin in secretions
    b. Increased in infectious diseases
    c. Mediates some types of hypersensitivity reactions
    d. Produced earliest in the immune response
19. The characteristic associated with IgD is:
    a. Predominant immunoglobulin in secretions
    b. Increase in infectious diseases, collagen disorders, and hematologic disorders
    c. Mediates some types of hypersensitivity reactions
    d. Primarily a cell membrane immunoglobulin
20. The characteristic associated with IgE is:
    a. Predominant immunoglobulin in secretions
    b. Increase in infectious diseases, collagen disorders, and hematologic disorders
    c. Mediates some types of hypersensitivity reactions
    d. Primarily a cell membrane immunoglobulin
21. A characteristic of an isotype is:
    a. Found on the immunoglobulins of some, but not all, animals of a species
    b. Dominant type found on immunoglobulins of all animals of a species
    c. Individual determinants characteristic of each antibody
    d. None of the above
22. A characteristic of an allotype is:
    a. Found on the immunoglobulins of some, but not all, animals of a species
    b. Dominant type found on immunoglobulins of all animals of a species
    c. Individual determinants characteristic of each antibody
    d. None of the above
23–26. Arrange the sequence of events of a typical antibody response.
23. _____
24. _____
25. _____
26. _____
    a. Plateau
    b. Lag phase
    c. Log phase
    d. Decline
27. Which of the following statements is false about an anamnestic response versus a primary response?
    a. Has a shorter lag phase
    b. Has a longer plateau
    c. Antibodies decline more gradually
    d. IgM antibodies predominate
28. Which type of antibody is capable of placental transfer from mother to fetus?
    a. IgM
    b. IgG
    c. IgA
    d. IgD
29. Specificity is defined as:
    a. Strength of a bond between a single antigenic determinant and an individual combining site
    b. Noncovalent combination of an antigen with its respective specific antibody
    c. Ability of an antibody to combine with one antigen instead of another
    d. Strength with which a multivalent antibody binds to a multivalent antigen

30. Affinity is defined as:
    a. Strength of a bond between a single antigenic determinant and an individual combining site
    b. Noncovalent combination of an antigen with its respective specific antibody
    c. Ability of an antibody to combine with one antigen instead of another
    d. Strength with which a multivalent antibody binds to a multivalent antigen
31. Avidity is defined as:
    a. Strength of a bond between a single antigenic determinant and an individual combining site
    b. Noncovalent combination of an antigen with its respective specific antibody
    c. Ability of an antibody to combine with one antigen instead of another
    d. Strength with which a multivalent antibody binds to a multivalent antigen
32. Immune complex is defined as:
    a. Strength of a bond between a single antigenic determinant and an individual combining site
    b. Noncovalent combination of an antigen with its respective specific antibody
    c. Ability of an antibody to combine with one antigen instead of another
    d. Strength with which a multivalent antibody binds to a multivalent antigen
33. The major types of bonding of antigen–antibody reactions include all of the following *except*:
    a. Hydrogen bonds
    b. Electrostatic bonds
    c. Van der Waals forces
    d. Covalent bonds
34. What section of an immunoglobulin molecule is responsible for the differences between immunoglobulin classes?
    a. Fc
    b. Fab
    c. Heavy chains
    d. Light chains
35. Which of the following is an accurate statement about monoclonal antibodies (MAbs) *except*?
    a. MAbs are antibodies engineered to bind to a single epitope
    b. MAbs are purified antibodies cloned from a single cell
    c. MAbs are used to classify and identify specific cellular membrane characteristics
    d. MAbs are formed in response to an infection in a patient
36. Antigens are characterized as:
    a. Not usually large organic molecules
    b. Usually lipids
    c. Can be glycolipids or glycoproteins
    d. Are also called immunoglobulins
37. The immunogenicity of an antigen depends greatly on:
    a. Its biochemical composition
    b. Being structurally unstable
    c. Its degree of foreignness
    d. Having a low molecular weight
38. Antibodies are also referred to as:
    a. Immunoglobulins
    b. Haptens
    c. Epitopes
    d. Gamma globulins
39. An appropriate description of IgM is:
    a. Accounts for 10% of the Ig pool, largely confined to the intravascular space
    b. Mediates some types of hypersensitivity
    c. Found in tears, saliva, colostrum, milk, and intestinal secretions
    d. Diffuses more readily into extravascular spaces, neutralizes toxins, and binds to microorganisms
40. An appropriate description of IgG is:
    a. Accounts for 10% of the Ig pool, largely confined to the intravascular space
    b. Mediates some types of hypersensitivity
    c. Found in tears, saliva, colostrum, milk, and intestinal secretions
    d. Diffuses more readily into extravascular spaces, neutralizes toxins, and binds to microorganisms
41. An appropriate description of IgA is:
    a. Accounts for 10% of the Ig pool, largely confined to the intravascular space
    b. Mediates some types of hypersensitivity
    c. Found in tears, saliva, colostrum, milk, and intestinal secretions
    d. Diffuses more readily into extravascular spaces, neutralizes toxins, and binds to microorganisms
42. An appropriate description of IgE is:
    a. Accounts for 10% of the Ig pool, largely confined to the intravascular space
    b. Mediates some types of hypersensitivity
    c. Found in tears, saliva, colostrum, milk, and intestinal secretions
    d. Diffuses more readily into extravascular spaces, neutralizes toxins, and binds to microorganisms
43. An appropriate description of IgD is:
    a. Accounts for 10% of the Ig pool, largely confined to the intravascular space
    b. Mediates some types of hypersensitivity
    c. Found in tears, saliva, colostrum, milk, and intestinal secretions
    d. Makes up less than 1% of total immunoglobulins
44. The properties of an antibody class are defined by the:
    a. Size of the immune complex
    b. Nature of the stimulating antigen
    c. Fab end of the antibody
    d. Fc end of the antibody
45. Which of the following characterizes IgM?
    a. Composed of five basic subunits
    b. Less efficient in the activation of the complement cascade and agglutination than IgG
    c. Less response in an initial antibody response
    d. Predominant in a secondary (anamnestic) response
46. The phase at the highest point in an antibody response curve is?
    a. Log
    b. Plateau
    c. Lag
    d. Decline
47. The phase at the lowest point in an antibody response curve is?
    a. Log
    b. Plateau
    c. Lag
    d. Decline
48. The phase at the ascending point in an antibody response curve is?
    a. Log
    b. Plateau
    c. Lag
    d. Decline

49. The phase at the descending point in an antibody response curve is?
    a. Log
    b. Plateau
    c. Lag
    d. Decline
50. What characteristic differentiates a secondary immune response from a primary immune response?
    a. IgM is the predominant type of antibody in a secondary response
    b. The IgG antibody titer is lower in a secondary response compared with a primary response
    c. The lag phase of antibody production is longer in the secondary immune response
    d. The IgG antibody titer is higher than the IgM titer in a secondary response
51. Bonding of antigen to antibody exists exclusively as:
    a. Hydrogen bonding
    b. Van der Waals forces
    c. Electrostatic forces
    d. Noncovalent bonding
52. The strongest bond of antigen and antibody chiefly results from the:
    a. Type of bonding
    b. Goodness of fit
    c. Antibody type
    d. Quantity of antibody
53. Monoclonal antibodies have the characteristic of:
    a. A diversified mixture of antibodies
    b. Cloned from a single cell
    c. Engineered to bind to a single specific antibody
    d. Frequent occurrence in nature
54. The normal reference ratio of kappa (κ) to lambda (λ) light chain of immunoglobulin (Ig) molecules is:
    a. Kappa (κ) 25% to 75% lambda (λ)
    b. Kappa (κ) 45% to 55% lambda (λ)
    c. Kappa (κ) 70% to 35% lambda (λ)
    d. Kappa (κ) 85% to 15% lambda (λ)
55. Each class or isotype of an antibody has distinct physical and biological properties and effector functions that are differentiated according to ____.
    a. Constant region of heavy chain
    b. Constant region of light chain
    c. Variable region of heavy chain
    d. Variable region of light chain

4

Cellular Activities and Clinical Disorders of Innate and Adaptive Immunity

LEARNING OUTCOMES

- Explain the process of phagocytosis.
- Describe the composition and function of neutrophil extracellular traps (NETs).
- Discuss the role of monocytes and macrophages in cellular immunity.
- Define and compare acute inflammation and sepsis.
- Briefly describe cell surface receptors.
- Compare the function of T lymphocytes and B lymphocytes in immunity.
- Explain the function of natural killer (NK) cells.
- Define the term *cluster of differentiation (CD)* and explain the purpose of detecting this marker.
- Differentiate the characteristics of T-lymphocyte subsets on the basis of antigen structures and function.
- Name and compare the signs and symptoms of disorders of neutrophil function.
- Compare the signs and symptoms of two monocyte or macrophage disorders.
- Describe states involving the leukocyte integrins.
- Explain the etiology, clinical findings, and laboratory assessment of chronic granulomatous disease (CGD) and leukocyte adhesion defect (LAD).
- Describe the evaluation of suspected lymphocytic or plasma cell defects.
- Name and compare disorders of immunologic (lymphocytic or plasma cell) origin.
- Analyze case studies related to defects of innate or adaptive immunity.
- Correctly answer case study–related questions.
- Describe the principal reporting of results, sources of error, clinical applications, and limitations of a phagocytic engulfment test.
- Assessment of cellular immune status.
- Correctly answer 80% of the end-of-chapter review questions.

OUTLINE

Innate Immunity, 68
Process of Phagocytosis, 68
    Chemotaxis, 68
    Adhesion, 69
    Engulfment, 70
    Digestion, 70
    Subsequent Phagocytic Activities, 71
Neutrophil Extracellular Traps, 71
Monocyte-Macrophage Host Defense Functions, 71
    Phagocytosis, 71
    Antigen Presentation and Induction of the Immune Response, 72
    Secretion of Biologically Active Molecules, 72
Cytokine Storm Syndromes, 72
Acute Inflammation, 73
Sepsis, 73
Cell Surface Receptors, 74
Disorders of Neutrophils, 74
    Noninfectious Neutrophil-Mediated Inflammatory Disease, 74
    Abnormal Neutrophil Function, 75
    Innate (Congenital) Neutrophil Abnormalities, 75
        Chédiak-Higashi Syndrome, 75
        Chronic Granulomatous Disease, 75
        Complement Receptor 3 Deficiency, 75
        Myeloperoxidase Deficiency, 76
        Specific Granule Deficiency, 76
Monocyte-Macrophage Disorders, 76
    Gaucher Disease, 76
    Niemann-Pick Disease, 77
Disease States Involving Leukocyte Integrins, 77
Adaptive Immunity, 77
Lymphoid and Nonlymphoid Surface Membrane Markers, 77
Development of T Lymphocytes, 79
    Early Cellular Differentiation and Development, 79
        Double-Negative Thymocytes, 79
        Double-Positive Thymocytes, 80
        Later Cellular Differentiation and Development of T Lymphocytes, 81
        T-Lymphocyte Subsets, 81
    CD4 Lymphocytes, 81
        Subsets of CD4+ Effector T Lymphocytes, 82
        CD8+ Cytotoxic T Lymphocytes, 84
    Antigen Recognition by T Cells, 86
        T-Cell Activation, 87
    T-Independent Antigen Triggering, 87
    Antigen Processing and Antigen Presentation to T Cells, 87
Innate Lymphoid Cells, 88
T-Regulatory Lymphocytes, 88
    Natural Killer Cells, 88
B Lymphocytes, 90
    Development and Differentiation of B Lymphocytes, 90
        Cell Surface Antigens, 90
Plasma Cell Biology, 92
Alterations in Lymphocyte Subsets, 92
    Changes with Aging, 92
Immunologic Disorders, 92
    Immune-Mediated Disease, 93
Case Study 4.1   History and Physical Examination, 93
Case Study 4.2   History and Physical Examination, 94
Case Study 4.3   History and Physical Examination, 94
Procedure: Screening Test for Phagocytic Engulfment, 96.e1

KEY TERMS

- anergy
- antigen-presenting cells (APCs)
- B lymphocytes
- bacteremia
- cell adhesion molecules (CAMs)
- cell surface markers
- cell surface receptors
- chemokines
- chemotaxis
- chronic granulomatous diseases (CGDs)
- cluster of differentiation (CD)
- complement receptor
- cytokines
- double-negative lymphocytes
- double-negative thymocytes
- double-positive thymocytes
- dyscrasias
- effector T cells
- endogenous pathway
- exogenous pathway
- extracellular matrix (ECM)
- extravasation
- Gaucher disease
- granzyme A-B
- immunophenotyping
- immunoproliferative
- immunoregulatory cells
- interferon
- interleukins
- leukocyte integrins
- ligands
- macrophages
- margination
- memory cells
- monoclonal antibody (MAb)
- natural killer (NK) cells
- natural T_{reg} cells
- neutrophil extracellular traps (NETs)
- opsonization
- plasma cells
- reactive oxygen species (ROS)
- selectin
- sepsis
- suppressor-cytotoxic lymphocytes
- surface immunoglobulin (sIg)
- T lymphocytes
- T-cell receptor (TCR)
- T-independent antigens

INNATE IMMUNITY

Polymorphonuclear neutrophils (PMNs) and monocytes-macrophages are the principal cells that defend the body against various types of microbial invasion and produce a localized inflammatory response. The granules of segmented neutrophils contain various antibacterial substances (Table 4.1). During the phagocytic process, powerful antimicrobial enzymes are released and disrupt the integrity of the cell itself.

> **KEY CONCEPTS: Neutrophilic Defense Activities**
> - The primary phagocytic cells are the neutrophilic leukocytes and the mononuclear monocytes-macrophages.
> - The neutrophilic leukocyte provides an effective host defense against bacterial and fungal infections.
> - Neutrophils are the principal leukocyte associated with phagocytosis and a localized inflammatory response.
> - Phagocytosis can be divided into the significant actions of movement of cells, engulfment of particles, and digestion/destruction.
> - Another innate defense mechanism involves neutrophil extracellular traps (NETs), which are produced after the release of the nuclear contents of PMNs into the extracellular space.

TABLE 4.1 Function and Types of Granules in Neutrophils

Function	Azurophilic (Primary) Granules	Specific (Secondary) Granules
Microbicidal	Myeloperoxidase	Cytochrome b558 and other respiratory burst components
	Lysozyme	Lysozyme
	Elastase	Lactoferrin
	α-Defensins	
	Cathepsin G	
	Proteinase-3	
	Bacterial permeability–increasing protein (BPI)	
Cell migration		Collagenase
		CD11b–CD18 (CR3)
		N-formulated peptides (e.g., N-formyl-methionyl-leucylphenylalanine receptor [FMLP-R])

Adapted from Peakman M, Vergani D: *Basic and clinical immunology*, ed 2, Edinburgh, 2009, Churchill Livingstone.

PROCESS OF PHAGOCYTOSIS

Phagocytosis can be divided into six stages: chemotaxis, adhesion, engulfment, phagosome formation, fusion, and digestion and destruction (Fig. 4.1). The physical occurrence of damage to tissues, whether by trauma or microbial multiplication, releases substances such as activated complement components and products of infection to initiate phagocytosis.

Chemotaxis

Various phagocytic cells continually circulate throughout the blood, lymph, gastrointestinal (GI) system, and respiratory tract. When trauma occurs, the neutrophils arrive at the site of injury and can be found in the initial exudate in less than 1 hour. Monocytes are slower in moving to the inflammatory site. Macrophages resident in the tissues of the body are already in place to deal with an intruding agent. Additional macrophages from the bone marrow and other tissues can be released in severe infections.

Recruitment of PMNs is an essential prerequisite in innate immune defense. Recruitment of PMNs consists of a cascade of events that allows for the capture, adhesion, and extravasation of the leukocyte. Activities such as rolling, binding, and diapedesis have been well characterized, but receptor-mediated processes, such as mechanisms attenuating the electrostatic repulsion between the negatively charged glycocalyx of leukocytes and endothelium, are poorly understood. Research has demonstrated that myeloperoxidase (MPO), a PMN-derived heme protein, facilitates PMN recruitment because of its positive surface charge.

Neutrophils have been shown to activate complement when stimulated by cytokines or coagulation-derived factors. Neutrophils activate the alternative complement pathway and release C5 fragments, which further amplify neutrophil proinflammatory responses. This mechanism may be relevant to complement involvement in neutrophil-mediated diseases.

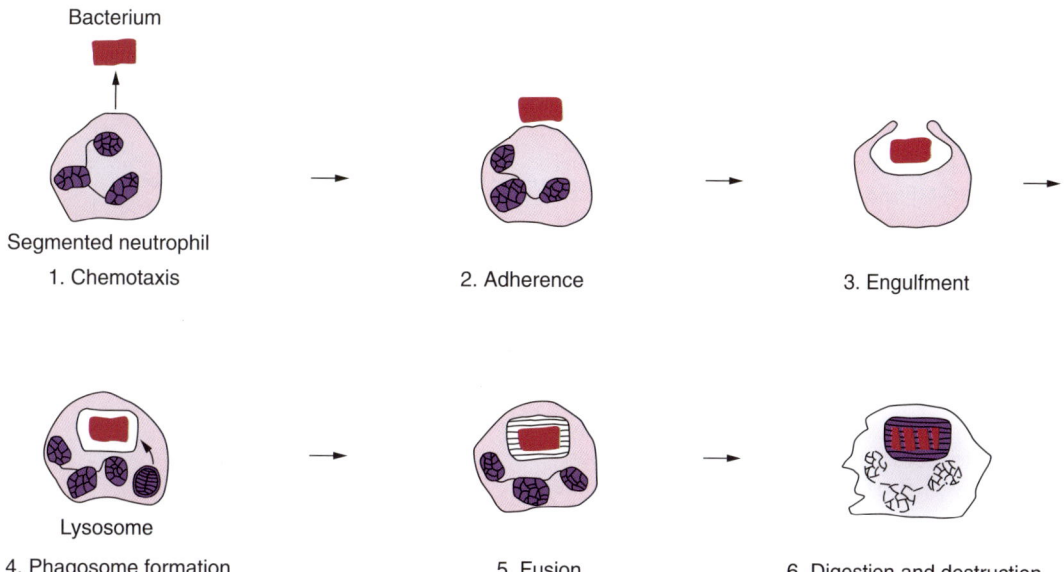

Fig. 4.1 Process of Phagocytosis. (Adapted from Turgeon ML: *Clinical hematology: theory and procedures,* ed 5, Philadelphia, 2012, Lippincott Williams & Wilkins.)

Segmented neutrophils are able to gather quickly at the site of injury because they are actively motile. Neutrophils are followed later by monocytes, macrophages, and dendritic cells. Macrophages and dendritic cells can also clean up injured or dead host cells. The marginating pool of neutrophils, adhering to the endothelial lining of nearby blood vessels, migrates through the vessel wall to the interstitial tissues. Mediators produced by microorganisms and by cells participating in the inflammatory process include interleukin-1 (IL-1), which is released by macrophages in response to infection or tissue injury. Another is histamine, released by circulating basophils, tissue mast cells, and blood platelets. Mediators cause capillary and venular dilation.

Cells are guided to the site of injury by an event called chemotaxis. Chemotaxis is defined as an increased directional migration of cells, particularly in response to concentration gradients of certain chemotactic factors (e.g., chemokines or chemoattractants). Chemokines are a group of at least 50 cytokines involved in cell migration, activation, and chemotaxis. The chemokines determine which cells will cross the endothelium and where they will move within the tissues.

Antigens can function as chemoattractants. Phagocytes detect antigens using various cell surface receptors. The speed of phagocytosis can be greatly increased by recruiting the following two attachment devices present on the surface of phagocytic cells:
- Fc receptor, which binds the Fc portion of antibody molecules, chiefly immunoglobulin G (IgG). The IgG attaches to the organism through its Fab site.
- Complement receptor, the third component of complement, C3, also binds to organisms and then attaches to the complement receptor.

This coating of the organisms by molecules that speed up phagocytosis is termed opsonization; the Fc portions of antibody and complement (C3) are called *opsonins*. The steps in opsonization are as follows:
1. Antibody attached to the surface of a bacterium minimally binds the Fc phagocyte receptor.
2. Complement C3b is attached to the surface of the bacterium and binds loosely to the phagocyte C3b receptor.
3. Both antibody and C3b are attached to the surface of the bacterium and bound tightly to the phagocyte, allowing greater opportunity for the phagocyte to engulf the bacterium.

Necrotic cells release an independent chemoattractant of necrotaxis signal, which directs PMN migration beyond the intravascular chemokine gradient. These intravascular danger-sensing and recruitment mechanisms have evolved to limit the collateral damage during a response to sterile injury. In this process, PMNs are allowed to migrate intravascularly as they navigate through healthy tissue to sites of injury. Necrotaxis signals promote localization of neutrophils directly into existing areas of injury to focus the innate immune response on damaged areas and away from healthy tissue, which provides an additional safeguard against collateral damage during sterile inflammatory responses. The innate immune system can clean up the dead by killing the living.

Adhesion

The leukocyte adhesion cascade is a sequence of adhesion and activation events that ends with the cell exerting its effects on the inflamed site (see the section Acute Inflammation later in the chapter). Adhesion is mediated by the granulocytes and ligands on the endothelial cells and is promoted by chemoattractants (e.g., interleukin-8 [IL-8]). The transit time through the microcirculation and, more specifically, the contact time during which the leukocyte is close to the endothelium, appears to be a key parameter in determining the success of the recruitment process, as reflected in firm adhesion.

A number of steps appear to be necessary for effective leukocyte adhesion:
1. Tethering
2. Triggering
3. Adhesion

After recruitment of phagocytic cells at the site of injury, the process known as capture (tethering) represents the first contact of a leukocyte with the activated endothelium. Tethering occurs after margination, which allows phagocytes to move in a position close to the endothelium. P-selectin, a carbohydrate ligand on endothelial cells, is a primary adhesion molecule for capture and the initiation of rolling. Other carbohydrate ligands are E-selectin and L-selectin. In tethering, a neutrophil is slowed in the circulation by interactions between E-selectin and carbohydrate groups on CD15, causing it to roll along the endothelial surface.

In the next step, triggering, the neutrophil is now prepared to receive signals from chemokines bound to the endothelial surface or by direct signaling from endothelial surface molecules. The longer a cell rolls along the endothelium, the longer it has to receive sufficient signal to trigger migration.

In the final step of leukocyte adhesion, upregulation of integrins (complement receptor 3 [CR3] and lymphocyte function–associated antigen 1 [LFA-1]) promotes the activity of cell adhesion molecules (CAMs) on the endothelium to initiate migration of leukocytes. Adhesion molecules fall into families that are structurally related. In addition to L-selectin, other CAMs interact with leukocyte integrins and selectins. Some CAMs have been implicated in capture (e.g., platelet/endothelial cell adhesion molecule-1 [PECAM-1], intercellular adhesion molecule-1 [ICAM-1], vascular endothelial [VE]-cadherin, LFA-1 [CD11a/CD18], integrin-associated protein [IAP, CD47], very late antigen-4 [VLA-4, α4β1–integrin]) but their level of actual involvement varies. It is important for CAMs to interact by binding to a cellular cytoskeleton to allow a cell to gain traction on another cell or on the extracellular matrix (ECM), which allows the cell to move through the tissues.

The inflammatory response begins with a release of inflammatory chemicals into the extracellular fluid. Sources of these inflammatory mediators, the most important of which are histamine, prostaglandins, and cytokines, are injured tissue cells, lymphocytes, mast cells, and blood proteins. The presence of these chemicals promotes the reactions to inflammation (redness, heat, swelling, and pain).

Engulfment

On reaching the site of infection, phagocytes engulf and destroy the foreign matter (Fig. 4.2). Eosinophils can also undergo this process, except that they kill parasites. After the phagocytic cells have arrived at the site of injury, the bacteria can be engulfed through active membrane invagination. Pseudopodia are extended around the pathogen, pulled by interactions between the Fc receptors and Fc antibody portions on the opsonized bacterium. Pseudopodia meet and fuse, thereby internalizing the bacterium and enclosing it in a phagocytic vacuole, or phagosome.

The principal factor in determining whether phagocytosis can occur is the physical nature of the surface of the bacteria and phagocytic cells. The bacteria must be more hydrophobic than the phagocyte. Some bacteria, such as *Streptococcus pneumoniae*, have a hydrophilic capsule and are not normally phagocytized. Most nonpathogenic bacteria are easily phagocytized because they are very hydrophobic. The presence of certain soluble factors such as complement, a plasma protein, coupled with antibodies and chemicals such as acetylcholine enhance the phagocytic process. Enhancement of phagocytosis through opsonization can speed up the ingestion of particles. If the surface tensions are conducive to engulfment, the phagocytic cell membrane invaginates. This invagination leads to the formation of an isolated vacuole (phagosome) within the cell.

Digestion

Digestion follows the ingestion of particles, with the required energy primarily provided by anaerobic glycolysis. Granules (see Table 4.1) in the phagocyte cytosol then migrate to and fuse with the phagosome to form the phagolysosome. These granules contain degradatory enzymes of the following three types:

1. Primary, or azurophilic, granules containing enzymes (e.g., lysozyme and MPO)
2. Secondary, or specific, granules containing substances such as lactoferrin
3. Tertiary granules containing substances such as caspases

Bacterial killing by neutrophils is associated with two general and frequently synergistic mechanisms: oxidative and nonoxidative (Box 4.1).

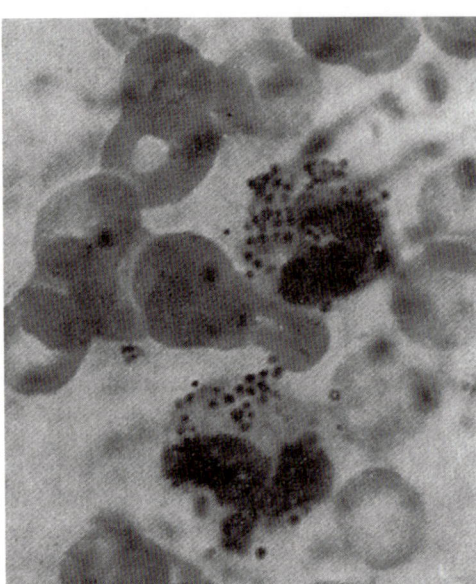

Fig. 4.2 Two Phagocytic Cells Have Engulfed Numerous *Staphylococcus aureus* Cells. (From Barrett JT: *Textbook of immunology*, ed 5, St. Louis, 1988, Mosby.)

The oxygen-dependent mechanism appears to be of major importance in bacterial killing, but other bactericidal mechanisms that do not require oxygen also operate within phagocytes.

Bacterial killing in the phagosome is augmented by the generation of superoxide. Activated neutrophils produce superoxide via a multicomponent *reduced nicotinamide-adenine dinucleotide phosphate* (NADPH)-dependent oxidase that is activated by neutrophil stimulation. In resting cells, oxidase components are found in the plasma membrane and intracellular stores. After stimulation, intracellular components are translocated to the plasma membrane and activated, producing superoxide. The resulting reactions result in the formation of hydrogen peroxide (H_2O_2) and hypochlorous acid (HOCl) that increases bacterial killing. Bacterial killing decreases under anaerobic conditions compared with phagocytosis that does not.

Degranulation of the neutrophil releases antibacterial substances (e.g., lactoferrin, lysozyme, and α-defensin) from the granules; released enzymes promote bactericidal activity by increasing membrane permeability. Elastase, one of several substances that can damage host tissues, is also released. The MPO granules are responsible for the action of the oxygen-dependent, MPO-mediated system. H_2O_2 and an oxidizable cofactor serve as major factors in the actual killing of bacteria within the vacuole. Other oxygen-independent systems, such as alterations in pH, lysozymes, lactoferrin, and the granular cationic proteins, also participate in the bactericidal process. Monocytes are particularly effective as phagocytic cells because of the large amounts of lipase in their cytoplasm. Lipase is able to attack bacteria with a lipid capsule, such as *Mycobacterium tuberculosis*. Monocytes are further able to bind and destroy cells coated with complement-fixing antibodies because of the presence of membrane receptors for specific components or types of Ig.

Release of lytic enzymes results in the destruction of neutrophils and their subsequent phagocytosis by macrophages. Macrophage digestion proceeds without risk to the cell unless the ingested material is toxic. If the ingested material damages the lysosomal membrane, however, the macrophage will also be destroyed owing to the release of lysosomal enzymes.

During phagocytosis, cells demonstrate increased metabolic activity, referred to as *respiratory burst*. The respiratory burst is important

> **BOX 4.1 Antimicrobial Systems of Neutrophils**
>
> **Oxygen Dependent**
> Myeloperoxidase mediated
> Myeloperoxidase independent
> Hydrogen peroxide
> Superoxide
>
> **Oxygen Independent**
> Acid
> Lysozymes
> Lactoferrin
> α-Defensins
> Bactericidal permeability–increasing protein
> Cationic granule proteins

to bactericidal activity. This results in the production by the phagocyte of large quantities of reactive oxygen species (ROS), which are released into the phagocytic vesicle. This phenomenon is achieved by the activity of the enzyme known as *reduced nicotinamide-adenine dinucleotide phosphate oxidase*. Together, the granule-mediated and NADPH oxidase–mediated effects elicit microbicidal results. NADPH oxidase forms the centerpiece of the phagocyte-killing mechanism and is activated in about 2 seconds. The NADPH oxidase generates ROS by generating the superoxide radical, $O_2^{\cdot-}$; the associated cyanide-insensitive increase in oxygen consumption is the respiratory burst.

The importance of the oxygen-dependent microbicidal mechanism is dramatically illustrated by patients with chronic granulomatous disease (CGD), a severe congenital deficit in bacterial killing that results from the inability to generate phagocyte-derived superoxide and related reactive oxygen intermediates (ROIs). The production of residual ROIs is predicted by the specific NADPH oxidase mutation, regardless of the specific gene affected. CGD results from defects in the genes encoding individual components of the enzyme system responsible for oxidant production. Acquisition of oxidase activity occurs in the course of myeloid cell maturation, and the genes for several of its components have been identified. This system also lends itself to analysis of the transcriptional and translational events that occur during cellular differentiation and under the influence of specific cytokines.

Subsequent Phagocytic Activities

If invading bacteria are not phagocytized at entry into the body, they may establish themselves in secondary sites such as the lymph nodes or various body organs. These undigested bacteria produce a secondary inflammation, where neutrophils and macrophages again congregate. If bacteria escape from secondary tissue sites, a bacteremia will develop. In patients who are unresponsive to antibiotic intervention, this situation can prove fatal.

Following phagocytosis, macrophages and dendritic cells process peptides from ingested pathogens for presentation to T lymphocytes. These T lymphocytes then interact with B lymphocytes to produce antibodies (see Chapter 3). Due to the fact that T lymphocytes cannot respond to intact pathogens, phagocytosis is an important link between the innate and adaptive immune systems.

NEUTROPHIL EXTRACELLULAR TRAPS

In addition to phagocytosis, including the release of antimicrobial molecules at the site of infection, another defense mechanism has been discovered. This mechanism is the formation of neutrophil extracellular traps (NETs), which are produced after the release of the nuclear contents of the neutrophil into the extracellular space. NETs function in innate immunity. They are composed of chromatin components, including histones, and neutrophil antimicrobial proteins. Microbes are trapped in NETs, where they encounter high concentrations of antimicrobial proteins.

> **KEY CONCEPTS: Monocytes-Macrophages**
> - Functionally, monocytes-macrophages have phagocytosis as their major role, but these cells perform at least three distinct but interrelated functions in host defense.
> - Macrophages carry out the fundamental function of ingesting and killing invading microorganisms.
> - Macrophages remove and eliminate extracellular pathogens, such as pneumococci, from the blood circulation.
> - Macrophages have the capacity to phagocytize particulate and internalized soluble materials, which supports increased microbicidal and tumoricidal ability of activated macrophages.
> - The phagocytic property of the macrophage is particularly important in the processing of antigens as part of the immune response.
> - Monocytes-macrophages release many factors associated with host defense and inflammation.
> - Cytokine storm syndromes are inflammatory disorders that result in an overwhelming systemic inflammation, unstable blood flow in the heart and vessels to perfuse normal organ functions, multiple-organ dysfunction, and potentially death.

MONOCYTE-MACROPHAGE HOST DEFENSE FUNCTIONS

Functionally, monocytes-macrophages have phagocytosis as their major role, but these cells perform at least three distinct but interrelated functions in host defense. The categories of host defense functions of monocytes-macrophages include:

1. Phagocytosis
2. Antigen presentation and induction of the immune response
3. Secretion of biologically active molecules

Phagocytosis

The principal functions of mononuclear phagocytes in body defenses result from the changes that take place in these functions when the macrophage is activated (Box 4.2). Macrophages carry out the fundamental function of ingesting and killing invading microorganisms such as intracellular parasites, *M. tuberculosis*, and some fungi. In addition, macrophages remove and eliminate such extracellular pathogens as pneumococci from the blood circulation. The macrophage also has the capacity to phagocytize particulate and aggregated soluble materials. This process is enhanced by the presence of receptors on the surface of the Fc portion of IgG and complement component, C3. The ability to internalize soluble substances supports the increased microbicidal and tumoricidal ability of activated macrophages. Activation of macrophages or monocytes can result in the release of parasiticidal mediators and in receptor-mediated phagocytosis during malaria infection. The most likely location for this innate immune response is within the spleen, which is crucial for development of immunity to malaria.

Another important phagocytic function of macrophages is their ability to dispose of damaged or dying cells. Macrophages lining the sinusoids of the spleen are particularly important in ingesting aging erythrocytes. They are also involved in removing tissue debris, repairing wounds, and removing debris as embryonic tissues replace one another.

> **BOX 4.2 Primary Functions of Macrophages**
>
> - Phagocytosis (microbicidal activity to digest and destroy bacteria, dead host cells, and cellular debris).
> - Mediation of antibody-dependent cellular cytotoxicity of antibody-coated bacteria.
> - Clearance of altered forms of lipoproteins, glycoproteins, or proteins with advanced glycan products.
> - Phagocytosis-associated respiratory burst.
> - Antigen processing and presentation of antigens to CD4 helper T lymphocytes.
> - Secretion of cytokines to promote acute-phase and T-cell responses.

Phagocytic activity increases when there is tissue damage and inflammation, which releases substances that attract macrophages. Activated macrophages migrate more vigorously in response to chemotactic factors and should enter sites of inflammation (e.g., locations of infection or cancer) more efficiently than resting macrophages. Migration of monocytes into different body tissues appears to be a random phenomenon in the absence of localized inflammation. An essential factor in the protective function of monocytes is the capacity of the cell to move through the endothelial wall of blood vessels (diapedesis) to the site of microbial invasion in tissues. The attracting forces for monocytes, chemotactic factors, include complement products and chemoattractants derived from neutrophils, lymphocytes, or cancer cells.

The activity of mononuclear phagocytes against cancer cells in humans is less well understood than the phagocytosis of microorganisms. Phagocytes are thought to suppress the growth of spontaneously arising tumors. The ability of these cells to control malignant cells may not involve phagocytosis but may be related to secreted cellular products, such as lysosomal enzymes, oxygen metabolites (e.g., H_2O_2), proteinases, and tumor necrosis factor α (TNF-α, cachectin). The proteolytic enzymes present on the surface membrane of monocytes also may play a role in tumor rejection.

Antigen Presentation and Induction of the Immune Response

The phagocytic property of the macrophage is particularly important in the processing of antigens as part of the immune response. Macrophages are believed to process antigens and physically present this biochemically modified and more reactive form of antigen to lymphocytes (particularly helper T cells) as an initial step in the immune response. Recognition of antigen on the macrophage surface by T lymphocytes, however, requires an additional match of the surface major histocompatibility complex (MHC) class II gene product. This gene product is the Ia product in the mouse and the D gene region product in humans. With proper recognition, the macrophage secretes a lymphocyte-activating factor (IL-1), lymphocyte proliferation ensues, and the immune response (T-cell–B-cell response) is facilitated.

Secretion of Biologically Active Molecules

Monocytes-macrophages release many factors associated with host defense and inflammation. These cells serve as supportive accessory cells to lymphocytes, at least partly by releasing soluble factors. In cellular immunity, monocytes assume a killer role in that they are activated by sensitized lymphocytes to phagocytize offending cells or antigen particles. This is important in fields such as tumor immunology.

In addition to their phagocytic properties, monocytes-macrophages are able to synthesize a number of biologically important compounds, including transferrin, complement, *interferon*, pyrogens, and certain growth factors. Approximately 100 distinct substances have been identified as being secreted by monocytes-macrophages.

Blood monocytes and tissue macrophages are primary sources of the polypeptide hormone called *IL-1*, which has a particularly potent effect on the inflammatory response. IL-1 also supports B-lymphocyte proliferation and antibody production, in addition to T-lymphocyte production of lymphokines. The increased synthesis of IL-1 by activated macrophages could contribute to enhancement of the immune response. Endotoxin also induces the synthesis of IL-1. This effect is achieved at least partly by stimulation of macrophages to release TNF-α, which then stimulates the production of IL-1 by endothelial cells and macrophages. Activated macrophages release much more TNF-α than resting macrophages exposed to endotoxin. Both TNF-α and IL-1 can induce the fever and synthesis of acute-phase reactants that characterize inflammation.

CYTOKINE STORM SYNDROMES

Cytokine storm syndromes (CSS, see Chapter 2, Cytokine Storm) are a group of disorders representing a variety of inflammatory disorders that result in an overwhelming systemic inflammation, unstable blood flow in the heart and vessels to perfuse normal organ functions, multiple-organ dysfunction, and potentially death. Macrophage activation syndrome (MAS) is classified as a CSS disorder. Macrophages are innate immune cells that sense and respond to microbial threats by producing inflammatory molecules that eliminate pathogens and promote tissue repair. However, a dysregulated macrophage response can be damaging to the host, as is seen in MAS with severe infections caused by SARS-CoV-2.

The main pathophysiologic feature of MAS is excessive activation and expansion of cytotoxic CD8+ T cells and macrophages. These activated immune cells produce large amounts of proinflammatory cytokines creating a cytokine storm. Nonspecific acute-phase reactants with an abrupt decrease in circulating peripheral blood cells and an acute drop in fibrinogen are associated with MAS but can be seen in any cytokine storm syndrome and often suggest active disseminated intravascular coagulopathy (DIC). The exact drivers of monocyte and macrophage activation in COVID-19 disease pathophysiology remain to be clarified. Severe COVID-19–associated pneumonia patients may exhibit features of systemic hyper inflammation response induced by SARS-CoV-2. The pathogenicity of infiltrating macrophages can extend beyond the promotion of acute inflammation and be associated with fibrotic complications.

> **KEY CONCEPTS: Inflammation**
>
> - Tissue damage results in inflammation, a series of biochemical and cellular changes that facilitate the phagocytosis of invading microorganisms or damaged cells and may be accompanied by an increase in the plasma concentration of acute-phase reactants.
> - Changes in inflamed tissue follow a well-defined cascade of events beginning with the capture of free-flowing white blood cells (WBCs) to the vessel wall and subsequent leukocyte rolling along and adhesion to the inflamed endothelial layer, and activation of integrins and the firm arrest of leukocytes.
> - Integrin-dependent signaling events prepare the attached leukocyte to spread and crawl in search for a way out of the vasculature into tissue.
> - The primary objective of inflammation is to localize and eradicate the irritant and repair the surrounding tissue.
> - If an inflammation overwhelms the whole body, severe sepsis and septic shock are progressively severe stages of systemic inflammatory response syndrome (SIRS).

CHAPTER 4 Cellular Activities and Clinical Disorders of Innate and Adaptive Immunity

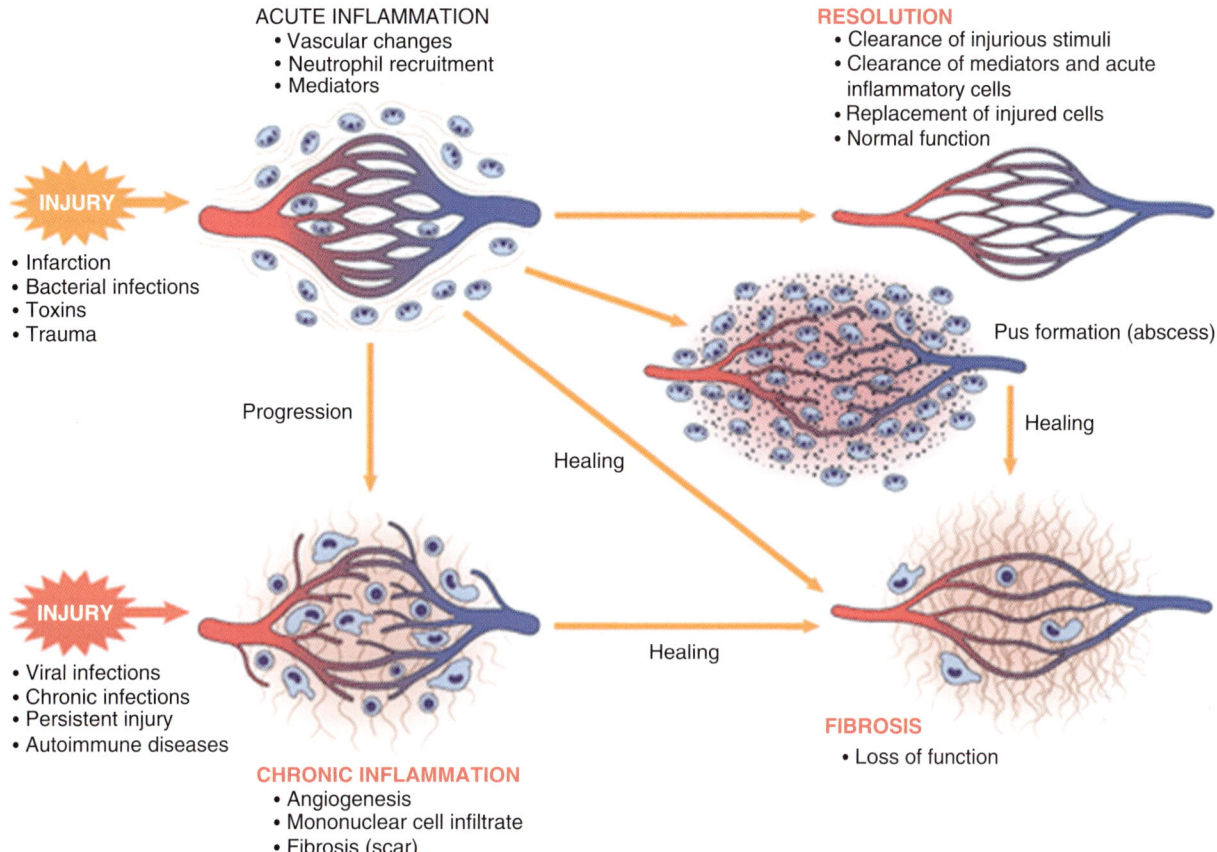

Fig. 4.3 Outcomes of Acute Inflammation: Resolution, Healing by Fibrosis, or Chronic Inflammation. (From Kumar V, Abbas AK, Fausto N: *Robbins and Cotran pathologic basis of disease*, ed 8, St. Louis, 2009, Elsevier.)

Patients with severe sepsis are considered to have defective adaptive immunity. Sepsis begins when the innate immune system responds aggressively to the presence of bacteria.

ACUTE INFLAMMATION

Acute inflammation is defined as an immune response resulting in complete elimination of a pathogen (sterile immunity), followed by resolution of tissue damage, disappearance of leukocytes from the tissue, and full regeneration of tissue function. Sites of acute inflammation have more neutrophils and activated T lymphocytes than chronic inflammation. With chronic inflammation, the immune system tries to contain an infection and minimize the tissue damage. Sites of chronic inflammation have an abundance of macrophages, cytotoxic T lymphocytes, and even B lymphocytes.

In acute inflammation, tissue damage results in inflammation, a series of biochemical and cellular changes that facilitate the phagocytosis of invading microorganisms or damaged cells (Fig. 4.3). If inflammation is sufficiently extensive, it is accompanied by an increase in the plasma concentration of acute-phase reactants (see Chapter 2). Leukocyte recruitment into inflamed tissue follows a well-defined cascade of events, beginning with the capture of free-flowing WBCs to the vessel wall and subsequent leukocyte rolling along and adhesion to the inflamed endothelial layer. During rolling, WBCs come into close contact with the endothelial surface, which allows endothelium-bound chemokines to interact with their specific receptors on the leukocyte surface. This triggers the activation of integrins, which leads to firm leukocyte arrest on the endothelium. In addition, integrin-dependent signaling events induce cytoskeletal rearrangements and cell polarization, modifications necessary to help prepare the attached leukocyte to spread and crawl in search of a way out of the vasculature into tissue.

Celsus, a practitioner of Greek medicine who was born in 25 BCE, is credited with recording the cardinal signs of inflammation: rubor (redness), calor (heat), dolor (pain), and tumor (swelling). The primary objective of inflammation is to localize and eradicate the irritant and repair the surrounding tissue. The inflammatory response involves the following three major stages:
1. Dilation of capillaries to increase blood flow
2. Microvascular structural changes and escape of plasma proteins from the bloodstream
3. Leukocyte transmigration through endothelium and accumulation at the site of injury

Hypoxia can induce inflammation. Inflammation in response to hypoxia is clinically relevant. Ischemia in organ grafts increases the risk of inflammation and graft failure or rejection. Hypoxia has multiple effects on the innate and adaptive immune systems.

Once inflammation is triggered, it must be appropriately resolved or pathologic tissue damage will occur. In some diseases, the body's defense system (immune system) inappropriately triggers an inflammatory response when no foreign substances are present. In these autoimmune disorders, the body's normally protective immune system causes damage to its own tissues (see Chapter 22).

SEPSIS

If an inflammation overwhelms the whole body, SIRS is diagnosed. **Sepsis**, severe sepsis, and septic shock are progressively severe stages of SIRS. The criteria for SIRS require two or more of the following conditions: alteration of body temperature (>38°C or <36°C), increased heart rate, increased respiratory rate, and a total leukocyte count >12 × 10^9/L (or >10% immature forms). Sepsis is defined as SIRS + infection; severe sepsis is defined as sepsis + evidence of organ dysfunction. Patients with severe sepsis are considered to have defective adaptive immunity.

Sepsis begins when the innate immune system responds aggressively to the presence of bacteria. Toll-like receptors (TLRs) cause the antigen-presenting cell (APC) to produce proinflammatory cytokines. Biochemical markers associated with sepsis include TNF and IL-1 and IL-6, a proinflammatory cytokine. Other proteins produced in response to infection and/or inflammation include procalcitonin and chemokines. Another consequence of inflammation is that the liver is stimulated to produce C-reactive protein (CRP, see Chapter 2).

> **KEY CONCEPTS: Cellular Interactions**
> - Interactions occur through cell surface receptors that mediate cell-to-cell binding (adhesion) of leukocytes.
> - Three protein families (immunoglobulin, integrin, and selectin) are associated in a network of cellular interactions in the immune system.

CELL SURFACE RECEPTORS

Cellular communication is essential to the development, tissue organization, and function of all multicellular organisms. Cells communicate with each other and their environment through soluble mediators and during direct contact (e.g., phagocytosis). An immunologic response is a result of the interactions of various leukocytes with each other and other cells in the body. These interactions occur through cell surface receptors that mediate cell-to-cell binding, or adhesion, of leukocytes.

The discovery of several cell surface receptors involved in cellular communication has been a key factor in understanding the mechanisms underlying inflammatory and immune phenomena. Three protein families—the immunoglobulin (Ig) family, integrin family, and the rather recently designated selectin family—form a network of cellular interactions in the immune system. Neutrophils tether to and roll on P- and E-selectin expressed on activated endothelial cells. Rolling neutrophils encounter immobilized chemokines. Chemokines activate integrins to their high-affinity states that enable interactions with ICAM-1, which promote arrest, adhesion strengthening, intraluminal crawling, and transendothelial migration. E-selectin directly triggers signals in rolling PMNs that cooperate with chemokine signals to minimize neutrophil recruitment during inflammation.

Members of the Ig superfamily include antigen-specific receptors (e.g., T-cell receptor [TCR] and surface immunoglobulin [sIg]), in addition to antigen-independent receptors and their counterreceptors, such as CD2 and lymphocyte function–associated antigen-3. Ig superfamily members function in cell activation, differentiation, and cell-to-cell interaction. In some cases, both an adhesion receptor and the counterreceptor to which it binds are members of the Ig superfamily.

Three selectin family molecules—endothelial CAM-1, leukocyte adhesion molecule (LAM-1, Mel-14), and CD62, also known as *platelet activation–dependent granule–external membrane protein* and *granule membrane protein of 140 kDa* (GMP-140)—have been implicated in a number of leukocyte adhesion phenomena, including leukocyte homing to lymphoid tissue. Selectins are expressed on leukocytes and endothelial cells. Mel-14 functions early in neutrophil–endothelium adhesion.

The integrin family consists of at least 14 alpha-beta heterodimers divided into subfamilies with distinct structural and functional characteristics. The subfamily of leukocyte integrins contains three members: LFA-1, Mac-1, and p150,95. These molecules are glycoproteins composed of noncovalently associated alpha and beta subunits. LFA-1 is expressed on all leukocytes, whereas Mac-1 and p150,95 are found primarily on granulocytes and monocytes.

The integrin family is phylogenetically ancient. Integrin family members engage in interactions with cell surface ligands and extracellular matrix (ECM) components. ECM components, including fibronectin, collagen, and laminin, have been shown to be ligands for members of the beta-1 and beta-3 subfamilies. Members of these subfamilies are of great significance in embryogenesis, growth and repair, and hemostasis. The leukocyte integrins, or beta-2 subfamily, have been shown to be involved in a diverse number of leukocyte adhesion–dependent phenomena, giving them a critical role in inflammatory and immune responses. The term *integrin* was initially used to emphasize that these receptors integrate signals from the extracellular environment with the intracellular cytoskeleton. A signal is transduced from outside to inside the cell.

In addition to the involvement of these receptors in a variety of immune functions, integrin molecules play a role in the spread of malignant cells. The major cause of death in malignant disease is not the primary tumor, but rather the metastasis of tumor cells to distant sites within the body. Metastasis is a complex multistep process that begins with the detachment of a few tumor cells from the primary tumor. The tumor cells then move into the circulatory system, where they can be transported to other organs. While in the circulatory system, tumor cells must survive the natural defense system of the body before attaching to and invading the tissues of another organ. A better understanding of the metastatic process could provide the basis for diagnostic and therapeutic strategies.

DISORDERS OF NEUTROPHILS

Noninfectious Neutrophil-Mediated Inflammatory Disease

Although neutrophils provide the major means of defense against bacterial and fungal infections, they can also be destructive to host tissues. The same oxidative and nonoxidative processes that destroy microorganisms can affect adjacent host tissues. A number of disease states correspond to inappropriate phagocytosis (Box 4.3), associated with prolonged activation of NADPH oxidase. This process occurs when phagocytes attempt to engulf particles that are too large. The phagocyte

> **BOX 4.3 Noninfectious Neutrophil-Mediated Diseases**
> 1. Autoimmune arthritis
> 2. Autoimmune vasculitis
> 3. Dermatologic disorders
>   a. Autoimmune bullous dermatoses
>   b. Behçet disease
>   c. Psoriasiform dermatoses
>   d. Pyoderma gangrenosum
>   e. Sweet syndrome
> 4. Glomerulonephritis
> 5. Gout
> 6. Inflammatory bowel disease
> 7. Malignant neoplasms at site of chronic inflammation
> 8. Myocardial infarction
> 9. Respiratory disorders—adult respiratory distress syndrome, asthma and allergic asthma, emphysema

> **BOX 4.4 Examples of Innate (Congenital) Neutrophil Abnormalities**
>
> Chédiak-Higashi syndrome (anomaly)
> Chronic granulomatous disease
> Complement receptor 3 deficiency
> Myeloperoxidase deficiency
> Specific granule deficiency

releases oxygen radicals and granule contents onto the particle, but these escape into the surrounding tissues, generating tissue damage. This is often observed in response to dust inhalation and smoking (e.g., nicotine), and in persistent infections such as cystic fibrosis.

In addition, many autoimmune diseases are thought to be caused by inappropriate activation of the process of phagocytosis or ineffective resolution of the inflammatory process, whereby the body attacks its own cells and tissues. Examples include rheumatoid arthritis, multiple sclerosis, and Graves disease.

Abnormal Neutrophil Function

Patients with quantitative or qualitative defects of neutrophils have a high rate of infection, which illustrates the importance of the neutrophil to body defenses. Individuals with a marked decrease of neutrophils (neutropenia) or severe defects in neutrophil function frequently have recurrent systemic bacterial infections (e.g., pneumonia), disseminated cutaneous pyogenic lesions, and other types of life-threatening bacterial and fungal infections.

Leukocyte mobility may be impaired in some diseases (e.g., rheumatoid arthritis, cirrhosis, and CGD). Defective locomotion or leukocyte immobility can also be seen in patients receiving steroids and in those with lazy leukocyte syndrome. A marked defect in the cellular response to chemotaxis, an important step in phagocytosis, can be seen in patients with diabetes mellitus, Chédiak-Higashi anomaly (syndrome), or sepsis, and also in those with high levels of antibody IgE, as in Job syndrome.

Innate (Congenital) Neutrophil Abnormalities

A small number of patients have congenital abnormalities of neutrophil structure and function (Box 4.4).

Chédiak-Higashi Syndrome

Chédiak-Higashi syndrome represents a qualitative disorder of neutrophils. It is a rare familial disorder inherited as an autosomal-recessive genetic trait. The responsible gene has been mapped to chromosomal locus 1q42.1-q42.2 and is known as the LYST gene. The abnormal gene affects the movement or transport of proteins within the neutrophils.

Chédiak-Higashi syndrome is characterized by very large granules. These gigantic, peroxidase-positive deposits represent abnormal fusion of primary and secondary granules during lysosomal development in neutrophils and other leukocytes. Neutrophils display impaired chemotaxis and delayed killing of ingested bacteria. Patients with this disorder suffer from frequent infections, which suggests that neutrophils with this defect are not efficient bactericidal cells.

Chronic Granulomatous Disease

A number of types of chronic granulomatous diseases (CGDs) have been described, including sex-linked (X chromosome-linked) in 66%, autosomal recessive in 34%, and autosomal dominant in less than 1% of cases. Patients with the autosomal-recessive form may have a less severe clinical course than patients with the X-linked form.

CGD is a defect of neutrophil microbicidal ROS generation resulting from gp91^{phox} deficiency. CGD is caused by a missense, nonsense, frameshift, splice, or deletion mutation in the genes for p22^{phox}, p40^{phox}, p47^{phox}, p67^{phox} (autosomal CGD), or gy91^{phox} (X-linked CGD), which results in variable production of the neutrophil-derived ROIs.

Patients with X-linked CGD (X-CGD) have a mutation in CYBB encoding the transmembrane gp91^{phox} subunit of phagocyte NADPH oxidase required for microbicidal ROS production by neutrophils and monocytes. As a result, patients have life-threatening infections and granulomatous complications. If a suitable hematopoietic stem cell donor is available, X-CGD can be cured, but graft-versus-host disease (see Chapter 25) is a significant risk.

The onset of CGD is during infancy, with one-third of patients dying before the age of 7 years because of infections. It was observed that in the presence of normal or elevated leukocyte counts, the neutrophilic granulocytes in vitro ingested and destroyed only streptococci, not staphylococci. Subsequent testing revealed that cells from patients with CGD can phagocytize non–H_2O_2-producing bacteria, such as *Staphylococcus aureus* and Gram-negative rods (e.g., Enterobacteriaceae), but it cannot destroy them. In the X-linked form, the defective leukocytes fail to exhibit increased anaerobic metabolism during phagocytosis because of a cytochrome b558 deficiency (which expresses itself as a defect in the 91,000-Da glycoprotein membrane anchor of the cytochrome complex), or these defective leukocytes produce H_2O_2 because of an MPO deficiency.

Patients with CGD have infections with catalase-positive bacteria and fungi affecting the skin, lungs, liver, and bones. They also develop granulomas resulting from a lack of resolution of inflammatory foci, even after the infection has been eliminated. This leads to extensive granuloma formation and, in some circumstances, impairment of physiologic processes (e.g., obstruction of the esophagus or urinary tract).

Laboratory evaluation of CGD begins with nonspecific testing to rule out other disorders. These assays include serum quantitative Ig, complement activity enzyme immunoassay, complete blood count (CBC) with differential, MPO stain, and a neutrophil receptor profile. The evaluation of neutrophil phagocytic function is best determined by the neutrophil oxidative burst assay via flow cytometry that can indicate CGD by the absence or significant alteration of activity. Other, less reliable tests include measurement of superoxide production, ferrocytochrome reduction, and the classic nitroblue tetrazolium (NBT) test.

Complement Receptor 3 Deficiency

CR3 deficiency is a rare condition inherited as an autosomal-recessive trait. A deficiency of CR3 on phagocytic cells presents as a leukocyte adhesion deficiency (LAD). Leukocyte adhesion deficiency type 1 (LAD-1) is caused by a deficiency of CD18. LAD-2 is caused by the absence of Sialyl–Lewis X (CD15s) blood group antigen.

A CR3 deficiency in neutrophils is associated with marked abnormalities of adherence-related functions, including decreased aggregation of neutrophils to each other after activation, decreased adherence of neutrophils to endothelial cells, poor adherence and phagocytosis of opsonized microorganisms, defective spreading, and decreased diapedesis and chemotaxis. Patients may also lack an intravascular marginating pool of neutrophils. Defects in T lymphocytes are characterized by faulty lymphocyte-mediated cytotoxicity, with poor adherence to target cells. Abnormalities of B lymphocytes have also been observed.

Clinically, a deficiency can manifest as delayed separation of the umbilical cord. Other signs and symptoms include early onset of bacterial infections, including skin infections, mucositis, otitis, gingivitis, and periodontitis. A depressed inflammatory response and neutrophilia can be observed.

Myeloperoxidase Deficiency

A deficiency of MPO is inherited as an autosomal-recessive trait on chromosome 17. Myeloperoxidase is an iron-containing heme protein responsible for the peroxidase activity characteristic of azurophilic granules; it accounts for the greenish color of pus. Human neutrophils contain many granules of various sizes that are morphologically, biochemically, and functionally distinct. The azurophilic granules normally contain MPO. In this disorder, azurophilic granules are present, but MPO is decreased or absent. If phagocytes are deficient in MPO, the patient's phagocytes manifest a mild-to-moderate defect in bacterial killing and a marked defect in fungal killing in vitro.

Persons with an MPO deficiency are generally healthy and do not have an increased frequency of infection, probably because of other microbicidal mechanisms compensating for the deficiency. Patients with diabetes and MPO deficiency, however, may have deep fungal infections caused by *Candida* spp.

Specific Granule Deficiency

Specific granule deficiency is believed to be an autosomal-recessive disease. It is caused by a failure to synthesize specific granules and some contents of other granules during differentiation of neutrophils in the bone marrow. Patients with specific granule deficiency have recurrent, severe bacterial infections of the skin and deep tissues, with a depressed inflammatory response.

> **KEY CONCEPTS: Disorders of Monocyte-Macrophages and Leukocyte Integrins**
> - Qualitative monocyte-macrophage disorders manifest as lipid-storage diseases, including a number of rare autosomal-recessive disorders.
> - Leukocyte adhesion deficiency ultimately leads to recurrent and often fatal bacterial and fungal infections.

MONOCYTE-MACROPHAGE DISORDERS

Monocytes-macrophages have been shown to be abnormal in a variety of diseases (Table 4.2). The abnormality is partial, and no related association with increased susceptibility to infection has been established. In cases of severely depressed migration of monocytes, however, it is likely that this dysfunction predisposes a patient to infection because other defects of host defense coexist in these disorders.

The signs and symptoms of abnormalities of monocyte-macrophage function are extremely evident in some conditions. The profound defect of phagocytic killing exhibited by patients with CGD results in the formation of subcutaneous abscesses and abscesses in the liver, lungs, spleen, and lymph nodes. Cancer patients with defective monocyte cytotoxicity may develop this defect because tumors have the ability to release factors that suppress the generation of toxic oxygen metabolites by macrophages. In newborn infants, depressed chemotaxis, killing, and decreased synthesis of the phagocytosis-promoting factors fibronectin, C3, and complement factor B have been observed. In addition, the newborn's macrophages may not respond effectively to infection because the lymphocytes have impaired the production of the macrophage activator interferon-α (IFN-α).

Qualitative disorders of monocytes-macrophages manifest as lipid-storage diseases, including a number of rare autosomal-recessive disorders. The expression in macrophages of a systemic enzymatic defect permits the accumulation of cell debris normally cleared by macrophages. The macrophages are particularly prone to accumulating undegraded lipid products. Resistance to infection can be impaired, at least partially, because of a defect in macrophage function. Disorders of this type include Gaucher disease and Niemann-Pick disease.

TABLE 4.2 Examples of Primary and Secondary Abnormalities of Monocyte-Macrophage Function

Abnormality	Condition/Group
Defect in phagocyte killing	Chronic granulomatous disease, corticosteroid therapy, newborn infants, viral infections
Defective monocyte cytotoxicity	Cancer, Wiskott-Aldrich syndrome
Defective release of macrophage-activating factors	AIDS, intracellular infections (e.g., lepromatous leprosy, tuberculosis, visceral leishmaniasis)
Depressed migration	AIDS, burns, diabetes, immunosuppressive therapy, newborn infants
Impaired phagocytosis	Congenital deficiency of CD11–CD18, monocytic leukemia, systemic lupus erythematosus

Gaucher Disease

Gaucher disease is a monocyte-macrophage disorder caused by a rare genetic defect. Scientists have identified more than 400 genetic mutations associated with Gaucher disease. It is important to genetically screen patients of Ashkenazi Jewish descent who are pregnant or considering pregnancy, because there is a high incidence of disease in this ethnic group. Approximately 1 in 10 Ashkenazi (Eastern European) Jewish people are carriers, which makes Gaucher disease the most common inherited Jewish genetic disease.

Gaucher disease is divided into two major types, neuronopathic and nonneuronopathic disease, based on the particular symptoms. In nonneuronopathic disease, most organs and tissues can be involved, but not the brain. In neuronopathic disease, the brain is also involved. The nonneuronopathic form, type I, is the most common form of the disease. Types II and III constitute the neuronopathic form of the disease. The prognosis varies; with mild disease, the patient may live a relatively normal life, whereas with severe disease the patient may die prematurely.

The disorder is expressed as a deficiency of α-glucocerebrosidase, the enzyme that normally splits glucose from its parent sphingolipid, glucosylceramide. As a result of this enzyme deficiency, cerebroside accumulates in histiocytes (macrophages). Gaucher cells are rarely found in the circulating blood; the typical cell is large, with one to three eccentric nuclei and a characteristically wrinkled cytoplasm (Fig. 4.4). These cells are found in the bone marrow, spleen, and other organs of the mononuclear phagocyte system. Production of erythrocytes and leukocytes decreases as these abnormal cells infiltrate the bone marrow.

In the past, treatment for type 1 Gaucher disease was only aimed at managing or relieving symptoms. Treatments included various pain-reduction therapies, blood transfusions, orthopedic surgery for bones and joints, and possible splenectomy. Although some of these measures may still have a place in the management of type 1 Gaucher disease, the focus of disease management shifted in the early 1990s to two major approaches:

- Enzyme-replacement therapy
- Substrate-reduction therapy

Enzyme-replacement therapy either supplements or replaces the missing α-glucocerebrosidase in type 1 Gaucher disease.

CHAPTER 4 Cellular Activities and Clinical Disorders of Innate and Adaptive Immunity

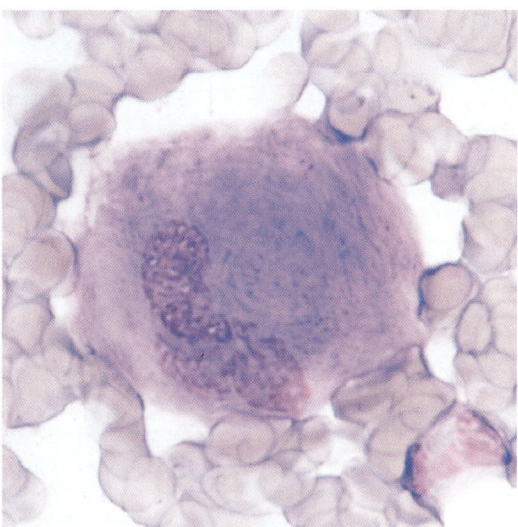

Fig. 4.4 Gaucher Cell. All photomicrographs are ×1000 with a Wright-Giemsa stain unless stated otherwise. (Carr JH, Rodak BF: *Clinical hematology atlas: cytoplasmic alterations of leukocytes*, St. Louis, 2009, Elsevier.)

Substrate-replacement therapy aims to minimize the amount of production and accumulation of excess material, or a particular substrate (glucosylceramide [GL1]), within cells. This allows the existing patient enzyme to better prevent GL1 from accumulating inside of cells.

In August 2014, the US Food and Drug Administration (FDA) approved a new orphan drug, eliglustat (Cerdelga), for the long-term treatment of adult patients with the type 1 form of Gaucher disease.

Niemann-Pick Disease

Niemann-Pick disease is a group of diseases similar to Gaucher disease. The characteristic cell in this disorder, the Pick cell, is similar in appearance to the Gaucher cell, although the cytoplasm of the cell is foamy.

There are three common forms of the disease: type A, type B, and type C. This disorder represents a rare autosomal-recessive deficiency of the enzyme sphingomyelinase in types A and B. These two types are characterized by a massive accumulation of sphingomyelin in the mononuclear phagocytes. An absence of enzyme challenges the normal functioning of an involved organ. Type A occurs in all races and ethnicities but is more common in the Ashkenazi (Eastern European) Jewish population.

Type C occurs when the body cannot properly break down cholesterol and other lipids. An accumulation of cholesterol results in an accumulation in the liver and spleen with an excess of other lipids in the brain. Type C is most common among Puerto Ricans of Spanish descent. Type C1 is a variant of type C. It involves a defect that interferes with the movement of cholesterol between brain cells. This type has only been seen in French Canadians in Nova Scotia.

DISEASE STATES INVOLVING LEUKOCYTE INTEGRINS

LAD ultimately leads to recurrent and often fatal bacterial and fungal infections. The cause of this very rare condition is mutations in the gene or chromosome; about 300 cases have been diagnosed worldwide.

There are several types of LAD based on genotypes and phenotypes. Two genotypes have been identified: LAD-1 and LAD-2. LAD-1 can affect people of all racial groups. LAD-2 has been reported only in people from the Middle East and Brazil. LAD-1 patients have a deficiency of the α_2-integrin subunit (CD18). The phenotypes are severe, moderate, and novel or variant. LAD-2 is described as the failure to convert guanosine diphosphate (GDP) mannose to fructose.

Patients have a history of delayed separation of the umbilical cord, gingivitis, recurrent and persistent bacterial or fungal skin infections, and impaired wound healing. A lack of pus formation has also been noted. Patients frequently develop severe life-threatening infections, although their neutrophil counts are usually elevated (25×10^9/L). Affected individuals do not have increased susceptibility to viral infections or malignant neoplasms. Patients with LAD-2 have a characteristic facial appearance, short stature, limb malformations, and severe developmental delay.

Adhesion defects can also be caused by two common drugs: epinephrine and corticosteroids. Both demarginate neutrophils from the peripheral vasculature, although the mechanism is not understood. Epinephrine acts by causing endothelial cells to release cyclic adenosine monophosphate (cAMP), which in turn interrupts adherence.

ADAPTIVE IMMUNITY

The principal cells of the adaptive immune system are T lymphocytes and B lymphocytes. These categories of lymphocytes recognize foreign antigens, directly destroy some cells, or produce antibodies as plasma cells. The total immune response involves the interaction of many different cell types and cell-mediated and antibody-mediated responses. T-lymphocyte subsets, including natural killer (NK) cells, together with classic innate immune cells, contribute significantly to the development and establishment of acute and chronic inflammatory diseases.

> **KEY CONCEPTS: Facts About Lymphocytes**
> - Lymphocytes represent the cellular components of the specific system of body defense. These cells function cooperatively in cell-mediated or humoral immunity.
> - Monoclonal antibody (MAb) testing led to the present identification of surface membrane markers (CDs).
> - Some CD markers are specific for cells of a particular lineage or maturational pathway.
> - Some markers vary in expression, depending on the state of activation or differentiation of the same cells.
> - In addition to using CD classification for the identification and separation of lymphocytes, CD antigens are involved in various lymphocyte functions.

LYMPHOID AND NONLYMPHOID SURFACE MEMBRANE MARKERS

The introduction of monoclonal antibody (MAb) testing (see Chapter 3) led to the present identification of surface membrane markers on lymphocytes and other cells. Surface markers can be used to identify and enumerate various lymphocyte subsets, establish lymphocyte maturity, classify types of leukemias and lymphomas, and monitor patients on immunosuppressive therapy.

Cell surface molecules recognized by MAbs are called *antigens* because antibodies can be produced against them. Originally, surface markers were named according to the antibodies that reacted with them, but a common nomenclature system, cluster of differentiation (CD), now exists (Fig. 4.5). CD numbers have been assigned to more than 320 unique clusters and subclusters of MAbs. The CD designation

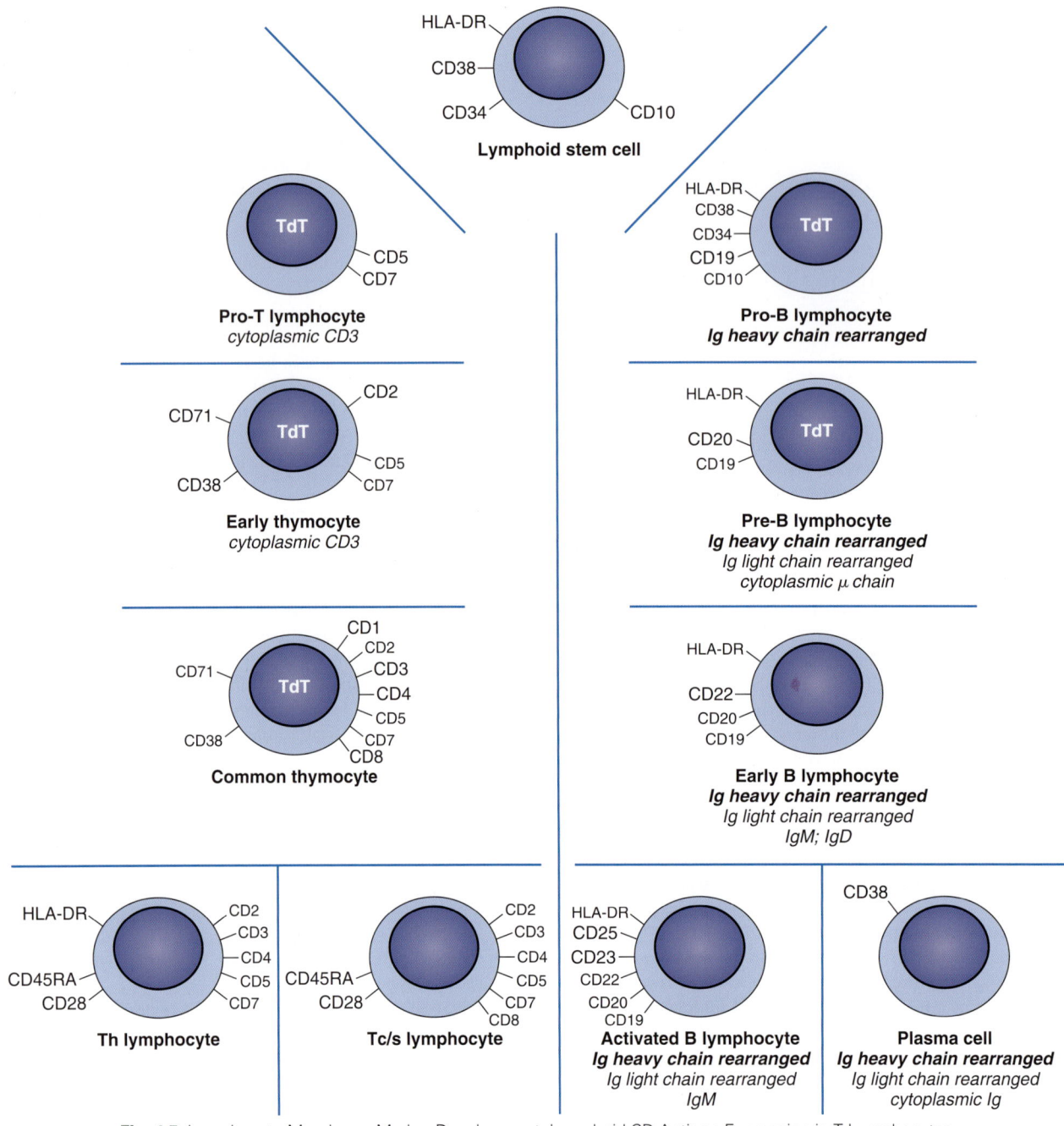

Fig. 4.5 Lymphocyte Membrane Marker Development: Lymphoid CD Antigen Expression in T Lymphocytes. *CD*, Cluster of differentiation; *HLA*, human leukocyte antigen; *Ig*, immunoglobulin; *TdT*, terminal deoxynucleotidyl transferase.

is now universally embraced as a label for the target molecule rather than just a grouping of MAbs with common reactivity.

The CD system can identify and discriminate between, or "mark" different cell populations or differentiate the maturational stages of lymphocytes. Cell membrane markers can be categorized as follows:
- Some markers are specific for cells of a particular lineage or maturational pathway.
- Some markers vary in expression, depending on the state of activation or differentiation of the same cells, such as when CD antigen identification is used to classify lymphocyte subsets such as CD4 or CD8.

In addition to the use of CD classification for the identification and separation of lymphocytes, CD antigens are involved in various lymphocyte functions, usually the following:
- Promotion of cell-to-cell interactions and adhesion
- Transduction of signals that lead to lymphocyte activation

Characterization of cell surface marker expression by normal and malignant T or B cells launched a new method of **immunophenotyping** for the classification of leukemias and lymphomas. Today, the use of MAbs in flow cytometry (see Chapter 11) represents the gold standard for the diagnosis and treatment of these malignancies.

> **KEY CONCEPTS: Functions of Lymphocytes**
> - When virgin lymphocytes encounter antigen, they proliferate and differentiate into effector T cells including CD4+ helper T cells and CD8+ T cells, and effector B lymphocytes.
> - Some of the progeny of antigen-activated T and B lymphocytes differentiate into **memory cells** that survive for long periods in a quiescent state.
> - Memory B cells carry surface IgG as their antigen receptor; memory T cells express the CD45RO variant of the leukocyte common antigen and increased levels of CAMs that function as chemical mediators involved in inflammatory processes throughout the body.
> - Persistent antigen-specific antibody titers are derived primarily from long-lived plasma cells.
> - Primary and secondary immune responses generate separate pools of long-lived plasma cells in the spleen, which migrate to the marrow where they occupy essential survival niches and can persist for the life of the host without the need for self-replenishment or turnover.
> - The marrow plasma cell pool does not require ongoing contributions from the memory B–cell pool for its maintenance. When depleted, plasma cells are replenished from the pool of memory B cells.
> - Persisting antigen, cytokines, or TLR signals may drive the memory B–cell pool to chronically differentiate into long-lived plasma cells for long-lived antibody production.

> **KEY CONCEPTS: Lymphocyte Characteristics**
> - Lymphocytes begin development in the thymus and experience an orderly rearrangement of the genes coding for an antigen receptor.
> - Lymphocyte maturation is a complicated process that lasts for a period of 3 weeks.
> - Early thymocytes lacking CD4 and CD8 surface membrane markers are referred to as double-negative thymocytes. These double-negative cells represent most of the population of T lymphocytes in the skin and intestinal and pulmonary epithelium.
> - The presence of low numbers of double-negative T cells in healthy individuals and the increase observed in association with lymphoproliferative disorders, graft-versus-host disease, and autoimmune diseases suggest a pathogenic or immunoregulatory role for this population of T lymphocytes.
> - Double-positive cells are lymphocytes with both CD4+ and CD8+ surface markers that represent the second stage of thymocyte development.
> - T cells must recognize foreign antigen in association with class I or II MHC molecules. Recognition of self-MHC is called *positive selection*. Without self-recognition, the cell will die without ever leaving the thymus gland.
> - A second selection process, negative selection, takes place among the surviving double-positive T cells.

DEVELOPMENT OF T LYMPHOCYTES

Virgin or naïve lymphocytes (Fig. 4.6) express high-molecular-weight variants of leukocyte common antigen. When these cells do encounter antigens, they proliferate and differentiate into effector lymphocytes that have functions related to protective immune responses. Effector T cells include cytokine-secreting CD4+ helper T cells and CD8+ cytotoxic T lymphocytes. Effector B lymphocytes are antibody-secreting plasma cells.

Some of the progeny of antigen-activated T and B lymphocytes differentiate into memory cells that survive for long periods in a quiescent state. These memory cells are responsible for the rapid and enhanced response to a previously encountered antigen. Memory B cells carry surface IgG as their antigen receptor; memory T cells express the CD45RO variant of the leukocyte common antigen and increased levels of CAMs that function as chemical mediators involved in inflammatory processes throughout the body. Persistent antigen-specific antibody titers are derived primarily from long-lived plasma cells. Primary and secondary immune responses generate separate pools of long-lived plasma cells in the spleen, which migrate to the marrow where they occupy essential survival niches and can persist for the life of the host without the need for self-replenishment or turnover. The marrow plasma cell pool does not require ongoing contributions from the memory B–cell pool for its maintenance. When depleted, plasma cells are replenished from the pool of memory B cells. Persisting antigen, cytokines, or TLR signals may drive the memory B–cell pool to chronically differentiate into long-lived plasma cells for long-lived antibody production.

Most lymphocytes found in the circulating blood are T cells derived from bone marrow progenitor cells that mature in the thymus gland (Table 4.3). These cells are responsible for cellular immune responses and are involved in the regulation of antibody reactions in conjunction with B lymphocytes.

During cellular development, T-lymphocyte function–associated antigens vary in expression. Some antigens appear early in cellular development and remain on mature T cells. Others appear at an early or intermediate stage of cellular maturation and are lost before maturity.

Early Cellular Differentiation and Development

Differentiation of a lymphocyte begins in the thymus, with the thymocyte. Early surface markers on thymocytes that are committed to becoming T cells include CD44 and CD25. As thymocytes develop, there is an orderly rearrangement of the genes coding for an antigen receptor.

Maturation is a complicated process that lasts for a period of 3 weeks. During this period, cells filter through the cortex to the medulla of the thymus. Thymic stromal cells include fibroblasts, macrophages, epithelial cells, and dendritic cells; all these cell types play a role in T-cell development.

Double-Negative Thymocytes

Early thymocytes lacking CD4 and CD8 surface membrane markers are referred to as double-negative thymocytes. These cells proliferate in the outer cortex of the thymus under the influence of interleukin-7 (IL-7). IL-7 is critical for this growth and differentiation.

Rearrangement of the genes that code for the antigen receptor, the T-cell receptor (TCR), begins at this developmental stage. CD3 constitutes the main part of the T-cell antigen receptor. The configuration of two of the eight chains of the receptor has variable regions that recognize specific antigens. These are coded for by selecting gene segments and deleting others.

Rearrangement of the beta (β) chain occurs first; the appearance of a functional β chain on the cell surface sends a signal to suppress any further β-chain gene rearrangements. The combination of the β chain with the CD3 forms the pre-TRC. Signaling by the β chain promotes the development of a CD4+ and CD8+ thymocyte.

Thymocytes that express gamma (γ) and delta (δ) chains follow a different developmental pathway. Cells expressing gamma-delta (γδ) chains typically remain both CD4– and CD8–. These double-negative cells represent most of the population of T lymphocytes in the skin and intestinal and pulmonary epithelium.

Double-negative lymphocytes circulating CD3+CD4–CD8– T cells are usually described as double-negative lymphocytes and are thought to represent a distinct T-cell lineage. The presence of low numbers of double-negative T cells in healthy individuals and the increase observed in association with lymphoproliferative disorders,

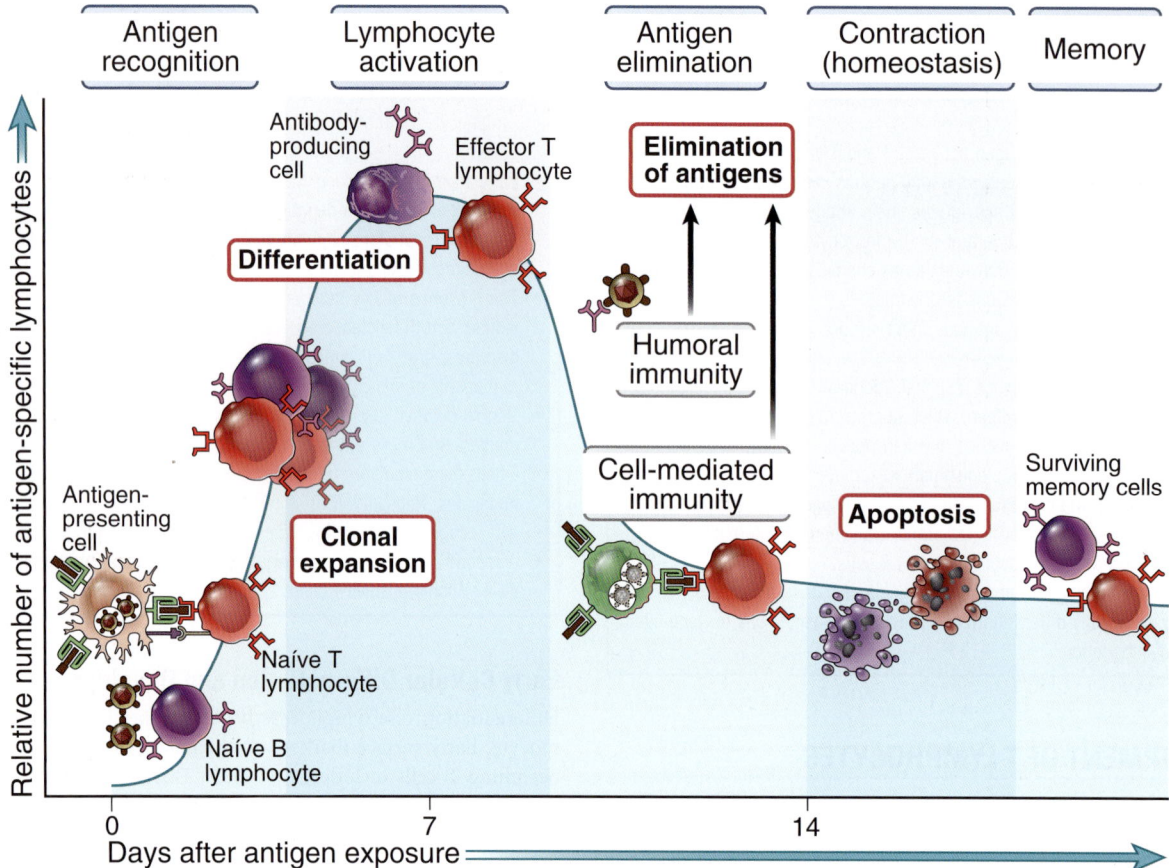

Fig. 4.6 Phases of an Adaptive Immune Response. An adaptive immune response consists of distinct phases; the first three are the recognition of antigens, activation of lymphocytes, and elimination of antigen (effector phase). The response declines as antigen-stimulated lymphocytes die by apoptosis, restoring homeostasis, and the antigen-specific cells that survive are responsible for memory. The duration of each phase may vary in different immune responses. The y-axis represents an arbitrary measure of the magnitude of the response. These principles apply to humoral immunity (measured by B lymphocytes) and cell-mediated immunity (mediated by T lymphocytes). (From Abbas AK, Lichtman AH: *Basic immunology: functions and disorders of the immune system*, ed 5, Philadelphia, 2016, Elsevier.)

TABLE 4.3	Lymphocyte Subset Characteristics		
Type	Function(s)	Phenotypic Marker	Peripheral Blood (% of Total)
Helper T (T$_h$) cells	Stimulate B-cell growth and differentiation (humoral immunity); macrophage activation by secreted cytokines (cell-mediated immunity)	CD3+, CD4+, CD8–	50–60
Cytotoxic T (Tc) cells	Lysis of virus-infected cells, tumor cells, and allografts (cell-mediated immunity); macrophage activation by secreted cytokines (cell-mediated immunity)	CD3+, CD4–, CD8+	20–25
Natural killer (NK) cells	Lysis of virus-infected cells (ADCC)	Fc receptor for IgG or CD16 cells	?10
B cells	Antibody production (humoral immunity)	Fc receptors, MHC class II, CD19, CD21	10–15

ADCC, Antibody-dependent cellular cytotoxicity; *MHC*, major histocompatibility complex; *?*, questionable.

graft-versus-host disease, and autoimmune diseases suggest a pathogenic or immunoregulatory role for this population of T lymphocytes.

Double-Positive Thymocytes

Cells with both CD4+ and CD8+, or double-positive, surface markers represent the second stage of thymocyte development. These thymocytes begin to demonstrate rearranged genes coding for the alpha (α) chain. When the CD3-αβ receptor complex (TCR) is expressed on the cell surface, a process known as *positive selection* permits only double-positive cells with functional TCR receptors to survive. T cells must recognize foreign antigens in association with class I or class II MHC molecules. Any thymocyte that is unable to recognize self-MHC dies without ever leaving the thymus gland. Functioning T lymphocytes must be able to recognize a foreign antigen along with MHC molecules. A second selection process, negative selection, takes place among the surviving double-positive T cells. Only 1% to 3% of **double-positive thymocytes** survive in the cortex.

Double-positive CD4 and CD8 Tαβ cells have been reported in normal individuals and also in different pathologic conditions, including inflammatory diseases, viral infections, and cancer, but their function remains to be elucidated. Double-negative cells may act like NK cells because they are capable of binding to many natural, unprocessed cell surface molecules. In addition, these cells are capable of recognizing antigens without being presented by MHC proteins. Consequently, NK cells may represent an important bridge between natural and adaptive immunity.

> **KEY CONCEPTS: Differentiation of CD4 and CD8 Lymphocytes**
> - When mature T cells leave the thymus, survivors of selection exhibit only one marker, CD4+ or CD8+, and migrate to the medulla and subsequently gain functional maturity with their entry into the peripheral blood circulation.
> - The repertoire of antigen receptors in the entire population of lymphocytes is extremely large and diverse. This increases the probability that an individual lymphocyte will encounter an antigen that binds to its receptor and triggers activation and proliferation of the cell. This process, clonal selection, accounts for most of the basic properties of the adaptive immune system.
> - T-lymphocyte subset divisions are not absolute, with considerable overlap or redundancy in function among the different subsets.
> - CD4 T lymphocytes represent a population of cells that are central to protection against a wide range of pathogens.
> - Two subsets of activated CD4 T cells are type 1 helper T (Th1) and type 2 helper T (Th2) cells.
> - Some CD4 T-cell populations are actually distinct lineages of cells already distinguished from one another when they emerge from the thymus, such as "natural" regulatory T (nT$_{reg}$) cells and NK T cells (NKT cells).
> - Several subtypes of lymphocytes represent alternative patterns of differentiation of naïve CD4 T cells; they are essential for the differentiation processes that are central to the mounting of effective and regulated immune responses.
> - Helper T lymphocytes, or helper T (Th) cells, play critical roles in orchestrating the adaptive immune responses and can be assigned to three major CD4+ effector subsets: Th1, Th2, and Th17.
> - Cytotoxic T lymphocytes, or cytotoxic T (Tc) cells, are effector cells found in the peripheral blood that are capable of directly destroying virally infected target cells.
> - Most Tc cells are CD8+ and recognize antigen on the target cell surface associated with MHC class I molecules (e.g., human leukocyte antigen [HLA] types A, B, and C) or MHC class I alone.
> - Suppressor T lymphocytes, or suppressor T (Ts) cells, are functionally defined T cells that downregulate the actions of other T and B cells. Ts cells have no unique markers.
> - Defining properties of memory CD8 T cells include being present in higher numbers than naïve CD8 T cells and the ability to mount a rapid secondary response with a lower response threshold.
> - T cells are clonally restricted, so that each T cell expresses a receptor that can interact with a given peptide. Each lymphocyte makes only one type of antigen receptor and can recognize only a very limited number of antigens. The entire lymphocyte population has an enormous number of different, specific antigen receptors.
> - APCs are a group of functionally defined cells capable of taking up antigens and presenting them to lymphocytes in a form that they can recognize. APCs take up antigens (e.g., dendritic cells, macrophages, B cells, even tissue cells) in various ways.
> - There are two major pathways of antigen processing for the APC and target cell: endogenous and exogenous. For both systems of antigen presentation, recognition of the antigen by the T cells is described as being MHC restricted, a process whereby T cells recognize only antigen presented by self-MHC molecules.
> - Innate lymphoid cells (ILCs) are lymphocyte-like cells that produce cytokines and perform similar functions to CD4+ or CD8+ effector cells but do not express a T-cell antigen receptor (TCR) that is specific for the peptide displayed by the MHC molecule.

Later Cellular Differentiation and Development of T Lymphocytes

When mature T cells leave the thymus, their TCRs are CD4+ or CD8+. Survivors of selection exhibit only one type of these two markers, CD4+ or CD8+, and migrate to the medulla. These cells gain functional maturity with their entry into the peripheral blood circulation.

T cells develop into a variety of clones. Each lymphocyte displays a single type of structurally unique receptor. The repertoire of antigen receptors in the entire population of lymphocytes is extremely large and diverse. This increases the probability that an individual lymphocyte will encounter an antigen that binds to its receptor, thereby triggering activation and proliferation of the cell. This process, clonal selection, accounts for most of the basic properties of the adaptive immune system.

Antigen receptors for common pathogens need to be reinvented by every generation of cells. Because the binding sites of antigen receptors arise from random genetic mechanisms, the receptor repertoire contains binding sites that can react not only with infectious microorganisms but also with innocuous environmental antigens and self-antigens.

T-Lymphocyte Subsets

T-lymphocyte subset divisions are not absolute, with considerable overlap or redundancy in function among the different subsets. This classification is based on the blends of cytokines that they produce. The following factors can influence the terminal differentiation of lymphocytes:
- Type of APC
- Affinity of the specific antigenic peptide
- Types of costimulatory molecules expressed by APCs
- Cytokines acting on T cells during primary activation through TCRs

A hierarchy is apparent among these factors and is determined by how they influence T-cell differentiation. Certain cytokines acting directly on T cells during primary activation appear to be the most proximal or direct mediators of CD4+ T-cell differentiation.

Certain T cells carry out delayed hypersensitivity reactions. These T cells react with antigen MHC class II on APCs and create their effects mainly through cytokine production. These cells generally are of the CD4+ phenotype.

CD4 Lymphocytes

CD4 T lymphocytes represent a population of cells that are central to protection against a wide range of pathogens. CD4 T cells act through their capacity to help B cells make antibodies; to induce macrophages to develop enhanced microbicidal activity; to recruit neutrophils, eosinophils, and basophils to sites of infection and inflammation; to produce cytokines and chemokines; and to coordinate a variety of immune responses.

In 1986, two subsets of activated CD4 T cells, Th1 and Th2 cells, were identified based on those that produced IFN-γ as their signature cytokine and those that produced IL-4. Th1 cells and Th2 cells also differ from each other in their functions. Since the identification of Th1 and Th2, the importance of the distinct differentiated forms of CD4 T cells and the knowledge of the mechanisms through which these cells achieve their differentiated state have greatly expanded. Naïve conventional CD4 T cells are open to various distinct fates that are determined by the pattern of signals they receive during their initial interaction with antigen.

Some CD4 T-cell populations are actually distinct lineages of cells already distinguished from one another when they emerge from the thymus, such as nT$_{reg}$ cells and NKT cells. Several subtypes of lymphocytes represent alternative patterns of differentiation of naïve CD4

T cells. The Jak/Stat pathways and a specific Stat in association with the master regulators, T-bet, GATA-3, RORγt, and Foxp3, are essential for the differentiation processes that are central to the mounting of effective and regulated immune responses.

In all processes of differentiation, whole sets of genes are activated or repressed during the transition of naïve CD4 T cells to Th1, Th2, Th17, and T-regulatory (T_{reg}) cells. These differentiated states are associated with changes in the conformation of key genes. Analysis of genome-wide epigenetic modification patterns of histone modification revealed that modifications are critical for regulation of gene expression in the major types of lymphocytes.

Subsets of CD4+ Effector T Lymphocytes

Initially immunologists believed that there were fundamentally two types of immune responses that require the action of CD4 T cells. One was cell mediated; the other was antibody mediated. As T-cell cloning technology developed in the early 1980s, many cytokines were discovered. Based on this evidence, mature CD4 T cells could be subdivided into two distinct populations with different sets of products and unique functions. Transcription factors are important during the process of Th differentiation. Transcription factors are either specifically expressed or function differently in each of the lineages.

Helper T lymphocytes, or Th cells, can be assigned to three major CD4+ effector subsets:

- Th1
- Th2
- Th17

These major subsets function in host defense against different types of infectious pathogens and are associated with different types of tissue injuries in autoimmune diseases. Th cells play critical roles in orchestrating the adaptive immune responses. They exert their influence mainly by secreting cytokines and chemokines that activate and/or recruit target cells.

Th1 and Th2 cells can promote the development of cytotoxic cells. Th1 cells interact most effectively with mononuclear phagocytes; Th2 cells release cytokines that are required for B-cell differentiation. Activation through the TCR is a requirement for initiating terminal differentiation, but the signals from the TCR appear to be phenotype neutral.

Properties of the Th1 subset. Th1 (Figs. 4.7 and 4.8) cells are responsible for cell-mediated effector mechanisms against intracellular pathogens. In humans, Th1 cells play a particularly important role in resistance to mycobacterial infections. Th1 cells are also responsible for the induction of some autoimmune diseases.

The principal cytokine products of Th1 cells are IFN-γ, lymphotoxin-α (LTα), and IL-2. IFN-γ produced by Th1 cells is important in activating macrophages to increase their microbicidal activity. Characterized by high IFN-γ production, Th1 responses promote the elimination of intracellular pathogens. The presence of IL-12 during primary T-cell activation leads to strong development of Th1 responses.

IL-2 production is important for CD4 T-cell memory. IFN-γ+ IL-2 cells are regarded as precursors of the Th1 memory cells. IL-2 stimulation of CD8 cells during their priming phase is critical for CD8 memory formation.

Properties of the Th2 subset. Th2 cells play a greater role in the regulation of antibody production (Figs. 4.9 and 4.10).

Th2 cells mediate host defense against extracellular parasites, including helminths. They are important in the induction and persistence of asthma and other allergic inflammatory diseases.

Th2 cells produce IL-4, IL-5, IL-9, IL-10, IL-13, IL-25, and amphiregulin. IL-4 is the positive-feedback cytokine for Th2 cell differentiation. Characterized by IL-4 and IL-5, Th2 responses promote a different type of effector response that involves IgE production and

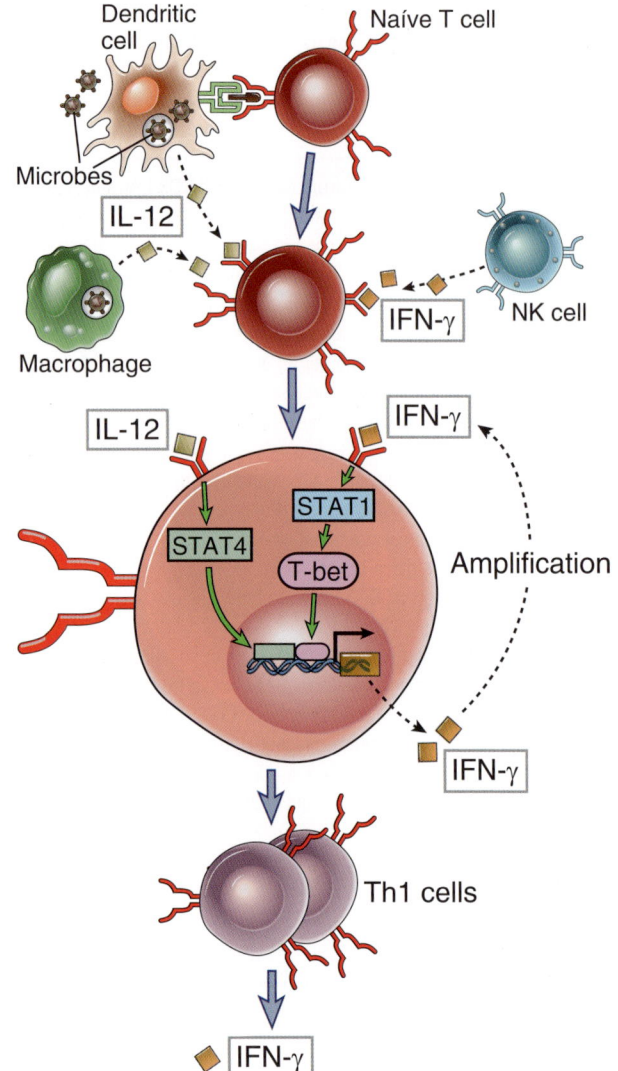

Fig. 4.7 Development of Type 1 Helper T (Th1) Cells. IL-12 produced by dendritic cells and macrophages in response to microbes, including intracellular microbes, and IFN-γ produced by NK cells (all part of the early innate immune response to the microbes) activate the transcription factors T-bet, STAT1, and STAT4, which stimulate the differentiation of naïve CD4+ T cells to the Th1 subset. IFN-γ produced by the Th1 cells amplifies this response and inhibits the development of Th2 and Th17 cells. *IFN-γ*, Interferon gamma; *IL-12*, interleukin 12; *NK*, natural killer; *STAT1*, signal transducer and activator of transcription 1; *STAT4*, signal transducer and activator of transcription 4. (From Abbas AK, Lichtman AH: *Cellular and molecular immunology,* ed 8, Philadelphia, 2015, Elsevier.)

eosinophils capable of eliminating larger extracellular pathogens, such as helminths. IgE binds to receptors on basophils and mast cells, which can lead to the secretion of active mediators such as histamine and serotonin, and to the production of several cytokines, including IL-4, IL-13, and TNF-α. IL-5 plays a critical role in recruiting eosinophils. In addition to its effect on mast cells and lymphocytes, IL-9 induces mucin production in epithelial cells during allergic reactions. IL-10, produced by Th2 cells, suppresses Th1 cell proliferation. IL-10 can also suppress dendritic cell function. IL-13 is the effector cytokine in the expulsion of helminths and in the induction of airway hypersensitivity.

When repeated pathogen exposure or persistent infections occur, the polarization of T-cell responses serves to focus the antigen-specific

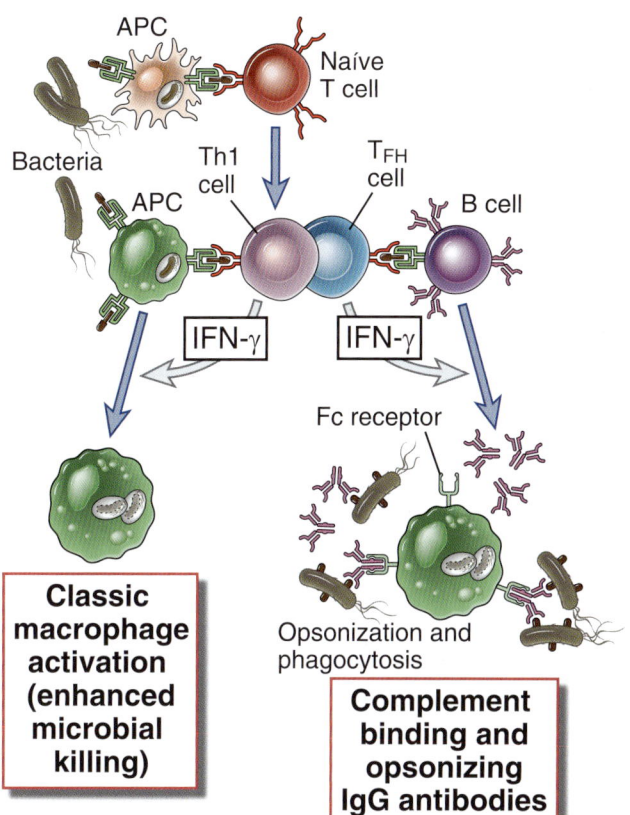

Fig. 4.8 Functions of Type 1 Helper T (Th1) Cells. Th1 cells secrete IFN-γ, which acts on macrophages to increase phagocytosis and killing of microbes in phagolysosomes and on B lymphocytes to stimulate production of immunoglobulin G (IgG) antibodies that opsonize microbes for phagocytosis. Help for antibody production may be provided, not by classic Th1 cells, most of which migrate out of lymphoid organs to sites of infection and inflammation, but by TFH cells that remain in lymphoid organs and produce IFN-γ. The role of IFN-γ in antibody production is established in mice but not in humans. Th1 cells also produce tumor necrosis factor, which activates neutrophils and promotes inflammation. *APC,* Antigen-presenting cell; *IFN-γ,* interferon gamma; *TFH,* follicular helper T; *Th1,* type 1 helper T. (From Abbas AK, Lichtman AH: *Cellular and molecular immunology,* ed 8, Philadelphia, 2015, Elsevier.)

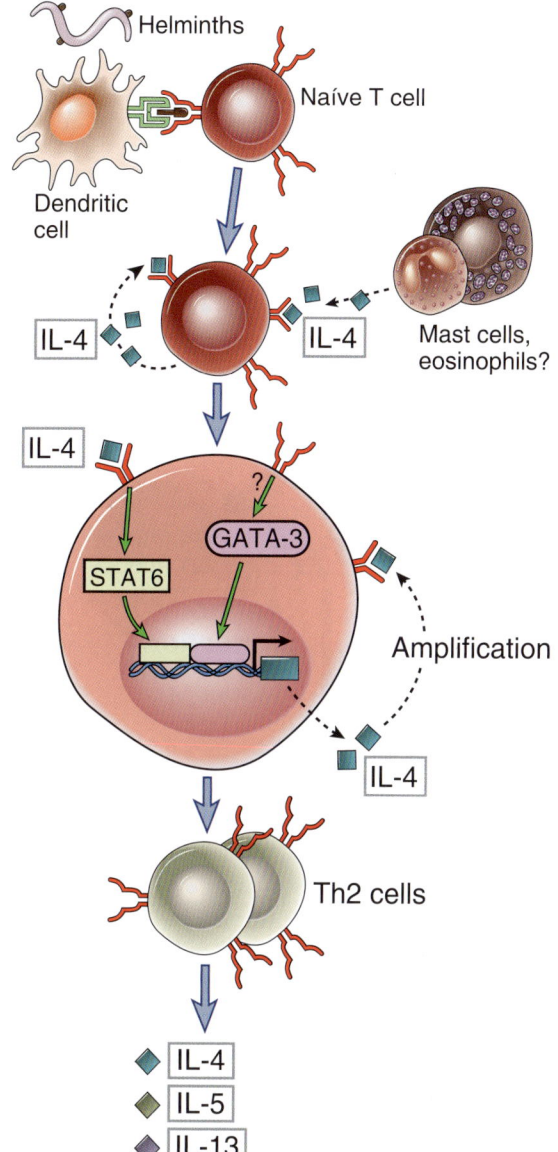

Fig. 4.9 Development of Type 2 Helper T (Th2) cells. IL-4 produced by activated T cells themselves or by mast cells and eosinophils, especially in response to helminths, activates the transcription factors GATA-3 and STAT6, which stimulate the differentiation of naïve CD4+ T cells to Th2 cells. IL-4 produced by the Th2 cells amplifies this response and inhibits the development of Th1 and Th17 cells. *GATA-3,* GATA binding protein 3; *IL-4,* interleukin 4; *IL-5,* interleukin 5; *IL-13,* interleukin 13; *STAT6,* signal transducer and activator of transcription 6; *Th2,* type 2 helper T. (From Abbas AK, Lichtman AH: *Cellular and molecular immunology,* ed 8, Philadelphia, 2015, Elsevier.)

response on a specific effector pathway, and IL-4 promotes Th2 development.

Amphiregulin is a member of the epidermal growth factor (EGF) family. In the absence of amphiregulin, the expulsion of the nematode *Trichuris muris* is delayed. Amphiregulin may also be important for the induction of airway hypersensitivity.

IL-25 (also known as *IL-17E*) is also a Th2 cytokine. IL-25, signaling through IL-17RB, enhances the production of IL-4, IL-5, and IL-13. IL-25 is also produced by lung epithelial cells in response to allergens. As a result, IL-25 serves as an initiation factor and as an amplification factor for Th2 responses. IL-25 can induce the production of chemokines, including RANTES (CCL5) and eotaxin (CCL11) that recruit eosinophils.

Properties of the Th17 subset. Th17 cells (Figs. 4.11 and 4.12) have been recognized much more recently, but there is now a growing body of research that indicates not only that these cells exist, but that they play a critical function in protection against microbial challenges, especially extracellular bacteria and fungi. Some of the autoimmune responses formally attributed to Th1 cells have now been demonstrated to be mediated, at least in part, by Th17 cells.

In addition to mediating immune responses against extracellular bacteria and fungi, Th17 cells are responsible for, or participate in, the induction of many organ-specific autoimmune diseases.

Th17 cells produce IL-17a, IL-17f, IL-21, and IL-22. Both IL-17a and IL-17f recruit and activate neutrophils during immune responses against extracellular bacteria and fungi. IL-21 made by Th17 cells is a stimulatory factor for Th17 differentiation and serves as a positive-feedback amplifier, as does IFN-γ for Th1 and IL-4 for Th2 cells. IL-21 also acts on CD8 T cells, B cells, NK cells, and dendritic cells.

IL-22 is produced by Th17 cells through IL-6– or IL-23–mediated Stat3 activation. transforming growth factor β (TGF-β) inhibits IL-22 expression. IL-22 mediates host defense against bacterial pathogens

84 PART I Basic Immunologic Mechanisms

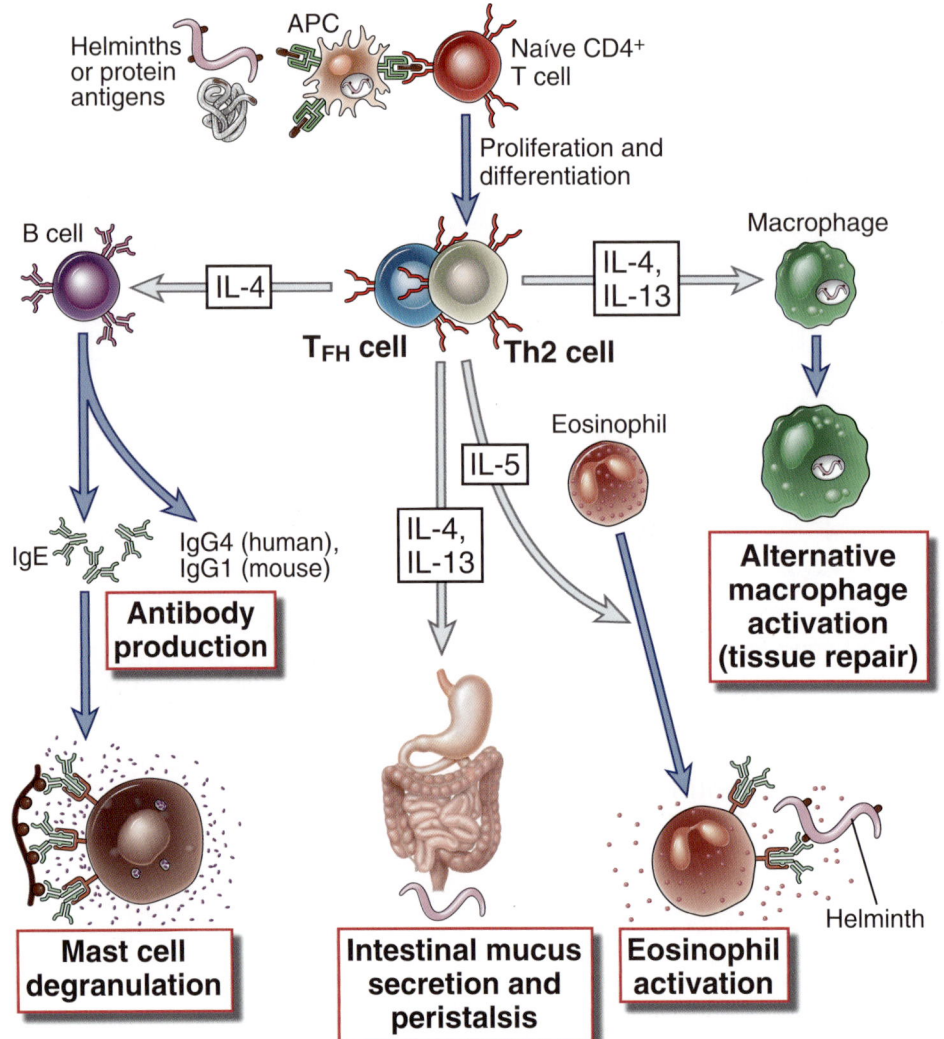

Fig. 4.10 **Functions of Type 2 Helper T (Th2) Cells.** CD4+ T cells that differentiate into Th2 cells secrete IL-4, IL-5, and IL-13. IL-4 and IL-13 act on B cells to stimulate production of antibodies that bind to mast cells, such as IgE. Help for antibody production may be provided by TNF cells that produce Th2 cytokines and reside in lymphoid organs, and not by classic Th2 cells. IL-4 is also an autocrine growth and differentiation cytokine for Th2 cells. IL-5 activates eosinophils, a response that is important for defense against helminthic infections. IL-4 and IL-13 are involved in immunity at mucosal barriers, induce an alternative pathway of macrophage activation, and inhibit classic Th1-mediated macrophage activation. *APC*, Antigen-presenting cell; *IgE*, immunoglobulin E; *IL-4*, interleukin 4; *IL-5*, interleukin 5; *IL-13*, interleukin 13; *TFH*, follicular helper T; *Th2*, type 2 helper T. (From Abbas AK, Lichtman AH: *Cellular and molecular immunology*, ed 8, Philadelphia, 2015, Elsevier.)

such as *Klebsiella pneumoniae* and *Citrobacter rodentium*, but these functions may essentially depend on IL-23 stimulation of innate cells to produce IL-22 rather than on the action of Th17 cells.

CD8+ Cytotoxic T Lymphocytes

Cytotoxic T lymphocytes, or Tc cells, are effector cells found in the peripheral blood that are capable of directly destroying virally infected target cells (Fig. 4.13). Most Tc cells are CD8+ and recognize antigens on the target cell surface associated with MHC class I molecules (e.g., HLA types A, B, and C) or MHC class I alone. This process is demonstrated by the immune response to virus-infected cells or tumor cells.

In a primary viral infection, naïve CD8+ T cells are primed in secondary lymph nodes and consequently proliferate and differentiate into effector CD8+ T cells to eliminate virus-infected cells. After clearance of the virus, most effector CD8+ T cells contract because of apoptosis, but a small number of these CD8+ T cells form a memory T-cell pool.

Studies have demonstrated that human CD8+ T cells undergo a change in the expression of costimulatory molecules (e.g., CD27, CD28, and CD45RA) on their surface, according to their differentiation and maturation. Cytolytic effector molecules, perforin, and **granzyme A-B** are considered markers for effector CD8+ T cells because they are the actual functional molecules for killing target cells.

Naïve and central memory CD8+ T cells express the membrane marker CCR7 for homing to secondary lymph nodes, but effector memory and effector CD8+ T cells express the chemokine receptors for inflammatory cytokines, which enable the cells to migrate toward infected and inflamed sites. A unique subset of the effector CD8+ T-cell population expresses CXCR1. These CXCR1 CD8+ T cells possess chemotactic activity toward the CDCR1 ligand IL-8, a potent inflammatory cytokine produced in inflamed tissues and in tissues infected with some viruses (Box 4.5), such as human cytomegalovirus (HCMV) or influenza A. This suggests that these CXCR1+ effector CD8+ T cells

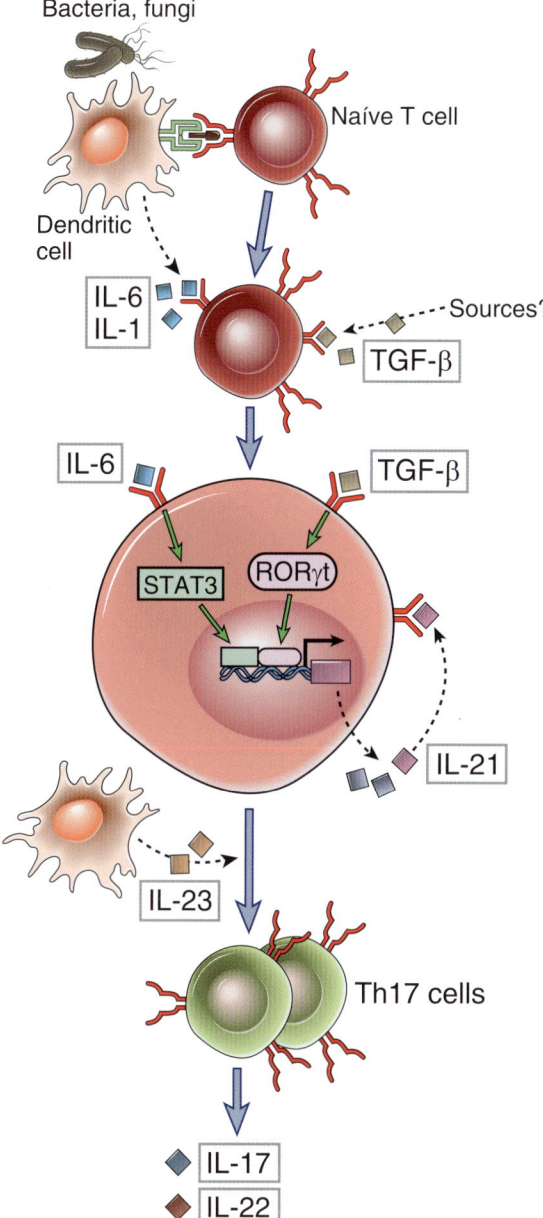

Fig. 4.11 Development of Type 17 Helper T (Th17) Cells. IL-1 and IL-6 produced by APCs and TGF-β produced by various cells activate the transcription factors RORγt and STAT3, which stimulate the differentiation of naïve CD4+ T cells to the Th17 subset. IL-23, which is also produced by APCs, especially in response to fungi, stabilizes the Th17 cells. TGF-β may promote Th17 responses indirectly by suppressing Th1 and Th2 cells, both of which inhibit Th17 differentiation. IL-21 produced by the Th17 cells amplifies this response. *APC,* Antigen-presenting cell; *IL-1,* interleukin 1; *IL-6,* interleukin 6; *IL-17,* interleukin 17; *IL-21,* interleukin 21; *IL-22,* interleukin 22; *IL-23,* interleukin 23; *STAT3,* signal transducer and activator of transcription 3; *TGF-β,* transforming growth factor-β; *Th1,* type 1 helper T; *Th2,* type 2 helper T; *Th17,* type 17 helper T. (From Abbas AK, Lichtman AH: *Cellular and molecular immunology,* ed 8, Philadelphia, 2015, Elsevier.)

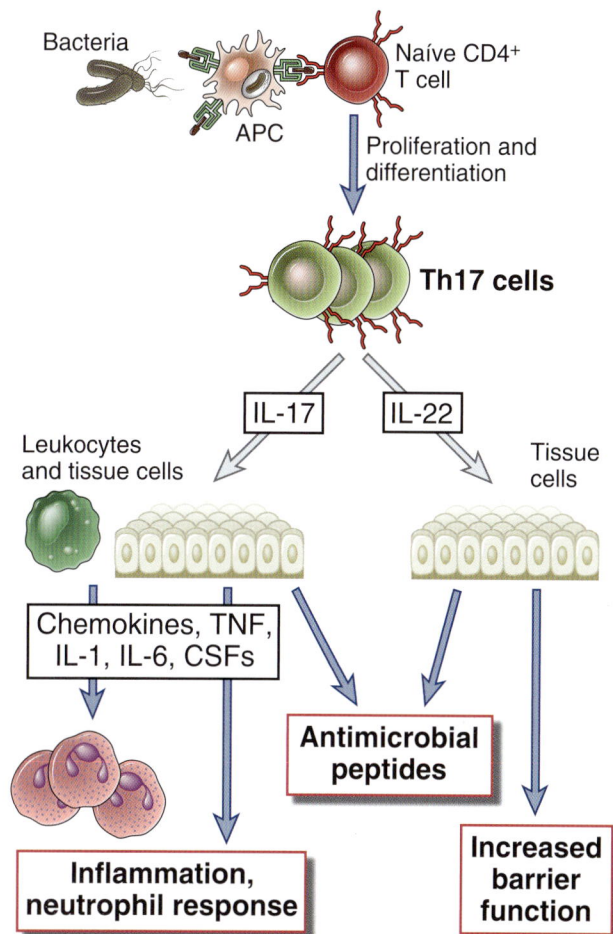

Fig. 4.12 Functions of Type 17 Helper T (Th17) Cells. Cytokines produced by Th17 cells stimulate local production of chemokines that recruit neutrophils and other leukocytes, increase production of antimicrobial peptides (defensins), and promote epithelial barrier functions. *APC,* Antigen-presenting cell; *CSF,* colony-stimulating factor; *IL-1,* interleukin 1; *IL-6,* interleukin 6; *IL-17,* interleukin 17; *IL-22,* interleukin 22; *Th17,* type 17 helper T; *TNF,* tumor necrosis factor. (From Abbas AK, Lichtman AH: *Cellular and molecular immunology,* ed 8, Philadelphia, 2015, Elsevier.)

immediately migrate to inflamed and infected sites to exert their effector function in the initial stage of an immune response. It is possible that effector CD8+ T-cell subsets are functionally distinct populations of T lymphocytes.

In addition to destruction of virally infected MHC class I–bearing targets, Tc cells are major effectors in allograft organ rejection. Tc cells express CD4 or CD8, depending on the MHC antigen restriction that governs their antigen recognition (i.e., class I or class II antigens [Fig. 4.14]).

Suppressor T lymphocytes, or Ts cells, are functionally defined T cells that downregulate the actions of other T and B cells. Ts cells have no unique markers. Although antigen-specific suppression was described in 1970, and many investigators believe that Ts cells are critical in various phases of immunoregulation, peripheral tolerance, and autoimmunity, their mode of action is unclear. Many Ts cells are CD8+ and may operate through secretion of free TCRs.

Memory T cells persist long term, can occur without specific antigen, and cycle in vivo even without antigen stimulation. Maintenance and turnover are dependent on IL-7 and IL-15 in the absence of antigen. Defining properties of memory CD8 T cells include:
- Present in higher numbers than naïve CD8 T cells
- Able to mount a rapid secondary response with a lower response threshold
- Stable, long-term, antigen-independent maintenance
- Homeostatic turnover and survival because IL-7 and IL-15 cytokines permit replenishment of pool

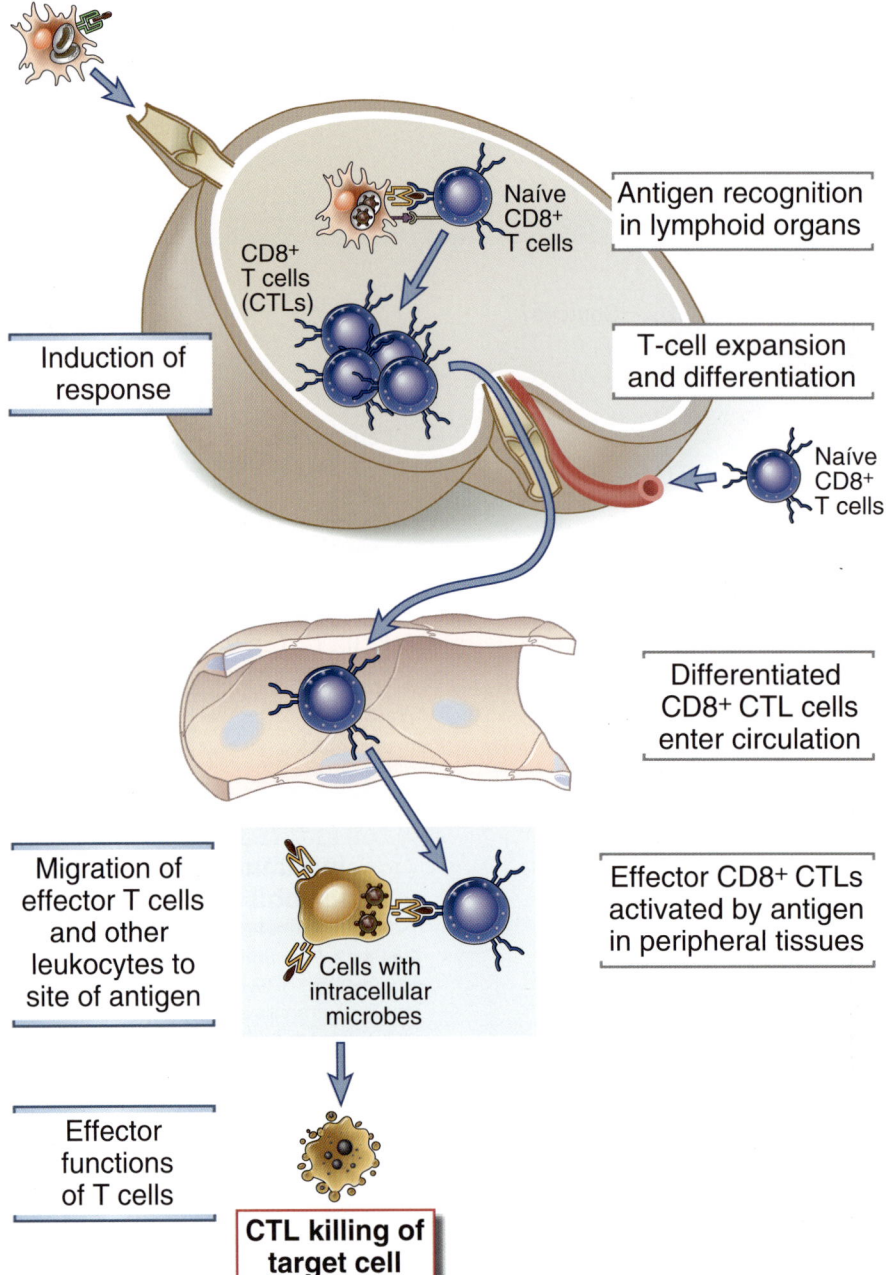

Fig. 4.13 Induction and Effector Phases of CD8+ T-Cell Responses. Induction of response: CD8+ T cells recognize peptides that are derived from protein antigens and resented by dendritic cells in peripheral lymphoid organs. The T lymphocytes are stimulated to proliferate and differentiate into CTLs and memory cells, which enter the circulation. Migration of effector T cells and other leukocytes to the site of antigen: Effector T cells migrate to tissues at sites of infection, tumor growth, or graft rejection. Effector functions of T cells: CD8+ CTLs recognize the antigen in the tissues and respond by killing the cells where the antigen is produced. *CTL*, Cytotoxic T lymphocyte. (From Abbas AK, Lichtman AH: *Cellular and molecular immunology*, ed 8, Philadelphia, 2015, Elsevier.)

Antigen Recognition by T Cells

There are different types of antigen recognition by T lymphocytes:
1. CD8+ T-cell cytoplasmic antigens
2. CD4+ T-cell phagolysosomal antigens

T cells are clonally restricted, so that each T cell expresses a receptor that can interact with a given peptide. Each lymphocyte makes only one type of antigen receptor and can recognize only a very limited number of antigens. Because receptors differ on each clone of cells, the entire lymphocyte population has an enormous number of different, specific antigen receptors.

The TCR of most T lymphocytes is composed of an α and a β polypeptide chain, with constant regions located close to the cell surface and the part that binds to the antigenic peptide of appropriate fit located away from the cell surface. The difference in structure of the distal regions of the alpha and beta chains allows the development of different clones of T cells. The TCR reacts with antigens in the context of MHC class I or II molecules on an APC.

T cells recognize protein antigens in the form of peptide fragments presented at the cell surface by MHC class I or class II molecules.

CHAPTER 4 Cellular Activities and Clinical Disorders of Innate and Adaptive Immunity

> **BOX 4.5 Viral Responses by Lymphocytes**
>
> **CD4+ T-Cell Responses to Viruses**
> - CD4+ T cells provide important help to B cells to synthesize antibodies.
> - CD4+ T cells induce macrophages to develop enhanced microbicidal activity.
> - CD4+ T cells recruit neutrophils, eosinophils, and basophils to sites of infection and inflammation; produce cytokines and chemokines; and coordinate a variety of immune responses.
>
> **CD8+ T-Cell Responses to Viruses**
> - CD8+ T cells expand in concentration dramatically during the first 1–2 weeks postinfection; for example, in infection with Epstein-Barr virus or HIV.
> - CD8+ T cells are critical for control of many viral infections because they directly destroy infected cells and produce high levels of antiviral cytokines such as interferon (IFN-γ) and tumor necrosis factor α.
> - Rapid effector functions and numerical expansion are the keys to viral control.
> - CD8+ T cells persist as memory cells for long-term protection.

cells and marker CD80 on APCs). This interaction also triggers several intracellular signaling pathways.

T-Cell Activation

T-cell activation requires a minimum of two signals:
- Signal 1 is delivered by the TCR-CD3 complex through interaction of the TCR α and β chains as they recognize peptide presented by a class I CD8+ T cell or a class II CD4+ T-cell MHC molecule.
- Signal 2 is usually provided by the engagement of CD28 on the T cell with the costimulatory molecule CD80 or CD86 on the APC. The surface markers CD137 and CD134 also provide costimulation to T cells.

The optimal combination of effector function, proliferation, and survival requires both signals. Delivery of signal 1 without costimulation, which often occurs in tumor-infiltrating lymphocytes, leads to **anergy** and apoptosis, which limits the antitumor response of the cells.

Activation of T cells can lead to the following:
- Cell division
- Cytokine secretion by T cells
- Expression by T cells of antigens associated with activated state

Activated T cells frequently express activation antigens (see Box 4.5). Expression of CD69 occurs within 12 hours of activation, followed by CD25 (IL-2 receptor) and CD71 (transferrin receptor) in 1 to 3 days. Alternatively, in the case of Tc cells, interaction with antigen through the specific TCR leads to destruction of target cells.

If a cell does not receive a full set of signals, it will not divide and may even become anergic. Peripheral T cells generally exist in a resting state (G0 or G1). T-cell activation is a complex reaction involving transmembrane signaling and intracellular enzyme activation steps. It is through soluble cytokines that T-cell regulation influences the action of other T cells, accessory cells, and nonimmune constituents. When activated by the proper signals, T cells may carry out one or more of the following functions:
1. Proliferation
2. Differentiation
3. Production of cytokines
4. Development of effector function

T-Independent Antigen Triggering

Some antigens, particularly polysaccharide polymers (e.g., dextran), can trigger B cells without help from T cells. These **T-independent antigens** generally are not strong, provoke mainly IgM responses, and induce minimal immunologic memory.

Antigen Processing and Antigen Presentation to T Cells

Antigen-presenting cells (APCs) are a group of functionally defined cells capable of taking up antigens and presenting them to lymphocytes in a form that they can recognize. APCs take up antigens (e.g., dendritic cells, macrophages, B cells, and even tissue cells) in various ways. Some are collected in the periphery and transported to the secondary lymphoid tissues; other APCs normally reside in lymphoid tissues and intercept antigens as it arrives. B cells recognize antigens in a native form.

There are two major pathways of antigen processing for the APC and target cell: endogenous and exogenous. The **endogenous pathway** processes proteins that have been internalized, processed into fragments, and reexpressed at the cell surface membrane in association with MHC molecules. In this pathway, proteins in the cytoplasm are cleaved into peptide fragments about 20 amino acids in length. These fragments are then transported into the lumen of the endoplasmic reticulum by the transporter associated with the antigen-processing complex, where the fragments encounter newly formed heavy-chain molecules of MHC class I and their associated beta$_2$-microglobulin (β_2m) light chains. The

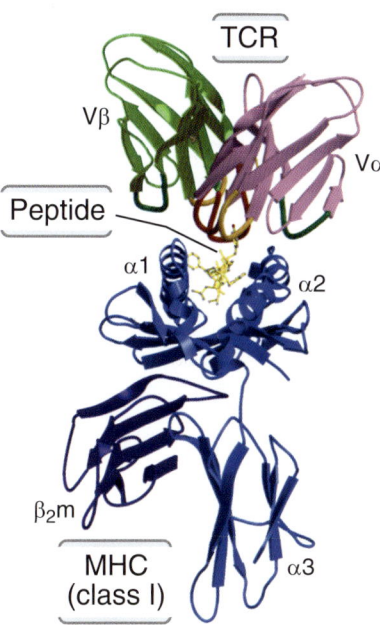

Fig. 4.14 Recognition of Peptide-Major Histocompatibility Complex (MHC) by the T-Cell Receptor (TCR). This ribbon diagram is drawn from the crystal structure of the extracellular portion of a peptide–MHC bound to a TCR that is specific for the peptide displayed by the MHC molecule. The peptide can be seen attached to the cleft at the top of the MHC molecule, and one residue of the peptide contacts the variable (V) region of a TCR. (Adapted from Bjorkman PJ: MHC restriction in three dimensions: a view of T cell receptor/ligand interactions, *Cell* 89:167–170, 1997.)

When the antigen-specific TCR on the T-cell surface (specifically the Z-β chains) of the CD3 complex interacts with the appropriate peptide–MHC complex, it triggers phosphorylation of the intracellular domains of the CD3 Z chains. Subsequently, the zeta-associated protein 70 (ZAP-70) binds to the phosphorylated Z chains and is activated.

Simultaneous colligation of the cell marker CD4 (or CD8) with the MHC class II (or class I) molecule results in the phosphorylation of particular kinases. These events stimulate the activation of at least three intracellular signaling cascades. T-cell activation also requires a second costimulatory signal (e.g., interaction between marker CD28 on T

heavy chain, light chain, and peptide form a trimeric complex, which is then transported to and expressed on the cell surface.

T cells that express the CD8+ cell–surface marker recognize antigens presented by MHC class I molecules. CD8+ functions as a coreceptor in this process, binding to an invariant region of the MHC class I molecule. Pathogen clearance requires that CD8+ effector cells produce inflammatory cytokines and develop cytolytic activity against infected target cells, after which a small number of memory cells survive that rapidly regain effector function in the event of rechallenge. During this process, a relatively homogeneous pool of naïve CD8+ T cells differentiates into heterogeneous pools of effector and memory CD8+ T cells.

In the exogenous pathway soluble proteins are taken up from the extracellular environment, generally by specialized or so-called professional APCs. The antigens are then processed in a series of intracellular acidic vesicles called *endosomes*. During this process, the endosomes intersect with vesicles that are transporting MHC class II molecules to the cell surface. CD4+ T cells recognize antigens that are presented by MHC class II molecules. As with CD8, the CD4 molecule functions as a coreceptor, increasing the strength of the interaction between the T cell and the APC.

For both systems of antigen presentation, recognition of the antigen by the T cells is described as being MHC restricted, a process whereby T cells recognize only antigen presented by self-MHC molecules.

INNATE LYMPHOID CELLS

ILCs are lymphocyte-like cells that produce cytokines and perform similar functions to CD4+ or CD8+ effector cells but do not express TCRs.

ILCs include several developmentally related subsets of bone marrow–derived cells with lymphoid morphology and effector functions similar to those of T cells, but lacking T-cell antigen receptors. The major functions of ILCs are to provide early defense against infectious pathogens, to recognize stress and damaged host cells, and to help eliminate these cells. ILCs also influence the nature of the subsequent adaptive immune response.

The first and best characterized ILCs are NK cells, which kill infected and damaged cells and secrete IFN-γ, a cytokine also produced by the Th1 subset of CD4+ effector T cells. Other subsets of ILCs secrete cytokines that are also produced by certain subsets of CD4+ Th cells, including IL-5, IL-13, IL-17, and IL-22.

> **KEY CONCEPTS: T-Regulatory Lymphocyte Facts**
> - T regulatory (T_{reg}) cells are immunoregulatory Th cells that control autoimmunity in the peripheral blood through dominant tolerance.
> - "Natural" regulatory T cells (nT_{reg}) cells that express the transcription factor Foxp3 and produce IL-10 are required for systemic immunologic tolerance.
> - Natural T_{reg} cells represent approximately 5% to 10% of the total CD4+ T-cell population.
> - "Induced" regulatory T cells (iT_{reg}) are nonredundant and essential for tolerance at mucosal surfaces, but their mechanisms of suppression and stability are unknown.
> - Other types of T_{reg} cells that can develop in the periphery are Tr1 and Th3 cells. Tr1 cells are CD4+ and are functionally induced by IL-10. Th3 progenitor cells are also CD4+.

T-REGULATORY LYMPHOCYTES

T_{reg} cells are immunoregulatory Th cells that control autoimmunity in the peripheral blood through dominant tolerance. nT_{reg} cells that express the transcription factor Foxp3 and produce IL-10 are required for systemic immunologic tolerance. "Induced" regulatory T cells (iT_{reg}) are nonredundant and essential for tolerance at mucosal surfaces, yet their mechanisms of suppression and stability are unknown.

Natural Treg cells, characterized by constitutive expression of CD25, are developed primarily in the thymus from positively selected thymocytes with a relatively high avidity for self-antigens. Natural T_{reg} cells represent approximately 5% to 10% of the total CD4+ T-cell population. The signal to develop into T_{reg} cells is thought to come from interactions between the TCR and MHC class II self-peptide complex expressed on the thymic stroma. In humans, natural T_{reg} cells express CD4 and CD25. An interesting subset of T_{reg} cells, those that express CD103, also known as *alpha E integrin*, is mainly found in the gut or at sites of inflammation.

Other types of T_{reg} cells that can develop in the periphery are Tr1 and Th3 cells. Tr1 cells are CD4+ and are functionally induced by IL-10. These T_{reg} cells, in turn, secrete IL-10 and regulate the immune system. Th3 progenitor cells are also CD4+. In vitro CD4+ cells have been shown to secrete TGF-β. CD8+ T_{reg} cells are less well characterized and are reportedly capable of suppressing CD4+ cells in vitro.

> **KEY CONCEPTS: Characteristics and Functions of Natural Killer Lymphocytes**
> - Natural killer (NK) lymphocytes have an associated effector function similar to T lymphocytes but lack T-lymphocyte antigen receptors.
> - NK cells belong to the innate immune system and unlike T or B lymphocytes of the adaptive or antigen-specific immune system, they do not rearrange TCR or Ig genes from their germline configuration.
> - Properties of NK cells include antigen specificity and clonal expansion.
> - NK cells express a variety of surface membrane markers, such as CD2, CD16, CD56^{dim}, CD56^{bright}, and CD57.
> - NK cells synthesize a number of cytokines involved in the modulation of hematopoiesis and immune responses, and in the regulation of their own activities. NK cells produce proinflammatory cytokines IL-12, IL-15, and IL-18; and cytokines IFN-α, TNF-α, and chemokines.
> - NK cells are able to bind and lyse antibody-coated nucleated cells through a membrane receptor that can recognize part of the heavy chain of Igs.
> - NK cells mediate antibody-dependent cellular cytotoxicity (ADCC) against sensitized IgG-coated targets.
> - NK cells are essential mediators of virus immunity with clonal expansion after viral exposure.

Natural Killer Cells

There are several developmentally related subsets of bone marrow–derived cells, including the natural killer lymphocyte, that have lymphoid morphology and associated effector function similar to T lymphocytes but lack T-lymphocyte antigen receptors. Natural killer (NK) cells are derived from CD34+ stem cells and belong to the innate immune system. Unlike T or B lymphocytes of the adaptive or antigen-specific immune system, NK cells do not rearrange TCR or Ig genes from their germline configuration. NK cells outnumber B cells in the circulation by a 3:1 ratio. They are believed to be relatively short-lived, but at any one time, there are likely more than 2 billion of them circulating in an adult.

A third major population of lymphocytes uses different strategies to discriminate self from nonself. The NK subpopulation of circulating lymphocytes (approximately 10%), NK lymphocytes, lacks conventional antigen receptors of T or B cells. Properties of NK cells include antigen specificity and clonal expansion, but they have a limited repertoire of NK cell receptors. Although these cells were previously classified as null cells, MAbs demonstrate that NK cells express a variety of surface membrane markers (Table 4.4). Most of these cells lack CD3 but express CD2, CD16, CD56^{dim}, CD56^{bright}, and CD57.

TABLE 4.4 T-Cell–Dependent and T-Cell–Independent Antigens

	T-Cell–Dependent Antigen	T-Cell–Independent Antigen
Structural properties	Complex	Simple
Chemical nature	Proteins, glycoproteins, lipoproteins	Polysaccharide; bacterial lipopolysaccharide
Antibody class induced	IgM, IgG, IgA, IgD, IgE	IgM
Activation model	MZ B cells shuttle between the MZ and follicles and transport antigens and pathogens to follicular DCs.	Type I activated by polysaccharide antigen
	DCs internalize antigen processes into peptides, present peptides together with MHC molecules to T cells.	Type II activated by dendritic/macrophages
	B cells bind antigens via surface Ig, transmit BCR signals and present peptides to T cells, and receive T-cell help (growth and differentiation factor that leads to plasma cell secretion of antibodies).	
Source of humoral antibody response	High-affinity antibodies, long-lived plasma cells	Short-lived plasma cells
Immunologic memory response	Yes	No
Present in most pathogenic microbes	Yes	No

BCR, B-cell receptor; *DC*, dendritic cell; *Ig*, immunoglobulin; *MHC*, major histocompatibility complex; *MZ*, marginal zone.
(Adapted from Abbas AK, Lichtman AH, Pillai S: *Cellular and molecular immunology*, ed 7, Philadelphia, 2012, Saunders.)

NK cells synthesize a number of cytokines involved in the modulation of hematopoiesis and immune responses, and in the regulation of their own activities. NK cells produce proinflammatory cytokines IL-12, IL-15, and IL-18; and cytokines IFN-α, TNF-α, and chemokines.

NK cells are classified as effector lymphocytes. The cells' surface marker, CD56, may mediate interactions between effector and target cells. NK cells are able to bind and lyse antibody-coated nucleated cells through a membrane receptor that can recognize part of the heavy chain of Igs. This enables NK cells to mediate ADCC against sensitized IgG-coated targets upon crosslinking of Fc(alpha) RIII. ADCC is remarkably similar to NK cells. Cytolytic function is activated by several mechanisms. Some, if not all, of the activation of NK cells is mediated by CD16, which exerts a regulatory role in their cytolytic function.

NK cells are essential mediators of virus immunity. Clonal expansion occurs after viral exposure. A deficiency in humans leads to uncontrolled viral replication and a poor clinical outcome. MHC class I is essential to NK and T-cell effector and surveillance functions. Human patients with selective NK cell deficiencies have recurrent, severe viral infections.

NK cells destroy target cells through an extracellular nonphagocytic mechanism referred to as a *cytotoxic reaction*. Target cells include tumor cells, some cells of the embryo, cells of the normal bone marrow and thymus, and microbial agents. A considerable number of NK cells may be present in other tissues, particularly in the lungs and liver, where they may play important roles in inflammatory reactions and in host defense, including defense against certain viruses (e.g., cytomegalovirus and hepatitis). NK cells will actively kill virally infected target cells, and, if this activity is completed before the virus has time to replicate, a viral infection may be stopped.

NK cells produce proinflammatory cytokines IL-12, IL-15, and IL-18; and cytokines IFN-α, TNF-α, and chemokines (discussed in Chapter 2). Several cytokines affect NK cell activation and proliferation. NK cells are highly responsive to IL-2, IL-7, and IL-12. These cytokines generate high cytokine–activated killer activity in these cells. Target cell recognition and the molecular identification and analysis of the involved NK cell receptors are undergoing intensive research. These molecules are mainly classified under the family of CAMs. The main class of effector CAMs shown to mediate NK cell functions is the leukocyte integrins, more specifically, the β_2 class of integrins.

Several NK cell surface molecules involved in target cell recognition and binding have been identified. NK cells recognize targets using several cell surface molecular receptors (e.g., CD2, CD69, NKR-P1) and a high density of the Fc receptor CD16 of IgG (FC-R III). They also receive inhibitory signals from MHC class I on potential target cells, transduced by a killer inhibitory receptor on the NK cell. CD56 may mediate interactions between effector and target cells. NK cells are able to bind and lyse antibody-coated nucleated cells through a membrane Fc receptor that can recognize part of the heavy chain of Igs. This enables NK cells to mediate ADCC activities. Some, if not all, of the activation of NK cells is mediated by CD16, which exerts a regulatory role in their cytolytic function. NK cells respond to crosslinking of CD16 and CD69 as follows:

- Increasing the rate of proliferation of NK cells
- Elevating the levels of TNF production within 4 hours of stimulation
- Increasing the expression of CD69 on the cell surface of NK cells
- Increasing the cytotoxicity activity against a normally resistant cell line (P815)

> **KEY CONCEPTS: Function and Characteristics of B Lymphocytes**
> - B cells mediate or regulate many other functions essential for immune homeostasis, including an antibody-independent pathogenic role of B cells, giving them the capability to present antigen.
> - The surface presentation of antigen, in the presence of various costimulatory molecules, elicits the assistance of T cells required to assist B-cell maturation, which in turns allows B cells to drive optimal T-cell activation and differentiation into memory subsets.
> - B cells also have the capacity to expand clonally, which allows them to become the numerically dominant APCs.
> - B cells regulate wound healing and transplanted tissue rejection, and also influence tumor development and tumor immunity.
> - One phenotypically distinct subset, designated B10 cells, has been shown to uniquely regulate T-cell–mediated inflammatory responses through the production of IL-10.
> - A subset of memory B cells in humans is not fully functional in children below 2 to 4 years of age. This is demonstrated by the high susceptibility of children to infections by encapsulated bacteria
> - B cells have **surface immunoglobulin (sIg)**, except for very immature lymphocytes and mature plasma cells.

B LYMPHOCYTES

The discovery of B cells began with the identification of an antibody that led to the eventual discovery of antibody-producing plasma cells. B cells represent a small proportion of the circulating peripheral blood lymphocytes. The unfavorable image of B lymphocytes in the pathogenesis of immune disease has been associated mainly with their capacity to produce harmful antibodies after differentiation into plasma cells.

Other roles have been discovered for B lymphocytes. B cells mediate or regulate many other functions essential for immune homeostasis, including an antibody-independent pathogenic role that gives B cells the capability to present antigens. On recognition of a specific antigen, the B-cell membrane is reorganized, resulting in an aggregation of B-cell receptors in an immunologic synapse that functions as a platform for internalization of the complex. Internalized antigen is degraded and subsequently exposed to the B-cell surface in association with MHC complex molecules for presentation to T cells. This surface presentation of antigen, in the presence of various costimulatory molecules, elicits the assistance of T cells required to assist B-cell maturation, which in turn allows B cells to drive optimal T-cell activation and differentiation into memory subsets.

B cells also have the capacity to expand clonally, which allows them to become the numerically dominant APCs. Activated B cells also produce a wide range of cytokines and chemokines that modulate the maturation, migration, and function of other immune effector cells. B cells regulate wound healing and transplanted tissue rejection and also influence tumor development and tumor immunity. One phenotypically distinct subset, designated B10 cells, has been shown to uniquely regulate T-cell–mediated inflammatory responses through the production of IL-10.

Development and Differentiation of B Lymphocytes

Mammalian B-cell development encompasses a continuum of stages that begin in primary lymphoid tissue, such as human fetal liver and fetal or adult marrow, with subsequent functional maturation in secondary lymphoid tissue, such as human lymph nodes and spleen. The functional or protective endpoint is antibody production by terminally differentiated plasma cells. At least 10 distinct transcription factors regulate the early stages of B-cell development.

B cells participate in the humoral immune response by reacting to antigenic stimuli through division and differentiation into plasma cells. Plasma cells or antibody-forming cells are terminally differentiated B cells. These cells are entirely devoted to antibody production.

A subset of memory B cells in humans is not fully functional in children below 2 to 4 years of age. This is demonstrated by the high susceptibility of children to infections by encapsulated bacteria. Today, pure polysaccharide vaccines (e.g., PNEUMOVAX 23) are approved for use in patients aged 2 years or older and in adults aged 50 years or older who are at increased risk for pneumococcal disease. PNEUMOVAX 23 will not prevent disease caused by capsular types of pneumococci other than those contained in the vaccine. Protein-conjugated vaccines (e.g., Prevnar 13) are for use in children aged 6 weeks to 5 years old and in adults aged 50 years or older (see Chapter 27, Vaccines). The specific antibodies produced are able to bind to infected cells and free organisms bearing the antigen and then inactivate those cells or organisms and destroy them. The condition of hyperacute rejection of transplanted organs is also mediated by B cells. In addition, antigenic stimulation prompts B cells to multiply.

The evolution of the humoral immune response includes:
1. Activation of B cells and migration into the germinal center
2. B-cell proliferation

TABLE 4.5 Cell Surface Cluster of Differentiation Molecules Preferentially Expressed by B Cells

Name	Structure
CD19	Ig superfamily
CD20	MS4A family
CD21	Complement receptor family
CD22	Ig superfamily
CD23	C-type lectin
CD24	GPI anchored
CD40	TNF receptor
CD72	C-type lectin
CD79a,b	Ig superfamily

CD, Cluster of differentiation; *GPI*, glycosylphosphatidylinositol; *Ig*, immunoglobulin; *TNF*, tumor necrosis factor.

3. Somatic hypermutation of IgV genes
4. B-cell recognition of antigen on follicular dendritic cells; selection of high-affinity B cells
5. B cells that encounter antigen on follicular dendritic cells are selected to survive; B cells that do not bind antigen die
6. Generation of memory and antibody-secreting cells

Cell Surface Antigens

Before 1980, the molecular architecture of the B-cell surface was known to consist of membrane-bound Ig, complement component receptors, and Fc receptors; beyond that, the molecular constitution of the cell surface was completely uncharacterized. MAb testing launched a new era of B-cell studies. The first B-cell–specific molecule described was termed *B1* and is now known as *CD20*.

Over the past 25 years, approximately 10 B-cell–specific cell surface molecules (Table 4.5) have been identified by MAbs, with non–B-cell expression identified for some.

B lymphocytes are best known to express CD19, but not CD3, surface membrane markers. During B-cell differentiation in the bone marrow, the surface molecule CD19 appears early and remains on the B-cell unit until it differentiates into a plasma cell. Four proteins on the surface of mature B cells—CD19, CD21, CD81, and CD225—form the CD19 complex. CD21 is the C3d and Epstein-Barr virus receptor that interacts with CD19 to generate transmembrane signals and inform the B cell of inflammatory responses within microenvironments.

Primitive B-cell precursors have δ chains in their cytoplasm and no Ig on their surface. More differentiated (but still immature) B cells have intact cytoplasmic IgM and surface IgM.

Mature B cells lose their cytoplasmic IgM and add surface IgD to the surface IgM. These changes appear to occur in the absence of antigen and depend on cytokines.

In humans, there is evidence of four types of B-**cell surface markers**:
1. The Ig receptor is the best studied B-cell surface marker. This receptor is actually an antibody molecule with antigenic specificity. According to the clonal selection theory, B cells exist in the body with Ig receptors specific for antigen before exposure to the antigenic substances. When specific antigen exposure does occur, the antigen will select the B cell having an Ig receptor with the best fit. The secreted antibody, in turn, has the same specificity as the Ig receptor on the B cell. Almost all the antibody produced by plasma

cells is secreted (plasma cells have few Ig receptors), but 90% of the antibody produced by B cells is expressed as surface Ig receptors. Some antigens (e.g., lipopolysaccharides from some gram-negative organisms) can bind to the Ig receptor and also stimulate an antibody response independent of T-cell cooperation (T-independent antigens). This type of response is generally of low intensity and is class restricted to the production of IgM antibody. B cells have sIg, except for very immature lymphocytes and mature plasma cells, that are normally polyclonal (i.e., kappa and lambda light chains are present on the cytoplasmic membrane of B cells). Mu and delta heavy chains are usually found with kappa or lambda chains on any one cell surface. Gamma and alpha chains are rarely found on the surface of properly prepared, normal lymphocytes.

2. An Fc receptor that specifically binds the Fc portion of IgG antibody may function to aid B cells in binding to antigen already bound to antibody.
3. Receptors that bind fragments of the cleaved complement component C3 have been reported on the surface of approximately 75% of B cells. This receptor binds C3b, iC3b (inactivated C3b), and C3d, but the function of these receptors is not completely understood.
4. B-cell surface antigens coded by the MHC class II genes are a fourth type of human B-cell marker.

B cells outside the marrow are morphologically homogeneous, but their cell surface phenotypes, anatomic localization, and functional properties have not been fully described. Immature B cells exiting the marrow acquire cell surface IgD, in addition to CD21 and CD22, with functionally important density changes in other receptors. Immature B cells respond to T-cell–independent type 1 antigens such as lipopolysaccharides, which elicit rapid antibody responses in the absence of MHC class II–restricted T-cell help.

B cells proliferate in response to bacterial DNA stimulation, indicating the existence of B-cell surface receptors for DNA. These are now known to represent TLRs that are expressed by multiple leukocyte lineages.

B-lymphocyte subsets. B1 and B2 cells are B-cell subsets. One phenotypically distinct subset, designated *B10 cells*, has been shown to uniquely regulate T-cell–mediated inflammatory responses through the production of IL-10. Further characterization of this B-cell subset is needed.

Bone marrow B lymphopoiesis generates naïve B cells. Peripheral B-cell subsets include B_{regs}, $CD21^{lo/-}$ B cells, B1, marginal zone (MZ) B cells, and B2 cells. $CD21^{lo/-}$ B cells have distinct populations: activated memory B cells, plasmablast precursors, and exhausted memory B cells. $CD21^{lo/-}$ B cells are increased in patients with autoimmune disease or chronic viral infections.

B-cell functions include:
1. A source of natural antibody and a major source of IgM
2. Host protection
3. Clearance of apoptotic cells
4. Possible negative selection of self-reactive B cells
5. Response to stress-induced antigens

B1 cells. B1 cells are distinguished by the CD5 marker, appear to form a self-renewing set, respond to a number of common microbial antigens, and occasionally generate autoantibodies. B1 cells constitutively produce natural Ig, primarily IgM, but some IgG and IgA. B1 cells have a special ability for self-renewal, but constant addition of new B1 cells from bone marrow ensures continuous natural IgM production throughout life.

B1 cells derived from hemogenic endothelial cells develop independently of hematopoietic stem cells (HSCs) in the fetal liver. Approximately 9.5 days later, bone marrow becomes peritoneal B cells. Peritoneal B1 cells subdivide into B1a and B1b. B1a cells produce natural antibody that provides innate protection against bacterial infection in naïve hosts. B1b cells are the primary source of long-term adaptive antibody responses to polysaccharides and other T-cell–independent type 2 antigens during infection.

B2 cells. B2 cells account for most of the B lymphocytes in adults. This subset generates a greater diversity of antigen receptors and responds effectively to T-dependent antigen. B2 cells arise from bone marrow in adults.

Marginal zone B cells. MZ B cells are specialized for quick responses to bloodborne pathogens and T-independent antibody. To generate a T-independent antibody response, MZ cells must establish interactions with other cellular components and respond to environmental cytokines in a controlled spatiotemporal manner.

B-lymphocyte activation. Early B-cell development is characterized by the ordered rearrangement of Ig H and L chain loci, and Ig proteins themselves play an active role in regulating B-cell development.

B cells can be stimulated in their resting state to enlarge, develop synthetic machinery, divide, mature, and secrete antibodies. The proper signals for this sequence depend on the type of triggers, which can be specific or nonspecific and polyclonal. Specific activation involves the antigen that is complementary to the particular Ig on the surface. Nonspecific activation occurs with B-cell mitogens.

Efficient antibody production to complex protein antigens requires T-cell help, which in turn develops from APCs presenting antigen to the T cell. Activated T cells secrete a variety of cytokines that, together with the specific antigen, trigger the B cell to develop into an antibody-secreting cell. This process also involves class switching.

In the immune response to a foreign protein, the first antibodies to appear are of the IgM class (or isotype). As the response proceeds, other isotypes (IgG, IgA, and IgE) emerge from Ig class switching. The isotype switch has considerable clinical importance because each of the four major isotypes has specialized biological properties. IgG is the principal class of antibody in interstitial fluids, and IgA is the protective antibody of mucosal surfaces. Isotype switching requires collaboration between antibody-synthesizing B cells and helper CD4+ T cells. The B cell uses IgM molecules on its surface to capture the antigen and present the antigen to the T cell.

Contact between the collaborating lymphocytes is enhanced by complementary pairs of CAMs. Some CAMs (e.g., CD4, MHC class II antigens) are constitutively expressed on the surface of T and B cells, whereas others are induced. For example, contact between B and T cells induces the T cell to express a ligand for the B-cell surface molecule CD40. In turn, CD40 interacts with the newly expressed CD40 ligand on the T cell, which leads to the expression of another B-cell surface molecule, B7. The latter's partner on the surface of the T lymphocyte is CD28. These cooperative and synergistic interactions between T and B cells induce the secretion of cytokines such as IL-2 and IL-4.

Isotype switching requires two signals. The first is delivered by an interleukin and the second by the binding of CD40 to its ligand on the T cell. In the process of switching from IgM synthesis to IgE synthesis, IL-4 makes the IgE gene in the B cell accessible to the switch machinery initiated when CD40 binds to its ligand. In this process, the gene that encodes the variable region (the part of the antibody molecule that contains the antigen-binding site) moves from its position near the gene that encodes for IgM to a position near the gene that encodes for IgE.

> **KEY CONCEPTS: Plasma Cell Facts**
> - After binding and cooperative interaction with T cells, B cells undergo transformation into plasma cells. Plasma cells arise as the end stage of B-cell differentiation into a large, activated plasma cell.
> - The function of plasma cells is the synthesis and excretion of immunoglobulins.

PLASMA CELL BIOLOGY

After binding and cooperative interaction with T cells, B cells undergo transformation into plasma cells. Plasma cells arise as the end stage of B-cell differentiation into a large, activated plasma cell. The function of plasma cells is the synthesis and excretion of Igs.

The pathway from the B lymphocyte to the antibody-synthesizing plasma cell forms when the B cell is antigenically stimulated and undergoes transformation because of the stimulation of various interleukins. The immune antibody response begins when individual B lymphocytes encounter an antigen that binds to their specific Ig surface receptors. After receiving an appropriate second signal provided by interaction with helper T cells, these antigen-binding B cells undergo transformation and proliferation to generate a clone of mature plasma cells that secretes a specific type of antibody.

An increase in plasma cells can be seen in a variety of nonmalignant disorders, such as viral disease (e.g., rubella and infectious mononucleosis), allergic conditions, chronic infections, and collagen diseases. In plasma cell dyscrasias, the plasma cells can be greatly increased or can infiltrate the bone marrow completely (e.g., multiple myeloma, Waldenström macroglobulinemia).

Antibody molecules secreted by plasma cells consist of four chains—two light chains and two heavy chains, based on molecular weight—and can be enzymatically cleaved into Fab (antigen-binding) and Fc (crystallizable) fragments. The Fab portion binds antigen and contains the light chains and their antigenic markers (kappa, lambda), in addition to heavy chains.

The Fc fragment contains the markers that distinguish the different classes of antibodies and sites that will bind and activate complement and bind to Fc receptors on cells. The amino acid sequence for most of the antibody protein is constant except for the antigen-binding portion of the molecule, which has a hypervariable region and accounts for the various antigenic specificities that the antibody is programmed to recognize.

> **KEY CONCEPTS: Lymphocyte Dysfunction**
> - The total number of T cells in the peripheral blood is relatively stable throughout adult life.
> - A change in the distribution of T-cell subpopulations with a decrease in the number of suppressor cells and an increase in the helper cell population are demonstrated in older adults.
> - Although variable, the immunologic response to disease is age related.
> - Functional deficits of T lymphocytes impair cell-mediated immunity and delayed hypersensitivity in older adults.
> - A decrease in Th cells is the primary cause of the impaired humoral response in older adults.

ALTERATIONS IN LYMPHOCYTE SUBSETS

The normal functioning of helper cells and suppressor cells in the immune response can be reversed under certain conditions. For example, the target cell for human T-cell leukemia or HIV is phenotypically a helper cell but functionally a suppressor cell. Functionally, the helper-inducer subset of cells signals B cells to generate antibodies, control production and switching of types of antibodies formed, and activate suppressor cells. The suppressor-cytotoxic lymphocytes control and inhibit antibody production by suppressing helper cells or by turning off B-cell differentiation. The normal ratio of helper cells and suppressor cells (± 2:1) can be reversed under certain conditions.

Changes with Aging

Alterations in the number and composition of lymphocytes and their subsets in blood are considered a hallmark of immune system aging. The rates of change of T, B, and NK cells are relatively stable throughout adulthood. T cells appear to demonstrate the greatest rate of individual variations. However, there is not complete agreement about the individual stability or variations of lymphocyte composition in extremely old adults.

Although the effect of aging on the immune response is highly variable, the ability to respond immunologically to disease is age related. Faulty immunologic reactions (e.g., aberrant functioning of immunoregulatory cells, effector T cells, and antibody-producing B cells) may contribute to poor immunity in older adults. Functional deficits of T lymphocytes have been identified with aging, causing impairment of cell-mediated immunity. In addition, skin testing reveals decreases in the intensity of delayed hypersensitivity in older adults. The proliferative response of T lymphocytes to mitogens or antigens such as *M. tuberculosis* or varicella-zoster virus is impaired. A decrease in Th cells is the primary cause of the impaired humoral response in older adults. Although the total number of B cells and total Ig concentration remain unchanged, the serum concentration of IgM is decreased and IgA and IgG concentrations are increased.

> **KEY CONCEPTS: Immunologic Disorders**
> - Immunologic disorders can be divided into primary processes (dysfunction in the immune organ itself) and acquired, or secondary, processes (disease or therapy causing an immune defect).
> - Another category, diseases mediated through immune mechanisms, can also be included.

IMMUNOLOGIC DISORDERS

Immunologic disorders can be divided into primary immunodeficiency disorders and acquired, or secondary, disorders. A third category, diseases mediated through immune mechanisms, can also be included. Because of their complexity and contemporary importance, primary and secondary immunodeficiency disorders are discussed separately in Chapter 19.

Alternatively, there are diseases characterized by an activation of the adaptive immune response, with T and B lymphocytes responding to self-antigen in the absence of any detectable microbial invasion or tumor invasion. Disruption of the delicate balance between activating and inhibitory signals that regulate normal B-cell activation and longevity can predispose to pathogenic autoantibody production and autoimmunity. It has become more obvious that B cells contribute substantially to multiple human autoimmune diseases. B cells may contribute to autoimmune pathogenesis by presentation of autoantigen to

T cells or through the production of proinflammatory cytokines. In most cases of human autoimmune disease, the combination of environmental factors and polygenic effects collectively dysregulate normal B-cell function and confer disease susceptibility. These diseases constitute the vast majority of diseases that are considered to be autoimmune in origin. Other *immunoproliferative* and autoimmune diseases are discussed in Chapters 21 and 22.

Immune-Mediated Disease

The immune system is normally efficient at eliminating foreign antigens. The nature of the antigen or the genetic makeup of the host, however, can cause alterations of the immune response that can be injurious and lead to immune-mediated disease (Table 4.6). In these disorders, the immune response is normal but the reactivity is heightened, prolonged, or inappropriate.

A major concern is allergic reactions, characterized by an immediate response on exposure to an offending antigen and the release of mediators (e.g., histamine, leukotrienes, prostaglandins) capable of initiating signs and symptoms (see Chapter 20). Although allergic reactions are associated with IgE, not all allergic reactions are IgE mediated. Complement activation by immune complexes or through the alternative complement pathway has been shown to release complement C3a and C5a anaphylatoxins, which are capable of producing similar reactions.

TABLE 4.6 Immune-Mediated Disease

Type	Cause, Disease
Allergic hypersensitivity	Foods, drugs, aeroallergens (dust, pollens, molds)
Contact hypersensitivity	Poison ivy, nickel, cosmetics
Transfusion or Transplantation	
Reactions involving blood or tissue cells	
Autoimmune disease	Systemic lupus erythematosus, rheumatoid arthritis, vasculitis syndromes, hemolytic anemia, idiopathic thrombocytopenia, pernicious anemia, Goodpasture syndrome, myasthenia gravis, Graves disease

CASE STUDY 4.1 History and Physical Examination

A family had a son who died at age 2 weeks because of overwhelming bacterial infection. When their newborn daughter began developing recurrent infections, she was immediately taken to a pediatrician.

Laboratory Data
Hemoglobin and hematocrit—within normal range
Total WBC count—62.0×10^9/L
Absolute leukocyte counts—above normal for each leukocyte type
Leukocyte differential—neutrophils 76%, lymphocytes 22%, eosinophils 2%

Flow Cell Cytometry
T lymphocytes—normal proportions of CD4+ and CD8+ cells
B lymphocytes (CD19+)—elevated
NK cells—elevated
CD15+ leukocytes—absent
Serum Ig fractions—within reference ranges

Treatment
The infant was given busulfan cyclophosphamide and antithymocyte serum for 10 days. She received mature T-lymphocyte–depleted bone marrow transplanted from her mother. This was followed by a short period of immunosuppressive therapy.

She recovered from the procedures and did well clinically.

Questions
1. What significant finding in flow cytometry suggests an immune deficiency?
   a. Elevated B lymphocytes (CD19+) count
   b. Normal CD4+ and CD8+ lymphocyte counts
   c. Elevated NK cell count
   d. Absence of CD15+ cells
2. What does the patient's family history suggest?
   a. Acute leukemia
   b. Immune antibody dysfunction
   c. Genetic leukocyte disorder
   d. Hereditary anemia

See Appendix A for the answers to these questions.

Critical-Thinking Group Discussion Questions
1. What laboratory test is of the greatest diagnostic value in diagnosing this patient?
2. What value in the reported flow cytometry results is diagnostic?
3. Can leukocyte adhesion deficiency be misdiagnosed?

CASE STUDY 4.2   History and Physical Examination

A 6-year-old White male patient was taken to a pediatrician because of recurring abscesses since the age of 1 month. The current abscesses were lanced, and he was placed on antibiotic therapy. The patient had two brothers who had died in infancy of infections. His parents and two sisters are healthy.

Laboratory Data
Hemoglobin and hematocrit—slightly decreased
Total leukocyte count—elevated
Differential leukocyte count—increased percentage of segmented neutrophils
Ig profile—polyclonal elevation of all Ig classes
Neutrophil oxidative burst assay (DHR) activity—absent
NBT test (automated)—reduction of unstimulated and stimulated neutrophils
Culture of abscess revealed *S. aureus*

Questions
1. What does the patient's family history suggest?
   a. A genetic disorder in male offspring
   b. A genetic disorder in female offspring
   c. Lack of leukocyte production
   d. Anemia producing an immune dysfunction
2. What laboratory assay is most helpful in the diagnosis of this case?
   a. Percentage of segmented neutrophils
   b. Immunoglobulin profile
   c. Neutrophil oxidative burst assay (DHR)
   d. Nitroblue tetrazolium (NBT) test (automated)

See Appendix A for the answers to these questions.

Critical-Thinking Group Discussion Questions
1. Does this boy's condition appear to be related to sex?
2. Why are the bacteria not killed?

CASE STUDY 4.3   History and Physical Examination

A 33-year-old man, the child of parents of Mexican descent, was examined because of a history of frequent sore throats and sinus headaches. Recently he had a severe bout of pneumonia and was just diagnosed with bacterial conjunctivitis and chronic gastritis caused by *Helicobacter pylori*.

Laboratory Data

Assay	Patient Results	Reference Range
Total leukocytes	7.2×10^9/L	$4.5-9.0 \times 10^9$/L
Total lymphocytes	3.2×10^9/L	$2.7-5.4 \times 10^9$/L
T lymphocytes	3.15×10^9/L	$2.7-5.3 \times 10^9$/L
B lymphocytes	Too low to count, almost undetectable	

Serum Immunoglobulins

Assay	Patient Results	Reference Range
IgM	0.03 g/L	3.0–15.8 g/L
IgG	0.31 g/L	0.4–2.2 g/L
IgA	Not detectable	0.15–1.3 g/L
IgE	Not detectable	<100 IU/mL
Assay	Patient Results	
Blood group	0	
Anti-A and anti-B titer	1:2, very low	

Assay	Patient Results	Reference Range
Serum immunoglobulin (mg/dL)		
IgM	45, low	
IgG	200, very low	
IgA	23, very low	

Questions
1. A laboratory result of significance to the diagnosis of this patient is:
   a. Low or absent immunoglobulin levels
   b. Extremely low B-lymphocyte count
   c. Low T-lymphocyte count
   d. Both a and b
2. When this man is vaccinated, his immune system should:
   a. Recognize the vaccine as a foreign antigen
   b. Mount a weak antibody response to a vaccine
   c. Fail to recognize the vaccine as a foreign antigen
   d. Both a and b

See Appendix A for the answers to these questions.

Critical-Thinking Group Discussion Questions
1. What abnormalities are evident in the laboratory assay results?
2. Does the patient's history suggest a genetic abnormality?
3. What kind of response would be expected from a vaccination?

REVIEW QUESTIONS

Questions 1–4. Arrange the steps of phagocytosis in the proper sequence.
1. _____
2. _____
3. _____
4. _____
   a. Digestion of bacteria
   b. Increase in chemoattractants at site of tissue damage
   c. Ingestion of bacteria
   d. Change in direction of movement due to a chemoattractant substance

5. Phagocytosis by cells of the mononuclear phagocytic system is greatly enhanced by which of the following?
   a. Hemolysins
   b. Opsonins
   c. Specific antitoxins
   d. Neutralizing antibodies

6. The function of polymorphonuclear neutrophil (PMN) leukocytes is:
   a. Primary phagocytic cells
   b. Antibody-synthesizing cells
   c. Recognition of foreign antigens and production of antibody
   d. Synthesize complement

7. Chronic granulomatous disease represents a defect of:
   a. Oxidative metabolism
   b. Abnormal granulation of neutrophils
   c. Diapedesis
   d. Chemotaxis
8. An alteration of phagocytic killing is associated with:
   a. Lazy leukocyte syndrome
   b. Burns or diabetes
   c. Systemic lupus erythematosus
   d. Corticosteroid therapy
9. A defective monocyte cytotoxicity is associated with:
   a. Wiskott-Aldrich syndrome
   b. Burns or diabetes
   c. Systemic lupus erythematosus
   d. Corticosteroid therapy
10. Diseases associated with a dysfunction of polymorphonuclear neutrophils (PMNs) include all of the following except:
    a. Gaucher syndrome
    b. Chédiak-Higashi syndrome
    c. Chronic granulomatous diseases
    d. Myeloperoxidase deficiency
11. A depressed migration is associated with:
    a. Rheumatoid arthritis
    b. Burns or diabetes
    c. Systemic lupus erythematosus
    d. Intracellular infections
12. Impaired phagocytosis is associated with:
    a. Lazy leukocyte syndrome
    b. Burns or diabetes
    c. Systemic lupus erythematosus
    d. Intracellular infections
13. A characteristic of chronic granulomatous disease is:
    a. Marked defect in cellular response to chemotaxis
    b. Failure to exhibit increased anaerobic metabolism during phagocytosis
    c. Mild-to-marked defect in bactericidal ability of neutrophils
    d. Defective leukocyte locomotion
14. A characteristic of lazy leukocyte syndrome is:
    a. Marked defect in cellular response to chemotaxis
    b. Failure to exhibit increased anaerobic metabolism during phagocytosis
    c. Mild-to-marked defect in bactericidal ability of neutrophils
    d. Defective leukocyte locomotion
15. A characteristic of Chédiak-Higashi anomaly (syndrome) is:
    a. Marked defect in cellular response to chemotaxis
    b. Failure to exhibit increased anaerobic metabolism during phagocytosis
    c. Mild-to-marked defect in bactericidal ability of neutrophils
    d. Defective leukocyte locomotion
16. A characteristic of myeloperoxidase deficiency is:
    a. Marked defect in cellular response to chemotaxis
    b. Failure to exhibit increased anaerobic metabolism during phagocytosis
    c. Mild-to-marked defect in bactericidal ability of neutrophils
    d. Defective leukocyte locomotion
17. Which statement about mast cells is correct?
    a. They have a low concentration of heparin in the granules
    b. They have a high concentration of histamine in the granules
    c. They react with two adjacent IgA molecules on mast cells
    d. They are not associated with anaphylactic shock
18. A function of the cell-mediated immune response *not* associated with humoral immunity is:
    a. Defense against viral and bacterial infection
    b. Initiation of rejection of foreign tissues and tumors
    c. Defense against fungal and bacterial infection
    d. Antibody production
19. All of the following are a function of T cells except:
    a. Mediation of delayed hypersensitivity reactions
    b. Mediation of cytolytic reactions
    c. Regulation of the immune response
    d. Synthesis of antibody
20. The function of T cells is:
    a. Antibody-dependent cellular cytotoxicity (ADCC) reaction
    b. Cellular immune response
    c. Cytotoxic reaction
    d. Humoral response
21. The function of B cells is:
    a. Antibody-dependent cellular cytotoxicity (ADCC) reaction
    b. Cellular immune response
    c. Cytotoxic reaction
    d. Humoral response
22. The function of natural killer (NK) cells is:
    a. Antibody-dependent cellular cytotoxicity (ADCC) reaction
    b. Cellular immune response
    c. Cytotoxic reaction
    d. Humoral response
23. Natural killer cells:
    a. Mediate viral immunity
    b. Participate in phagocytosis
    c. Do not synthesize cytokines
    d. Are conventional antigen receptors
24. The surface membrane marker for CD4 is:
    a. All or most T lymphocytes
    b. Helper-inducer T cells
    c. Suppressor-cytotoxic T cells
    d. T-regulatory lymphocytes
25. The surface membrane marker for CD8 is:
    a. All or most T lymphocytes
    b. Helper-inducer T cells
    c. Suppressor-cytotoxic T cells
    d. T-regulatory lymphocytes
26. The surface membrane marker for CD3 is:
    a. All or most T lymphocytes
    b. Helper-inducer T cells
    c. Suppressor-cytotoxic T cells
    d. T-regulatory lymphocytes
27. All of the following are B-cell surface membrane markers *except*:
    a. sIg
    b. Fc receptor
    c. C3 receptor
    d. CD4
28. The process of aging causes the thymus to:
    a. Decrease in size
    b. Not change over time
    c. Lose cellularity
    d. Both a and c
29. T lymphocytes can also be referred to as:
    a. Mast cells
    b. Memory cells
    c. Phagocytic cells
    d. Short-lived cells

30. Which of the following is *not* a characteristic of T lymphocytes?
    a. Can form a suppressor-cytotoxic subset
    b. Can be helpers-inducers
    c. Can be CD4+ or CD8+
    d. Can synthesize and secrete immunoglobulin
31. The appropriate function of T lymphocytes is:
    a. Cellular immune response
    b. Humoral immune response
    c. Phagocytosis
    d. Antibody production
32. The appropriate function of B lymphocytes is:
    a. Cellular immune response
    b. Humoral antibody response
    c. Destruction of foreign particles
    d. Phagocytosis
33. The appropriate function of cytotoxic T cells is related to/associated with all of the following *except*:
    a. Directly destroying target cells
    b. Transplanted organ rejection
    c. CD4+ marker
    d. Directly destroying virally infected target cells
34. The primary characteristic of T_{reg} cells is:
    a. Control of autoimmunity in peripheral blood
    b. Control of autoimmunity in bone marrow stem cells
    c. Expression of CD25
    d. Secretion of IL-3
35. Which subset of effector lymphocytes is predominantly responsible for regulation of antibody production?
    a. Th1
    b. Th2
    c. Th17
    d. CD8+

PART II
The Theory of Immunologic and Serologic Procedures

Chapter 5: Basic Safety in the Immunology-Serology Laboratory, 98

Chapter 6: Basic Quality Control and Quality Assurance Practices, 107

Chapter 7: Basic Serologic Laboratory: Techniques and Clinical Applications, 117

Chapter 8: Precipitation and Particle Agglutination Methods, 128

Chapter 9: Electrophoresis Techniques and Chromatography, 143

Chapter 10: Labeling Techniques in Immunoassay, 150

Chapter 11: Flow Cytometry, 159

Chapter 12: Molecular Laboratory Techniques, 168

5

Basic Safety in the Immunology-Serology Laboratory

LEARNING OUTCOMES

- Assess risk assessment and strategies to enhance laboratory safety.
- Name the federal or national agencies responsible for safety issues.
- Discuss patient safety: compliance and improvement actions
- Discuss the occupational transmission of hepatitis B virus (HBV) and human immunodeficiency virus (HIV).
- Name and describe Standard Precautions and additional COVID-19 safety requirements.
- Compare various methods to reduce the risk of surface-based infections
- Explain the proper handling of hazardous material and waste management, including infectious waste, chemicals, and radioactive waste.
- Describe the basic aspects of infection-control policies, including the use of personal protective equipment (PPE) or devices (gowns, gloves, masks, goggles) and the purpose of Standard Precautions.
- Demonstrate the proper decontamination of a work area at the start and completion of work and after a hazardous spill.
- Explain the process of properly segregating and disposing of various types of waste products generated in the clinical laboratory.
- Describe the role of a laboratory safety team to reduce risks and promote patient safety.
- Correctly answer 80% of end-of-chapter review questions.

OUTLINE

Risk and Risk Management, 98
Safety Standards and Agencies, 99
Safety Manual, 99
Patient Safety, 100
Prevention of Transmission of Infectious Diseases, 100
Safe Work Practices for Infection Control, 101
Protective Techniques for Infection Control, 101
    Selection and Use of Gloves, 101
    Facial Barrier Protection and Occlusive Bandages, 101
    Laboratory Coats or Gowns as Barrier Protection, 101
Hand Sanitizing and Handwashing, 101
Other Safety Practices, 103
    Nail Care, 103
    Shoes, 103
    Electronic Devices, 103

Reducing Risk of Surface-Based Infection, 103
    Traditional Decontamination of Work Surfaces, 103
    Traditional Decontamination of Nondisposable Equipment, 103
    Traditional Decontamination of Spills, 103
    Guidance for SARS-CoV-2 Decontamination, 104
Disposal of Infectious Laboratory Waste, 104
    Containers for Waste, 104
        Biohazard Containers, 104
        Biohazard Bags, 104
    Final Decontamination of Waste Materials, 104
Disease Prevention, 104
    COVID-19, 104
        Essential Vaccines for Healthcare Providers, 105
Case Study 5.1, 105
Procedure: Test Your Safety Knowledge, 106.e1

KEY TERMS

autoclaving
biosafety policies
COVID-19
human immunodeficiency virus (HIV)
nonintact
nosocomial transmission
occlusive
percutaneous (parenteral)
personal protective equipment (PPE)
phlebotomy
skin lesions

Over the years, multiple pandemic preparedness reviews warned that America's healthcare system was woefully unprepared for a fast-moving infectious disease outbreak. Since the fury of COVID-19 slammed into the United States in early March 2020, safety practices were challenged to effectively manage the pandemic. Today, traditional safety practices have been expanded to include additional COVID-19 safety practices to protect laboratory staff against viral aerosol contamination and exposure to solid-surface contamination.

RISK AND RISK MANAGEMENT

Risk is defined as the probability that a health effect will occur after an individual has been exposed to a specified amount of a hazard.

In the immunology-serology laboratory, precautions must be taken to prevent accidental exposure to infectious diseases and other laboratory hazards. Clinical laboratory personnel are routinely exposed to potential hazards in their daily activities. The importance of safety cannot be overemphasized. Many accidents do not just happen; they are caused by carelessness or lack of proper communication. For this reason, the practice of safety should be uppermost in the mind of every laboratory staff member in a clinical laboratory, particularly in the post-COVID era.

During the COVID-19 pandemic, the World Health Organization (WHO) launched its first-ever global report on infection prevention and control (IPC). The COVID-19 pandemic and other recent large disease outbreaks have highlighted the extent to which healthcare settings can contribute to the spread of infections, harming patients, health workers, and visitors if insufficient attention is paid to IPC. The COVID-19 pandemic has exposed many challenges and gaps in IPC in all countries.

Laboratories should perform a risk assessment to determine if there are certain procedures or specimens that may require higher levels of biocontainment. The WHO advises that all procedures must be performed based on risk assessment and only by personnel with demonstrated capability, in strict observance of any relevant protocols at all times. Risk assessment is an important part of biosafety. Primary risks that determine levels of containment are:

1. infectivity,
2. severity of disease,
3. transmissibility, and
4. the nature of the work conducted.

> **KEY CONCEPTS: Safety Issues**
> - Clinical laboratories have Standard Blood and Body Fluid Precautions, or Standard Precautions, to prevent parenteral, mucous membrane, and non-intact skin exposures of healthcare workers to bloodborne pathogens such as HIV or HBV.
> - Additional COVID-19 safety practices have been published to protect laboratory staff against virus aerosol contamination and exposure to solid-surface contamination.
> - Risk assessment is an important part of biosafety.

SAFETY STANDARDS AND AGENCIES

Safety standards for clinical laboratories are initiated, governed, and reviewed by several agencies or committees. These include the following:

- College of American Pathologists (CAP)
- The Joint Commission (TJC)
- US Centers for Disease Control and Prevention (CDC), part of the US Department of Health and Human Services Public Health Service (HHS)
- US Department of Labor, Occupational Safety and Health Administration (OSHA)
- US Food and Drug Administration (FDA)
- US National Institutes of Health
- World Health Organization (WHO)

The primary purpose of OSHA standards is to ensure that workers have safe and healthful working conditions. The federal government passed the Occupational Safety and Health Act of 1970 and, in 1988, expanded the Hazard Communication Standard to apply to hospital staff. Occupational Safety and Health Act regulations apply to all businesses with one or more employees and are administered by the US Department of Labor through OSHA.

In 1991 OSHA mandated that all clinical laboratories must implement a chemical hygiene plan and an exposure-control plan. As part of the chemical hygiene plan, a copy of the safety data sheets (SDSs, previously called *Material Safety Data Sheets*) must be on file and readily accessible and available to all employees at all times. The SDS describes the hazards, safe handling, storage, and disposal of hazardous chemicals. Information is provided by chemical manufacturers and suppliers about each chemical and accompanies the shipment of each chemical. Each SDS contains basic information about the specific chemical or product, including its trade name, chemical name and synonyms, chemical family, manufacturer's name and address, emergency telephone number for further information about the chemical, hazardous ingredients, physical data, fire and explosion data, and health hazard and protection information. The SDS describes the effects of overexposure or exceeding the threshold limit value of allowable exposure for an employee in an 8-hour day. The SDS also describes protective personal clothing and equipment requirements, first-aid practices, spill information, and disposal procedures.

In 2006, the CDC introduced the National Healthcare Safety Network (NHSN). This voluntary system integrates a number of surveillance systems and provides data on devices, patients, and staff. Many hospitals have reorganized the physical layout of handwashing stations (see later, Handwashing) to prevent the spread of pathogens.

Most recently, from 2019 to 2020, OSHA has developed interim guidance to help prevent occupational exposure to SARS-CoV-2, the virus that causes COVID-19. Measures for protecting laboratory staff from exposure to, and infection with, SARS-CoV-2 depend on the type of laboratory work being performed and exposure risk, including potential for interaction with people with suspected or confirmed COVID-19 and contamination of the laboratory.

According to the joint guidance of OSHA and the HHS, infection-control strategies should be based on a thorough hazard assessment, engineering and administrative controls, safe work practices, and PPE to prevent staff exposures (see Safe Work Practices for Infection Control below). Some OSHA standards that apply to preventing occupational exposure to SARS-CoV-2 also require employers to train workers on elements of infection prevention, including PPE.

SAFETY MANUAL

All laboratories should perform a site-specific and activity-specific risk assessment to identify and mitigate risks. Risk assessments and mitigation measures are dependent on a number of variables:

- The procedures performed
- Identification of the hazards involved in the process and/or procedures
- The competency level of the personnel who perform the procedures
- The laboratory equipment and facility
- The resources available

For most types of laboratory staff, the risk of infection with SARS-CoV-2 is similar to that of the general American public. Staff who do not have contact with people known to be, or suspected of being, infected with SARS-CoV-2, nor frequent closer contact within 6 feet, are considered to be at lower risk of occupational exposure. Certain laboratory employees, including phlebotomists, are likely to perform job duties that may involve medium, high, or even very high occupational exposure risks. Staff in close contact[a] with COVID-19 patients require additional engineering and administrative controls, safe work practices, and PPE. If a laboratory staff member has an increased susceptibility

---

[a]The CDC defines close contact as being within about 6 feet of an infected person while not wearing recommended PPE. Close contact also includes instances where there is direct contact with infectious secretions while not wearing recommended PPE.

for SARS-CoV-2 infection or complications from COVID-19, consideration should be given to adjusting their work responsibilities or locations to minimize exposure. Other flexibilities, if possible, can help prevent potential exposures among workers who have diabetes, heart or lung issues, or other immunocompromising health conditions.

Each laboratory must have an up-to-date safety manual. This manual should contain a comprehensive listing of approved policies, acceptable practices, and precautions, including Standard Blood and Body Fluid Precautions. Specific standards that conform to current state and federal requirements (e.g., OSHA regulations with COVID-19 updates [see Appendix D]) must be included in the manual.

PATIENT SAFETY

The newest Institute of Medicine's Improving Diagnosis in Health Care stresses the importance of the need for laboratory staff to work as a team and collaborate with other healthcare personnel. The desired outcome is that increased collaboration, including the ordering of appropriate tests, analysis and interpretation, reporting, and communicating of results, enhances clinical decision-making.

The TJC's Laboratory: 2024 *National Patient Safety Goals®* are part of the overall quality-improvement requirements for accreditation of hospitals by TJC. Applicable goals include:
1. *Correct patient identification.* At least two methods of patient identification are required. For example, use the patient's name and date of birth.
2. *Improved staff communication.* Get important test results to the right staff person on time falls.
3. *Prevent infection*
   One of the most important ways to address healthcare-acquired infections (HAIs) is by improving the hand hygiene of healthcare staff.
   Compliance with WHO and/or CDC hand hygiene guidelines to reduce the transmission of infectious agents by staff to patients to decrease HAIs.
   Ensure compliance with National Patient Safety Goal by assessing compliance with the CDC and/or the WHO guidelines through a comprehensive program that:
   1. provides a hand hygiene policy,
   2. fosters a culture of hand hygiene,
   3. monitors compliance, and
   4. provides feedback.

A recent report from the WHO shows that where good hand hygiene and other cost-effective practices are followed, 70% of those infections can be prevented.

> **KEY CONCEPTS: Infection Control**
> - Medical personnel should be aware that HBV, HIV, and SARS-CoV-2 are different diseases caused by unrelated viruses. The control of infectious, chemical, and radioactive waste is regulated by various governmental agencies (e.g., OSHA, US FDA).
> - The TJC's Laboratory Services: 2024 *National Patient Safety Goals* are part of the overall quality-improvement requirements for accreditation of hospitals by the TJC.

PREVENTION OF TRANSMISSION OF INFECTIOUS DISEASES

Transmission of various bloodborne pathogens has always been a concern for laboratory staff but with the identification of the **human immunodeficiency virus (HIV)** a new awareness was created. Specific regulations in regard to the handling of blood and body fluids from patients suspected or known to be infected with a bloodborne pathogen were originally issued in 1983.

According to the CDC's concept of **Standard Precautions**, all human blood and other body fluids are treated as potentially infectious for HIV, HBV, and other bloodborne microorganisms that can cause disease in human beings. Compliance with the OSHA Bloodborne Pathogens (BBP) Standard and the Occupational Exposure Standard is required to provide a safe work environment. OSHA mandates that the employer do the following:
- Educate and train all healthcare workers in Standard Precautions and in preventing bloodborne infections
- Provide proper equipment and supplies (e.g., gloves)
- Monitor compliance with protective **biosafety policies**

Blood is the most important source of HIV, HBV, and other bloodborne pathogens in the occupational setting. HBV can be present in extraordinarily high concentrations in blood, but HIV is usually found in lower concentrations. HBV may be stable in dried blood and blood products at 25°C for up to 7 days. HIV retains infectivity for more than 3 days in dried specimens at room temperature and for more than 1 week in an aqueous environment at room temperature.

Both HBV and HIV may be transmitted indirectly. Viral transmission can result from contact with inanimate objects, such as work surfaces or equipment contaminated with infected blood or certain body fluids. If the virus is transferred to the skin or mucous membranes by hand contact between a contaminated surface and **nonintact** skin or mucous membranes, it can produce viral exposure.

Medical personnel must remember that HBV and HIV are different diseases caused by unrelated viruses. The most feared hazard of all, the transmission of HIV through occupational exposure, is among the least likely to occur. The modes of transmission for HBV and HIV are similar, but the potential for transmission in the occupational setting is greater for HBV than HIV.

The transmission of hepatitis B can also be fatal if contracted, and it is more probable than transmission of HIV. The number of cases of acute hepatitis among healthcare workers because of occupational exposure has sharply declined since the hepatitis B vaccine became available in 1982. The likelihood of infection in healthcare workers after exposure to blood infected with HBV or HIV depends on the following factors:
1. Concentration of HBV or HIV; viral concentration is higher for HBV than HIV
2. Duration of the contact
3. Presence of **skin lesions** or abrasions on the hands or exposed skin of the healthcare worker
4. Immune status of the healthcare worker for HBV

Both HBV and HIV may be directly transmitted by various portals of entry. In the occupational setting, however, the following situations may lead to infection:
1. **Percutaneous (parenteral)** inoculation of blood, plasma, serum, or certain other body fluids from accidental needlesticks
2. Contamination of the skin with blood or certain body fluids without overt puncture, caused by scratches, abrasions, burns, weeping, or exudative skin lesions
3. Exposure of mucous membranes (oral, nasal, or conjunctival) to blood or certain body fluids, as the direct result of pipetting by mouth, splashes, or spattering
4. Centrifuge accidents or the improper removal of rubber stoppers from test tubes, producing droplets. If these aerosol products are infectious and come into direct contact with mucous membranes or nonintact skin, direct transmission of virus can result

The risk varies not only with the type of exposure but also with the amount of infected blood in the exposure, the length of contact with the infectious material, and the amount of virus in the patient's blood or body fluid or tissue at exposure. Studies have reported that the average risk of HIV transmission is approximately 0.3% after percutaneous exposure to HIV-infected blood and 0.09% after mucous membrane exposure.

SAFE WORK PRACTICES FOR INFECTION CONTROL

The use of CDC Standard Precautions is an approach to infection control that prevents occupational exposures to bloodborne pathogens. It eliminates the need for separate isolation procedures for patients known or suspected to be infectious. The application of Standard Precautions also eliminates the need for warning labels on specimens.

Safe work practices for the control of contracting an infectious disease are regulated by several US government regulations. These are the Bloodborne Pathogens (BBP) standard (29 CFR 1910.1030), Personal Protective Equipment (29 CFR 1910.132), Eye and Face Protection (29 CFR 1910.133), Hand Protection (29 CFR 1910.138), and Respiratory Protection (29 CFR 1910.134) standards. The use of these standards is in association with the July 2, 2020 Guidance for General Laboratory Safety Practices during the COVID-19 pandemic document (Appendix D).

PROTECTIVE TECHNIQUES FOR INFECTION CONTROL

OSHA requires laboratories to have a **personal protective equipment (PPE)** program. Comprehensive compliance with this regulation includes a workplace hazard assessment with a written hazard certification; proper equipment selection, employee information and training with written competency certification; and a regular reassessment of work hazards.

Laboratory personnel should not rely solely on PPE to protect themselves against hazards. They should also apply PPE standards when using various forms of safety protection.

The risk of **nosocomial transmission** of pathogens can be minimized if laboratory personnel are aware of and adhere to essential safety guidelines. Laboratory personnel should adhere to current PPE safety precautions when conducting routine laboratory activities. Staff must wear PPE that should be selected based on the results of an employer's hazard assessment and specific job duties of laboratory staff. PPE consists of gloves, a laboratory coat, and in the era of COVID-19, a face covering in laboratory spaces that do not have specific requirements for respiratory PPE and where other social-distancing measures are difficult to maintain.

Selection and Use of Gloves

Gloves for medical use are sterile surgical or nonsterile examination gloves made of vinyl or latex. There are no reported differences in barrier effectiveness between intact latex and intact vinyl gloves. Tactile differences have been observed between the two types of gloves, with latex gloves providing more tactile sensitivity; however, either type is usually satisfactory for **phlebotomy** and as a protective barrier during technical procedures. Latex-free gloves should be available for personnel with sensitivity to usual glove material. Rubber household gloves may be used for cleaning procedures.

General guidelines related to the selection and use of gloves include the following:
1. Use sterile gloves for procedures involving contact with normally sterile areas of the body or during procedures in which sterility has been established and must be maintained.
2. Use nonsterile examination gloves for procedures that do not require the use of sterile gloves. Gloves must be worn when receiving phlebotomy training. The National Institute of Occupational Safety and Health mandates the use of gloves for phlebotomy.
3. Gloves should be changed between each patient contact.
4. Wear gloves when processing blood specimens, reagents, or blood products, including reagent red blood cells.
5. Gloves should be changed frequently and immediately if they become visibly contaminated with blood or certain body fluids, or if physical damage occurs.
6. Do not wash or disinfect latex or vinyl gloves for reuse. Washing with detergents may cause increased penetration of liquids through undetected holes in the gloves. Rubber gloves may be decontaminated and reused, but disinfectants may cause deterioration. Rubber gloves should be discarded if they have punctures, tears, or evidence of deterioration or if they peel, crack, or become discolored.

Gloves should be properly removed (Fig. 5.1) or covered with an uncontaminated glove or paper towel before answering the telephone, handling laboratory equipment, or touching doorknobs.

Facial Barrier Protection and Occlusive Bandages

Facial barrier protection was originally required to be used if there was a potential for splashing, spraying, or mucous membrane contact with blood or certain body fluids could occur.

Additional PPE, in the era of COVID-19, is a face covering in laboratory spaces that do not have requirements for respiratory PPE and where other social-distancing measures are difficult to maintain. Facial barrier protection should be used if there is a reasonably anticipated potential for splattering or splashing blood, body fluids, or any other potentially infectious agents.

The CLSI advises that plastic face splash guards do not offer enough protection against an aerosol such as SARS-CoV-2.

Standard Precautions require that all disruptions of exposed skin, including defects on the arms, face, and neck, should be covered with a water-impermeable **occlusive** bandage.

Laboratory Coats or Gowns as Barrier Protection

A color-coded, two–laboratory coat or equivalent system should be used whenever laboratory personnel are working with potentially infectious specimens. The garment worn in the laboratory must be changed or covered with an uncontaminated coat when leaving the immediate work area. Garments should be changed immediately if grossly contaminated with blood or body fluids to prevent seepage through to street clothes or skin. Contaminated coats or gowns should be placed in an appropriately designated biohazard bag for laundering. Disposable plastic aprons are recommended if blood or certain body fluids may be splashed. Aprons should be discarded into a biohazard container.

The introduction of water-retardant gowns has been the greatest change in many PPE practices.

HAND SANITIZING AND HANDWASHING

Standard Precautions are intended to supplement rather than replace handwashing recommendations for routine infection control. Frequently wash your hands with soap and water for at least 20 seconds. Whenever possible, wash your hands if they are visibly soiled, visibly soiled with blood or other body fluids, or after using the toilet before using a hand sanitizer. If exposure to potential spore-forming pathogens is strongly suspected or proven, including outbreaks of *Clostridium difficile*, handwashing with soap and water is the preferred means.

Alternatively, frequent handwashing should be performed after contact with patients and laboratory specimens (Box 5.1). Gloves should be

> When the hand hygiene indication occurs before a contact requiring glove use, perform hand hygiene by rubbing with an alcohol-based handrub or by washing with soap and water.

I. How to don gloves:

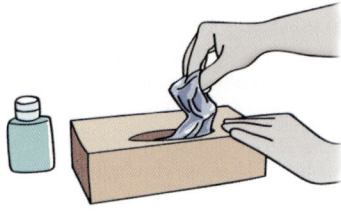
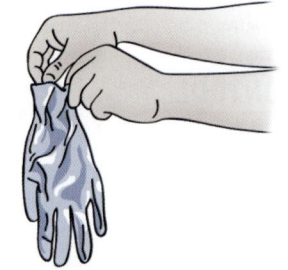
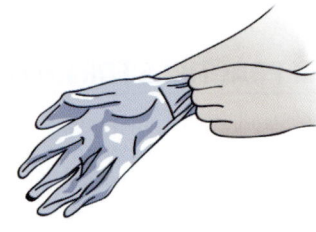

1. Take out a glove from its original box.
2. Touch only a restricted surface of the glove corresponding to the wrist (at the top edge of the cuff).
3. Don the first glove.

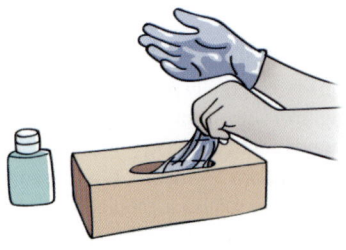
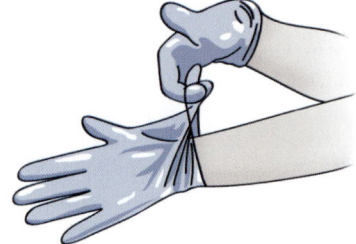
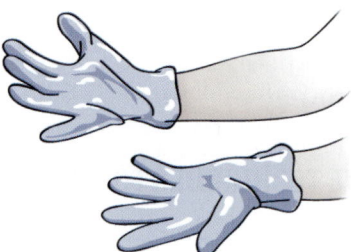

4. Take the second glove with the bare hand and touch only a restricted surface of the glove corresponding to the wrist.
5. To avoid touching the skin of the forearm with the gloved hand, turn the external surface of the glove to be donned on the folded fingers of the gloved hand, thus permitting gloving of the second hand.
6. Once gloved, hands should not touch anything else that is not defined by indications and conditions for glove use.

II. How to remove gloves:

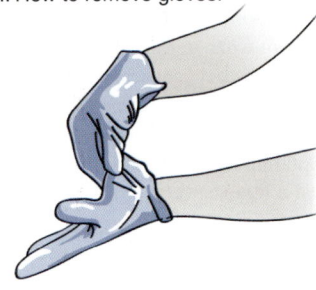
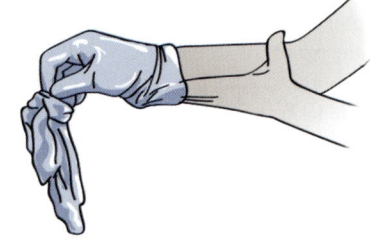
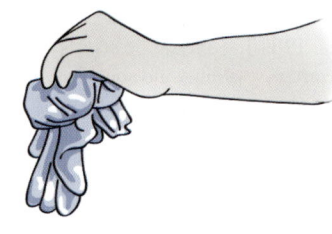

1. Pinch one glove at the wrist level to remove it, without touching the skin of the forearm, and peel away from the hand, thus allowing the glove to turn inside out.
2. Hold the removed glove in the gloved hand and slide the fingers of the ungloved hand inside between the glove and the wrist. Remove the second glove by rolling it down the hand and fold into the first glove.
3. Discard the removed gloves.

> 4. Then, perform hand hygiene by rubbing with an alcohol-based handrub or by washing with soap and water.

Fig. 5.1 Technique for Donning and Removing Nonsterile Examination Gloves. (From World Health Organization: Glove use information leaflet, Geneva, Switzerland, 2009, WHO.)

> **BOX 5.1 Guidelines for Handwashing and Hand Antisepsis in Healthcare Settings**
>
> 1. Wash hands with a nonantimicrobial soap and water or an antimicrobial soap and water when hands are visibly dirty or contaminated with proteinaceous material.
> 2. If hands are not visibly soiled, use an alcohol-based, waterless antiseptic agent for routinely decontaminating hands in all other clinical situations.
> 3. Waterless antiseptic agents are highly preferable, but hand antisepsis using an antimicrobial soap may be considered in settings in which time constraints are not an issue and easy access to hand hygiene facilities can be ensured, or in rare cases when a caregiver is intolerant of the waterless antiseptic product used in the institution.
> 4. Decontaminate hands after contact with a patient's intact skin.
> 5. Decontaminate hands after contact with body fluids or excretions, mucous membranes, nonintact skin, or wound dressings, as long as hands are not visibly soiled.
> 6. Decontaminate hands if moving from a contaminated body site to a clean body site during patient care.
> 7. Decontaminate hands after contact with inanimate objects in the immediate vicinity of the patient.
> 8. Decontaminate hands before caring for patients with severe neutropenia or other forms of severe immune suppression.
> 9. Decontaminate hands after removing gloves.

used as an adjunct to, not a substitute for, handwashing. After removing PPE, always wash hands with soap and water, if available, for at least 20 seconds. Ensure that hand hygiene facilities (e.g., sink or alcohol-based hand rub) are readily available at or adjacent to the PPE-removal area.

According to the WHO and CDC, clean your hands by rubbing them with an alcohol-based sanitizer with a formulation of at least 60% alcohol or 70% isopropanol as the preferred means for routine hygienic hand antisepsis if hands are not visibly soiled. It is faster, more effective, and better tolerated by your hands than washing with soap and water.

OTHER SAFETY PRACTICES

Nail Care
According to the CDC, to promote infection control, nails should be no longer than 1/4 inch beyond the tip of the finger. Longer nails do not fit into gloves properly and can cause problems with blood collection and analysis. In addition, in many healthcare organizations, artificial nails are not allowed.

Shoes
According to CLSI document GP17-A2, shoes worn in the clinical laboratory and phlebotomy services should be rubber soled and cover the entire foot. Unless covered with shoe covers, canvas shoes are not recommended. Fluid-impermeable material (e.g., leather or synthetic) is recommended.

Electronic Devices
Electronic devices (e.g., mobile phones, iPods, MP3 players, and tablet computers) should not be exposed to potential sources of infectious contamination.

REDUCING RISK OF SURFACE-BASED INFECTION
Surface-based pathogens are one of the leading causes of HAIs. Surfaces are a complex issue with currently no regulatory requirements or standards for testing and validating surface materials and products.

It is important to note that surface compatibility with chemical disinfectants can impact the safety of patients and healthcare personnel.

Guidance from the CDC, the National Institutes of Health, and other partners suggests that SARS-CoV-2 can survive on certain types of surfaces, for example, plastic and stainless steel, for 2 to 3 days.

Traditional Decontamination of Work Surfaces
The CDC provides instructions for environmental cleaning and disinfection for various types of workplaces. Cleaning solutions must be EPA-registered disinfectants with label claims to be effective against SARS-CoV-2.

WHO advises that a concentration of either 0.1% sodium hypochlorite, hydrogen peroxide ≥0.5%, or 70% to 90% ethanol may be used in healthcare settings, while remaining effective against other clinically relevant pathogens after a minimum contact time of 1 minute.

Prior to new additional COVID-19 guidelines, a sodium hypochlorite solution was an inexpensive and effective broad-spectrum germicidal solution for decontamination in the laboratory. Generic sources of sodium hypochlorite include household chlorine bleach. This type of solution is inexpensive and an effective broad-spectrum germicidal solution. Concentrations of 1:10 to 1:100 free chlorine are effective, depending on the amount of organic material present on the surface to be cleaned and disinfected. Many chlorine bleaches (available at grocery stores) are not registered by the US Environmental Protection Agency (EPA) for use as surface disinfectants and are unacceptable surface disinfectants. The EPA encourages the use of registered products because the agency reviews them for safety and performance when the products are used according to label instructions. When unregistered products are used for surface disinfection, users do so at their own risk. EPA-registered chemical germicides may be more compatible with certain materials that could be corroded by repeated exposure to sodium hypochlorite, especially the 1:10 dilution.

While wearing gloves, personnel should clean and sanitize all work surfaces at the beginning and end of the shift with a 1:10 dilution of household bleach. Instruments such as scissors or centrifuge carriages should be sanitized daily with a diluted solution of bleach. It is equally important to clean and disinfect work areas frequently during the workday and before and after each shift. Studies have demonstrated that HIV is inactivated rapidly after being exposed to common chemical germicides at concentrations much lower than used in practice. Diluted household bleach prepared daily inactivates HBV in 10 minutes and HIV in 2 minutes. Disposable materials contaminated with blood must be placed in containers marked "Biohazard" and properly discarded.

Hepatitis C virus (HCV), HBV, and HIV have never been documented as being transmitted from a housekeeping surface (e.g., countertops). However, an area contaminated by blood or body fluids needs to be treated as potentially hazardous and requires prompt removal and surface disinfection.

Traditional Decontamination of Nondisposable Equipment
Decontaminate nondisposable equipment by soaking overnight in a dilute (1:10) bleach solution and rinsing with methyl alcohol and water before reuse. Disposable glassware or supplies that have come into contact with blood should be autoclaved or incinerated. Staff should receive training on environmental surface and infection-control strategies and procedures as part of an overall infection-control and safety program.

Traditional Decontamination of Spills
Strategies differ for decontaminating spills of blood and other body fluids, based on the setting. The cleanup procedure depends on the

porosity of the surface and volume of the spill. The following protocol is recommended for managing spills in a clinical laboratory:

1. Wear gloves and a laboratory coat.
2. Absorb the blood with disposable towels. Bleach solutions are less effective in the presence of high concentrations of protein. Remove as much liquid blood or serum as possible before decontamination.
3. Using a diluted bleach (1:10) solution, clean the spill site of all visible blood.
4. Wipe down the spill site with paper towels soaked with diluted bleach.
5. Place all disposable materials used for decontamination into a biohazard container.

Guidance for SARS-CoV-2 Decontamination

Guidance from the CDC, the National Institutes of Health, and other partners suggests that SARS-CoV-2 can survive on certain types of surfaces (e.g., plastic and stainless steel), for 2 to 3 days. However, the transmissibility of SARS-CoV-2 from contaminated environmental surfaces and objects is still not fully understood. Laboratory managers should carefully evaluate whether or not work areas occupied by patients during the COVID-19 pandemic may have been contaminated and whether or not these patient areas need to be decontaminated in addition to routine cleaning and other housekeeping practices in any healthcare settings in which aerosol-generating procedures are performed.

The CDC provides instructions for environmental cleaning and disinfection for various types of workplaces. Cleaning solutions must be EPA-registered disinfectants with label claims to be effective against SARS-CoV-2. Those who perform cleaning tasks must be protected from exposure to hazardous chemicals used in these tasks. In these cases, the PPE (29 CFR 1910 Subpart I) and Hazard Communication (29 CFR 1910.1200) standards may apply, and workers may need appropriate PPE to prevent exposure to the chemicals. If workers need respirators, they must be used in the context of a comprehensive respiratory protection program that meets the requirements of OSHA's Respiratory Protection standard (29 CFR 1910.134) and includes medical exams, fit testing, and training. In addition, SDSs and other manufacturer instructions can provide additional guidance about what resources PPE workers need to use for their safety.

DISPOSAL OF INFECTIOUS LABORATORY WASTE

The control of infectious, chemical, and radioactive waste is regulated by a variety of government agencies, including OSHA and the FDA. Laboratories should implement applicable federal, state, and local laws that pertain to hazardous material and waste management by establishing safety policies. Laboratories with multiple agencies should follow the guidelines of the most stringent agency. Safety policies should be reviewed and signed annually or whenever a change is instituted. Employers are responsible for ensuring that personnel follow the safety policies.

Containers for Waste

Containers must be easily accessible to personnel needing them and must be located in the laboratory areas in which they are typically used. They should be constructed so that their contents will not spill out if the container is tipped over accidentally.

Biohazard Containers

Body fluid specimens, including blood, must be placed in well-constructed biohazard containers with secure lids to prevent leakage during transport and for future disposal. Contaminated specimens and other materials used in laboratory tests should be decontaminated before reprocessing for disposal or should be placed in special impervious bags for disposal in accordance with established waste-removal policies. If outside contamination of the bag is likely, a second bag should be used.

Hazardous specimens and potentially hazardous substances should be tagged and identified as such. The tag should read "Biohazard," or the biological hazard symbol should be used. All persons working in the laboratory area must be informed about the meaning of these tags and precautions to take for each.

Contaminated equipment must be placed in a designated area for storage, washing, decontamination, or disposal. With the increased use of disposable PPE (e.g., gloves), the volume of waste for disposal will increase.

Biohazard Bags

Although rigid impermeable containers are used for the disposal of sharps and broken glassware, plastic bags are appropriate for the disposal of most infectious waste materials. Plastic bags with the biohazard symbol and lettering prominently visible can be used in secondary metal or plastic containers. These containers can be decontaminated or disposed of regularly, or immediately when visibly contaminated. These biohazard bags should be used for all blood, body fluids, tissues, and other disposable materials contaminated with infectious agents and should be handled with gloves.

If the primary infectious waste containers are red plastic bags, they should be kept in secondary metal or plastic cans. Extreme care should be taken not to contaminate the exterior of these bags. If they do become contaminated on the outside, the entire bag must be placed into another red plastic bag. Secondary plastic or metal cans should be decontaminated regularly, and immediately after any grossly visible contamination, with an agent such as a 1:10 solution of household bleach.

Final Decontamination of Waste Materials

Terminal disposal of infectious waste should be by incineration; an alternative method is terminal sterilization by autoclaving. If incineration is not done in the healthcare facility or by an outside contractor, all contaminated disposables should be autoclaved before leaving the facility for disposal with routine waste. Disposal of medical waste should be carried out by licensed organizations to ensure that no environmental contamination or esthetic problem occurs. Congress has passed various acts and regulations regarding the proper handling of medical waste to assist the EPA to carry out this process in the most prudent manner.

DISEASE PREVENTION

A well-planned and properly implemented healthcare employee immunization program is an important component of a healthcare organization's IPC program. Vaccination of healthcare personnel protects against potentially dangerous diseases such as COVID-19 and influenza, and protects healthcare staff as well as patients and the community.

COVID-19

According to the CDC Interim Guidance for Managing Healthcare Personnel with SARS-CoV-2 Infection or Exposure to SARS-CoV-2, individual states and healthcare facilities may set their own COVID-19 vaccine requirements for healthcare workers. Healthcare providers who have higher risk exposure are generally not restricted from working, regardless of vaccination status, unless they test positive or develop symptoms.

Essential Vaccines for Healthcare Providers

As of August 2023, the Advisory Committee on Immunization Practices (ACIP) recommends six up-to-date vaccinations for healthcare workers in addition to COVID-19 vaccinations. These vaccinations are:

1. Chickenpox vaccine (varicella)
2. Flu vaccine (influenza)
3. Hepatitis B vaccine
4. Meningococcal vaccine—especially lab workers who work with *Neisseria meningitidis*
5. MMR vaccine (measles, mumps, and rubella)
6. Tdap (tetanus, diphtheria, and whooping cough) or Td (tetanus and diphtheria)

Healthcare workers should make sure they are up to date on any other vaccines routinely recommended for them based on age or other factors. These vaccinations may include:

- HPV vaccine (human papillomavirus)—recommended for adults aged 18 through 26 years and adults aged 27 through 45 years based on shared clinical decision-making
- Shingles vaccine (zoster)—recommended for all adults 50 years of age and older

Screening is available for the detection of many occupationally acquired bloodborne pathogens. Clinical laboratory staff need to demonstrate antibody immunity to various pathogens including rubella and hepatitis.

THE LABORATORY SAFETY TEAM: The laboratory director and various laboratory safety officers, coaches, and staff comprise the critical "safety eyes" and "safety ears" of a laboratory safety program.

Laboratory Director

The laboratory director is the person who is ultimately responsible for overall laboratory safety including a safety manual with the details of all aspects of the laboratory safety program. This manual should contain adequate policies, procedures, and practices to ensure the safety of laboratory employees, patients and visitors.

Safety Coaches

Safety coaches are volunteers who assume additional job responsibilities. These volunteers represent all laboratory departments and shifts, and job roles. Safety coaches have six important functions:

1. Communicator of safety habits
2. Educator of safety habits
3. Role model of safety habits
4. Observer of safety habits
5. Storyteller to implement positive change
6. Change agent for maximum compliance with correct safety habits

Safety coaches can facilitate safety habits for prevention of errors by paying attention to details, communicating clearly, and having a questioning attitude.

These volunteers must recognize that barriers such as peer resistance and time constraints need to be overcome.

CASE STUDY 5.1

When a new employee in a rural laboratory started to work, she wiped down the workbench with 5% bleach and donned latex gloves that she had rinsed off the night before. When she opened up a specimen (a red-top tube), a small amount of serum spilled out of the tube. She promptly wiped it up with a sterile paper towel and discarded the paper towel into a cardboard box marked "Biohazard." When it was lunchtime, she removed her gloves, discarded them in the biohazard container, and left the laboratory to go to the cafeteria. Her laboratory coat was clean, so she did not remove it to go to lunch. On returning from lunch, she put on clean gloves and worked until the end of the shift. She discarded her gloves into the biosafety box and hung her laboratory coat on a hook in the laboratory.

Questions

1. A safety violation in the case study is:
   a. Use of freshly prepared 10% bleach on the countertops
   b. Use of new latex-free gloves
   c. Washing hands before donning gloves
   d. Not washing hands after removing gloves
2. Wearing a laboratory coat to do testing and then back home to wash it is:
   a. Acceptable if the coat is washed when stained
   b. Always acceptable
   c. Never acceptable
   d. OK if only done once in a while

See Appendix A for the answers to these questions.

Critical-Thinking Group Discussion Questions

1. Name all the safety violations that occurred in this case study.
2. State the corrective action for each of the violations.
3. How can these violations be avoided?

REVIEW QUESTIONS

1. Which of the following is the government agency primarily responsible for safeguards and regulations to ensure a safe and healthful workplace throughout the United States?
   a. Occupational Safety and Health Administration (OSHA)
   b. Clinical Laboratory Improvement Amendments of 1988 (CLIA '88)
   c. Centers for Disease Control and Prevention (CDC)
   d. City ordinances

2. The term *Standard Precautions* refers to:
   a. Treating all specimens as if they are infectious
   b. Assuming that every direct contact with a body fluid is infectious
   c. Treating only blood or blood-tinged specimens as infectious
   d. Both a and b

3. The CDC's Bloodborne Pathogen Requirement mandates:
   a. Education and training of all healthcare workers in Standard Precautions
   b. Proper handling of chemicals
   c. Calibration of equipment
   d. Fire extinguisher maintenance

4. The single most common source of HIV in the occupational setting is:
   a. Saliva
   b. Urine
   c. Blood
   d. Cerebrospinal fluid

5. When using gloves for phlebotomy or blood specimen processing, laboratory staff should:
   a. Use sterile gloves
   b. Wash hands after removing gloves
   c. Not wash hands before leaving the laboratory
   d. Not wash hands before and after using the bathroom
6. Gloves for medical use may be:
   a. Sterile or nonsterile
   b. Latex or vinyl
   c. Used only once
   d. All of the above
7. Diluted bleach for disinfecting work surfaces, equipment, and spills should be prepared daily by preparing a (7) _____ dilution of household bleach. This dilution requires (8) _____ mL of bleach diluted to 100 mL with H_2O.
   a. 1:5
   b. 1:10
   c. 1:20
   d. 1:100
8. Diluted bleach for disinfecting work surfaces, equipment, and spills should be prepared daily by preparing a (7) _____ dilution of household bleach. This dilution requires (8) _____ mL of bleach diluted to 100 mL with H_2O.
   a. 1
   b. 10
   c. 25
   d. 50
9. Infectious waste must be discarded into containers with all of the following features *except*:
   a. Marked "Biohazard"
   b. Has a standard biohazard symbol
   c. Orange, orange and black, or red
   d. Made of sturdy cardboard for landfill disposal
10. Clinical laboratory personnel need to have demonstrable immunity to:
    a. Rubella
    b. Polio
    c. Hepatitis B
    d. Both a and c

6

Basic Quality Control and Quality Assurance Practices

LEARNING OUTCOMES

- Identify the regulatory and accrediting organizations that influence quality assessment in clinical laboratories.
- Describe the eight nonanalytic factors related to testing accuracy.
- Identify and give examples of the three categories of errors related to the phase of testing.
- Define the terms *accuracy, precision, reproducibility,* and *reliability.*
- Describe the use of the coefficient of variation and give the formula.
- Define true positive, true negative, false positive, and false negative.
- Provide the equations for calculating percentage sensitivity and percentage specificity.
- Define positive predictive value and negative predictive value.
- Describe the process of proficiency testing.
- Explain the use of control specimens.
- Cite seven causes for a control value being out of the acceptable range or out of control.
- Define the terms *mean, median, mode, standard deviation,* and *reference range.*
- Discuss issues related to testing outcomes.
- Describe parallel testing of test kits.
- Describe how a new procedure is validated.
- Write and evaluate a procedural write-up using Clinical and Laboratory Standards Institute (CLSI) requirements.
- Correctly answer case study–related multiple-choice questions.
- Be prepared to participate in a discussion of critical-thinking questions.
- Correctly answer end-of-chapter review questions.

OUTLINE

Clinical Laboratory Regulatory and Accrediting Organizations, 108
Nonanalytic Factors Related to Testing Accuracy, 108
    Qualified Personnel, 108
    Established Laboratory Policies, 108
    Laboratory Procedure Manual, 108
    Test Requisitioning, 108
    Patient Identification, Specimen Procurement, and Labeling, 108
    Preventive Maintenance of Equipment, 109
    Appropriate Testing Methods, 109
    Inaccurate Results, 109
Errors Related to Phase of Testing, 109
Quality Descriptors, 109
    Definitions, 110
    Coefficient of Variation, 110
    Sensitivity and Specificity, 110
    Sensitivity, 110
    Specificity, 110
    Sensitivity and Specificity Related to SARS-CoV-2, 110
    Limits of Detection, 111
    Predictive Values, 111
    Positive and Negative Predictive Values Related to SARS-CoV-2, 111
Monitoring Quality, 111
    Proficiency Testing, 111
    Control Specimens, 112
Reference Range Statistics, 112
Testing Outcomes, 112
Validating New Procedures, 113
    Parallel Testing of Test Kits, 113
Case Study 6.1, 115
Procedure: Validation of a New Procedure Write-Up, 116.e1

KEY TERMS

accuracy
aliquots
biometrics
coefficient of variation (CV)
confidence limits
control specimen
gaussian curve
hemolyzed specimens
limits of detection

mean
median
mode
nonwaived assays
normal values
precision
predictive value (PV)
proficiency testing (PT)
quality assurance (QA)

quality control (QC)
reference range
reliability
reproducibility
sensitivity
specificity
standard deviation (SD)
systematic

The introduction of routine quality assurance (QA) programs and quality control (QC) in the clinical laboratory was a major advance in improving the accuracy and reliability of testing. This process assures the clinician ordering the test that the testing method has been done in the best possible way to provide the most useful information in diagnosing or managing a patient. QA indicators and QC are tools to ensure that reported laboratory results are of the highest quality.

> **KEY CONCEPTS: Quality Regulators**
> - QA indicators and QC are tools to ensure that reported laboratory results are of the highest quality.
> - The Clinical Laboratory Improvement Amendments of 1988 (CLIA '88) established a minimum threshold for all aspects of clinical laboratory testing.
> - Voluntary QC standards have been set by The Joint Commission (TJC), the Commission on Office Laboratory Accreditation (COLA), and the College of American Pathologists (CAP).

CLINICAL LABORATORY REGULATORY AND ACCREDITING ORGANIZATIONS

The US Congress enacted the Clinical Laboratory Improvement Amendments of 1988 (CLIA '88) in response to concerns about laboratory testing errors. The final CLIA rule, Laboratory Requirements Relating to Quality Systems and Certain Personnel Qualifications, was published in the *Federal Register* in January 2003. Enactment of the CLIA established a minimum threshold for all aspects of clinical laboratory testing.

Voluntary standards have been set by TJC, the COLA, and the CAP.

A more recent development in voluntary accreditation aimed at improving quality was the introduction of International Organization for Standardization (ISO) 15189. The ISO is the world's largest nongovernmental developer and publisher of international standards. ISO standards and certification are widely used by industry, but ISO 15189 has now been formulated for clinical laboratories. ISO 15189 has gained some standing abroad as a mandatory accreditation, such as in Australia, Ontario, and many European countries. In the United States, ISO 15189 accreditation remains optional. Requirements for quality and competence in ISO 15189 are unique because they take into consideration the specific requirements of the medical environment and the importance of the medical laboratory to patient care. CAP 15189 is a voluntary, nonregulated accreditation to the ISO 15189:2007 standard as published by ISO. CAP 15189 does not replace CAP's CLIA-based Laboratory Accreditation Program but complements CAP accreditation and other quality systems by optimizing processes to improve patient care, strengthen the deployment of quality standards, reduce errors and risk, and control costs.

> **KEY CONCEPTS: Quality Methods**
> - Nonanalytic factors related to testing accuracy include the following: qualified personnel; established policies; procedure manual; test requisitioning; patient identification; specimen procurement and labeling; preventive maintenance of equipment; appropriate testing methods; and inaccurate results.
> - The Institute for Quality Laboratory Medicine has developed measures to evaluate quality in the laboratory based on the phase of testing: preanalytic, analytic, and postanalytic.

NONANALYTIC FACTORS RELATED TO TESTING ACCURACY

Qualified Personnel

The competence of personnel is an important determinant of the quality of the laboratory result. Only properly certified personnel can perform nonwaived assays (see Chapter 7) for levels of laboratory testing.

Established Laboratory Policies

Laboratory policies should be included in a laboratory reference manual that is available to all hospital personnel. Each laboratory must have an up-to-date safety manual. This manual contains a comprehensive listing of approved policies, acceptable practices, and precautions, including Standard Blood and Body Fluid Precautions. Specific regulations that conform to current state and general requirements, such as Occupational Safety and Health Administration (OSHA) regulations, must be included in the manual.

Laboratory Procedure Manual

A complete laboratory procedure manual for all procedures performed in the laboratory must be provided. The manual must be reviewed regularly, in some cases annually, by the supervisory staff and updated as needed. The Clinical and Laboratory Standards Institute (CLSI) recommends that these manuals follow a specific pattern for how procedures are organized (Box 6.1).

Test Requisitioning

A laboratory test request must include the following: (1) patient identification data, (2) time and date of specimen collection, (3) source of the specimen, and (4) analyses to be performed. The information on the accompanying specimen container must exactly match the patient identification on the test request.

Patient Identification, Specimen Procurement, and Labeling

Patients must be carefully identified. For outpatients, identification may be validated with two forms of identification. Using established specimen-processing information, the clinical specimens must be properly labeled or identified once obtained from the patient. An important rule is that the analytic result can only be as good as the specimen. Specimens must be efficiently transported to the laboratory.

> **BOX 6.1   Written Procedural Protocol**
> - Procedure name
> - Name of the test method
> - Principle and purpose of the test
> - Specimen collection and storage
> - Quality control
> - Reagents, supplies, and equipment
> - Procedural protocol
> - Expected or normal (reference) values
> - Procedural notes
>   - Sources of error
>   - Limitations
>   - Clinical applications

Adapted from Clinical and Laboratory Standards Institute: *Clinical laboratory technical procedure manual: approved guideline*, ed 4, Wayne, PA, 2002, CLSI Document GP2-A4.

For elimination of the most frequent source of pretesting error, a patient must be positively identified when a blood specimen is obtained. This specimen must be properly collected and labeled. In general, hemolyzed specimens should not be used for serologic testing.

Preventive Maintenance of Equipment

Microscopes, centrifuges, and other pieces of equipment need to be cleaned and checked for accuracy. A preventive maintenance schedule should be followed for all automated equipment. Failure to monitor equipment regularly can produce inaccurate test results and lead to expensive repairs.

Appropriate Testing Methods

Each laboratory must have an assessment routine for all procedures performed on a daily, weekly, or monthly basis to detect problems. When such problems are indicated, they must be corrected as soon as possible.

Another part of a QC program concerns the way new procedures are validated before they are included in the methods routinely used by the laboratory. Each laboratory must determine the reproducibility (or confidence limits) for each procedure used and establish acceptable limits of variation for control specimens.

Inaccurate Results

Inaccuracies in testing can be systematic or sporadic. Systematic errors can be eliminated by a program that monitors equipment, reagents, and other supplies. Sporadic or isolated errors in technique can produce false-positive and false-negative results, depending on the technique used for testing (Box 6.2).

An important aspect of quality is documentation of results. CLIA regulations mandate that any problem or situation that might affect the outcome of a test result be recorded and reported. These incidents can involve specimens that are improperly collected, labeled, or transported to the laboratory or problems concerning prolonged turnaround times for test results. There must be a reasonable attempt to correct the problems or situation, and all steps in this process must be documented.

ERRORS RELATED TO PHASE OF TESTING

The Institute for Quality Laboratory Medicine has developed measures to evaluate quality in the laboratory based on the preanalytic, analytic, and postanalytic phases of testing.

> **BOX 6.2 Possible Causes of General Technical Errors in Serology**
>
> **False-Positive Errors**
> Overcentrifugation of serum–cell mixture
> Dirty glassware
> Hemolyzed patient serum
> Inadequate dispersal of centrifuged serum–cell mixture
> Extended incubation
>
> **False-Negative Errors**
> Omitting patient serum from test mixture
> Omitting reagent from test mixture
> Undercentrifugation of serum–cell mixture
> Vigorous shaking of centrifuged serum–cell mixture
>
> **False-Positive or False-Negative Errors**
> Incorrect labeling of test tubes
> Addition of wrong reagent to test tube
> Erroneously reading or interpreting results
> Inaccurately recording results
> Expired or improperly stored reagents

Errors occurring during the analytic phase of testing in clinical laboratories are now relatively rare. Currently, most laboratory errors are related to the preanalytic and postanalytic phases of testing. To guarantee the highest-quality laboratory results and to comply with CLIA regulations, various preanalytic factors need to be considered (Boxes 6.3 and 6.4).

QUALITY DESCRIPTORS

QC activities include monitoring the performance of laboratory instruments, reagents, other testing products, and equipment. A written record of QC activities for each procedure or function should include details of deviation from the usual results, problems, or failures in functioning or in the analytic procedure and any corrective action taken in response to these problems. All solutions and kits used in testing must be carefully checked before actually being used for testing patient samples.

> **KEY CONCEPTS: Quality Metrics**
> - QC monitors the accuracy and reproducibility of results through control specimens.
> - *Accuracy* describes how close a test result is to the true value.
> - *Precision* describes how close the test results are to one another when repeated analyses of the same specimen are performed. It is possible to have great precision, but without accuracy if the answer does not represent the actual value tested.
> - The precision of a test, its *reproducibility*, may be expressed as a standard deviation (SD) or the derived coefficient of variation (CV), which is used to compare the SDs of two samples. A procedure may be extremely accurate but so difficult that values are not clinically meaningful.
> - Assessing the sensitivity and specificity of a test involves tests positive, tests negative, disease present (positive), and disease absent (negative). *Clinical sensitivity* is the proportion of subjects with a specific disease or condition who have a positive test result. *Clinical specificity* is the proportion of subjects without the specific disease or condition who have a negative test result.
> - Assessing the predictive value (PV) requires knowledge of the sensitivity, specificity, and disease prevalence. *Prevalence* is the proportion of a population that has the disease. *Incidence* is the number of subjects who have the disease within a defined period per 100,000 population.
> - Proficiency testing (PT) is incorporated into the CLIA requirements. In addition to internal QC programs, each laboratory should participate in an external PT program to verify laboratory accuracy.
> - A *control specimen* has a known value and is similar in composition to the patient's blood. A control value out of the acceptable range (out of control) may result from the deterioration of reagents, faulty equipment, dirty glassware, lack of attention to timing or temperature, use of inappropriate methods, or poor technique.

> **BOX 6.3 Preanalytic Errors**
> - Incorrect test request
> - Specimen obtained from wrong patient
> - Specimen procured at wrong time
> - Specimen collected in wrong tube or container
> - Blood specimens collected in wrong order
> - Incorrect labeling of specimen
> - Improper processing of specimen

> **BOX 6.4 Postanalytic Errors**
> - Recording results inaccurately
> - Verbally reporting results for wrong patient

Definitions

QC consists of procedures used to detect errors that result from test system failure, adverse environmental conditions, and differences between technologists, in addition to the monitoring of the accuracy and precision of test performance over time. Accrediting agencies require monitoring and documentation of QA records. Documentation of QC includes preventive maintenance records, temperature charts, and QC charts for specific assays.

QC monitors the accuracy and reproducibility of results through the use of control specimens. The diagnostic usefulness of a test and its procedure is assessed by using statistical evaluations, such as descriptions of the accuracy and reliability of the test and its methodology.

The terms *accuracy* and *precision* are often used to describe quality. **Accuracy** describes how close a test result is to the true value. **Precision** describes how close the test results are to one another when repeated analyses of the same specimen are performed. It is possible to achieve great precision, with all laboratory personnel who perform the same procedure arriving at the same answer, but without accuracy if the answer does not represent the actual value being tested. Accuracy can be improved by the following:

- Use of properly standardized procedures
- Statistically valid comparisons of new methods with established reference methods
- Use of samples of known values (controls)
- Participation in PT programs

The precision of a test, its **reproducibility**, may be expressed as the **standard deviation (SD)** or derived **coefficient of variation (CV)**. A procedure may be extremely accurate, yet so difficult to perform that individual laboratory personnel are unable to arrive at values that are close enough to be clinically meaningful.

Precision can be ensured by the proper inclusion of standards, reference samples, and/or control solutions; statistically valid, replicate determinations of a single sample; or duplicate determinations of sufficient numbers of unknown samples. Within-run (day-to-day) precision and between-run precision are measured by the inclusion of blind samples and control specimens.

Coefficient of Variation

The CV can be used to compare the SDs of two samples. SDs cannot be compared directly without considering the mean. The CV can be used to compare a day's work with that of a similar day or to compare test results from one laboratory with the same type of test results from another laboratory. The CV (%) is equal to the SD divided by the mean, as follows:

$$CV\,(\%) = \frac{SD}{Mean} \times 100$$

Sensitivity and Specificity

Laboratory results should provide medically useful information, including the sensitivity and specificity of the tests being ordered and reported.

Sensitivity

Analytic sensitivity and analytic specificity. Practically, analytic sensitivity represents how much of a given substance is measured; the more sensitive the test, the smaller the amount of assayed substance that is measured. Analytic specificity represents what is being measured. A highly specific test measures only the assay substance in question; it does not measure interfering or similar substances.

Clinical sensitivity and clinical specificity. Assessing the sensitivity and specificity of a test requires four factors: tests positive, tests negative, disease present (positive), and disease absent (negative). True positives are subjects who have a positive test result and who also have the disease in question. True negatives represent those who have a negative test result and do not have the disease. False positives are those who have a positive test result but do not have the disease. False negatives are those who have a negative test result but do have the disease. Both specificity and sensitivity are desirable characteristics for a test, but in different clinical situations, one is generally preferred over the other.

The clinical **sensitivity** of a test is defined as the proportion of subjects with the specific disease or condition who have a positive test result (i.e., assay correctly predicts with a positive result):

$$Sensitivity\,(\%) = \frac{True\ positives}{True\ positives + False\ negatives} \times 100$$

Practically, analytic sensitivity represents how much of a given substance is measured; the more sensitive the test, the smaller the amount of assayed substance that is measured.

Specificity

The clinical **specificity** of a test is defined as the proportion of subjects without the specific disease or condition that has a negative test result (i.e., assay correctly excludes with a negative result):

$$Sensitivity\,(\%) = \frac{True\ negatives}{False\ positives + True\ negatives} \times 100$$

Practically, analytic specificity represents what is being measured. A highly specific test measures only the assay substance in question; it does not measure interfering or similar substances.

Sensitivity and Specificity Related to SARS-CoV-2

During a public health emergency, the US Food and Drug Administration (FDA) can use its **Emergency Use Authorization (EUA)** authority to allow the use of unapproved medical products, or unapproved uses of approved medical products, to diagnose, treat, or prevent serious or life-threatening diseases when certain criteria are met, including that there are no adequate, approved, or available alternatives. Before the FDA can issue an EUA, the Department of Health and Human Services (HHS) must make a declaration of emergency or threat justifying authorization of emergency use for a product. If an EUA request is not submitted by a commercial manufacturer of a diagnostic test within a reasonable period of time, or if significant problems are identified with such a test that cannot be or have not been addressed in a timely manner, the FDA will remove the manufacturer and test from the FDA.gov notification list.

When the emergency is over, the EUA declaration is terminated, and all EUAs issued based on that declaration will no longer remain in effect.

Since the beginning of the SARS-CoV-2 pandemic testing in early 2020, the quality of laboratory EUA assays approved by the FDA for emergency use of in vitro diagnostics for the detection and/or diagnosis of COVID-19 (February 4, 2020) has been of concern, primarily due to higher than expected false-positive or false-negative patient results. As of July 22, 2020, the FDA has authorized 187 tests under EUAs; these include 154 molecular tests, 31 antibody tests, and 2 antigen tests.

The principal issues related to the quality of test results are assay sensitivity, specificity, and PV. The sensitivity or ability to identify patients with antibodies to SARS-CoV-2 (true positive rate), and the specificity or their ability to identify patients without antibodies to SARS-CoV-2 (true negative rate) failures have caused recalls of many testing procedures.

A test's sensitivity can be estimated by determining whether or not it is able to detect SARS-CoV-2 antibodies in blood samples from patients who have been confirmed to have COVID-19 with a nucleic acid amplification test (NAAT). In some validation studies of these tests, like the ones performed by the FDA conducted in partnership with the National Institutes of Health (NIH), Centers for Disease Control and Prevention (CDC), and Biomedical Advanced Research and Development Authority (BARDA), the samples used came from patients confirmed to have COVID-19 by a NAAT and could also be confirmed to have antibodies present using other serology tests.

A test's specificity can be estimated by testing large numbers of samples collected and frozen before SARS-CoV-2 is known to have circulated to demonstrate that the test does not produce positive results in response to the presence of other causes of a respiratory infection, such as other coronaviruses. These estimates of sensitivity and specificity include 95% confidence intervals, which are the range of estimates that a test's sensitivity and specificity will fall within given acceptable ranges.

Limits of Detection

The best SARS-CoV-2 virus assays demonstrate a **limit of detection** (LoD) of ~100 copies of viral RNA per milliliter of transport media. The LoD is a measure of analytic sensitivity as opposed to clinical sensitivity, which measures the fraction of infected people detected by a given test. For molecular diagnostic assays, the LoD is generally considered the lowest concentration of target that can be detected in ≥95% of repeat measurements. However, LoDs of the currently approved EUA nucleic acid amplification and antigen detection tests for SARS-CoV-2 vary up to 10,000 fold and are associated with significant differences in clinical sensitivity for these tests. Assays with higher LoDs will miss more infected patients and result in more false-negative test results. Each 10-fold increase in LoD is expected to increase the false-negative test rate by 13% or one in eight infected patients. When various EUA-approved methods on the market were evaluated, the majority of infected patients were missed, with false-negative rates as high as 70%.

LoDs are sometimes reported in units other than copies of viral genomic RNA per milliliter of transport media (copies/mL), such as tissue culture infectious dose 50% (TCID50), copies/microliter, copies per reaction volume, or molarity of assay target. LoDs are quantitative (e.g., RT-PCR tests), but in practice results for SARS-CoV-2 testing are generally reported qualitatively as positive or negative, even though viral load may provide both clinically and epidemiologically important information. qPCR cycle threshold (Ct) values are repeatable with acceptably low variance and a reliable means of converting from Ct value to viral load. There have been reports demonstrating how appropriate measurements, based on the principles of RT-PCR, can be used as an alternative for reliable conversion of Ct values to viral loads. Viral loads vary widely among infected individuals, from individuals with extremely high viral loads, potential "super-spreaders" who presumably would be detected by even the least sensitive assays, to those whose viral loads are near, at, or even below the LoD of many assays.

Predictive Values

To assess the **predictive value (PV)** for a test, the sensitivity, specificity, and prevalence of the disease in the population being studied must be known. The prevalence of a disease is the proportion of a population that has the disease. The incidence is the number of subjects found to have the disease within a defined period, such as 1 year, in a population of 100,000.

A positive predictive value (PPV) for a test indicates the number of patients with an abnormal test result who have the disease compared with all patients with an abnormal result:

$$\text{Positive PV} = \frac{\text{Number of patients with disease and with abnormal test results}}{\text{Total number of patients with abnormal test results}}$$

$$\text{Positive PV} = \frac{\text{True positives}}{\text{True positives} + \text{False positives}}$$

A negative predictive value (NPV) for a test indicates the number of patients with a normal test result who do not have the disease compared with all patients with a normal (negative) result:

$$\text{Negative PV} = \frac{\text{True negatives}}{\text{True negatives} + \text{False negatives}}$$

Positive and Negative Predictive Values Related to SARS-CoV-2

Tests are also described by their PPVs and NPVs. These measures assume the percentage about the percentage (prevalence) of individuals in the population who have antibodies to SARS-CoV-2. Every test returns some false-positive and false-negative results. The PPV and NPV help individuals who are interpreting these tests understand how likely it is that a person who receives a positive result from a test truly does have antibodies to SARS-CoV-2 and how likely it is that a person who receives a negative result from a test truly does not have antibodies to SARS-CoV-2.

According to the FDA, the prevalence of SARS-CoV-2 antibody-positive individuals in the US population has not been firmly established. The prevalence may change based on the duration the virus is in the country and the effectiveness of mitigations. Prevalence may vary widely between geographic locations and between different groups of people (e.g., healthcare workers) due to different rates of infection. In low-prevalence populations (e.g., many asymptomatic patients in the general population), the result of a single antibody test is not likely to be sufficiently accurate to make an informed decision regarding whether or not an individual has had a prior infection or truly has antibodies to the virus. A second test to assess the presence of antibodies to a different viral protein would usually be needed to increase the accuracy of the overall testing results.

The FDA has summarized the expected performance of the tests it has authorized based on the information it reviewed when deciding whether or not to grant these tests an EUA and assuming a prevalence of 5% for PPV and NPV calculations. For tests that had multiple validation studies or where the tests showed variable performance in samples collected at different times after symptom onset, FDA experts selected the results they considered to be most representative of expected test performance. This is an incomplete representation of the performance of these tests. It is always important to refer to the complete instructions for use in a specific assay to put estimates into the proper context and to understand how to use and interpret these tests. The FDA also allows users to see the estimated performance of a single test or two independent tests based on their performance characteristics and the estimated prevalence of SARS-CoV-2 antibodies in the target population.

MONITORING QUALITY

Proficiency Testing

Proficiency testing (PT) is incorporated into the CLIA requirements. In addition to the use of internal QC programs, each laboratory should participate in an external PT program as a means of verification of laboratory accuracy. Periodically, a laboratory tests a specimen that has been provided by a government agency, professional society, or commercial company. Identical samples are sent to a group of laboratories participating in the PT program. Each laboratory analyzes the specimen, reports the results to the agency, and is evaluated and graded on those results compared with results from other laboratories. In this way, QC between laboratories is monitored.

Control Specimens

A QC program for the laboratory uses a **control specimen**, a specimen with a known value that is similar in composition to the patient's blood. A control specimen must be carried through the entire test procedure and treated in exactly the same way as any unknown specimen; it must be affected by all the variables that affect the unknown specimen. Control specimens are used because repeated determinations on the same or different portions (or **aliquots**) of the same sample will not give identical values. Many factors can produce variations in laboratory analyses. With a properly designed control system, it is possible to monitor testing variables.

If the control value in a determination is out of the acceptable range (out of control), one or more of the following factors may be responsible:
- Deterioration of reagents or standards
- Faulty instrument or equipment
- Dirty glassware
- Lack of attention to timing or incubation temperature
- Use of a method not suited to the needs and facilities of the laboratory
- Use of poor technique by the technologist doing the test

> **KEY CONCEPTS: Performance Indicators**
> - The reference range for a particular measurement is usually a normal, bell-shaped curve.
> - *Mean* is the mathematical average of the values. *Median* is the middle value. *Mode* is the most frequently occurring value. *SD* is the square root of the variance of the values.
> - *Reference range* is the range of values that includes 95% of the test results for a healthy reference population, formerly referred to as *normal values* or *normal range*.
> - *Biometrics* attempts to describe statistical variations in biological observation.
> - Each laboratory must determine the reproducibility for each new procedure and establish acceptable limits of variation for control specimens.

REFERENCE RANGE STATISTICS

In analytic immunology and serology testing, using methods such as enzyme immunoassay and quantitative reference range statistics can be used. Statistically, the **reference range** for a particular measurement is usually related to a normal, bell-shaped curve (Fig. 6.1). This **gaussian curve** has been shown to be correct for almost all types of biological, chemical, and physical measurements. A statistically valid series of individuals who are thought to represent a normal healthy group are measured, and the average value is calculated. This mathematical average is defined as the mean (called the *X-bar*). The distribution of all values around the average for the particular group measured is described statistically by SD.

Mean: Mathematical average calculated by dividing the sum of all individual values by the number of values.

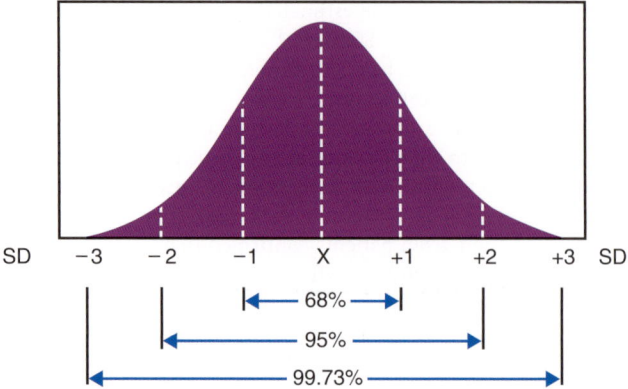

Fig. 6.1 Normal, Bell-Shaped Gaussian Curve. *SD,* Standard deviation. (From Turgeon ML: Linné and Ringsrud's clinical laboratory science: the basics and routine techniques, ed 6, St. Louis, 2012, Mosby.)

Median: Middle value in a body of data; if all the variables are arranged in order of increasing magnitude, the median is the variable that falls halfway between the highest and lowest variables.

Mode: Value that occurs most frequently in a mass of data.

Use of the mean, median, and mode is explained in the following example:
1. A series of results reported for a laboratory test on seven different specimens is 7, 2, 3, 6, 5, 4, and 2.
2. The mean is the mathematical average and is calculated by taking the sum of the values (29) and dividing by the number of values (7) in the list. The mean is 4.1 (rounded off to 4).
3. The median equals the middle value. To find the median, the list of numbers must first be ranked according to magnitude: 2, 2, 3, 4, 5, 6, 7. There are seven values in the list, and the median is the middle value, 4.
4. The mode is the most frequently occurring value, or 2 in this example.

The SD is the square root of the variance of the values in any one observation or in a series of test results. In a normal population, 68% of the values will be clustered above and below the average and defined statistically as falling within the first SD (±1 SD; see Fig. 6.1). The second SD (±2 SD) represents 95% of the values falling equally above and below the average, and 99.73% is included within the third SD (±3 SD). (Again, variations occur equally above and below the average value [or mean] for any measurement.) Thus in determining reference values for a particular measurement, a statistically valid series of people is chosen and assumed to represent a healthy population. These people are then tested, and the results are averaged.

The reference range is the range of values that includes 95% of the test results for a healthy reference population. The term replaces **normal values**, or normal range. The limits (or range) of normal are defined in terms of the SD from the average value. Thus normal or reference values are stated as a range of values in terms of SD units.

TESTING OUTCOMES

Before physicians can determine whether a patient has a disease, they must know what is acceptable for a representative population of similar patients (e.g., same age, same gender, and same ethnicity), in addition to the analytic method used for an assay. Furthermore, an individual may show daily, circadian, and physiologic variations.

Biometrics, the science of statistics applied to biological observations, has been a rapidly expanding field that attempts to describe these variations. The selection of a group on whom to base reference groups is another problem confronting the individual laboratory.

To develop reference values (normal values), the proper statistical tools of sampling, selection of the comparison group, and analysis of data must be used by the manufacturer of testing kits or individual laboratories.

Although generally accepted values are published, reference values will vary, especially between laboratories and between geographic locations. Each laboratory must give the physician information concerning the range of reference values for that particular laboratory.

VALIDATING NEW PROCEDURES

The QC program also determines how new procedures are validated (Table 6.1) before being included as one of the methods routinely used by the laboratory. Each laboratory must determine the reproducibility (or confidence limits) for each procedure used and establish acceptable limits of variation for control specimens. The QC program includes calculation of the mean (or average value) and SD, and the preparation of control charts for each procedure.

Parallel Testing of Test Kits

The requirements for the parallel testing of test kits differ depending on the accreditation agency. For example, CAP and CLIA have slightly different requirements. There is also a difference in the requirements depending on the circumstances. Are you changing manufacturers and test kits, or are you only changing lot numbers for the same kit?

The CAP asserts that CLIA-waived assays are not recognized and the laboratory must treat all tests the same way. It is best to check the immunology checklist at the CAP website (www.cap.org) for the latest revisions to questions related to kits. Currently, CAP checklist question IMM.33150 (phase II) is "Are new reagent lots checked against old reagent lots, or with suitable reference material before, or concurrently with, being placed in service?"

TABLE 6.1 Procedure Validation Checklist Example: Traditional Screening Test for Infectious Mononucleosis

	Procedure Details	Evaluation of Write-Up	Acceptable: Yes/No (Add Comments as Needed)
1. Format			
Title	Paul-Bunnell Screening Test for Infectious Mononucleosis	Is the title defined and specific?	
Purpose or principle of assay	The Paul-Bunnell test is a hemagglutination test designed to detect heterophil antibodies in patient serum when mixed with antigen-bearing sheep erythrocytes. Dilutions of inactivated patient serum are mixed with sheep erythrocytes, incubated, centrifuged, and macroscopically examined for agglutination. Positive reactions are preliminarily associated with the manifestation of infectious mononucleosis.	Is the principle or purpose of the assay clearly stated?	
2. Specimen Collection and Preparation			
Preliminary specimen preparation	No special preparation of the patient is required before specimen collection. The patient must be positively identified when the specimen is collected. The specimen should be labeled at the bedside and include the patient's full name, date the specimen is collected, patient's hospital identification number, and phlebotomist's initials. Blood should be drawn by aseptic technique. The required specimen is a minimum of 2 mL of clotted blood (red-top evacuated tube). Centrifuge the tube of blood and remove an aliquot of clear serum. The presence of hemolysis makes the specimen unsuitable for testing. Inactivate the serum at 56°C for 30 min before testing.	Are the specimen collection requirements clearly stated? Are any special specimen-processing requirements stated?	
3. Reagents, Supplies, and Equipment			
Reagents, supplies, and equipment	Two percent suspension of washed sheep cells in normal saline (prepared by pipetting 0.2 mL of packed erythrocytes into 9.8 mL of saline). 0.9% sodium chloride (normal physiologic saline) 12 × 75-mm test tubes. Note: The cell should be no more than 1 week old. Graduated serologic pipettes. Centrifuge 37°C incubator (optional).	Are all of the necessary reagents, supplies, and equipment listed?	
4. Quality Control			
Positive control serum; negative control serum	A known positive controls should be run concurrently.	Are the QC requirements stated?	

Continued

TABLE 6.1 Procedure Validation Checklist Example: Traditional Screening Test for Infectious Mononucleosis—cont'd

Procedure Details		Evaluation of Write-Up	Acceptable: Yes/No (Add Comments as Needed)
5. Procedural Steps			
Steps	1. Label two sets of test tubes. Each set should consist of 10 tubes. 2. Pipette 0.5 mL of saline into tube 1 and 0.25 mL of saline into each of the remaining nine tubes. 3. To the first set of tubes, add 0.1 mL of patient's inactivated serum to the first tube; mix and transfer 0.25 mL of the dilution to the second tube; mix and transfer 0.25 mL of the dilution to the third tube. Repeat this process to tube 10. Discard 0.25 mL from the final tube, tube 10. 4. To the second set of tubes, add 0.1 mL of the control serum and proceed to dilute it as in step 3. 5. Add 0.1 mL of 2% sheep cells to each tube. 6. Gently shake the tubes until mixed. 7. Incubate the tubes at 37°C for 1 hour or overnight at room temperature. 8. Centrifuge the tubes for 1 min at 1500 rpm. 9. Gently shake each tube and examine macroscopically for agglutination. 10. Record the results.	Are the steps in the procedure understandable? Can the procedure be performed as described?	
6. Reporting Results			
Positive reaction	A titer >1:56 is considered to be a positive presumptive test.		
Negative reaction	The antigens on sheep erythrocytes are associated with infectious mononucleosis, serum sickness, and the Forssman antigen.		
7. Procedural Notes			
Sources of error	False-positive reactions have been observed in conditions such as hepatitis infection and Hodgkin disease. An improperly inactivated serum will produce hemolysis.	Are the criteria for acceptable results clearly defined?	
Limitations	The test is only indicative of the presence or absence of heterophil antibodies. Demonstrating agglutination by using sheep erythrocytes does not make a distinction between antibodies associated with infectious mononucleosis, serum sickness, or the Forssman antigen. Heterophil antibody assay lacks sensitivity as a diagnostic criterion for infectious mononucleosis. Sheep erythrocytes are less sensitive than erythrocytes from other species such as the horse. A patient may take as long as 3 months to develop a detectable heterophil titer.		
Clinical applications	The Paul-Bunnell test is a useful screening test for the presence of heterophil antibodies because it is simple and inexpensive. Although the specificity of the heterophil assay is rated as good, negative results are demonstrated in individuals who do not produce infectious mononucleosis heterophil antibodies. If negative results are displayed, however, Epstein-Barr virus serology may be indicated.		
8. References			

General question: Are all necessary fields of the CLSI format addressed?
Additional general comments:
Evaluation of write-up validation by: _____ Date _____ Supervisory reviewer: _____ Date _____

Adapted from Paul JR, Bunnell WW: The presence of heterophil antibodies in infectious mononucleosis, *Am J Med Sci* 183:90–104, 1932; and Sumaya CV: Infectious mononucleosis and other EBV infections: diagnostic factors, *Lab Manage* 24:37–45, 1986.

CASE STUDY 6.1

A new employee was asked to examine a CLSI procedural protocol worksheet and rate the write-up. She noted the following entries:

Title	Entry
Title	Test for *Staphylococcus*
Quality Control	No positive or negative controls available

Questions

1. Is the title acceptable as written?
   a. Yes
   b. No
2. Is the quality control requirement acceptable?
   a. Yes
   b. No

See Appendix A for the answers to these questions.

Critical-Thinking Group Discussion Question

1. Why are positive and negative controls essential to the accuracy of a test result?

See instructor site for the discussion of this question.

A CLIA inspection focuses on the following:

- If the test is moderate or of high complexity and the change is to a new kit manufacturer, the new test kit must be validated for accuracy and precision. This can be done with controls, other known samples, or comparison with an old kit. If the laboratory is receiving a new lot shipment of the same test kit, only controls need to be done, or whatever the manufacturer requires.
- If the test is a waived test, a laboratory only needs to follow the manufacturer's directions if a new test is put into use or if there is a lot change of a current test. This rule is also applicable if the waived test is being performed in a moderate- or high-complexity laboratory. If an assay is waived anywhere, it is performed under CLIA requirements.

REVIEW QUESTIONS

1. An example of a factor in preanalytic testing is:
   a. Accuracy in testing
   b. Patient identification
   c. Critical value reporting
   d. Age of specimen
2. An example of a factor in analytic testing is:
   a. Accuracy in testing
   b. Patient identification
   c. Critical value reporting
   d. Specimen label
3. An example of a factor in postanalytic testing is:
   a. Accuracy in testing
   b. Patient identification
   c. Critical value reporting
   d. Type of specimen
4. Blood from the wrong patient is an example of an error classified as:
   a. Preanalytic
   b. Analytic
   c. Postanalytic
5. A specimen collected in the wrong evacuated tube is an example of an error classified as:
   a. Preanalytic
   b. Analytic
   c. Postanalytic
6. A quality control value outside of an acceptable limit is an example of an error classified as:
   a. Preanalytic
   b. Analytic
   c. Postanalytic
7. The term *accuracy* means:
   a. How close results are to one another when repeatedly analyzed
   b. How close a test result is to the true value
   c. Specimen similar to patient's blood; known concentration of constituent
   d. Comparison of an instrument measure or reading to a known physical constant
8. The term *control* means:
   a. How close results are to one another when repeatedly analyzed
   b. How close a test result is to the true value
   c. Specimen similar to patient's blood; known concentration of constituent
   d. Comparison of an instrument measure or reading to a known physical constant
9. The term *precision* means:
   a. How close results are to one another when repeatedly analyzed
   b. How close a test result is to the true value
   c. Specimen similar to patient's blood; known concentration of constituent
   d. Comparison of an instrument measure or reading to a known physical constant
10. The term *sensitivity* means:
    a. Subjects with a specific disease or condition produce a positive result
    b. Subjects without a specific disease or condition produce a negative result
11. The term *specificity* means:
    a. Subjects with a specific disease or condition produce a positive result
    b. Subjects without a specific disease or condition produce a negative result
12. The type of error caused by omitting patient serum or reagent from a test mixture is a:
    a. False-positive error
    b. False-negative error
    c. False-positive or false-negative error
13. The type of error caused by using dirty glassware is a:
    a. False-positive error
    b. False-negative error
    c. False-positive or false-negative error
14. The type of error caused by addition of the wrong reagent is a:
    a. False-positive error
    b. False-negative error
    c. False-positive or false-negative error

15. The type of error caused by inaccurately recording results is a:
    a. False-positive error
    b. False-negative error
    c. False-positive or false-negative error
16. The type of error caused by using hemolyzed patient serum is a:
    a. False-positive error
    b. False-negative error
    c. False-positive or false-negative error
17. The quality control term used to describe the number of patients with an abnormal test result who have a disease being tested for by a specific assay compared with all patients with an abnormal results is:
    a. Positive predictive value
    b. Negative predictive value
    c. Specificity
    d. Sensitivity
18. In a written procedural protocol, the _____ should follow the specimen collection and storage information.
    a. Reagents, supplies, and equipment
    b. Sources of error
    c. Principle and purpose of the test
    d. Procedural protocol
19. In a written procedural protocol, the _____ should follow the list of reagents, supplies, and equipment.
    a. Quality control
    b. Sources of error
    c. Principle and purpose of the test
    d. Procedural protocol
20. In a written procedural protocol, the _____ should follow the reference values and procedural notes.
    a. Quality control
    b. Sources of error
    c. Principle and purpose of the test
    d. Procedural protocol

Basic Serologic Laboratory: Techniques and Clinical Applications

LEARNING OUTCOMES

- Explain the purpose of a procedures manual.
- Describe the preparation of blood specimens for testing.
- Provide examples of the types of specimens that can be tested using immunologic procedures.
- Explain how complement is inactivated in a serum sample.
- Describe and demonstrate pipetting techniques using manual and automatic pipettes.
- Define the term *dilution*.
- Calculate the concentration of a substance using the dilution factor.
- Calculate the concentration of a single dilution.
- Compare the characteristics of the acute and chronic phases of illness.
- Define the term *antibody titer*.
- Explain and be able to prepare a serial dilution.
- Define point-of-care testing (POCT).
- Cite some advantages and disadvantages of POCT.
- Differentiate among the four different types of testing categories.
- Discuss the immunology techniques used in rapid testing for human immunodeficiency virus (HIV), and pregnancy.
- Analyze case studies with interpretation of the assay results.
- Correctly answer case study–related multiple-choice questions.
- Discuss the critical-thinking questions.
- Correctly answer 80% of the end-of-chapter review questions.

OUTLINE

Procedures Manual, 118
Blood Specimen Preparation, 118
  Types of Specimens Tested, 118
  Inactivation of Complement, 118
  Pipettes, 118
    Micropipettors, 119
    Automatic Dispensers or Syringes, 120
    Diluter-Dispensers, 120
  Dilutions, 120
    Diluting Specimens, 120
    Dilution Factor, 120
    Single Dilutions, 121
    Serial Dilutions, 121
  Antibody Testing, 122
  Serial Dilution, 122
    Principle, 122

Interpretation of Results, 122
Antibody Titer, 122
Rapid Point-of-Care Testing, 122
  Testing Categories, 123
    Waived Testing, 123
    Quality Control, 123
  Quality Control Standards for Moderate- and High-Complexity Testing, 123
  Examples of Non–Instrument-Based Testing, 123
    HIV Testing, 123
    Pregnancy Testing, 123
Case Study 7.1, 124
Case Study 7.2, 124
Procedure: Card Pregnancy Test, 127.e1

KEY TERMS

acute phase
aliquot
antibody titer
chyle
colorimetric reactions
convalescent phase
cytopathology
diluent
dilution
ectopic pregnancy
follicle-stimulating hormone (FSH)
hemagglutination
hemagglutination assays
hematology
human chorionic gonadotropin (hCG)
icteric
immunochromatographic
immunohematology
immunologic
in vitro
inactivation
lipemia
luteinizing hormone
microbial antigens
microbiology
monoclonal
nontrophoblastic neoplasms
passive agglutination assays
point-of-care testing (POCT)
preanalytic
serial dilutions
serologic
spectrophotometrically
toxicology
trophoblastic neoplasms
turbid

Serologic testing has long been an important part of diagnostic tests in the clinical laboratory for viral and bacterial diseases. Immunologic testing is done in many areas of the clinical laboratory—microbiology, chemistry, toxicology, immunology, hematology, surgical pathology, cytopathology, immunohematology (blood banking)—and a great variety of specimens are tested. Rapid testing is typically used in the laboratory and in home testing kits.

The advent of monoclonal antibody technology has led to the development of highly specific and sensitive immunoassays. Common serologic and immunologic tests include pregnancy tests for human chorionic gonadotropin (hCG) and tests for infectious mononucleosis and syphilis.

> **KEY CONCEPTS: Basics of Serologic Testing**
> - Traditional serologic tests have been done for viral and bacterial diseases. Other common tests include pregnancy tests for hCG and immunologic tests for infectious mononucleosis and syphilis.
> - The procedures manual describes current techniques (in Clinical and Laboratory Standards Institute [CLSI] format) and approved policies, and is always available to laboratory personnel.
> - After a blood sample has clotted, serum should be promptly removed for testing or frozen at –20°C. Standard Precautions must be followed when blood specimens are handled.
> - Lipemia, hemolysis, and bacterial contamination can make the specimen unacceptable. Icteric or turbid serum may give valid results or may interfere. Blood specimens should be collected before a meal to avoid chyle. Contamination with alkali or acid must be avoided.
> - Some procedures require inactivated serum. Complement can be inactivated by heating to 56°C for 30 minutes or, after 4 hours, reinactivated by heating for 10 minutes.

PROCEDURES MANUAL

The procedures manual must be a complete document of current techniques and approved policies that is available at all times in the immediate bench area of laboratory personnel. It is extremely important that all personnel review this manual periodically. The manual should comply with the Clinical and Laboratory Standards Institute (CLSI) format for a procedure. The procedural format found in this text generally follows these guidelines.

Alternative techniques can be included with each procedure if more than one technique is acceptable. New pages must be dated and initialed when inserted, and removed pages must be retained for 5 years, with the date of removal and the reason for removal indicated. It may be legally necessary to identify the procedure followed for a particular reason.

Procedures used in immunology apply many techniques common to other scientific disciplines, such as chemistry. In the field of immunology, different serologic techniques are used to detect the interaction of antigens with antibodies. These methods (see Chapters 7–11) are suitable for the detection and quantitation of antibodies to infectious agents, in addition to microbial antigens and nonmicrobial antigens.

BLOOD SPECIMEN PREPARATION

After blood has been obtained from a patient in a plain evacuated tube, without anticoagulant, it should be allowed to clot and the serum should be promptly removed for testing. Clotting and clot retraction should take place at room temperature or in the refrigerator, depending on the protocol for the specific procedure. Complete clot retraction normally takes about 1 hour. After clot retraction, the clot should be loosened from the sides of the test tube with an applicator stick. The tube should be centrifuged for 10 minutes at a moderate speed.

After centrifugation, serum can be transferred to a labeled tube with a Pasteur pipette and rubber bulb. If the serum is contaminated with erythrocytes, it should be recentrifuged. The serum-containing tube should be sealed.

Excessive heat and bacterial contamination are avoided. Heat coagulates the proteins and bacterial growth alters protein molecules. If the test cannot be performed immediately, the serum should be refrigerated. In most cases, if the testing cannot be done within 72 hours, a serum specimen must be frozen at –20°C. Standard Precautions must be followed when blood specimens are handled.

For some testing, the serum complement must first be inactivated (see the following discussion). If the protein complement is not inactivated, it will promote lysis of the red blood cells (RBCs) and other types of cells, and can produce invalid results. Complement is also known to interfere with certain tests for syphilis.

Types of Specimens Tested

Most immunology tests are done on serum, although body fluids may also be tested. Lipemia, hemolysis, or any bacterial contamination can make the specimen unacceptable. Icteric or turbid serum may yield valid results for some tests but may interfere with others. Blood specimens should be collected before a meal to avoid the presence of chyle, an emulsion of fat globules that often appears in serum after eating, during digestion. Contamination with alkali or acid must be avoided because these substances have a denaturing effect on serum proteins and make the specimens useless for serologic testing.

Other specimens include urine for pregnancy tests and tests for urinary tract infection. It is important that the urine specimen be collected after thorough cleaning of the external genitalia to prevent contamination of microbiological assays. Urine for the hCG assay (pregnancy test) must be collected at a suitable time interval after fertilization to allow the concentration of the hCG hormone to rise to a significantly detectable level.

Any specimen must be collected into a suitable container to prevent in vitro changes that could affect the assay results. Proper handling and storage of the specimen until testing are essential. Immunologic assays are also carried out on cerebrospinal fluid (CSF), other body fluids, and swabs of various body exudates and discharges. The established protocol for each specific assay must be followed in terms of specimen-collection requirements and conditions for the assay itself.

Inactivation of Complement

Some procedures require the use of inactivated serum. Inactivation is the process that destroys complement activity. Complement is known to interfere with the reactions of certain syphilis tests and complement components (e.g., C1q). It can agglutinate latex particles and cause a false-positive reaction in latex passive agglutination assays. Complement may also cause lysis of the indicator cells in hemagglutination assays.

Complement in body fluids can be inactivated by heating to 56°C for 30 minutes. When more than 4 hours have elapsed since inactivation, a specimen can be reinactivated by heating it to 56°C for 10 minutes.

Pipettes

Pipettes are used in the immunology-serology laboratory for the quantitative transfer of reagents and the preparations of serial dilutions of specimens such as serum (Fig. 7.1). Although semiautomated pipettes have replaced traditional glass pipettes, traditional methods may be needed at times (Box 7.1).

Automatic pipettes allow fast, repetitive measurement and delivery of solutions of equal volumes. The sampling-diluting type measures the substance in question and then adds the desired diluent. The

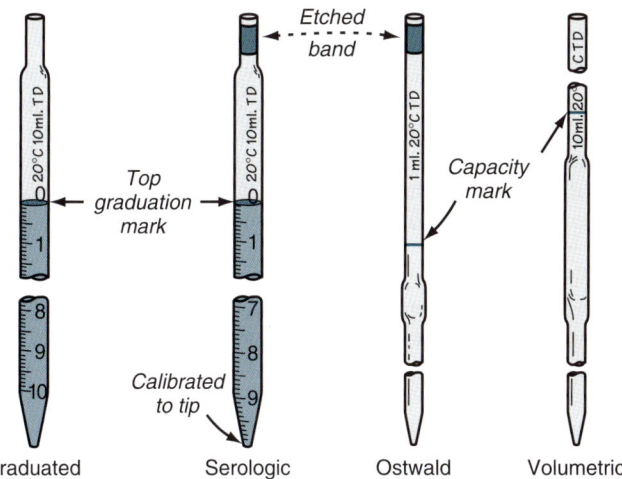

Fig. 7.1 Types of Manual Pipettes. *TD*, To deliver. (From Turgeon ML: *Linné & Ringsrud's clinical laboratory science: the basics and routine techniques,* ed 6, St. Louis, 2012, Mosby.)

BOX 7.1 Pipetting With Manual Pipettes

1. Check the pipette to ascertain its correct size, being careful to also check for broken delivery or suction tips.
2. Wearing protective gloves, hold the pipette lightly between the thumb and the last three fingers, leaving the index finger free.
3. Place the tip of the pipette well below the surface of the liquid to be pipetted.
4. Using mechanical suction or an aspirator bulb, carefully draw the liquid up into the pipette until the level of the liquid is well above the calibration mark.
5. Quickly cover the suction opening at the top of the pipette with the index finger.
6. Wipe the outside of the pipette dry with a piece of Kimwipe tissue to remove excess fluid.
7. Hold the pipette in a vertical position with the delivery tip against the inside of the original vessel. Carefully allow the liquid in the pipette to drain by gravity until the bottom of the meniscus is exactly at the calibration mark. To do this, do not entirely remove the index finger from the suction hole end of the pipette; rather, by rolling the finger slightly over the opening, allow slow drainage to take place.
8. While still holding the pipette in a vertical position, touch the tip of the pipette to the inside wall of the receiving vessel. Remove the index finger from the top of the pipette to permit free drainage. Remember to keep the pipette in a vertical position for correct drainage. In TD (to deliver) pipettes, a small amount of fluid will remain in the delivery tip.
9. To be certain that the drainage is as complete as possible, touch the delivery tip of the pipette to another area on the inside wall of the receiving vessel.

sampling-diluting type of automatic pipette is mechanically operated and uses a piston-operated plunger. These are adjustable so that varying amounts of reagent or sample can be delivered with the same device. Disposable and exchangeable tips are available for these pipettes. Automatic pipettes and micropipettors must be calibrated before use. Micropipettors must be checked yearly and recalibrated if necessary.

Micropipettors

Automatic micropipetting devices allow rapid repetitive measurements and delivery of predetermined volumes of reagents or specimens. The most common type of micropipette used in many laboratories is one that is automatic or semiautomatic, called a *micropipettor*. These are piston-operated devices that allow repeated, accurate, reproducible delivery of specimens, reagents, and other liquids requiring

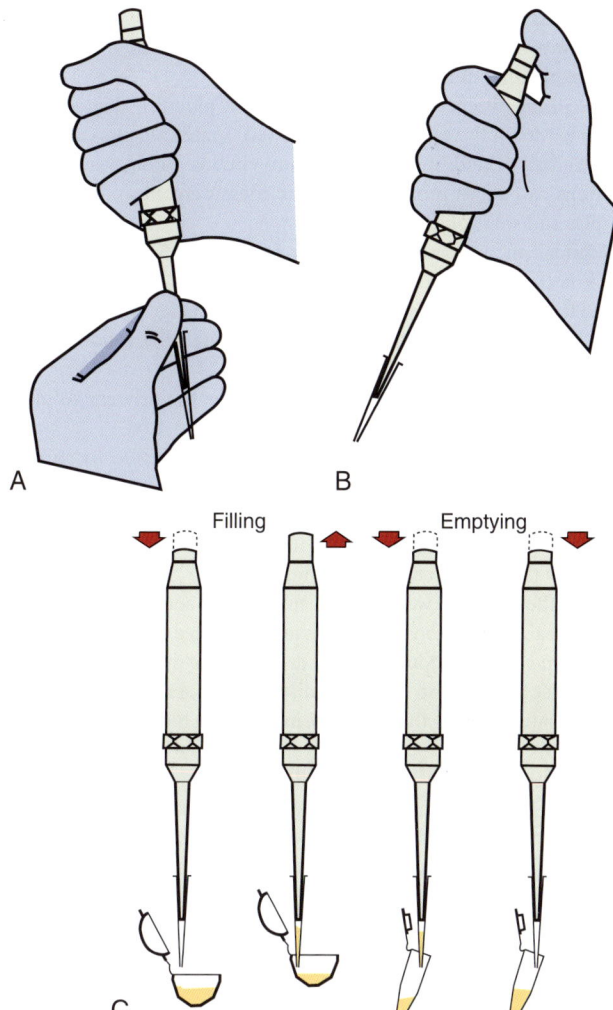

Fig. 7.2 Steps for Using a Piston-Type Automatic Micropipette. (A) Attaching the proper tip size for the range of pipette volume and twisting the tip as it is pushed onto the pipette to give an airtight, continuous seal. (B) Holding the pipette before use. (C) Follow instructions for filling and emptying the pipette tip. (From Kaplan LA, Pesce A: *Clinical chemistry: theory, analysis, correlation,* ed 5, St. Louis, 2010, Mosby.)

measurement in small amounts. Many micropipettors are continuously adjustable so that variable volumes of liquids can be dispensed with the same device. Delivery volume is selected by adjusting the settings. Different types or models are available that allow volume delivery ranging, for example, from 0.5 to 5000 µL. The calibration of these micropipettes should be checked periodically.

The piston, usually in the form of a thumb plunger, is depressed to a stop position on the pipetting device. The tip is placed in the liquid to be measured, and then the plunger is slowly allowed to rise back to the original position (Fig. 7.2). This will fill the tip with the desired volume of liquid. The tips are usually drawn along the inside wall of the vessel from which the measured volume is drawn so that any adhering liquid is removed from the end of the tip. These pipette tips are not usually wiped, as is done with the manual pipettes, because the plastic surface is considered nonwettable. The tip of the pipette device is then placed against the inside wall of the receiving vessel, and the plunger is depressed. When the manufacturer's directions for the device being used are followed, sample delivery volume is judged to be extremely accurate.

The pipette tips are usually made of disposable plastic, so no cleaning is necessary. Various types of tips are available. Some pipetting devices automatically eject the tip after use. These will also allow the user to insert a new tip and remove the used tip without touching it, minimizing infectious biohazard exposures.

The problems encountered with automatic pipetting depend largely on the nature of the solution to be pipetted. Some reagents cause more bubbles than others, and some are more viscous. Bubbles and viscous solutions can cause problems with the measurement and delivery of samples and solutions.

Manual micropipettors contain or deliver 1 to 500 µL of solution, which is the same volume as automated pipettors. It is important to follow the individual manufacturer's instructions for the device being used; each may be slightly different. In general, the following steps apply for use of a micropipettor:

1. Attach the proper tip to the pipettor, and set the delivery volume.
2. Depress the piston to a stop position on the pipettor.
3. Place the tip into the solution, and allow the piston to rise back slowly to its original position (this fills the pipettor tip with the desired volume of solution).
4. Some tips are wiped with a dry gauze at this step, and some are not. Follow the manufacturer's directions.
5. Place the tip on the wall of the receiving vessel and depress the piston, first to a stop position where the liquid is allowed to drain and then to a second stop position where full dispensing of the liquid takes place.
6. Dispose of the tip in the waste-disposal receptacle. Some pipettors automatically eject the used tips, minimizing biohazard exposure.

Automatic Dispensers or Syringes

Many types of automatic dispensers or syringes are used in the laboratory for repetitively adding multiple doses of the same reagent or diluent. These devices are used for measuring serial amounts of relatively small volumes of the same liquid. The volume to be dispensed is determined by the pipettor setting. Dispensers are available with a variety of volume settings. Some are available as syringes and others as bottle-top devices. Most of these dispensers can be cleaned by autoclaving.

Diluter-Dispensers

In automated instruments, diluter-dispensers are used to prepare a number of different samples for analysis. These devices pipette a selected aliquot of sample and diluent into the instrument or receiving vessel. They are primarily of the dual-piston type, with one used for the sample and the other for the diluent or reagent.

KEY CONCEPTS: Facts About Dilutions
- Automatic pipettes allow fast repetitive measurement and delivery of solutions of equal volumes.
- All dilutions are a ratio. Dilution is an indication of relative concentration.
- A dilution factor is used to correct for having used a diluted sample in a determination rather than the undiluted sample. The result (answer) using the dilution must be multiplied by the reciprocal of the dilution made.
- When the concentration is too high or less specimen is available for analysis, the original specimen may be diluted or the initial dilution (or filtrate) further diluted. These single dilutions are usually expressed as a ratio (1:2, 1:5, 1:10) or a fraction (½, 1/5, {1/10}).
- A dilution is the volume or number of parts of the substance to be diluted in the total volume, or parts, of the final solution. A dilution is an expression of concentration, the relative amount of substance in solution. Dilutions can be made singly or in series.
- In a dilution series, all dilutions, including or following the first one, are the same, called *serial dilutions*.
- A complete dilution series usually contains 5 or 10 tubes, although any single dilution may be made directly from an undiluted specimen or substance.

Dilutions

It is often necessary to make dilutions of specimens being analyzed or to make weaker solutions from stronger solutions in various laboratory procedures. Clinicians must be able to work with various dilution problems and dilution factors. They often need to determine the concentration of antibodies in each solution, the actual amount of material in each solution, and the total volume of each solution. All dilutions are a form of ratio. **Dilution** is an indication of relative concentration.

Diluting Specimens

In most laboratory determinations, a small sample is taken for analysis and the final result is expressed as concentration per some convenient standard volume. In a certain procedure, 0.5 mL of blood is diluted to a total of 10 mL with various reagents, and 1 mL of this dilution is then analyzed for a particular chemical constituent. The final result is to be expressed in terms of the concentration of that substance per 100 mL of blood.

Dilution Factor

A dilution factor is used to correct for having used a diluted sample in a determination rather than the undiluted sample. The result (answer) using the dilution must be multiplied by the reciprocal of the dilution made. For example, a dilution factor by which all determination answers are multiplied to give the concentration per 100 mL of sample (blood) may be calculated as follows.

First, determine the volume of blood that is actually analyzed in the procedure. Using a simple proportion, it is evident that 0.5 mL of blood diluted to 10 mL is equivalent to 1 mL of blood diluted to 20 mL:

$$\frac{0.5 \text{ mL blood}}{10 \text{ mL solution}} = \frac{1 \text{ mL blood}}{x \text{ mL solution}}$$

$$x = \frac{1 \text{ mL blood} \times 10 \text{ mL}}{0.5 \text{ mL}} = 20 \text{ mL}$$

The concentration of specimen (blood) in each milliliter of solution may be determined by the use of another simple proportion to be 0.05 mL of blood per milliliter of solution:

$$\frac{1 \text{ mL blood}}{20 \text{ mL solution}} = \frac{x \text{ mL blood}}{1 \text{ mL solution}}$$

$$x = \frac{1 \text{ mL} \times 1 \text{ mL}}{20 \text{ mL}} = 0.05 \text{ mL}$$

Because 1 mL of the 1:20 dilution of blood is analyzed in the remaining steps of the procedure, 0.05 mL of blood is actually analyzed (1 mL of the dilution used × 0.05 mL/mL = 0.05 mL of blood analyzed).

To relate the concentration of the substance measured in the procedure to the concentration in 100 mL of blood (the units in which the result is to be expressed), another proportion may be used:

$$\frac{100 \text{ mL (volume of blood desired)}}{0.05 \text{ mL (volume of blood used)}} = \frac{\text{concentration desired}}{\text{concentration used or determined}}$$

$$\text{Concetrationon desired} = \frac{100 \text{ mL} \times \text{concentration determined}}{0.05 \text{ mL}}$$

$$\text{Concentration desired} = 2000 \times \text{value determined}$$

The concentration of the substance being measured in the volume of blood actually tested (0.05 mL) must be multiplied by 2000 to report the concentration per 100 mL of blood.

The preceding material may be summarized by the following statement and equations. In reporting results obtained from laboratory determinations, one must first determine the amount of specimen actually analyzed in the procedure and then calculate the factor that will express the concentration in the desired terms of measurement. Thus in the previous example, the following equations may be used:

$$\frac{0.5 \text{ mL (volume of blood used)}}{10 \text{ mL (volume of total dilution)}} = \frac{x \text{ mL (volume of blood analyzed)}}{1 \text{ mL (volume of dilution used)}}$$

$x = 0.05$ mL (volume of blood actually analyzed)

$$\frac{100 \text{ mL (volume of blood required or expression of result)}}{0.05 \text{ mL (volume of blood actually analyzed)}} = 2000 \text{ (dilution factor)}$$

Single Dilutions

When the concentration of a particular substance in a specimen is too great to be determined accurately, or when there is less specimen available for analysis than the procedure requires, it may be necessary to dilute the original specimen or further dilute the initial dilution (or filtrate). These single dilutions are usually expressed as a ratio (e.g., 1:2, 1:5, or 1:10) or as a fraction (e.g., ½, 1/5, or {1/10}). These ratios or fractions refer to 1 unit of the original specimen diluted to a final volume of 2, 5, or 10 units, respectively. A dilution, therefore, refers to the volume or number of parts of the substance to be diluted in the total volume, or parts, of the final solution. A dilution is an expression of concentration, not volume; it indicates the relative amount of substance in solution. Dilutions can be made singly or in series.

To calculate the concentration of a single dilution, multiply the original concentration by the dilution expressed as a fraction.

Example of calculation of concentration of a single dilution. A specimen contains 500 mg of substance per deciliter of blood. A 1:5 dilution of this specimen is prepared by volumetrically measuring 1 mL of the specimen and adding 4 mL of diluent. The concentration (C) of substance in the dilution is calculated as follows:

$$C = 500 \frac{\text{mg/dL} \times 1}{5} = 100 \text{ mg/dL}$$

Note that the concentration of the final solution (or dilution) is expressed in the same units as that of the original solution.

To obtain a dilution factor that can be applied to the determination answer and express it as a concentration per standard volume, proceed as follows. Rather than multiply by the dilution expressed as a fraction, multiply the determination value by the reciprocal of the dilution fraction. In the case of a 1:5 dilution, the dilution factor applied to values obtained in the procedure would be 5, because the original specimen was five times more concentrated than the diluted specimen tested in the procedure.

Use of dilution factors. A 1:5 dilution of a specimen is prepared, and an **aliquot** (one of a number of equal parts) of the dilution is analyzed for a particular substance. The concentration of the substance (C) in the aliquot is multiplied by 5 to determine its concentration in the original specimen. If the concentration of the dilution is 100 mg/dL, the concentration of the original specimen is:

$C = 100 \text{ mg/dL} \times 5$ (dilution factor) $= 500 \text{ mg/dL}$ in blood

TABLE 7.1 Example of Preparation of a Serial Dilution

	1	2	3	4	5	6
Saline (mL)	1	1	1	1	1	1
Patient serum or preceding dilution (mL)	1	1 of 1:2	1 of 1:4	1 of 1:8	1 of 1:16	1 of 1:32
Final dilution	1:2	1:4	1:8	1:16	1:32	1:64

Serial Dilutions

Dilutions can also be made in series, in which the original solution is further diluted. A general rule for calculating the concentrations of solutions obtained by dilution in series is to multiply the original concentration by the first dilution (expressed as a fraction), this by the second dilution, and so on, until the desired concentration is known.

Several laboratory procedures, especially serologic methods, make use of a dilution series in which all dilutions, including or following the first one, are the same. Such dilutions are referred to as **serial dilutions** (Table 7.1). A complete dilution series usually contains 5 or 10 tubes, although any single dilution may be made directly from an undiluted specimen or substance. In calculating the dilution or concentration of a substance or serum in each tube of the dilution series, the rules previously discussed apply.

A twofold dilution may be prepared as follows (Fig. 7.3). A serum specimen is diluted 1:2 with buffer. A series of five tubes are prepared, in which each succeeding tube is rediluted 1:2. This is accomplished by placing 1 mL of diluent into each of four tubes (tubes 2–5). Tube 1 contains 1 mL of undiluted serum. Tube 2 contains 1 mL of undiluted serum plus 1 mL of diluent, resulting in a 1:2 dilution of serum. A 1-mL portion of the 1:2 dilution of serum is placed in tube 3, resulting in a 1:4 dilution of serum (½ × ½ × ¼). A 1-mL portion of the 1:4 dilution from tube 3 is placed in tube 4, resulting in a 1:8 dilution (¼ × ½ × {⅛}). Finally, 1 mL of the 1:8 dilution from tube 4 is added to tube 5, resulting in a 1:16 dilution ({⅛} × ½ ×{1/16}). One milliliter of the final dilution is discarded so that the volumes in all the tubes are equal.

Note that each tube is diluted twice as much as the previous tube and that the final volume in each tube is the same. The undiluted serum may also be given a dilution value, 1:1.

The concentration of serum in terms of milliliters in each tube is calculated by multiplying the previous concentration (mL) by the succeeding dilution. In this example, tube 1 contains 1 mL of serum; tube 2 contains 1 mL × ½ × 0.5 mL of serum; and tubes 3 to 5 contain 0.25, 0.125, and 0.06 mL of serum, respectively.

Other serial dilutions might be fivefold or tenfold; that is, each succeeding tube is diluted 5 or 10 times. A fivefold series would begin with 1 mL of serum in 4 mL of diluent and a total volume of 5 mL in each tube. A tenfold series would begin with 1 mL of serum in 9 mL of diluent and a total volume of 10 mL in each tube.

> **KEY CONCEPTS: Significant Antibody Applications**
> - When antibody levels are tested for a specific infectious organism, blood should be drawn during both the acute and convalescent phases.
> - A difference in the amount of antibody present, or the antibody titer, may be noted when two different samples are tested concurrently. A rise in titer is central to serologic testing.
> - The antibody titer is defined as the reciprocal of the highest dilution of the patient's serum in which the antibody is still detectable.

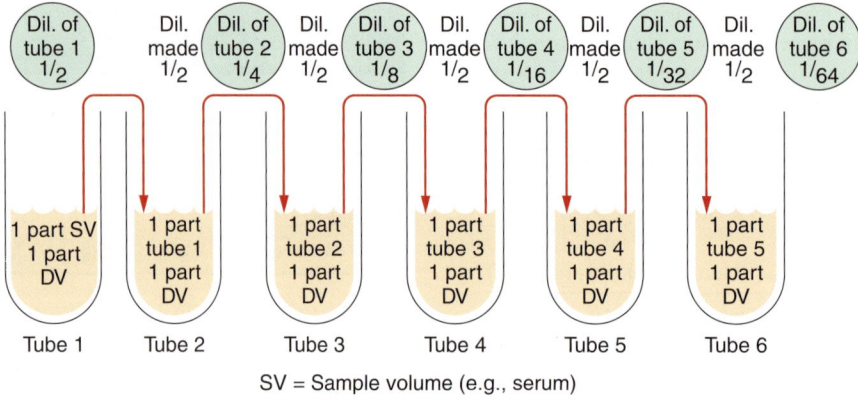

Fig. 7.3 Schematic of a Twofold Serial Dilution. (From Turgeon ML: *Linné & Ringsrud's clinical laboratory science: the basics and routine techniques,* ed 6, St. Louis, 2012, Mosby.)

Antibody Testing

In obtaining specimens for serologic testing, it is important to consider the phase of the disease and the condition of the patient at the time of specimen collection. This is especially important in assays for diagnosis of infectious diseases. If serum is being tested for antibody levels with a specific infectious organism, generally the blood should be drawn during the acute phase of the illness (when the disease is first discovered or suspected) and another sample drawn during the convalescent phase, usually about 2 weeks later. Accordingly, these samples are called *acute* and *convalescent serum*. A difference in the amount of antibody present, or the antibody titer, may be noted when the two different samples are tested concurrently. Some infections, such as legionnaires' disease or hepatitis, may not manifest a rise in titer until months after the acute infection.

Serial Dilution
Principle
Serial dilutions are a method for determining the concentration of a substance (e.g., antibody). The greatest dilution of the sample that yields a positive result is the endpoint. This endpoint dilution can be expressed as a fraction. The reciprocal of that fraction is called the *titer* of the antibody.

A series of dilutions of a sample are necessary for determining an antibody titer. In serial dilution, each dilution is prepared from the previous dilution. Dilutions can be in large test tubes (i.e., macrotitration) or in a miniaturized version (i.e., microtitration).

Microtitration is valuable for any procedure in which dilutions are made and RBCs are used as indicator cells (e.g., hemagglutination). Colorimetric reactions can be performed (e.g., enzyme immunoassay [EIA]) and quantitated spectrophotometrically with specialized instruments for microtiter plates.

Interpretation of Results
In clinical immunology, the titer of an antibody in an individual's serum can have clinical significance, depending on the antibody in question. Antibody titers are sometimes used to evaluate a person's immune status. Titers may be obtained over time, as with acute and convalescent specimens for infectious diseases or monitoring a mother's titer for blood group antibodies during pregnancy.

Antibody Titer
A central concept of serologic testing is the manifestation of a rise in titer, or concentration, of an antibody. The antibody titer is defined as the reciprocal of the highest dilution of the patient's serum in which the antibody is still detectable. That is, the titer is read at the highest dilution of serum that gives a positive reaction with the antigen. If a serum sample has been diluted 1:64 and reacts positively with the antigen suspension used in the testing process, and if the next highest dilution of 1:128 does not give a positive reaction, the titer is read as 64. A high titer indicates that there is a relatively high concentration of the antibody present in the serum.

Determination of the concentration of antibody (titer) for a specific antigen involves the following two steps:
1. Preparing a serial dilution of the antibody-containing solution (e.g., serum)
2. Adding an equal volume of antigen suspension to each dilution

A high titer indicates that a considerable amount of antibody is present in the serum. For most pathogenic infections, an increase in the patient's titer of two doubling dilutions, or from a positive result of 1:8 to a positive result of 1:32 over several weeks, is an indication of a current infection. This is known as a *fourfold rise in the antibody titer.*

> **KEY CONCEPTS: Characteristics of Point-of-Care Testing**
> - Point-of-care testing (POCT) involves laboratory assays performed near the patient and includes home test kits and handheld monitors.
> - The major advantage of POCT is the rapidity of assay results; the major drawback is cost.
> - Testing can be divided into waived, moderately complex, highly complex, and provider-performed microscopy tests. POCT is in the waived or moderately complex category.

RAPID POINT-OF-CARE TESTING

Point-of-care testing (POCT) is defined as laboratory assays performed near the patient. The development of new POCT assays has been increasing at a rapid rate. POCT testing can include home test kits and handheld monitors. The major advantage is the rapidity of obtaining quality results if the procedure is performed by an appropriate patient or healthcare provider. The major drawback is cost, particularly if a large volume of testing is done. Other areas of concern include maintenance of quality control (QC) and quality assurance (QA).

Testing Categories

The Clinical Laboratory Improvement Amendments of 1988 (CLIA '88) subjects all clinical laboratory testing to federal regulation and inspection. According to CLIA '88, test procedures are grouped into one of the four following categories:

1. *Waived tests.* Simple procedures with little chance of negative outcomes if performed inaccurately.
2. *Moderately complex tests.* More complex than waived tests but usually automated (e.g., EIAs).
3. *Highly complex tests.* Usually nonautomated or complicated tests requiring considerable judgment (e.g., serum protein electrophoresis).
4. *Provider-performed microscopy tests.* Slide examinations of freshly collected body fluids.

Test complexity is determined by criteria that assess knowledge, training, reagent and material preparation, operational technique, QC-QA characteristics, maintenance and troubleshooting, and interpretation and judgment. Any over-the-counter test approved by the US Food and Drug Administration (FDA) is automatically placed into the "waived" category. POCT falls within the "waived" or "moderately complex" category.

Waived Testing

Waived testing is defined by CLIA '88 as tests that have the following characteristics:

- They use methodologies that are so simple and accurate as to render the likelihood of erroneous results negligible.
- They pose no reasonable risk of harm to the patient if the test is performed incorrectly.
- They have been cleared by the FDA for home use.

These tests are "waived" from certain federal requirements. The most commonly used waived tests are glucose testing, urine pregnancy screens, rapid strep screens, and urine drug screens. Any organization that performs waived testing needs a CLIA certificate to do so. Tests approved by the FDA for home use only should not be used for professional purposes. For example, glucose meters cleared for home use should not be used in a hospital setting by nursing staff unless they are being used for patient education only.

The Joint Commission standards for waived testing standards require the following:

1. Identification of tests that will be performed
2. Procedures for each test
3. Confirmatory testing
4. Instrument maintenance
5. QC checks

In addition, staff competency and QC are required aspects of waived testing.

Staff competency. Staff must be trained in each waived test they perform with documentation required.

- Competency for each waived test must be assessed at orientation and annually with documentation required.
- Competency must be assessed using *two* of the following methods:
  - Performance of a test on a blind specimen
  - Periodic observation of work by a supervisor
  - Monitoring of each user's QC performance
  - Written test

Quality Control

For instrument-based waived testing, QC checks must be performed on the instrument per manufacturer's instructions. Before 2012, testing was required each day the instrument was used. In 2012 the requirement was changed to be per "manufacturer's instructions." For instrument-based waived testing, QC checks must include two levels of control, if commercially available.

Quality Control Standards for Moderate- and High-Complexity Testing

All laboratory testing must meet the same quality standards, regardless of where it is performed. State and city governments may enact mandatory regulations, including qualifications of personnel performing the test, which may be more (but not less) stringent than federal regulations. Voluntary participation in QA programs is also available.

Ultimate responsibility and control of POCT reside within the CLIA-certified laboratory and require a minimum of one laboratory staff member to be responsible for each POCT program. Written policies and procedures must be available to all laboratory personnel for patient preparation, specimen collection and preservation, instrument calibration, policies for QC and remedial actions, equipment performance evaluations, procedures for test performance, result reports, and recording. The greatest source of error is preanalytic error, such as patient identification and specimen collection.

Examples of Non–Instrument-Based Testing

Most POCT is done by manual rapid test methods. More tests continue to be developed for the rapid laboratory testing in emergency departments, hospital settings, and even at home. Numerous POCT tests are referenced throughout this book in various chapters. Several examples of rapid testing are presented as examples in this chapter.

HIV Testing

Various CLIA-waived rapid HIV tests are presented in (Fig. 7.4). These POCTs can be used in settings such as community-based organizations, field testing, outreach activities, sexually transmitted disease (STD) or other clinics, mobile clinics, nontraditional testing, or community/college clinics. Currently, confirmation of POCT, if positive, should reflex to a fourth-generation antigen–antibody test (HIV-1, HIV-2). A disadvantage of rapid tests includes lower sensitivity than third- and fourth-generation EIAs.

Pregnancy Testing

The first type of rapid POCT testing was for the detection of pregnancy. The original test kits relied on an antigen–antibody reaction for the detection of a condition of pregnancy. Although this method is still available, it has been replaced by POCT testing such as the OSOM procedure (described in detail next).

The OSOM Card Pregnancy Test is a solid-phase, sandwich-format, immunochromatographic assay for the qualitative detection of human chorionic gonadotropin (hCG).

Urine is added to the sample well and the sample migrates through reaction pads, where hCG, if present in the sample, binds to a monoclonal anti-hCG dye conjugate. The sample then migrates across a membrane toward the "results window," where the labeled hCG complex is captured at a test line region containing immobilized rabbit anti-hCG. Excess conjugate will flow past the test line region and will be captured at a control line region containing an immobilized antibody directed against the anti-hCG dye conjugate (with or without hCG complexed to it).

The appearance of two black bands in the results window, one at T (test) and the other at C (control), indicates the presence of hCG in the sample. If a detectable level of hCG is not present, only the control band will appear in the results window.

CASE STUDY 7.1

A 9-year-old boy was taken to the emergency department with a sore throat. On examination, he had redness of the throat and slightly swollen glands. The physician assistant ordered a throat culture and blood drawn for an antistreptolysin-O antibody (ASO). An antibiotic was prescribed for a 10-day period. His mother was told to make an appointment with his pediatrician for a follow-up.

At the follow-up visit 2 weeks later, the results of the laboratory test revealed a throat culture with a few colonies of β-streptococci. The qualitative ASO test result was reported as positive. The acute serum was frozen at the time of testing. The pediatrician ordered a convalescent specimen to be tested semiquantitatively in parallel with the acute specimen for an ASO titer.

The acute and convalescent specimens were prepared as twofold serial dilutions of each specimen (see the following table).

	TUBE					
	1	2	3	4	5	6
Saline (µL)	–	50	50	50	50	50
Serum (µL)	50	50	50 (1:2)	50 (1:4)	50 (1:8)	50 1:16)
Mix and transfer to next tube		50	50	50	50	50
Dilution/titer	1:1	1:2	1:4	1:8	1:16	1:32
IU/mL	200	4008	800	1600	3200	6400

The results of the parallel testing of the acute and convalescent specimens revealed the following:
- Acute specimen positive, 1:1 dilution/titer (IU/mL 200)
- Convalescent specimen positive, 1:4 dilution/titer (IU/mL 800)

Questions
1. The convalescent specimen demonstrated:
   a. No evidence of streptococci infection
   b. A possibility of streptococci infection
   c. Significant evidence of streptococci infection
   d. Evidence of a chronic streptococci infection
2. Comparing acute and chronic patient specimens can:
   a. Distinguish acute from chronic infection
   b. Diagnose the cause of the infection
   c. Demonstrate at least a twofold dilution rise that is significant for an acute infection
   d. Demonstrate at least a twofold dilution rise that is significant for a chronic infection

See Appendix A for the answers to these questions.

Critical-Thinking Group-Discussion Questions
1. Is the difference between the acute and convalescent titers significant?
2. What does a rise in titer mean?

CASE STUDY 7.2

A 28-year-old woman has been trying to get pregnant for the past 6 months. Although she has no health problems, conceiving a child is proving to be difficult. She is considering fertility treatment. Her period was 10 days late, and she was experiencing pain in her side. She performed an at-home pregnancy test, but it was negative.

Questions
1. A false-negative hCG test can be the result of all of the following examples *except*:
   a. hCG concentration being below the sensitivity threshold of the assay
   b. Delayed ovulation
   c. Delayed implantation
   d. A high concentration of hCG
2. The earliest marker of fertilization is:
   a. Early pregnancy factor (EPF)
   b. hCG latex agglutination procedure
   c. Serum progesterone
   d. Serum estrogen

See Appendix A for the answers to these questions.

Critical-Thinking Group-Discussion Questions
1. Is a negative test result conclusive for the lack of conception?
2. Would a serum progesterone level be helpful in determining her status?
3. What is early pregnancy factor? Would it be helpful in establishing a diagnosis?

Rapid HIV tests suitable for use in non-clinical settings (CLIA-waived)[a]

[For use with finger stick or venipuncture whole blood or oral fluid]

Test Name	Time to test result	Indications for use	Sensitivity for established HIV-1 infection, % (95% CI)[b]	Specificity % (95% CI)[b]	Approved specimen types and volumes	Test kit shelf life	Manufacturer web site
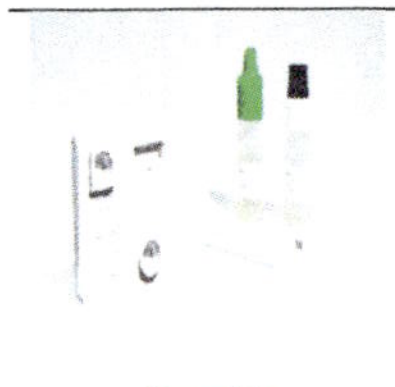 Chembio DPP HIV-1/2	15 min	Antibodies to HIV-1 and 2	Finger stick whole blood 99.8 (99.2–99.9) oral fluid 98.9 (98.0–99.4) Venous whole blood 99.9 (99.4–99.9)	Finger stick whole blood 100 (99.8–100) oral fluid/ venous whole blood 99.9 (99.7–99.9)	Finger stick or venous whole blood 10 μl Or oral fluid swab	23 months	http://chembio.com/products/human-diagnostics/dpp-hiv-12-assay/
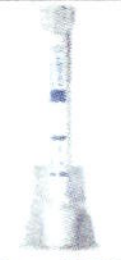 Clearview COMPLETE HIV 1/2	15 min	Antibodies to HIV-1 and 2	Finger stick or venous whole blood 99.7 (98.9–100.0)	Finger stick or venous whole blood 99.9 (99.6–100.0)	Finger stick or venous whole blood 2.5 μL	24 months	http://www.alere.com/us/en/product-details/clearview-complete-hiv-1-2.html
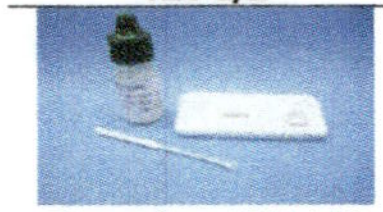 Clearview HIV 1/2 STAT-PAK	15 min	Antibodies to HIV-1 and 2	Finger stick or venous whole blood 99.7 (98.9–100)	Finger stick or venous whole blood 99.9 (99.6–100.0)	Finger stick or venous whole blood 5 μL	24 months	http://www.alere.com/us/en/product-details/clearview-hiv-1-2-stat-pak.html

Continued

Fig. 7.4 HIV CLIA-Waived Tests. (From US Department of Health and Human Services, Clinical Laboratory Improvement Amendments, https://www.cdc.gov, retrieved February 5, 2017.)

Test	Time	Detects	Specimen & Sensitivity% (95% CI)	Specificity% (95% CI)	Shelf life	Website
Determine HIV-1/2 Ag/Ab Combo Test	20 min	Antibodies to HIV-1 and HIV-2, Detects HIV-1 p24 Antigen	Venous/finger stick whole blood 99.9 (99.4–100)	Venous whole blood: Low risk subjects 100 (99.6–100) High risk subjects: 99.2 (98.2–99.7) Finger stick whole blood: Low risk subjects 100 (99.5–100), High risk subjects 99.7 (98.9–100)	Finger stick or venous whole blood 50 µL	14 months	http://www.alere.com/content/alere/us/en/product-details/determine-1-2-ag-ab-combo-us.html.html
INSTI HIV-1/HIV-2 Antibody Test	<2 min	Antibodies to HIV-1 and 2	Finger stick whole blood 99.8 (99.3–99.9), venous whole blood 99.9 (99.5–100)	Finger stick whole blood 99.0 (97.9–99.6), venous whole blood 100 (99.7–100)	Finger stick or venous whole blood 50 µl	12 months	http://www.biolytical.com/products/tiHIV
OraQuick ADVANCE Rapid HIV-1/2 Antibody Test	20 min	Antibodies to HIV-1 and 2	Oral fluid 99.3 (98.4–99.7) finger stick whole blood (venous whole blood not evaluated) 99.6 (98.5–99.9)	Oral fluid 99.8 (99.6–99.9), finger stick whole blood (venous whole blood not evaluated) 100 (99.7–100)	Finger stick or venous whole blood 5 µl or oral fluid swab	12 Months	http://www.orasure.com/products-infectious/products-infectious-oraquick.asp
Uni-Gold Recombigen HIV-1/2	10 min	Antibodies to HIV-1 and HIV-2	Finger stick or venous whole blood 100 (99.5–100.0)	Finger stick or venous whole blood 99.7 (99.0–100)	Finger stick or venous whole blood 50 µL	12 months	http://www.trinitybiotech.com/area/uni-gold/

Fig. 7.4, cont'd

[a] CLIA-waived rapid tests can be used in settings such as: community-based organizations, field testing, outreach activities, STD or other clinics, mobile clinics, non-traditional testing, or community/college clinics. The Clinical Laboratory Improvement Amendments (CLIA) sets criteria based on complexity levels of tests. Briefly, there are three levels of complexity: 1) Waived – simple, low-risk tests that can be performed with minimal training that do not require centrifugation of specimens for testing, 2) Moderate Complexity – simple tests that use plasma or serum specimens (must participate in an external proficiency testing program), 3) High Complexity – tests that require trained laboratory personnel, involve multiple-step protocols, frequent quality control, and participation in an external proficiency testing program. For more information about CLIA regulations go to http://www.cms.gov/Regulations-and-Guidance/Legislation/CLIA/CLIA_Regulations_and_Federal_Register_Documents.html.

[b] Sensitivity is a measure of the test's ability to correctly identify persons with a disease. Specificity is the test's ability to correctly identify persons without the disease.

CHAPTER 7 Basic Serologic Laboratory: Techniques and Clinical Applications

REVIEW QUESTIONS

1. A condition that does not denature, coagulate, or alter protein molecules is:
   a. Heat
   b. Strong acid solution
   c. Strong alkali solution
   d. Refrigerated specimen storage

2. In most cases, if testing cannot be done within _____ hours of collection, a serum specimen should be frozen at –20°C.
   a. 24
   b. 48
   c. 72
   d. 96

3. Complement can be inactivated in human serum by heating to _____ °C.
   a. 25
   b. 37
   c. 45
   d. 56

4. A specimen should be reinactivated when more than _____ hour(s) has (have) elapsed since inactivation of complement.
   a. 1
   b. 2
   c. 4
   d. 8

5. Manual micropipettes can deliver _____ of solution.
   a. Less than 1 µL
   b. Between 10 and 50 µL
   c. Between 1 and 500 µL
   d. More than 500 µL

6. Automatic pipettes have the disadvantage of:
   a. Being fast
   b. Allowing repetitive measurement of solutions
   c. Delivering equal volumes of solutions
   d. Inaccurate measurements of viscous serum or bubbly solutions

7. A dilution is a(n):
   a. Ratio of volume or parts, of the final solution
   b. Indication of relative concentration
   c. Indication of absolute concentration
   d. Both a and b

8. If a serial dilution is prepared in 1:2 dilutions, the final dilution in tube 6 is:
   a. 1:25
   b. 1:32
   c. 1:64
   d. 1:256

9. To prepare 10 mL of a diluted serum specimen 1:10, _____ part of serum is needed.
   a. 1.0
   b. 0.75
   c. 0.50
   d. 0.20

10. To prepare 10 mL of a diluted serum specimen 1:10, _____ part(s) of distilled water is (are) needed to reach the total volume.
    a. 10
    b. 9
    c. 4.5
    d. 0.1

11. Serum for detection of antibodies should be drawn during the:
    a. Acute phase of illness only
    b. Acute and convalescent phases of illness
    c. Convalescent phase of illness only
    d. Acute and convalescent phases, and also 6 months after an illness

12. A central concept of serologic testing is:
    a. Antigen–antibody interaction
    b. Determination of antibody composition
    c. Quantitation of antigen titer
    d. Manifestation of a rise in antibody titer

13. A major advantage of rapid POCT testing is:
    a. Faster turnaround time
    b. Lower cost
    c. Better quality than traditional testing
    d. None of the above

14. Rapid testing assays are usually in the _____ CLIA category:
    a. Waived
    b. Provider-performed microscopy
    c. Moderately complex
    d. Highly complex

15. Over-the-counter test kits are in the _____ CLIA category:
    a. Waived
    b. Provider-performed microscopy
    c. Moderately complex
    d. Highly complex

8
Precipitation and Particle Agglutination Methods

LEARNING OUTCOMES

- Define the terms precipitation and agglutination.
- Name and describe various types of precipitation assays.
- Describe the principles of particle agglutination.
- Identify and compare the characteristics of particle agglutination methods.
- Explain methods for enhancing agglutination.
- Describe the characteristics of graded agglutination reactions.
- Discuss the principles of classic latex pregnancy testing, including sources of error.
- Describe the principle, advantages, and disadvantages of nephelometry.
- Discuss the analysis and clinical implications of cryoglobulins.
- Analyze a case study.
- Correctly answer case study–related multiple-choice questions.
- Participate in a discussion of critical thinking questions.
- Explain agglutination reactions of the ABO blood group procedure.
- Describe the principle and sources of error of the ABO blood group procedure.
- Correctly answer end-of-chapter review questions.

OUTLINE

Principles of Precipitation and Particle Agglutination Assays, 129
    Precipitation Assays, 129
    Particle Agglutination Assays, 130
Latex Agglutination, 130
Pregnancy Testing, 131
    Human Chorionic Gonadotropin, 131
    Agglutination Inhibition, 131
Alternative Procedural Protocols, 131
Flocculation Tests, 132
Direct Bacterial Agglutination, 132
Hemagglutination, 134
    Mechanisms of Agglutination, 134
        Sensitization, 134
        Lattice Formation, 135

Methods of Enhancing Agglutination, 136
    Graded Agglutination Reactions, 136
    Microplate Agglutination Reactions, 136
Nephelometry, 138
    Principle, 138
    Physical Basis, 139
    Optical System, 139
    Measuring Methods, 139
    Advantages and Disadvantages, 139
    Clinical Application: Cryoglobulins, 139
Case Study 8.1   ABO Testing Results, 140
Procedure: Pregnancy Latex Slide Agglutination, 142.e1
Procedure: ABO Blood Grouping (Reverse Grouping), 142.e2

KEY TERMS

- agglutination
- antibovine antibodies
- antigenic determinants
- antihuman globulin (AHG)
- antisera
- chimerism
- classic Ouchterlony gel diffusion
- coagglutination
- conjugated
- cryoglobulins
- cuvette
- double immunodiffusion
- denaturation
- elution
- flocculation tests
- Heidelberger curve
- hemagglutination
- human chorionic gonadotropin (hCG)
- in vitro agglutination inhibition
- isoagglutinins
- lattice hypothesis
- liposome-enhanced
- macromolecular complex
- photometrically
- postzone phenomenon
- precipitation
- precipitins
- prozone phenomenon
- pseudoagglutination
- reagents
- rouleaux formation
- steric hindrance
- zeta potential
- zone of equivalence

PRINCIPLES OF PRECIPITATION AND PARTICLE AGGLUTINATION ASSAYS

> **KEY CONCEPTS: Precipitation and Particle Agglutination Assays**
> - Precipitation and agglutination are unlabeled immunoassays. These assay methods produce a visible expression of the aggregation of antigens and antibodies.
> - *Precipitation* is the combination of soluble antigen with soluble antibody to produce a visible insoluble complex.
> - *Agglutination* is the process whereby specific antigens (e.g., red blood cells [RBCs]) aggregate to form larger visible clumps when the corresponding specific antibody is present in the serum.
> - Immune precipitation methods in gel can be classified as passive methods or those using electrophoresis. Precipitation assays include the Ouchterlony double-diffusion technique, based on the visualization of lines of identity or precipitin lines for reaction results, and radial immunodiffusion (RID), in which antigen passively diffuses through agar with a precipitate forming at the zone of equivalence that is directly proportional to the concentration of the antigen.
> - Flocculation tests used for antibody detection are based on the interaction of soluble antigen with antibody, which results in the formation of a precipitate of fine particles.

Precipitation and agglutination are unlabeled immunoassays. These assay methods produce a visible expression of the aggregation of antigens and antibodies through the formation of a framework in which antigen particles or molecules alternate with antibody molecules (Fig. 8.1). *Precipitation* is the term for the aggregation of soluble test antigens. Precipitation is the combination of soluble antigen with soluble antibody to produce a visible insoluble complex. Agglutination is the process whereby specific antigens (e.g., red blood cells [RBCs]) aggregate to form larger visible clumps when the corresponding specific antibody is present in the serum.

The immunoglobulin M (IgM) class of antibodies is the best at agglutination and precipitation. Furthermore, IgM classes are almost exclusively used as reagents, and this class of antibodies is the one that is most commonly detected in patients as an analyte, for example, rheumatoid factor.

Precipitation Assays

A precipitation reaction involves the diffusion of soluble antigen and antibody. Precipitation reactions can be measured by light refraction using a nephelometer.

Precipitation reactions in gel are not as commonly performed in the clinical laboratory today. Both radial and Ouchterlony immunodiffusion methods discussed in this chapter are restricted to detecting high-abundance serum proteins such as antibodies after an immune response and antigens such as complement.

Immune precipitation methods in gel can be classified as passive methods or those using electrophoresis (Table 8.1). Examples of precipitation assays discussed in this chapter include the Ouchterlony technique or radial immunodiffusion (RID). Agarose gel produces the most stable precipitation reaction.

Flocculation tests used for antibody detection are based on the interaction of soluble antigen with antibody, which results in the formation of a precipitate of fine particles.

Double immunodiffusion (classic Ouchterlony gel diffusion) (Fig. 8.2) is the simplest and least sensitive method. Today, most laboratories have replaced this method with enzyme-linked immunoassays (ELISAs), except in the identification of fungal diseases.

The Ouchterlony double-diffusion technique (Fig. 8.3) performed on a gel medium is based on visualization of lines of identity

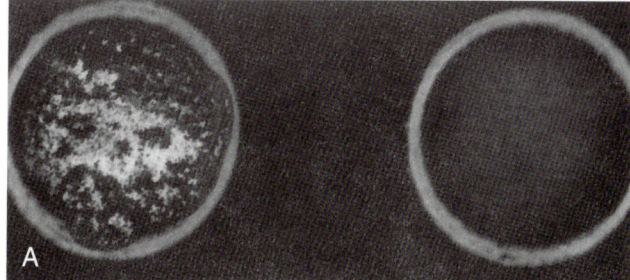
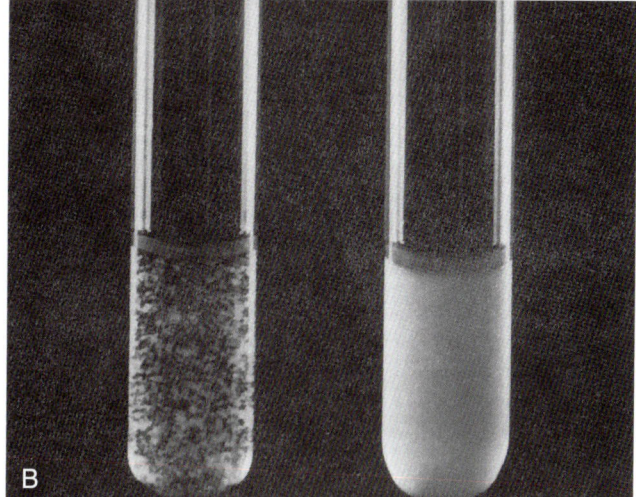

Fig. 8.1 Agglutination Patterns. (A) Slide agglutination of bacteria with known antisera or known bacteria. *Left*, Positive reaction; *right*, negative reaction. (B) Tube agglutination. *Left*, Positive reaction; *right*, negative reaction. (From Barrett JT: *Textbook of immunology*, ed 5, St. Louis, 1988, Mosby.)

or precipitin lines for reaction results. The reaction of the antigen–antibody combination occurs by means of diffusion. The size and position of precipitin bands provide information regarding equivalence or antibody excess. Proteins are differentiated not only by their electrophoretic mobility, but also by their diffusion coefficient and antibody specificity. Although double immunodiffusion produces a separate precipitation band for each antigen–antibody system in a mixture, it is often difficult to determine all the components in a complex mixture.

In this technique, cylindrical wells are cut out of agarose gel and spaced appropriately in a Petri dish. For the detection of antibody, a known crude or purified antigen is placed in one well of the agar plate, and the patient's serum is added to an adjacent well. Because this method relies on passive diffusion, it is a slow process. Reactions take from 48 to 72 hours to develop.

The antigen and antibody molecules in solution diffuse out of the wells and through the porous agar. If antibody specific for the antigen is present, the antigen and antibody combine at a point of optimal concentration called the **zone of equivalence** and produce a visible precipitin band or line of precipitation. A pattern of identity confirms the presence of the antibody in an unknown specimen. Patterns of partial identity and nonidentity are ambiguous.

This procedure is used for looking at immune responses (antibodies) produced in patients in response to various diseases, especially fungal ones. Today, most of these antibodies are detected by ELISAs or multiplex bead array systems (e.g., Luminex), but some large laboratories continue to use the Ouchterlony method for detection of fungal antibodies.

In RID (Fig. 8.4) antibody is uniformly distributed in the gel medium, and antigen is added to a well cut into the gel. The antigen

TABLE 8.1 Summary of Unlabeled Immune Reactions

Technique	Principle
Passive	
Double-diffusion (Ouchterlony technique) gel precipitation	Allow antiserum and antigens in gel wells across from one another. Allow time for diffusion in the gel. Observe and interpret reactions as identity, nonidentity, or partial identity.
Single-diffusion (radial immunodiffusion) gel precipitation	Allow antigen in a gel well to diffuse into the gel. Visualize and interpret. Draw a standard curve using D^2 for Fahey or Marcini, or use semilog paper with D versus concentration on the y-axis.
Electrophoresis	A method of separating macromolecules such as proteins on the basis of their net electrical charge and size (molecular weight). Serum electrophoresis is a technique for separating ionic molecules, principally proteins, into five fractions on a medium such as paper, cellulose acetate, or gel. The separation is based on the rate of migration, depending on the size and ionic charge of the individual components in an electrical field. The components can be visualized by staining and quantitated using a densitometer.
Counterimmunoelectrophoresis	Oppositely charged antigen and antibody are propelled toward each other by an electrical field. This allows detection of concentrations of antigens and antibodies 10-times smaller than the lowest concentrations measurable by immunodiffusion or double diffusion.
Immunofixation electrophoresis	Specific antibodies help produce sensitive and specific qualitative visual identification of paraproteins by electrophoretic position.
Soluble Phase	
Nephelometry	Antigen and antibody are added to a tube. Light scattered at 10 degrees to 90 degrees (usually 70 degrees) is visualized. Concentration is determined using a standard curve.
Turbidometry	Antigen and antibody are added to a tube. Light is visualized that is directly across from the light source. Concentration is determined using a standard curve.

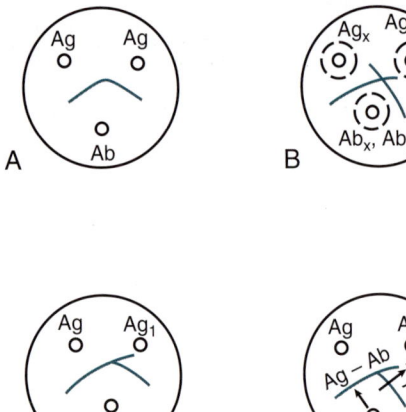

Fig. 8.2 Double Immunodiffusion in Two Dimensions by the Ouchterlony Technique (A) Reaction of identity. (B) Reaction of nonidentity. (C) Reaction of partial identity. (D) Scheme for spur formation. *Ab*, Antibody; *Ag*, antigen. (From Burtis CA, Ashwood ER, Bruns DB: *Tietz fundamentals of clinical chemistry*, ed 6, St. Louis, 2008, Saunders.)

passively diffuses through the agar and, at the zone of equivalence with the antibody, forms a precipitate. The diameter of the zone of precipitation is directly proportional to the concentration of the antigen. This infrequently used procedure is used to quantify antigen concentration.

> **KEY CONCEPTS: Agglutination Concepts**
> - Agglutination of particles to which soluble antigen has been adsorbed is a serum method of demonstrating **precipitins**.
> - Examples of artificial carriers include latex particles and colloidal charcoal. Cells unrelated to the antigen, such as erythrocytes coated with antigen in a constant amount, can be used as biological carriers.
> - In latex agglutination procedures, antibody molecules can be bound to the surface of latex beads. If an antigen is present in a test specimen, the antigen will bind to the combining sites of the antibody exposed on the surface of the latex beads, forming visible crosslinked aggregates of latex beads and antigen.

Particle Agglutination Assays

Artificial carrier particles may be needed to indicate visibly that an antigen–antibody agglutination reaction has taken place; examples include latex particles and colloidal charcoal. Cells unrelated to the antigen, such as erythrocytes coated with antigen in a constant amount, can be used as biological carriers. Whole bacterial cells can contain an antigen that will bind with antibodies produced in response to that antigen when it is introduced into the host (Table 8.2).

The quality of test results depends on the following technical factors:
- Time of incubation with the antibody source (e.g., patient serum)
- Amount and avidity (see Chapter 3) of an antigen **conjugated** to the carrier
- Conditions of the test environment (e.g., pH, protein concentration)

Agglutination tests are easy to perform and, in some cases, are the most sensitive tests currently available. It is important to note that quality results are dependent on the proper training of the person performing the assay and adherence to strict quality-control regulations (e.g., positive and negative control sera). Agglutination-type tests (Table 8.3) have a wide range of applications in the clinical diagnosis of noninfectious immune disorders and infectious diseases.

LATEX AGGLUTINATION

In latex agglutination procedures (Box 8.1), antibody molecules can be bound to the surface of latex beads. Many antibody molecules can be bound to each latex particle, increasing the potential number of exposed antigen-binding sites. If an antigen is present in a test specimen such as C-reactive protein, the antigen will bind to the combining sites of the antibody exposed on the surface of the latex beads, forming visible crosslinked aggregates of latex beads and antigen (Fig. 8.5). In some procedures (e.g., rheumatoid arthritis testing), latex particles can be coated with antigen. In the presence of serum antibodies, these particles agglutinate into large visible clumps. Latex agglutination methods can yield qualitative or semiquantitative results.

Procedures based on latex agglutination must be performed under standardized conditions. The amount of antigen–antibody binding is influenced by factors such as pH, osmolarity, and ionic concentration

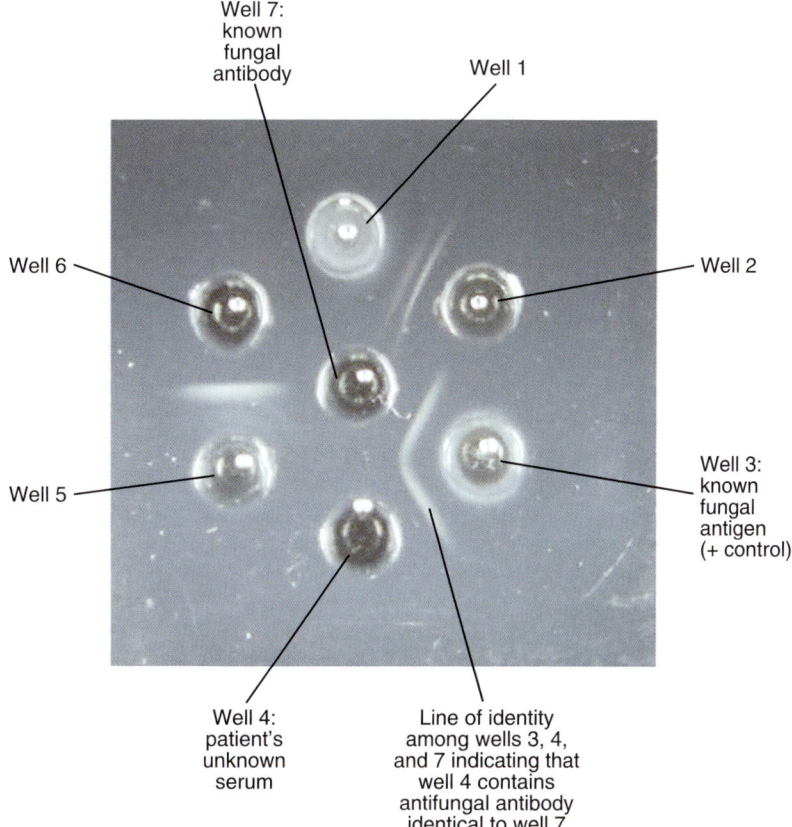

Fig. 8.3 Ouchterlony Plate. A serum specimen containing an unknown antibody is placed in one well (e.g., well 4), a known antigen of interest is placed in an adjacent well (well 3—positive control), and a known antiserum to the antigen (well 7—positive control) is placed in another adjacent well. The antigen and antibody molecules in the solution diffuse from the wells and through the porous agarose. If the unknown serum contains antibody to the known antigen, a precipitin band forms at a point of optimal concentration of each component. This precipitin band is called a *line of identity*. (From Mahon C, Lehman D, Manuselis G: *Textbook of diagnostic microbiology*, ed 5, St. Louis, 2015, Elsevier.)

of the solution. A variety of conditions can produce false-positive or false-negative reactions in agglutination testing (Table 8.4).

Coagglutination and liposome-enhanced testing are variations of latex agglutination (Fig. 8.6). Coagglutination uses antibodies bound to a particle to enhance the visibility of agglutination. It is a highly specific method but may not be as sensitive as latex agglutination for detecting small quantities of antigen.

PREGNANCY TESTING

The principle of antigen and antibody interaction was applied to classic pregnancy testing since the first agglutination tests were developed in the 1960s, before the development and availability of lateral flow techniques for testing. These assays originally replaced animal testing.

Human Chorionic Gonadotropin

Pregnancy tests are designed to detect minute amounts of human chorionic gonadotropin (hCG), a glycoprotein hormone secreted by the trophoblast of the developing embryo that rapidly increases in the urine or serum during the early stages of pregnancy.

This glycoprotein hormone consists of two noncovalently linked subunits, alpha (α) and beta (β). The α unit is identical to that found in luteinizing hormone, follicle-stimulating hormone, and thyroid-stimulating hormone. The β subunit has a unique carboxy-terminal region. Using antibodies made against the β subunit will cut down on cross-reactivity with the other three hormones. Accordingly, many pregnancy test kits contain monoclonal antibody (MAb) directed against the β subunit to increase the specificity of the reaction.

For the first 6 to 8 weeks after conception, hCG helps maintain the corpus luteum and stimulate the production of progesterone. As a general rule, the level of hCG should double every 2 to 3 days. Pregnant women usually attain serum concentrations of 10 to 50 mIU/mL of hCG in the week after conception. If a test is negative at this stage, the test should be repeated within a week. Peak levels are reached approximately 2 to 3 months after the last menstrual period.

Agglutination Inhibition

The determination of in vitro agglutination inhibition depends on the incubation of the patient's specimen with anti-hCG, followed by the addition of latex particles coated with hCG. If hCG is present, it neutralizes the antibody; thus no agglutination of latex particles is seen. If no hCG is present, agglutination occurs between the anti-hCG and hCG-coated latex particles.

ALTERNATIVE PROCEDURAL PROTOCOLS

Latex agglutination slide tests have been replaced in many situations by one-step chromatographic color-labeled immunoassays for the qualitative detection of hCG in urine (e.g., Clearview hCG II and Clearview hCG Easy, Wampole Laboratories, Princeton, NJ). Another variation is a one-step chromatographic color-labeled immunoassay for use with urine or serum (e.g., Wampole PreVue hCG Stick or Cassette, Status hCG).

> **KEY CONCEPTS: Alternate Test Principles**
> - Flocculation tests for antibody detection are based on the interaction of soluble antigen with antibody, which results in the formation of a precipitate of fine particles.
> - Direct bacterial agglutination can be used to detect antibodies directed against pathogens.

FLOCCULATION TESTS

Flocculation tests for antibody detection are based on the interaction of soluble antigen with antibody, which results in the formation of a precipitate of fine particles. These particles are macroscopically or microscopically visible only because the precipitated product is forced to remain in a confined space.

Flocculation testing can be used in syphilis serologic testing (see Chapter 15). These tests are the classic Venereal Disease Research Laboratories (VDRL) and rapid plasma reagin (RPR) tests. In the VDRL test, an antibody-like protein, reagin, binds to the test antigen, cardiolipin-lecithin–coated cholesterol particles, and produces the particles that flocculate. In the RPR test, the antigen, cardiolipin-lecithin–coated cholesterol with choline chloride, also contains charcoal particles that allow for macroscopically visible flocculation.

> **KEY CONCEPTS: Direct Bacterial Agglutination**
> - Direct agglutination of whole pathogens can be used to detect antibodies directed against pathogens.
> - The most basic tests measure the antibody produced by the host to antigen determinants on the surface of a bacterial agent in response to infection with that bacterium.
> - This type of agglutination is called *bacterial agglutination*.

DIRECT BACTERIAL AGGLUTINATION

Direct agglutination of whole pathogens can be used to detect antibodies directed against the pathogens. The most basic tests measure the

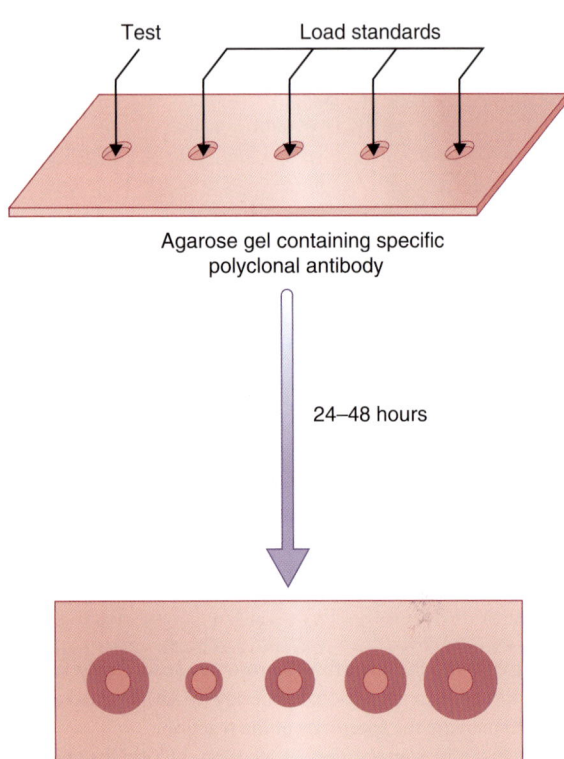

Fig. 8.4 Measurement of Immune-Related Proteins by Radial Immunodiffusion. (From Peakman M, Vergani D: *Basic and clinical immunology*, ed 2, Edinburgh, 2009, Churchill Livingstone.)

TABLE 8.3 Summary of Particle Agglutination Reactions

Technique	Detects
Direct agglutination	Antibody, antigen[a]
Passive agglutination	Antibody
Inhibition agglutination	Antigen
Reverse passive agglutination	Antigen
DAT	Specific antibody coating specific antigens on RBCs
Indirect antiglobulin test	The presence of antibody capable of reacting with specific antigens on RBCs

[a]Direct agglutination to detect antigen, such as rapid strep testing, uses antibodies to *Streptococcus* to detect antigen *Streptococcus* in a patient sample.
DAT, Direct antiglobulin test; *RBC*, red blood cell.

TABLE 8.2 Examples of Carriers

Type (Reagent)	Type of Assay	Principle	Result
Latex particles	CRP	A suspension of polystyrene latex particles of uniform size is coated with the IgG fraction of an antihuman CRP-specific serum.	If CRP is present in the serum, an antigen–antibody reaction takes place. This reaction causes a change in the uniform appearance of the latex suspension, and a clear agglutination results.
Stabilized sheep erythrocytes sensitized with rabbit gamma globulin suspended in buffer solution	RF	RF acts like antibodies against gamma globulin, which acts as the antigen.	If gamma globulin is attached to a particular carrier (e.g., red blood cells or latex particles), the reaction of RF with gamma globulin becomes a visible agglutination.

CRP, C-reactive protein; *IgG*, immunoglobulin G; *RF*, rheumatoid factor.

CHAPTER 8 Precipitation and Particle Agglutination Methods

BOX 8.1 Immunologic Assays Performed by Latex Particle Agglutination

- C-reactive protein
- Immunoglobulin G rheumatoid factors
- Immunoglobulin M rheumatoid factors
- Rubella antibody

antibody produced by the host to antigen determinants on the surface of a bacterial agent in response to infection with that bacterium. In a thick suspension of the bacteria, the binding of specific antibodies to surface antigens of the bacteria causes the bacteria to clump together in visible aggregates. This type of agglutination is called *bacterial agglutination*.

The formation of aggregates in solution is influenced by electrostatic and other forces; therefore certain conditions are usually necessary for satisfactory results. The use of sterile physiologic saline with free positive ions in the agglutination procedure enhances the aggregation of bacteria because most bacterial surfaces exhibit a negative charge that causes them to repel each other. Because it allows more time for the antigen–antibody reaction, tube testing is considered more sensitive than slide testing. The small volume of liquid used in slide testing requires rapid reading before the liquid evaporates.

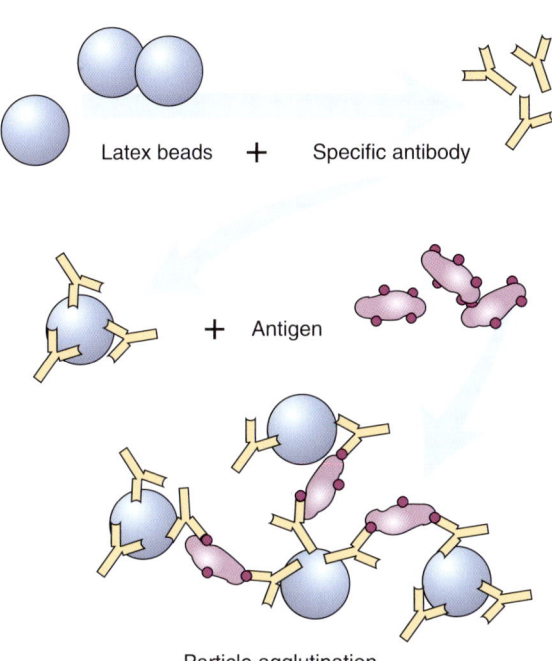

Fig. 8.5 Alignment of Antibody Molecules Bound to Surface of a Latex Particle and Latex Agglutination Reaction. (Adapted from Forbes BA, Sahm DF, Weissfeld AS: *Bailey and Scott's diagnostic microbiology*, ed 12, St. Louis, 2007, Elsevier.)

KEY CONCEPTS: Hemagglutination

- The hemagglutination method of testing detects physical attachment of antibodies to erythrocyte antigens.
- Binding different antigens to the RBC surface in indirect hemagglutination or passive hemagglutination (PHA), the hemagglutination technique can be extended to detect antibodies to antigens other than those present on the cells.
- Some antibodies (e.g., IgG) do not directly agglutinate erythrocytes, but this incomplete or blocking type of antibody may be detected by using an enhancement medium such as antihuman globulin (AHG) reagent. The use of AHG forms cross-links between antibody molecules that have bound to the surface of RBCs. This promotes the formation of agglutination and allows for visual observation of an antigen–antibody reaction.
- Agglutination is influenced by a number of factors and is believed to occur in two stages: sensitization and lattice formation.
- Inert particles such as latex, RBCs, and bacteria have a net negative surface charge called the *zeta potential*. These charges can be overcome by centrifugation, addition of charged molecules (e.g., albumin, low ionic-strength saline [LISS]), or enzyme pretreatment to permit the cross-linking that results in agglutination.

TABLE 8.4 Causes of False-Positive and False-Negative Agglutination Test Reactions

Cause	Correction
False-Positive Reactions	
Contaminated equipment or reagents may cause particles to clump	Store equipment and reagent in a clean, dust-free environment, and handle with care. Use negative QC steps.
Autoagglutination	Use a control with saline and no antibody as a negative control. If positive, patient's result is invalid.
Delay in reading slide reactions results in drying out of mixture	Follow procedural directions and read reactions exactly as specified
Overcentrifugation causes cells or particles to clump too tightly	Calibrate centrifuge to proper speed and time
False-Negative Reactions	
Inadequate washing of red blood cells in AHG testing may result in unbound immunoglobulins neutralizing the reagent	Wash cells according to directions. Use positive and negative QC steps.
Failure to add AHG reagent	Use positive QC steps
Contaminated or expired reagents	Use positive and negative QC steps
Improper incubation	Follow procedural protocol exactly. Use positive and negative QC steps.
Delay in reading slide reactions	Follow procedural protocol exactly. Use positive and negative control steps.
Undercentrifugation	Calibrate centrifuge to proper speed and time
Prozone phenomenon	Dilute patient serum containing antibody, and repeat the procedure.

AHG, Antihuman globulin; *QC*, quality control.

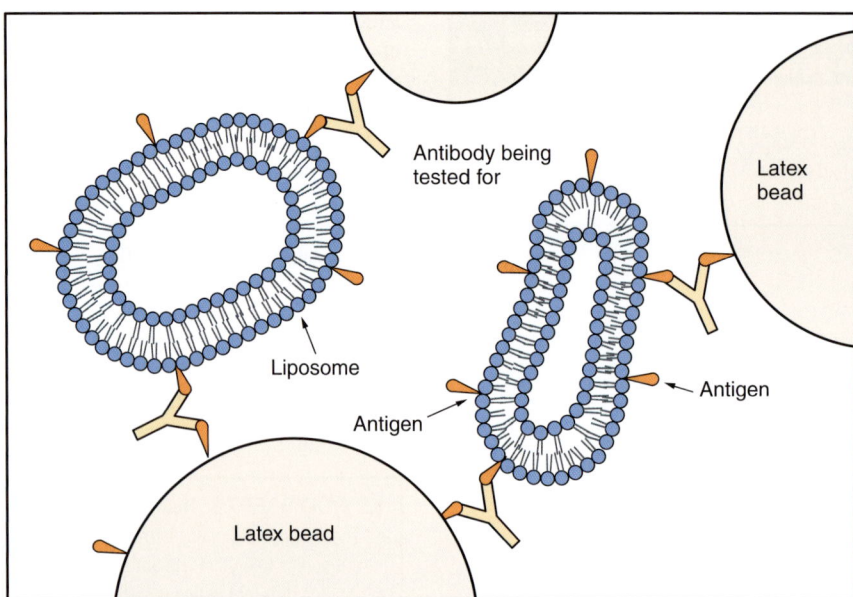

Fig. 8.6 Diagram of Liposome-Enhanced Latex Agglutination Reactions. (Adapted from Neo-Planotest Ducoclox slide test, Organon Teknika, Durham, NC.)

HEMAGGLUTINATION

The **hemagglutination** method of testing detects antibodies to erythrocyte antigens. The antibody-containing specimen can be serially diluted and a suspension of RBCs added to the dilutions. If a sufficient concentration of antibody is present, the erythrocytes are crosslinked and agglutinated. If nonreacting antibody or an insufficient quantity of antibody is present, the erythrocytes will fail to agglutinate.

By binding different antigens to the RBC surface in indirect hemagglutination or PHA, the hemagglutination technique can be extended to detect antibodies to antigens other than those present on the cells. Chemicals such as chromic chloride, tannic acid, and glutaraldehyde can be used to crosslink antigens to the cells.

Some antibodies (e.g., immunoglobulin G [IgG]) do not directly agglutinate erythrocytes. This incomplete or blocking type of antibody may be detected by using an enhancement medium such as **antihuman globulin (AHG)** reagent (previously known as *Coombs reagent*). If AHG reagent is added, this second antibody binds to the antibody present on the erythrocytes.

Mechanisms of Agglutination

Agglutination is the clumping of particles that have antigens on their surface, such as erythrocytes, by antibody molecules that form bridges between the **antigenic determinants**. This is the endpoint for most tests involving erythrocyte antigens. Agglutination is influenced by a number of factors and is believed to occur in two stages: sensitization and lattice formation.

Sensitization

The first phase of agglutination, sensitization, represents the physical attachment of antibody molecules to antigens on the erythrocyte membrane. The combination of antigen and antibody is a reversible chemical reaction. Altering the physical conditions can result in the release of antibody from the antigen-binding site. When physical conditions are purposely manipulated to break the antigen–antibody complex, with subsequent release of the antibody into the surrounding medium, the procedure is referred to as an **elution**.

The amount of antibody that will react is affected by the equilibrium constant, or affinity constant, of the antibody. In most cases, the higher the equilibrium constant, the higher the rate of association and the slower the rate of dissociation of antibody molecules. The degree of association between antigen and antibody is affected by a variety of factors and can be altered in some cases in vitro by altering some of the factors that influence antigen–antibody association, including the following:

- Particle charge
- Electrolyte concentration and viscosity
- Antibody type
- Antigen-to-antibody ratio
- Antigenic determinants
- Physical conditions (e.g., pH, temperature, duration of incubation)

Particle charge. Inert particles such as latex, RBCs, and bacteria have a net negative surface charge called the **zeta potential** (Fig. 8.7). The concentration of salt in the reaction medium has an effect on antibody uptake by the membrane-bound erythrocyte antigens. Sodium (Na^+) and chloride (Cl^-) ions in a solution have a shielding effect. These ions cluster around and partially neutralize the opposite charges on antigen and antibody molecules, which hinders antibody–antigen association. By reducing the ionic strength of a reaction medium (e.g., using LISS), antibody uptake is enhanced. Charges can be overcome by centrifugation, addition of charged molecules (e.g., albumin, LISS), or enzyme pretreatment to permit the cross-linking that results in agglutination (Table 8.5).

> **KEY CONCEPTS: Antigen–Antibody Ratio Characteristics**
> - Precipitation reactions depend on a zone of equivalence, the zone in which optimum precipitation occurs. In the zone of equivalence, each antibody or antigen binds to more than one antigen or antibody, respectively, forming a stable lattice or network.
> - The lattice hypothesis is based on the assumptions that each antibody molecule must have at least two binding sites and that an antigen must be multivalent.
> - If excessive antibody concentration is present, the phenomenon known as the **prozone phenomenon** occurs and can result in a false-negative reaction.
> - If an excess of antigen occurs, the postzone phenomenon occurs and small aggregates are surrounded by excess antigen and no lattice formation is established. A repeat blood specimen should be collected 1 or more weeks later to increase the likelihood that detectable antibody will be observed.

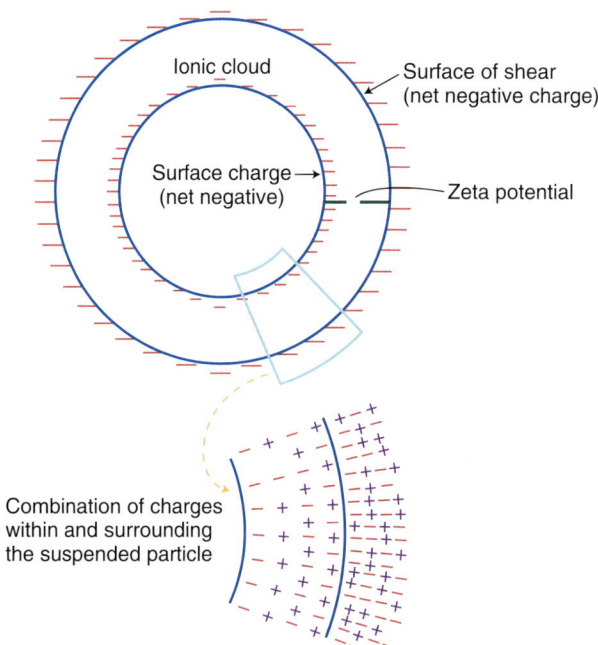

Fig. 8.7 Zeta Potential. Difference in electrostatic potential between net charge at cell membrane and charge at surface of shear. (From Turgeon ML: *Fundamentals of immunohematology*, ed 2, Baltimore, 1995, Williams & Wilkins.)

TABLE 8.5	Techniques to Reduce Zeta Potential
Technique	**Action**
Enzyme pretreatment of red blood cells	Removes negatively charged sialic acid residues from cell surface membrane
Addition of colloids (e.g., albumin)	Increases electrical conductivity of the environment
Centrifugation	Mechanical process to force red blood cells closer together

Antibody type. IgM antibodies are more efficient at agglutination because their large size and multivalency permit more effective bridging of the space between cells caused by zeta potential. IgG antibodies are too small to overcome electrostatic forces between cells. The use of AHG forms cross-links between antibody molecules that have bound to the surface of RBCs. This promotes this formation of agglutination and allows for visual observation of an antigen–antibody reaction.

Antigen–antibody ratio. Under conditions of antibody excess, there is a surplus of molecular antigen-combining sites not bound to antigenic determinants. Precipitation reactions depend on a zone of equivalence, the zone in which optimum precipitation occurs because the number of multivalent sites of antigens and antibodies is approximately equal. For a precipitation reaction to be detectable, the reaction must occur in the zone of equivalence. In this zone, each antibody or antigen binds to more than one antigen or antibody, respectively, forming a stable lattice or network (see section Lattice Formation). This lattice hypothesis is based on the assumption that each antibody molecule must have at least two binding sites and that an antigen must be multivalent.

On either side of the zone of equivalence, precipitation is prevented because of an excess of antigen or antibody. If excessive antibody concentration is present, a phenomenon known as the prozone phenomenon (Table 8.6) occurs, which can result in a false-negative reaction. In this case, antigen combines with only one or two antibody molecules and no cross-linkages are formed. This phenomenon can be overcome by serially diluting the antibody-containing serum until optimum amounts of antigen and antibody are present in the test system.

If an excess of antigen occurs, the postzone phenomenon occurs, in which small aggregates (clumps) are surrounded by excess antigen and no lattice formation is established. Excess antigen can block the presence of a small amount of antibody. To correct the postzone phenomenon, a repeat blood specimen should be collected 1 or more weeks later. If an active antibody reaction is occurring in vivo, the titer of antibody will increase and should be detectable. Repeated negative results generally suggest that the patient has the specific antibody being tested for by the procedure.

Antigenic determinants. The placement and number of antigenic determinants both affect agglutination. For example, the A blood group antigen has more than 1.5 million sites per RBC, whereas the Kell blood group antigen has about 3500 to 6000 sites per RBC. If the number of antigenic sites is small or if the antigenic sites are buried deeply in the cell membranes, antibodies will be physically unable to contact antigenic sites.

Steric hindrance is an important physiochemical effect that influences antibody uptake by cell surface antigens. If dissimilar antibodies with approximately the same binding constant are directed against antigenic determinants located close to each other, the antibodies will compete for space in reaching their specific receptor sites. The effect of this competition can be mutual blocking or steric hindrance, and neither antibody type will be bound to its respective antigenic determinant. Steric hindrance can occur whenever there is a conformational change in the relationship of an antigenic receptor site to the outside surface. In addition to antibody competition, competition with bound complement, other protein molecules, or the action of agents that interfere with the structural integrity of the cell surface can produce steric hindrance.

pH. The pH of the medium used for testing should be near physiologic conditions or an optimum pH of 6.5 to 7.5. At a neutral pH, high electrolyte concentrations act to neutralize the net negative charge of particles.

Temperature and length of incubation. The optimum temperature needed to reach equilibrium in an antibody–antigen reaction differs for different antibodies. IgM antibodies are cold reacting (thermal range, 4°C to 22°C [39°F to 72°F]), and IgG antibodies are warm reacting, with an optimum temperature of reaction at 37°C (98.6°F).

The duration of incubation required to achieve maximum results depends on the rate of association and dissociation of each specific antibody. In laboratory testing, incubation times range from 15 to 60 minutes. The optimum time of incubation varies, depending on the class of immunoglobulin and how tightly an antibody attaches to its specific antigen.

Lattice Formation

Lattice formation, or the establishment of cross-links between sensitized particles (e.g., erythrocytes) and antibodies resulting in aggregation, is a much slower process than the sensitization phase. The formation of chemical bonds and resultant lattice formation depend on the ability of a cell with attached antibody on its surface to come close enough to another cell to permit the antibody molecules to bridge the gap and combine with the antigen receptor site on the second cell. As antigens and antibodies combine, a multimolecular lattice increases in size until it precipitates out of solution as a solid particle. Cross-linking is influenced by factors such as the zeta potential.

TABLE 8.6 Prozone and Postzone Phenomena

	Prozone	Prozone	E	E	E	E	E	E	E	Postzone
Serum dilution	None	1:2	1:4	1:8	1:16	1:32	1:64	1:128	1:256	1:512
Strength of agglutination	Neg	Neg	1+	2+	3+	4+	3+	2+	1+	Neg

E, Equivalence zone.
From Turgeon ML: *Linné and Ringsrud's clinical laboratory science,* ed 7, St. Louis, 2015, Elsevier.

Methods of Enhancing Agglutination

Techniques used to enhance agglutination include the following:
- Centrifugation
- Treatment with proteolytic enzymes
- Use of colloids
- AHG testing

Treatment with proteolytic enzymes and the use of colloids or AHG techniques could be applied in the immunology laboratory.

Centrifugation attempts to overcome the problem of distance by subjecting sensitized cells to a high gravitational force that counteracts the repulsive effect and physically forces the cells together.

Enzyme treatment alters the zeta potential or dielectric constant to enhance the chances of demonstrable agglutination. Mild proteolytic enzyme treatment can strip off some of the negative charges on the cell membrane by removing surface sialic acid residues (cleaving sialoglycoproteins from the cell surface), which reduces the surface charge of cells, lowers the zeta potential, and permits cells to come closer together for chemical linking by specific antibody molecules.

Some IgG antibodies will agglutinate if the zeta potential is carefully adjusted by the addition of colloids and salts.

In some cases, antigens may be so deeply embedded in the membrane surface that the previous techniques will not bring the antigens and antibodies close enough to cross-link. The AHG test is frequently incorporated into the protocol of many laboratory techniques to facilitate agglutination. The direct AHG test can be used to detect disorders such as hemolytic disease of the newborn, transfusion reactions, and differentiation of immunoglobulin from complement coating of erythrocytes.

Graded Agglutination Reactions

Observation of agglutination is initially made by gently shaking the test tube containing the serum and cells and viewing the lower portion, the button, with a magnifying glass as it is dispersed. Because agglutination is a reversible reaction, the test tube must be treated delicately and hard shaking must be avoided; however all the cells in the button must be resuspended before an accurate observation can be determined. Attention should also be given to whether discoloration of the fluid above the cells, the supernatant, is present. Rupture or hemolysis of erythrocytes is as important a finding as agglutination.

The strength of agglutination (Table 8.7 and Figs. 8.8 and 8.9), called *grading*, uses a scale of 0, or negative (no agglutination), to 4+ (all erythrocytes clumped). Pseudoagglutination, or the false appearance of clumping, may rarely occur because of rouleaux formation. Rouleaux formation can be encountered in patients with high or abnormal types of globulins in their blood, such as in multiple myeloma or after receiving dextran as a plasma expander. On microscopic examination, the erythrocytes appear as rolls resembling stacks of coins. To disperse the pseudoagglutination, a few drops of physiologic NaCl (saline) can be added to the reaction tube, remixed, and reexamined. This procedure, saline replacement, should be performed carefully after pseudoagglutination is suspected. It should never be done before the initial testing protocol is followed; a false-negative result may occur from the dilutional effect of the saline.

TABLE 8.7 Grading Agglutination Reactions

Grade	Description
Negative	No aggregates
Mixed field	A few isolated aggregates; mostly free-floating cells; supernatant appears red
Weak (±)	Tiny aggregates barely visible macroscopically; many free erythrocytes; turbid and reddish supernatant
1+	A few small aggregates just visible macroscopically; many free erythrocytes; turbid and reddish supernatant
2+	Medium-sized aggregates; some free erythrocytes; clear supernatant
3+	Several large aggregates; some free erythrocytes; clear supernatant
4+	All erythrocytes are combined into one solid aggregate; clear supernatant

Adapted from Lehman CA: *Saunders' manual of clinical laboratory science,* Philadelphia, 1998, Saunders.

Microplate Agglutination Reactions

Serologic testing has usually been performed by slide or test tube techniques, but the increased emphasis on cost containment has stimulated interest in microtechniques as an alternative to conventional methods. Micromethods for RBC antigen and antibody testing include hemagglutination and solid-phase adherence assays. These methods are also considered to be easier to perform. The use of microplates allows for the performance of a large number of tests on a single plate, which eliminates time-consuming steps such as labeling test tubes.

A microplate is a compact plate of rigid or flexible plastic with multiple wells. The wells may be U shaped or have a flat-bottom configuration. The U-shaped well has been used most often in immunohematology. The volume capacity of each well is approximately 0.2 mL, which prevents spilling during mixing. Samples and reagents are dispensed with small-bore Pasteur pipettes. These pipettes are recommended because they deliver 0.025 mL, which prevents splashing. After the specimens and reagents are added to the wells, they are mixed by gentle agitation of the plates. The microplate is then centrifuged for an immediate reading.

Countertop or floor-model centrifuges are suitable if they are equipped with special rotors that can accommodate microplate centrifuge carriers and are capable of speeds of 400 to 2000 rpm. Smaller plates can be centrifuged in serologic centrifuges with an appropriate adapter.

After centrifugation, the cell buttons are resuspended by gently tapping the microplate or by using a flat-topped mechanical shaker. A shaker provides a more consistent and standard resuspension of the cells than manual tapping. After the cells are resuspended, the wells are examined with an optical aid or over a well-lit surface. A positive reaction will settle in a diffuse uneven button; negative reactions are manifested by a smooth compact button. Detection of weakly positive reactions is enhanced by allowing the RBCs to settle.

READING AGGLUTINATION

GRADE	DESCRIPTION		APPEARANCE	
	Cells	Supernate	Macroscopic[a]	Microscopic[b]
0	No agglutinates	Dark, turbid, homogeneous	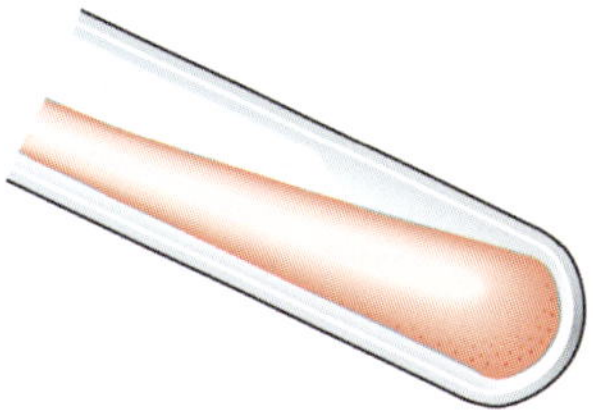	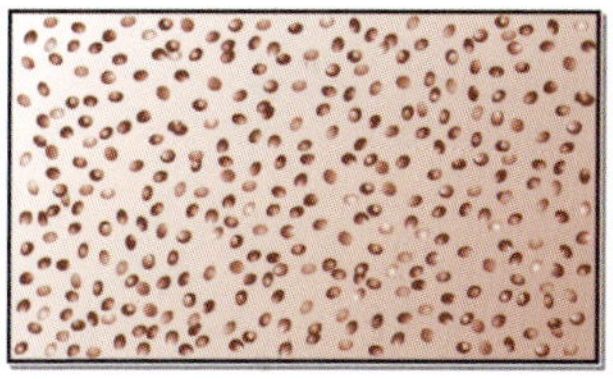
w+	Many tiny agglutinates Many free cells May not be visible without microscope	Dark, turbid	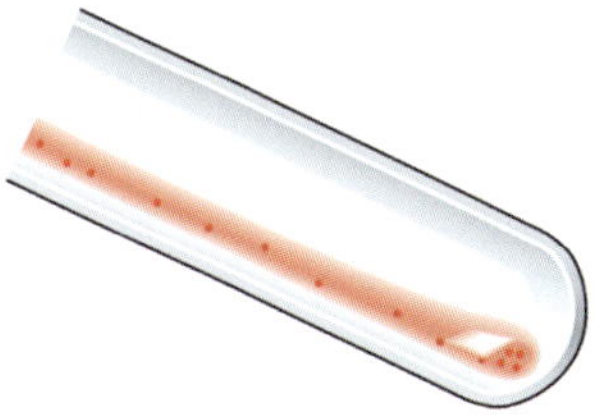	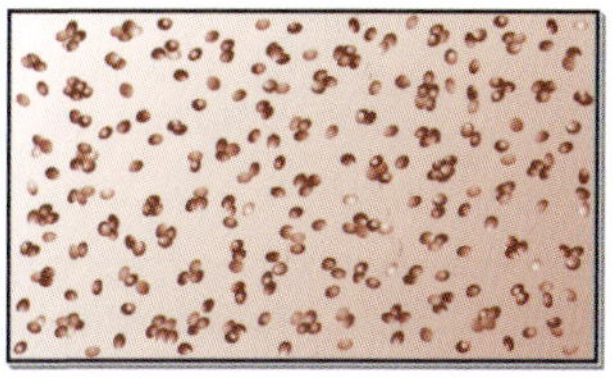
1+	Many small agglutinates Many free cells	Turbid	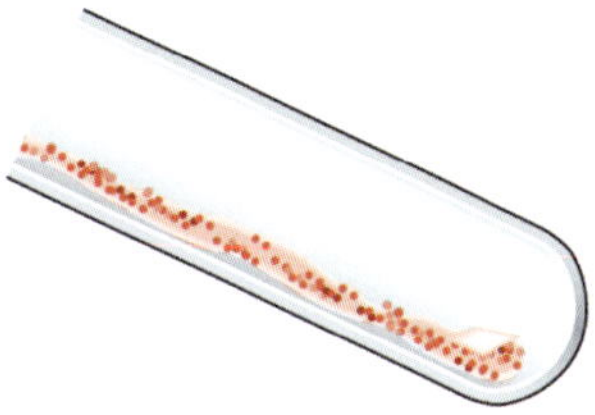	
2+	Many medium-sized agglutinates Moderate number of free cells	Clear	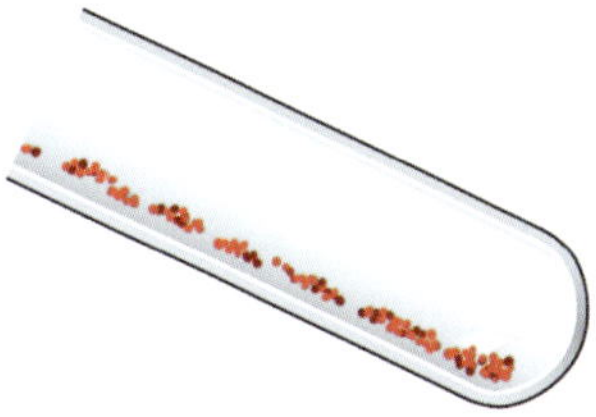	
3+	Several large agglutinates Few free cells	Clear	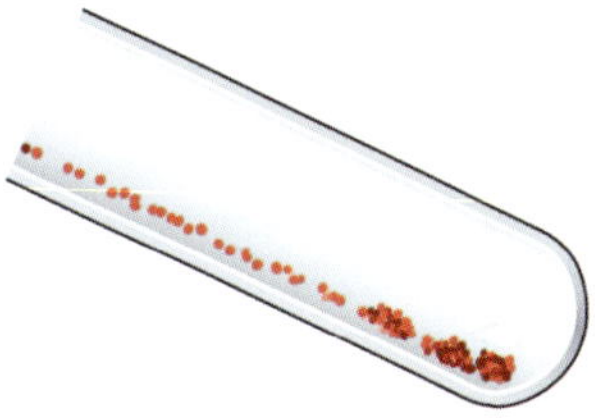	
4+	One large, solid agglutinate No free cells	Clear	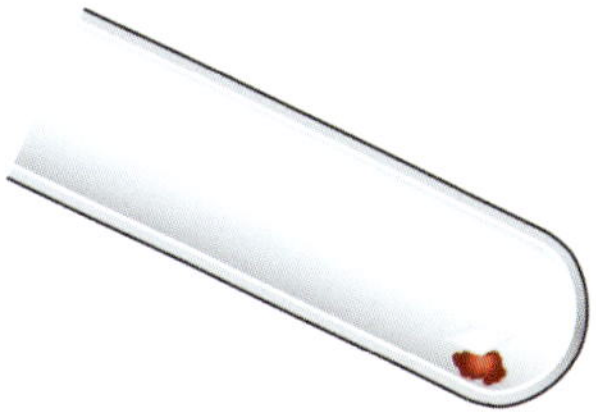	

[a]For any one grade, readings can be on a scale from weak + to strong + (e.g., grade 2 can be stored as 2+w, 2+, or 2+s, depending on the number and size of agglutinates).
[b]Microscopic readings are generally performed to differentiate pseudoagglutination (rouleaux) from true agglutination, to detect mixed-field reactions, and to confirm a negative reaction.

Fig. 8.8 Reading Red Blood Cell Agglutination Reactions. (From Lehman CA: *Saunders' manual of clinical laboratory science,* Philadelphia, 1998, Saunders.)

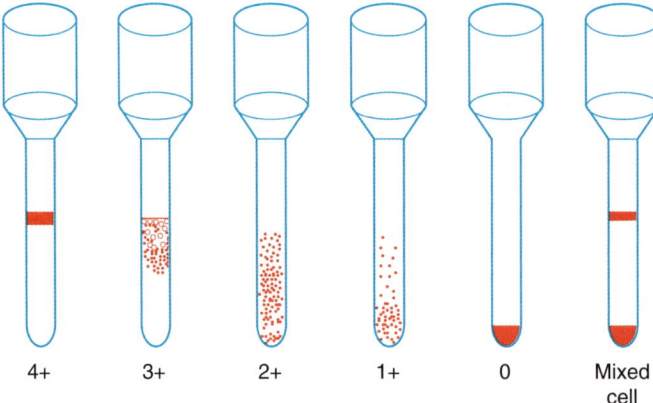

Fig. 8.9 Appearance of Reaction Patterns and Grading for Gel or Column Agglutination Technology. (From McPherson RA, Pincus MR: Henry's clinical diagnosis and management by laboratory methods, immunohematology, St. Louis, 2007, Elsevier.)

> **KEY CONCEPTS: Nephelometry**
> - Nephelometry depends on the light-scattering properties of antigen–antibody complexes based on the formation of a macromolecular complex.
> - Nephelometry is based on the principle that light is scattered by a homogeneous particulate solution at a variety of angles.
> - In immunology, nephelometry is used to measure complement components, immune complexes, and the presence of a variety of antibodies.
> - The disadvantages of nephelometry include high initial equipment cost and interfering substances such as microbial contamination, which may cause protein denaturation and erroneous test results.
> - Newer methods of testing use nephelometry with cold treatment for analysis of cryoglobulins.
> - Cryoglobulins are classified into three types. In type I, cryoprecipitate is a monoclonal IgG, IgA, or IgM; in type II, cryoprecipitate is mixed, containing two classes of immunoglobulins, at least one of which is monoclonal; and in type III, cryoprecipitate is mixed and no monoclonal protein is found.

> **BOX 8.2 Immunologic Assays Performed by Nephelometry**
>
> Acid α_1-glycoprotein
> Albumin
> α_1-Antitrypsin
> α_2-Macroglobulin
> C1 esterase inhibitor (C1 inhibitor)
> C3
> C3b inhibitor (C3b inactivator)
> C3PA (C3 proactivator, properdin factor B)
> C4
> C6
> C7
> C8
> Ceruloplasmin
> Complement components (C1r, C1s, C2, C3, C4, C5, C6, C7, C8)
> C-reactive protein (CRP)
> Cryofibrinogen
> Cryoglobulins
> Haptoglobin
> Hemopexin
> Immunoglobulins
> Properdin factor B
> Transferrin

NEPHELOMETRY

The quantity of cloudiness or turbidity in a solution can be measured **photometrically**. When specific antigen-coated latex particles acting as reaction intensifiers are agglutinated by their corresponding antibody, the increased light scatter of a solution can be measured by nephelometry as the macromolecular complexes form. The use of polyethylene glycol (PEG) enhances and stabilizes the precipitates, thus increasing the speed and sensitivity of the technique by controlling the particle size for optimal light angle deflection. The kinetics of this change can be determined when the photometric results are analyzed by computer.

In immunology, nephelometry is used to measure complement components, immune complexes, and the presence of a variety of antibodies (Box 8.2).

Principle

Formation of a **macromolecular complex** is a fundamental prerequisite for nephelometric protein quantitation. The procedure is based on the reaction between the protein being assayed and a specific antiserum. Protein in a patient's specimen reacts with specific nephelometric antiserum to human proteins and forms insoluble complexes. When light is passed through such a suspension, the resulting complexes of insoluble precipitants scatter incident light in solutions (Fig. 8.10). The scattered light can be detected with a photodiode. The amount of scattered light is proportional to the number of insoluble complexes and can be quantitated by comparing the unknown patient values with standards of known protein concentration.

The relationship between the quantity of antigen and measuring signal at a constant antibody concentration is expressed by the **Heidelberger curve**. If antibodies are present to excess, a proportional relationship exists between the antigen and resulting signal. If the antigen overwhelms the quantity of antibody, the measured signal drops.

By optimizing the reaction conditions, the typical antigen–antibody reactions as characterized by the Heidelberger curve are effectively shifted in the direction of high concentration. This ensures that these high concentrations will be measured on the ascending portion of the

CHAPTER 8 Precipitation and Particle Agglutination Methods

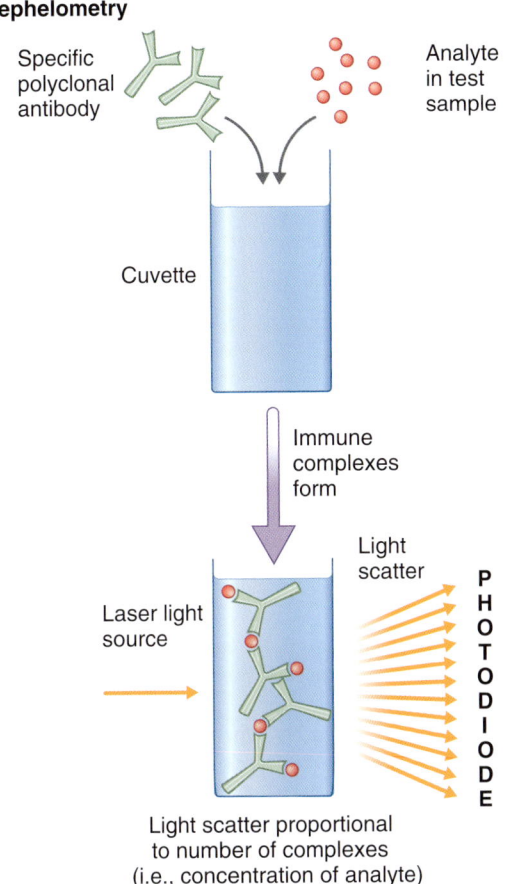

Fig. 8.10 Principle of Nephelometry for the Measurement of Antigen–Antibody Reactions. Light rays are collected in a focusing lens and can ultimately be related to the antigen or antibody concentration in a specimen.

curve. At concentrations higher than the reference curve, the instrument will transmit an out-of-range warning.

Physical Basis
Nephelometry is based on the principle that light is scattered by a homogeneous particulate solution at a variety of angles. Three types of scatter can occur: (1) scatter around the particles, (2) forward scatter caused by out-of-phase backscatter, and (3) forward scatter exceeding backscatter.

Optical System
In the nephelometric method, an infrared high-performance, light-emitting diode (LED) is used as the light source. Because an entire solid angle is measured after convergence of this light through a lens system, an intense measuring signal is available when the primary beam is blocked off. In connection with the lens system, this produces a light beam of high collinearity. The wavelength is 840 nm. Light scattered in the forward direction in a solid angle to the primary beam ranges between 13 and 24 feet and is measured by a silicon photodiode with an integrated amplifier. The electrical signals generated are digitized, compared with reference curves, and converted to protein concentrations.

Measuring Methods
A fixed-time method is used routinely for precipitation reactions. Ten seconds after all reaction components have been mixed, a cuvette reading (initial blank measurement) is taken. A second measurement is taken 6 minutes later and, after subtraction of the original 1-second blanking value, a final answer is calculated against the multiple-point or single-point calibration in the computerized program memory for the assay.

Advantages and Disadvantages
Nephelometry represents an automated system that is rapid, reproducible, relatively simple to operate, and common in higher volume laboratories. It has many applications in the immunology laboratory. Currently, instruments using a rate method and fixed time approach are commercially available with tests for IgG, IgA, IgM, C3, C4, properdin, C-reactive protein (CRP), rheumatoid factor, ceruloplasmin, α_1-antitrypsin, apolipoproteins, and haptoglobins.

The disadvantages of nephelometry include high initial equipment cost and interfering substances such as microbial contamination, which may cause protein denaturation and erroneous test results. Intrinsic specimen turbidity or lipemia may exceed the preset limits. In these cases, a clearing agent may be needed before an accurate assay can be performed. In addition, low-molecular-weight immunoglobulins, monoclonal immunoglobulins, and antibovine antibodies also may produce spurious results in nephelometry.

Clinical Application: Cryoglobulins
Cryoglobulin analysis is frequently requested when patient symptoms such as pain, cyanosis, Raynaud phenomenon, and skin ulceration on exposure to cold temperatures are present. Cryoglobulins are proteins that precipitate or gel when cooled to 0°C (32°F) and dissolve when heated. In most cases, monoclonal cryoglobulins are IgM or IgG. Occasionally, the macroglobulin is both cryoprecipitable and capable of cold-induced anti-I–mediated agglutination of RBCs.

Cryoglobulins with a detected monoclonal protein component normally prompt a clinical investigation to determine whether an underlying disease exists. Cryoglobulins are classified as follows:
- Type I: Cryoprecipitate is a monoclonal IgG, IgA, or IgM.
- Type II: Cryoprecipitate is mixed, containing two classes of immunoglobulins, at least one of which is monoclonal.
- Type III: Cryoprecipitate is mixed and no monoclonal protein is found.

To test for the presence of cryoglobulins, blood is collected, placed in warm water, and centrifuged at room temperature. The serum is then put into a graduated centrifuge tube and placed in a 4°C (39°F) environment for 7 days. If a gel or precipitate is observed, the tube is centrifuged and the precipitate is washed at 4°C (39°F), redissolved at 37°C (98.6°F), and evaluated by double diffusion and immunoelectrophoresis for the content of the cryoglobulin. Newer methods use nephelometry with cold treatment for analysis.

CASE STUDY 8.1 ABO Testing Results

An 85-year-old man had a discrepancy between his forward grouping (ABO antigens) and reverse grouping (ABO antibodies).

	Patient RBCs	Patient Serum
Anti-A typing sera	Negative	
Anti-B typing sera	Negative	
A_1 RBCs		2+
B RBCs		Negative

Questions
1. The discrepancy between ABO antigen and antibody (forward and reverse testing) can be caused by:
   a. Too much A antigen on RBCs
   b. Too much B antigen on RBCs
   c. False-positive antibody to A antigen
   d. False-negative antibody to B antigen
2. The cause of the discrepancy between this patient's ABO antigen and antibody testing can be caused by all of the following examples *except*:
   a. Deteriorated reagent RBCs
   b. Hypogammaglobulinemia
   c. Age of the patient
   d. Alloantibodies

See Appendix A for the answers to these questions.

Critical Thinking Group Discussion Questions
1. What is the most likely cause of the discrepancy between ABO antigens and antibodies in this patient?
2. How can the discrepancy be resolved?

REVIEW QUESTIONS

1. The quality of test results in an agglutination reaction depends on all of the following *except*:
   a. Duration of incubation
   b. Amount of antigen conjugated to the carrier
   c. Avidity of antigen conjugated to the carrier
   d. Whether the carrier is artificial or biological

2. Flocculation procedures differ from latex agglutination procedures because:
   a. Antigen is bound to a carrier
   b. Antibody is bound to a carrier
   c. Soluble antigen reacts with antibody
   d. Flocculation procedures are only qualitative

3. In the hemagglutination technique, antihuman globulin is used as an enhancement medium to detect _____ antibodies.
   a. IgM
   b. IgG
   c. IgD
   d. IgE

4. The prozone phenomenon can result in a(an):
   a. False-positive reaction
   b. False-negative reaction
   c. Enhanced agglutination
   d. Diminished antigen response

5. The effect of competing antibodies seeking to attach to antigen sites is called:
   a. Prozone phenomenon
   b. Ionic strength
   c. Steric hindrance
   d. Sensitization

6. Which class of antibody can agglutinate erythrocytes (RBCs) after antihuman globulin (AHG) is added to the test tube?
   a. IgA
   b. IgE
   c. IgG
   d. IgM

7. The description of a mixed-field graded agglutination reaction is:
   a. All erythrocytes are combined into one solid aggregate; clear supernatant
   b. Few isolated aggregates; supernatant appears red
   c. Medium-sized aggregates; clear supernatant
   d. A few small aggregates; turbid and reddish supernatant

8. The description of a 1+ graded agglutination reaction is:
   a. All erythrocytes are combined into one solid aggregate; clear supernatant
   b. Few isolated aggregates; supernatant appears red
   c. Medium-sized aggregates; clear supernatant
   d. A few small aggregates; turbid and reddish supernatant

9. The description of a 2+ graded agglutination reaction is:
   a. All erythrocytes are combined into one solid aggregate; clear supernatant
   b. Few isolated aggregates; supernatant appears red
   c. Medium-sized aggregates; clear supernatant
   d. A few small aggregates; turbid and reddish supernatant

10. The description of a 4+ graded agglutination reaction is:
    a. All erythrocytes are combined into one solid aggregate; clear supernatant
    b. Few isolated aggregates; supernatant appears red
    c. Medium-sized aggregates; clear supernatant
    d. A few small aggregates; turbid and reddish supernatant

11. A classic technique for the detection of viral antibodies is:
    a. Passive hemagglutination
    b. Indirect hemagglutination
    c. Hemagglutination inhibition
    d. Latex particle agglutination

12. If the principle of a laboratory procedure is based on testing for an antigen in an infectious entity, it is classified as:
    a. passive agglutination
    b. reverse passive agglutination
    c. direct agglutination
    d. indirect agglutination

13. The definition of precipitation is:
    a. Aggregation of particulate test antigens
    b. Aggregation of soluble test antigens
    c. Uses antibodies bound to a particle to enhance visibility of agglutination
    d. Agglutination of erythrocytes in tests for antibody detection

14. The definition of agglutination is:
    a. Aggregation of particulate test antigens
    b. Aggregation of soluble test antigens
    c. Uses antibodies bound to a particle to enhance visibility of agglutination
    d. Agglutination of erythrocytes in tests for antibody detection

15. The definition of coagglutination is:
    a. Aggregation of particulate test antigens
    b. Aggregation of soluble test antigens
    c. Uses antibodies bound to a particle to enhance visibility of agglutination
    d. Based on the interaction of soluble antigen with antibody, resulting in formation of a precipitate of fine particles
16. The definition of flocculation is:
    a. Aggregation of particulate test antigens
    b. Aggregation of soluble test antigens
    c. Uses antibodies bound to a particle to enhance visibility of agglutination
    d. Based on the interaction of soluble antigen with antibody, resulting in formation of a precipitate of fine particles
17. The definition of hemagglutination is:
    a. Aggregation of particulate test antigens
    b. Aggregation of soluble test antigens
    c. Uses antibodies bound to a particle to enhance visibility of agglutination
    d. Agglutination of erythrocytes in tests for antibody detection
18. Artificial or biological carriers that can be used in an agglutination reaction include all of the following *except*:
    a. Latex particles
    b. Colloidal charcoal
    c. Erythrocytes coated with antigen in a constant amount
    d. Radioactive metals

Identify the components (a and b) of a latex agglutination reaction in the figure below:

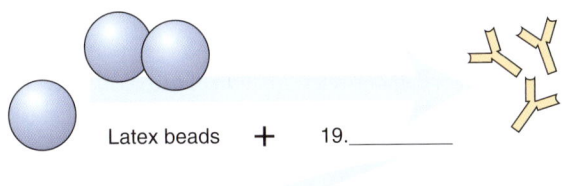

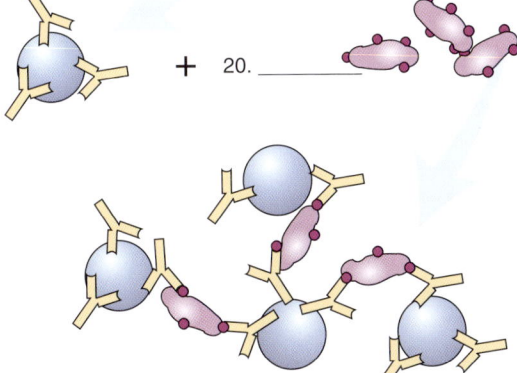

Particle agglutination

(Adapted from Forbes BA, Sahm DF, Weissfeld AS: *Bailey and Scott's diagnostic microbiology,* ed 12, St. Louis, 2007, Elsevier.)

19. Identify____
    a. Antigen
    b. Specific antibody
20. Identify____
    a. Antigen
    b. Antibody

21. Sensitization:
    a. Is the first phase of agglutination
    b. Represents the physical attachment of antibody molecules to antigens on the RBC membrane
    c. Is an irreversible reaction
    d. Both a and b
22. Agglutination can be used to enhance reactions by all of the following means *except*:
    a. Decreasing the ionic strength of the reaction
    b. Centrifugation
    c. Increasing the pH of the reaction
    d. Using colloids and antihuman globulin
23. A negative latex agglutination reaction would appear as:
    a. Tiny aggregates that are barely visible macroscopically
    b. Several large aggregates
    c. All erythrocytes combined into one solid aggregate
    d. No aggregates
24. A weak (1+ or 2+) latex agglutination reaction would appear as:
    a. Tiny aggregates that are barely visible macroscopically
    b. Several large aggregates
    c. All erythrocytes combined into one solid aggregate
    d. No aggregates
25. A 3+ latex agglutination reaction would appear as:
    a. Tiny aggregates that are barely visible macroscopically
    b. Several large aggregates
    c. All erythrocytes combined into one solid aggregate
    d. No aggregates
26. All of the following statements are correct regarding human pregnancy testing *except*:
    a. Tests detect human chorionic gonadotropin (hCG)
    b. hCG is secreted by the trophoblast of the developing embryo
    c. The presence of hCG rapidly increases in urine or serum
    d. The presence of hCG in maternal urine or serum persists throughout pregnancy
27. All of the following statements are correct regarding hCG *except*:
    a. It helps maintain the corpus luteum
    b. It stimulates production of progesterone
    c. It is detectable within 102 hours after the last expected menstrual period
    d. It reaches peak levels at 2 to 3 months after the last menstrual period
28. The original, nonanimal laboratory method for detecting hCG is:
    a. Latex or hemagglutination
    b. Enzyme-linked immunosorbent assay
    c. Immunofluorescence
    d. Antibody titration
29. In the latex agglutination method for the detection of hCG, no agglutination indicates the:
    a. Absence of hCG
    b. Presence of hCG
    c. Absence of hCG, a positive test
    d. Presence of hCG, a negative test
30. A false-positive reaction in a latex agglutination test for hCG can be caused by all of the following *except*:
    a. Chorioepithelioma
    b. Hydatidiform mole
    c. Taking oral contraceptives
    d. Excessive ingestion of aspirin
31. The difference between gel precipitation reactions and flocculation:
    a. Is a soluble reaction
    b. Involves red blood cell indicators
    c. Is agarose based
    d. Is based on latex antigen-coated particles

32. If soluble antigen is added to soluble antibody, the kind of antigen–antibody reaction that is expected is:
    a. Precipitation
    b. Agglutination
    c. Complement fixation
    d. Hemagglutination
33. Nephelometry is based on the principles of:
    a. Turbidity resulting from specific antigen-coated latex particles agglutinated by corresponding antibody.
    b. Agglutination from physical attachment of antibody molecules to antigens on an erythrocyte membrane.
    c. Agglutination of host antibody to antigenic determinants on a bacterial agent.
    d. Precipitation of immune-related protein in agarose gel.
34. Cryoglobulins are proteins that precipitate or gel when cooled to:
    a. −18°C (−0.4°F)
    b. 0°C (32°F)
    c. 4°C (39°F)
    d. 18°C (64°F)
35. A characteristic of type I cryoglobulins is:
    a. Two classes of immunoglobulins, at least one of which is monoclonal
    b. Mixed, no monoclonal protein found
    c. Monoclonal IgG, IgA, or IgM
    d. Five classes of immunoglobulins
36. A characteristic of type II cryoglobulins is:
    a. Two classes of immunoglobulins, at least one of which is monoclonal
    b. Mixed, no monoclonal protein found
    c. Monoclonal IgG, IgA, or IgM
    d. Five classes of immunoglobulins
37. A characteristic of type III cryoglobulins is:
    a. Five classes of immunoglobulins, at least one of which is monoclonal
    b. Mixed, no monoclonal protein found
    c. Monoclonal IgG, IgA, or IgM
    d. Five classes of immunoglobulins
38. Cryoglobulin analysis can be useful in the diagnosis of:
    a. Hypothermia
    b. Raynaud phenomenon
    c. Hepatitis C
    d. Rheumatoid arthritis

Questions 39–40

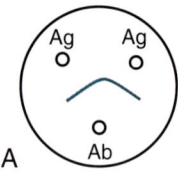
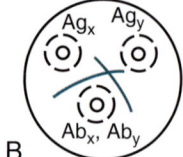
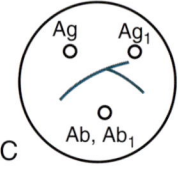
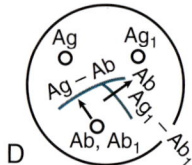

39. Which pattern demonstrates a pattern of identity?
    a. Fig. A
    b. Fig. B
    c. Fig. C
    d. Fig. D
40. Which pattern demonstrates a pattern of non-identity?
    a. Fig. A
    b. Fig. B
    c. Fig. C
    d. Fig. D
41. Which pattern demonstrates a pattern of partial-identity?
    a. Fig. A
    b. Fig. B
    c. Fig. C
    d. Fig. D

9

Electrophoresis Techniques and Chromatography

LEARNING OUTCOMES

- Define the term *electrophoresis*.
- Describe the electrophoresis technique.
- Identify the fractions into which serum proteins can be divided by electrophoresis.
- Draw and label a serum electrophoresis pattern.
- Describe the principle, expected results, reference values, and clinical interpretation of the serum protein electrophoresis procedure.
- Explain the principle of immunofixation electrophoresis (IFE).
- Describe various observations of IFE.
- Discuss the clinical applications of IFE.
- Explain follow-up laboratory testing.
- Compare capillary electrophoresis and microchip capillary electrophoresis.
- Describe two electrophoresis separation methods.
- Explain the principles of immunochromatography.
- Analyze a patient history and laboratory data, and answer the multiple-choice and critical thinking questions related to serum electrophoresis.
- Correctly answer case study–related multiple-choice questions.
- Participate in a discussion of critical thinking questions.
- Describe the principle of the immunofixation electrophoresis procedure.
- Correctly answer 80% of end-of-chapter review questions.

OUTLINE

Electrophoresis, 143
Serum Protein Electrophoresis, 144
    Principle, 144
    Results, 144
        Reference Values, 144
    Clinical Interpretation, 144
Immunofixation Electrophoresis, 144
    Principle, 146
    Interpretation, 146

    Clinical Applications, 147
    Follow-Up Laboratory Testing, 147
Capillary Electrophoresis, 147
Chromatography and Immunochromatography, 147
    Types of Chromatographic Methods, 147
    Lateral or Vertical Flow Immunoassays (Immunochromatography), 147
Case Study 9.1   History and Physical Examination, 148
Procedure: Immunofixation Electrophoresis, 149.e1

KEY TERMS

buffer
capillary electrophoresis
electrophoresis

immunofixation electrophoresis (IFE)
isoelectric focusing
M protein

monoclonal gammopathy
multiple myeloma

KEY CONCEPTS: Facts About Electrophoresis

- Serum electrophoresis results in the separation of proteins into five fractions on agarose gel based on the rate of migration of these individual components in an electrical field.
- Electrophoresis is used to identify the presence or absence of aberrant proteins and to determine when different groups of proteins are increased or decreased in serum or urine.
- Immunofixation electrophoresis (IFE) or immunofixation, has replaced the older technique of immunoelectrophoresis (IEP) because of its rapidity and ease of interpretation.
- The primary use of IFE in clinical laboratories is for the characterization of monoclonal immunoglobulins.
- IFE has two stages: agarose gel protein electrophoresis and immunoprecipitation.
- Capillary electrophoresis is a molecular method in which high electrical field strengths are used to separate molecules based on differences in charge, size, and hydrophobicity.

ELECTROPHORESIS

Using the principle of **electrophoresis**, migration of charged solutes or particles in an electrical field, charged molecules can be made to move. As a consequence, different molecules can be separated if they have different velocities in an electrical field. Many electrophoresis-based technologies are commonly used (Table 9.1) as nucleic acid detection techniques to separate nucleic acids based on molecular size and shape.

The electrical field is applied to a solution with oppositely charged electrodes. Charged particles in this solution begin to migrate. Positively charged particles (cations) move to the negatively charged (−) electrode; negatively charged particles (anions) migrate to the positively charged (+) electrode (Fig. 9.1). Nondenaturing electrophoresis takes place from a mechanistic standpoint, including proteins having charge in the pH 9.6 buffer based on their isoelectric point. This is why a pH such as 9.6 is used.

143

TABLE 9.1 Examples of Commonly Used Electrophoresis-Based Techniques

Technique	Abbreviation	Primary Application
Polymerase chain reaction (or reverse transcriptase polymerase chain reaction) length	PCR (or RT-PCR)	Detection
Polymerase chain reaction/restriction fragment length polymorphism	PCR/RFLP	Detection
Southern blotting		Detection
Northern blotting		Detection
Dideoxy-termination sequencing (Sanger)		Sequencing
Single-nucleotide extension assay	SNE	Genotyping
Oligonucleotide ligation assay	OLA	Genotyping
Multiplex ligation-dependent probe amplification	MLPA	Quantification
Heteroduplex migration assay	HAD	Scanning
Confirmation-sensitive gel electrophoresis	CSGE	Scanning
Single-strand conformation polymorphism analysis	SSCP, SSCA	Scanning
Denaturing gradient gel electrophoresis	DGGE	Scanning
Temperature gradient electrophoresis	TGGE, TGCE	Scanning
Temperature cycling capillary electrophoresis	TCCE	Scanning

From Rifai N, Horvath AR, Wittwer CT: *Tietz textbook of clinical chemistry and molecular diagnostics,* St. Louis, 2018, Elsevier.

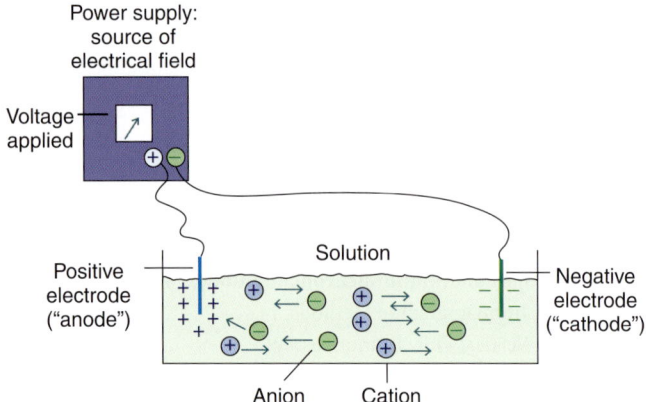

Fig. 9.1 Application of Electrical Field to a Solution of Ions Makes the Ions Move. (From Kaplan LA, Pesce AJ: *Clinical chemistry: theory, analysis, correlation,* ed 5, St. Louis, 2009, Elsevier.)

Note: A buffer solution or pH buffer is an acid or a base aqueous solution consisting of a mixture of a weak acid or base and its conjugate base. The pH changes very little when a small amount of strong acid or base is added to it. Buffer solutions resist pH change.

SERUM PROTEIN ELECTROPHORESIS

Principle

Serum protein electrophoresis is used to separate and quantitate serum proteins based on electrophoretic mobility on cellulose acetate or, more commonly, gel agar. Serum proteins are often separated by electrophoresis. Serum electrophoresis results in the separation of proteins into five fractions using cellulose acetate or agarose gel as a support medium. This separation is based on the rate of migration of these individual components in an electrical field.

Electrophoresis (Fig. 9.2) is a versatile analytic technique. Immunoglobulins are separated by electrophoresis using agarose as a support medium. The immunologic applications of electrophoresis include identification of monoclonal proteins in serum or urine.

Proteins are large molecules composed of amino acids. Depending on electron distributions resulting from covalent or ionic bonding of structural subgroups, proteins have different electrical charges at a given pH. Based on electrical charge, serum proteins can be fractionated into five fractions: albumin, alpha-1 (α_1), alpha-2 (α_2), beta (β), and gamma (γ) proteins (Fig. 9.3). For the following method, the pH is 9.9. After the proteins are separated, the plate is placed in a solution of sulfosalicylic acid and Ponceau S to stain the protein bands. The intensity of the stain for each band is related to protein concentration.

Results

The fastest moving band, and normally the most prominent, is the albumin band found closest to the anodic edge of the plate. The faint band next to this is α_1 globulin, followed by α_2, β, and γ globulins. Prealbumin is seldom visible with this system.

Reference Values

Each laboratory should establish its own range. The following reference values are for illustrative purposes only.

Protein Fraction	Concentration (g/dL)
Albumin	3.63–4.91
Alpha-1	0.11–0.35
Alpha-2	0.65–1.17
Beta	0.74–1.26
Gamma	0.58–1.74

Clinical Interpretation

Electrophoresis is used to identify the presence or absence of aberrant proteins and to determine when different groups of proteins are increased or decreased in serum (Fig. 9.4) or urine. It is frequently ordered to detect and identify monoclonal proteins, often excessive production of one specific immunoglobulin.

Protein and immunofixation electrophoresis are ordered to help detect, diagnose, and monitor the course and treatment of conditions associated with these abnormal proteins (e.g., multiple myeloma).

IMMUNOFIXATION ELECTROPHORESIS

Immunofixation electrophoresis (IFE), or simply immunofixation, has replaced the older technique of immunoelectrophoresis (IEP) because of its rapidity and ease of interpretation (Table 9.2).

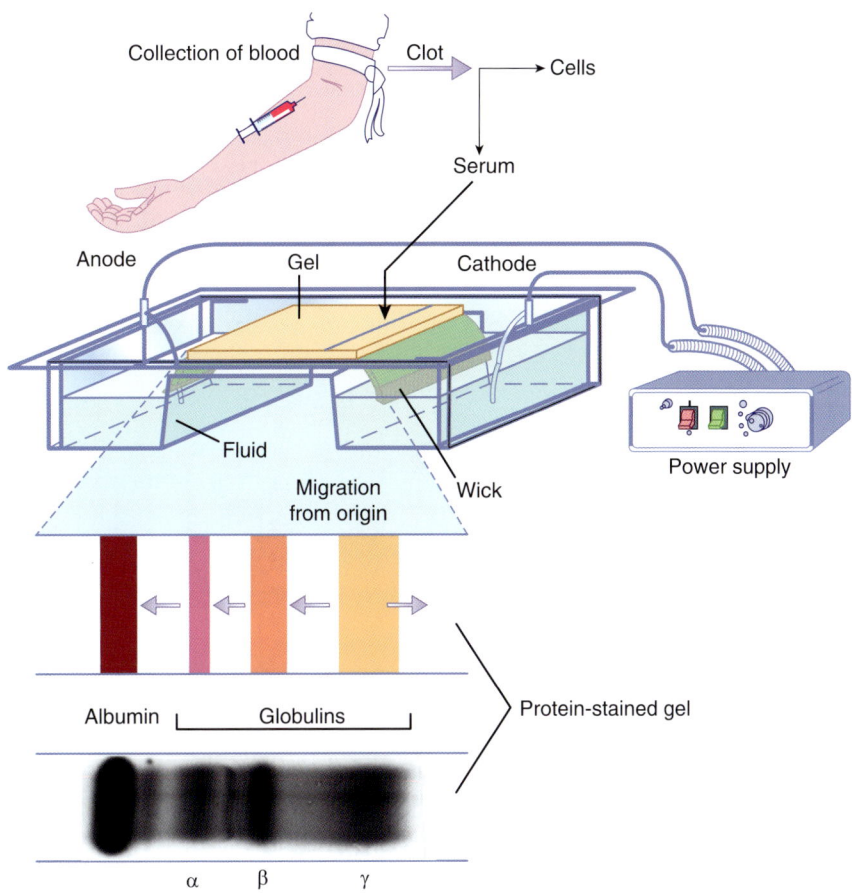

Fig. 9.2 Separation of Serum Proteins by Electrophoresis. (Adapted from Peakman M, Vergani D: *Basic and clinical immunology*, St. Louis, 2009, Elsevier.)

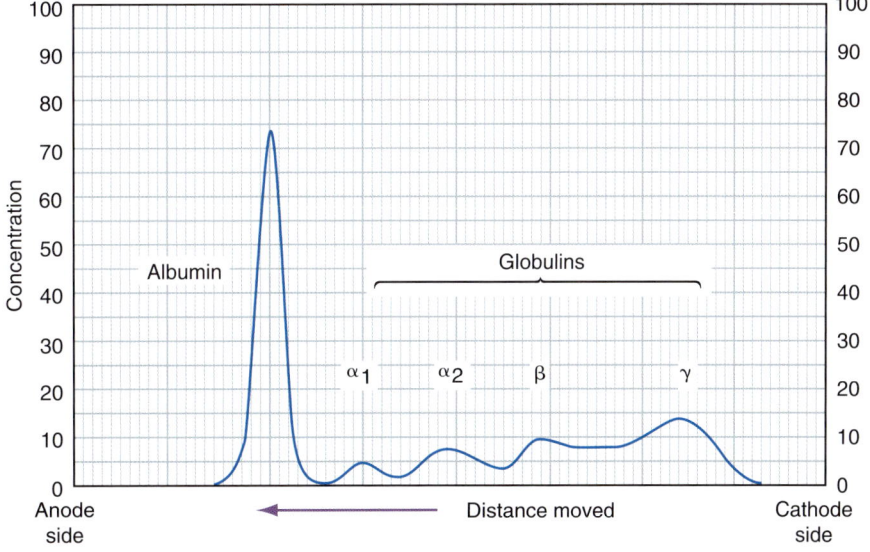

Fig. 9.3 Tracing of Electrophoretic Pattern of Normal Serum. (Adapted from Kaplan LA, Pesce AJ, Kazmierczak SC, editors: *Clinical chemistry theory, analysis, correlation*, ed 4, St. Louis, 2003, Mosby.)

The primary use of IFE in clinical laboratories is for the characterization of monoclonal immunoglobulins. The test specimen for IFE may be serum, urine, cerebrospinal fluid (CSF), or other body fluids.

Although IFE was first described in 1964, it wasn't introduced as a procedure for the study of immunoglobulins until 1976. The laboratory protocol for ruling out **monoclonal gammopathy** should include high-resolution electrophoresis, IEP of both serum and urine, and a quantitative immunoglobulin assay. These procedures are usually sufficient to detect and characterize monoclonal proteins with a serum concentration of 1 g/dL or more.

PART II The Theory of Immunologic and Serologic Procedures

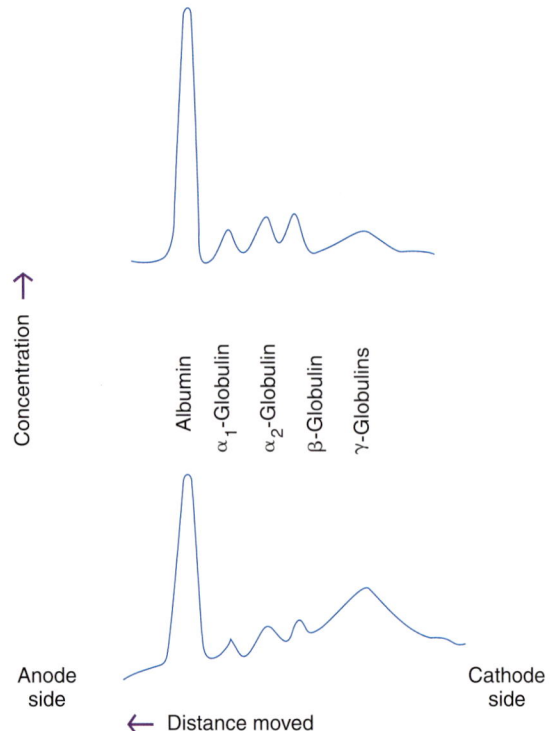

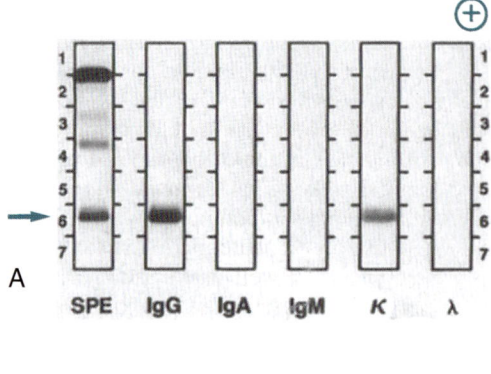

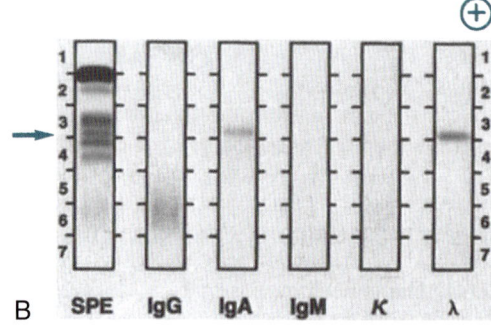

Fig. 9.4 *Upper profile,* Protein distribution characteristic of healthy people. *Lower profile,* Example of the effect of disease on a serum protein electrophoresis pattern. (Upper profile from Kaplan LA, Pesce AJ: *Clinical chemistry: theory, analysis, correlation,* ed 5, St. Louis, 2010, Mosby.)

Fig. 9.5 Immunofixation Electrophoresis (IFE). (A), Patient specimen with an IgG (κ) monoclonal protein, as identified by IFE. Note the position of the monoclonal protein *(arrow).* After electrophoresis, each track except serum protein electrophoresis (SPE) is reacted with its respective antiserum; then, all tracks are stained to visualize the respective protein bands. IgG, IgA, IgM; κ; and λ indicate antiserum used on each track. (B) Patient specimen with an IgA (λ) monoclonal protein identified by the IFE procedure, as described in (A). κ, Kappa; *IgA,* immunoglobulin A; *IgG,* immunoglobulin G; *IgM,* immunoglobulin M; λ, lambda; *SPE,* serum protein electrophoresis.

TABLE 9.2	Characteristics of Immunofixation Electrophoresis (IFE)
Feature	**IFE**
Ease of use	More complex than older techniques
Sensitivity	More sensitive than older techniques
Monoclonal gammopathies	Used for difficult-to-characterize anomalous proteins
Interpretation	Easier than older techniques

From Burtis CA, Ashwood ER, Bruns DB: *Tietz fundamentals of clinical chemistry,* ed 6, St. Louis, 2008, Saunders.

The following three protein variables can be determined using IFE:
1. Antigenic specificity
2. Electrophoretic mobility
3. Quantity or ratio of test and control proteins

Principle
IFE is a two-stage procedure. Immunofixation consists of an electrophoresis phase and a fixation phase. Serum is applied to an agarose gel, and the negatively charged serum proteins move toward the cathode under the influence of an electric current. The speed of movement is dictated by their charge. During the fixation phase, antiserum containing anti-IgG, anti-IgA, anti-IgM, anti–light-chain kappa, or anti–light-chain lambda is inoculated with the serum proteins. The gel is washed away with saline to remove all unprecipitated proteins and then stained, destained, and dried.

Interpretation
IFE is not a quantitative test. Therefore when an IFE pattern is interpreted, the results are based on visual observation. Immunofixation can either reveal a normal pattern or identify a monoclonal protein or a polyclonal immunoglobulin pattern (Fig. 9.5). Serum or urine immunofixation negative for a monoclonal protein or a polyclonal pattern is considered to be normal. CSF immunofixation that does not reveal oligoclonal bands is also considered normal.

A normal result includes a darker immunoglobulin G (IgG) lane, a lighter immunoglobulin A (IgA), an absent immunoglobulin M (IgM), and a denser kappa compared with lambda lane, with a ratio of 2:1. In a normal result, the lanes are broad and there is a gradual and smooth reduction in the intensity of color toward the edges of the lane, with no narrow dense band, with sharp borders identified within the lane. In some cases, all the lanes are homogeneously darkened to the same degree.

A negative urine or serum immunofixation result does not always rule out a plasma cell dyscrasia, because a nonsecretory or oligosecretory **multiple myeloma** can present with a negative immunofixation finding in both the urine and the serum. A serum-free light-chain ratio is indicated in the case of a negative immunofixation result when the suspicion for multiple myeloma is still high.

A polyclonal immunoglobulin pattern in the serum or urine immunofixation is considered to be nonspecific. In a polyclonal increase, the pattern displays an increased intensity of color in all five lanes. A polyclonal pattern does not exclude the possibility of the presence of an **M protein**.

Most of the M proteins will be IgG because IgG is the most prevalent immunoglobulin. IgA frequently will polymerize and display two or even three bands. IgA is often very elevated with a distorted pattern and can undergo posttranslational modification, such as glycosylation. IgM is the most troublesome protein to interpret. It is the largest immunoglobulin, often exists as a pentamer, and can polymerize. It can remain at the application point, making it impossible to identify. IgM,

IgG, and IgA comprise 99% of all M proteins seen in the laboratory. Only 1% will be IgD, and IgE is rarely observed. Depending on the patient population, many M proteins will be monoclonal gammopathy of unknown or undetermined significance (MGUS).

Clinical Applications

Immunofixation is clearly indicated upon clinical or laboratory evidence of a plasma cell dyscrasia for the diagnosis of multiple myeloma, Waldenström macroglobulinemia, or amyloid light-chain (AL) amyloidosis. If serum and urine protein electrophoresis results are negative, immunofixation is indicated as a more sensitive test if the clinical suspicion is high. In addition, when protein electrophoresis assays are positive for a monoclonal protein, serum and urine immunofixation are indicated for the appropriate identification of the immunoglobulin and the corresponding light chain. Most patients with a monoclonal protein will be diagnosed with MGUS rather than any of the malignant plasma cell dyscrasias.

If there is a suspicion of multiple sclerosis, immunofixation using CSF for the detection of oligoclonal bands is indicated. However, the presence of oligoclonal bands does not necessarily confirm the diagnosis, as other conditions can present with oligoclonal bands in the CSF.

Follow-Up Laboratory Testing

IFE of urine and serum samples should be performed for all patients with multiple myeloma, Waldenström macroglobulinemia, and AL amyloidosis every 3 months after the completion of treatment in order to evaluate for response or to document a relapse.

For surveillance of patients with MGUS or smoldering (asymptomatic) multiple myeloma, IFE of the urine and serum should be included in a battery of tests 2 to 3 months after diagnosis of smoldering myeloma, then every 4 to 6 months for 1 year, and, finally, every 6 to 12 months if the results are stable. Surveillance for multiple myeloma in patients with MGUS and favorable prognostic factors (i.e., low levels of monoclonal protein and IgG type) should include monitoring at 6 months and then every 2 to 3 years thereafter. For patients with MGUS and a high risk for progression to multiple myeloma, surveillance should be performed at 6 months and then yearly thereafter.

CAPILLARY ELECTROPHORESIS

In **capillary electrophoresis (CE)**, a molecular method, the classic separation techniques of zone electrophoresis, isotachophoresis, **isoelectric focusing**, and gel electrophoresis are performed in small-bore (10–100-μm), fused silica capillary tubes 20 to 200 cm in length (Box 9.1). Two distinct advantages of CE include the ability to apply much higher voltages than in traditional electrophoresis and the ease of automation. High electrical field strengths are used to separate molecules based on differences in charge, size, and hydrophobicity. Sample introduction is accomplished by immersing the end of the capillary into a sample vial and applying pressure, vacuum, or voltage.

Microchip CE was developed in the early 1990s. The advantages of microchip CE include high speed, reduced reagent consumption, integration analysis, and miniaturization. The applications of microchip CE are diverse and include immune disorders.

Conventional CE revolutionized DNA analysis and was vital to the Human Genome Project. Applications of CE are extensive and include the separation of many entities, including low–molecular-weight ions, proteins and other macromolecules, inorganic ions, amino acids, drugs, vitamins, and DNA fragments.

CHROMATOGRAPHY AND IMMUNOCHROMATOGRAPHY

The word *chromatography* comes from the Greek words *chromatos*, "color," and *graphein*, "to write." In chromatography, the solvent is the

> **BOX 9.1 Separation Techniques Used in Capillary Electrophoresis**
>
> **Capillary Zone Electrophoresis**
> Capillary zone electrophoresis (CZE) is the most widely used type of capillary electrophoresis (CE) because of its simplicity and versatility. As long as a molecule is charged, it can be separated by CZE. In addition, CZE is simple to perform because the capillary is only filled with buffer. Separation occurs as solutes migrate at different velocities through the capillary. Another advantage of CZE is that it separates anions and cations in the same run, which is not done in other CE methods. However, CZE cannot separate neutral molecules.
>
> **Isotachophoresis**
> Isotachophoresis (ITP) is a focusing technique based on the migration of sample components between the leading and terminating electrolytes. Solutes with mobilities intermediate to those of the leading and terminating electrolytes stack into sharp focused zones. Although used as a mode of separation, transient ITP has been used primarily as a sample concentration technique.
>
> **Capillary Isoelectric Focusing**
> Capillary isoelectric focusing (CIEF) is a separation method that allows amphoteric molecules, such as proteins, to be separated by electrophoresis in a pH gradient generated between the cathode and anode. A solute will migrate to a point at which its net charge is zero. At the solute's isoelectric point (pI), migration stops, and the sample is focused into a tight zone. In CIEF, once a solute has focused at its pI, the zone is mobilized past the detector by either pressure or chemical means. CIEF is often used in protein characterization as a mechanism to determine a protein's pI.

first phase that is mobile and carries the mixture of solutes through the second phase. The second phase is a fixed or stationary phase. The variations of chromatographic techniques as well as their applications to clinical assays have grown rapidly.

Types of Chromatographic Methods

The two main categories of chromatography are gas chromatography, in which the solute phase is in a gaseous state, and liquid chromatography, in which the solute phase is a solution or liquid. Liquid chromatography is subdivided into flat and column methods. Flat chromatography is the stationary phase that is supported on a flat sheet, such as cellulose paper (paper chromatography), or in a thin layer on a mechanical backing, such as glass or plastic (thin-layer chromatography). Column methods are classically liquid chromatography. Gas chromatography is done by a column method.

Lateral or Vertical Flow Immunoassays (Immunochromatography)

Immunochromatography is a combination of chromatography (separation of components of a sample based on differences in their movement through a substance which has the property of collecting molecules of another substance) by absorption and adsorption as a single process and immunochemical reactions. Immunochromatography is divided into lateral or vertical flow immunoassays.

The lateral or vertical flow immunoassay is an extremely versatile and rapid method for visual detection of antigen in a blood sample on a test strip. The probes used in lateral or vertical flow assays are commonly based on gold nanoparticle–antibody conjugates. Due to the optical properties of gold, a noble metal, nanoparticle detection with the naked eye can be achieved with excellent sensitivity. The assay is simple to perform.

The basic technology that underlies lateral flow immunoassays was first described in the 1960s. The first real commercial

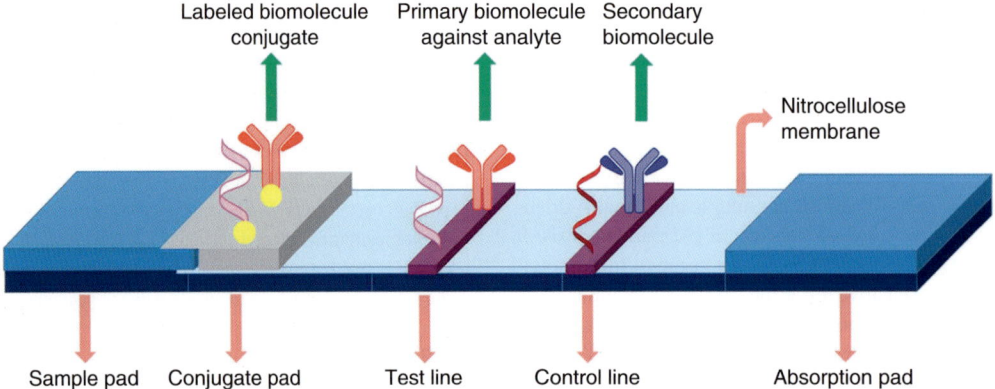

Fig. 9.6 Lateral Flow Immunoassay. (From Bahadır EB, Sezgintürk MK: Lateral flow assays: principles, designs and labels, *Trends Anal Chem* 82:286–306, 2016.)

application was an over-the-counter home pregnancy test launched in 1988. Since then, this technology has been employed to develop a wide and ever-growing range of assays. Strip assays are extremely versatile and are available for an extensive range of analytes from blood proteins to mycotoxins, and from viral pathogens to bacterial toxins.

A typical lateral flow rapid test strip consists of the following components:
- Sample pad—an adsorbent pad onto which the test sample is applied.
- Conjugate or reagent pad—this contains antibodies specific to the target analyte conjugated to colored particles (usually colloidal gold nanoparticles or latex microspheres).
- Reaction membrane—typically a nitrocellulose or cellulose acetate membrane onto which antitarget analyte antibodies are immobilized in a line that crosses the membrane to act as a capture zone or test line (a control zone will also be present, containing antibodies specific for the conjugate antibodies).
- Wick or waste reservoir—a further absorbent pad designed to draw the sample across the reaction membrane by capillary action and collect it.

The components of the strip are usually fixed to an inert backing material and may be presented in a simple dipstick format or within a plastic casing with a sample port and reaction window showing the capture and control zones (Fig. 9.6).

Vertical flow immunoassays rely on the same basic principles as the common lateral flow immunoassay format with some modifications, the most apparent difference between the two methods being the vertical and lateral flow of fluid. Vertical flow technology has reduced assay time (<5 minutes). As with lateral flow, vertical flow immunoassays rely on the immobilization of a capture antibody on a reagent pad to which the sample of interest (with or without antigen to be detected) is applied. Detection of the bound antigen is subsequently achieved through the binding of an antigen-specific antibody–gold conjugate. This step completes a sandwich consisting of a capture antibody, an antigen, and finally the gold conjugate, and results in a direct and permanent visually detectable red-colored dot indicating the presence of the antigen.

CASE STUDY 9.1 History and Physical Examination

A 40-year-old woman with a long history of alcohol abuse comes to the emergency department complaining of difficulty breathing. Physical examination reveals a slightly jaundiced appearance, icteric sclera, hepatomegaly, and splenomegaly. She has decreased breathing sounds and swollen legs (edema). Laboratory tests are ordered and show the following results:

Hematology	Patient's Results	Reference Range
Hemoglobin	12.5 g/dL	12–16.0 g/dL
Hematocrit	42%	36%–45%
Mean corpuscular volume	100 fL	80–96 fL
Total leukocyte count	13.5×10^9/L	$4.5–11.0 \times 10^9$/L
Platelets	95.0×10^9/L	$150–450 \times 10^9$/L
Coagulation—prothrombin time	17 seconds	10–14 seconds
Urinalysis		
Occult blood	1+	Negative
Bilirubin	Moderate	Negative
Clinical Chemistry		
Bilirubin	2.5 mg/dL	0.3–1.2 mg/dL
Liver enzymes (alanine aminotransferase [ALT])	55 IU/L	10–35 IU/L
Total protein	5.5 g/dL	6.4–8.3 g/dL
Albumin	2.5 g/dL	3.9–5.g/dL

Laboratory Results
- Serum protein electrophoresis interpretation—normal electrophoretic migration
- Decreased prealbumin, alpha lipoprotein, and transferrin levels
- α_2-Macroglobulin level—markedly increased
- Questionable increase in IgG and IgA because of a diffuse increase in background staining in the beta and gamma immunoglobulin regions

Questions
1. The organ system dysfunction in this patient is:
   a. Renal
   b. Hepatic
   c. Respiratory
   d. Urinary
2. The acute-phase reactant that is the most sensitive indicator of hepatocellular disease is:
   a. C-reactive protein (CRP)
   b. α_1-Antitrypsin
   c. Prothrombin time
   d. Bilirubin

See Appendix A for the answers to these questions.

Critical Thinking Group Discussion Questions
1. What is the cause of the abnormal laboratory results?
2. What does a decrease in prealbumin suggest?
3. What is the diagnostic significance of α_1-antitrypsin?

REVIEW QUESTIONS

1. Protein can be separated into _____ fractions by use of serum electrophoresis.
   a. Three
   b. Four
   c. Five
   d. Six
2. Buffers used in electrophoresis function to:
   a. Effect protein configuration
   b. Stabilize electrolytes
   c. Maintain an alkaline pH
   d. Act as a carrier for ions
3. Immunofixation electrophoresis (IFE) is primarily used in the:
   a. Workup of a polyclonal gammopathy
   b. Detection of a monoclonal immunoglobulins
   c. Screening for circulating immune complexes
   d. Identification of hypercomplementemia
4. Immunofixation electrophoresis (IFE) can test:
   a. Serum and urine
   b. Cerebrospinal fluid
   c. Whole blood
   d. Both a and b
5. The primary use of IFE is:
   a. Determination of molecular weight
   b. Characterization of monoclonal immunoglobulins
   c. Characterization of polyclonal immunoglobulins
   d. Both b and c
6. IFE can be used to detect the protein variable of:
   a. Electrophoretic mobility
   b. Molecular weight
   c. Total protein
   d. Monoclonal protein serum in a concentration of <1 g/dL
7. Most M proteins are:
   a. IgM
   b. IgG
   c. IgE
   d. IgD
8. The **basis** of a chromatography **technique is:**
   a. Temperature
   b. Gravity
   c. Differential solubility
   d. Separated molecules

10

Labeling Techniques in Immunoassay

LEARNING OUTCOMES

- Compare heterogeneous and homogeneous immunoassays.
- Name and cite applications of at least three types of labels that can be used in an immunoassay.
- Describe chemiluminescence.
- Describe and compare chemiluminescence, enzyme immunoassay (EIA), and immunofluorescence techniques.
- Briefly compare direct immunofluorescent, inhibition immunofluorescent, and indirect immunofluorescent assays.
- Describe the advantages, disadvantages, and application of signal-amplification technology and magnetic labeling technology, time-resolved fluoroimmunoassay, and fluorescent polarization assay.
- Analyze a case study related to immunoassay.
- Correctly answer case study–related multiple-choice questions.
- Be prepared to participate in a discussion of critical thinking questions.
- Describe the principle of pregnancy testing.
- Describe the direct fluorescent antibody test for *Neisseria gonorrhoeae.*
- Correctly answer 80% of end-of-chapter review questions.

OUTLINE

Immunoassay Formats, 150
Types of Labels, 151
   Immunoassays, 151
      Radioimmunoassay, 151
      Solid-Phase Immunoassays, 151
   Antigen Detection, 153
   Antibody Detection, 153
      Noncompetitive Enzyme Immunoassay, 153
      Competitive Enzyme Immunoassay, 153
      Capture Enzyme Immunoassay, 153
   Multiple and Portable Enzyme-Linked Immunosorbent Assay, 153
   Enzyme Immunoassay Modification, 153
Chemiluminescence, 153
   Direct Labels, 154
   Indirect Labels, 154
   Specific Clinical Applications, 154

Immunofluorescence, 154
   Stage 1: Excitation, 154
   Stage 2: Excited-State Lifetime, 155
   Stage 3: Fluorescent Emission, 155
   Direct Immunofluorescent Assay, 155
   Inhibition Immunofluorescent Assay, 155
   Indirect Immunofluorescent Assay, 156
Alternative Labeling Technologies, 156
   Signal-Amplification Technology, 156
   Magnetic Labeling Technology, 156
   Time-Resolved Fluoroimmunoassay, 157
   Fluorescence Polarization Immunoassay, 157
   Fluorescence In Situ Hybridization, 157
Case Study 10.1, 157
Procedure: Pregnancy Testing, 158.e1
Procedure: Direct Fluorescent Antibody Test for *Neisseria gonorrhoeae,* 158.e1

KEY TERMS

antinuclear antibodies (ANAs)
capture enzyme immunoassay
chemiluminescence
competitive enzyme immunoassay
competitive immunoassay
conjugated antibody
direct fluorescent antibody (DFA)

enzyme immunoassay (EIA)
fluorescence in situ hybridization (FISH)
fluorescence polarization immunoassay
fluorescent antibody (FA)
immunofluorescent assay
indirect fluorescent assay (IFA)
inhibition immunofluorescent assay

noncompetitive enzyme immunoassay
photomultiplier tube
radioimmunoassay (RIA)
sandwich immunoassay
time-resolved fluoroimmunoassay

> **KEY CONCEPTS: Immunoassay Format Facts**
> - Heterogeneous immunoassays have a solid phase (microwell, bead) and require washing steps to remove unbound antigens or antibodies.
> - Homogeneous immunoassays are faster and easier to automate because they have only a liquid phase and do not require washing steps.
> - The ideal immunoassay label should be measurable by several methods, including visual inspection.

IMMUNOASSAY FORMATS

Immunoassays can be divided into two types, heterogeneous and homogeneous immunoassays. Heterogeneous immunoassays involve a solid phase (microwell, bead) and require washing steps to remove unbound antigens or antibodies. Heterogeneous immunoassays can have a competitive or noncompetitive format. Variations can exist in heterogeneous assays, including the following:

- Use of a label with an antigen or antibody
- Direct detection of an antigen–antibody complex
- Use of a second, labeled anti-immunoglobulin
- Capture of antigen or antibody to a solid phase using a capture molecule and detection using a second molecule
- Use of an inhibition step in which labeled and unlabeled reactants compete

Homogeneous immunoassays consist only of a liquid phase and do not require washing steps. The binding of an antigen and antibody in homogeneous assays produces a change in the compound used for visualization that can be measured. Homogeneous assays are used to assess small molecules such as therapeutic drugs and drugs of abuse. This method is less sensitive than the heterogeneous method. Homogeneous immunoassays are faster and easier to automate than heterogeneous immunoassays. In addition, homogeneous immunoassays have competitive formats.

> **KEY CONCEPTS: Facts About Enzyme Immunoassay**
> - Enzyme immunoassay (EIA) uses a nonisotopic label.
> - EIA is safer than but shares the advantages of specificity, sensitivity, and rapidity with radioimmunoassay (RIA).
> - Specificity is linked to the antibody used in immunoassay procedures. In fact, the most highly rated advantage of a labeled immunoassay procedure compared with an unlabeled immunoassay procedure is sensitivity.
> - In EIA antibody detection, the antigen in question is firmly fixed to a solid matrix (microplate well, outside of bead); this is called a *solid-phase immunosorbent assay*.

TYPES OF LABELS

The principles and applications of enzyme immunoassays (EIA), chemiluminescence, and fluorescent substances as labels are presented in Table 10.1. The first published EIA and enzyme-linked immunosorbent assay (ELISA) systems differed in assay design, but both techniques are based on the principle of immunoassay with an enzyme. EIAs with fluorescent or chemiluminescent products are the most sensitive labels.

The original technique of using antigen-coated cells or particles in agglutination techniques may be considered the earliest method for labeling components in immunoassays. Ideal characteristics of a label include the quality of being measurable by several methods, including visual inspection. The properties of a label used in an immunoassay determine how detection is possible. For example, coated latex particles can be detected by various methods, such as visual inspection, light scattering (nephelometry), and particle counting. The conversion of a colorless substrate into a colored product in EIA allows for two methods of detection, colorimetry and visual inspection.

Immunoassays

Radioimmunoassay

Yalow and Berson developed the radioimmunoassay (RIA) method in 1959 using a radioactive label that could identify an immunocomponent at very low concentrations. In the 1960s, researchers began to search for a substitute for the successful RIA method due to the inherent drawbacks of using radioactive isotopes as labels (e.g., radioactive waste and short shelf life). Because of the safety concerns regarding the use of radioactivity, RIA was modified by replacing the radioisotope with an enzyme.

Solid-Phase Immunoassays

Solid-phase quantitative immunoassays are some of the most commonly used diagnostic tests to measure the presence of antigens or antibodies in clinical specimens. A large proportion of modern immunoassays involve the use of synthetic solid phases to immobilize one of the reactants.

EIA/ELISA uses the basic immunology concept of an antigen binding to its specific antibody, which allows detection of very small quantities of antigens such as proteins, peptides, hormones, or antibodies. They use enzyme-labeled antigens and antibodies to detect the biological molecules. Several variations of the method exist; the sandwich assay is the most commonly used version.

The key step is the direct or indirect detection of antigen by adhering or immobilizing the antigen or antigen-specific capture antibody, respectively, directly onto the testing well surface. For sensitive selectivity, antigen can be specifically selected out from a sample of mixed antigens via a "capture" antibody. The antigen is thus sandwiched between the capture antibody and a detection antibody.

The EIA/ELISA method offers many advantages (Box 10.1) including the use of a nonisotopic label that offers the advantage of safety. Some procedures provide diagnostic information and measure immune status (e.g., detect total antibody immunoglobulin M [IgM] or immunoglobulin G [IgG]).

The EIA/ELISA method uses the catalytic properties of enzymes to detect and quantitate immunologic reactions. An enzyme-labeled antibody or enzyme-labeled antigen conjugate is used in immunologic assays. The enzyme, with its substrate, detects the presence and quantity of antigen or antibody in a patient specimen. In some tissues, an enzyme-labeled antibody can identify antigenic locations.

TABLE 10.1 Types of Immunoassays

Type	Antigen or Antibody	Comments
Radioimmunoassay (RIA)	Antigen or antibody labeled with a radioisotope	Limited use in clinical laboratories but used in research laboratories
Enzyme immunoassay (EIA); enzyme-linked immunosorbent assay (ELISA)	Enzyme-labeled antibody (e.g., horseradish peroxidase)	Competitive ELISA Noncompetitive (e.g., direct ELISA, indirect ELISA)
Chemiluminescence	Chemiluminescent molecule–labeled antibody (e.g., isoluminol or acridinium ester labels)	Competitive or sandwich immunoassay
Electrochemiluminescence	Electrochemiluminescent molecule–labeled antibody (e.g., ruthenium label)	—
Fluoroimmunoassay	Fluorescent molecule–labeled antigen (e.g., europium or fluorescein label)	Heterogeneous (e.g., time-resolved immunofluoroassay) Homogeneous (e.g., fluorescence polarization immunoassay)

Various enzymes are used in EIA (Table 10.2). Common enzyme labels are horseradish peroxidase, alkaline phosphatase, glucose-6-phosphate dehydrogenase, and beta-galactosidase. To be used in an EIA/ELISA, an enzyme must fulfill the following criteria:
- High degree of stability
- Extreme specificity
- Absence from the antigen or antibody
- No alteration by an inhibitor within the system

Most commercially developed EIA/ELISA applications require physical separation of the specific antigens from nonspecific complexes found in clinical samples. If the antibody directed toward the agent being assayed is fixed firmly to a solid matrix, either to the inside of the wells of a microdilution tray or to the outside of a spherical plastic or metal bead or some other solid matrix, the system is termed a *solid-phase immunosorbent assay (SPIA)*. A modification of SPIA uses a disposable plastic cassette consisting of the antibody-bound membrane and a small chamber to which the specimen can be added. An absorbent material is placed below the membrane to wick the liquid reactants through the membrane. This helps separate nonreacted components from the antigen–antibody complexes being studied.

In a representative solid-phase EIA/ELISA test, a plastic bead or plastic plate is coated with antigen (e.g., virus; Fig. 10.1). The antigen reacts with antibody in the patient's serum. The bead or plate is then

BOX 10.1 Advantages and Disadvantages of EIA/ELISA Methods

Advantages
- Detection at very low concentrations of antigen or antibody
- Multiple and portable enzyme-linked immunosorbent assays (ELISAs) are available for large population screening in low-resource situations

Disadvantages
- False-positive results if sample is overincubated
- False-positive results if nonspecific binding of antigen or antibody to reaction well occurs
- To detect an antigen or antibody, a known reciprocal antigen or antibody must be generated

Adapted from Gan SD, Patel KR: Enzyme immunoassay (EIA) and enzyme-linked immunosorbent assay (ELISA). *J Invest Dermatol* 133(9):e12, 2013.

TABLE 10.2 Enzymes Used in Enzyme Immunoassays

Enzyme	Source
Acetylcholinesterase	*Electrophorus electricus*
Alkaline phosphatase	*Escherichia coli*
Beta-galactosidase	*Escherichia coli*
Glucose oxidase	*Aspergillus niger*
Glucose-6-phosphate dehydrogenase (G6PD)	*Leuconostoc mesenteroides*
Lysozyme	Egg white
Malate dehydrogenase	Pig heart
Peroxidase	Horseradish

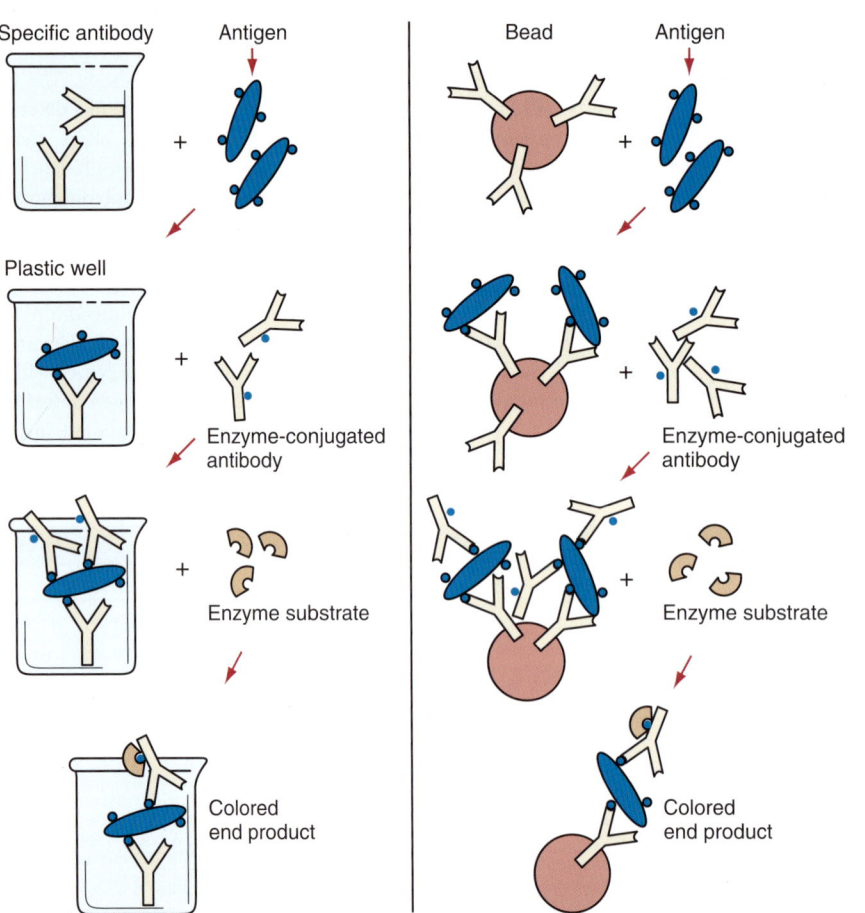

Fig. 10.1 Principle of Solid-Phase Enzyme Immunosorbent Assay. (From Forbes BA, Sahm DF, Weissfeld AS: *Bailey and Scott's diagnostic microbiology*, ed 12, St. Louis, 2007, Mosby.)

incubated with an enzyme-labeled antibody conjugate. If antibody is present, the conjugate reacts with the antigen–antibody complex on the bead or plate. The enzyme activity is measured spectrophotometrically after the addition of the specific chromogenic substrate. For example, peroxidase cleaves its substrate, *o*-dianisidine, causing a color change. In some cases, the test can be read subjectively.

The results of a typical test are calculated by comparing the spectrophotometric reading of the patient's serum to that of a control or reference serum. The advantage of an objective enzyme test is that results are not dependent on a technician's interpretations. In general, the EIA procedure is faster and requires less laboratory work than comparable methods.

Antigen Detection

EIA/ELISAs for antigen detection (Box 10.2) (e.g., hepatitis B surface antigen [HBsAg]) have four steps. Antigen-specific antibody is attached to a solid-phase surface (e.g., plastic beads). The patient's serum that may contain the antigen is added. Next, an enzyme-labeled antibody specific to the antigen (conjugate) is added. Finally, a chromogenic substrate is added, which changes color in the presence of the enzyme. The amount of color that develops is proportional to the amount of antigen in the patient specimen.

Antibody Detection

There are three types of methods for antibody detection: noncompetitive, competitive, and capture.

Noncompetitive Enzyme Immunoassay

The noncompetitive enzyme immunoassay takes place when a specific antigen is attached to a solid-phase surface, such as a plastic bead or microtiter well. The patient's serum that could contain antibody (e.g., cytomegalovirus [CMV] IgG and HIV antibody) is added to the solid-phase surface, followed by an enzyme-labeled antibody specific to the test antibody. The added chromogenic substrate changes color if the enzyme is present. The amount of color that develops is proportional to the amount of antibody in the patient's serum.

Competitive Enzyme Immunoassay

Competitive enzyme immunoassay involves using a solid-phase surface to which a specific antigen is attached. If the antigen to be measured is small or has only one epitope for antibody binding, a competitive method is used in which either the antigen is labeled and competes for the unlabeled antigen–antibody complex formation or the antibody is labeled and competes for the bound antigen and antigen in the sample.

The patient's specimen potentially containing antibody (e.g., hepatitis B core antibody) and an enzyme-labeled antibody specific to the test antibody (conjugate) are mixed. Chromogenic substrate is then added, which changes color in the presence of the enzyme. The amount of color that develops is inversely proportional to the amount of antibody in the patient's serum.

Capture Enzyme Immunoassay

Capture enzyme immunoassay is designed to detect a specific type of antibody, such as IgM or IgG, CMV IgM, rubella IgM, or *Toxoplasma* IgM. Antibody specific for IgM or IgG is attached to a solid-phase surface (e.g., plastic bead and microtiter well). The patient specimen potentially containing IgM or IgG is added. Specific antigen is then added. Finally, chromogenic substrate is added, which changes color in the presence of the enzyme. The amount of color that develops is proportional to the amount of antigen-specific IgM or IgG in the patient's serum.

> **BOX 10.2 Examples of Enzyme Immunoassays**
>
> - *Borrelia burgdorferi* (IgG and IgM)
> - Cytomegalovirus (IgG and IgM)
> - Cytomegalovirus (Ag)
> - Hepatitis A virus (total Ab)
> - Hepatitis B virus (HBV)
> - Hepatitis delta virus (total Ab)
> - HIV Ab
> - HIV Ag
> - HTLV-I Ab
> - HTLV-II Ab
> - Human B-lymphotropic virus Ab
> - Rubella virus (IgG and IgM)
> - *Toxoplasma gondii* (IgG and IgM)
>
> *Ab*, Antibody; *Ag*, antigen; *HTLV*, human T-lymphotropic (leukemia-lymphoma) virus; *Ig*, immunoglobulin.

Multiple and Portable Enzyme-Linked Immunosorbent Assay

Multiple and portable ELISA is a new technique that uses a device with 8 or 12 immunosorbent protruding pins on a central stick that can be immersed into a specimen. The washings and incubation with enzyme-conjugated antigens and chromogens are performed by dipping the pins in microwells prefilled with reagents.

The main advantage of these ready-to-use laboratory kits is that they are relatively inexpensive, can be used for large population screening, and do not require skilled personnel or laboratory equipment, making them an ideal tool for low-resource settings. Clinical applications include point-of-care detection of infectious diseases, bacterial toxins, oncologic markers, and drug screening.

Enzyme Immunoassay Modification

A recent modification of the basic EIA takes advantage of the phenomenon of grating-coupled surface plasmon resonance (GCSPR) to provide a label-free real-time variant of this solid-phase immunoassay. Using GCSPR, similar assessments of antigen–antibody interactions can be done with smaller sample sizes and in a microarray format that enables the simultaneous measurement of large numbers of antibody–antigen interactions on the same sensor chip. These measurements allow for a highly refined and sensitive determination of the effects that toxins can have on biological systems, and they can be applied to a variety of immune and nonimmune protein, cell, and tissue evaluations.

CHEMILUMINESCENCE

> **KEY CONCEPTS: Chemiluminescence Facts**
> - Chemiluminescence is the technology of choice of most immunodiagnostics manufacturers.
> - In competitive and sandwich immunoassays, chemiluminescent labels can be attached to an antigen or antibody.

Chemiluminescence refers to light emission (photons) produced during a chemical reaction; it is used extensively in automated immunoassays In immunoassays, chemiluminescent labels can be attached to an antigen or antibody. Chemiluminescent labels are used to detect proteins, viruses, oligonucleotides, and genomic nucleic acid sequences in an immunoassay. This method has excellent

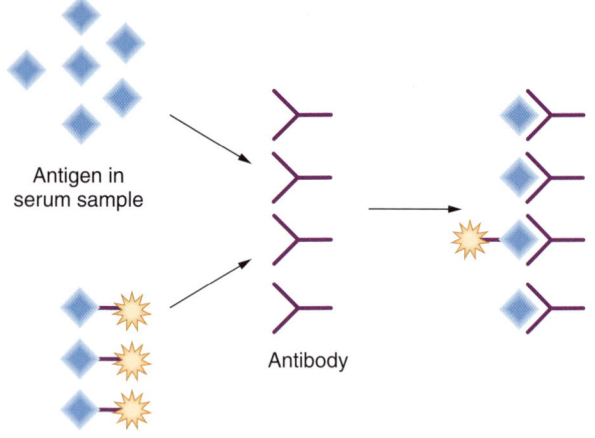

Fig. 10.2 Format for Competitive Immunoassays. (Adapted from Jandreski MA: Chemiluminescence technology in immunoassays, *Lab Med* 29[9]:555–560, 1998.)

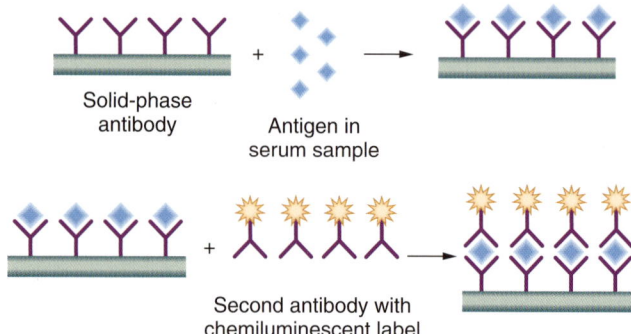

Fig. 10.3 Format for Sandwich Immunoassays. (Adapted from Jandreski MA: Chemiluminescence technology in immunoassays, *Lab Med* 29[9]:555–560, 1998.)

sensitivity and dynamic range. It does not require sample radiation, and nonselective excitation and source instability are eliminated. Most chemiluminescent reagents and conjugates are stable and relatively nontoxic.

Direct Labels

Chemiluminescent labels can be divided into five major groups:
1. Luminol
2. Acridinium esters
3. Peroxyoxalates
4. Dioxetanes
5. Tris(2,2′–bipyridyl)-ruthenium (II)

These labels are attached directly to antigens, antibodies, or DNA probes, depending on the assay format. Two formats are used, competitive and sandwich immunoassays.

In a *competitive immunoassay*, a fixed amount of labeled antigen competes with unlabeled antigen from a patient specimen for a limited number of antibody-binding sites (Fig. 10.2). The amount of light emitted is inversely proportional to the amount of analyte (antigen) measured.

In a *sandwich immunoassay*, the sample antigen binds to an antibody fixed onto a solid phase; a second antibody, labeled with a chemiluminescent label, binds to the antigen–antibody complex on the solid phase (Fig. 10.3). In the sandwich assay, the emitted light is directly proportional to the analyte concentration. The detection device for analysis is a simple *photomultiplier tube* used to detect the emitted light.

Indirect Labels

Enzymes are typically used for indirect labels. Indirect labels are attached to antibodies, antigens, and DNA probes, depending on the assay format. Enzyme labels often used in indirect procedures include the following:
- Alkaline phosphatase (ALP)
- Horseradish peroxidase (HRP)
- Beta-galactosidase (β-galactosidase)

An interesting label is native or recombinant apoaequorin (from the bioluminescent jellyfish *Aequorea*). It is activated by reaction with coelenterazine. Light emission at 469 nm is triggered by reaction with calcium chloride.

Specific Clinical Applications

One of many clinical applications of chemiluminescence is a third-generation serum immunoglobulin E (sIgE) method, Immulite 2000 (Siemens Healthcare Diagnostics, Tarrytown, NY), a solid-phase (bead), two-step chemiluminescent EIA. Allergens are covalently lined on a soluble polymer-ligand matrix, allowing immunochemical reactions to occur in liquid phases for random-access automation.

Using the $Ru(bpy)_3^{+}$ complex label, various assays have been developed in a flow cell using magnetic beads as the solid phase. Beads are captured at the electrode surface, and unbound label is washed out of the cell by a wash buffer. Label bound to the bead undergoes an electrochemiluminescent reaction and the emitted light is measured by an adjacent photomultiplier tube.

IMMUNOFLUORESCENCE

> **KEY CONCEPTS: Immunofluorescence**
> - Fluorescent labeling (direct and indirect) also demonstrates the complexing of antigens and antibodies.
> - Fluorescent antibodies are used as substitutes for radioisotope or enzyme labels.
> - Fluorescence is the result of a three-stage process: excitation, excited-state lifetime, and fluorescent emission.
> - Fluorescent conjugates are used in the basic methods of direct, inhibition, and indirect immunofluorescent assay. In direct immunofluorescence, a conjugated antibody is used to detect antigen–antibody reactions. In the indirect method, antibodies react with homologous antigens but also can act as antigens.

Fluorescent labeling is another method used to demonstrate the complexing of antigens and antibodies to a specific region of a cell to allow for identification, such as in flow cytometry analysis of blood cells (see Chapter 12) (Fig. 10.4). Fluorescent molecules, fluorophores, are used as substitutes for radioisotope or enzyme labels. Fluorescent techniques are extremely specific and sensitive.

Fluorescence is the result of a three-stage process that occurs in certain molecules called *fluorophores* or *fluorescent dyes*.

Stage 1: Excitation

A photon of energy is supplied by an external source such as a laser and absorbed by the fluorophore, creating an excited electronic singlet state. This process distinguishes fluorescence from chemiluminescence, in which the excited state is populated by a chemical reaction.

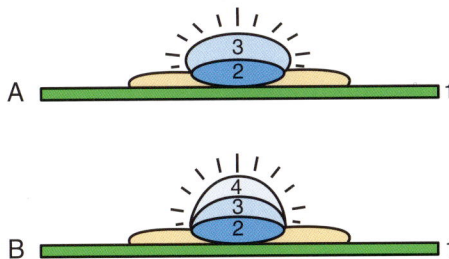

Fig. 10.4 Principles of Direct and Indirect Fluorescent Techniques. (A) Direct fluorescence. (B) Indirect fluorescence. *1*, Microscopic slide; *2*, cell (cytoplasm and nucleus); *3*, antiserum (conjugate in [A], unconjugate in [B]); *4*, conjugated antiglobulin serum.

Stage 2: Excited-State Lifetime

The excited state exists for a finite time (typically 1 to 10 nanoseconds). During this time, the fluorophore undergoes conformational changes and is exposed to many possible interactions with its molecular environment. These processes have two important consequences:
1. The energy of excitation is partially dissipated, yielding a relaxed singlet excited state from which fluorescence emission originates.
2. Not all of the molecules initially excited by absorption return to the ground state by fluorescence emission. Other processes may also interfere.

Stage 3: Fluorescent Emission

A photon of energy is emitted, returning the fluorophore to its ground state. Because of energy dissipation during the excited-state lifetime, the energy of this photon is lower and of a longer wavelength than in the excitation photon. The difference in energy or wavelength is called the *Stokes shift*. The Stokes shift is essential to the sensitivity of fluorescence techniques because it allows emission photons to be detected against a low background, isolated from excitation photons. In comparison, absorption spectrophotometry requires measurement of transmitted light relative to high incident light levels at the same wavelength.

Fluorescent signals can be amplified using the following:
1. Avidin-biotin or antibody-hapten secondary detection techniques
2. Enzyme-labeled secondary detection reagents in conjunction with fluorogenic substrates
3. Probes that contain multiple fluorophores

If multiple fluorophores are used for detection, the fluorescence signals, signal amplification, will be enhanced. A limitation of antibodies labeled with more than four to six fluorophores per protein may produce reduced specificity and reduced binding affinity. With a high degree of substitution, the extra fluorescence obtained per added fluorophore typically decreases as a result of self-quenching. As these limitations have been resolved, flow cytometry output has continued to increase the number of colors used in analysis.

Antibodies may be conjugated to other markers in addition to fluorescent dyes; the use of these markers is called *colorimetric immunologic probe detection*. The use of the original enzyme-substrate marker systems has been expanded. HRP, ALP, and avidin-biotin conjugated enzyme labels have all been used as visual tags for the presence of antibody. These reagents have the advantage of requiring only a standard light microscope.

Fluorescent conjugates are used in the following basic **immunofluorescent assay** methods, which are widely used:
- Direct immunofluorescent assay
- Inhibition immunofluorescent assay
- Indirect immunofluorescent assay

Direct Immunofluorescent Assay

In the **direct fluorescent antibody (DFA)** technique, a **conjugated antibody** is used to detect antigen–antibody reactions at a microscopic

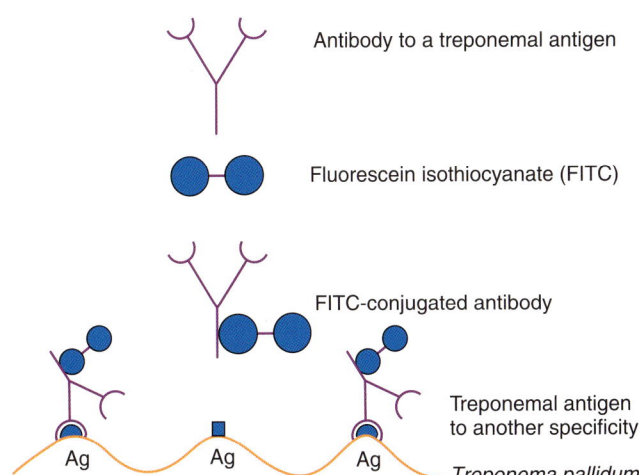

Fig. 10.5 Direct Fluorescent Antibody (DFA) Technique. After a specific antibody is labeled with fluorescein isothiocyanate (FITC), it can be reacted with its antigen and identified microscopically. *Ag*, Antigen.

level (Fig. 10.5). DFA can be applied to tissue sections or in smears for microorganisms. In addition, clinical immunophenotyping is done through direct fluorescence assays.

Fluorescein-conjugated antibodies bound to the fluorochrome fluorescein isothiocyanate (FITC) are used to visualize many bacteria in direct specimens (see Procedure: Direct Fluorescent Antibody Test for *Neisseria gonorrhoeae*). HRP conjugated to antibody, the immunoperoxidase stain, can be used to detect CMV, other viruses, or nucleic acids in cells. In biotin–avidin enzyme-conjugated methods, single-stranded nucleic acid probes, antimicrobial antibodies, or antibiotin antibodies can be bound to the small biotin molecule. These molecules have a strong affinity for the protein avidin, which has four binding sites. Biotin bound to avidin or antibody can be complexed to fluorescent dyes or to color-producing enzymes to form specific detector systems. This system can be applied to the detection of nucleic acids in organisms such as CMV, hepatitis B virus (HBV), Epstein-Barr virus (EBV), and *Chlamydia*.

The chemical manipulation in labeling antibodies with fluorescent dyes to permit detection by direct microscopic examination does not seriously impair antibody activity, the ability of fluorescent antibody (FA) conjugate to react specifically with its homologous antigen. Monoclonal antibodies (MAbs) have also been successfully conjugated to fluorescein for the detection of chlamydiae, rabies virus, and other pathogens in directly stained specimens.

When absorbing light of one wavelength, a fluorescent substance emits light of another (longer) wavelength. In **fluorescent antibody (FA)** microscopy, the incident or exciting light is often blue-green to ultraviolet. The light is provided by a high-pressure mercury arc lamp with a primary (e.g., blue-violet) filter between the lamp and the object that passes only fluorescein-exciting wavelengths. The color of the emitted light depends on the nature of the substance. Fluorescein gives off yellow-green light, and the rhodamines fluoresce in the red portion of the spectrum. The color observed in the fluorescence microscope depends on the secondary or barrier filter used in the eyepiece. A yellow filter absorbs the green fluorescence of fluorescein and transmits only yellow. Fluorescein fluoresces an intense apple-green color when excited.

Inhibition Immunofluorescent Assay

The **inhibition immunofluorescent assay** is a blocking test in which an antigen is first exposed to unlabeled antibody and then to labeled antibody and is finally washed and examined. If the unlabeled and labeled antibodies are both homologous to the antigen, there should be no fluorescence. This result confirms the specificity of the FA technique. Antibody in an unknown serum can also be detected and identified by the inhibition test.

Indirect Immunofluorescent Assay

The basis for indirect fluorescent assay (IFA) is that antibodies (immunoglobulins) not only react with homologous antigens but also can act as antigens and react with anti-immunoglobulins (Box 10.3). IFA is the serologic method that can be used for the detection of diverse antibodies, primarily in research laboratories. Immunofluorescence is used extensively in the detection of autoantibodies and antibodies to tissue and cellular antigens. For example, antinuclear antibodies (ANAs) are a heterogeneous group of circulating immunoglobulins that react with the whole nucleus or nuclear components (e.g., nuclear proteins, DNA, histones) in host tissues and are frequently assayed by indirect fluorescence. By using tissue sections that contain a large number of antigens, it is possible to identify antibodies to several different antigens in a single test. The antigens are differentiated according to their different staining patterns.

Immunofluorescence can also be used to identify specific antigens on live cells in suspension (flow cytometry), as discussed in Chapter 11. When a live stained cell suspension is put through a fluorescence-activated cell sorter (FACS), which measures its fluorescent intensity, the cells are separated according to their particular fluorescent brightness. This technique permits the isolation of different cell populations with different surface antigens (e.g., CD4+ and CD8+ lymphocytes; see Chapter 4).

In the IFA, the antigen source (e.g., whole *Toxoplasma* microorganism and virus in infected tissue culture cells) to the specific antibody being tested is affixed to the surface of a microscope slide. The patient's serum is diluted and placed on the slide to cover the antigen source. If antibody is present in the serum, it will bind to its specific antigen. Unbound antibody is then removed by washing the slide. In the second phase, antihuman globulin (AHG; directed specifically against IgM or IgG) conjugated to a fluorescent substance that will fluoresce when exposed to ultraviolet light is placed on the slide. This conjugated marker for human antibody will bind to the antibody already bound to the antigen on the slide and will serve as a marker for the antibody when viewed under a fluorescence microscope.

A major problem in interpreting IFA results is background staining. For most IFAs, laboratories must choose a screening dilution, because undiluted specimens will show background staining resulting from nonspecific binding or clinically insignificant levels of circulating autoantibodies. The screening dilution plays a critical role; the more dilute the specimen becomes, the less sensitive but more specific the procedure.

An example of a changing clinical situation is that many laboratories have replaced indirect immunofluorescence, once the standard for ANA testing, with the EIA. Less labor and technical experience are cited as reasons for switching from indirect immunofluorescence. However, the trade-off may not be valuable if patients have antibody titers of less than 1:160.

ALTERNATIVE LABELING TECHNOLOGIES

> **KEY CONCEPTS: Alternative Labeling Techniques**
> - Signal amplification can be used for various fluorescent and colorimetric applications (e.g., cytokines).
> - Magnetic labeling is a magnetic recording technology that can be used for DNA analysis.
> - Time-resolved fluoroimmunoassay has a direct format that is heterogeneous with a direct format sandwich assay.
> - Fluorescence polarization immunoassay is a competitive fluoroimmunoassay.
> - Fluorescence in situ hybridization (FISH) is both a labeling method and a molecular technique.

> **BOX 10.3 Examples of Immunologic Assays Performed by Indirect Fluorescent Antibody Technique**
> - Antiadrenal antibodies
> - Antibody (histone-reactive [HR]–ANA)
> - Anticentriole antibodies
> - Anticentromere antibodies
> - Anti–glomerular basement membrane antibodies
> - Anti–islet cell antibodies
> - Anti–liver-kidney microsomal (LKM) antibodies
> - Antimitochondrial
> - Antimyelin
> - Antimyocardial
> - Antinuclear antibody
> - Anti–parietal cell
> - Antiplatelet
> - Antireticulin
> - Antiribosome
> - Antiskin (dermal-epidermal)
> - Antiskin (intraepithelial)
> - Anti–smooth muscle
> - Antistriational
> - Cytomegalovirus (IgM antibody)
> - Histone-reactive antinuclear antibody (HR-ANA)
> - Human immunodeficiency virus (total and IgM antibody)
> - Immunoglobulin M (IgM) antibodies (antigen-specific)
> - Lymphocyte typing
> - Rubella virus antibody
> - *Toxoplasma gondii* antibody

Signal-Amplification Technology

Tyramide signal amplification (TSA) can be used in various fluorescent and colorimetric detection applications. TSA protocols are simple and require few changes to standard operating procedures. TSA provides an mRNA in situ hybridization protocol that is effective in detecting B-cell clonality in plastic-embedded tissue specimens. Immunoglobulin light-chain mRNA molecules can be detected directly in paraffin-embedded tissue using fluorescein-labeled oligonucleotide probes. TSA amplification enables B cells to be detected in tissue sections without additional processing steps and specially prepared sections. Similar in situ hybridization technology can also be used for the detection of cytokines, such as interferon-gamma (IFN-γ) and interleukin-4 (IL-4).

Magnetic Labeling Technology

Magnetic labeling technology is an application of the high-resolution magnetic recording technology developed for the computer disk drive industry. Increased density of microscopic, magnetically labeled biological samples (e.g., nucleic acid on a biochip) translates directly into reduced sample-processing times. Magnetic labeling can be applied to automated DNA sequences, DNA probe technology, and gel electrophoresis (Fig. 10.6). Compared with other nonradioactive labeling systems, magnetic labels are inherently safe, instrumentation is less expensive, signals are almost permanent, and spatial resolution is increased.

In a magnetic label–based gel electrophoresis application sphere, DNA is analyzed. DNA is separated into bands using electrophoresis and magnetic labels are bound to the DNA in each band. By applying and then removing a magnetic field, the magnetic domains in each label are oriented in the same direction, resulting in a net magnetic field near the bands in the direction of the applied field (Fig. 10.7).

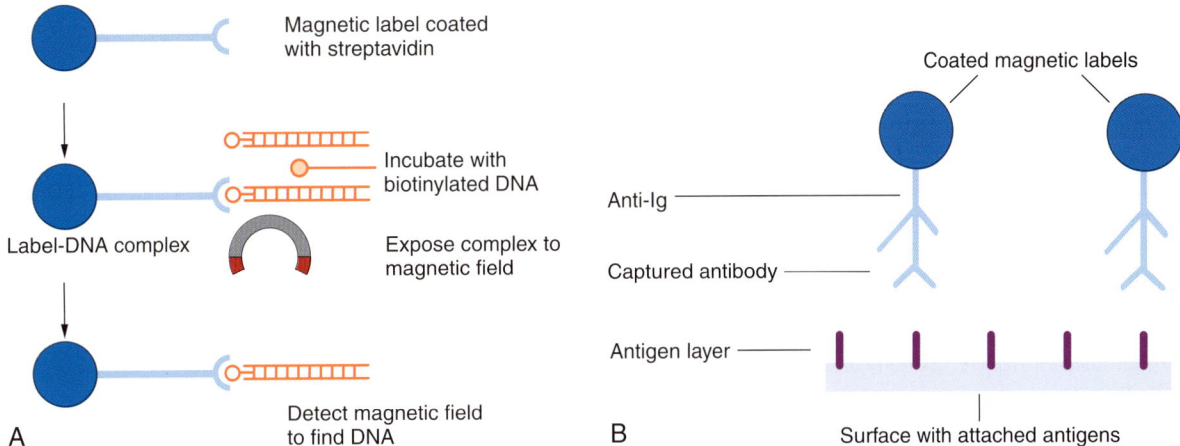

Fig. 10.6 Magnetic Labeling Techniques. (A) Detection of DNA. (B) Detection of antibodies. (Adapted from Adelman L: Laboratory technology: magnetic labeling technology, *Adv Med Lab Admin* 11:131, 1991.)

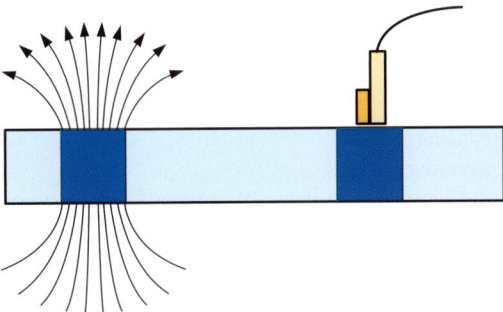

Fig. 10.7 Cross-Sectional Schematic of a Small Region of Sequencing Gel or Nylon Membrane with Magnetic Labels Bound to DNA, Separated into Two Bands. *Left*, Arrows on the band represent the magnetic field resulting from the magnetized labels. *Right*, The band has a sensor near the surface. (Adapted from Adelman L: Laboratory technology: magnetic labeling technology, *Adv Med Lab Admin* 11:131, 1991.)

Time-Resolved Fluoroimmunoassay

In a time-resolved assay, fluorescence is measured after a certain period to exclude background interference fluorescence. This form of immunoassay is heterogeneous with a direct format (sandwich assay), similar to direct ELISA. The **time-resolved fluoroimmunoassay** uses europium-labeled antibodies. If excited at 340 nm, europium fluoresces at 620 nm. The fluorescence is measured and is directly proportional to the concentration of the substance.

Fluorescence Polarization Immunoassay

In the **fluorescence polarization immunoassay**, a homogeneous competitive fluoroimmunoassay, the polarization of the fluorescence from a fluorescein–antigen conjugate is determined by its rate of rotation during the lifetime of the excited state in solution. Binding to a large antibody molecule slows down the rate of rotation and increases the degree of polarization, and the fluorescence emitted is polarized.

Fluorescence In Situ Hybridization

Fluorescence in situ hybridization (FISH) is both a labeling method and a molecular technique. FISH is discussed in Chapter 12, Molecular Laboratory Techniques.

CASE STUDY 10.1

A 25-year-old woman missed her menstrual period 3 weeks earlier. She suspected pregnancy and went to her primary care provider for confirmation.

Questions
1. Failure to develop a colored line with a quality-control specimen in a lateral flow chromatographic immunoassay for pregnancy indicates:
   a. A weakly positive result
   b. A strongly positive result
   c. An invalid test result
   d. A negative result
2. A negative human chorionic gonadotropin (hCG) level can be observed in a lateral flow chromatographic immunoassay for pregnancy if:
   a. The specimen contains hCG at a level close to or greater than 24 mIU/mL
   b. hCG in the specimen binds to sites on the antihCG antibody–gold conjugate to form a complex, the complex binds to the capture antibody coated on the test line, and a burgundy red–colored band develops
   c. No color develops at the test line of the test strip
   d. Both a and b

See Appendix A for the answers to these multiple-choice questions.

Critical Thinking Group Discussion Questions
1. When the primary care provider read the test result after the specified limit of 7 minutes, no colored lines appeared on the strip. What does this mean?
2. If the test had resulted in a negative result, should the test be repeated?
3. Can a woman have a positive pregnancy test after delivering a baby?

REVIEW QUESTIONS

1. Chemiluminescence:
   a. Has excellent sensitivity and dynamic range
   b. Does not require sample radiation
   c. Uses unstable chemiluminescent reagents and conjugates
   d. Both a and b
2. The description of a competitive immunoassay is:
   a. A fixed amount of labeled antigen competes with unlabeled antigen from the patient specimen for a limited number of antibody-binding sites
   b. A sample antigen binds to antibody fixed onto solid phase; chemiluminescent-labeled antibody binds to the antigen–antibody complex
3. The description of a sandwich immunoassay is:
   a. A fixed amount of labeled antigen competes with unlabeled antigen from the patient specimen for a limited number of antibody-binding sites.
   b. A sample antigen binds to antibody fixed onto solid phase; chemiluminescent-labeled antibody binds to the antigen–antibody complex.
4. Enzyme labels often used in indirect procedures include the following *except*:
   a. Alkaline phosphatase
   b. Horseradish peroxidase
   c. Beta-galactosidase
   d. Radioactive labels
5. The description of the enzyme immunoassay (EIA) is that it:
   a. Uses a nonisotopic label
   b. Uses antibody labeled with fluorescein isothiocyanate (FITC)
   c. Uses colloidal particles consisting of a metal or insoluble metal compound
   d. Is restricted to noncompetitive situations
6. The description of the immunofluorescent technique assay is that it:
   a. Uses a nonisotopic label
   b. Uses antibody labeled with fluorescein isothiocyanate (FITC)
   c. Uses colloidal particles consisting of a metal or insoluble metal compound
   d. Is restricted to noncompetitive situations
7. The description of the direct immunofluorescent assay is that:
   a. It is based on antibodies acting as antigens and reacting with anti-immunoglobulins
   b. It uses conjugated antibody to detect antigen–antibody reactions
   c. Antigen is first exposed to unlabeled antibody, then to labeled antibody
   d. It is restricted to noncompetitive situations
8. The description of inhibition immunofluorescent assay is that:
   a. It is based on antibodies acting as antigens and reacting with anti-immunoglobulins
   b. It uses conjugated antibody to detect antigen–antibody reactions
   c. Antigen is first exposed to unlabeled antibody, then to labeled antibody
   d. It is restricted to noncompetitive situations
9. The description of indirect immunofluorescent assay is that:
   a. It is based on antibodies acting as antigens and reacting with anti-immunoglobulins
   b. It uses conjugated antibody to detect antigen–antibody reactions
   c. Antigen is first exposed to unlabeled antibody, then to labeled antibody
   d. It is restricted to noncompetitive situations
10. For an enzyme to be used in an enzyme immunoassay (EIA), it must meet all the following criteria *except*:
    a. High amount of stability
    b. Extreme specificity
    c. Presence in antigen or antibody
    d. No alteration by inhibitor with the system
11. A fluorescent substance is one that _____ light of one wavelength.
    a. Emits
    b. Absorbs
    c. Generates bright
    d. Generates dull
12. A fluorescent substance has the dual characteristic of _____ light of another longer wavelength.
    a. Emitting
    b. Absorbing
    c. Reducing
    d. Increasing
13. What is the major advantage of enzyme-linked immunosorbent assay (ELISA) compared with other quantification labeling methods?
    a. Detection of an antigen or antibody at a low concentration
    b. Low specificity
    c. Readily available
    d. Inexpensive, rapid testing
14. Fluorescence labeling (direct and indirect) demonstrates the complexing of:
    a. Antigens
    b. Antibodies
    c. Enzymes
    d. Both a & b
15. The most highly rated advantage of chemiluminescence is:
    a. Sensitivity
    b. Lower supplies cost
    c. Faster to conduct the assay
    d. Easier to report results

11

Flow Cytometry

LEARNING OUTCOMES

- Identify and give examples of the three phases in automated instrumentation.
- Define the term *fluorophore*.
- Explain the conjugation of antibody to a fluorophore.
- Describe the flow process.
- Explain the use of monoclonal antibodies.
- Summarize the characteristics of tandem dyes in flow cytometry.
- Explain the process of the Luminex system.
- Analyze the case study, and discuss the answers to the related questions.
- Discuss questions related to videos about flow cytometry.
- Correctly answer end-of-chapter review questions.

OUTLINE

Characteristics of Instrumentation, 159
Flow Cell Cytometry, 160
    Fundamentals of Laser Technology, 160
    Principles of Cell Cytometry, 160
    Fluorophores, 160
    Fluorochromes and Conjugated Antibodies, 160
    Factors to consider for fluorophore selection, 160
    The Flow Process, 161
    The Use of Monoclonal Antibodies, 161
    Immunofluorescence, 162

    Tandem Dyes for Flow Cytometry, 162
    A Multicolor System, 163
    The Luminex Flow Cytometry System, 163
    Sample Preparation, 163
    Clinical Immunology Applications, 163
    Lymphocyte Subsets, 164
    Other Cellular Applications, 165
Case Study 11.1   History and Physical Examination, 166
Procedure: Laboratory Activities, 167.e1

KEY TERMS

cluster of designation (CD)
flow cell cytometry
fluorophores
Förster resonance energy transfer (FRET)

harmonization
immunofluorescence
immunophenotyping
laser

photon
Stokes shift

CHARACTERISTICS OF INSTRUMENTATION

Laboratory automation can be separated into preanalytic, analytic, and postanalytic phases. Accuracy in each of these phases is critical to quality results. The preanalytic phase includes specimen labeling (bar coding preferred), accessioning, and tracking, along with proper test ordering.

The analytic phase involves the following areas:
- Automated results entry
- Quality control
- Validation of results
- Networking to laboratory information systems

Automated analyzers link each specimen to its specific test request. Any results generated must be verified (approved or reviewed) by the operator before the data are released to the patient report. Useful data for this verification process include flags, signifying results outside the reference range; critical or panic values (possibly life-threatening), or values that are out of the technical range for the analyzer; and failures in other checks and balances built into the system.

The postanalytic phase includes adding to patient cumulative reports, workload recording, and networks to other systems. Quality assurance (QA) procedures, including the use of quality control (QC) solutions, are part of the analytic functions of the analyzer and its interfaced computer. The Clinical Laboratory Improvement Amendments of 1988 (CLIA '88) regulations require the documentation of all QC data associated with any test results reported (see Chapter 6). Harmonization of analytes has been gaining momentum as an essential component of the outcomes of analysis. In the future, harmonized or normalized results may be mapped together and presented numerically and graphically to reduce data output.

> **KEY CONCEPTS: Flow Cytometry Basics**
> - Laser light ranges from the ultraviolet (UV) and infrared (IR) spectrum through all the colors of the rainbow.
> - Laser light is concentrated in contrast to other diffuse forms of radiation.
> - The photon is the basic unit of all radiation.
> - Laser light is the most common light source used in flow cytometers.
> - Flow cytometry is based on cells being stained in suspension with an appropriate fluorochrome dye that stains a specific component.

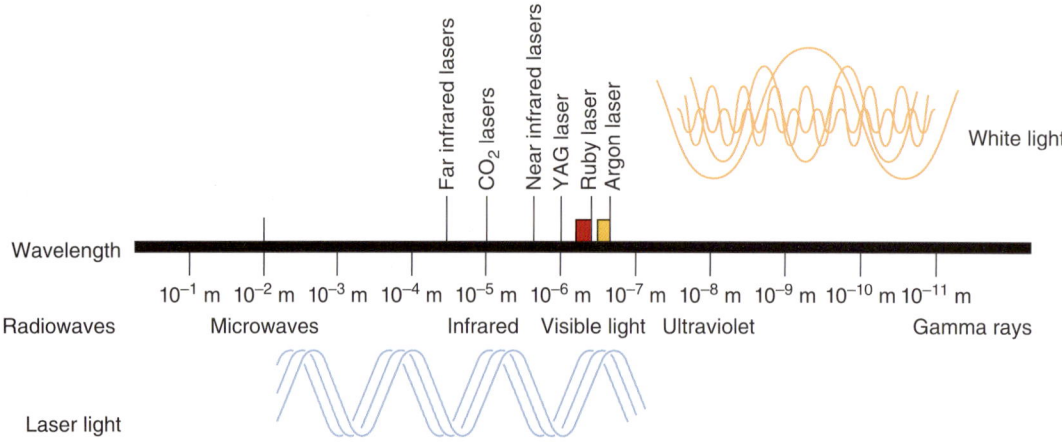

Fig. 11.1 The Electromagnetic Spectrum. *YAG*, Yttrium-aluminum-garnet. (From Turgeon ML: *Clinical hematology: theory and procedures,* ed 5, Philadelphia, 2012, Lippincott Williams & Wilkins.)

FLOW CELL CYTOMETRY

Fundamentals of Laser Technology

Flow cytometry is a powerful high-throughput technique that is widely used for laboratory applications, such as immunophenotyping, cell sorting and isolation, cell cycle analysis, cell proliferation and cytotoxicity assays, biomarker detection, and protein engineering.

In 1917, Einstein speculated that under certain conditions, atoms or molecules could absorb light or other radiation and then be stimulated to shed this gained energy. Lasers have been developed with numerous medical and industrial applications.

The electromagnetic spectrum ranges from long radiowaves to short, powerful gamma rays (Fig. 11.1). Within this spectrum is a narrow band of visible or white light composed of red, orange, yellow, green, blue, and violet light. **Laser** (*l*ight *a*mplification by *s*timulated *e*mission of *r*adiation) light ranges from the UV and IR spectrum through all the colors of the rainbow. In contrast to other diffuse forms of radiation, laser light is concentrated. It is almost exclusively of one wavelength or color, and its parallel waves travel in one direction. Through the use of fluorescent dyes, laser light can occur in numerous wavelengths. Types of lasers include glass-filled tubes of helium and neon (most common), yttrium-aluminum-garnet (YAG; an imitation diamond), argon, and krypton.

Lasers sort the energy in atoms and molecules, concentrate it, and release it in powerful waves. In most lasers, a medium of gas, liquid, or crystal is energized by high-intensity light, an electrical discharge, or even nuclear radiation. When an atom extends beyond the orbits of its electrons or when a molecule vibrates or changes its shape, it instantly snaps back, shedding energy in the form of a photon. The **photon** is the basic unit of all radiation. When a photon reaches an atom of the medium, the energy exchange stimulates the emission of another photon in the same wavelength and direction. This process continues until a cascade of growing energy sweeps through the medium.

Photons travel the length of the laser and bounce off mirrors. First a few and eventually countless photons synchronize themselves until an avalanche of light streaks between the mirrors. In some gas lasers, transparent disks referred to as *Brewster windows* are slanted at a precise angle that polarizes the laser's light. The photons, which are reflected back and forth, finally gain so much energy that they exit as a powerful beam. The power of lasers to transmit energy and information is rated in watts.

Principles of Cell Cytometry

The basic principles of flow cell cytometry have changed little in the past decade, but the applications of this technology have evolved a great deal. The foundations of flow cytometry have been consistent with its primary function, which is to analyze individual cells or particles in a stream with a laser as the cells move past a set of stationary detectors. Increasingly, more colors of fluorescence are being used by cytometers, along with high speed sorting and analytical function[8]

Flow cell cytometry, developed in the 1960s, combines fluid dynamics, optics, laser science, high-speed computers, and fluorochrome-conjugated monoclonal antibodies (MAbs) that rapidly classify groups of cells in heterogeneous mixtures. The principle of flow cytometry is based on cells being stained in suspension with an appropriate fluorochrome, such as an immunologic reagent, a dye that stains a specific component, or some other marker with specific reactivity. Fluorescent dyes used in flow cytometry must bind or react specifically with the cellular component of interest (e.g., reticulocytes, peroxidase enzyme, DNA content).

Fluorophores

Fluorophores reemit light after exposure to a light particle, a photon. With fluorophores, the terms *excitation* and *emission wavelengths* are used. The shorter wavelength light is the light that is used as the excitation light for fluorophores. The shorter wavelength light is absorbed by an electron of the fluorophore and, as a result, this higher energy photon excites the fluorophore. Excitation does not last long because the natural state of the fluorophore is the ground state. In returning to this ground state, the fluorophore emits a photon at a longer wavelength (lower energy) and returns once more to a relaxed state. In the fluorophores used in the clinical laboratory, the cycle of excitation and emission typically happens in about 0.5 to 20 nanoseconds. Recurrent cycles will continue, if there is continued exposure to the excitation light, until photobleaching occurs.

The unit of wavelength is the nanometer (nm). The **Stokes shift** is the difference, in nanometers, between the peak excitation and peak emission wavelengths. Each fluorophore has a distinct and individual Stokes shift.

Fluorochromes and Conjugated Antibodies

Immunolocalization of antigens with fluorescence requires that fluorochromes be linked either to a primary or secondary antibody to provide a fluorescent signal that marks the site of antibody–antigen binding. A primary antibody method is generally more useful and practical. Fluorochromes can be covalently conjugated to antibodies through reactions with thiol or amine groups. Typically, fluorochromes containing isothiocyanate, succinimidyl ester, or sulfonyl chloride reactive groups are conjugated to amines on the antibody molecules.

Factors to consider for fluorophore selection

Spectral profile—the excitation and emission maxima should be compatible with the instrument's lasers and detectors, and with other fluorophores in a multiplexed panel; selecting fluorophores with narrow spectral bandwidths can help to reduce spillover.

Brightness—useful when assigning fluorophores to cellular markers based on target abundance.

Stokes shift—the difference between the excitation and emission maxima, which can be exploited when the number of available lasers becomes limiting.

Fluorophore size—smaller fluorophores may be preferred for penetration of thick tissues or into the nuclei of cells.

Photostability—especially critical for fluorescent microscopy, including live-cell imaging applications.

Heat stability—important in long-term and time-lapse live-cell imaging.

Fixation stability—fluorescent proteins may be more susceptible to alcohol-based fixation methods than small molecule or polymer dyes.

Stability over time and from batch-to-batch—tandem dyes can be especially prone to variability.

Specificity—non-specific binding of fluorophores can be due to chemical properties such as charge, hydrophobicity, and fluorophore type; for example, cyanine dyes and their tandems are known to bind non-specifically to monocytes.

Toxicity—fluorophores used in live-cell imaging should have minimal toxicity and not affect cellular health or function.

Autofluorescence of biological samples—fluorophores with red or far-red emissions, or narrow emission spectra, are useful when working with samples that have high autofluorescence.

Membrane permeability—this will determine whether there is a need for fixation and permeabilization if detecting intracellular targets.

Water solubility—high water solubility helps to prevent aggregation or precipitation of fluorophores and fluorophore-labeled reagents out of solution, as well as facilitates a greater degree of labeling for increased brightness.

Staining buffer requirements for multiplexing—some fluorophores require specific buffer conditions to prevent aggregation when combined with other fluorophores.

Compatibility with mounting media—some fluorophores are not compatible with certain antifade reagents.

Ability to pre-mix—useful to reduce pipetting errors between samples (and can save time/money) if building large panels and having samples arrive over an extended period.

Reference www.biocompare.com. *Gude to Flow Cytometry Fluorophore Selection.* Accessed July 15, 2024.

The Flow Process

A suspension of stained cells is pressurized using gas and transported through plastic tubing to a flow chamber within the instrument (Fig. 11.2). In the flow chamber, the specimen is injected through a needle into a stream of physiologic saline called the *sheath*. The sheath and specimen both exit the flow chamber through a 75-μm orifice. This laminar flow design confines the cells to the center of the saline sheath, with the cells moving in single file.

Most new cytometers have three or more lasers, selected from ultraviolet (355 nm), violet (405 nm), blue (488 nm), yellow (561 nm), and red (640 nm).

The stained cells then pass through the laser beam. The laser activates the dye, and the cell fluoresces. Although the fluorescence is emitted throughout a 360-degree circle, the amount of scattered light is measured from each cell by two optical detectors at two different angles. Forward scatter light (FSC) detects scattered light along the path of the laser and side scatter light (SSC) measures scatter at a 90-degree angle relative to the laser.

Hydrodynamic focusing is a technique that enables users of flow cytometry to measure the size of particles in a flow channel. As particles enter the chamber, they pass through a laser beam that causes an instrument to be able to measure the particle's dimensions.

The intensity of FSC primarily due to light refraction around the cell is proportional to the diameter of a cell (cell size). By comparison, the SSC reveals information about cellular internal complexity such as granularity based on reflected or refracted light at the interface between the laser and intracellular structures.

The fluorescence information is then transmitted to a computer that controls all decisions regarding data collection, analysis, and cell sorting.

The Use of Monoclonal Antibodies

Cluster of differentiation (CD) is a nomenclature system for identifying and classifying antigens on the surface of immune system cells. CD molecules are cell surface markers that are highly specific to each cell, which permits identification and isolation of immune cell populations, subsets, and differentiation stages. CD molecules are composed of a mixture of proteins, glycoproteins, and glycolipids, and some can be transmembrane while others are extracellular. BD FACS instruments can detect different numbers of colors depending on the model.

Monoclonal antibodies, identified by a cluster of designation (CD), are used in most flow cytometry immunophenotyping (Table 11.1).

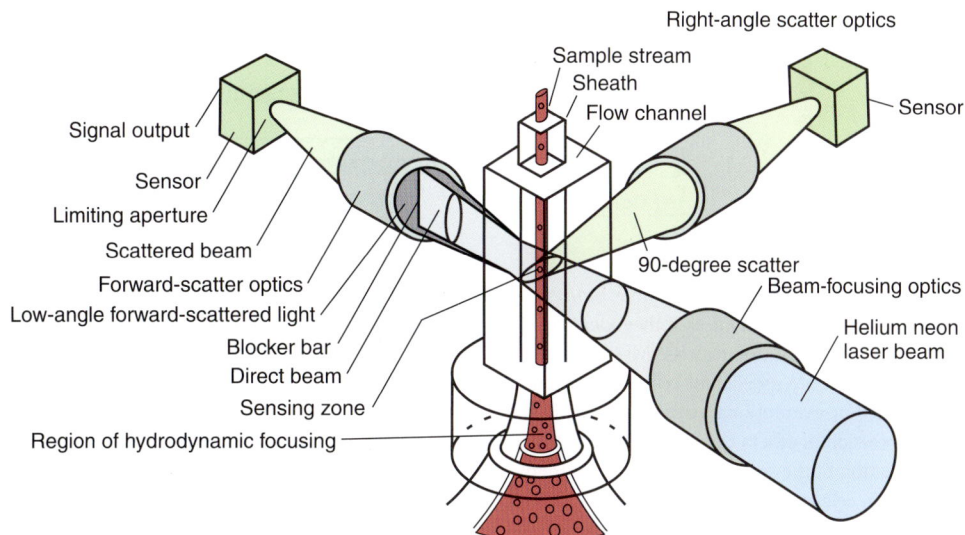

Fig. 11.2 Laser Flow Cytometry. (Courtesy Ortho Diagnostics, Raritan, NJ.)

TABLE 11.1 Commonly Used Monoclonal Antibodies in Flow Cytometry.

CD Designation	Cell Type
CD2	Thymocytes, T lymphocytes, NK cells
CD3	Thymocytes, T lymphocytes
CD4	T lymphocytes (helper subset), monocytes (dimly expressed), macrophages
CD5	Mature T lymphocytes, thymocytes, subset of B lymphocytes (B1)
CD8	T lymphocytes (cytotoxic), macrophages
CD10	T- and B-lymphocyte precursors, bone marrow stromal cells
CD19	B lymphocytes, follicular dendritic cells
CD21	B cells, follicular dendritic cells, subset of immature thymocytes
CD23	B cells, monocytes, follicular dendritic cells
CD25	Activated T lymphocytes, B cells, monocytes
CD34	Progenitor (hematopoietic stem) cells
CD44	Most leukocytes
CD45	All hematopoietic cells
CD56	Subsets of T lymphocytes, NK cells
CD94	Subsets of T lymphocytes, NK cells

DiaSorin tests not available on other manufacturers' analyzers: *Borrelia burgdorferi*; varicella-zoster virus (VZV) immunoglobulin G (IgG); herpes virus type 1 (HSV-1) type-specific IgG; HSV-2 type-specific IgG; Epstein-Barr virus (EBV) IgM; Epstein-Barr nucleic acid (EBNA) IgG; viral capsid antigen (VCA) IgG; early antigen (EA) IgG.
This is a partial list of immunology assays. It includes autoimmune, cancer-related, and infectious disease antibodies and/or antigens. Other analytes are not included in the list.
CD, Cluster of differentiation; *NK*, Natural killer.

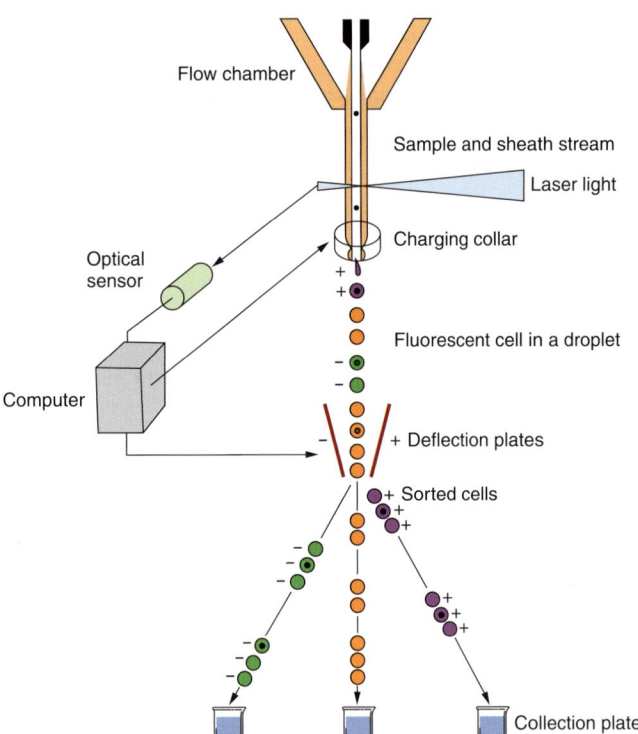

Fig. 11.3 Laser and Cell-Sorting Schematic.

Any fresh specimen that can be placed into a single-cell suspension is a valid candidate for immunophenotyping (e.g., T cells, B cells, CD34+ stem cells; detection of minimal residual disease in leukemia). Sorting is accomplished using stored computer information.

When the laser strikes a stained cell, the dye creates distinctive colored light that the cytometer recognizes. This fluorescent intensity is recorded and analyzed by the computer, and cells are sorted according to a preprogrammed selection. If the particular cell in the laser beam is of interest, the computer waits for the appropriate time for the cell to reach the droplet break-off point within the charging collar. At that point, the computer signals the charging collar to administer an electrostatically positive or negative charge to the stream containing the target cell. A droplet containing this cell is then removed from the main stream before the charge has time to redistribute.

This action produces the cell of interest within a liquid drop that has an electrostatic charge on its surface (only the droplet is charged). The droplet falls between a set of deflection plates, which creates an electrical field. The charged droplets are deflected to the left or right, depending on their polarity, and collected for further analysis.

Immunofluorescence

> **KEY CONCEPTS: Flow Cytometry: Tags and Colors**
> - Color immunofluorescence uses MAbs, each directly conjugated to a different fluorochrome. Eight-color immunofluorescence offers the advantages of greater sensitivity and specificity.
> - Newer systems in immunoassay automation use chemiluminescent labels and substrates rather than fluorescent labels and detection systems.

Tandem Dyes for Flow Cytometry

Tandem dyes consist of two different covalently bonded fluorophores, a donor and an acceptor molecule. The spectral properties of tandem dyes are that they exhibit the characteristics of the donor fluorophores and the emission characteristics of the acceptor molecule. These

Cell surface molecules recognized by MAbs are called either *antigens*, if antibodies can be produced against them, or *markers*, if they identify and discriminate between (mark) different cell populations. Markers can be grouped into several categories. Some are specific for cells of a particular lineage (e.g., CD4+ lymphocytes) or maturational pathway (e.g., CD34+ progenitor stem cells); the expression of others can vary according to the state of activation or differentiation of the same cells. In flow cytometry, cells can be sorted from the main cellular population into subpopulations for further analysis (Fig. 11.3).

properties are the result of Förster resonance energy transfer (FRET) or fluorescence resonance energy transfer. In this process, energy is passed from an excited donor to a nearby acceptor molecule that subsequently emits a photon of light.

Multiple tandem dyes can be used in the design of panels of eight or more colors. There are both laser excitation and single fluorophore limitations that make it necessary for a single laser to excite the maximum number of fluorophores possible.

Particular precautions need to be observed when working with tandem dyes, because they are highly susceptible to photobleaching. The dyes always need to be protected from light. Tandem dye antibody conjugates should never be frozen as it could denature the donor fluorophores, which can result in either reduced staining or no staining. Tandem dyes have high batch-to-batch variability and need to be reoptimized.

A Multicolor System

Current fluorescent methods (e.g., BD FACSCanto II: Can be configured with two or three lasers to detect up to eight colors.

BD FACSLyric: Can be configured with four, six, eight, ten, or twelve colors.

BD FACS ymphony A3: Can simultaneously measure up to 28 colors.

BD FACS Celesta: Can detect up to 12 colors, depending on the configuration.

In the flow cytometry the goal is to identify specific cell types and quantify the expression levels of certain antigens/proteins associated with cells/particles. However, in luminex the goal is to quantify analytes (such as cytokines) in your samples.

The four most common fluorochromes are fluorescein isothiocyanate (FITC), phycoerythrin (PE), peridinin chlorophyll protein (PerCP), and allophycocyanin (APC). The first three fluorochromes are excited by the 488-nm line of an argon laser; the fourth fluorochrome is excited by the 633-nm line of a helium-neon or diode laser.

Multiple-color immunofluorescence offers the advantages of greater sensitivity and specificity, with increased ability to identify and subclassify individual cells. Improvements in methods and probes may lead to fluorescence in situ hybridization (FISH) in suspension as a routine protocol and enable flow cytometry to operate on a molecular level simultaneously to identify chromosomal abnormalities.

The Luminex Flow Cytometry System

In the flow cytometry the goal is to identify specific cell types and quantify the expression levels of certain antigens/proteins associated with cells/particles. However, in luminex the goal is to quantify analytes (such as cytokines) in your samples.

A system that uses a flow cytometer, specific data analysis software, and fluorescent latex particles—the Luminex 100 Total System—has been developed by Luminex Technology (Austin, TX). This system combines advances in computing and optics with a new concept in color coding to create a simple, cost-effective analysis system (Fig. 11.4). Latex beads are coupled to various amounts of two different fluorescent dyes, which are analyzed by the flow cytometer and software to allow the distinct separation of up to 64 slightly different colored bead sets. The color-coded microspheres identify each unique reaction. Hundreds of microsphere sets can be identified at once in a single sample. Optical technology recognizes each microsphere and provides a precise, quantitative measure simply and in real time.

Currently, up to 64 microsphere sets are recognized. The current FlowMetrix system is compatible with the BD FACS Vantage SE System and BD FACSCalibur, the most widely used flow cytometers for cellular analysis. Because the Luminex 100 Total System requires fewer steps to assess multiple parameters with a high level of sensitivity and accuracy, it is significantly more cost-effective than current methods of analysis. Some immunologic applications already demonstrated with FlowMetrix are HIV and hepatitis B seroconversion; multicytokine measurement, multiplexed allergy testing; DNA–based tissue typing; herpes simplex viral load; immunoglobulin G (IgG), immunoglobulin A (IgA), and immunoglobulin M (IgM) assays; IgG subclassification; autoimmunity panel; epitope mapping; human chorionic gonadotropin (hCG) and alpha-fetoprotein; HIV viral load; and the TORCHS (*t*oxoplasmosis, *o*ther [viruses], *r*ubella, *c*ytomegalovirus [CMV], *h*erpesviruses, *s*yphilis) panel.

Sample Preparation

Specimens that can be used for flow cell analysis include whole blood, bone marrow, and aspirates of body fluids. For whole blood, ethylenediaminetetraacetic acid (EDTA) is the preferred anticoagulant if specimens are processed within 30 hours of collection. Heparin is an alternative anticoagulant for whole blood and bone marrow, and can provide stability of specimens more than 24 hours old.

Blood specimens should be stored at room temperature (20°C to 25°C [68°F to 77°F]) before processing. Specimens need to be well mixed before delivery into staining tubes. Unsuitable specimens include hemolyzed or clotted samples. For the efficient analysis of white blood cells, whole blood, bone marrow, or aspirates should have the bulk of red blood cells removed before analysis. Tissue specimens (e.g., lymph nodes) should be collected and transported in a tissue culture medium at room temperature or at 4°C (39°F) if analysis is delayed. Such a specimen requires disaggregation by enzymatic or mechanical methods to form a single-cell suspension. After proper specimen processing, antibodies are added to the cellular preparation and analyzed. MAbs, tagged with different fluorescent tags, are used for analysis.

Clinical Immunology Applications

> **KEY CONCEPTS: Clinical Applications of Flow Cytometry**
>
> - Immunophenotyping has diverse clinical applications distributed throughout the workload: cancer diagnosis (80%), monitoring patients who have AIDS (10%), and quantifying CD34+ cells for hematopoietic stem cell (HSC) transplantation (10%).
> - A six-color flow cytometry diagnostic application can determine the absolute counts of mature T, B, and natural killer (NK) lymphocytes, in addition to CD4+ and CD8+ T-cell subsets in human peripheral blood, in a single tube.
> - Immunophenotyping for cancer diagnosis is about 80% of what most flow cytometric equipment does daily in clinical laboratories. Another 10% of the workload may be monitoring patients who have AIDS, and another subset of specimens are focused on quantifying CD34+ cells for HSC transplantation.
> - The quantitation of T and B cells using monoclonal surface markers can be performed using flow cytometry. Using MAbs, T- and B-cell populations can be divided into subpopulations with specific functions. T cells are divided into two functional subpopulations, helper T (Th) cells and suppressor T (Ts) cells.
> - A basic lymphocyte screening panel can detect and quantify CD3, CD4, CD8, CD19, and CD16/56. Anti–CD45/CD14 is included to assist in distinguishing lymphocytes from monocytes. This type of panel reveals the frequency of T cells (CD3+), B cells (CD19+), and NK cells (CD3–, CD16+, CD56+).
> - Human leukocyte antigen B27 (HLA-B27) can be detected by flow cytometry. This application of flow cytometry is clinically relevant to the evaluation of seronegative spondyloarthropathies.

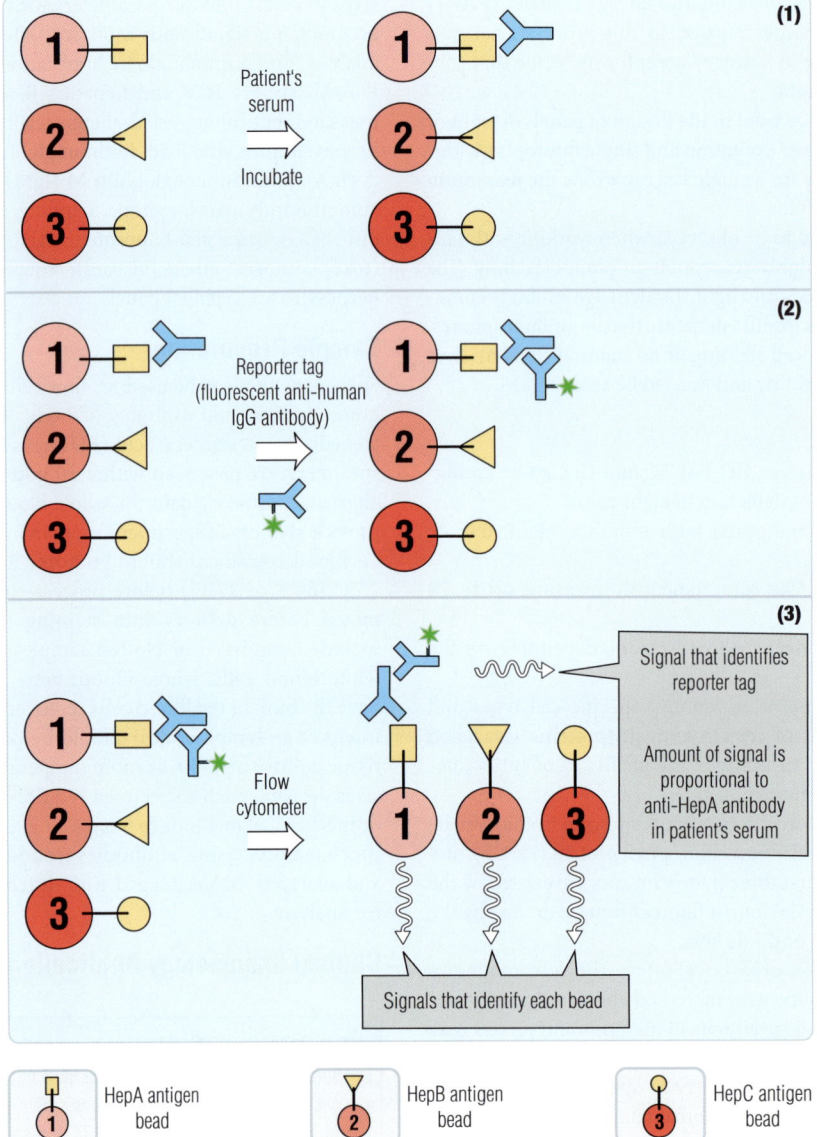

Fig. 11.4 Fluorescent Microsphere–Based Immunoassay for Antibodies to Hepatitis Virus (Luminex xMAP Technology). This approach is especially valuable when multiple tests must be done. It uses aspects of enzyme-linked immunosorbent assay (ELISA) and flow cytometry. Polystyrene microspheres are internally color coded with two fluorescent dyes that can be detected after laser illumination. *HepA*, Hepatitis A; *HepB*, hepatitis B; *HepC*, hepatitis C; *IgG*, immunoglobulin G. (From Nairn R, Helbert M: *Immunology for medical students*, ed 2, St. Louis, 2007, Mosby.)

One of the main principles of using flow cytometry is the ability to analyze the complete cell cycle and analyze DNA content in different phases. Monitoring the natural events of the cell cycle can provide information for disease diagnosis and therapy prognosis. The different phases of the cell cycle can reveal altered DNA content and other anomalies indicated tumor presence or signs of advanced cell death.

Immunophenotyping for cancer diagnosis is about 80% of what most flow cytometric equipment does daily in clinical laboratories. Another 10% of the workload may be monitoring patients who have AIDS, and another subset of specimens are focused on quantifying CD34+ cells for hematopoietic stem cell (HSC) transplantation.

Flow cytometry can detect cancers such as:
- Acute myeloid leukemia
- Acute lymphoblastic leukemia
- Chronic lymphocytic leukemia'-Multiple myeloma
- Non-Hodgkins lymphoma

Another cellular function, apoptosis, can be studied using flow cytometry. Apoptosis, also called programmed cell death, is a highly regulated cellular process that plays roles in development, stress response, and cancer. It involves the activities of many protein players. Specific antibodies may serve as useful markers when studying the complex apoptosis pathways.

Lymphocyte Subsets

A six-color flow cytometry diagnostic application uses the BD FACS-Canto II flow cytometer and BD Multitest six-color TBNK with BD Trucount tubes to determine the absolute counts of mature T, B, and NK lymphocytes (Fig. 11.5), in addition to CD4+ and CD8+ T-cell subsets in human peripheral blood, in a single tube.

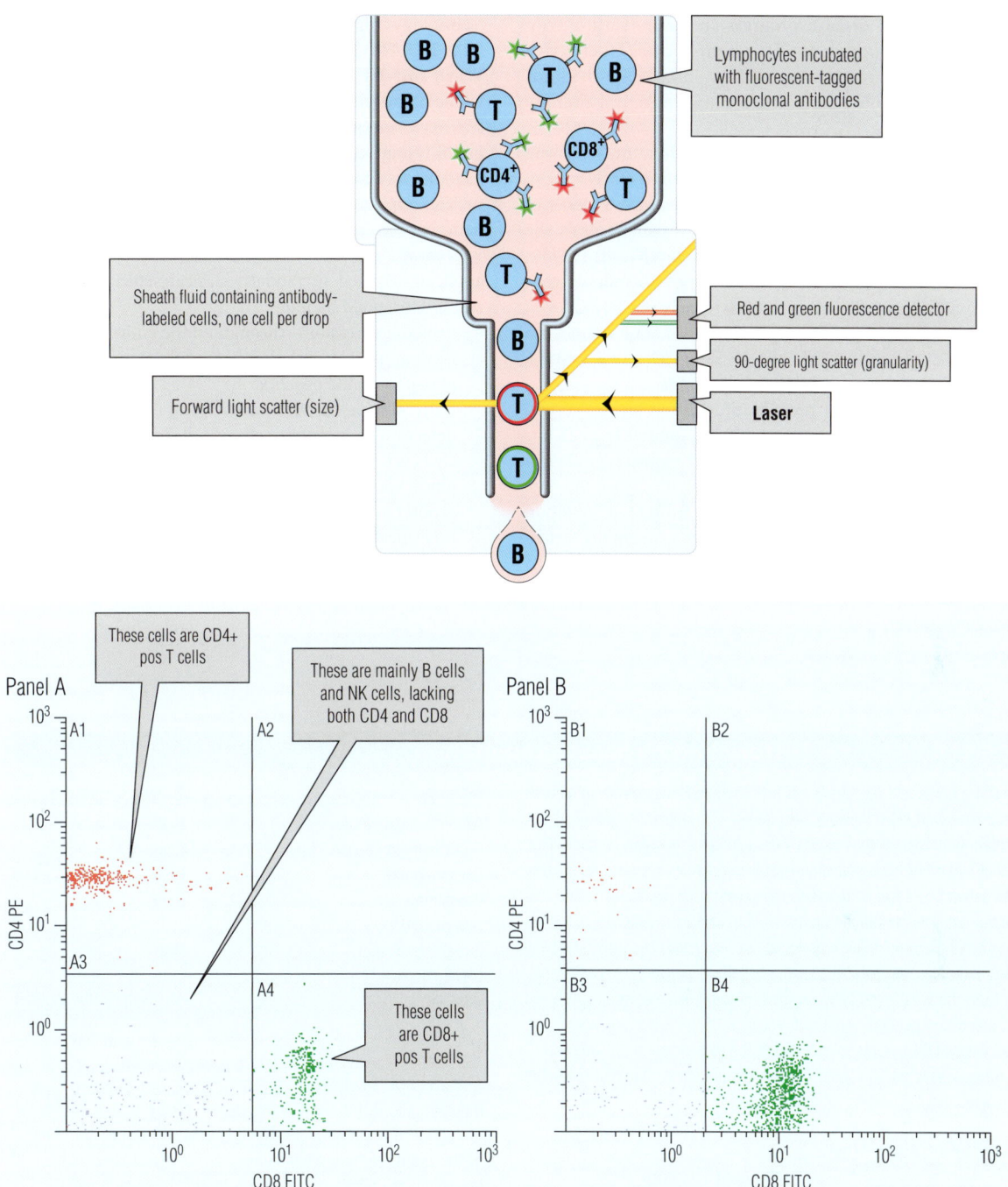

Fig. 11.5 Flow Cell Cytometry Dot Plots. (A) Cells stained with the red CD4 antibody account for 59% of all lymphocytes; this is a normal sample. (B) There is a reduction in the number of red-staining CD4+ T cells; this sample is from a patient with HIV infection. *FITC*, Fluorescein isothiocyanate (emits green light); *NK*, natural killer; *PE*, phycoerythrin (emits red light). (From Nairn R, Helbert M: *Immunology for medical students*, ed 2, St. Louis, 2007, Mosby.)

Other Cellular Applications

Measuring T cells for AIDS analysis. The quantitation of T and B cells using monoclonal surface markers can be performed using flow cytometry. With the flow cytometer, 10,000 cells can be assayed into subsets in 1 minute with multiparameter analysis. Through the use of MAbs, T- and B-cell populations can be divided into subpopulations with specific functions. T cells are divided into two functional subpopulations, helper T (Th) cells and suppressor T (Ts) cells.

Normal individuals have a Th/Ts ratio of 2:1 to 3:1. This ratio is inverted in certain disorders and diseases, including the acute phase of CMV mononucleosis, after bone marrow transplantation, and AIDS.

CD4 lymphocytes. The CD4 (helper subset) T-lymphocyte cell count is one of the standard measures for diagnosing AIDS and the management of disease progress in patients with HIV infection. The absolute number of CD4+ lymphocytes is reflective of the degree of immunodeficiency in HIV-infected individuals and may be used as a guide for initiating antiretroviral therapy and monitoring therapy.

Basic lymphocyte screening panel. A basic immune screening panel typically consists of the detection and quantitation of CD3, CD4, CD8, CD19, and CD16/56. Anti–CD45/CD14 is included to assist in distinguishing lymphocytes from monocytes. This panel reveals the frequency of T cells (CD3+), B cells (CD19+), and NK cells (CD3–, CD16+, CD56+). It also provides the frequency of Th inducer cells (CD3+, CD4+) and T suppressor or cytotoxic cells (CD3+, CD8+). Typical percentage ranges for lymphocyte subsets in adult donors are as follows: CD3, 56% to 86%; CD4, 33% to 58%; CD8, 13% to 39%; CD16+ and CD56, 5% to 26%; and CD19, 5% to 22%.

However, this panel does not provide information on cell activation or signaling pathway receptors, frequency of T subsets (e.g., Th1 or Th2), stem or blast cells, B lymphocytes (e.g., immunoblasts or plasma cells), or nonlymphoid elements.

HLA-B27 antigen. The automated BD FACSCanto, BD FACSCalibur, BD FACSort, and BD FACScan flow cytometers can rapidly detect HLA-B27 antigen expression in erythrocyte-lysed whole blood (LWB) using a qualitative two-color direct immunofluorescence method. This technology compares the intensity of T lymphocytes stained with anti–HLA-B27 FITC to a predetermined decision marker during analysis. When anti–HLA-B27 FITC/CD3 PE MAb reagent is added to human whole blood, the fluorochrome-labeled antibodies bind specifically to leukocyte surface antigens. The stained samples are treated with BD FACS lysing solution to lyse erythrocytes and are then washed and fixed before flow cytometric analysis.

This application of flow cytometry is clinically relevant to the evaluation of seronegative spondyloarthropathies.

Therapeutic and Research Applications. A few of the major applications used in modern clinical settings both therapeutic and research oriented include:

- Protein expression—throughout the entire cell, even the nucleus
- Protein post translational modifications—includes cleaved and phosphorylated proteins
- RNA—including both miRNA, and mRNA transcripts
- detection of apoptotic cells or cell death
- Cell cycle status—providing a powerful tool to assess cells in G0/G1 phase versus S phase, G2, or polyploidy, including analysis of cell proliferation and activation
- Identification and characterization of distinct subsets of cells within a heterogeneous sample—including distinguishing central effector memory cells from exhausted T cells or regulatory T cells

---

CASE STUDY 11.1 History and Physical Examination

The parents of a 6-year-old boy brought him to the hospital complaining of back pain and refusal to walk since falling a week earlier. Consequently, he walked less and slept more than usual; 3 days earlier, after taking a few steps, he had fallen. His family took him to see his pediatrician. His temperature was normal. No organomegaly was detected. He had tenderness in the lower back region, with more tenderness on the left side than on the right side. Pain increased with sitting and leg flexion. The neurologic examination was normal. He was prescribed aspirin for pain. A radiograph of his hips was prescribed and was subsequently reported as normal.

One day later, he was found lying on the bathroom floor, crying. He refused to walk or stand and needed assistance because of the lower back pain. The pediatrician advised his parents to take him to the local hospital. He was admitted. Laboratory assays and a repeat hip radiograph, chest film, and magnetic resonance imaging (MRI) studies were prescribed.

Admission Laboratory Data

Assay	Patient Results
Hematology	
Hemoglobin	Within reference range
Hematocrit	Within reference range
White blood cell count (WBC)	Within reference range
Differential WBC	90% immature mononuclear cells; reference range, no immature mononuclear cells
Erythrocyte sedimentation rate (ESR)	High
Chemistry	
Glucose	N
Total protein	N
Albumin	N
Globulin	N
Bilirubin (total)	N

Assay	Patient Results
Alkaline phosphatase	High
Lactic dehydrogenase (LDH)	High
Calcium (total)	High
Phosphorus	High
Serology	
C-reactive protein	High
Urinalysis	
Dipstick	All results within normal limits

Follow-Up
Diagnostic Imaging
Radiographs of the chest were normal. MRI scans of the lumbar spine with the administration of gadolinium were considered to be normal. MRI studies of the brain, without gadolinium, were interpreted as normal. MRI scans of the spine and pelvis revealed deformities of several vertebral bodies of the thoracic and lumbar spine.

Hematology
A bone marrow biopsy was ordered. Samples of the bone marrow aspirate were sent for morphologic examination, flow cytometry, and cytogenetic analysis.

Hematology (4 days after admission):

Assay	Patient Results
Peripheral Blood	
Hemoglobin	Low
Hematocrit	Low
White blood cell count (WBC)	Low
Differential WBC	90% immature mononuclear cells; reference range, no immature mononuclear cells

CASE STUDY 11.1 History and Physical Examination—cont'd

Assay	Patient Results
Bone Marrow	
Microscopic examination	Predominant population of small-to-medium–size immature mononuclear cells; nucleoli present

Flow Cytometry (4 days after admission):

Cell surface markers	Reactivity
CD34	Positive
Terminal deoxynucleotidyl transferase (TdT)	Positive
CD19	Positive
CD10	Positive
CD45	Weakly positive

Cytogenetic Analysis
A normal male karyotype (46,XY) was found. Fluorescence in situ hybridization showed normal numbers of chromosomes 4, 10, and 17 and no evidence of rearrangements involving *TEL*, *AML1*, *BCR*, *ABL1*, or *MLL* and normal leukocytes, platelets, and red cells.

Questions
1. The CD34+ surface membrane marker is exhibited by:
   a. Stem cells
   b. Mature T lymphocytes
   c. Mature B lymphocytes
   d. Mature plasma cells
2. The classic marker for mature B lymphocytes is:
   a. CD4
   b. CD8
   c. CD10
   d. CD20

Answers to these questions can be found in Appendix A.

Critical Thinking Group Discussion Questions
1. What is the significance of positive reactivity of CD45?
2. What is the significance of positive reactivity of CD34?
3. What is the significance of positive reactivity of CD19 and CD20?
4. What is the significance of a normal cytogenetic profile?

REVIEW QUESTIONS

1. *Laser* is an acronym for:
   a. Light amplification by stimulated emission of radiation
   b. Light augmentation by stimulated emitted radiation
   c. Light amplified by stimulated energy radiation
   d. Large-angle stimulation by emitted radiation
2. All of the following are descriptive characteristics of laser light *except*:
   a. Intensity
   b. Stability
   c. Polychromaticity
   d. Monochromaticity
3. A photon is a:
   a. Basic unit of light
   b. Basic unit of all radiation
   c. Component of an atom
   d. Component of laser light
4. A major application of flow cell technology is:
   a. Identification of cells
   b. Cell sorting before further analysis
   c. Diagnosis of autoimmune disease
   d. Both a and b
5. Four-color immunofluorescence typically uses all of the following labels *except*:
   a. Fluorescein isothiocyanate (FITC)
   b. Phycoerythrin (PE)
   c. Peridinin chlorophyll protein (PerCP)
   d. Color-emitting radioactive substances
6. A fluorophore:
   a. Reemits light after exposure to photons
   b. Is excited by shorter wavelength light
   c. Stays excited for a long period of time
   d. Both a and b
7. The Stokes shift is:
   a. The difference between peak excitation and peak emission wavelengths
   b. The same for each fluorophore
   c. Protective against photobleaching
   d. Both b and c
8. The name of the immunological method used in flow cytometry is:
   a. Radioimmunoassay
   b. Immunofluorescence
   c. ELISA
   d. Hemagglutination
9. In flow cytometry, forward-scattered light assists with identification of:
   a. Cell size
   b. Cellular granularity
   c. Ability to absorb fluorescence
   d. Both a and b
10. In flow cytometry, side-scattered light assists with identification of:
    a. Cellular granularity
    b. Cell size
    c. Ability to absorb fluorescence
    d. Both a and b
11. The step of centering the sample core within the sheath fluid is called:
    a. Isoelectric focusing
    b. Hydrodynamic focusing
    c. Liquid focusing
    d. Light focus

12

Molecular Laboratory Techniques

LEARNING OUTCOMES

- Describe the composition of DNA and RNA.
- Compare the functions of DNA and various forms of RNA.
- Define the terms *mutation* and *polymorphism*.
- Describe the polymerase chain reaction (PCR) amplification technique.
- Describe the technique and clinical applications of real-time PCR.
- Identify other amplification techniques.
- Describe dideoxy-termination sequencing (Sanger sequencing).
- Compare the genome-sequencing approaches of conventional Sanger, shotgun Sanger, and massively parallel sequencing/next-generation sequencing (NGS).
- Describe single-nucleotide polymorphisms (SNPs).
- Describe the principle, advantages, and disadvantages of fluorescence in situ hybridization (FISH).
- Explain various types of microarrays and the clinical applications of microarray testing.
- Outline the generalized steps in massively parallel sequencing (next-generation sequencing [NGS]).
- Discuss additional applications of molecular diagnostic testing.
- Analyze a case study related to immunoassay.
- Describe a molecular testing procedure.
- Correctly answer 80% of the end-of-chapter review questions.

OUTLINE

Characteristics of Nucleic Acids, 169
    How Does DNA Replicate?, 169
    Forms of Ribonucleic Acid, 169
        Mutations and Polymorphisms, 169
Molecular Amplification Methods, 170
    Amplicons, 170
    Amplification Methods, 171
        Target Amplification Methods, 171
        Polymerase Chain Reaction, 171
        Modified Polymerase Chain Reaction Techniques, 173
        Real-Time Polymerase Chain Reaction, 173
        Transcription-Mediated Amplification (TMA), 174
        Nucleic Acid Sequence–Based Amplification (NASBA), 174
        Signal Amplification Methods, 174
        Serial Invasive Signal Amplification, 175
        Probe Amplification Methods, 175
        Strand Displacement Amplification, 175
    Alternative Target Amplification Techniques, 175
Molecular Analysis of Amplification Products, 175
    Electrophoresis-Based Techniques, 176
        Polymerase Chain Reaction Product Length, 176
        Real-Time Fluorescent Methods, 176
    TaqMan Assays and SYBR Green Dye–Based Assays, 176
        TaqMan Method, 176
        SYBR Green, 178
        Sanger (Chain Termination) Sequencing, 178
    Alternatives to Electrophoresis, 179
        Pyrosequencing, 179
        Hybridization Assays, 179
    Fluorescence In Situ Hybridization, 179
        Principle of the Fluorescence In Situ Hybridization Technique, 179
        Use of Fluorescence In Situ Hybridization in the Clinical Laboratory, 179
    Microarrays, 180
        Spotted Arrays on Glass, 180
        Self-Assembled Arrays, 181
        DNA Methylation Analysis, 183
        Illumina assays, 183
        Advantages and Disadvantages of Array-Based Methods, 183
Massively Parallel Sequencing/Next-Generation Sequencing Technology, 183
    Target Enrichment Strategies, 184
        Steps of Next-Generation Sequencing, 185
    Adaptation of DNA Methylation Detection Technologies for NGS, 185
Case Study 12.1   **History and Physical Examination, 186**
Procedure: Molecular Testing Group A *Streptococcus* Direct Test, 187.e1

KEY TERMS

amplicon
anneal
deoxynucleotide
deoxyribonucleic acid (DNA)
exome
fluorescence in situ hybridization (FISH)

fluorophore quencher
fluorophore reporter
massively parallel sequencing/next-generation sequencing (NGS)
nosocomial
nucleic acid probe

nucleotides
oligonucleotides
polymerase chain reaction (PCR)
primer
purine

pyrimidine
reverse transcriptase (RT)
ribonucleic acid (RNA)

single-nucleotide polymorphism (SNP)
thermocycler
transcription

translation
tumorigenesis

Molecular diagnostic testing is under the umbrella of the clinical laboratory. In industry, molecular diagnostics can also be referred to as *biotechnology*. Molecular testing has the following basic advantages:
- Faster turnaround time
- Smaller required sample volumes
- Increased specificity and sensitivity

Molecular testing is no longer confined to high-volume reference laboratories. Molecular diagnostic techniques have continued to advance in precision, accuracy, turnaround testing speed, detection, and lower cost. The clinical applications of molecular diagnostic testing using nucleic acid–based methods range from detection of infectious diseases (e.g., See COVID-19 testing in Chapter 13, Infectious Disease) to cellular and tissue antigens.

New automated systems focus on pathogen detection and multidrug-resistant organisms, particularly healthcare-acquired (e.g., nosocomial) infections. Developing countries have expanded their use of molecular diagnostics in HIV diagnosis and viral load testing. Genomic testing permits the increased collection of data on large populations in disease research studies.

> **KEY CONCEPTS: DNA and RNA Essentials**
> - The two main types of nucleic acid are deoxyribonucleic acid (DNA) and ribonucleic acid (RNA).
> - Nucleotides of DNA have a deoxyribose sugar with one of the following bases: adenine (A), guanine (G), thymine (T), or cytosine (C). The genetic code is redundant, the 3-base code can have 64 different combinations, but only 20 amino acids are recognized.
> - RNA is composed of a ribose sugar with a nitrogen base similar to DNA, except thymine (T) is replaced with uracil (U).
> - DNA is double strand; RNA is typically single strand.
> - DNA arranged in a double helix has the bases A with T, and G with C.
> - The two strands of DNA are bound together by hydrogen bonds and stacking forces that can be broken and reformed without damage to the DNA. This property is exploited by many molecular diagnostic methods.
> - RNA pairing of bases substitutes U for T.
> - DNA is the template for messenger RNA that codes for proteins. Only 1.2% to 1.5% of the human genome is translated into protein. Much more of the genome is made into RNA.
> - Mutations and polymorphisms reflect changes in nucleotide sequences that can impact specific protein sequences.

CHARACTERISTICS OF NUCLEIC ACIDS

Nucleic acids are of two main types, deoxyribonucleic acid (DNA) and ribonucleic acid (RNA). New studies suggest that humans have about 19,000 genes. Genes are sequences of DNA carried on chromosomes that encode information for the translation of nucleic acid sequences into amino acid sequences that result in the production of proteins. In comparison, RNA acts as an intermediate nucleic acid structure that helps convert the DNA-encoded genetic information into proteins. DNA is the template for the synthesis of RNA.

DNA and RNA are polymers made up of repeating nucleotides or bases that are linked together (Fig. 12.1). DNA and RNA have the same two purine bases, adenine (A) and guanine (G), but the pyrimidine bases differ. DNA has cytosine (C) and thymine (T); RNA substitutes uracil (U) for T. DNA is predominantly a double-strand molecule with specific base pairs linked together (Fig. 12.2). Nucleotides are bonded together, and two strands are twisted into an alpha helix (Figs. 12.3 and 12.4).

How Does DNA Replicate?

DNA is a very stable molecule, and replication is straightforward. The process of replication (Fig. 12.5) involves one strand of the molecule acting as a template for the creation of a complementary strand. As a result of this process, two identical daughter molecules are produced. In the laboratory, the hydrogen bonds that hold the strands of the double helix can be broken apart or denatured. If complementary strands of DNA are denatured in the laboratory, they can spontaneously rejoin, or anneal. The process of denaturation and annealing (see later discussion) can be used effectively in molecular testing.

The genetic code is required to convert a nucleic acid sequence; for example, UCU, UCC, UCA, and UCG all code for the amino acid serine. One hallmark of the genetic code is redundancy, usually in the third base of the codon. Production of functional protein from genetically encoded DNA is achieved by two processes, transcription and translation. Francis Crick originated the concept of the central dogma of biology, which describes the transfer of genetic information into functional macromolecules. This was generally depicted to show the movement of genetic information from DNA to RNA via transcription.
- Transcription is a process of generating a strand of messenger RNA (mRNA) that encodes for the gene and is expressed as a protein.
- Translation occurs when the mRNA moves from the nucleus of a cell into the cellular cytoplasm to the ribosomes. mRNA is translated into an amino acid sequence on the ribosome.

This process manufactures a protein that was originally encoded in DNA in the cellular nucleus.

Forms of Ribonucleic Acid

RNA can be easily replicated and is used in molecular laboratory testing. The forms of RNA exist as single-strand polymers.

There are different forms of RNA with various overall functions. These include RNAs involved in protein synthesis, RNAs involved in post-transcriptional modification or DNA replication, and regulatory RNAs. In both prokaryotes and eukaryotes, there are three main types of RNA associated with protein synthesis: mRNA, transfer RNA (tRNA), and ribosomal RNA (rRNA).

The function of each form of RNA in protein synthesis differs, as follows:
- mRNA: Translates DNA coding into functional proteins (Fig. 12.6)
- tRNA: Transports various amino acids to manufacture proteins
- rRNA: Site of protein synthesis directed by mRNA

Mutations and Polymorphisms

A *mutation* is defined as a change in the nucleotide sequence. A *polymorphism* or *variant*, as the name implies, is the term used to express frequent changes in the nucleotide sequence.

Variations in the nucleotide sequence can extend from a single base pair, a single-nucleotide polymorphism (SNP), to chromosomal alterations involving millions of base pairs. SNPs are the most abundant source of genetic variation in the human genome. Since

the decoding of the human genome (and thus more than 3 million SNPs), laboratory techniques have been able to associate disease states and pharmacologic responses with individual SNPs. SNPs have some important characteristics:
- They are not completely synonymous with point mutation.
- They often cause a premature stop codon or a missense codon.
- They are the most common clinically significant DNA polymorphism.
- They can be studied by allele-specific polymerase chain reaction (PCR), melt curve analysis, and microarrays.
- They occur at specific regions in the genome.
- They can vary between populations or ethnic groups.

Many SNPs are studied in pharmacogenetics, in which pharmacodynamics is monitored by a biomarker or a clinical parameter (e.g., international normalized ratio [INR] or blood pressure). Multiple laboratory methods can be used to detect mutations. Polymorphisms that create, destroy, or impact restriction enzyme sites are detected as restriction fragment length polymorphisms (RFLPs) (discussed later in this chapter).

The major histocompatibility complex (MHC) on chromosome 6 is an area that has frequent nucleotide sequence changes (polymorphic). Another highly polymorphic section in the MHC is the area of gene coding for antigen-receptor proteins in T lymphocytes and antibody synthesis in B lymphocytes.

In addition to the genome located in the nucleus of a cell, mitochondria have their own genome. Mutations in the mitochondrial genome can impact the immune system, particularly in the defense against frequent or prolonged infections and other disorders, such as type 2 diabetes.

> **KEY CONCEPTS: General Characteristics of Amplification Methods**
> - Nucleic amplification methods can amplify the target, the signal, or the probe.
> - Nucleic amplification techniques may be isothermal or may cycle through different temperature ranges.
> - Nucleic acid techniques can be qualitative, quantitative, or digital.
> - Amplification is the copying of a specific nucleic acid sequence in order to obtain enough to identify the sequence of interest.
> - PCR allows for exponential amplification of a DNA segment from the genome, allowing multiple analytical procedures on a single, pure sequence.

MOLECULAR AMPLIFICATION METHODS

Molecular diagnostics requires techniques to detect extremely low concentrations of nucleic acids (NAs) in a background of complex genomic structure. Techniques that increase the amount of the NA target, the detection signal, or the probe are referred to as *amplification*. The selection of one technique over another is often based on factors such as sensitivity and specificity profiles, cost, turnaround time, and local experience.

Amplicons

An **amplicon** is a piece of genetic material, such as DNA, that can be formed as the product of a natural event or artificial amplification technique. A molecular diagnostic laboratory that performs in vitro amplification reactions needs to practice techniques to control contamination. This is especially true if a high number of thermal cycles is used for **polymerase chain reaction (PCR)**. PCR is highly sensitive, but a disadvantage to the use of this method is that it is

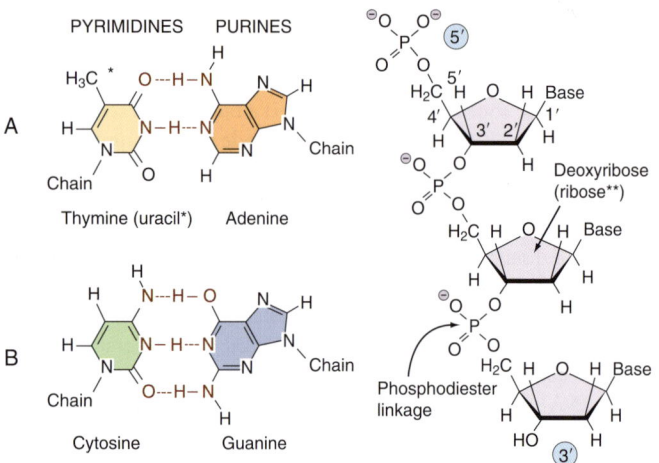

Fig. 12.1 (A) Purine and pyrimidine bases and the formation of complementary base pairs. Dashed lines indicate the formation of hydrogen bonds. (B) A single-strand DNA chain. Repeating nucleotide units are linked by phosphodiester bonds that join the 5′ carbon of one sugar to the 3′ carbon of the next. Each nucleotide monomer consists of a sugar moiety, a phosphate residue, and a base. *In RNA, thymine is replaced by uracil, which differs from thymine only in its lack of the methyl group. **In RNA, the sugar is ribose, which adds a 2′-hydroxyl to deoxyribose. (Adapted from Piper MA, Unger ER: *Nucleic acid probes: a primer for pathologists*, Chicago, 1989, ASCP Press.)

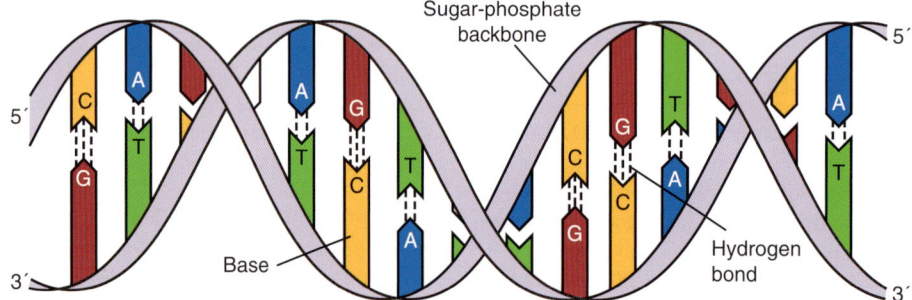

Fig. 12.2 Structure of DNA. The DNA molecule is a double helix that consists of two sugar-phosphate backbones with four bases—cytosine (*C*), guanine (*G*), adenine (*A*), and thymine (*T*)—attached. *C* and *G* residues and *A* and *T* residues on opposite strands pair through hydrogen bonding. (From LeGrys V, Leinbach SS, Silverman L: Clinical applications of DNA probes in the diagnosis of genetic diseases, *Crit Rev Clin Lab Sci* 25[4]:255–274, 1987.)

amplicons, which can then adhere to laboratory coats and objects in the room.

> **KEY CONCEPTS: Facts about Amplifications Methods**
> - Amplification methods to increase the target DNA include PCR adaptations involving the most popular point-of-care technique, real-time PCR.
> - PCR is an in vitro method that multiplies low levels of specific DNA sequences in a sample to higher levels suitable for further analysis. PCR, an enzymatic process, is carried out in cycles. Each repeated cycle consists of DNA denaturation, primer annealing, and extension of the primed DNA sequence. Each cycle theoretically doubles the amount of specific DNA sequence present and results in an exponential accumulation of the DNA fragment being amplified (amplicons).
> - PCR analysis can lead to the identification of viral DNA associated with specific cancers and detection of genetic mutations.
> - Branched DNA represents a signal amplification method in which multiple probes attach to the original target sequence DNA.
> - Probe-based DNA detection systems provide sequence specificity and lower detection limits.

Amplification Methods

Three categories of amplification methods (Table 12.1) are:
1. **Target amplification**, in which a well-defined segment of nucleic acid, the target sequence, is copied many times by in vitro methods. Areas outside of the target are not amplified.
2. **Signal amplification**, which produces the same amount of target, but the signal is increased by one of several methods, including sequential hybridization of branching nucleic acid structures and continuous enzyme action on substrate that may be recycled.
3. **Probe amplification**, which takes place when the probe or a product of the probe is amplified only in the presence of the target.

Target Amplification Methods

The gold standard for target amplification is PCR that exponentially amplifies DNA. Associated versions of PCR are real-time (RT-PCR) and multiplex PCR. Other non-PCR target amplification techniques include transcription-mediated amplification (TMA) and nucleic acid sequence–based amplification (NASBA).

Polymerase Chain Reaction

Qualitative PCR detects the presence or absence of specific DNA product. Qualitative PCR is a good technique to use when PCR is performed for cloning purposes or for pathogen identification. Quantitative PCR provides more information beyond just detection of DNA. Quantitative PCR can indicate how much of a specific DNA or gene is present in a specimen.

PCR (Fig. 12.7) is an in vitro method that amplifies low levels of specific DNA sequences in a sample to higher levels suitable for further analysis. To use this technology, the target sequence to be amplified must be known. Typically, a target sequence ranges from 100 to 1000 base pairs (bp) in length. Two short DNA primers typically are used; these are short pieces of single-strand DNA (ssDNA), typically 16 to 20 bp in length. Two primers are used in each PCR reaction, and they are designed so that they flank the target region (region that should be copied). A technologist needs to design primers that are complementary to the template region of DNA. They are synthesized chemically by joining nucleotides together.

The oligonucleotides (small portions of a single DNA strand) act as a template for the new DNA. These primer sequences are complementary to the 3′ ends of the sequence to be amplified.

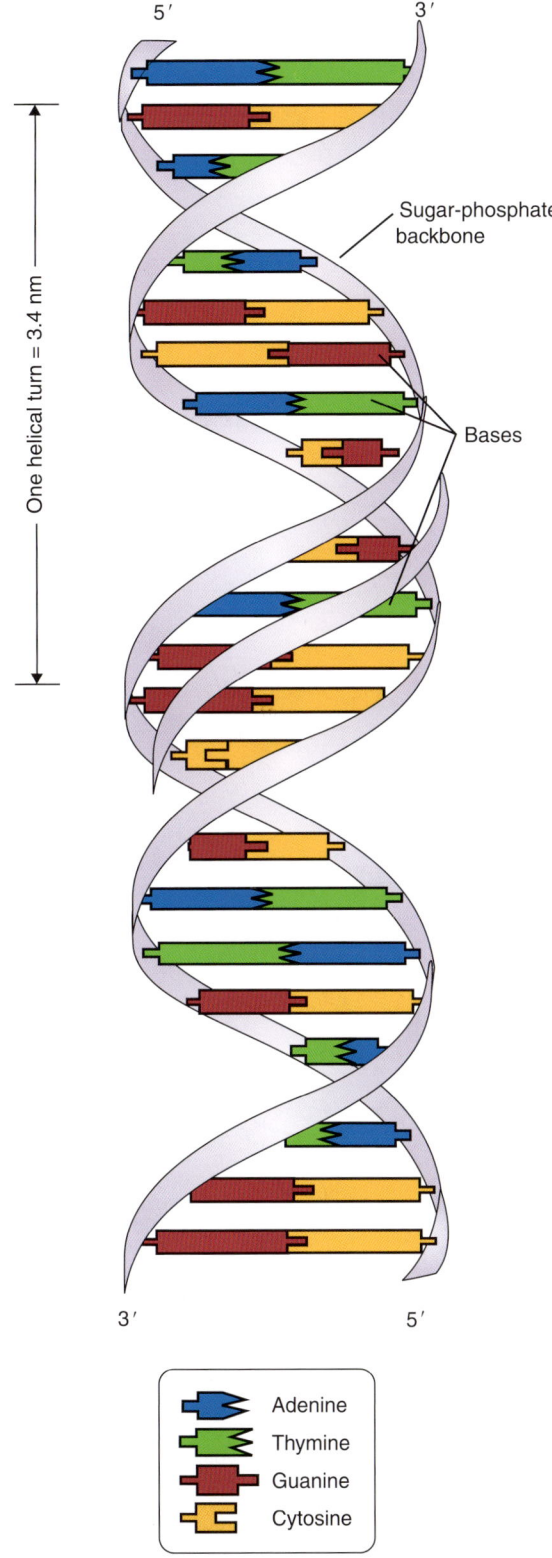

Fig. 12.3 The DNA Double Helix, With a Sugar-Phosphate Backbone and Pairing of the Bases in the Core Forming Planar Structures. (From Jorde CB, Carey JC, Bamshead MJ et al, editors: *Medical genetics*, ed 3, St. Louis, 2006, Mosby.)

prone to producing false-positive results (Box 12.1). In laboratories in which PCR is performed frequently, any false positives are generally caused by amplicon contamination. A broken capillary tube or a PCR plate left carelessly at the edge of a table can aerosolize those

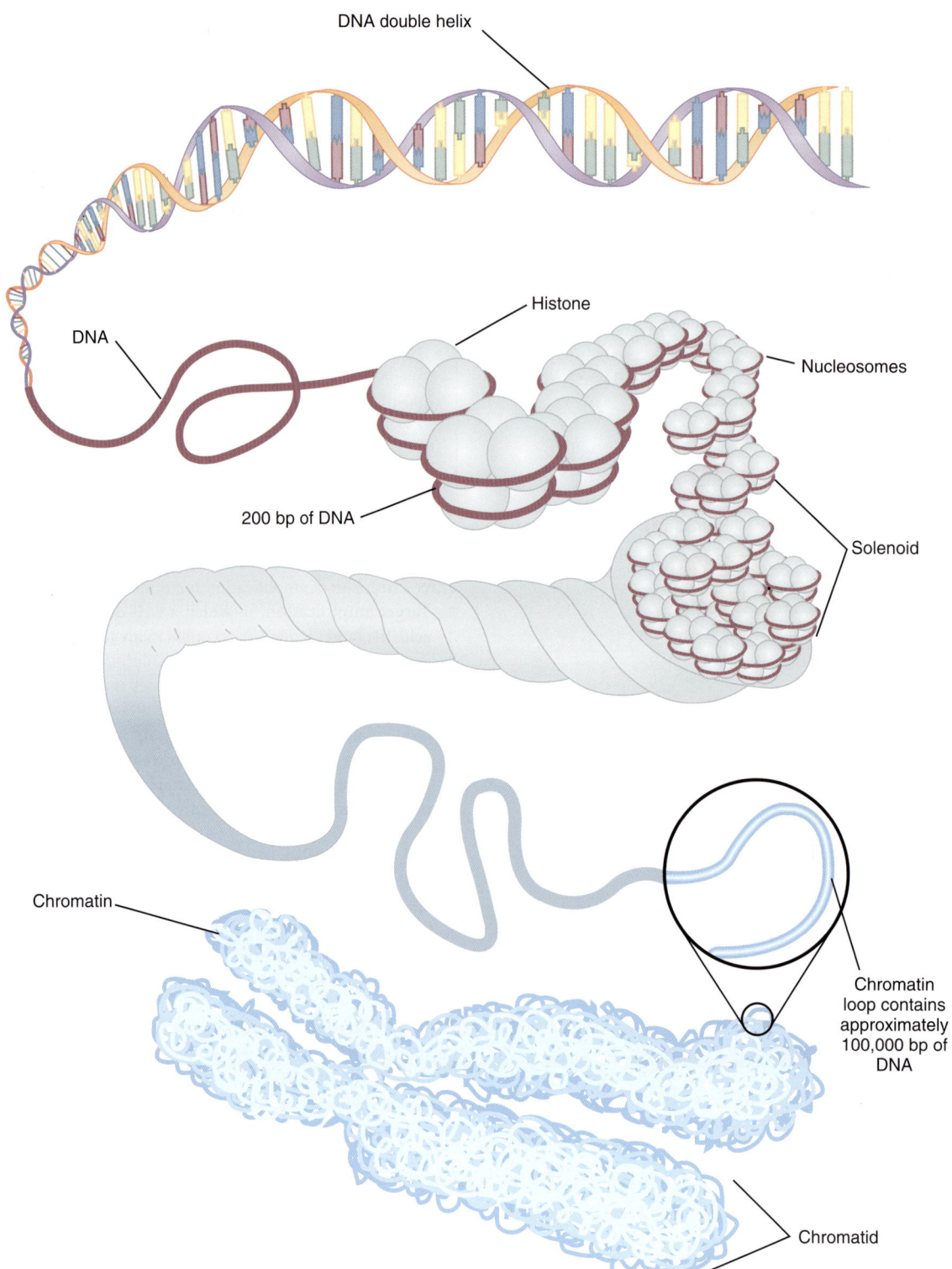

Fig. 12.4 Structural Organization of Human Chromosomal DNA. Double-strand DNA is wound around the octamer core of histone proteins to form nucleosomes, which are further compacted in a helical structure called a *solenoid*. Nuclear DNA in conjunction with its associated structural proteins is known as *chromatin*. Chromatin in its most compact state forms chromosomes. The primary construction of a chromosome is the centromere, and the chromosome's ends are the telomeres. (From Jorde L, Carey JC, Bamshad MJ, editors: *Medical genetics*, ed 6, St. Louis, 2020, Elsevier.)

This enzymatic process is carried out in cycles. Each repeated cycle consists of the following:
- DNA denaturation. The double DNA strands are separated into two single strands through the use of heat.
- Primer annealing. The oligonucleotide primers are recombined with the single-strand original DNA.
- Extension of the primed DNA sequence. The enzyme DNA polymerase synthesizes new complementary strands by the extension of primers.

CHAPTER 12 Molecular Laboratory Techniques

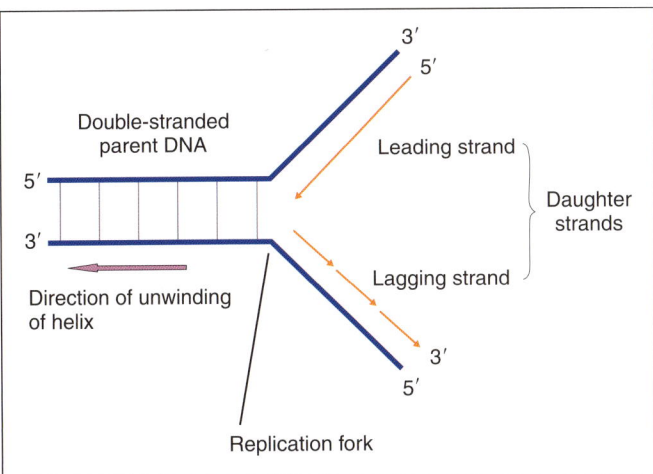

Fig. 12.5 DNA Replication. Double-strand DNA is separated at the replication fork. The leading strand is synthesized continuously, whereas the lagging strand is synthesized discontinuously but joined later. (From Burtis CA, Ashwood ER, Bruns DB: *Tietz fundamentals of clinical chemistry,* ed 6, St. Louis, 2008, Saunders.)

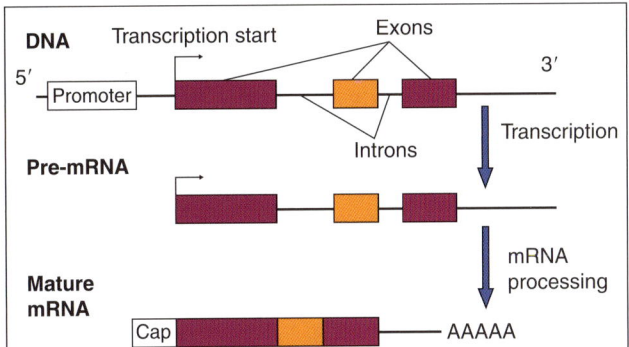

Fig. 12.6 DNA Transcription and Messenger RNA (mRNA) Processing. A gene that encodes for a protein contains a promoter region with a variable number of introns and exons. Transcription commences at the transcription start site. Pre-mRNA is processed by capping, polyadenylation, and intron splicing and becomes a mature mRNA. (From Burtis CA, Ashwood ER, Bruns DB: *Tietz fundamentals of clinical chemistry,* ed 6, St. Louis, 2008, Saunders.)

BOX 12.1 Some Weaknesses of the Polymerase Chain Reaction Technique

1. Contamination is possible.
2. Only short sequences can be amplified (generally).
3. Large deletions in the sequence produce no location for primer binding.
4. Polymerase chain reaction (PCR) should not be used for a mutation search unless it is known that the mutation does not involve large deletions or that PCR can amplify across from an identified deletion from an adjacent site.

Each cycle (Fig. 12.8) theoretically doubles the amount of specific DNA sequence present and results in an exponential accumulation of the DNA fragment being amplified (amplicons). In general, this process is repeated approximately 30 times. At the end of 30 cycles, the reaction mixture should contain about 2^{30} molecules of the desired product. Potential problems with PCR at this stage can result from assuming that the process is 100% efficient with each cycle, but amplification in the second phase may not be truly exponential. There is variation in efficiency of amplification of sequences due to conditions that cannot be fully controlled. The required number of cycles is difficult to determine because exponential amplification is very rapid and very low amounts of starting material may fail to amplify.

After cycling is complete, the amplification products can be analyzed in various ways. Typically, the contents of the reaction vessel are subjected to gel electrophoresis. This allows visualization of the amplified gene segments (e.g., PCR products and bands) and determination of their specificity. Additional product analysis by probe hybridization or direct DNA sequencing is often performed to verify the authenticity of the amplicon further.

The three important applications of PCR are:
1. Amplification of DNA
2. Identification of a target nucleotide sequence
3. Synthesis of a labeled antisense probe

PCR analysis can lead to a variety of positive outcomes, such as detection of gene mutations in the early stages of cancer; identification of viral DNA associated with specific cancers (e.g., human papillomavirus [HPV]); and detection of genetic mutations associated with various diseases, such as coronary artery disease associated with mutations of the gene that encodes for the low-density lipoprotein receptor (LDLR).

The PCR technique has undergone modifications. One subtype uses nested primers in a two-step amplification process. First, a broad region of the DNA surrounding the sequence of interest is amplified, followed by another round of amplification to amplify the specific gene sequence to be studied.

Modified Polymerase Chain Reaction Techniques

Multiplex PCR uses numerous primers in a single reaction tube to amplify nucleic acid amplicons, segments of chromosomal DNA that undergo amplification and contain replicated genetic material, from different targets. Specific nucleic acid amplification should occur if the appropriate target DNA is present in the sample tests. Detection may be accomplished by the traditional Southern transfer method and subsequent nucleic acid probe, normally a short sequence of nucleotide bases that will bind to specific regions of a target sequence of nucleotides, by enzyme immunoassay (EIA) methods, or by gene chip analysis. This technology is limited by (1) the number of primers that can be included in a single reaction, (2) primer-primer interference, and (3) nonspecific nucleic acid amplification.

Real-Time Polymerase Chain Reaction

Conventional PCR is used to detect the presence or absence of certain genomic fragments, but RT-PCR is used to detect the expression level of that fragment in the organism. Conventional PCR is more time-consuming because it uses agarose gel electrophoresis to detect the amplified PCR products.

For diagnostic purposes, traditional PCR has been replaced by RT-PCR in many circumstances, particularly in point-of-care testing (e.g., Abbott Laboratories and ID NOW COVID-19 assay for SARS-CoV-2 coronavirus). RT-PCR is used for many qualitative and quantitative applications, including gene expression analysis, microRNA analysis for identification of cancer biomarkers, SNP genotyping, copy number variation (CNV) analysis, and even protein analysis.

Quantitative RT-PCR can determine the quantity of virus and extent of mRNA expression. Specific examples include detection of influenza virus strains and coronavirus disease 2019 (COVID-19). In March 2020, the US Food and Drug Administration (FDA) issued Emergency Use Authorization to Abbott Laboratories for a fluorescent coronavirus test, ID NOW. This test delivers positive results in as little as 5 minutes and negative results in 13 minutes. The test runs on the

TABLE 12.1 Examples of Amplification Techniques

Technique	Type	Definition
Polymerase chain reaction (PCR)	Target	An in vitro method for exponentially amplifying DNA.
Transcription-mediated amplification (TMA)	Target	An amplification method that uses RNA polymerase and DNA reverse transcriptase to produce RNA amplicon from a target nucleic acid. TMA is used to amplify both RNA and DNA.
Nucleic acid sequence–based amplification (NASBA)	Target	Process similar to TMA, but only RNA is targeted for amplification.
Strand displacement amplification (SDA)	Target	An amplification technique that uses two types of primers, DNA polymerase, and a restriction endonuclease to exponentially produce single-strand amplicons asynchronously.
Branched-chain signal amplification DNA (bDNA)	Signal	A molecular probe technique that uses branched DNA (bDNA) as a means to amplify the hybridization signal.
Serial invasive signal amplification	Signal	A signal-enhancing technique that combines two invasive signal amplification reactions in series in a single tube. The cleaved 5′-arm from the target-specific primary reaction is used to drive a secondary invasive reaction, resulting in a total signal amplification of more than seven orders of magnitude in about 4 hours.
Ligase chain reaction (LCR)	Probe	A process that amplifies probes rather than the target DNA. LCR is one of many techniques developed to detect specific nucleic acid sequences by amplificatin of nucleic acid targets.

Modified from Wittwer CT, Makrigiorgos GM: Important terms and definitions, in *Tietz textbook of clinical chemistry and molecular diagnostics,* ed 6, Chapter 47, Nucleic Acid Techniques, pp. 960–961.

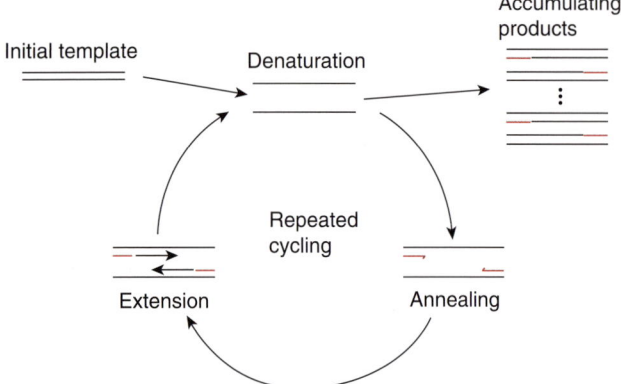

Fig. 12.7 Simple Schematic of the Polymerase Chain Reaction. Amplification of the initial template requires denaturation by heat, allowing primers to anneal at a lower temperature, followed by primer extension at an intermediate temperature. In each cycle, a doubling of the DNA product occurs. After 20 to 40 cycles, the product accumulates more than 1 million-fold. (From Rifai N: *Tietz textbook of clinical chemistry and molecular diagnostics,* ed 6, St. Louis, 2018, Elsevier.)

company's ID NOW platform, a 6.6-pound portable device the size of a small toaster. There are currently about 18,000 ID NOW instruments in the United States and this is the most widely available molecular point-of-care testing platform in the nation.

RT-PCR uses the same basic reagents and techniques as the original PCR method but with the addition of fluorescently labeled sequence-specific probes. As the name suggests, RT-PCR is a technique used to monitor the progress of a PCR reaction in real time. Note that RT-PCR involves conversion of RNA to complementary DNA (cDNA) via reverse transcription, followed by several rounds of PCR to amplify and detect the genes of interest. The products can be detected in "real time" by using SYBR Green or TaqMan probes. RT-PCR data is collected throughout the PCR cycles instead of at the end of a fixed number of PCR cycles. The higher the starting copy number of the nucleic acid target, the sooner a significant increase in fluorescence is observed. A relatively small amount of PCR product (DNA, cDNA, or RNA) can be quantified.

The first step in an RT-PCR reaction is the conversion of RNA to cDNA; this process is known as *reverse transcription* (Fig. 12.9). The next step uses fluorescent reporters and a PCR reaction to amplify and detect specific genes. RT-PCR uses fluorescence-resonance energy transfer to quantitate specific DNA sequences of interest and identify point mutations, a mutation altering only one or very few nucleotides in a gene sequence. It is particularly appealing because the procedure is less susceptible to amplicon contamination and is more accurate in quantifying the initial copy number.

RT-PCR is increasingly being adopted for RNA quantification and genetic analysis. At present the most popular RT-PCR assay is based on the hybridization of a dual-labeled probe to the PCR product, and the development of a signal by loss of fluorescence quenching as PCR degrades the probe. The TaqMan approach has proved easy to optimize in practice, but the dual-labeled probes are relatively expensive.

Transcription-Mediated Amplification (TMA)

TMA (Fig. 12.10) is an amplification method that starts with a target of RNA and exponentially produces RNA amplicons. A cDNA copy is made using the original RNA and is used to produce millions of copies of RNA. TMA is an isothermal assay that is used to detect microorganisms (e.g., *Mycobacterium tuberculosis*).

Nucleic Acid Sequence–Based Amplification (NASBA)

NASBA is similar to TMA, but only RNA is targeted for amplification. Its applications include the detection and quantitation of HIV and detection of cytomegalovirus (CMV).

Signal Amplification Methods

Branched DNA. Branched DNA (bDNA) is a quantitative test that uses signal amplification instead of target amplification to amplify the hybridization signal. Target DNA or RNA is hybridized at different sites by two types of probes. Branched DNA assays are used to measure the viral load of hepatitis B virus (HBV), hepatitis C virus (HCV), HIV-1, CMV, and microbial organisms (e.g., *Trypanosoma brucei*).

The Versant HIV-1 RNA 3.0 assay (Bayer, Berkeley, CA) uses bDNA technology. It is the only viral load assay specifically designed to target multiple sequences of the HIV-1 genome with more than 80 nucleic acid probes.

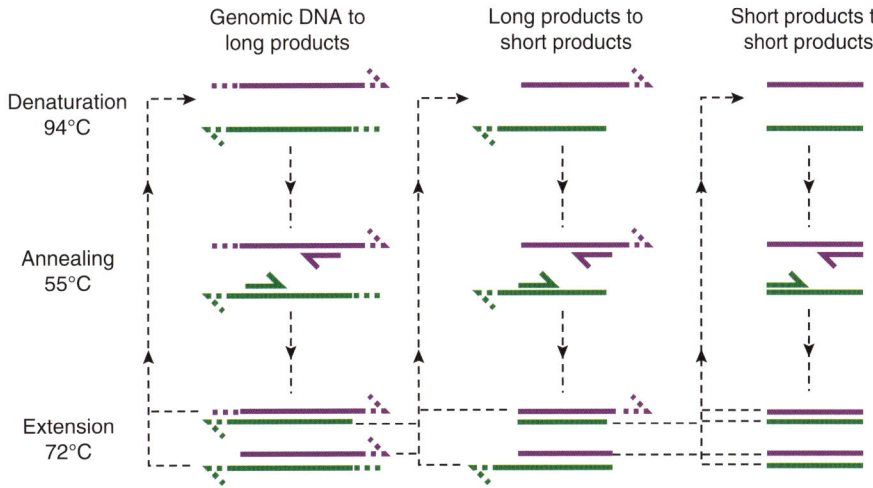

Fig. 12.8 Polymerase Chain Reaction. Repetitive cycles of denaturation, annealing, and extension are paced by temperature cycling of the reaction. Two primers indicated as short segments anneal to opposite template strands *(long line)* to define the region to be amplified. Extension occurs from the 3′ ends *(half-arrowheads)*. In each cycle, genomic DNA is denatured and annealed to primers that extend in opposite directions across the same region, producing long products of undefined length. Long products generated by extension of one of the primers anneal to the other primer during the next cycle, producing short products of defined length. Any short products present also produce more short products. After *n* cycles, up to 2*n* new copies of the amplified region are present—*n* long products and (2*nn* − *n*) short products plus one original genomic copy. A similar approach can be used to amplify RNA targets by initial reverse transcription of the RNA template to produce the DNA template. (From Burtis CA, Ashwood ER, Bruns DB: *Tietz fundamentals of clinical chemistry,* ed 6, St. Louis, 2008, Saunders.)

Serial Invasive Signal Amplification

Serial invasive signal amplification is a signal-enhancing technique that combines two invasive signal amplification reactions in series in a single tube. The cleaved 5′-arm from the target-specific primary reaction is used to drive a secondary invasive reaction, resulting in a total signal amplification of more than seven orders of magnitude in about 4 hours.

Probe Amplification Methods

Probe-based DNA detection systems (e.g., ligase chain reaction [LCR]) have the advantage of providing sequence specificity and lower detection limits.

The LCR amplifies probes rather than the target DNA. LCR is one of many techniques developed in recent years to detect specific nucleic acid sequences by amplification of nucleic acid targets. Simple LCR consists of two complementary oligonucleotide pairs (four oligonucleotides, 20–35 nucleotides each) that are homologous to adjacent sequences on the target DNA, as opposed to two used in the PCR assay. The adjacent pairs are ligated when they hybridize to the complementary sequence next to each other in a 32 to 52 orientation on the same strand of the target DNA. The 52 nucleotides of the ends of the primers to be ligated must be phosphorylated. Newly ligated oligonucleotides become targets in subsequent cycles, so logarithmic amplification occurs. At low frequency, the two complementary pairs can also be blunt-end ligated to each other and serve as a template for amplification, even though no target sequence was present in the original sample.

LCR has been used for genotyping studies to detect tumors and identify the presence of specific genetic disorders. LCR is now recognized as the method of choice for detection of urogenital infections due to its greater sensitivity compared with traditional cell culture, nonamplified DNA probes, or antigen-detection assays.

Strand Displacement Amplification

Strand displacement amplification (SDA) amplifies a probe instead of the original target DNA. SDA is a fully automated method that amplifies target nucleic acid without the use of a thermocycler, an instrument most commonly used in the laboratory to amplify segments of DNA (fragments) in PCR by raising and lowering the temperature in preprogrammed steps. A double-strand DNA (dsDNA) fragment is created and becomes the target for exponential amplification. This amplification technique uses two types of primers, DNA polymerase and a restriction endonuclease, to exponentially produce single-strand amplicons asynchronously.

Alternative Target Amplification Techniques

Other techniques are used as variations of amplification techniques. These include:

- Target loop-mediated isothermal amplification (LAMP). A single tube technique for the amplification of DNA that uses a single temperature incubation.
- Target whole-genome amplification (WGA). A nonspecific amplification technique that produces an amplified product representative of the initial starting material (whole genome).
- Target antisense RNA amplification (asRNA). A single-strand RNA that is complementary to an mRNA strand transcribed within a cell.

MOLECULAR ANALYSIS OF AMPLIFICATION PRODUCTS

Molecular genetic analysis focuses on the examination of nucleic acids (DNA or RNA) by special techniques to determine whether a specific nucleotide base sequence is present. The analysis of PCR amplification products (amplimers) is an essential step in determining the quality (i.e., the presence or absence of nonspecific amplimers) and quantity (relative values or exact values) of the DNA target that has been amplified.

Molecular diagnostics detection techniques use both generic and specific methods of nucleic detection. Specific methods of detection and quantification usually use sequence-specific primers or probes

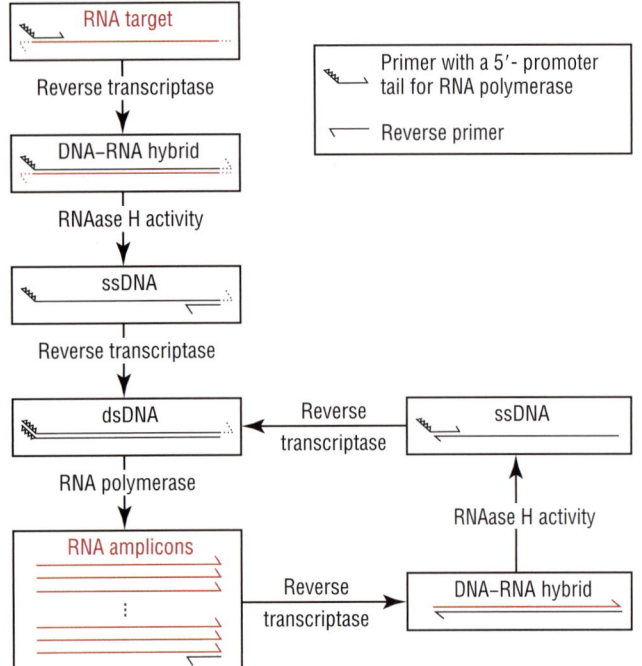

Fig. 12.9 Schematic Diagram of Transcription-Mediated Amplification (TMA). Starting with a single-strand RNA target, a primer with an RNA polymerase promoter on its 5′ end is extended by reverse transcriptase to form a DNA–RNA hybrid. The reverse transcriptase also has RNAase H activity that subsequently degrades the RNA strand to leave single-strand DNA (ssDNA). A second primer then binds to the ssDNA, and an extension forms double-strand DNA (dsDNA) with the attached RNA polymerase promoter. RNA polymerase then makes 100 to 1000 copies of RNA, some of which are again primed by the second primer. Repeated cycles of reverse transcription, DNA–RNA hybrid degradation by RNAase H activity, dsDNA formation by reverse transcriptase, and further transcription by RNA polymerase exponentially produce ssRNA amplicons. Single-strand targets are amplified isothermally, and double-strand targets are first denatured to single strands. (From Rifai N: *Tietz textbook of clinical chemistry and molecular diagnostics,* ed 6, St. Louis, 2018, Elsevier.)

with fluorescent or electronic detection. Many of the revolutionary changes that have occurred in research in the biological sciences, particularly the Human Genome Project, can be directly attributed to the ability to manipulate DNA in defined ways.

Examples of molecular methods that are nucleic acid discrimination techniques include:

1. Electrophoresis methods that physically separate nucleic acids based on molecular size or shape (Table 12.2). Primary applications can be detection, sequencing, genotyping, quantification, or scanning.
2. Pyrosequencing, or sequencing by a synthesis method that does not require dideoxy-termination or electrophoresis.
3. Hybridization assays that identify specific NAs by annealing or melting of complementary NAs.

Note: Some methods use both electrophoresis and hybridization.

Electrophoresis-Based Techniques
Polymerase Chain Reaction Product Length

Detection of DNA products by PCR is used frequently to determine product size and specificity. If the nucleic acid of interest is RNA rather than DNA, the PCR procedures can be modified to include the conversion of RNA to DNA using reverse transcriptase (RT) in the initial steps.

There are two main methods of visualizing the PCR products: (1) staining of the amplified DNA product with a chemical dye (e.g., ethidium bromide), which intercalates between the two strands of the duplex, or (2) labeling the PCR primers or nucleotides with fluorescent dyes (fluorophores) prior to PCR amplification. The latter method allows the labels to be directly incorporated into the PCR product. The most widely used method for analyzing the PCR product is the use of agarose gel electrophoresis, which separates DNA products on the basis of size and charge. Agarose gel electrophoresis is the easiest method of visualizing and analyzing the PCR product. It allows for determination of the presence and size of the PCR product. A predetermined set of DNA products with known sizes are run simultaneously on the gel as standardized molecular markers to help determine the size of the product.

PCR products can be visualized by staining the gel with a fluorescent DNA-binding dye, such as ethidium bromide. Ethidium bromide is a dye that intercalates into nucleic acids and will fluoresce with an orange color under ultraviolet (UV) irradiation. An image analyzer uses UV light to capture computer images of the PCR products. This technique is simply an extra step after a PCR assay has been run. DNA and other biomolecules can be separated based on charge, size, and shape. DNA has a net negative charge and will migrate toward the anode (positive pole) with an appropriately buffered solution.

Small insertions, deletions, rearrangements, and changes in the number of repeated sequences can be detected by monitoring PCR product length on gels. Length differences may be large and easily seen using agarose gel electrophoresis, but they may be small and require a denaturing polyacrylamide matrix. Fluorescent primers may be added to the product during PCR to simplify detection of fragment lengths.

Real-Time Fluorescent Methods

The presence of an amplification product may be directly diagnostic if a detected sequence is found only in a virus, bacteria, or fungus in a human specimen. RT-PCR is useful in the identification of RNA viral agents, such as coronaviruses, influenza A and B viruses, HIV, and HCV. The technique also can be used in the diagnosis of genetic disorders and in identity assessment.

TaqMan Assays and SYBR Green Dye–Based Assays

Many real-time fluorescent PCR methods exist, but the most widely used are the 5′ nuclease assays, such as TaqMan assays and SYBR Green dye–based assays.

TaqMan Method

TaqMan is one of the most frequently used probes because of the ease of probe design and low levels of background fluorescence. TaqMan probes are hydrolysis probes that are designed to increase the specificity of quantitative PCR. The TaqMan probe principle relies on the 5′–3′ exonuclease activity of Taq polymerase to cleave a dual-labeled probe during hybridization to the complementary target sequence and fluorophore-based detection. TaqMan functions to amplify the DNA for the production of multiple copies of it. In addition, Taq DNA polymerase is a thermostable DNA polymerase that can work at a high temperature.

There are three steps in the detection of PCR products by TaqMan probes (Fig. 12.10):

1. The TaqMan probe is composed of about 20 bases of DNA complementary to a specific region of the target gene. This technique uses a fluorophore reporter and a fluorophore quencher. A fluorophore reporter is a genetically encoded fluorescent tag that

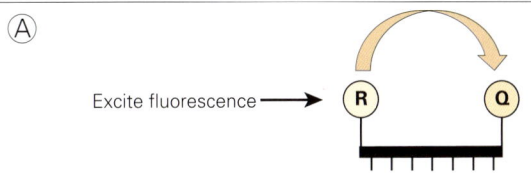

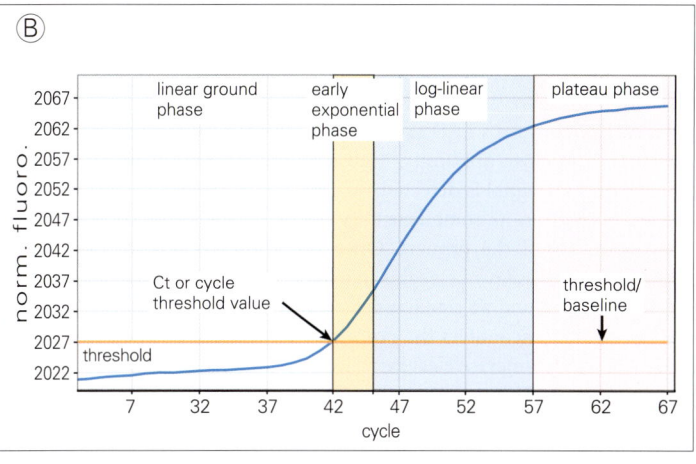

Step 1: The intact TaqMan probe consists of approximately 20 bases of DNA complementary to a specific region of the target gene. A reporter (R) fluorophore and a quencher fluorophore (Q) are attached to the 5' and 3' ends respectively. When fluorescence is excited by the thermal cycler's LED, the quencher, due to its close proximity, absorbs fluorescence from the reporter and no signal is detected.

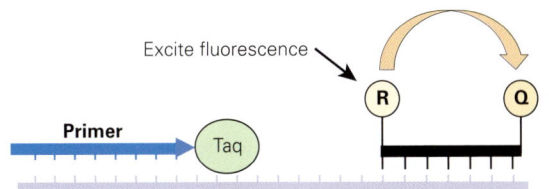

Step 2: The probe binds to its complementary region on the target strand, together with one of the primers. Now that the primer is bound, the Taq polymerase begins to extend it, moving towards the probe, which is still intact and so no signal is detected.

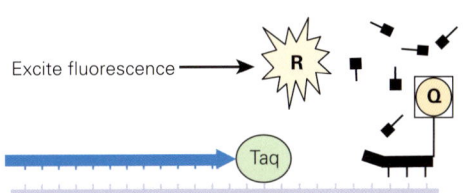

Step 3: As the Taq encounters the probe, the inherent 5'-3' nuclease activity of the polymerase cleaves nucleotides and releases the reporter fluorophore. The reporter is now free from quenching and able to fluoresce and its signal detected.

Fig. 12.10 Real-Time Polymerase Chain Reaction (PCR). (A) The steps involved in real-time detection of PCR products by TaqMan probes. (B) A typical S-shaped real-time PCR amplification curve. The number of cycles in the reaction is shown on the x-axis, and the levels of fluorescence, derived from the TaqMan probe and representing the accumulating amplicon, are shown on the y-axis. The threshold or baseline value can be set by the user. The cycle threshold (Ct) value represents the PCR cycle number as the exponential phase of amplification begins. P.l-time PCR amplification curve. (From Goering RV, Dockrell HV, Zuckerman M, Chiodini PL: *Mims' medical microbiology and immunology*, ed 6, 2019, Elsevier, p. 432.)

TABLE 12.2 Examples of Electrophoresis-Based Techniques

Technique	Abbreviation	Primary Application
Polymerase chain reaction (PCR) for reverse transcriptase PCR length	PCR for RT-PCR	Detection
Southern blotting	–	Detection
Dideoxy-termination sequencing (Sanger)	–	Sequencing
Single-nucleotide extension assay	SNE	Genotyping
Oligonucleotide ligation assay	OLA	Genotyping
Multiplex ligation-dependent probe amplification	MLPA	Quantification
Temperature-cycling capillary electrophoresis	TCCE	Scanning
Temperature gradient electrophoresis	TGGE, TGCE	Scanning
Single-strand conformation polymorphism analysis	SSCP, SSCA	Scanning
Denaturing gradient gel electrophoresis	DGGE	Scanning

Adapted from Wittwer CT, Makrigiorgos GM: Important terms and definitions, in *Tietz textbook of clinical chemistry and molecular diagnostics*, ed 6, Chapter 47, Nucleic Acid Techniques, Table 47.2, p. 973.

178 PART II The Theory of Immunologic and Serologic Procedures

is composed of protein sequences that can be fused to a protein of interest to render it fluorescent. A fluorophore quencher absorbs fluorescence. The fluorophore reporter and the fluorophore quencher are attached to the 5′ and 3′ ends of the target gene. A thermocycler's LED excites the fluorescence. Because the quencher is in close proximity, it absorbs fluorescence from the reporter and no signal is detected.

2. The probe binds to its complementary region on the target strand along with one of the primers. Once the primer is bound, the TaqMan polymerase probe begins to extend it, moving toward the still-intact probe, and no signal is detected.

3. As the TaqMan encounters the probe, the inherent 5′–3′ nuclease activity of the polymerase cleaves nucleotides and releases the fluorophore reporter. The reporter is now free from quenching and able to fluoresce, thus allowing its signal to be detected.

SYBR Green

SYBR Green is a green fluorescent cyanine dye that has a high affinity for dsDNA in agarose and polyacrylamide gels. The mode of binding is believed to be a combination of DNA intercalation and external binding. When bound, SYBR absorbs at a wavelength around 497 nm and emits fluorescence around 520 nm.

SYBR Green nucleic acid gel stain is considered to be one of the most sensitive methods available for detecting dsDNA. It is especially useful for assays in which the presence of contaminating RNA or ssDNA might obscure results. This method has exceptionally low background fluorescence and spectral characteristics that closely match light sources and filter sets in existing instruments. It is ideal for use with laser scanners.

Sanger (Chain Termination) Sequencing

The Human Genome Project was completed using first-generation deoxyribonucleic acid (DNA) sequencing. Currently, massive parallel sequencing is used for genome sequencing, but this method developed out of earlier sequencing using the conventional Sanger method developed in 1975. It can be used to confirm nucleotide changes seen with the newer massively parallel sequencing/next-generation sequencing (NGS) technology.

The conventional Sanger sequencing (Fig. 12.11) of genomes was the technology used for the initiation of the Human Genome Project. Members of the genome sequencing consortium methodically sequenced in 700 base reactions. Each round of sequencing depends on the sequencing data from the prior round. Assembly of data by conventional sequencing is not as computationally intensive as massively parallel or shotgun sequencing.

Shotgun sequencing was the key to the speedy completion of the Human Genome Project. This method relied on random shearing of DNA and subcloning of the fragments into plasmids. The plasmids were sequenced in parallel, separate reactions. The evolutionary roots of massively parallel sequencing technology can be traced back to shotgun sequencing.

Since the completion of the Human Genome (sequence) Project in 2003, new horizons have opened up, especially massively parallel sequencing/NGS. Second-generation sequencing, or NGS, analyzes

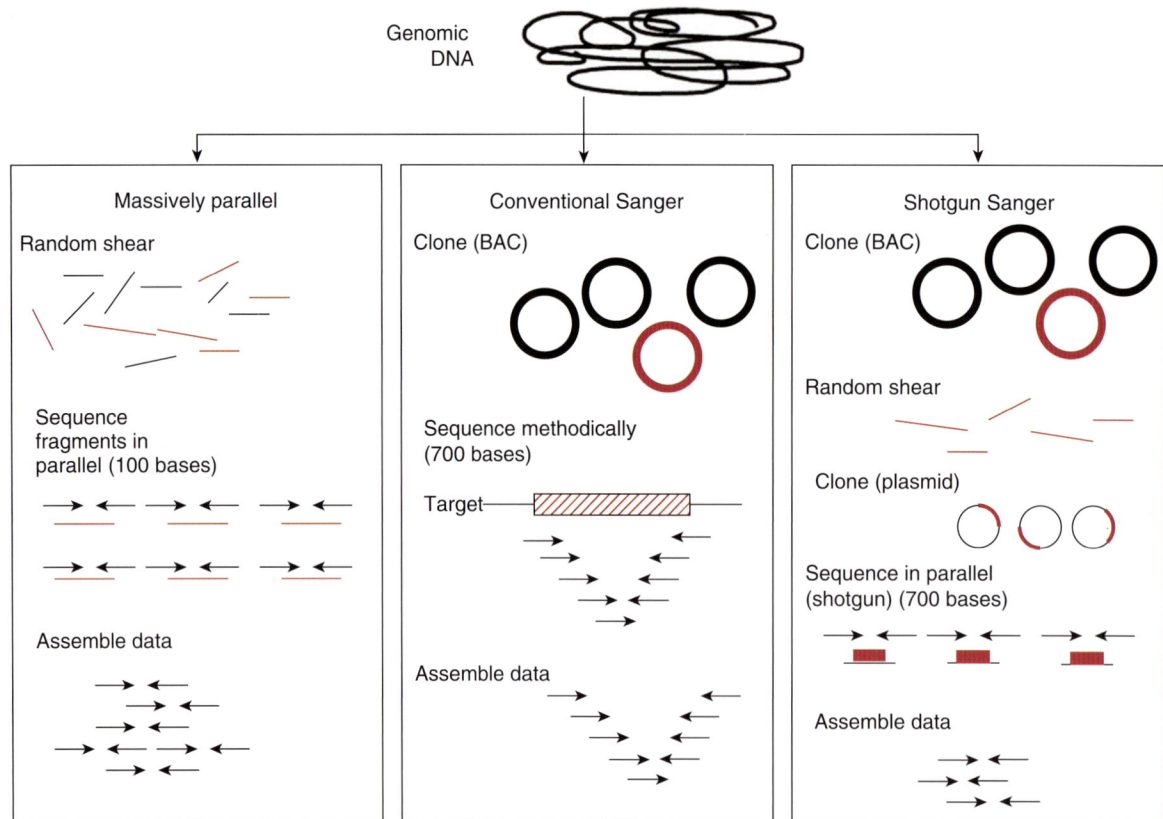

Fig. 12.11 Genome-Sequencing Approaches. Massively parallel sequencing *(left panel)* is the current technology used for genome sequencing, but it evolved out of earlier conventional Sanger *(middle panel)* and shotgun Sanger *(right panel)* sequencing methods. *BAC,* Bacterial artificial chromosomes. (From Rifai N: *Tietz textbook of clinical chemistry and molecular diagnostics,* ed 6, St. Louis, 2018, Elsevier.)

millions of fragments of DNA in sequenced unison from a single patient specimen. The creation of NGS platforms has made sequencing accessible to many laboratories and has expanded the clinical use of nucleic acid sequencing. However, there can be errors using NGS, because the human genome is still not 100% mapped and there are several gaps that need to be completed.

DNA sequencing is considered to be the gold standard to which other molecular methods are compared. DNA sequencing displays the exact nucleotide or base sequence of a fragment of DNA that is targeted. The Sanger method, which uses a series of enzymatic reactions to produce segments of DNA complementary to the DNA being sequenced, is the most commonly used method for DNA sequencing. Automated sequencing techniques use primers with four different fluorescent labels.

1. The first step in sequencing a target is usually to amplify it by cloning or in vitro amplification, usually through PCR. Once the amplified DNA is purified from the clinical specimen (the target DNA), it is heat-denatured to separate the dsDNA into ssDNA.
2. The second step involves adding primers to the ssDNA. Primers are short synthetic segments of ssDNA that contain a nucleotide sequence complementary to a short strand of target DNA. The patient's DNA serves as a template to copy. DNA polymerase catalyzes the addition of the appropriate nucleotides to the preexisting primer. DNA synthesis is terminated when the di-deoxynucleotide is incorporated into a growing DNA chain.

Alternatives to Electrophoresis

Scanning methods have mostly been replaced with direct dideoxy-sequencing and massively parallel sequencing or NGS. Both of these methods not only identify that a variant is present but also provide the variant sequence. However, alternatives do exist that do not require electrophoresis.

Pyrosequencing

Pyrosequencing is based on a technique in which a sequencing primer is hybridized to a single-strand template generated by PCR. As the process is repeated by adding one of the four individual **deoxynucleotides** (dNTPs), the generation of visible light occurs. The light produced is proportional to the number of nucleotides incorporated. A nucleotide-degrading enzyme continuously degrades adenosine triphosphate (ATP) and unincorporated dNTP in the mixture. This switches off the light prior to the next dNTP addition. Through the process of repeatedly adding one dNTP at a time, the complementary strand is built and the nucleotide sequence is determined.

Pyrosequencing is a useful technique because it is a quick and cost-effective method for quantifying point mutations and indels. The three types of DNA mutations can be base substitutions, deletions, or insertions. SNPs, or point mutations (e.g., sickle cell disease), are the most common type of mutation. SNPs and indels represent the two other types of DNA mutations, insertions and deletions, respectively. Pyrosequencing is additionally useful in methylation analysis. Methylation can be involved in regulation of gene expression, regulation of protein function, and RNA metabolism.

Hybridization Assays (Box 12.2)

Hybridization reactions can be divided into the solid phase type, in which either probe or target is tethered to a solid support while the other is in solution, and the solution phase type, in which both are in solution.

Many forms of probe hybridization assays involve the complementary pairing of a probe with a DNA or RNA strand derived from the patient's specimen. The common feature of probe hybridization assays

---

BOX 12.2 Examples of Hybridization Assays

Solid-Phase Hybridization
Dot blot and line probe assays
Arrays (microarrays and medium-density arrays)
Micro-bead assays
In situ hybridization
Southern and Northern blotting assays
Massively parallel sequencing on beads or planar flow cells

Solution-Phase Hybridization
Real-time (for homogeneous) polymerase chain reaction
Melting analysis
Single-molecule sequencing

---

is the use of a labeled nucleic acid probe to examine a specimen for a specific, homologous DNA or RNA sequence. Clinical probes are usually labeled with nonradioisotopic molecules (e.g., digoxigenin, alkaline phosphatase, or biotin) or a fluorescent compound. The detection systems are conjugate dependent and include chemiluminescent, fluorescent, and calorimetric methodologies.

In the liquid-phase hybridization (LPH) assay, the target nucleic acid and labeled probe interact in solution. Specific homologous hybrids are subsequently separated from the remaining nucleic acid component, and the hybrids are identified by an appropriate detection system. LPH is used extensively in many assays now because it can be multiplexed and automated, and is a high-throughput technique for tests such as human leukocyte antigen (HLA) typing.

Fluorescence In Situ Hybridization

Fluorescence in situ hybridization (FISH) is a tissue-based molecular diagnostic assay that uses fluorescent molecules to brightly "paint" genes or chromosomes. The FISH molecular cytogenetic technique uses recombinant DNA technology. Probes are short sequences of ssDNA that are complementary to the DNA sequences to be examined. Probes hybridize, or bind, to the cDNA, and labeled fluorescent tags indicate the location of the sequences. Probes can be locus specific, centromeric repeat probes, or whole-chromosome probes.

Principle of the Fluorescence In Situ Hybridization Technique

In the FISH technique, a probe is a specifically designed sequence of nucleic acid—usually DNA—that is labeled with a fluorescent compound, and the target is DNA or RNA from the patient being tested. In metaphase FISH, a specific probe is bound to the homologous segment on a metaphase chromosome or, more commonly, on interphase nuclei affixed to a glass slide. Metaphase chromosomes are more open and receptive to probes. Uniquely, the existence of a region-specific DNA sequence in a nondividing cell can be detected using interphase FISH.

After exposure of the patient sample to the probe and a washing step, the presence of the fluorochrome in the sample indicates that the target sequence is present. Because fluorescence microscopy is required, the target may have a weak fluorescent counterstain to permit it to be seen, but the primary fluorescent material is the probe.

Use of Fluorescence In Situ Hybridization in the Clinical Laboratory

FISH is generally better for detection of deletions and inversions than PCR. It can be used to assess DNA or mRNA. FISH is in essence the next generation of cytogenetic techniques after banding. The results of FISH can be correlated with microscopic tissue morphology.

The FISH technique requires a fluorescent microscope. Probes must be specifically designed, because FISH can only be used to detect the presence or absence of previously identified chromosomal aberrations. FISH cannot be used to identify new abnormalities. Limitations of FISH include only being able to look for larger amplifications and deletions. Additionally, with rearrangements, only detection of those specific breakpoints that flank the primer being used can be discovered. Therefore the possibility of missing infrequent translocation sites exists. FISH is labor intensive and does not have a high throughput of testing.

Clinical applications of FISH include the detection of inherited and acquired chromosomal mutations, including monosomy, polysomy, large deletions, insertions, rearrangements, and inversions. One of the primary uses is in detecting specific gene rearrangements. It has a resolution of about 10 million base pairs and can detect gene amplifications and deletions. Many genetic syndromes have been recognized through this technique. DiGeorge syndrome is an example of a chromosomal deletion leading to the loss of several genes. In addition, the FISH technique can detect and identify the species of *Mycobacterium* and *Candida* organisms.

Microarrays

Technology changed dramatically during the 12-year span of The Cancer Genome Atlas (TCGA) project. At the program's close, TCGA used microarrays for profiling copy number variants, methylation, and protein expression and high-throughput sequencing for characterizing DNA and RNA.

Microarray technology (Box 12.3) is very cost-effective and, along with massively parallel sequencing/NGS, it is at the forefront of molecular oncology. Microarrays are divided into three types based on the mode of preparation of the array:

1. **Spotted arrays** on glass are arrays made on glass microscope slides. This provides binding of high-density DNA by using slotted pins. It allows fluorescent labeling of the sample.
2. **Self-assembled arrays** are fiber-optic arrays made by the deposition of DNA synthesized on small polystyrene beads. The beads are deposited on the etched ends of the array. Different DNA can be synthesized on different beads, and applying a mixture of beads to the fiber-optic cable will make a randomly assembled array.
3. **In situ synthesized arrays** are made by chemical synthesis on a solid substrate. Chemical synthesis arrays are used in expression analysis, genotyping, and sequencing.

Microarray (DNA chip) technology has accelerated genetic analysis (Fig. 12.12). The DNA microarray is a tool used to determine whether the DNA from a particular individual contains an inherited mutation in genes such as *BRCA1* and *BRCA2*. Sometimes microarrays are also used to determine which drugs might be best prescribed for particular individuals because genes determine how our bodies handle the chemistry related to those drugs. With the advent of new DNA sequencing technologies, some of the tests for which microarrays were used in the past now use DNA sequencing instead. Because microarray testing still tends to be less expensive than NGS, microarrays may be used for very large studies and for some clinical testing.

Spotted Arrays on Glass

Originally, commercially available microarray technology was manufactured by Affymetrix (Santa Clara, CA). In 1995, the first study that used the term *microarray* explained how the expression

---

BOX 12.3 Types of Microarrays Based on the Types of Probes Used

1. **DNA microarrays** (gene chip, DNA chip, or biochip) measures DNA or uses DNA as a part of its detection system. Four different types of DNA microarrays: complementary DNA (cDNA) microarrays, oligo DNA microarrays, bacterial artificial chromosome (BAC) microarrays, and single-nucleotide polymorphism (SNP) microarrays.
2. **MM Chips study** interactions between DNA and protein. Chromatin immunoprecipitation + array hybridization or chromatin immunoprecipitation + next-generation sequence/massively parallel sequencing are the two techniques used.
3. **Protein microarrays** characterize hundreds of thousands of proteins. There are three types: analytic protein microarrays, functional protein microarrays, and reverse-phase protein microarrays.
4. **Peptide microarrays** are used for detailed analyses or optimization of protein–protein interactions, which helps in antibody recognition.
5. **Tissue microarrays** are mainly used in pathology.
6. **Cellular microarrays** (transfection microarrays, living cell microarrays) are used for screening large-scale chemical and genomic libraries and investigating the local cellular microenvironment.
7. **Chemical compound** microarrays are used for drug screening and drug discovery.
8. **Antibody microarrays** (antibody array or antibody chip) are protein-specific microarrays containing a collection of capture antibodies placed inside a microscope slide and used to detect antigens.
9. **Carbohydrate arrays** (glycoarrays) are used in screening proteomes that are carbohydrate binding, calculating protein binding affinities and automization of solid support synthesis for glycans.
10. **Phenotype microarrays** (PM) are mainly used in drug development, but they are also used in functional genomics and toxicologic testing.
11. **Reverse-phase protein microarrays** are mostly used in clinical trials, especially in the field of cancer, but they also have pharmaceutical uses and can be used in the study of biomarkers.
12. **Interferometric reflectance imaging sensor (IRIS)** is a biosensor that is used to analyze protein–protein, protein–DNA, and DNA–DNA interactions.

Adapted from https://www.ncbi.nlm.nih.gov. Accessed March 31, 2020.

---

of many genes could be monitored in parallel through the use of this new technology. A DNA microarray (also commonly known as a *DNA chip* or *biochip*) is easily performed and readily automated. Arrays are basically the product of bonding or direct synthesis of numerous microscopic DNA spots attached to a solid surface, often silicon-based support. The chip may be tailored to particular disease processes. These chips are used to examine the gene activity of thousands or tens of thousands of gene fragments and to identify genetic mutations using a hybridization reaction between the sequences on the microarray and a fluorescent sample. After hybridization, the chips are scanned with high-speed fluorescent detectors, and the intensity of each spot is quantitated (Fig. 12.13). The identity and amount of each sequence are revealed by the location and intensity of fluorescence displayed by each spot. Computers are used to analyze the data (Fig. 12.14). If the patient has a mutation, the individual's DNA will not bind properly to the DNA sequences on the chip that represent the "normal" sequence, but instead will bind to the sequence on the chip that represents the mutated DNA.

The Human Genome GeneChip set (HG-U133A, Affymetrix), consisting of two GeneChip arrays, contains almost 45,000 probe sets representing more than 39,000 transcripts derived from approximately 33,000

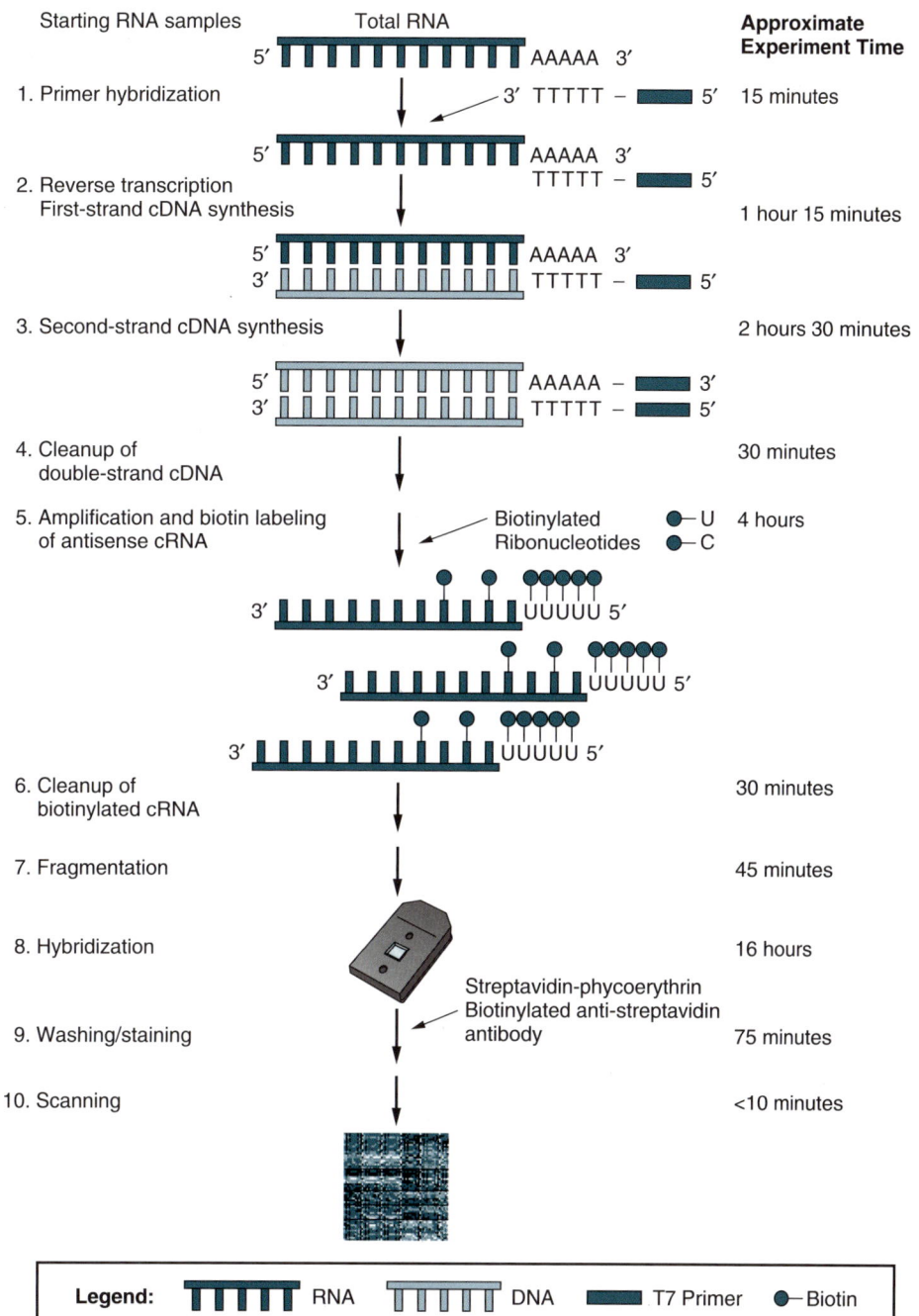

Fig. 12.12 Overview of Eukaryotic Target Labeling for GeneChip Expression Arrays. *cDNA*, Complementary DNA; *cRNA*, complementary RNA. (Courtesy Affymetrix, Santa Clara, CA.)

well-substantiated human genes. The sequence clusters were created from the UniGene database and then refined by analysis and comparison with a number of other publicly available databases (e.g., Washington University expressed sequence tag [EST] trace repository and University of California, Santa Cruz, Golden Path human genome database).

The HG-U133A array includes representation of the RefSeq database sequences and probe sets related to sequences previously represented on the Human Genome U95Av2 array. The HG-U133B array contains primarily probe sets representing EST clusters. The applications of this array include defining tissue and cell type–specific gene expression and investigating cellular and tissue responses to the environment (e.g., heat shock, interactions with other cells, exposure to chemical compounds, growth factors, or other signaling molecules). In addition, this array helps elucidate human cell differentiation by (1) determining which transcripts are increased or decreased during distinct stages in cellular differentiation, and (2) detecting which genes are uniquely expressed during different stages of **tumorigenesis**, the creation or formation of a mass of cells (i.e., a tumor).

Self-Assembled Arrays

An example of a self-assembled genomic microarray is the one manufactured by Illumina (San Diego, CA). This company offers high-density silica bead–based microarray technology. Bead array microarray technology is based on 3-micron silica beads that self-assemble in

182 PART II The Theory of Immunologic and Serologic Procedures

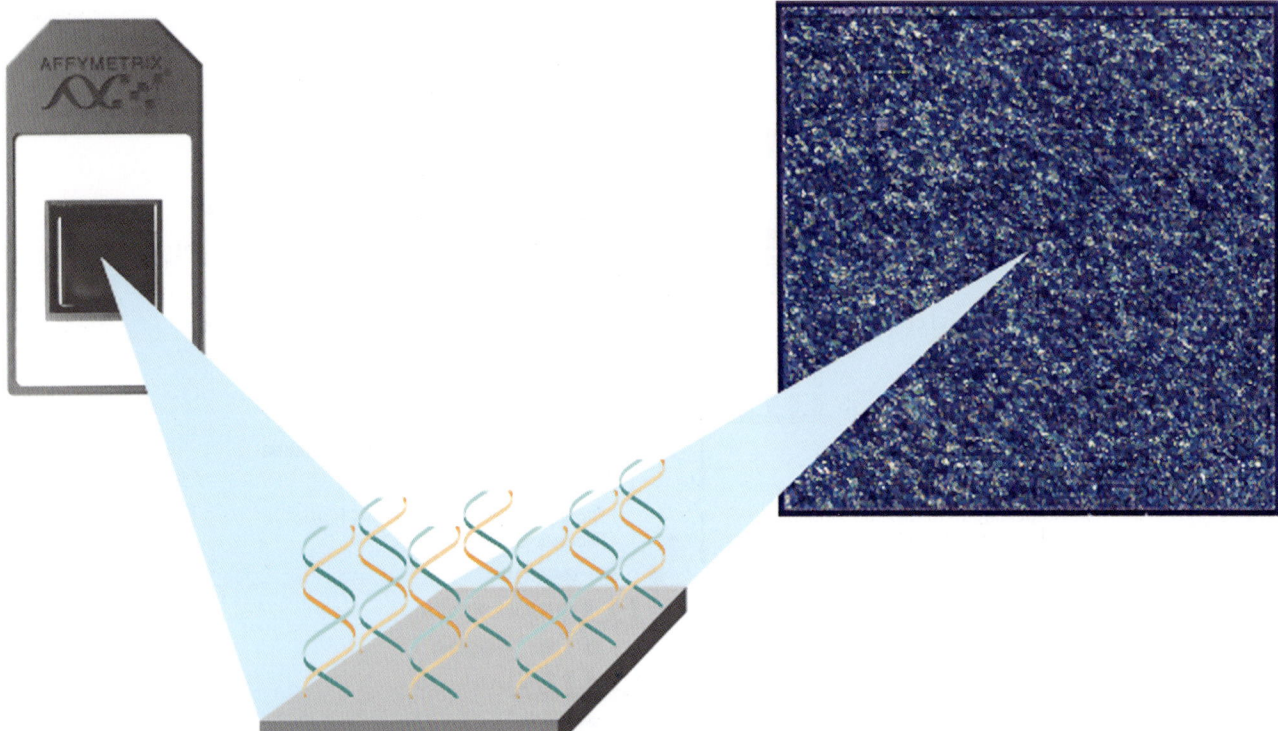

Fig. 12.13 Data from an Experiment Showing the Expression of Thousands of Genes on a Single GeneChip Probe Array.

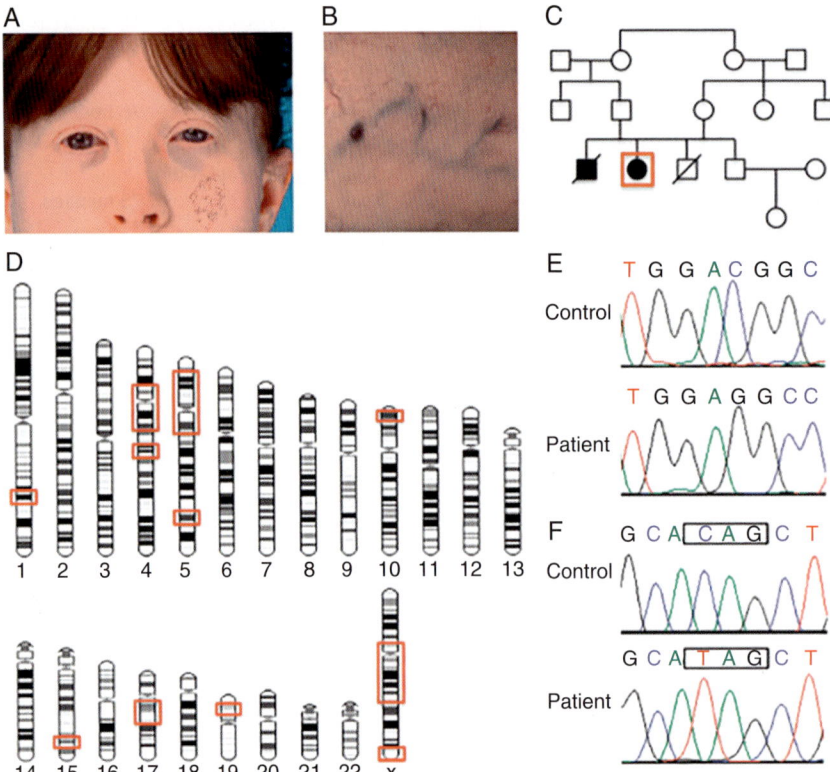

Fig. 12.14 Clinical Application of Whole-Exome Sequencing. This figure depicts the use of homozygosity mapping, followed by whole-exome sequencing, to identify two disease-causing mutations in a patient with oculocutaneous albinism and congenital neutropenia. (A and B) The common phenotypic traits. (C) A pedigree of the patient's family, both the affected and unaffected individuals. (D) Graphic chromosome map that highlights the areas of genetic homozygosity. These regions were identified by single-nucleotide polymorphism (SNP) analysis and were identified as possible locations for the disease-causing mutation(s). (E and F) Chromatograms for the two disease-causing mutations identified by whole-exome sequencing. (E) The mutation in SLC45A2. (F) The mutation in G6PC3. (From Grada A, Weinbrecht K: Next-generation sequencing: methodology and application, *J Invest Dermatol* 133[8]:1–4, 2013.)

microwells on either of two substrates: fiber-optic bundles or planar silica slides. When randomly assembled on one of these two substrates, the beads have a uniform spacing of about 5.7 microns. Each bead is covered with hundreds of thousands of copies of a specific oligonucleotide that act as the capture sequences in a given Illumina assay. This methodology uses target DNA hybridization with single-base extension enzymology. It allows copy number analysis by SNP analysis, molecular oncology, and genome-wide DNA methylation analysis.

DNA Methylation Analysis

Array-based methodologies have evolved to enable genome-scale DNA methylation analysis through advances in methylation detection methods and development of new high-density arrays. Affymetrix and Illumina produce methylation detection devices.

Affymetrix arrays. Affymetrix provides several array platforms that have been used in a number of methylation studies. The *Arabidopsis* tiling 1.0 array method showed improved sensitivity and resolution over the traditional methylated DNA immunoprecipitation (MeDIP) method. It is highly sensitive and has a low incidence of false positives. The major advance with the bioconductor immunoprocessing (BiMP) approach is the reduced amplification bias in the bisulfite-converted DNA, which enables preparation of genome-wide probes for high-density tiling arrays. Because a small amount of DNA can be used for whole genome–wide DNA methylation analysis using BiMP, this is a new opportunity for genome-wide DNA methylation analysis from small tissue samples or analysis of DNA methylation during embryogenesis.

Illumina assays

Illumina bead arrays provide one of the most advanced array-based approaches for large-scale DNA methylation analysis. The Illumina platform for DNA methylation analysis using the GoldenGate genotyping assay is implemented on a bead array platform. The bead array enables probes to be specifically designed for most CpG sites (a site where cytosine [C] lies next to guanine [G] in the DNA sequence). The p indicates that C and G are connected by a phosphodiester bond. This matrix bead array has 99.9% accuracy. In the future, this technology might be useful for identifying DNA methylation signatures in different cancers and other pathologic conditions.

Advantages and Disadvantages of Array-Based Methods

Compared with deep sequencing approaches (i.e., sequencing a genomic region multiple times, sometimes hundreds or even thousands of times), a major advantage to using array-based platforms for DNA methylation analysis is the ease of performing assays with limited expertise. The data obtained from array-based platforms is easier to interpret through the use of many easy-to-operate software programs. There are several drawbacks to array-based methods compared with NGS. These drawbacks include the fact that arrays have lower resolution, and designing specific probes that can distinguish one repetitive sequence from another in a hybridization-based method is not easy.

MASSIVELY PARALLEL SEQUENCING/NEXT-GENERATION SEQUENCING TECHNOLOGY

An important recent use of NGS technology has been in the discovery of novel human coronaviruses (e.g., SARS-CoV-2). In addition to detection, the other applications of NGS include:
- Performing surveillance screening and epidemiology
- Tracking mutations
- Analyzing human response to disease

Other clinical applications of NGS include high-resolution sequencing of HLA alleles, targeted oncology panels, and inherited disease panels.

Advances in optical data processing, bioinformatics, and computer power have stimulated increased demand for NGS. Cost, turnaround time, and convenience are factors that also contribute to increased demand for NGS. NGS methods have different underlying technical features, such as biochemistries and sequencing protocols.

Compared with dideoxy-termination, massively parallel sequencing/NGS technology generates more bases of sequence data in one test run at a lower cost per base. High-throughput sequencing technologies are capable of sequencing multiple DNA molecules in parallel, enabling hundreds of millions of DNA molecules to be sequenced at a time. Manufacturers of first- through third-generation high-throughput sequencing technologies include Fisher Scientific, Life Technologies (Waltham, MA), Illumina, Applied Biosystems (San Diego, CA), and Pacific Biosciences (Menlo Park, CA). Recent advances in NGS technology have unveiled a more comprehensive view of the transcriptome, enabling identification of both small and large RNAs, splice isoforms, and novel transcripts from unannotated genes. However, the amount of possible data generated presents challenges. There is a need for better methods of NGS data analysis, including RNA-Seq bias correction and improved isoform quantification.

Clonal sequencing methods replicate a single DNA strand to form a clonal template in order to generate sufficient signal for detection. Characteristics of massively parallel sequencing methods are summarized in Table 12.3. In emulsion PCR, one strand of a library element is captured on one bead and is clonally amplified inside a water-in-oil

TABLE 12.3 Characteristics of Next-Generation Sequencing (NGS) or Massively Parallel Sequencing Methods

Method	Principle	Detection	Clonal	Read Length (bp)
Synthesis	Pyrophosphate release	Chemiluminescence	Emulsion PCR	400–700
Synthesis	pH change	Electronic CMOS	Emulsion PCR	125–400
Synthesis	Reversible terminator	Fluorescence	Bridge amplification	200–600[a]
Ligation	Multiple ligation events	Fluorescence	Emulsion PCR	110
Single molecule	Zeta-mode waveguide	Fluorescence	No	10 kb
Single molecule	Conductivity	Electronic	No	5 kb

[a]Includes both paired-end reads (sequencing from both ends).
CMOS, Complementary metal oxide semiconductor; *PCR*, polymerase chain reaction.
Adapted from Wittwer CT, Makrigiorgos GM: Important terms and definitions, in *Tietz textbook of clinical chemistry and molecular diagnostics*, ed 6, Chapter 47, Nucleic Acid Techniques, Table 47.2, p. 973.

droplet; this generates a bead cover with single-strand PCR products. In contrast, bridge amplification generates clusters of single-strand PCR products tethered to a flat surface flow cell. Sequencing by synthesis can be detected by three different methods.

These clonal amplification methods allow parallel observation of thousands to millions of strand extensions, which increases signal strength. Sequencing by ligase uses a ligase mixture of probes about eight bases long. The template is either a clonal bead formed by emulsion PCR or a colony formed by isothermal amplification directly on a flat surface. Although the ligase method is massively parallel, the read length averages less than 75 bases.

Target Enrichment Strategies

NGS technologies have been developed in the past decade. This approach overcomes the limitations of traditional Sanger sequencing by providing highly parallel sequencing with a separate sequence result for every sequence of interest. This has positioned NGS as the method of choice for targeted resequencing of regions of the human genome (Fig. 12.15).

Molecular characterization of tumors typically includes Sanger sequencing (described previously) of a limited number of genes known to harbor mutations with well-described clinical appearances. If several genes need to be studied, Sanger sequencing can be costly and time-consuming. NGS technologies (Box 12.4) have the potential to be more cost-effective and be able to simultaneously sequence complete genomes of patients to deliver personalized medicine. NGS can produce thousands to millions of genome sequences at once, compared with the 96 sequences processed by the traditional Sanger method. Although sequencing of the entire human genome is possible, physicians are typically interested in only the protein-coding regions of the genome, the exome. The exome comprises slightly more than 1% of the genome. Exome sequencing is helpful in the identification of disease-causing mutations when the genetic cause is unknown.

NGS technologies permit analysis of mutations (see Fig. 12.15), rearrangement, amplifications, and deletions (DNA sequencing), or

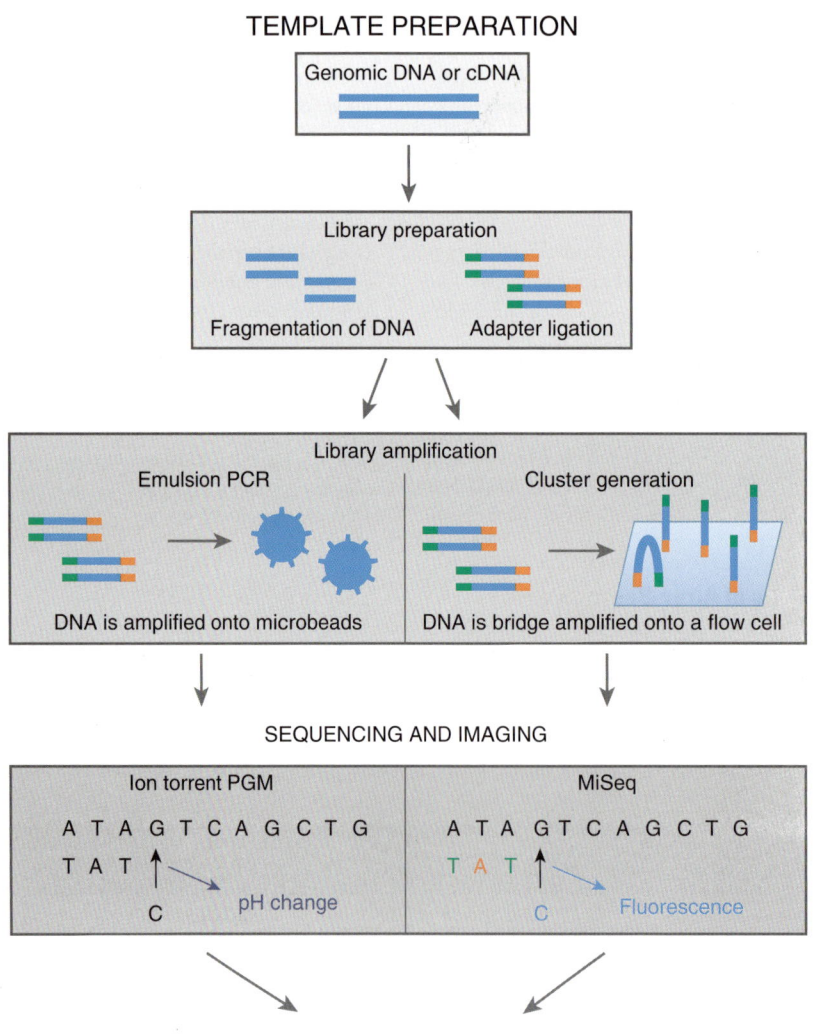

Fig. 12.15 Next-Generation Sequencing (Massively Parallel Sequencing): Methodology and Application. This is an overview of the sequencing methodology. Within each generalized step, the individual platforms have unique aspects. *cDNA*, Complementary DNA; *PCR*, polymerase chain reaction. (From Grada A, Weinbrecht K: Next-generation sequencing: methodology and application, *J Invest Dermatol* 133[8]:1–4, 2013.)

BOX 12.4 Advantages and Disadvantages of Massively Parallel Sequencing/Next-Generation Sequencing

Advantages
- Faster alternative to first-generation sequencing DNA than the traditional method.
- Targeted sequencing of the human genome provides identification of the disease-causing mutation.
- RNA sequencing can provide information on the entire transcriptome of a single specimen in one analysis without previous knowledge of the genetic sequence of an organism.
- A strong alternative to the use of microarrays in gene expression studies.

Disadvantages
- Expensive to establish next-generation sequencing (NGS) platforms.
- Potentially inaccurate results if spans of repeating nucleotides, homopolymer regions, occur.
- Short sequencing read lengths (average 200–500 nucleotides) can produce sequence errors.
- Challenging data analysis.

Other techniques include the hybridization protection assay, DNA enzyme immunoassay (EIA), automated DNA sequencing technology, single-strand conformational polymorphism, and restriction fragment length polymorphism (RFLP) analysis.

From Grada A, Weinbrecht K: Next-generation sequencing: methodology and application, *J Invest Dermatol* 133(8):1–4, 2013.

---

coding and noncoding RNA (RNA sequencing). Most clinically used assays are based on DNA sequencing. Commercial panels available through the Life Technologies' Ion Torrent Personal Genome Machine (PGM) One Touch system and Illumina are popular; some laboratories design their own panels based on genes of interest. NGS permits analysis of all the exomes or even entire genes. This has led to an expansion of the number of genes that can be analyzed at one time and identification of patients at risk.

NGS has various applications:
1. Identification of actionable mutations in cancer (usually a panel specific to that tumor site). Actionable mutation identification can potentially help patients with metastatic cancer who are resistant to standard therapies.
2. Risk assessment by looking for inherited disease mutations (point mutations or small indels). For example, NGS panels can analyze genes associated with an increased risk of breast cancer, including *BRCA1* and *BRCA2*.

Steps of Next-Generation Sequencing

Each NGS platform is unique in how sequencing is accomplished, but the generalized sequencing protocol for the two commercially available NGS platforms includes three steps:
1. Template preparation
2. Sequencing and imaging
3. Data analysis

Template preparation. This step consists of building a DNA or cDNA library and amplification of that library. A sequencing library is constructed by fragmenting the DNA or cDNA specimen and attaching adapter sequences, synthetic oligonucleotides of a known sequence, to the ends of the DNA fragments. A constructed library is clonally amplified in preparation for sequencing. Amplification of a single library fragment onto microbeads is unique to the Ion Torrent PGM One Touch system; bridge amplification is used to form template clusters on a flow cell by the Illumina MiSeq system.

Sequencing and imaging. For the next step, the two commercial systems rely on sequencing by synthesis. The library fragments act as a template from which a new DNA fragment is synthesized. Sequencing occurs through a cycle of washing and flooding the fragments with the known nucleotides in a sequential order. As nucleotides incorporate into a growing DNA strand, they are digitally recorded as a sequence. One system, PGM, carries out semiconductor sequencing that relies on detection of pH changes induced by the release of a hydrogen ion upon the incorporation of a nucleotide into a growing strand of DNA. The Illumina MiSeq relies on detection of fluorescence generated by the incorporation of fluorescently labeled nucleotides into the growing strand of DNA.

Data analysis. The final step after sequencing is complete is analysis of the raw sequence data, which requires several steps. Preprocessing of data removes adapter sequences and low-quality read; it also provides mapping of data to a reference genome or de novo alignment of the sequence reads and analysis of the compiled sequence. Analysis can include identification of somatic and germline mutations.

With NGS technology, the process begins with template preparation by shearing of DNA (or cDNA) to create fragment libraries. Adaptor sequences are added to these fragments and serve as primers for amplification, usually by emulsion PCR or bridge PCR methods. The resulting amplified signal beads or clusters are analyzed using a variety of platform-specific chemical analyses, but all are based on the addition of labeled nucleotides. Digital images are captured and analyzed to determine the sequence of the target DNA. The impact of NGS on cancer treatment is presented in Chapter 26, Tumor Immunology.

Adaptation of DNA Methylation Detection Technologies for NGS

Most NGS technologies provide very short DNA sequence reads. This makes genome-scale alignments and analysis of data a challenge, but NGS produces huge data files. Appropriate computational resources and bioinformatics tools are extremely important to facilitate alignment, assembly, and visualization of NGS data.

DNA methylation marks or processes not directly governed by the genetic code include methylation of DNA that is an important regulator of many different biological processes in a wide range of living organisms. However, many diseases that are regulated through epigenetic changes in organisms caused by modification of gene expression, rather than alteration of the genetic code itself, cannot be identified using regular DNA sequencing that does not enrich the methylated genomic compartment. Consequently, there is a need for future development of technologies (e.g., genome-wide RNA interference [RNAi] screens) to explore the mechanisms and consequences of different DNA methylation–associated changes and the regulation of numerous epigenetically silenced genes. Multiple types of cancers have been studied in large-scale genome-wide DNA methylation analysis with the goal of understanding the processes in stem cells and cancer, in addition to bacterial virulence.

CASE STUDY 12.1   History and Physical Examination

A 38-year-old man drove himself to the emergency department because of a worsening condition of shortness of breath. He felt tired and had a fever, sore throat, nonproductive cough, and mild chest pain. He had no history of serious medical conditions and was a lifelong nonsmoker.

During the past 5 years, he had been diagnosed with genital herpes and gonorrhea. He reported having persistent diarrhea for the past several months. He also noted a weight loss during the same period. He and his male partner had unprotected intercourse for several years. There was no history of intravenous drug use.

Physical examination revealed an underweight man with palpable lymph nodes. Plaques of *Candida albicans* were seen in the back of his throat. His chest sounds had diffuse crackles in both lungs.

Laboratory assays and a chest x-ray were ordered. He was referred to counseling because of his high-risk status for HIV and AIDS.

Laboratory Results

Assay	Patient Results	Reference Range
Hemoglobin	10.5 g/dL	13.5–16.5 g/dL
Hematocrit	29%	40%–50%
Total leukocyte count	7.0×10^9/L	$4.5–10.0 \times 10^9$/L
Total lymphocyte count	0.80×10^9/L	$1–3.5 \times 10^9$/L
CD4+ T cells	0.04×10^9/L	$0.7–1.1 \times 10^9$/L
CD8+ T cells	0.41×10^9/L	$0.5–0.9 \times 10^9$/L
B lymphocytes	0.09×10^9/L	$0.2–0.5 \times 10^9$/L
ELISA HIV test	Positive	Negative

On the chest x-ray, bilateral diffuse interstitial shadowing was seen.

Follow-Up
A bronchoscopy with bronchoalveolar lavage was performed. Microscopic examination revealed the presence of *Pneumocystis jirovecii* (formerly called *Pneumocystis carinii*).

Questions
1. Diagnosis of suspected HIV infection is made with:
   a. Real-time PCR
   b. Antibody to HIV-1
   c. Antibody to HIV-2
   d. CD4 and CD8 cell counts
2. Monitoring the course of HIV infection includes:
   a. Viral load monitoring
   b. CD4+ absolute lymphocyte count
   c. Monitoring CD34+ cell counts
   d. Both a and b

See Appendix A for the answers to these questions.

Critical Thinking Group Discussion Questions
1. Which molecular assays can be used to detect Kaposi sarcoma in a suspected HIV infection?
2. Which serologic or cellular assays can be used to monitor the course of an HIV infection?
3. Which molecular assays could be used to monitor drug therapy?

REVIEW QUESTIONS

1. Each repeated cycle of the PCR process contains these three steps:
   a. Denaturation, transcription, annealing
   b. Annealing, denaturation, transcription
   c. Denaturation, annealing, extension of primed sequence
   d. Transcription, annealing, denaturation
2. A significant source of a false-positive error when carrying out PCR testing is?
   a. Poor quality of amplification
   b. Performing too many amplification cycles
   c. Amplification of probes
   d. Amplicon contamination
3. The traditional PCR technique:
   a. Extends the length of the genomic DNA
   b. Alters the original DNA nucleotide sequence
   c. Copies the target region of DNA
   d. Amplifies the target region of RNA
4. Extension in each PCR cycle consists of the following steps except:
   a. Enzymatic DNA denaturation
   b. Primer annealing
   c. Extension of primed DNA sequence
   d. Analysis of PCR product
5. The enzyme reverse transcriptase converts:
   a. mRNA to cDNA
   b. tRNA to mRNA
   c. dsDNA to ssDNA
   d. Mitochondrial DNA to nuclear DNA
6. DNA polymerase catalyzes:
   a. Primer annealing
   b. Primer extension
   c. Hybridization of DNA
   d. Hybridization of RNA

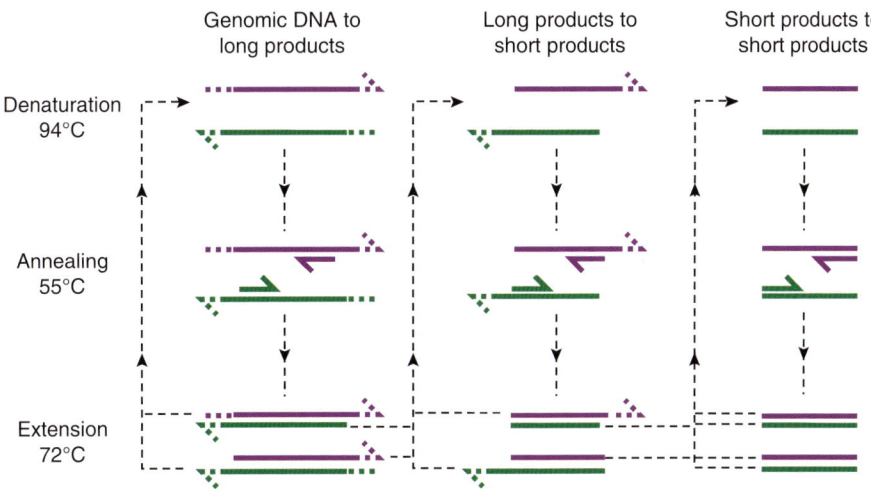

(From Burtis CA, Ashwood ER, Bruns DB: *Tietz fundamentals of clinical chemistry*, ed 6, St. Louis, 2008, Saunders.)

7. The preceding figure depicts:
   a. PCR
   b. Nested primer PCR
   c. RT-PCR
   d. Sanger analysis
8. Which of the following techniques uses signal amplification?
   a. bDNA
   b. TMA
   c. NASBA
   d. RT-PCR
9. Which of the following nucleic acid amplification techniques does *not* require the use of a thermocycler?
   a. PCR
   b. SDA
   c. NASBA
   d. TMA
10. The most common type of probe used for FISH is:
    a. DNA
    b. SNPs
    c. Antibodies
    d. Chromosome
11. A characteristic of FISH is:
    a. Semiconductor nanocrystals
    b. Method of tagging antibodies with super paramagnetic particles
    c. Technology based on two different 200-nm latex particles
    d. Molecular cytogenetic technique
12. Which of the following are the basic steps in performing massively parallel sequencing/next-generation sequencing?
    a. Template preparation, emulsion PCR, sequencing, data analysis
    b. Template preparation, sequencing and imaging, data analysis
    c. Template amplification, sequencing and imaging, data analysis
    d. DNA fragmentation, sequencing, data analysis
13. Clinical applications of NGS include:
    a. Identification of actionable gene mutations
    b. Risk assessment
    c. Identification of virulence factors in bacteria and viruses
    d. Both a and b
14. What molecular technique is appropriate for HIV-1 genotyping?
    a. Reverse transcriptase PCR
    b. Multiplex PCR
    c. Real-time PCR
    d. Strand displacement amplification (SDA)
15. Important applications of PCR include the following with the general exception of:
    a. Searching for mutations with large deletions
    b. Amplification of DNA
    c. Identification of a target sequence
    d. Synthesis of an antisense probe
16. Which modified PCR technique or other method of amplification is used to detect *Mycobacterium tuberculosis*?
    a. Transcription-mediated amplification
    b. Reverse transcriptase PCR
    c. Real-time PCR
    d. Nucleic acid sequence–based amplification
17. The generalized basic steps in next-generation sequencing (NGS) include the following except:
    a. Template preparation and data analysis
    b. Template preparation and sequencing
    c. Template amplification and imaging
    d. Sequencing of the entire genome and data analysis

PART III

Immunologic Manifestations of Infectious Diseases

Chapter 13: Infectious Diseases: Overview and TORCH Diseases, 190

Chapter 14: Streptococcal Infections, 221

Chapter 15: Syphilis, 228

Chapter 16: Vector-Borne Diseases, 240

Chapter 17: Infectious Mononucleosis, 267

Chapter 18: Viral Hepatitis, 273

13

Infectious Diseases: Overview and TORCH Diseases

LEARNING OUTCOMES

- Describe important characteristics of the acquisition and development of infectious diseases.
- Explain the major characteristics of dengue fever.
- Describe the principle, interpretation, and limitations of the TORCH procedure.
- Explain the signs and symptoms of acquired and congenital toxoplasmosis infection.
- Discuss the immunologic manifestations and diagnostic evaluation of toxoplasmosis, including the quantitative determination of IgM antibodies to *Toxoplasma gondii*.
- Explain the signs and symptoms of acquired and congenital rubella infection.
- Compare the immunologic manifestations of acquired and congenital rubella infection.
- Explain the laboratory diagnostic evaluation of rubella infection.
- Explain the signs and symptoms of acquired and congenital cytomegalovirus (CMV) infections.
- Identify and explain the serologic markers and diagnostic evaluation of CMV.
- Explain various diseases in the herpes category.
- Briefly describe the alternate immunology laboratory techniques.
- Analyze the case studies related to infectious diseases.
- Correctly answer case study–related multiple-choice questions.
- Participate in a discussion of critical thinking questions.
- Correctly answer end-of-chapter review questions.

OUTLINE

Characteristics of Infectious Diseases, 191
Development of Infectious Diseases, 192
Traditional Infectious Disease Laboratory Testing, 192
Bacterial Diseases, 192
    Mycobacterium Tuberculosis, 192
        Etiology, 192
        Pathophysiology, 192
Parasitic Diseases, 193
Fungal Diseases, 193
    Histoplasmosis, 194
    Aspergillosis, 194
    Coccidioidomycosis, 194
    North American Blastomycosis, 195
    Sporotrichosis, 195
    Cryptococcosis, 195
Viral, Rickettsial, and Mycoplasmal Diseases, 195
COVID-19 (SARS-CoV-2 Virus), 196
    Etiology, 196
    Epidemiology, 196
    Signs and Symptoms, 196
    Immunologic Manifestations, 196
    Diagnostic Laboratory Evaluation, 196
        Hematology and Coagulation Laboratory, 196
        Immunology-Serology Laboratory, 196
        Clinical Chemistry Laboratory, 197
    Severe Clinical Complications, 197
    Molecular and Serologic Laboratory Testing, 197
        Molecular-Based Techniques, 197
        Serologic-Based Techniques, 198
        Qualitative Chemiluminescent Immunoassay, 199
        Pooled Testing, 199
    Treatment and Prevention, 199
        Convalescent Plasma, 199
        Monoclonal Antibodies, 199
        Additional Types of Treatments, 199
Dengue Fever, 199
    Etiology, 199
    Epidemiology, 199
    Signs and Symptoms, 199
    Laboratory Diagnostic Testing, 199
Torch Test Panel, 200
Toxoplasmosis, 200
    Etiology, 200
    Epidemiology, 200
    Transplacental Transmission, 201
    Seroprevalence, 201
    Signs and Symptoms, 201
        Acquired Infection, 201
        Congenital Infection, 201
    Immunologic Manifestations, 203
    Diagnostic Evaluation, 203
        Serologic Tests, 204
        Sabin-Feldman Dye Test, 205
        Indirect Fluorescent Antibody Test, 205
        Polymerase Chain Reaction, 205
    Histologic Diagnosis, 205
    Cell Culture, 205

Rubella, 205
- Etiology, 205
- Epidemiology, 205
  - *Pregnant Women,* 206
  - *Healthcare Personnel,* 206
- Signs and Symptoms, 206
  - *Acquired Rubella Infection,* 206
- Immunologic Manifestations, 208
  - *Acquired Rubella Infection,* 208
  - *Congenital Rubella Syndrome,* 208
- Diagnostic Evaluation, 208

Rubeola (Measles), 208
- Epidemiology, 208
- Prevention, 208
- Laboratory Testing, 209

Cytomegalovirus, 210
- Etiology, 210
- Epidemiology, 210
- Transmission, 211
  - *Infection From Blood Transfusion,* 211
  - *Infection From Breast Milk,* 211
  - *Other Aspects of Infection,* 211
  - *Latent Infection,* 211
  - *Congenital Infection,* 211
- Signs and Symptoms, 211
  - *Acquired Infection,* 211
  - *Congenital Infection,* 212
- Immunologic Manifestations, 212
  - *Immune System Alterations,* 212
  - *Serologic Markers,* 213
- Laboratory Evaluation, 213
- Diagnostic Laboratory Testing, 213
  - *Diagnostic Testing for Congenital CMV in Newborns,* 213
  - *Virus Detection,* 214

Herpes Viruses, 214
- Herpes Simplex Virus, 214
  - *Congenital and Neonatal Infection,* 215
  - *Laboratory Diagnosis,* 215
- Varicella-Zoster Virus, 215
  - *Epidemiology and Etiology,* 215
  - *Signs and Symptoms,* 215
  - *Laboratory Diagnosis,* 215
  - *Prevention,* 216
- Human Herpes Virus 6, 216

Alternate Immunology Laboratory Techniques, 216
- Immunohistochemistry, 216
- Use of Immunohistochemistry in Infectious Diseases, 216
- Traditional Immunohistochemistry Protocols, 216
- Polymer-Based Immunohistochemistry Methods, 217
- Newer Molecular Testing Approaches, 217
  - *Respiratory Virus Panels,* 217

Case Study 13.1, 218
Case Study 13.2, 218
Case Study 13.3, 218
Case Study 13.4, 219
Procedure: Rapid TORCH Testing, 220.e1
Procedure: Passive Latex Rubella Agglutination Test, 220.e1
Procedure: Passive Latex Agglutination for Detection of Antibodies to Cytomegalovirus, 220.e2
Procedure: Quantitative Determination of Antibodies to Cytomegalovirus, 220.e3
Procedure: Immunohistochemistry in Infectious Diseases, 220.e3

KEY TERMS

clinical manifestations
complement fixation (CF)
congenital
COVID-19
definitive host
dengue fever
early antigens
endotoxins
enzyme immunoassay (EIA)
epidemic
etiologic agent
herd immunity
immediate-early antigens
immunocompromised
immunoperoxidase
latent infection
plaque-reduction neutralization tests (PRNT)
primary infection
prodromal
reactivated infection
serodiagnostic tests
seropositivity
seroprevalence
stillbirths
titers
TORCH
transplacental
zoonoses

CHARACTERISTICS OF INFECTIOUS DISEASES

The acquisition of an infectious disease (e.g., viral, bacterial, parasitic, and fungal) is influenced by factors related to the microorganism and host. The following factors can influence exposure to and development of an infectious disease:
- Immune status of an individual (immunocompromised individuals have a much higher rate of microbial disease)
- Overall incidence of an organism in the population
- Pathogenicity or virulence of the agent
- Presence of a sufficiently large dose of the agent or organism to produce an infection
- Appropriate portal of entry

In many cases, the successful dissemination of a microorganism results from spread of the microorganism over long distances by insect vectors or rapidly from country to country by global travelers, such as occurred with the Zika virus. Some microorganisms are able to multiply in an intracellular habitat, such as in macrophages, and others can display antigen variation, which makes normal immune mechanism control difficult.

Host factors, such as the general health and age of an individual, influence the likelihood of developing an infectious disease and are important determinants of its severity. The very young and older populations develop infectious diseases more frequently than individuals in other age groups. In addition, a history of previous exposure to a disease or harboring of an organism such as a virus in a dormant condition is also a determining factor in disease development.

> **KEY CONCEPTS: Innate Body Defenses Against Infectious Diseases**
> - For an infectious disease to be acquired by a host, the microorganism must penetrate the skin or mucous membrane barrier and survive other natural and adaptive body defense mechanisms.
> - The mechanism of body defense most effective in a healthy host depends on the microorganism.
> - Defenses such as phagocytosis are highly effective in bacterial immunity.
> - Phagocytosis and complement activation may be initiated within minutes of the invasion of a microorganism, but unless primed by previous contact with the same or a similar antigen, antibody and cell-mediated responses do not become activated for several days.

DEVELOPMENT OF INFECTIOUS DISEASES

For an infectious disease to develop in a host, the organism must penetrate the skin or mucous membrane barrier (first line of defense) and survive other natural or adaptive body defense mechanisms. These mechanisms include phagocytosis, antibody and cell-mediated immunity or complement activation, and associated interacting effector mechanisms. Phagocytosis and complement activation may be initiated within minutes of invasion by a microorganism; however, unless primed by previous contact with the same or a similar antigen, antibody and cell-mediated responses do not become activated for several days. Complement and antibodies are the most active constituents against microorganisms that are free in the blood or tissues, whereas cell-mediated responses are most active against microorganisms associated with cells.

The most effective mechanism of body defense in a healthy host depends on factors such as an appropriate portal of entry and the characteristics of each microorganism. The routes of infection or portals of entry can include transmission through oral routes (e.g., foodborne or waterborne contamination), maternal-fetal transmission, insect vectors, sexual transmission, parenteral routes (e.g., injection or transfusion of infected blood), and respiratory transmission. Development of an infectious disease occurs only if a microorganism can evade, overcome, or inhibit normal body defense mechanisms.

TRADITIONAL INFECTIOUS DISEASE LABORATORY TESTING

In many diseases, infected individuals show a spectrum of responses. Some patients may develop and manifest antibodies from a subclinical infection or after colonization of an agent without actually developing disease. In these patients, the presence of antibody in a single serum specimen or a comparative titer of antibody in paired specimens may merely indicate past contact with the agent; the presence of antibodies cannot be used for the accurate diagnosis of a recent disease. In comparison, some patients may respond to an antigenic stimulus by producing antibodies that can crossreact with other antigens. These antibodies are nonspecific and may lead to misinterpretation of serologic tests.

> **KEY CONCEPTS: The Body's Immune Defenses Against Infectious Diseases**
> - T cells are commonly involved in body defenses against parasites.
> - Sequestration of microorganisms is a classic T-cell–dependent hypersensitivity response.
> - Immunoglobulin M (IgM) is usually produced in significant quantities after the first exposure to an infectious agent. This is important in diseases that do not manifest decisive clinical signs and symptoms or under conditions requiring a rapid therapeutic decision.
> - TORCH procedures evaluate the presence of IgM to detect *Toxoplasma*, other viruses, rubella, CMV, and herpes.

In most cases, serologic diagnosis of recent infection using acute and convalescent specimens is the method of choice. The testing of a single specimen is not recommended.

Serologic diagnosis of recent infection should use acute and convalescent specimens. In some circumstances, when only a single specimen is tested to determine immune status, antibody to past infection or to immunization can be determined.

BACTERIAL DISEASES

The presence of key substances (e.g., lysozyme) and the process of phagocytosis represent major immunologic defense mechanisms against bacteria. A microorganism, however, can survive phagocytosis if it has a capsule that impedes attachment or a cell wall that interferes with the digestion and release of exotoxins, which damage phagocytic and other cells. Most capsules and toxins are strongly antigenic, but antibodies can overcome many of their effects; this is the basis of most antibacterial vaccines.

Mycobacterium Tuberculosis
Etiology
Mycobacterium tuberculosis can be a cause of bacterial infection of the lower respiratory tract. This infection is in the grouping of community-acquired pneumonia. Patients who have AIDS with reduced CD4 T-cell numbers and function have dramatically increased susceptibility to *M. tuberculosis* infection. In addition, AIDS and diabetes mellitus are important risk factors that can lead to a loss of immunologic control of *M. tuberculosis* infection.

Pathophysiology
Chronic infections can trigger persistent monocyte recruitment and macrophage activation that can result in granuloma formation. Granulomas cells are rich in macrophages, macrophage-derived multinucleated giant cells, and T cells.

Hypersensitivity reaction testing is an immunological form of testing. Tuberculin-type hypersensitivity testing is a form of type IVa reaction (see Chapter 20). Koch originally described this procedure. The tuberculin skin test (TST) reaction involves monocytes and lymphocytes. It is an example of the recall response to soluble antigen previously encountered during infection.

Following the challenge of intradermal tuberculin testing after a previous infection, mycobacterium memory-specific T cells are recruited and activated to secrete interferon-gamma (IFN-γ), which activates macrophages to secrete tumor necrosis factor gamma (TNF-α) and interleukin 1 (IL-1). A series of cellular interactions leads to these molecules binding receptors on leukocytes and recruiting them to the site of the reaction (Fig. 13.1). Additional information regarding the type I cell-mediated reaction is presented in Chapter 20.

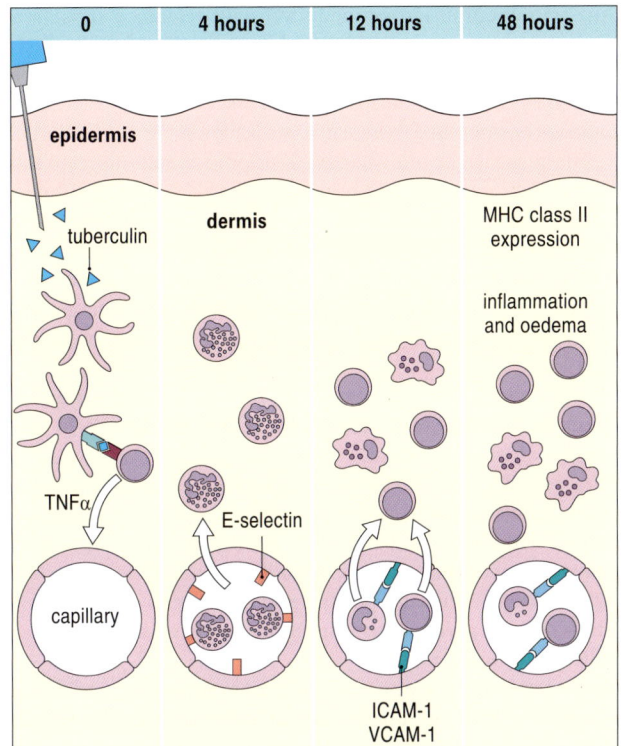

Fig. 13.1 Tuberculin type hypersensitivity. *ICAM-1*, Intercellular adhesion molecule-1; *MHC*, major histocompatibility complex; *TNF-α*, tumor necrosis factor alpha; *VCAM-1*, vascular cell adhesion molecule. (From Male D, Peebles, Jr RS. Male V: Immunology ed.9, Elsevier 2021, Table 26.3.)

Skin and blood testing. There are two types of tests for tuberculosis (TB) infection: the TB skin test and the TB blood test.

TB skin test. The TB skin test is also called the Mantoux TST. The TB skin test is the preferred TB test for children under the age of 5 years.

This test is performed by injecting a small amount of the fluid, tuberculin, into the skin on the lower part of the arm. Within 48 to 72 hours, the skin must be observed for the appearance of swelling or a raised hard area at the site of the injection, which indicates a positive reaction. A negative result in the injection area indicates that the patient is unlikely to have a latent TB infection or TB disease.

TB blood test. TB blood tests are IFN-γ release assays, or IGRAs, that measure the cell-mediated immune response to specific TB antigens in whole blood. The TB blood test is preferred for patients who have received the TB vaccine bacille Calmette–Guérin (BCG).

Two TB blood tests are US Food and Drug Administration (FDA) approved for use in the United States. These tests are:
- QuantiFERON®-TB Gold Plus (QFT-Plus), and
- T-SPOT® TB test (T-Spot).

Additional examples of representative bacterial diseases of importance in the study of immunology are presented in Chapter 14, Streptococcal Infections, and Chapter 15, Syphilis.

PARASITIC DISEASES

Parasites are relatively large, may have resistant body walls, and may avoid being phagocytized because of their ability to migrate away from an inflamed area. These differences set parasitic infections apart from bacterial and viral infections to which some forms of natural and adaptive immunity afford protection. Toxoplasmosis is a representative disease (discussed in the section TORCH Test Panel).

Immune responses (effectors) to parasitic infections include immunoglobulins, complement, antibody-dependent and cell-mediated cytotoxicity, and cellular defenses such as eosinophils and T cells. Some cestodes, especially in their larval stages, may be eradicated by complement-fixing immunoglobulin G (IgG) antibodies. In addition, some antibodies may crossreact with other parasitic antigens. Increased levels of immunoglobulin E (IgE) may be noted in many helminth infections. Activation of the classic and alternate complement pathways may occur in some cases of schistosomiasis, and the alternate pathway of complement activation may kill larvae in the absence of antibody.

Phagocytosis may have some direct activity against parasitic organisms, but the most effective protection in some parasitic infections is provided by antibody-dependent, cell-mediated cytotoxicity. Macrophages, neutrophils, and eosinophils may demonstrate direct toxicity or phagocytosis toward parasites. The actual attachment of the cytotoxic cells is usually mediated by IgG, although IgE may be effective. The role of eosinophils is complex. They may phagocytize immune complexes and act as effector cells in mediating local (type I) reactions, primarily in tissue-stage parasites. T cells are commonly involved in body defenses against parasites. Sequestration of microorganisms is a classic T-cell–dependent hypersensitivity response. In addition, helper T cells may sensitize B cells to specific parasitic antigens.

Other nonspecific factors (e.g., nonstimulated monocytes) are a major protective mechanism against parasites such as *Giardia* spp. Natural killer (NK) cells also have a direct activity against cancer cells and some parasites. Delayed hypersensitivity may be helpful in preventing some parasitic infections but may cause disease in other cases. Deposition of antigen-antibody complexes is responsible for severe pathologic lesions in some parasitic infections. In addition, high levels of circulating IgE may cause hypersensitivity reactions in helminth and cestode infections. Anaphylaxis is a clear risk in echinococcal infections, especially with spontaneous or surgical rupture of a hydatid cyst.

FUNGAL DISEASES

Fungal, or mycotic, infections are normally superficial, but a few fungi can cause serious systemic disease, usually entering through the respiratory tract in the form of spores. Disease manifestation depends on the degree and type of immune response elicited by the host. Fungi are common and harmless inhabitants of skin and mucous membranes under normal conditions (e.g., *Candida albicans*). In immunocompromised hosts, *Candida* spp. and other fungi become opportunistic agents that take advantage of the host's weakened resistance. Manifestations of fungal disease may range from unnoticed respiratory episodes to rapid, fatal dissemination of a violent hypersensitivity reaction.

Survival mechanisms of fungi that successfully invade the body are similar to bacterial characteristics and include the following:
1. Presence of an antiphagocytic capsule
2. Resistance to digestion within macrophages
3. Destruction of phagocytes (e.g., neutrophils)

Some types of yeast activate complement through the alternative pathway, but it is unknown whether this activation has any effect on the microorganism's survival.

Fungal infections are increasing worldwide for a variety of reasons, including the use of immunosuppressive drugs and the development of diseases that result in an immunocompromised host (e.g., AIDS). Serologic tests often play an important role in the diagnosis of these fungal infections (Table 13.1).

TABLE 13.1	Testing Methods for Fungal Disease.
Disease	Procedure
Aspergillosis	Gel immunodiffusion, EIA; IgG to *Aspergillus fumigatus* (≤110 mg/L) present in 85% of farmers and some persons with no evidence of disease
Blastomycosis	Complement fixation (>50% positive in proven cases); immunodiffusion (test is positive in about 80% of cases)
Coccidioidomycosis	Complement fixation using coccidioidin (blood, CSF)
Cryptococcosis	Latex agglutination (serum, CSF), EIA, IFA
Histoplasmosis	Complement fixation, immunodiffusion, PCR (sputum, blood, tissue); *Histoplasma capsulatum* antigen by EIA (urine); nucleic acid probe
Sporotrichosis	Latex particle agglutination

CSF, Cerebrospinal fluid; *EIA*, enzyme immunoassay; *IFA*, immunofluorescence assay; *IgG*, immunoglobulin G; *PCR*, polymerase chain reaction.

Several species of fungi are associated with respiratory disease in human beings. These diseases are acquired by inhaling spores from exogenous reservoirs, including dust, bird droppings, and soil.

Histoplasmosis

Histoplasma capsulatum can be found in soil contaminated with chicken, bird, or bat excreta. Spore-laden dust is the source of histoplasmosis, caused by inhalation.

Histoplasmosis can be difficult to diagnose and can range from asymptomatic to chronic pulmonary disease. In addition, a disseminated form manifesting hepatosplenomegaly with diffuse lymphadenopathy is usually present in varying degrees of severity because of the propensity of the fungus to invade the cells of the mononuclear phagocyte system. Disseminated disease is characterized by fever, anemia, leukopenia, weight loss, and lassitude.

Definitive diagnosis requires isolation in culture and microscopic identification of the fungus, in addition to serologic evidence. If an immunodiffusion technique is used, H and M bands appearing together indicate active infection. If only an M band is present, it indicates early infection, chronic infection, or a recent reactive skin test. An H band appears later than the M band and disappears earlier. Disappearance of an H band suggests regression of the infection.

Delayed hypersensitivity skin testing is confirmed by a rise in complement-fixing antibodies to *Histoplasma* antigens. Titers of 1:8 or 1:16 are highly suggestive of infection. A titer of 1:32 or higher usually indicates active infection. A rising titer indicates progressive infection; a decreasing titer suggests regression. Some disseminated infections are nonreactive in complement fixation (CF) tests. In addition, recent skin tests in individuals with prior exposure to *H. capsulatum* will produce a rise in the CF titer in 17% to 20% of patients. Crossreactions in the CF test occur in patients with aspergillosis, blastomycosis, or coccidioidomycosis, but the titers are usually lower. Several follow-up serum samples should be tested at 2- to 3-week intervals.

Aspergillosis

Another opportunistic mycotic infection that occurs in human beings is aspergillosis, which can be allergic, invasive, or disseminating, depending on pathologic findings in the host. Aspergillosis is usually secondary to another disease. Allergic bronchopulmonary aspergillosis is characterized by allergic reactions to the toxins and endotoxins of *Aspergillus* spp.

Species identification of aspergillosis can be made microscopically. Serologically, skin reactions and immunodiffusion are useful tools for identification, especially if the culture is negative.

The immunodiffusion antibody test with reference antisera and known antigen is a commonly used test for the identification of *Aspergillus* spp. in almost all clinical types of aspergillosis. Precipitin formation by immunodiffusion is useful for identifying patients with pulmonary eosinophilia, severe allergic aspergillosis, and aspergillomas. The presence of one or more precipitin bands suggests active infection. The precipitin bands correlate with CF titers. In this test, the greater the number of bands, the higher is the titer. In general, immunodiffusion measures IgG, and a positive result may suggest past infection. The test is positive in about 90% of sera from patients with aspergilloma and 50% to 70% of patients with allergic bronchopulmonary aspergillosis. A negative test result does not exclude aspergillosis.

In addition, the enzyme immunoassay (EIA) can be used to detect IgE and IgG antibodies. ImmunoCAP is a method used to detect *Aspergillus niger* IgE in serum.

EIA is used to detect *Aspergillus galactomannan* antigen in serum. Negative results do not exclude the diagnosis of invasive aspergillosis. A single positive test result should be confirmed by testing a separate serum specimen. Many agents (e.g., antibiotics and food) can crossreact with the assay. The false-positive rate is higher in children than in adults. If invasive aspergillosis is suspected in high-risk patients, serial sampling is recommended.

Hypersensitivity testing is characterized by immediate and delayed-type hypersensitivity reactions as a result of the presence of *Aspergillus*-specific immunoglobulin. IgE titers are greatly increased in allergic bronchopulmonary aspergillosis.

Coccidioidomycosis

Coccidioidomycosis is also known as *desert fever*, *San Joaquin fever*, or *valley fever*. The disease may assume several forms, including primary pulmonary, primary cutaneous, and disseminated. The disease is contracted from inhalation of soil or dust containing the arthrospores of *Coccidioides immitis*.

Hypersensitivity testing using intradermal injections is useful in screening for *C. immitis*. It is usually the first immunologic test to be positive in asymptomatic and symptomatic cases. Skin testing does not differentiate between recent and past exposures to *C. immitis*. A positive skin test should be followed by other serodiagnostic tests. A negative test in a previously positive person can indicate a disseminated infection and a state of anergy.

The fluorescent antibody (FA) test can be applied directly to clinical specimens. This procedure is invaluable for making a rapid and specific identification of fungal structures. In addition to culturing the organism, serologic tests used to confirm the diagnosis of coccidioidomycosis include the tube precipitin test, immunodiffusion, CF, and latex agglutination. The CF test is the most widely used quantitative serodiagnostic test to identify infection with *C. immitis*. It is very effective in detecting disseminated disease. The tube precipitin test is positive in more than 90% of primary symptomatic cases.

Immunodiffusion is equivalent to CF; it can be used as a screening test, but the results should be confirmed by CF. Latex agglutination is not usually a recommended method because it lacks specificity, which leads to many false-positive results.

Two antigens have been developed for the serologic identification of circulating antibodies to *C. immitis*. IgM appears 1 to 3 weeks after infection in 90% of symptomatic patients. IgG develops 3 to 6 months after the onset of symptoms. Titers of 1:2 to 1:4 are presumptive evidence of an early infection and should be repeated in 3 to 4 weeks. Titers of 1:8 to 1:16 are evidence of active infection, particularly when accompanied by a positive immunodiffusion test. Titers higher than 1:16 occur in 90% to 95% of patients with disseminated coccidioidomycosis.

North American Blastomycosis

Blastomycosis is a chronic fungal disease that is usually secondary to pulmonary involvement. *Blastomyces dermatitidis* causes tumors in the skin or lesions in the lungs, bones, subcutaneous tissues, liver, spleen, and kidneys.

Serologic diagnosis is problematic because of high crossreactivity with antigenic components of the organism. Although immunodiffusion and CF are used, immunodiffusion is considered the better method. CF titers of 8 and 16 are highly suggestive of active infection and titers of 32 or higher are diagnostic. A decreasing titer indicates regression, however, most patients with blastomycosis have negative CF tests.

Sporotrichosis

Sporotrichosis is a chronic, progressive, subcutaneous lymphatic mycosis caused by *Sporothrix schenckii*. The disease takes three forms—lymphatic (the most common), disseminated, and respiratory. It is characterized by a sporotrichotic chancre at the site of inoculation, followed by the development and formation of subcutaneous nodules along the lymphatics draining the primary lesions. Infection is associated with injuries caused by thorns or splinters. Handlers of peat moss are particularly susceptible to the disease, especially when working in rose gardens.

Laboratory methods of identification include cultures, serologic techniques, and the FA staining technique. Two of the most sensitive tests are yeast cell and latex agglutination. Titers of 80 or higher usually indicate active infection.

Skin testing is also available. Patients with cutaneous infections usually demonstrate negative tests; patients with extracutaneous infections have positive tests.

Cryptococcosis

Cryptococcus neoformans is the etiologic agent of cryptococcosis. Infected pigeons are the chief vector. Cryptococcosis is acquired by inhaling the fungus, which grows in culture as yeast. It may initially be asymptomatic or may develop as a symptomatic pulmonary infection. Any organ or tissue of the body may be infected, but localization outside the lungs or brain is relatively uncommon. The disease can be serious in immunocompromised or debilitated patients.

Antigen tests take less time to perform and are more specific than antibody detection. Latex agglutination antigen tests can be performed on serum or cerebrospinal fluid (CSF). Titers of 1:2 suggest infection, although such findings have been found in individuals with no evidence of cryptococcosis. Titers of 1:4 or higher are evidence of an active infection. Higher titers also indicate more severe infections. Positive titers are found in the CSF in 95% of patients with involvement of the central nervous system.

The indirect FA test detects antibodies to *C. neoformans*. It is most valuable when antigen tests are negative and can even be combined with an antigen test to determine a patient's prognosis. A positive test result suggests a present or recent infection.

CF is the most specific antibody detection test but is very insensitive. Tube agglutination, using serum or CSF that demonstrates a titer of 1:2 or higher, suggests a current or recent infection with *C. neoformans*.

As cryptococcosis progresses, antigens begin to appear, along with a decrease in antibody production. After treatment, a decrease in antigen titer and reappearance of antibodies indicate a good prognosis.

VIRAL, RICKETTSIAL, AND MYCOPLASMAL DISEASES

The characteristic process associated with viral infections is cellular replication, which may or may not lead to cell death. Interferon plays a major role in body defenses against viral infections. Antibodies are valuable in preventing the entry and bloodborne spread of some viruses, but the ability of other viruses to spread from cell to cell places the burden of adaptive immunity on the T-cell system, which specializes in recognizing altered self-histocompatibility antigens (histocompatibility leukocyte antigen [HLA]). Macrophages may also play a role in immunity. Some of the most virulent viruses for human beings are zoonoses (e.g., rabies). Other viruses, however, can persist for years without symptoms and can then be reactivated to cause serious disease, possibly including tumors.

Representative examples of the immunologically important viral diseases are presented in this chapter. Chapters related to other viral infections include Chapter 17, Infectious Mononucleosis; Chapter 18, Viral Hepatitis; and Chapter 19, Acquired Immunodeficiency Syndrome. The mutation rates of viruses, especially RNA viruses, such as HIV, are extraordinarily high. Consequently, RNA viruses evolve much more rapidly under selective conditions than their hosts, and contemporary RNA viruses may have descended from a common ancestor only relatively recently. The survival of influenza A and B viruses as new viruses depends on a continual evolution of mutants. These mutant forms are not recognized by the body as being variations of past viral exposures. The most common cause of new viral infections is old viruses that are not natural infections of human beings but rather are accidentally transmitted from other species as zoonoses.

Organisms intermediate between viruses and bacteria are obligatory intracellular organisms with cell walls (e.g., rickettsiae) and without cell walls but capable of extracellular replication (e.g., *Mycoplasma*). Immunologically, the former are closer to viruses and the latter are closer to bacteria.

> **KEY CONCEPTS: Infectious Diseases: COVID-19**
>
> - The virus severe acute respiratory syndrome coronavirus 2 (SARS-Co-V-2) causes COVID-19 infectious disease. COVID-19 is an acronym for *coronavirus disease of 2019*.
> - A high rate of viral transmission, especially due to the surge of delta or other variants, is due to unvaccinated individuals or the density of individuals who are asymptomatic or have only mild symptoms and are not aware that they are actually spreading the virus.
> - A significant minority of COVID patients require hospitalization.
> - Vaccinated individuals can contract COVID infection but it is usually milder than the infection in an unvaccinated patient. Although COVID vaccination does not prevent infection, the vaccine is intended to reduce the severity of infection and avoid hospitalization and death.
> - Molecular testing and serologic (antibody) assays are also needed for epidemiologic studies to assess the extent of virus spread in communities and to determine the infection-related fatality rate.
> - The majority of patients known to be infected with SARS-CoV-2 appear to exhibit a typical immune response.
> - Nonspecific laboratory tests can produce abnormal results in COVID-19.
> - The deadliest manifestations of an abnormal immunologic response is the cytokine storm syndrome (CSS).
> - Emergency Use Authorized (EUA) assays for viral testing include those that detect SARS-CoV-2 nucleic acid (nucleic acid amplification testing [NAAT]) or antigen using nasal or throat swabs to determine whether infection with SARS-CoV-2 has occurred.
> - The Centers for Disease Control and Prevention (CDC) does not currently recommend the use of antibody testing as the sole basis for diagnosis of acute infection.

COVID-19 (SARS-COV-2 VIRUS)

Etiology

The World Health Organization (WHO) declared the SARS-CoV-2 coronavirus outbreak a global pandemic in March 2020. This novel SARS-CoV-2 virus is a member of the Coronaviridae family of respiratory viruses. It is the cause of the infectious disease COVID-19. COVID-19 is an acronym for *corona virus disease of 2019*. SARS-CoV-2 is the third and latest coronavirus to jump over to humans since acute respiratory syndrome coronavirus (SARS-CoV-1) in 2003 and the Middle East respiratory syndrome coronavirus (MERS-CoV) in 2012.

Epidemiology

SARS-CoV-2 has exhibited a more rapid global spread than SARS-CoV-1 or MERS-CoV. Because it is a novel virus for which there is no widespread immunity, transmissibility of SARS-CoV-2 is high, with each infected individual expected to infect statistically about 2 to 2.5 others if no attempts are made to mitigate the spread of the virus. The high rate of transmission is due to the density of individuals who are asymptomatic or who have only mild symptoms and are not aware that they are actually spreading the virus. Active virus shedding appears to be transmissible several days before symptoms are manifested, and individuals might remain contagious for as long as 2 to 4 weeks after infection.

Adults of any age with cancer, chronic kidney disease, chronic obstructive pulmonary disease, cardiac condition, immunocompromised state, overweight, obese, severely obese, sickle cell disease, smoking or a history of smoking, and type 2 diabetes mellitus are at increased risk of severe SARS-CoV-2 infection. Adults of any age with other conditions (e.g., asthma) might be at risk for severe COVID-19 as well.

Children with the following conditions might be at increased risk for severe COVID-19 illness: obesity, medical complexity, severe genetic disorders, severe neurologic disorders, inherited metabolic disorders, congenital heart disease, diabetes, asthma, and other chronic lung disease, and immunosuppression due to malignancy or immune-weakening medications. COVID-19 mortality is high in patients with underlying medical conditions and those aged 85 years of age or older. Black/African Americans, Hispanic/Latinos, and indigenous Native Americans have a disproportionately higher mortality rate than White Americans.

Molecular testing and serologic (antibody) assays are needed for epidemiologic studies to assess the extent of virus spread in communities and to determine the infection-related fatality rate. The SARS-CoV-2 viral spike protein uses the angiotensin-converting enzyme II (ACE2) receptor to enter epithelial cells. Alveolar cells lining the lungs, gastrointestinal (GI) tract, heart, and kidneys all strongly express the ACE2 receptor and the membrane TMPRSS2 serine protease that is needed to cleave the viral spike protein and facilitate cell entry. It is not known definitively if organs other than the lungs are directly targeted.

Signs and Symptoms

Symptomatic patients exhibit symptoms from 2 to 14 days after viral exposure. The majority of cases of COVID-19 are mild, but a significant number of patients do require hospitalization. Clinical presentation ranges from asymptomatic infection to mild, acute upper respiratory symptoms to more severe flulike illness. SARS-CoV-2 can cause both upper and lower respiratory tract infections but predominantly causes infection of the lower respiratory tract. Frequently reported symptoms of patients admitted to the hospital include fever, cough, and shortness of breath. Prolonged symptom duration and disability are common in adults of all ages who have been hospitalized with severe COVID-19 and have survived.

Limited information is available about the spectrum of clinical illness related to COVID-19 in children, although they do appear to present with more mild signs and symptoms than adults. Infants may be at a higher risk for severe illness from COVID-19 compared with older children.

Asymptomatic people can be in any age range. When a group of asymptomatic Chinese citizens was studied, researchers showed that the median duration of viral shedding was 19 days, which was longer when compared to a group of symptomatic patients.

Immunologic Manifestations

The majority of patients known to be infected with SARS-CoV-2 appear to exhibit a typical immune response. In a normal immune response, various types of immune cells and cytokines cause a mild inflammatory state. The first cytokines released are interleukin-1 beta (IL-1β) and TNF-α. Another soluble mediator, complement, is involved. Cells of the innate immune system—neutrophils, monocytes, macrophages, and NK cells—are associated with the immune response. These cells directly attack the invading virus and release additional cytokines (e.g., interleukin-6 [IL-6]). IL-6 stimulates further recruitment, proliferation, and activation of macrophages.

In addition, IL-6 is essential for invoking the adaptive immune response, which involves T cells, B cells, and helper T (Th) cells. Like NK cells, T cells destroy viral-infected cells but are much more specific for the infecting virus. B cells produce antibodies that specifically target viral antigens and mark them for elimination. Th cells also release IL-6 and other cytokines, which assist in the process of recruiting and maintaining T- and B-cell activation and proliferation.

IL-6 and other cytokines directly cause endothelial cells lining the vasculature and organs to become slightly permeable, which facilitates movement of immune cells and complement into infected tissues. When an infection resolves, anti-inflammatory cytokines help to turn off the proinflammatory response and return the immune system to a nonactivated but vigilant state. Without this regulatory function, the immune system would continue to escalate the proinflammatory response, causing increasing damage to healthy cells and tissues.

Diagnostic Laboratory Evaluation

Various laboratory tests produce abnormal results in COVID-19. The following three sections present the most frequent abnormal clinical laboratory results.

Hematology and Coagulation Laboratory

- Increased white blood cell count, increased neutrophil count, decreased lymphocyte count (lymphopenia)
- Decreased hemoglobin
- Increased erythrocyte sedimentation rate (ESR)
- Increased D-dimers (worsening of these parameters, specifically the D-dimer, indicates progressive severity of the virus infection)
- Increased fibrin/fibrinogen degradation products
- Prothrombin time (PT), partial thromboplastin time, and platelet counts (abnormalities are relatively uncommon in initial patient presentations)
- Positive lupus-like inhibitors

Immunology-Serology Laboratory

- Increased C-reactive protein (CRP)—elevates due to stimulation by IL-6
- Increased IL-1β, TNF-α, and IFN-γ
- Detection of SARS-CoV-2 antigen and antibody

Clinical Chemistry Laboratory

- Increased lactic dehydrogenase (LDH)
- Serum amyloid A (SAA) proteins (sensitive markers of the acute-phase inflammatory response and also appear to correlate with disease severity)
- Decreased serum albumin
- Increased transaminase (ALT, AST)
- Increased bilirubin
- Increased creatinine
- Presence of cardiac troponin (cTn)
- Increased ferritin

Severe Clinical Complications

What is a cytokine storm? A simple definition of a cytokine storm is a severe immune reaction characterized by the rapid release of a high concentration of cytokines into the peripheral blood circulations. An important molecular factor is associated with overproduction of the kinetics of cytokine and chemokine gene expression.

The deadliest manifestation of an abnormal immunologic response is *cytokine storm syndrome (CSS)*. CSSs are a group of disorders such as macrophage activation syndrome, representing a variety of inflammatory disorders that result in an overwhelming systemic inflammation, unstable blood flow, multiple-organ dysfunction, and potentially death.

CSS is characterized by continuous activation and expansion of macrophage and lymphocyte populations, which secrete large amounts of cytokines. Systemic symptoms and signs are derived from the massive and uncontrolled inflammatory response caused by proinflammatory and anti-inflammatory cytokine dysregulation (see Chapter 4, Cytokine Storm Syndrome).

Acute respiratory distress coronavirus syndrome (ARDS) can rapidly degrade to septic shock and multiple-organ dysfunction within 12 to 24 hours of hospital admission. These patients require critical care measures, including the use of vasopressors, mechanical ventilation, and other interventions, such as dialysis. ARDS causes greater than 50% mortality in these COVID-19–associated fatalities. Complications established by autopsy examination include sepsis, acute cardiac injury and heart failure, acute kidney injury, hypoxic encephalopathy, alkalosis, and hyperkalemia. Microscopic examination of tissues has revealed focal hemorrhage in the kidney, inflammatory cell infiltration from an enlarged liver, edema, myocardial injury, and scattered degeneration of neurons in the brain.

Reduced vascular tone can mimic vasculitis, and the resulting hypercoagulability is a consequence of both vascular endothelial and liver dysfunction. Patients with serious infection are more likely to have COVID-19–associated coagulopathy than patients with mild infection, and those who die from COVID-19 are more likely to have met the criteria established by the International Society on Thrombosis and Haemostasis for disseminated intravascular coagulation (DIC) compared with survivors. The development of DIC is reported in 71% of nonsurvivors of COVID-19.

Lupus anticoagulants are not associated with bleeding unless they are masking an underlying bleeding tendency or have associated hypoprothrombinemia, in which case the PT will be prolonged. An elevated D-dimer upon hospital admission and a significantly increasing D-dimer level (threefold to fourfold increase) over time are associated with high mortality, which likely reflects coagulation activation from infection/sepsis, cytokine storm, and impending organ failure.

Molecular and Serologic Laboratory Testing

Serologic tests are important in coronavirus testing. Indirect diagnosis of past exposure to COVID-19 can be based on lateral flow immunochromatography (see Fig. 13.1) in point-of-care testing (POCT).

Vertical flow immunoassays rely on the same basic principles as the common lateral flow immunoassay format with some modifications, the most apparent difference between the two methods being the vertical and lateral flow of fluid. Vertical flow technology has reduced assay time (<5 minutes). As with lateral flow, vertical flow immunoassays rely on the immobilization of a capture antibody on a reagent pad to which the sample of interest (with or without antigen to be detected) is applied. Detection of the bound antigen is subsequently achieved through the binding of an antigen-specific antibody–gold conjugate. This step completes a sandwich consisting of a capture antibody, an antigen, and finally the gold conjugate, and results in a direct and permanent visually detectable reaction indicating the presence of the antigen (positive reaction).

Other types of SARS-CoV-2 testing are available: diagnostic, screening, and surveillance testing. Diagnostic testing is intended to identify currently infected individuals with signs and symptoms of COVID-19, patients identified through contact tracing, or individuals who are asymptomatic but have had recent or suspected exposure to SARS-CoV-2. Screening testing for SARS-CoV-2 is intended to identify infected asymptomatic patients without known exposure to SARS-CoV-2. Surveillance testing is used to gain information at a population level to monitor infection and disease, including the rate of positivity in geographic areas.

Molecular and antigen tests are types of viral testing that include SARS-CoV-2 nucleic acid (NAAT) or antigen tests using nasal or throat swabs to determine whether infection with SARS-CoV-2 exists. Currently, rapid antigen tests that have received EUAs from the FDA are authorized for diagnostic testing on symptomatic persons within the first 5 to 7 days of symptom onset. Viral tests are recommended to diagnose acute COVID-19 virus infection. Some tests are POCTs; other tests must be sent to a laboratory for analysis. Negative antigen diagnostic test results are considered presumptive; the CDC recommends confirming negative antigen test results with a reverse-transcriptase polymerase chain reaction (RT-PCR) when the pretest probability is relatively high, especially if the patient is symptomatic or has a known exposure to a person confirmed to have COVID-19. Ideally PCR retesting should be performed within 2 days of the initial testing.

The CDC does not currently recommend the use of antibody testing as the sole basis for diagnosis of acute infection. In certain situations serologic assays may be used to confirm clinical assessment of patients who seek treatment late in their illnesses when used in conjunction with viral detection tests. If a patient is suspected of suffering from postinfectious syndrome (e.g., multisystem inflammatory syndrome in children) caused by SARS-CoV-2 infection, serologic assays may be used.

The US Department of Health and Human Services (HHS) has announced that the US FDA will not require premarket review of laboratory-developed tests (LDTs) for SARS-CoV-2. Therefore the FDA will not review EUA requests for any LDTs. Clarification of the agency's priorities for reviewing EUA submissions for SARS-CoV-2 testing can be found at www.fda.gov/medical-devices/.

Frequently COVID-19 and influenza can be difficult to distinguish based on symptoms during the flu season. Today molecular methods for SARS-COV-2 and influenza are also available. These test systems manufactured by BioFire Diagnostics, the CDC, and QIAGEN are nonwaived testing according to Clinical Laboratory Improvement Act (CLIA) regulations. The BioFire Diagnostics and QIAGEN test systems are rated as moderate complexity by the CLIA; the CDC method is rated as high complexity.

Molecular-Based Techniques

Current molecular methods to diagnose COVID-19 detect either viral RNA or viral antigens. The SARS-CoV-2 genome consists of a single strand of positive-sense RNA surrounded by a lipid-bilayer membrane studded with transmembrane proteins. A positive result indicates the detection of nucleic acid from the relevant virus.

Direct qualitative pathogen detection of the novel coronavirus SARS-CoV-2 using real-time RT-PCR is the method of choice for detecting acute COVID-19. It allows for detection of SARS-CoV-2 for a few days after infection as well as in subclinical/asymptomatic infections. However, molecular false-negative results can be observed with PCR when the viral replication time window is missed.

RT-PCR assay of two specific gene targets detects SARS-CoV-2 and reliably distinguishes it from the other coronaviruses. However, PCR does have a high rate of false negativity because detection of virus relies on an adequate viral load in the specimen for sensitivity. The positivity rate for the different types of samples differs.

The highest positivity rate is seen in bronchoalveolar lavage (BAL) fluid specimens, and the lowest rate (between one-half to three-fourths of nasal swabs and throat swabs, particularly if the specimen is collected 8 days or longer after the onset of symptoms). The incubation period is in the range of 5 to 6 days (up to 14 days maximum). The rate of positivity is about 60% at about 11 days after symptoms are apparent and rapidly declines afterward.

Due to the high specificity of NAAT, a positive result based on an upper respiratory tract specimen is generally adequate to establish a COVID-19 diagnosis. If the initial upper respiratory sample result is negative and the suspicion for disease remains high, some recommend collecting a lower respiratory tract sample rather than collecting another upper respiratory sample.

The CDC's Influenza SARS-CoV-2 (Flu SC2) Multiplex Assay is an RT-PCR test that detects and differentiates RNA from SARS-CoV-2, influenza A virus, and influenza B virus in upper or lower respiratory specimens. The assay provides a sensitive, nucleic acid–based diagnostic tool for evaluation of specimens from patients in the acute phase of infection.

Serologic-Based Techniques

Detection of antibodies against SARS-CoV-2 virus complements PCR swab testing that detects the virus to help diagnose acute infection status. Antibody detection in combination with RT-PCR expands the detection window of SARS-CoV-2 infection and minimizes false-negative RT-PCR results. Serology testing can be used to complement direct antigen testing.

Unlike virus direct antigen testing methods (e.g., NAAT) or antigen detection tests that can detect acutely infected individuals, antibody tests help determine whether the individual being tested was previously infected, even if that person never showed symptoms. Additionally, antibody testing can help to identify individuals who have been exposed to SARS-CoV-2 in order to qualify potential convalescent plasma donors. COVID-19 convalescent plasma is being researched not only as a treatment for individuals who are critically ill with COVID-19, but also for use as a prophylactic means of protecting individuals at high risk of exposure. Serologic assays can also be used to select patients for clinical trials for vaccine or therapy development.

What are neutralizing antibodies (NAbs)? NAbs are a subset of antibodies that are an important specific defense against viral invaders. NAbs are a hallmark of various viral infections including SARS-CoV-2, where the human immune system develops broadly neutralizing antibodies (b-NAbs) and nonneutralizing antibodies (n-NAbs). NAbs are an essential component of the human immune response, with a complicated relationship between the innate and adaptive immune systems to prevent viral infection.

The concentration of NAbs against SARS-CoV-2 can be determined in the clinical laboratory, but this is not a replacement for serology testing for COVID-19 to determine prior or current infection. Routine total antibody testing for detection of specific isotypes (IgM, IgG, and immunoglobulin A [IgA]) does not directly assess the virus-neutralizing capacity of NAbs (see Chapter 3, Neutralizing Antibodies). However, a NAb test is not a replacement for overall antibody detection. NAbs primarily target the S protein in coronaviruses to prevent viral entry into the host cell. The presence of NAbs plays an important role in resolving viral infection, but alone these antibodies do not indicate that a person is immune to potential reinfection. In vitro **plaque-reduction neutralization tests (PRNT)** are considered the gold standard for determining the ability of antibodies to neutralize virus and prevent viral replication.

The humoral immune response to an antigen begins with the production of IgM antibodies. Patients with symptomatic SARS-CoV-2 infection will generally not have detectable antibodies to SARS-CoV-2 within the first 7 days of the onset of symptoms. The IgG class of antibodies appears next and gradually replaces the IgM antibodies, which is the seroconversion process. This process of switching to IgG antibodies appears in the blood circulation within 2 to 4 weeks after initial infection. At about 2 weeks after the development of symptoms, detection of IgM and/or IgG should be 100%. IgM and IgG antibodies are commonly detected using serologic tests due to their important role in tackling the viral infection.

IgG antibodies persist longer in the body and could contribute to long-term immune memory against SARS-CoV-2. However, it is currently unknown whether the presence of antibodies to SARS-CoV-2 is sufficient to confer protective immunity in vivo in infected individuals. SARS-CoV-2 is a novel pathogen, and there is no prior information regarding the duration or long-term effectiveness of these antibodies in recovered patients. Longitudinal studies are required to further understand the potential role of SARS-CoV-2–specific antibodies in patients.

IgA is a third class of antibodies that interacts with immune effector cells to initiate inflammatory reactions. However, in many respiratory infections, in addition to IgM antibodies, IgA antibodies are produced in high titers during the early acute phase of the infection. In fact, during the first week after symptoms appear, the acute phase, IgA antibodies were more commonly observed compared with IgM antibodies. This suggests that IgA antibodies could serve as a marker for acute infection.

Numerous SARS-CoV-2 antibody tests have recently been approved for use through the Emergency Use Authorization issued by the US FDA (see Chapter 6, Quality Assurance and Quality Control). These serologic tests are for indirect diagnosis of past exposure to the COVID-19 virus. They are typically based on lateral flow immunochromatography (see Chapter 9, Electrophoresis Techniques and Chromatography) that can be used near POCT as a complementary tool to the direct detection methods of enzyme-linked immunosorbent assays (ELISAs) or qualitative chemiluminescent immunoassay (see Chapter 10, Labeling Techniques in Immunoassay).

Coronavirus has four main structural proteins: nucleocapsid (N), spike (S), membrane (M), and envelope (E). The detection of IgG antibodies against the spike protein (S1) of SARS-CoV-2 in serum and plasma is used to evaluate exposure. Both N and S proteins could be potential targets for the antibody-based detection of SARS-CoV-2. The S1 subunit of the spike structural proteins could be the specific target antigen for detecting SARS-CoV-2 antibodies. The N protein plays an important role in the transcription and replication of viral RNA, packaging the encapsidated genome into virions and inhibiting the cell cycle process of the host cell. The N protein is abundantly expressed during infections and also has high immunogenic activity. A disadvantage of the N protein is that it could potentially demonstrate greater crossreactivities among the endemic coronaviruses.

Currently available tests predominantly target antibodies to two main surface proteins of the novel coronavirus:
- Nucleocapsid protein (N)
- Spike protein (S)

Several assays particularly focus on the S1 subunit of the spike protein, which is somewhat more specific to each coronavirus strain. Because the S1 subunit is highly immunogenic and its affinity for the ACE2 receptor appears to correlate with infectivity, it has been used as the target for SARS-CoV-2 serologic assays with reportedly high sensitivity and specificity. S1 subunits host the binding domain for the ACE2 receptor, which is thought to be the mechanism by which SARS-CoV-2 gains entry into cells.

Qualitative Chemiluminescent Immunoassay

Qualitative chemiluminescent immunoassay is used for the detection of IgG antibodies against the nucleocapsid protein of the SARS-CoV-2 virus to evaluate exposure. In order to reduce the likelihood of a false-positive result, the CDC's Interim Guidelines for COVID-19 Antibody Testing suggest using alternate testing so that individuals positive by one antibody test are retested with a second antibody test. A negative result indicates that SARS-CoV-2 RNA was not present in the specimen above the limit of detection. However, a negative result does not exclude the possibility of COVID-19 and should not be used as the sole basis for treatment or patient management. The possibility of a false-negative result should be considered if the patient's recent exposures or clinical presentation suggest that COVID-19 is likely. Retesting may be advisable in symptomatic individuals with an intermediate or high clinical suspicion of COVID-19.

Pooled Testing

Basically in pooled testing, multiple patient samples (from 2 to 100) are mixed together as a pool and tested. Negative results for a pool can be reported for each individual patient without further testing. If a pool has a positive result, then the individual specimens need to be retested individually to determine which sample(s) generated the positive pool result.

A disadvantage of using pooled serum is when the disease prevalence in a community rises above a certain level depending on the size of the pool. As disease prevalence rises, and optimal pool size decreases, at some point pooled testing is no longer possible.

Treatment and Prevention
Convalescent Plasma

The National Institute of Health's COVID-19 Treatment Guidelines Panel wants further investigation of convalescent plasma's effectiveness. Only randomized clinical trials could confirm any benefit. This treatment may provide a modest benefit but only to patients who get treated early in their disease with plasma with high levels of antibodies. The ultimate prevention of SARS-CoV-2 is immunization (see Chapter 27, Vaccines).

Monoclonal Antibodies

According to the Pasteur Institute, the protective efficacy of monoclonal antibodies depends primarily, but not solely, on their neutralizing antibody capability. Some monoclonal antibodies can also induce a key immune defense mechanism known as antibody-dependent cellular cytotoxicity (ADCC), which kills cells infected with SARS-CoV-2. In the case of COVID-19, natural killer (NK) cells in the immune system recognize the antibodies that bind to antigens on the surface of infected cells and then specifically lyse those cells. These antibodies are described as "polyfunctional."

Additional Types of Treatments

Interferons, steroids (e.g., dexamethasone, cytokine inhibitors, and cytokine blood filtration systems), and stem cells represent various methods of tamping down inflammation or cytokine storms, or secretion of anti-inflammatory molecules.

DENGUE FEVER

The rapidly expanding global footprint of dengue fever is a public health challenge.

Etiology

Dengue can be caused by one of four single-strand, positive-sense RNA viruses (serotypes dengue virus type 1 to dengue virus type 4) of the *Flavivirus* genus. After an incubation period of 3 to 7 days, signs and symptoms start suddenly and follow three phases—an initial febrile phase, a critical phase at about the time the fever subsides (defervescence), and the final spontaneous recovery phase.

Epidemiology

An estimated 50 million infections occur every year in about 100 countries, with the potential to spread further. The current data reported for 2024 by the CDC was a total of 2559 cases of Dengue fever. The number of locally acquired cases is currently 1732 cases. According to the WHO and the Centers for Disease Control and Prevention, Florida and the coastal areas of Texas are included in the geographic areas that have high suitability for dengue transmission.

Dengue fever is becoming more prevalent as locally acquired in the United States. The major areas of disease are endemic tropical and subtropical latitudes (e.g., India and Southeast Asia). The primary vector is the urban-adapted *Aedes aegypti* mosquito. Global trade, with the unintentional transport of mosquitoes, and increased travel by viremic people, urban crowding, and ineffective mosquito control are all factors in this modern pandemic.

Signs and Symptoms

Most dengue virus infections are asymptomatic, with a wide variety of clinical manifestations. Signs and symptoms range from mild febrile illness to severe and fatal disease.

Laboratory Diagnostic Testing

Laboratory diagnostic testing is by detection of viral components in serum or directly by serologic testing. Diagnostic tests are as follows:
- Viral component testing
- Detection of viral nucleic acid in serum by RT-PCR
- Serologic testing
- Detection of IgM seroconversion by ELISA

Currently no effective antiviral agents are available to treat dengue infection. Treatment is supportive. If patients have severe bleeding, a blood transfusion can be lifesaving. Clinical research with potential drugs or vaccines is ongoing.

TORCH TEST PANEL

The TORCH tests have been grouped under the acronym: *Toxoplasma gondii*, **o**ther (viruses, such as HIV [Chapter 18], hepatitis [Chapter 15], varicella, parvovirus), **r**ubella, **c**ytomegalovirus, and **h**erpes simplex virus [HSV] (Tables 13.2 and 13.3). Syphilis (Chapter 15) may be added to this list of infections that can result in congenital disorders, producing the acronym TORCHS.

The TORCH test panel is a group of tests for detecting infections in pregnant women suspected of having any of the TORCH infections. In addition a TORCH panel may be used in pregnant women to assess past exposure or immunization to *Toxoplasma*, rubella, CMV, and HSV. The test panel is not recommended for diagnosing congenital infections in newborns; tests should be selected individually to target the most likely infectious agents.

Antibody testing will help diagnose an infection that may be harmful to the fetus. Because IgM is usually produced in significant quantities during the first exposure of a patient to an infectious agent, the detection of specific IgM can be of diagnostic significance. This immunologic characteristic is particularly important in diseases that do not manifest decisive clinical signs and symptoms, such as toxoplasmosis, or under conditions in which a rapid therapeutic decision may be required, such as with rubella.

> **KEY CONCEPTS: Characteristics of Toxoplasmosis**
> - Toxoplasmosis is a widespread disease in human beings and animals caused by *T. gondii*, often found in cat feces.
> - Fecal contamination of food or water, soiled hands, inadequately cooked or infected meat, and raw milk are sources of human infection. All mammals, including human beings, can transmit the infection transplacentally.
> - In adults and children other than newborns, the disease is usually asymptomatic. A generalized infection probably occurs.
> - Although spontaneous recovery follows acute febrile disease, the organism can multiply in any organ of the body or circulatory system.
> - Congenital toxoplasmosis can result in central nervous system (CNS) malformation or prenatal mortality.

TOXOPLASMOSIS

Etiology

Toxoplasmosis is a widespread disease in human beings and animals. This infection is caused by *T. gondii*, recognized as a tissue coccidian.

Epidemiology

T. gondii was first discovered in a North African rodent and has been observed in numerous birds and mammals worldwide, including human beings. It is a parasite of cosmopolitan distribution, able to develop in a wide variety of vertebrate hosts.

Human infections are common in many parts of the world. According to the CDC, in the United States it is estimated that 22.5% of the population aged 12 years or older has been infected

TABLE 13.2 TORCH Antibodies: IgM.

Infectious Agent	Interpretation of Assay
Cytomegalovirus (CMV)	Negative
	Questionable—repeat testing in 10–14 days may be helpful. Low levels of IgM antibodies may persist for more than 12 months postinfection.
	Positive—IgM antibody to may indicate a current or recent infection.
Herpes simplex virus type 1 and/or type 2	Negative
	Questionable—repeat testing in 10–14 days may be helpful. Low levels of IgM antibodies may persist for more than 12 months postinfection.
	Positive—IgM antibody to HSV detected, which may indicate a current or recent infection.
Rubella, IgM	Negative
	Questionable—repeat testing in 10–14 days may be helpful. Low levels of IgM antibodies may persist for more than 12 months postinfection.
	Positive—IgM antibody to rubella detected, which may indicate a current or recent infection or immunization.
Toxoplasma gondii, IgM	Negative
	Questionable—repeat testing in 10–14 days may be helpful.
	Positive—significant level of *T. gondii* IgM

2024 Infectious Diseases Laboratory Testing. https://www.cdc.gov/laboratory/specimen-submission. Accessed on September 24, 2024.

TABLE 13.3 TORCH Antibodies: IgG.

Infectious Agent	Interpretation of Assay
Cytomegalovirus (CMV)	Negative
	Questionable—repeat testing in 10–14 days may be helpful.
	Positive IgG antibody may indicate a current or recent infection.
HSV-1 and/or HSV-2, IgG	Negative
	Questionable—repeat testing in 10–14 days may be helpful.
	Positive IgG antibody may indicate a current or recent infection
Rubella, IgG	Negative
	Questionable—repeat testing in 10–14 days may be helpful.
	Positive IgG antibody may indicate a current or recent infection
Toxoplasma gondii, IgG	Negative
	Questionable—repeat testing in 10–14 days may be helpful.
	Positive IgG antibody may indicate a current or recent infection

HSV, Herpes simplex virus; *TORCH*, toxoplasma, other (viruses), rubella, cytomegalovirus, herpes.
2024 Infectious Diseases Laboratory Testing. https://www.cdc.gov/laboratory/specimen-submission. Accessed on September 24, 2024.

with *Toxoplasma*. In various places throughout the world, it has been shown that up to 95% of some populations have been infected with *Toxoplasma*. Infection is often highest in areas of the world that have hot, humid climates and lower altitudes.

Toxoplasmosis is considered to be a leading cause of death attributed to foodborne illness in the United States. More than 60 million men, women, and children in the United States carry the *Toxoplasma* parasite, but very few individuals have symptoms because the immune system usually keeps the parasite from causing illness. Women who are newly infected with *Toxoplasma* during pregnancy and anyone with a compromised immune system can have severe consequences as the result of infection. Toxoplasmosis is considered one of the neglected parasitic infections, a group of five parasitic diseases that have been targeted by the CDC for public health action.

Toxoplasmosis is not passed from person to person, except in cases of mother-to-child (congenital) transmission and blood transfusion or organ transplantation. People typically become infected by three principal routes of transmission:
- Foodborne
- Animal to human (zoonotic)
- Mother to child (congenital)

The definitive host is the house cat and other members of the Felidae family (Fig. 13.2). Domestic cats are a source of the disease because oocysts are often present in their feces. Accidental ingestion of oocysts by human beings and animals, including the cat, produces a proliferative infection in the body tissues. Fecal contamination of food or water, soiled hands, inadequately cooked or infected meat, and raw milk can be major sources of human infection. The risk for infection is higher in many developing and tropical countries, especially when people eat undercooked meat, drink untreated water, or are extensively exposed to soil.

Organ transplant recipients can become infected by receiving an organ from a *Toxoplasma*-positive donor. Transfusion-transmitted toxoplasmosis has been associated with the use of leukocyte concentrates. Patients at risk are those receiving immunosuppressive agents or corticosteroids. Laboratory workers who handle infected blood can also acquire infection through accidental inoculation.

Transplacental Transmission

All mammals, including human beings, can transmit the infection transplacentally. Transplacental transmission usually takes place in the course of an acute but inapparent or undiagnosed maternal infection. Evidence has shown that the number of infants born in the United States each year with congenital *T. gondii* infection is considerably higher than the 3000 previously estimated. It is estimated that 6 of 1000 pregnant women in the United States will acquire primary infection with *Toxoplasma* during a 9-month gestation. Approximately 45% of women who acquire the infection for the first time and who are not treated will give birth to congenitally infected infants. Consequently, the expected incidence of congenital toxoplasmosis is 2.7 per 1000 live births.

It is recommended that all pregnant women be tested for toxoplasmosis immunity. If a patient is susceptible, screening should be repeated during pregnancy and at delivery. Prevention of infection in pregnant women should be practiced to avert congenital toxoplasmosis (Box 13.2). To further prevent infection of the fetus, women at risk should be identified by serologic testing, and pregnant women with primary infection should receive drug therapy.

Seroprevalence

Seroprevalence (antibody to *T. gondii*) varies considerably in the general population. It ranges from 96% in Western Europe to 10% to 40% in the United States. Of patients with AIDS who are seropositive for *T. gondii*, approximately 25% to 50% will develop toxoplasmic encephalitis (meningoencephalitis). In areas with a lower seroprevalence, such as the United States, the percentage of patients with AIDS who develop toxoplasmic encephalitis is lower (5% to 10%).

Signs and Symptoms

In adults and children other than newborns, toxoplasmosis is usually asymptomatic. A generalized infection probably occurs. Although spontaneous recovery follows acute febrile disease, the organism can localize and multiply in any organ of the body (Fig. 13.3) or the circulatory system.

Toxoplasma can be harmful to individuals with suppressed immune systems. Toxoplasmic encephalitis in patients with AIDS may result in death, even when treated. Persons at risk can be identified by screening patients who test positive for HIV for antibody to *T. gondii*.

Acquired Infection

When present, symptoms are commonly mild. Toxoplasmosis can simulate infectious mononucleosis, with chills, fever, headache, lymphadenopathy, and extreme fatigue. Primary infection may be promoted by immunosuppression. A chronic form of toxoplasmic lymphadenopathy exists. *T. gondii* presents a special problem in immunosuppressed or otherwise compromised hosts. Some of these patients have experienced reactivation of a latent toxoplasmosis. These patients have included those with Hodgkin and non-Hodgkin lymphoma and recipients of organ transplants.

Reactivation of cerebral toxoplasmosis is not uncommon in patients with AIDS, in whom toxoplasmic meningoencephalitis is almost always a reactivation of a preexisting latent infection, most often occurring when the total CD4 count falls below 100×10^9/L. *T. gondii*–seropositive, HIV-infected patients may develop toxoplasmic encephalitis because of (1) genetic susceptibility in the human immune response to *T. gondii*; (2) subtle differences in patients' immunocompromised status; (3) differences in the virulence of individual strains of *T. gondii*; (4) possible recurrent infections with different strains; and (5) variable coinfections with other opportunistic pathogens.

Congenital Infection

Toxoplasma can be harmful to fetuses whose mothers become infected during pregnancy. Congenital toxoplasmosis can result in CNS malformation or prenatal mortality. Many infants who are serologically positive at birth fail to display neurologic, ophthalmic, or generalized illness at birth. Toxoplasmosis acquired in utero can result in blindness, encephalomyelitis, intellectual disability, convulsions, and death in infected neonates.

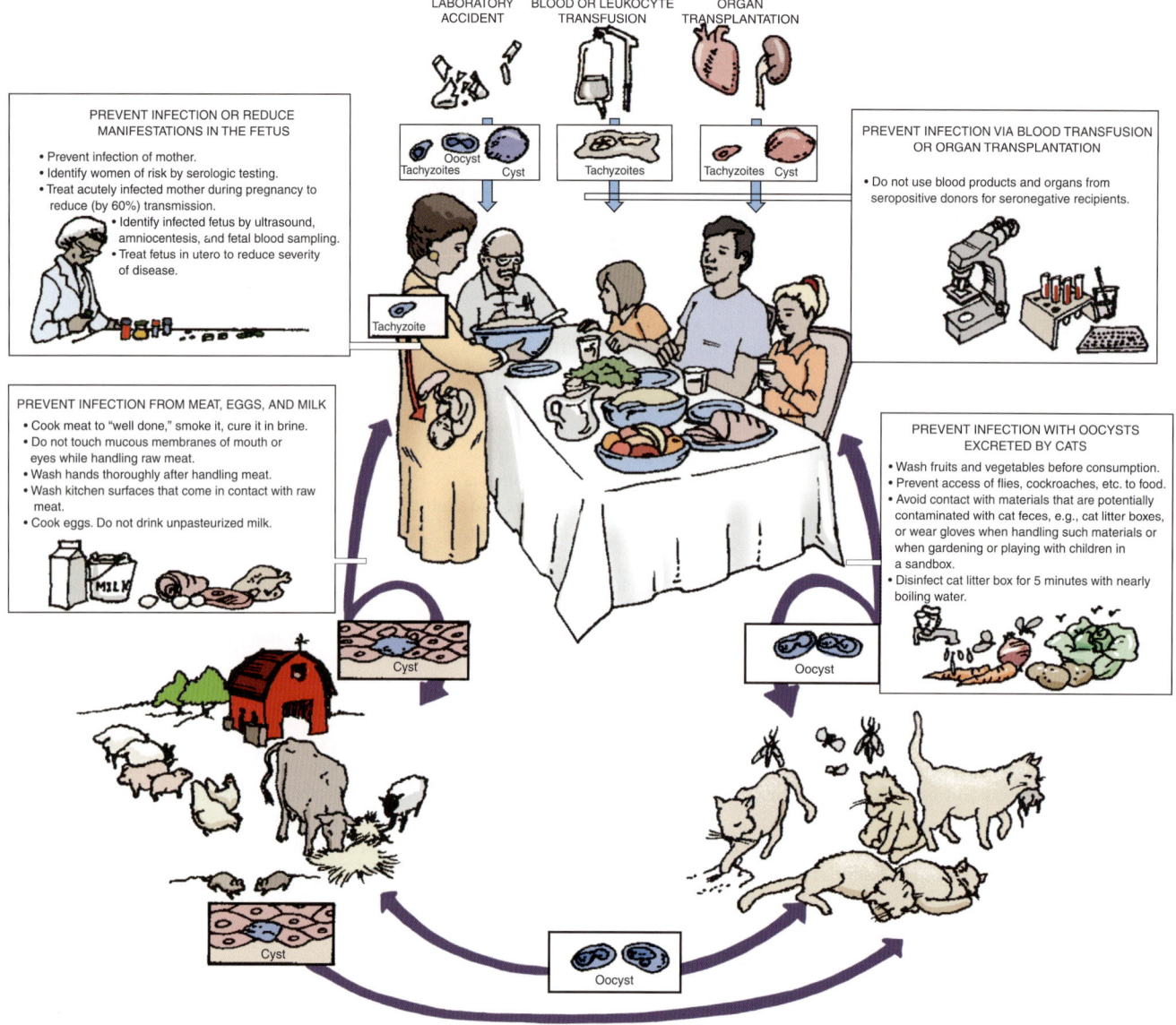

Fig. 13.2 Life cycle of *Toxoplasma gondii*. (Adapted from Katz SL, Gershon AA, Wilfert CM, Krugman S, editors: *Infectious diseases of children*, ed 9, St. Louis, 1992, Mosby.)

BOX 13.1 Lateral or Vertical Flow Immunoassays (Immunochromatography)

- The lateral or vertical flow immunoassays, immunochromatography assay, is an extremely versatile and rapid method for visual detection of antigen in a blood sample on a test strip (see Fig. 13.1).
- The basic technology of lateral flow immunoassays commercial application was an over-the-counter home pregnancy test launched in 1988. Since then, this technology has been employed to develop a wide and ever-growing range of assays including COVID-19. An assay is simple to perform.
- The probes used in lateral or vertical flow assays are commonly based on gold nanoparticle antibody conjugates. Due to the optical properties of gold, a noble metal, nanoparticles detection with the naked eye can be achieved with excellent sensitivity.
- A typical lateral flow rapid test strip consist of components:
  1. Sample pad—an adsorbent pad onto which the test sample is applied.
  2. Conjugate or reagent pad—this contains antibodies specific to the target analyte conjugated to colored particles (usually colloidal gold nanoparticles or latex microspheres).
  3. Reaction membrane—typically a nitrocellulose or cellulose acetate membrane onto which antitarget analyte antibodies are immobilized in a line that crosses the membrane to act as a capture zone or test line (a control zone will also be present, containing antibodies specific for the conjugate antibodies).
  4. Wick or waste reservoir—a further absorbent pad designed to draw the sample across the reaction membrane by capillary action and collect it.
- The components of the strip are usually fixed to an inert backing material and may be presented in a simple dipstick format or within a plastic casing with a sample port and reaction window showing the capture and control zones.

(From Turgeon, ML: *Linne & Ringsrud's clinical laboratory science,* ed 8, St. Louis, 2020;198–199, Elsevier.)

In as many as 75% of congenitally infected newborns not serologically diagnosed at birth, the disease remains dormant, only to be discovered when other symptoms become apparent, such as chorioretinitis, unilateral blindness, and severe neurologic sequelae.

> **KEY CONCEPTS: Laboratory Testing for Toxoplasmosis**
> - *T. gondii* is difficult to culture, and the diagnosis must be supported by serologic methods to determine levels of IgM and IgG antibodies to *T. gondii*.
> - The presence of IgM antibodies to *T. gondii* in an adult indicates active infection. Detection of IgM also suggests active infection in the newborn.
> - Serologic tests include immunofluorescence assay (IFA), chemiluminescent immunoassay, and polymerase chain reaction (PCR).

> **BOX 13.2 Methods for Prevention of Congenital Toxoplasmosis**
> - Avoid touching the mucous membranes of the mouth and eye while handling raw meat.
> - Wash hands thoroughly after handling raw meat.
> - Wash kitchen surfaces that come in contact with raw meat.
> - Cook meat to at least 18.8°C (65.8°F); smoke it or cure it in brine.
> - Wash fruits and vegetables before consumption.
> - Prevent access of flies, cockroaches, and other insects to fruits and vegetables.
> - Avoid contact with or wear gloves when handling materials that are potentially contaminated with cat feces (e.g., cat litter boxes) and when gardening.

Immunologic Manifestations

Both clinical and laboratory findings in toxoplasmosis resemble those of infectious mononucleosis. An increased number of variant lymphocytes can be seen on a peripheral blood smear.

The diagnosis can be established serologically by detecting a marked elevation of *Toxoplasma* antibodies. Antibodies are demonstrable within the first 2 weeks after infection, rising to high levels early in the infection and then falling slightly, but persisting at an elevated level for many months before declining to low levels after many years. The best evidence for current infection is a significant change on two appropriately timed specimens (paired acute and convalescent specimens), in which both tests are done in the same laboratory at the same time.

If a significant level of *T. gondii* IgM antibody is detected, it may indicate a current or recent infection. The presence of IgM to *T. gondii* in an adult indicates an infection, but low levels of IgM antibodies occasionally may persist for more than 12 months after infection. The CDC recommends that any equivocal or positive result should be retested using a different assay from another reference laboratory specializing in toxoplasmosis testing.

Diagnostic Evaluation

The diagnosis of toxoplasmosis is typically made by serologic testing. A test that measures IgG is used to determine whether a person has been infected. If it is necessary to try to estimate the time of infection, which is of particular importance for pregnant women, a test that measures IgM is also used along with other tests, such as an avidity test.

Diagnosis can be made by direct observation of the parasite in stained tissue sections, CSF, or other biopsy material. These techniques are used less commonly because of the difficulty of obtaining these specimens.

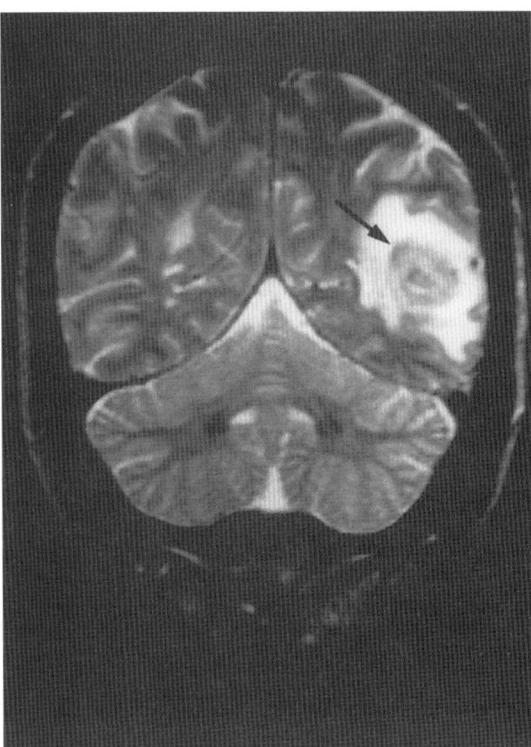 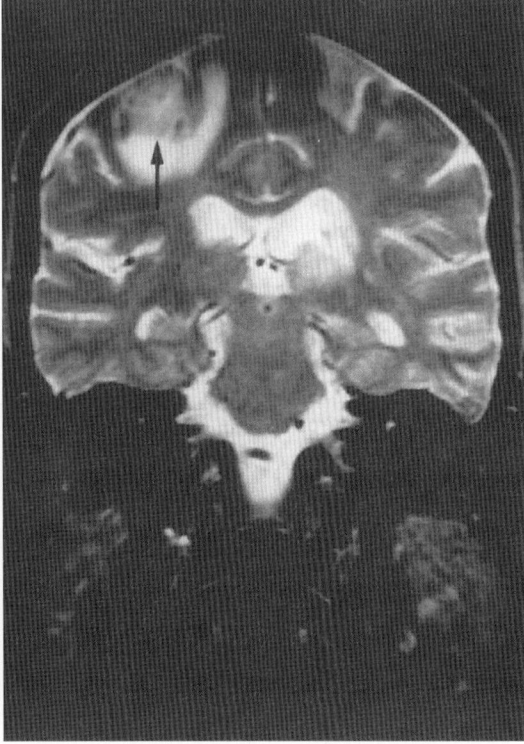

Fig. 13.3 Toxoplasmic Meningoencephalitis. Magnetic resonance imaging (MRI) brain scans of two different patients with acquired immune deficiency syndrome (AIDS). *Arrows* indicate areas infected with toxoplasmosis.

Parasites can also be isolated from blood or other body fluids (e.g., CSF), but this process can be difficult and requires considerable time. Molecular techniques that can detect the parasite's DNA in the amniotic fluid can be useful in cases of possible mother-to-child (congenital) transmission.

The diagnosis of toxoplasmosis can be established by the following:
- Serologic tests (Table 13.4)
- PCR
- IFA
- Isolation of the organism
- Histologic examination of infected tissue (immunohistochemistry [IHC]; provides a definitive diagnosis)

Serologic Tests

The mainstay of diagnosis of *T. gondii* infection is serologic testing. A relatively high proportion of people have antibodies to *T. gondii*, which makes interpretation of serologic test results difficult. Assays for different isotypes of antibodies have been developed to support the diagnosis of an acute or chronic *T. gondii* infection.

For the detection of IgM antibodies to *T. gondii* a variety of procedures are available, such as IFA, automated ELISA, and chemiluminescent immunoassay for IgM and IgG antibodies.

IgM antibodies. The IgM assay was widely used in the past, but this is not recommended for routine use in adults, because it may yield frequent false-positive or false-negative results, particularly in pregnant women, immunocompromised patients, and patients from areas in which *Toxoplasma* infection is highly endemic. IgM antibodies tend to appear earlier and decline more rapidly than IgG antibodies. Persistently elevated IgM-specific antibody titers after the initial infection can lead to false-positive results and difficulty in interpreting these tests.

In patients with recently acquired infection, IgM *T. gondii* antibodies are detected initially and, in most cases, these titers become negative within a few months. In some patients, however, positive IgM *T. gondii*–specific titers can be observed during the chronic stage of the infection. IgM antibodies have been reported to persist as long as 12 years after the acute infection. However, their persistence does not seem to be clinically relevant, and these patients should be considered chronically infected.

Clinicians should be cautious when using IgM antibody levels in prenatal screening. Any positive result in a pregnant patient confirmed positive by a second reference laboratory should be evaluated by amniocentesis and PCR testing for *T. gondii*. A negative result does not rule out the presence of PCR inhibitors in the patient specimen or *T. gondii* DNA concentrations below the level of detection of the assay.

The US FDA has recommended that sera with positive IgM test results obtained at nonreference laboratories should be sent to a *Toxoplasma* reference laboratory. After IgM-positive sera undergo confirmatory testing, the results are interpreted as (1) a recently acquired infection; (2) an infection acquired in the past; or (3) a false-positive result.

IgG antibodies. IgG antibodies appear 1 to 2 weeks after the initial infection, peak after about 6 to 8 weeks, and decline gradually over the next 1 to 2 years; in some cases, IgG antibodies persist for life.

Avidity test. The functional affinity of specific IgG antibodies is initially low after primary antigenic challenge and increases during subsequent weeks and months. Protein-denaturing reagents are used to dissociate the antibody-antigen complex. The avidity result is determined using the ratios of antibody titration curves of urea-treated and untreated serum.

The specialized avidity test can be used as an additional confirmatory diagnostic tool in patients with a positive or equivocal IgM test. Its highest value is observed when laboratory test results reveal high–IgG avidity antibodies, and the serum is obtained during the time window of exclusion of acute infection for a particular method (range, 12–16 weeks). Low- or equivocal-IgG avidity antibody results should not be interpreted as diagnostic of recently acquired infection. Low- or equivocal-avidity antibodies can persist for months to 1 year or longer.

Measurement of the avidity of the IgG provides information to differentiate a current from a past infection. Low-avidity IgG antibody indicates that the patient has experienced a *T. gondii* infection within the past 8 months. The presence of high-avidity antibody indicates that the patient experienced a *T. gondii* infection 5 or more months before this assay was performed. The discovery of a past versus a present *T. gondii* infection is diagnostically important for pregnant women. The low- and high-avidity antibody screening by EIA is performed in parallel.

Studies of the avidity of IgG in pregnant women who have seroconverted during gestation have shown that women with high-avidity test results were infected with *T. gondii* at least 3 to 5 months earlier (time to conversion from low- to high-avidity antibodies varies with the

TABLE 13.4 Serologic Evaluation of Toxoplasmosis.

Test	Method	Recommended Use
IgM		Usually detectable 5 days after infection, and at their highest levels 1–2 months after infection
IgG only		Detectable 1–2 weeks after infection, and at their highest levels 3–6 months after infection
Toxoplasma gondii antibodies, [a]Both IgG and IgM	Chemiluminescent immunoassay	Infection within the last year first-line test in endemic areas for identifying *T. gondii* infection in pregnant women; diagnosis of opportunistic infections in immunocompromised hosts
T. gondii by polymerase chain reaction (PCR)	PCR	Confirmation of toxoplasmosis infection in immunocompromised hosts

[a]The Centers for Disease Control and Prevention (CDC) suggests that equivocal or positive results be retested using a different assay from another reference laboratory specializing in toxoplasmosis testing (IgG Sabin dye test, IgM enzyme-linked immunosorbent assay [ELISA], reflex to avidity, and/or other tests such as chemiluminescent immunoassay).

IgG, Immunoglobulin G; *IgM,* immunoglobulin M.

https://www.cdc.gov/toxoplasmosis (Accessed on September 24, 2024).

method used). Because low-avidity antibodies may persist for many months, their presence does not necessarily indicate recently acquired infection.

Sabin-Feldman Dye Test

In the past, IgG antibodies were measured by the Sabin-Feldman dye test (DT), which was considered the gold standard. The DT is a sensitive and specific neutralization test in which live organisms are lysed in the presence of complement and the patient's IgG *T. gondii*–specific antibody. IgG antibodies usually appear within 1 to 2 weeks of the infection, peak within 1 to 2 months, fall at variable rates, and usually persist for life. The titer does not correlate with the severity of illness. This test is available mainly in reference laboratories.

A negative test result practically rules out prior *T. gondii* exposure, unless the patient is hypogammaglobulinemic. In a small number of patients, IgG antibodies might not be detected within 2 to 3 weeks after initial exposure to the parasite. Rare cases of toxoplasmic chorioretinitis and toxoplasmic encephalitis have been documented in immunocompromised patients who test negative for *T. gondii*–specific IgG antibodies.

Indirect Fluorescent Antibody Test

The IFA test uses killed organisms as a substrate, with patient serum assayed for activity against them. The IFA test is used widely because it measures the same antibodies as the Sabin-Feldman DT and results parallel DT results. False-positive results may occur with sera that contain antinuclear antibodies; false-negative results may occur when using sera from patients with low titers of IgG antibody.

Polymerase Chain Reaction

PCR amplification is used to detect *T. gondii* DNA in body fluids and tissues. The PCR assay can be used to detect the presence or absence of *T. gondii* DNA in fresh or frozen biopsy tissue, CSF, amniotic fluid, serum, or plasma. A negative result does not rule out the presence of PCR inhibitors in the specimen or *T. gondii* DNA concentrations below the level of detection by the assay.

A PCR test performed on amniotic fluid has revolutionized the diagnosis of fetal *T. gondii* infection by enabling an early diagnosis to be made, which prevents the use of more invasive procedures on the fetus.

Histologic Diagnosis

Demonstration of tachyzoites in tissue sections or smears of body fluid (e.g., CSF, amniotic fluid, and BAL fluid) establishes the diagnosis of acute infection. The immunoperoxidase method is applicable to unfixed or formalin-fixed paraffin-embedded tissue sections.

A rapid and technically simple method is the detection of *T. gondii* in air-dried, Wright-Giemsa–stained slides of centrifuged (e.g., cytocentrifuged) sediment of CSF or of brain aspirate, or in impression smears of biopsy tissue. Multiple tissue cysts near an inflammatory necrotic lesion indicate acute infection or reactivation of latent infection.

Cell Culture

Detection of *T. gondii* in the blood may represent a major advance in the diagnosis of toxoplasmosis in patients with AIDS. A cell culture method for the growth of *T. gondii* has been developed using monocytes. After 4 days, parasites in the culture are revealed by immunofluorescence with an anti-P30 monoclonal antibody. A quantitative and qualitative analysis by cytofluorometry can then be performed on the cultured cells.

> **KEY CONCEPTS: Characteristics of Rubella**
> - Acquired rubella (German, or 3-day, measles) is caused by an enveloped, single-strand RNA virus of the Togaviridae family.
> - Acquired rubella is endemic to human beings, highly contagious, and transmitted through respiratory secretions.
> - Contracting rubella infection and vaccinating against rubella are the only ways to develop immunity.
> - A diagnosis of acquired rubella is not based solely on clinical manifestations; signs and symptoms vary widely.
> - Although usually mild and self-limiting, with rare complications in children and adults, rubella infections in pregnant women, especially in the first trimester, can result in fetal death or congenital rubella syndrome.

RUBELLA

Etiology

The rubella virus was first isolated in 1962. Acquired rubella, also known as *German measles* or *3-day measles*, is caused by an enveloped, single-strand RNA virus of the Togaviridae family. Because the virus is endemic to human beings, the disease is highly contagious and is transmitted through respiratory secretions. Before widespread rubella immunization, this viral infection usually occurred in childhood, although it also affected adults.

Epidemiology

Three strains of live, attenuated rubella vaccine virus were developed and first licensed for use in the United States in 1969. Before widespread rubella immunization in the United States and Canada, rubella infections occurred in epidemic proportion at 6- to 9-year intervals. In 1964 more than 20,000 cases of congenital rubella syndrome (CRS) and an unknown number of stillbirths occurred in the United States as the result of an epidemic that year.

The Pan American Health Organization (PAHO) has made historic achievements in the elimination of measles (rubeola) and has announced a new effort to eliminate German measles (rubella). Many countries in the regions of the Americas have already made great progress in reducing the incidence of CRS through accelerated rubella control programs. Costa Rica, Honduras, Brazil, and Chile, in addition to the member countries of the Caribbean, have rubella elimination initiatives under way. In countries where vaccination is uncommon, the incidence of rubella infection is high and epidemics are common.

Because measles has not been eradicated worldwide, immunization must be maintained in a very high percentage of the population to prevent its reappearance. Subacute sclerosing panencephalitis (SSPE) is a late consequence of measles infection in a few patients. When measles was prevented in the United States, SSPE disappeared 15 to 20 years later.

In 2024 the CDC reported that there have been 13 outbreaks (defined as 3 or more related cases) . Sixty six percent of the reported cases of rubella infections (110 of 167) are outbreak-associated.

In 2000, the United States was declared measles free. This status means there is no measles spreading within the country and new cases are only found when someone contracts measles abroad and returns to the country. Achieving measles elimination status in the United States was a historic public health achievement. The national average for measles as a combined measles, mumps, and rubella (MMR) vaccination in the United States is about 92%, but pockets of undervaccinated children are breeding grounds for outbreaks.

This status means there is no measles spreading within the country and new cases are only found when someone contracts measles abroad and returns to the country. Achieving measles elimination status in the United States was a historic public health achievement. Because measles is so contagious, a high level of vaccination coverage is necessary to prevent outbreaks. **Herd immunity** occurs when most of a population has been vaccinated for an infectious disease. This provides some protection for people who are not vaccinated, but if herd immunity erodes, the most contagious diseases emerge first.

Primarily two types of outbreaks have occurred in the United States in the past, affecting the following groups:
- Unvaccinated preschool-age children
- Highly vaccinated school-age children

The epidemiology of measles reveals two major impediments to measles elimination: (1) unvaccinated preschool-age children, a factor that allows large outbreaks; and (2) vaccine failures, which accounts for outbreaks in highly vaccinated school-age populations. On US college and university campuses, the susceptibility to rubella infection among students is estimated to be as high as 20%. Many cases of rubella infection have been unrecognized or unreported because these cases are mild or subclinical.

Contracting the infection and vaccinating against rubella are the only routes to developing immunity. Individuals should be immune to rubella if they have a dated record of rubella vaccination on or after their first birthday, or if they have demonstrable rubella antibody. Even when antibody titers fall to relatively low levels, previous infection or successful vaccination appears to confer permanent immunity to rubella, except in cases of congenital rubella. The only proof of immunity is a positive serologic screening test result for rubella antibody. A history of rubella infection, even if verified by a physician, is not acceptable evidence of immunity.

It is critical to continue to determine the rubella immune status of women of childbearing age and to vaccinate those who are not immune. If a woman is not rubella immune, she should be vaccinated and advised not to become pregnant for 3 months because of the remote possibility that the vaccination could lead to an infected fetus. Individuals requiring rubella immune status determination include those in the following groups:
- Preschool- and school-age children
- All females at or just before childbearing age
- Women about to be married
- Married women

Pregnant Women

A positive test result confirms immunity, but to rule out any possibility of unsuspected current infection, an IgM screening procedure may also be ordered. If the patient is not rubella immune, she should be cautioned to avoid exposure to rubella infection. Vaccination is contraindicated in pregnant women; however, a woman should be vaccinated immediately after termination of the pregnancy.

Healthcare Personnel

Men and women should be vaccinated to prevent possible spread of nosocomial infection to pregnant patients.

Adverse reactions to rubella vaccine have been reported. The Institute of Medicine has determined that a causal relationship exists between rubella vaccine and acute arthritis in adult females. There is weak but consistent evidence for a causal relationship between rubella vaccine and chronic arthritis in adult women. Incidence rates are estimated to average 13% to 15% in adult women after vaccination. Much lower levels of arthritic adverse reactions were noted in children, adolescents, and adult males. Reliable estimates of excess risk of chronic arthritis after rubella vaccination are not available.

Signs and Symptoms

A diagnosis of acquired rubella is not based solely on **clinical manifestations**. The signs and symptoms of rubella vary widely from person to person and may not be recognized in some cases, especially if the characteristic rash is light or absent, as may occur in a substantial number of cases. Rubella infection also may resemble other disorders, such as infectious mononucleosis and drug-induced rashes.

Acquired Rubella Infection

The incubation period of acquired rubella infection varies from 10 to 21 days, and 12 to 14 days is typical. Infected persons are usually contagious for 12 to 15 days, beginning 5 to 7 days before the appearance (if present) of a rash. Acute rubella infection lasts from 3 to 5 days and generally requires minimal treatment. Permanent effects are extremely rare in acquired infections.

The clinical presentation of acquired rubella is usually mild. The clinical manifestations of infection usually begin with a prodromal period of catarrhal symptoms, followed by involvement of the retroauricular, posterior cervical, and postoccipital lymph nodes, and finally by the emergence of a maculopapular rash on the face and then on the neck and trunk (Figs. 13.4 and 13.5). A temperature less than 34.4°C (94°F) is usually present. In older children and adults, self-limiting arthralgia and arthritis are common.

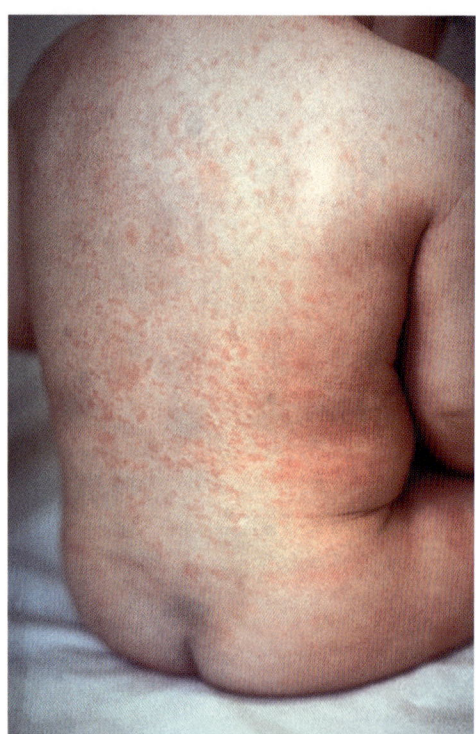

Fig. 13.4 Rubella. (From Marx JA, Hockberger RS, Walls RM: *Rosen's emergency medicine*, ed 6, St. Louis, 2006, Mosby/Elsevier.)

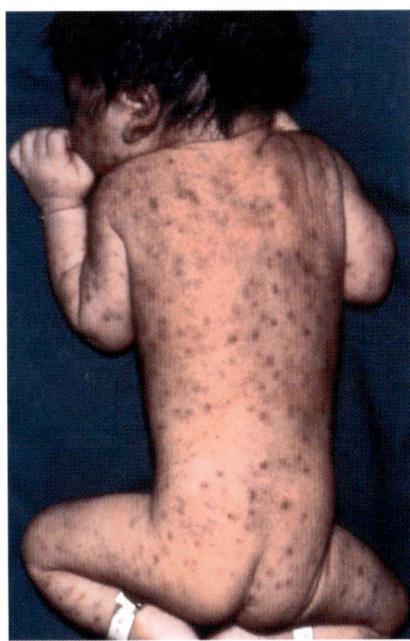

Fig. 13.5 Congenital rubella syndrome and "blueberry muffin" rash. (From Jong EC, Stevens DL, Netter FH: *Netter's infectious diseases*, Philadelphia, 2012, Elsevier/Saunders.)

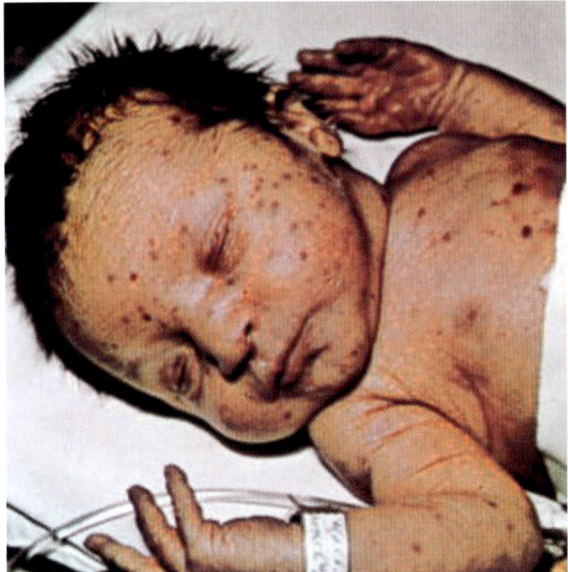

Fig. 13.6 Congenital malformations of rubella. (From Krugman S, Katz SL, Gershon AA, Wilfert CM: *Infectious diseases of children*, ed 8, St. Louis, 1985, Mosby.)

Congenital rubella infection. Rubella infection is usually a mild, self-limiting disease with only rare complications in children and adults. In pregnant women, however, especially those infected in the first trimester, rubella can have devastating effects on the fetus (Fig. 13.6). In utero infection can result in fetal death or manifest as rubella syndrome, a spectrum of congenital defects. About 10% to 20% of infants infected in utero fail to survive beyond 18 months.

The point in the gestation cycle at which maternal rubella infection occurs greatly influences the severity of CRS (Table 13.5); the extent of congenital anomalies varies from one infant to another. Some infants manifest almost all the defects associated with rubella, whereas others exhibit few, if any, consequences of infection. Clinical evidence of congenital rubella infection may not be recognized for months or even years after birth.

Rubella syndrome encompasses a number of congenital anomalies. In addition to stillbirth, fetal abnormalities associated with maternal rubella infection include encephalitis, hepatomegaly, bone defects, intellectual disability, cataracts, thrombocytopenic purpura, cardiovascular defects, splenomegaly, and microcephaly. Severely affected children are likely to have multiple defects in different organ systems. In neonates with CRS, low birth weight and failure to thrive are common.

Rubella immunity develops in almost all children who have had congenital rubella. In late childhood, however, about one-third of these patients lose antibody and become susceptible to acquired rubella. If acquired rubella occurs, it follows a typically benign course. Children with congenital rubella should be screened for rubella immunity in late childhood and vaccinated if necessary.

TABLE 13.5 Manifestation of Anomalies in Maternal Rubella.

Period of Gestation	Risk of Anomaly
Prospective Studies	
First trimester	Approximately 25%
First month	>1%
Second month	≥25%
Third month	≥10%
Serologically Confirmed Cases of Maternal Infection	
Before 11 wk	90%
11–12 wk	33%
13–14 wk	11%
15–16 wk	24%
After 16 wk	0%

> **KEY CONCEPTS: Laboratory Testing for Rubella Infection**
> - In primary rubella infection, the appearance of IgG and IgM antibodies is associated with clinical signs and symptoms, when present. IgM antibodies are detectable a few days after onset of symptoms, reach peak levels at 7 to 10 days, and persist but decrease rapidly in concentration over the next 4 to 5 weeks, until no longer clinically detectable.
> - IgM antibody in a single specimen suggests a recent rubella infection.
> - An unequivocal increase in IgG antibody concentration between the acute and convalescent specimens suggests a recent primary infection or an anamnestic antibody response to rubella in an immune individual.
> - Negative IgM and IgG test results indicate that the patient has never had rubella infection or been vaccinated. These patients are susceptible to infection. If no IgM is demonstrable but IgG is present in paired specimens, the patient is immune.
> - IgM does not cross an intact placental barrier, so its demonstration in a single neonatal specimen is diagnostic of CRS. Rubella infection can be confirmed serologically by IgM antibody testing for at least the first 6 months of life, especially when clinical evidence of congenital rubella is slow in emerging or has an uncertain origin.
> - Laboratory confirmation of measles (rubeola) is made by the detection of measles-specific IgM antibodies in serum, isolation of measles virus, or detection of measles virus RNA by nucleic acid amplification in an appropriate clinical specimen.

Immunologic Manifestations

Acquired Rubella Infection

In a patient with primary rubella infection, the appearance of both IgG and IgM antibodies is associated with the appearance of clinical signs and symptoms, when present.

The IgM antibodies become detectable a few days after the onset of signs and symptoms and reach peak levels at 7 to 10 days. These antibodies persist but rapidly diminish in concentration over the next 4 to 5 weeks, until antibody is no longer clinically detectable. The presence of IgM antibody in a single specimen suggests that the patient has recently experienced a rubella infection. In most cases, the infection probably occurred in the preceding month.

Production of IgG is also associated with the appearance of clinical signs and symptoms. Antibody levels increase rapidly for the next 7 to 21 days and then level off or even decrease in strength. IgG antibodies, however, remain present and protective indefinitely. Detection of IgG antibody is a useful indicator of rubella infection only when the acute and convalescent blood specimens are drawn several weeks apart. Optimum timing for paired testing in the diagnosis of a recent infection is 2 or more weeks apart, with the first (acute) specimen taken before or at the time signs and symptoms appear, or within 2 weeks of exposure.

Paired specimen testing may demonstrate that the antibody levels are the same. In these cases, either the patient was previously immunized or the acute sample was taken after the antibody had already reached maximum levels. Demonstration of an unequivocal increase in the IgG antibody concentration between the acute and convalescent specimens suggests a recent primary infection or a secondary (anamnestic) antibody response to rubella in an immune individual. In cases of an anamnestic response, IgM antibodies are not demonstrable, but IgG production begins quickly. No other signs or symptoms of disease are exhibited.

If both IgM and IgG test results are negative, the patient has never had rubella infection or been vaccinated. Such patients are susceptible to infection. If no IgM is demonstrable but IgG is present in paired specimens, the patient is immune.

In the evaluation of the immune status of patients, IgG antibodies present in a dilution of 1:8 or higher indicate past infection with rubella virus and clinical protection against future rubella infection. The clinical significance of lower levels is not currently known. Titers of 1:16, 1:64, 1:512, or higher may be found in acute and past infections; however, the diagnosis of acute infection requires an IgM antibody titer on the same specimen or a paired specimen comparison. It should be noted that IgM also appears for a transient period after vaccination.

Congenital Rubella Syndrome

Because IgG antibody is capable of crossing the placental barrier, there is no way of distinguishing between IgG antibody of fetal origin and IgG antibody of maternal origin in a neonatal blood specimen (Fig. 13.7).

Testing for IgM antibody is invaluable for the diagnosis of CRS in the neonate. IgM does not cross an intact placental barrier; therefore demonstration of IgM in a single neonatal specimen is diagnostic of CRS. In the newborn, serologic confirmation of rubella infection can be made by testing for IgM antibody for at least the first 6 months of life. This is especially useful when clinical evidence of congenital rubella is slow in emerging or is of uncertain origin.

Diagnostic Evaluation

Several screening methods are available, including the TORCH procedure. The assays for the determination of immune status and evidence of recent infection are presented in Table 13.6.

Persons with infectious mononucleosis sometimes have rubella-specific IgM in low concentrations. Crossreactions of rubella

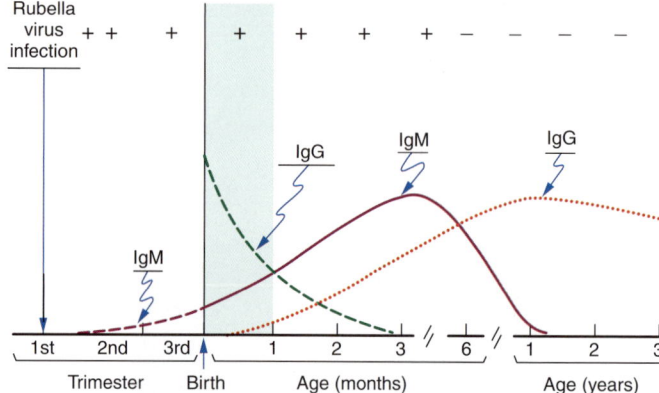

Fig. 13.7 Natural history of congenital rubella: pattern of virus excretion and antibody response. *IgG*, Immunoglobulin G; *IgM*, immunoglobulin M. (Adapted from Krugman S, Katz SL, Gershon AA, Wilfert CM, editors. *Infectious diseases of children*, ed 9, St. Louis, 1992, Mosby Year Book.)

IgM-positive sera can result from parvovirus IgM. Occasionally, pregnant women will demonstrate IgM antibodies not only to rubella but also to CMV, varicella-zoster virus, and measles virus. In these patients, diagnosis of rubella can be made only by the assessment of rubella-specific IgG antibodies supported by a detailed clinical history.

RUBEOLA (MEASLES)

Rubella and rubeola are two distinctly different infections. Rubeola is referred to as *measles*. Measles is a highly contagious disease caused by the rubeola virus. Rubella and rubeola — also known as German measles and measles, respectively — are both contagious viral infections.. The names and symptoms of these infections are similar and can be difficult to tell the difference beween them. Both infections are less common now because of vaccines developed in the 1960s.

Epidemiology

Endemic or sustained measles transmission has not occurred in the United States since the late 1990s. The minimal number of cases yearly in the United States is a result of the high rate of vaccination. Occasional small outbreaks from imported cases of measles primarily infects unvaccinated individuals.

Even though the ongoing transmission of endemic (native) measles was declared to be eliminated in the United States in 2000, the disease is still common in many other countries and can be imported into the United States by foreign visitors or returning travelers who are not fully protected against the disease. From 2001 to 2008, a median of 56 cases of measles was reported to the CDC annually. However, during the first 19 weeks of 2011, 118 cases of measles were reported, the highest number reported for this period since 1996. Of these cases, 87% were imported from the WHO European and Southeast Asia regions; 89% of these patients were unvaccinated.

Measles are caused by a single-strand RNA virus, the only member of the genus *Morbillivirus* (Paramyxoviridae family). Human beings are the only natural reservoirs of this virus, which is spread by respiratory droplets. It is highly contagious, with more than a 90% transmission rate among nonimmunized individuals.

Prevention

Prevention includes MMR vaccine administered to 12- to 15-month-old children, with revaccination between 4 and 12 years

TABLE 13.6 Rubella—CDC Recommendations for Testing.

Preference	Test	Specimen	Indication	Timing
Preferred test	RT-PCR Ideally performed within 10 days of rash onset	A specimen for detection of virus should be collected as soon as possible upon suspicion of rubella. Nasopharyngeal (NP) or throat (OP) swab should be collected within 3 days of rash onset but can be collected up to 7 days. Urine can be collected in addition to swab.	Acute disease	Specimen collection should be as soon as possible upon suspicion of rubella. RT-PCR should be performed for all suspected rubella cases identified within 7 days of rash onset. If specimen collection is >7 days, PCR testing is generally not recommended. Collecting a urine specimen along with NP or OP swab may improve test sensitivity.
Preferred test	IgM (with IgG)	Serum	Acute disease	In addition to RT-PCR, IgM serology testing can be obtained. IgM is most sensitive 4+ days after rash onset and may be negative 0–3 days after rash onset. IgM can be detected for 30 days after acute rubella. Testing IgG in acute cases can provide evidence of pre-existing immunity which can help to differentiate rare instances of vaccine failure. Rubella testing in asymptomatic, unexposed pregnant patients is inappropriate.
Only test for immunity	IgG only	Serum	Evidence of immunity	IgM testing is not appropriate testing for immunity. IgG can be detected approximately 2 weeks after measles vaccination. The presence of rubella specific IgG indicates a recent or prior exposure to measles virus or measles vaccine.

Notes
NP/OP swab collection (separated by at least 2 weeks) to demonstrate a 4-fold increase in IgG titer can confirm measles infection but is generally not required to confirm measles infection.
Viral culture is a valid way to confirm cases of acute rubella disease; however, is not generally recommended as it takes longer to receive results than RT-PCR, which is widely available. Specimen collection and timing is similar to that for RT-PCR.
Acute and convalescent phase serum specimen collection (separated by at least 2 weeks) to demonstrate a 4-fold increase in IgG titer can confirm rubella infection but is generally not required.
Rubella is a mandatory, immediately notifiable disease. Please report confirmed and probable cases of rubella to your local health department.
Adapted from Centers for Disease Control and Prevention. www.CDC.gov. Accessed on August 19, 2024.

of age. A high fever and pulmonary infiltrates can occur in patients exposed to measles who were vaccinated with MMR from 1964 to 1967. Because the vaccine is a live attenuated virus, it should not be used in pregnant women or those with significant immunosuppression.

Laboratory Testing

Laboratory confirmation of measles is made by the detection of measles-specific IgM antibodies in serum, isolation of measles virus, or detection of measles virus RNA by nucleic acid amplification in an appropriate clinical specimen (e.g., nasopharyngeal or oropharyngeal swabs, nasal aspirates, throat washes, or urine; Table 13.7).

Serum testing for antibodies is done for the following reasons:
- Can confirm acute infection with measles using IgM and IgG serial testing
- Can confirm seroconversion after vaccination using IgG testing

TABLE 13.7 Measles (Rubeola) Antibody Testing.

Test Name	Recommended Use	Comments
Viral culture method—cell culture, immunofluorescence	Gold standard procedure	Nasopharyngeal aspirate, washing, throat swab, lung tissue, CSF or urine samples
Serology testing	Measles (rubeola) antibody IgM	Detection of specific IgM antibodies in a serum specimens collected within the first few days of rash onset can provide presumptive evidence of a current or recent measles virus infection. Serology
Real-time RT-PCR	Real-time RT-PCR uses nasopharyngeal, throat swabs, and urine specimens. RT-PCR is available at many state public health laboratories and through the APHL/CDC Vaccine Preventable Disease Reference Centers	Real-time RT-PCR has the greatest diagnostic sensitivity when specimens are collected at first contact with a suspected case. If the acute-phase serum specimen collected ≤3 days after rash onset is negative, and the case has a negative (or not done) result for real-time RT-PCR (rRT-PCR), a second serum specimen collected 3–10 days after symptom onset is recommended. This is because the IgM response is not detectable in some cases until 3 days after symptom onset.

CDC Measles (Rubeola) https://www.cdc.gov/measles Accessed on September 24, 2024.

- IgM and IgG CSF testing to identify subacute sclerosing panencephalitis, which may occur years after the original infection using IgG testing
- Viral culture
- Nasopharyngeal and blood cultures; most sensitive if collected during prodrome up to 1 to 2 days after onset of rash
- Virus can be isolated from urine culture up to 1 week or more after onset of rash
- Difficult to isolate from CSF and brain tissue

CYTOMEGALOVIRUS

Etiology

CMV is a ubiquitous human viral pathogen. The first descriptive report of histologic changes characteristic of those now associated with CMV infection was originally published in 1904, when protozoan-like cells in the lungs, kidneys, and liver of a syphilitic fetus were seen. It was not until 1956 and 1957 that CMV was isolated in the laboratory. Actual isolation of the virus after transfusion, and observation of elevated antibody titers, occurred in 1966.

Human CMV is classified as a member of the herpes family of viruses (herpes viruses). All the herpes viruses are relatively large, enveloped DNA viruses that undergo a replicative cycle involving DNA expression and nucleocapsid assembly within the nucleus. The viral structure gains an envelope when the virus buds through the nuclear membrane, which in turn is altered to contain specific viral proteins.

Although the herpes viruses produce diverse clinical diseases, they share the basic characteristic of being cell associated. The requirements for cell association vary, but herpes viruses may spread from cell to cell, presumably via intercellular bridges and in the presence of antibody in the extracellular phase. CMV spreads to the lymphoid tissues and proceeds to circulate to systemic lymph nodes. The virus finally comes to rest in the epithelial cells of many tissues. This common characteristic may play a role in the ability of these viruses to produce subclinical infections that can be reactivated under appropriate stimuli.

> **KEY CONCEPTS: Characteristics of Cytomegalovirus**
> - CMV is a herpes virus. All the herpes viruses are relatively large, enveloped DNA viruses that undergo a replicative cycle involving DNA expression and nucleocapsid assembly within the nucleus. Although the herpes virus family causes various clinical diseases, herpes viruses share the basic feature of being cell associated.
> - CMV may produce subclinical infections that can be reactivated under appropriate stimuli. Dissemination of the virus may occur by the oral, respiratory, or venereal route, in addition to parenterally by organ transplantation or by transfusion of fresh blood.
> - The incidence of primary CMV infections during childhood is low. Patients at highest risk of mortality from CMV infections are allograft transplant, seronegative patients who receive tissue from a seropositive donor. Most of these infections are transmitted by the donor organ or from reactivation of the recipient's latent virus.
> - Transmission of CMV through transfusion of blood and blood components containing white blood cells (WBCs) is increasingly important in immunocompromised patients who require supportive therapy. Low-birth-weight neonates are also at high risk from CMV infections from infected blood products.
> - Persistent infections characterized by periods of reactivation of CMV (latent infections) have not been clearly defined for CMV.
> - CMV is a major cause of congenital viral infections in the United States because primary and recurrent maternal CMV infections can be transmitted in utero.

Epidemiology

CMV infection is endemic worldwide, with most urban adults demonstrating evidence of infection; 50% to 80% of adults in the United States are infected with CMV by age 40 years. The prevalence of CMV seropositivity increases steadily with age. CMV is found in all geographic and socioeconomic groups, but in general it is more widespread in developing countries and areas of lower socioeconomic conditions.

CMV is a major health risk because a large proportion of women, particularly White women, entering their childbearing years lack antibody to CMV. Those at greatest risk of infection are fetuses and immunocompromised persons.

Transmission

Transmission of CMV may be by the oral, respiratory, or venereal route. The virus has been isolated in urine, saliva, feces, breast milk, blood, cervical secretions, virus-infected grafts from a donor, semen, vaginal fluid, and respiratory droplets. It may also be transmitted by the transfusion of fresh blood. Transmission of CMV appears to require intimate contact with secretions or excretions. CMV can be transmitted from a pregnant woman to her fetus during pregnancy.

Infection From Blood Transfusion

Peripheral blood leukocytes and transplanted tissues have been strongly incriminated as sources of CMV. Transmission of CMV by transfusion of blood or blood components containing WBCs has assumed increased importance in patients with severely impaired immunity who require supportive therapy. In the United States CMV screening is required for all units of blood collected from donors. Preventive methods in these patients include effective donor screening, leukocyte-depleted or irradiated blood products, and immunoglobulin containing passively acquired CMV antibodies. The use of irradiated blood products has become more popular.

Infection From Breast Milk

Postnatal CMV infection can cause serious morbidity and mortality in very-low-birth-weight (VLBW) infants. The primary sources of postnatal CMV infection in this population are breast milk and blood transfusion. Transfusion of CMV-seronegative and leukoreduced blood products effectively prevents transmission of CMV to VLBW infants. However, among infants whose care is managed with this transfusion approach, maternal breast milk is the primary source of postnatal CMV infection.

Other Aspects of Infection

Once in a person's body, CMV stays there for life. Most CMV infections are silent, causing no signs or symptoms. Individuals who are CMV positive (infected with CMV in the past) usually do not have the virus in their urine or saliva, so the risk of acquiring a CMV infection from casual contact is negligible.

Women who are pregnant or planning a pregnancy should follow hygienic practices (e.g., careful handwashing) to prevent CMV infection. Because young children are more likely to have CMV in their urine or saliva than older children or adults, pregnant women who have or work with young children should be especially careful.

Healthcare professionals represent a group that has become increasingly concerned about the risks associated with exposure to CMV. Nosocomial transmission from patients to healthcare workers has not been documented, but observance of good personal hygiene and handwashing offer the best measures for preventing transmission.

Latent Infection

Persistent infections characterized by periods of reactivation are commonly termed latent infections. CMV can persist in a latent state, and active infections may develop under a variety of conditions (e.g., pregnancy; immunosuppression; after organ, bone, or stem cell transplantation). Of immunosuppressed patients, only seronegative patients appear to be at a significant risk of developing CMV infection. Patients at the highest risk of mortality from CMV infections are allograft transplant, seronegative patients who receive tissue from a seropositive donor. The great majority of infections in allograft recipients are transmitted by a donated organ or arise from the reactivation of the recipient's latent virus.

True viral latency is defined by the presence of the genetic information in an unexpressed state in the host cell. An operational definition of latency can include the conditions of a dynamic relationship between the virus and host, along with evidence of latency and reactivation of a latent infection. As with any herpes virus, CMV reactivation is possible at any time but rarely manifests in immunocompetent individuals.

Congenital Infection

Primary and recurrent maternal CMV infection can be transmitted in utero. CMV is the most common virus transmitted to the fetus. Approximately 1 in 150 children is born with congenital CMV infection, and about 1 in 5 babies with congenital CMV infection will be ill from the virus or will have long-term health problems.

The presence of maternal antibody to CMV before conception provides substantial protection against damaging, congenital CMV infection in the newborn.

Signs and Symptoms
Acquired Infection

Acquired CMV infection is usually asymptomatic and can persist in the host as a chronic or latent infection. The incubation period is believed to be 3 to 12 weeks.

In most patients, CMV infection is asymptomatic. Occasionally a self-limited, heterophile-negative, mononucleosis-like syndrome results. CMV hepatitis can also develop.

Symptoms include a sore throat and fever, swollen glands, chills, profound malaise, and myalgia. Lymphadenopathy and splenomegaly may be observed. Infections occurring in healthy immunocompetent individuals usually result in seroconversion. Virus may be excreted in the urine during primary and recurrent CMV infections; it can persist sporadically for months or years. Persons experiencing acquired infection, reinfection with the same or different strains of CMV, or reactivation of a latent infection can excrete the virus in titers as high as 10^6 infective units per milliliter in the urine or saliva for weeks or months.

Normal adults and children usually experience CMV infection without serious complications. Uncommon complications of CMV infection in previously healthy individuals, however, include interstitial pneumonitis, hepatitis, Guillain-Barré syndrome, meningoencephalitis, myocarditis, thrombocytopenia, and hemolytic anemia.

CMV infection can be life-threatening in immunosuppressed patients. Infections in these patients may result in disseminated multisystem involvement, including pneumonitis, hepatitis, GI ulceration, arthralgias, meningoencephalitis, and retinitis. Retinitis and encephalitis are common manifestations of disseminated CMV. Ulcerative damage of tissues (e.g., esophagus) is another demonstration of the cytopathic effects of CMV. Interstitial pneumonitis, which is commonly associated with CMV infection, is a major cause of death after allogeneic bone marrow transplantation. In premature infants, acquired CMV infection can result in atypical lymphocytosis, hepatosplenomegaly, pneumonia, or death.

Transfusion-acquired CMV infections may cause not only a mononucleosis-like syndrome, but also hepatitis and increased rejection of transplanted organs. Three types of CMV infections are possible in blood transfusion recipients:

1. **Primary infection** occurs when a previously unexposed (seronegative) recipient is transfused with blood from an actively or latently infected donor. This type of infection is accompanied by the presence of virus in the blood and urine, an immediate antibody response, and eventual seroconversion. Patients with primary infections may be symptomatic, but the great majority are asymptomatic.
2. **Reactivated infection** can occur when a seropositive recipient is transfused with blood from a CMV antibody–positive or CMV antibody–negative donor. Donor leukocytes are believed to trigger an allograft reaction, which in turn reactivates the recipient's latent infection. These infections may be accompanied by significant increases in CMV-specific antibody. Some reactivated infections exhibit viral shedding as their only manifestation. Reactivated infections are largely asymptomatic.
3. Reinfection can occur by a CMV strain in the donor's blood that differs from the strain that originally infected the recipient. A significant antibody response is observed, and viral shedding occurs. Although it is difficult to differentiate a reactivated infection if the patient and donor are CMV antibody positive before transfusion, reinfections can be documented if isolates can be obtained from the donor and recipient.

Congenital Infection

The classic congenital CMV syndrome is manifested by a high incidence of neurologic symptoms, in addition to neuromuscular disorders, jaundice, hepatomegaly, and splenomegaly. Skin eruptions, the most common clinical sign, are seen in about 50% of CMV-infected infants.

Congenitally infected newborns, especially those who acquire CMV during a maternal primary infection, are more prone to develop severe cytomegalic inclusion disease (CID). The severe form of CID may be fatal or can cause permanent neurologic sequelae, such as intracranial calcifications (Fig. 13.8), intellectual disability, deafness, vision defects, microcephaly, and motor dysfunction. Psychomotor impairment is seen in 51% to 75% of survivors. Hearing loss is observed in 20% to 50% and visual impairment in 20% of patients. Infants without symptoms at birth may develop hearing impairment and neurologic impairment later.

Immunologic Manifestations
Immune System Alterations

CMV infection is known to alter the immune system and to produce overt manifestations of infection. Infection interferes with immune responsiveness in normal and immunocompromised individuals. This diminished responsiveness results in a decreased proliferative response to the CMV antigen, which persists for several months. In patients with CMV mononucleosis-like syndrome, alterations of T-lymphocyte subsets result, producing an increase in the absolute number of CD8+ lymphocytes and a decrease in CD4+ lymphocytes. These subset abnormalities persist for months.

Questions have been raised regarding CMV as a potentially oncogenic virus because viral antigens and nucleic acids have been found in human malignancies, including adenocarcinoma of the colon, carcinoma of the cervix, cancer of the prostate, and Kaposi sarcoma. CMV does have transforming properties in vitro. Although considerable circumstantial evidence exists linking CMV to human malignancies, especially Kaposi sarcoma, a direct cause and effect relationship has not been established.

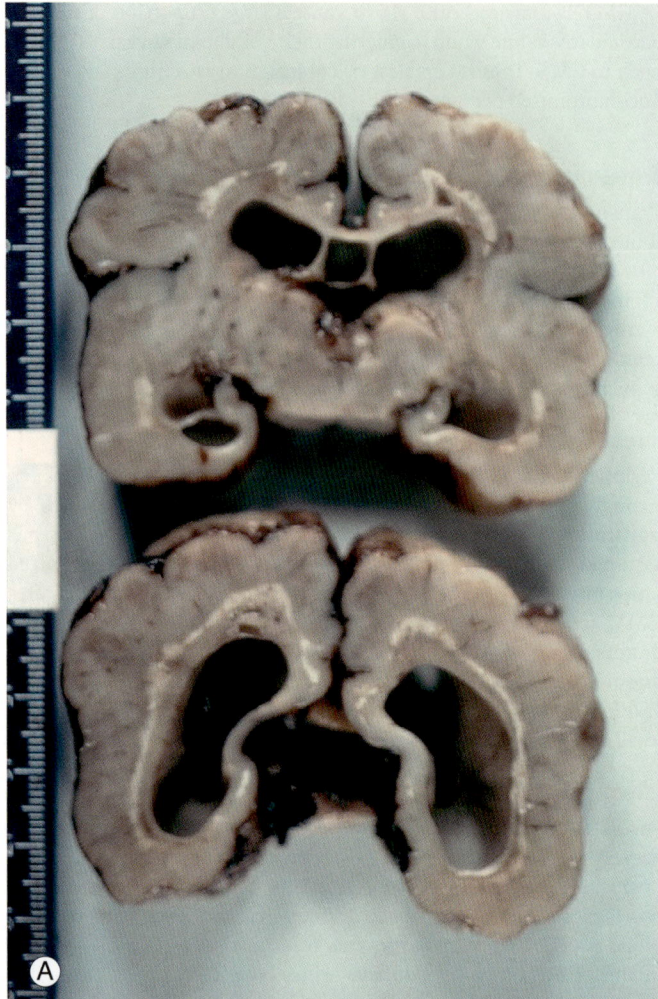

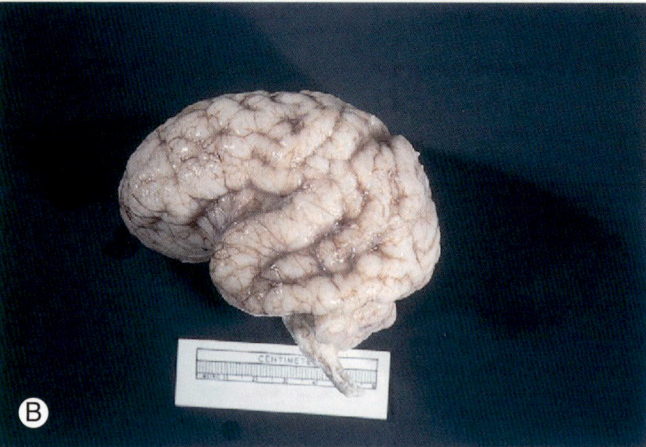

Fig. 13.8 Cytomegalovirus (CMV) Infection. (A) Coronal sections of the brain show a periventricular ring of calcifications and enlarged ventricles. (B) Microencephaly with polymicrogyria secondary to CMV. (From Gilbert-Barness E, Kapur RP, Oligny LL: *Potter's pathology of the fetus, infant and child,* ed 2, St. Louis, 2007, Elsevier.)

> **KEY CONCEPTS: Immunologic Characteristics of Cytomegalovirus Infection**
> - In CMV-infected cells, antigens appear at various times after infection, before the replication of viral DNA. Immediate-early antigens appear within 1 hour of cellular infection and early antigens within 24 hours. At about 72 hours or the end of the viral replication cycle, late antigens appear.
> - The presence of antibodies against immediate-early and early antigens is associated with active infection, primary or reactivated.
> - Primary infection is demonstrated by a transient, virus-specific IgM antibody response and eventual seroconversion to produce IgG antibodies to the virus.
> - Reactivation of latent CMV infection in seropositive (IgG) individuals may be accompanied by a significant increase in IgG antibodies to the virus, but no detectable IgM response.
> - Reinfection by a different CMV strain than the original infecting strain results in a significant IgG antibody response but unknown IgM response.
> - Serologic methods (e.g., EIA) to detect CMV-specific IgM can represent primary infection or rare reactivation. Detection of significant increases in CMV-specific IgG antibody suggest, but do not prove, recent infection or reactivation of latent infection.

Serologic Markers

In cells infected by CMV, several antigens appear at varying times after infection. Before replication of viral DNA takes place, *immediate-early antigens* and *early antigens* are present in the nuclei of infected cells. Immediate-early antigens appear within 1 hour of cellular infection, and early antigens are present within 24 hours. At about 72 hours after infection, or the end of the viral replication cycle, late antigens are demonstrable in the nucleus and cytoplasm of infected cells.

The immune antibody response to these various antigens differs in incidence and significance. The presence of antibodies against immediate-early and early antigens is associated with active infection, either primary or reactivated. New CMV infections can be identified by testing for IgG antibodies on blood samples taken at different times. If the first sample is negative and the second sample is positive, the patient became infected with CMV between the two blood samples.

A newer method, called *IgG avidity testing*, which measures antibody maturity, has been shown to detect recent primary CMV infection reliably. This test is available on a limited basis in the United States.

Antibody to early antigen undergoes a relatively rapid decline after recovery but can persist for up to 250 days and may identify patients with recent, in addition to active, infection. The presence of antibody to early antigen is strongly associated with viral shedding. Antibodies to late antigens persist in high titer long after the recovery from an active infection.

The incidence of viral exposure and subsequent antibody formation (seropositivity) varies greatly, depending on the socioeconomic status and living conditions of the population surveyed. The prevalence of CMV antibody varies with age and geographic location but ranges from 40% to 100%.

The characteristic antibody responses associated with infection are as follows:
- Primary infection, demonstrated by a transient virus-specific IgM antibody response and eventual seroconversion to produce IgG antibodies to the virus.
- Reactivation of latent infection in seropositive (IgG) individuals, which may be accompanied by significant increases in IgG antibodies to the virus, but elicits no detectable IgM response.
- Reinfection by a strain of CMV different from the original infecting strain. A significant IgG antibody response is demonstrated. It is not known whether an IgM response occurs.

There is no vaccine currently available for preventing congenital CMV disease (present at birth). A few CMV vaccines are being tested in humans, including live attenuated (weakened) virus vaccines and vaccines that contain only pieces of the virus.

In CMV infection, hematologic examination of the blood usually reveals a characteristic leukocytosis. A slight lymphocytosis with more than 20% variant lymphocytes is common. CMV infection is possible in the following situations:
- The patient has mononucleosis-like symptoms but exhibits a negative Epstein-Barr virus (EBV) test result.
- The patient manifests hepatitis symptoms but does not demonstrate any positive results when tested for common hepatitis viruses.

In affected infants, the most common laboratory abnormality is a low platelet count (thrombocytopenia). Clinical chemistry assays may demonstrate abnormal liver function. Presence of infection is also demonstrated by inclusion bodies in leukocytes in urine sediment.

Laboratory Evaluation

In immunocompromised patients, CMV serology is not recommended. Key facts about diagnostic testing include:
1. The enzyme-linked immunosorbent assay is the most common serologic test for measuring antibody to CMV.
2. Congenital CMV infection cannot be diagnosed with antibody testing (IgG and IgM).
3. The standard laboratory test for diagnosing congenital CMV infection is a PCR on saliva, with a confirmatory test on urine (Table 13.8).

Diagnostic Laboratory Testing

According to the CDC, tests for patients older than 12 months of age can include serologic tests that detect CMV antibodies (IgM and IgG). The enzyme-linked immunosorbent assay (ELISA) is the most common serologic test for measuring antibody to CMV.

Diagnostic Testing for Congenital CMV in Newborns

Polymerase chain reaction (PCR) testing using saliva is the standard laboratory test for diagnosing congenital CMV infection. Urine is usually collected and tested for confirmation. The reason for the confirmatory test on urine is that most CMV seropositive mothers shed CMV in their breast milk. This can cause a false-positive CMV result on saliva collected shortly after the baby has breast fed.

Currently, testing of newborns for CMV is not routinely performed, though some states perform targeted CMV testing of newborns who fail the hearing screening. CDC is currently studying whether dried blood spots (DBS), which are already collected on almost all newborns, can identify the majority of children who are most likely to suffer long-term health problems from congenital CMV.

The CDC guidelines for CMV testing in newborns has specific steps for appropriate collection of saliva samples from a baby:

Collect a saliva specimen more than 1 hour after breastfeeding and within 3 weeks of birth. Detection of CMV after 3 weeks could be the result of post-partum infection.

Insert a sterile cotton or polyester swab into the baby's mouth between the gum and cheek, and swirl for several seconds.

Remove the swab and place into a buffer formulated for PCR diagnostic testing. If CMV is present, it will leach from swab to the liquid.

The liquid is processed according to manufacturer's instructions, and PCR testing is performed according to the protocol in the laboratory. Specific procedures and interpretation of tests vary according to the laboratory.

TABLE 13.8 Laboratory Diagnosis of Cytomegalovirus Infection.[a]

Method	Test Method	Recommended Use
Cytomegalovirus (CMV) rapid culture	Cell culture, immunofluorescence	Rapid diagnosis of CMV infection Gold standard test for tissue
CMV by polymerase chain reaction (PCR) Blood, bone marrow, amniotic fluid	Qualitative PCR	Rapid test for diagnosing CMV in immunocompromised patients or solid organ donors. Amniotic fluid from a fetus of >20 weeks' gestation can be analyzed.
CMV PCR	Quantitative PCR	Diagnosing CMV infection Monitoring disease state in solid organ transplant and HIV patients
CMV antibodies: IgM and IgG	Latex agglutination	Screen pregnant women and infants possibly infected with CMV. Infants may test positive during first 6 months because of maternal antibodies. Discriminate between current (IgM) and prior infections (IgG).
CMV antibodies: total	Solid-phase agglutination	Screen organ donors.
CMV by immunohistochemistry	Immunohistochemistry	Histologic diagnosis of CMV based on tissue from affected site

[a] A negative result (less than 2.6 log copies per milliliter, or less than 390 copies per milliliter) does not rule out the presence of PCR inhibitors in the patient specimen or CMV nucleic acid in concentrations below the assay's level of detection. Inhibition may also lead to underestimation of viral quantitation.

HIV, Human immunodeficiency virus; *IgG*, immunoglobulin G; *IgM*, immunoglobulin M.

Adapted from Associated Regional and University Pathologists (ARUP) Laboratories: ARUP's laboratory test directory, 2012, https://www.aruplab.com.

Virus Detection

CMV IgM Testing. The presence of CMV IgM cannot be used by itself to diagnose primary CMV infection because IgM can also be present during secondary CMV infection. IgM positive results in combination with low IgG avidity results are considered reliable evidence for primary infection.

CMV IgG Testing. A positive test for CMV IgG in a patient older than 12 months of age indicates that the patient was infected with CMV at some time during their life but does not indicate when a patient was infected. This applies for people 12 months or older when maternal antibodies are no longer present.

Measurement of CMV IgG in paired samples taken one to three months apart can be used to diagnose primary CMV infection. Seroconversion (1st sample IgG negative, 2nd sample IgG positive) is documented evidence of a recent primary infection.

Avidity Testing. IgG avidity assays measure the binding strength between IgG antibodies and virus that can help distinguish a primary CMV infection from a past infection. Following primary CMV infection, IgG antibodies have low binding strength (low avidity), then over 2 to 4 months they mature to high binding strength (high avidity). Commercial tests for CMV avidity are available in the United States, however they are not FDA-approved and require further standardization and thus need to be used and interpreted with caution.

> **KEY CONCEPTS: Herpes Virus Facts**
> - All the human herpes viruses are large, enveloped DNA viruses that replicate within the cell's nucleus. The virus gains an envelope when the virus buds through the nuclear membrane, which has been altered to contain specific viral proteins.
> - Herpes viruses cause a number of different clinical diseases, and they share the basic characteristic of being cell associated.

HERPES VIRUSES

In addition to two members of the human herpes viruses CMV (previously presented in this chapter) and EBV (discussed in Chapter 17, Infectious Mononucleosis). Other members of the human herpes virus family associated with congenital infections (i.e., HSV, varicella-zoster virus [VZV], and human herpes virus-6 [HHV-6]) are briefly described in this section.

All the human herpes viruses are large, enveloped DNA viruses that replicate within the cell's nucleus. The virus gains an envelope when the virus buds through the nuclear membrane, which has been altered to contain specific viral proteins.

The herpes viruses cause a number of clinical diseases, although they share the basic characteristic of being cell associated, which may partly account for their ability to produce subclinical infections that can be reactivated under appropriate stimuli.

> **KEY CONCEPTS: Herpes Simplex Virus Facts**
> - HSV can be cultured from the oropharynx in about 1% of healthy adults and from the genital tract of slightly less than 1% of asymptomatic adult women who are not pregnant.
> - The incidence of HSV seropositivity rises to almost 100% in some populations by the age of 45 years, but antibody prevalence in adults varies greatly with socioeconomic class.
> - The most common manifestation of HSV infection is the common cold sore or fever blister.
> - Neonatal HSV infections may be acquired in the antenatal or perinatal period.
> - Methods for the laboratory diagnosis of HSV include isolation of the virus and direct detection of antigen in tissues or cytologic preparation through the use of immunofluorescence or immunoenzyme methods. In addition, detection of the virus using monoclonal antibodies can be performed with immunoassays or immunoblot techniques.

Herpes Simplex Virus

HSV can be cultured from the oropharynx in about 1% of healthy adults and from the genital tract of slightly less than 1% of asymptomatic adult women who are not pregnant. HSV is widespread. Human beings are the only natural hosts or known reservoir of infection. The incubation period is 2 to 12 days. The incidence of seropositivity rises to almost 100% in some populations by the age of 45 years. Antibody prevalence in adults varies greatly with socioeconomic class; 30% to 50% of upper socioeconomic class adults have detectable antibody to HSV compared with 80% to 100% of adults in lower socioeconomic groups.

The most common manifestation of HSV infection is the common cold sore or fever blister. HSV has been shown to be related to a wide variety of clinical syndromes and to subclinical infection, occurring with primary or recurrent disease. Recurrent HSV disease usually results from the reactivation of latent virus resting in paraspinal or cranial nerve ganglia that innervate the site of primary infection. Distant sites may be involved. Activated virus presumably travels down the axon to the skin (or other site) and induces disease. In some cases, exogenous reinfection can occur. Recurrence with cell-to-cell spread of virus occurs in the presence of serum-neutralizing antibodies.

Two crossreacting antigen types of HSV have been identified, type 1 (HSV-1) and type 2 (HSV-2). HSV-1 is generally found in and around the oral cavity and in skin lesions that occur above the waist. HSV-2 is isolated primarily to the genital tract and skin lesions below the waist.

Congenital and Neonatal Infection

Malnutrition, severe illness, many acute childhood illnesses, and prematurity predispose infants and young children to disseminated primary infection. Neonatal HSV infections may be acquired in the antenatal or perinatal period. Active lesions in the mother's genital tract at birth present the greatest risk of infection to the newborn. The spectrum of disease in an infected newborn varies from subclinical to severe. In cases of overwhelming generalized infection, the infant may develop encephalitis and respiratory failure; hepatic failure, with increasing jaundice and adrenal insufficiency, may occur. Infants who survive severe infection are frequently left with some neurologic damage and may have recurrent vesicular skin lesions for many years.

Laboratory Diagnosis

Methods for the laboratory diagnosis of HSV include isolation of the virus and direct detection of antigen in tissues or cytologic preparation through the use of immunofluorescence or immunoenzyme methods. In addition, detection of the virus in body fluids (using monoclonal antibodies) can be performed with immunoassays or immunoblot techniques. Serologic diagnosis of primary infections can be demonstrated when a fourfold or higher RNA viruses rise in titer occurs. Titers may rise significantly in early recurrent infection but usually become stable at moderately high levels after multiple recurrences.

> **KEY CONCEPTS: Varicella-Zoster Virus Facts**
> - The name varicella-zoster virus reflects two associated diseases: varicella (chickenpox) and zoster (shingles).
> - Varicella primarily affects children aged 2 to 5 years; zoster occurs most commonly in older individuals.
> - Reactivation of VZV is associated with a depressed immune response. High-risk patients include older adults and immunocompromised patients.
> - Neonatal varicella may be acquired in utero or in the perinatal period and can result in congenital abnormalities.
> - Laboratory diagnosis of VZV is similar to methods used to diagnose HSV. Serologic methods include indirect immunofluorescence, which detects antibodies to specific membrane antigens, and EIA.

Varicella-Zoster Virus

VZV is the cause of two different types of clinical diseases resulting from the same virus infection. Primary infection with the virus results in the clinical manifestations of chickenpox. After a primary infection, the virus enters a latent phase, presumably within nuclei in the dorsal root ganglia. Reactivation of the virus results in the characteristic clinical manifestation of zoster, known as *shingles*.

Epidemiology and Etiology

Human beings are the only natural hosts of VZV. Varicella primarily affects children aged 2 to 5 years. The virus is endemic and highly contagious. Periodic epidemics do occur. The presumed route of transmission is through the respiratory tract.

Zoster is less communicable than varicella. This sporadic disease occurs most commonly in older individuals. Antibodies to varicella do not protect against reactivation or clinical zoster. The reactivation of VZV is associated with a depressed immune response. Patients with AIDS, older adults, and immunocompromised persons are at high risk of developing disease. In addition manipulation of the spinal cord, local radiation therapy, and therapy that suppresses cellular immunity have been associated with triggering the onset of zoster.

Varicella has an incubation period of 14 to 17 days. There may be a 1- to 3-day prodromal period of fever, headache, and malaise. This precedes the eruption of the characteristic red macular rash, which progresses to papules, vesicles, and pustules that crust over and shed without scarring. Successive crops of lesions continue to appear for 2 to 6 days; therefore multiple lesions in various stages of development are present at any one time.

The name of the virus reflects two associated diseases – varicella (chickenpox) and zoster (shingles). Primary infection with the virus results in the clinical manifestation of chickenpox. After this, the virus enters a latent phase, presumably within nuclei of neurons in dorsal root ganglia or cranial nerve sensory ganglia. The reactivity of the virus results in the clinical manifestations characteristic of zoster.

Signs and Symptoms

Complications of VZV include pneumonitis, encephalitic conditions, nephritis, hepatitis, myocarditis, arthritis, and Reye syndrome. Susceptible individuals who are immunosuppressed have a greater risk of complications after VZV exposure. Another complication can include febrile purpura, which can occur a few days after the onset of the rash and is seen in children and adults. This complication is characterized by thrombocytopenia and hemorrhage into the vesicles. Postinfection purpura, which begins 1 to 2 weeks after the appearance of the rash, is characterized by thrombocytopenia with GI, genitourinary, cutaneous, and mucous membrane hemorrhage. More severe hemorrhagic complications include malignant varicella with purpura and purpura fulminans.

Neonatal varicella infection. Neonatal varicella may be acquired in utero or in the perinatal period and can result in congenital abnormalities. The infant is at greatest risk if the mother's illness occurs 4 days or less before delivery.

Laboratory Diagnosis

The laboratory diagnosis of VZV is similar to methods used to diagnose HSV. Serologic methods include indirect immunofluorescence, which detects antibodies to specific membrane antigens, and EIA.

Rapid preliminary diagnosis can also be made by direct immunofluorescence to detect viral antigens in vesicular lesions. A smear of cells taken from lesions enables direct examination. A presumptive diagnosis can be made by examining scrapings from the base of a vesicular lesion and histologically observing multinucleated giant cells containing intranuclear inclusion bodies, or by observing virus particles on electron microscopy. The best way to confirm VZV infection is to recover the virus in human diploid fibroblast cell cultures.

Antibodies to varicella are detectable within several days of the onset of rash and peak at 2 to 3 weeks. Antibodies to zoster increase more rapidly and are detectable at the onset of clinical symptoms. Because of the rapid turnaround time and correlation with clinical symptoms, serologic methods are preferable to viral isolation methods. In addition ELISA methods are valuable for assessing the immune status of adults.

Prevention

A vaccine is available for those in high-risk groups. The vaccine can be administered before an infection or to prevent reinfection because of waning immunity.

> **KEY CONCEPTS: Characteristics of Human Herpes Virus-6**
> - A new virus classified as a herpes virus because of its shape, size, and in vitro behavior has been identified as human herpes virus-6 (HHV-6).
> - Laboratory methods include direct examination by immunofluorescence or immunoperoxidase staining of cells taken from lesions.
> - In addition, PCR, DNA probes, and serologic methods (e.g., ELISA, radioimmunoassay, indirect immunofluorescence, and latex agglutination) can be used.
> - Culture methods include cocultivation of the patient's peripheral blood cells with cord blood mononuclear cells and examination of these cultures after 5 to 10 days by electron microscopy. Anticomplement immunofluorescence of an infected cell culture has also been used for antibody detection and titration.

Human Herpes Virus 6

One percent of newborns have congenital HHV-6 infection. Most of these congenital infections result from chromosomally integrated HHV-6. The remainder of HHV-6 congenital infections are presumed to be due to maternal HHV-6 reactivation or reinfection with subsequent transplacental infection of the fetus. The integration of the viral genome into human chromosomes is a unique mode of congenital infection.

HHV-6 is the same agent that has been implicated as the cause of roseola infantum (exanthema subitum). Up to 75% of infants develop antibody to HHV-6 by age 10 to 11 months, which suggests a high rate of seropositivity in the general population.

Specimens such as cord blood, peripheral blood, saliva, or urine samples can be analyzed for evidence of HHV-6. These assays include nested PCR assays with virus-specific typing with oligonucleotide probes specific for HHV-6 variants A and B, nested RT-PCR assay to amplify the gp82 to gp105 mRNA of HHV-6, and quantitative PCR assay for the HHV-6 *U38* gene. Serologic assays for HHV-6 antibody include indirect IFA using a clinical HHV-6 isolate that contains HHV-6A and HHV-6B genomes.

> **KEY CONCEPTS: Diversity of Alternate Laboratory Testing Methods**
> - IHC combines anatomic, immunologic, and biochemical characteristics to detect antigens in cells of a tissue section by applying the idea of antibody binding specifically to antigen.
> - The Infectious Disease Pathology Branch (IDPB) of the CDC uses a variety of diagnostic techniques in the evaluation of tissue specimens, including morphologic, antigenic, and nucleic acid methodologies.
> - The CDC currently has diagnostic PCR-based IHC assays for more than 100 etiologic agents, including viral, bacterial, parasitic, and fungal organisms.
> - The traditional direct and indirect IHC methods are the most widely used. Newly developed methods do not rely on antibody labeling, but rather use multiple secondary antibodies and enzymes linked to a polymer backbone.
> - The FDA has approved the FilmArray system from BioFire Diagnostics, which has set a new standard in molecular diagnostics. The system is a panel-based multiplex PCR-based assay for viral and bacterial testing.

ALTERNATE IMMUNOLOGY LABORATORY TECHNIQUES

Immunohistochemistry

In the clinical laboratory IHC plays a significant role in the diagnosis of certain infectious diseases and malignant disorders by testing tissues. IHC offers several distinct advantages compared with traditional identification methods. This technique is rapidly expanding the diagnostic capability of laboratory testing.

IHC combines anatomic, immunologic, and biochemical characteristics to detect antigens in cells of a tissue section by applying the idea of antibody binding specifically to antigen. In IHC an antigen-antibody construct is visualized through light microscopy by means of a color signal. One advantage of IHC over immunofluorescence techniques is the visible morphology of the tissue around the specific antigen by counterstaining (e.g., with hematoxylin [blue]).

IHC is estimated to be the most widely used technique at the protein level in dermatologic diagnostics. It complements morphologic histopathology, especially for the precise diagnosis of skin tumors and skin lymphoma, and for the detection of infectious microorganisms. Protein expression profiles detected through IHC—on the cell surface, intracellularly, and in the nucleus—enable the characterization of cell lineage, tumor, lymphoma, and inflammatory cell infiltrate. Intracellular and extracellular pathogens—bacteria, parasites, and viruses (e.g., *M. tuberculosis*, leishmaniasis, and human herpes viruses)—can be directly detected. Examples of the use of IHC for malignancies (e.g., melanoma and lymphoma) are discussed in Chapter 26.

Use of Immunohistochemistry in Infectious Diseases

IHC is a sensitive and specific test methodology for many microorganisms, and unlike some traditional staining methods, IHC can result in direct, highly interpretable visual evidence of the presence of an infectious agent within tissues. In addition IHC rapidly detects organisms that are difficult to culture and those that cannot be cultured. For some infectious agents, IHC tests may provide the only reliable methods of detection.

The IDPB uses a variety of diagnostic techniques in the evaluation of tissue specimens, including morphologic, antigenic, and nucleic acid methodologies. Molecular tests at the IDPB have been optimized for formalin-fixed paraffin-embedded tissues. The technique uses specific antibodies, which localize to the antigens of the etiologic agent of interest. Currently the IDPB has diagnostic PCR-based IHC assays for more than 100 etiologic agents, including viral, bacterial, parasitic, and fungal organisms. Specific monoclonal antibodies effectively distinguish viral infections caused by several agents:

- HSV-1
- HSV-2
- VZV
- EBV
- CMV

Traditional Immunohistochemistry Protocols

An IHC procedure can be performed in three steps:
1. Tissue processing and epitope retrieval
2. Antigen-antibody interaction
3. Visualization through different detection systems.

For the direct method, labeled monospecific antibody is directly applied to the tissue section (Fig. 13.9). The antibody is most commonly conjugated with biotin. Biotin then binds to labeled avidin

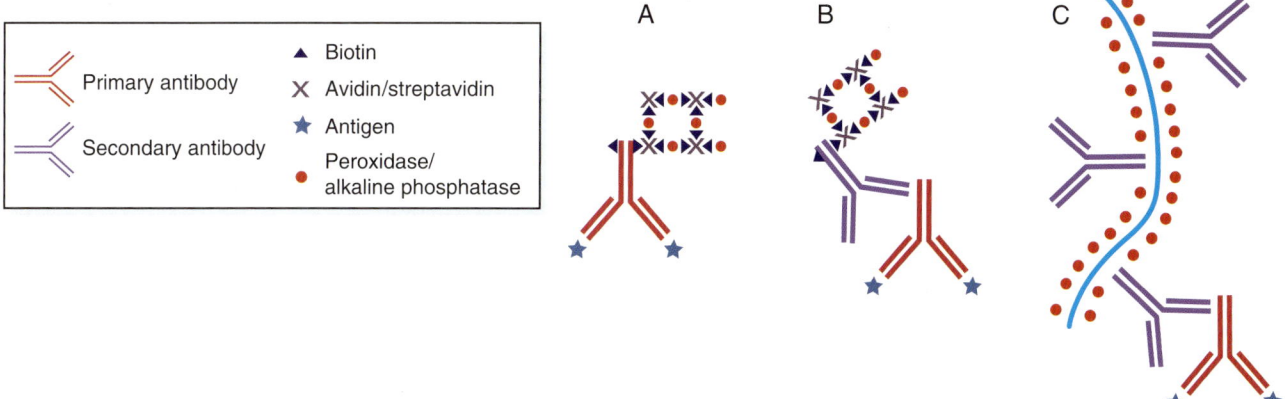

Fig. 13.9 Immunohistochemical Techniques. (A) Direct method. The antigen-specific primary antibody is biotin labeled. Biotin binds to avidin/streptavidin. Color visualization is achieved through enzymatic reaction of horseradish peroxidase/alkaline phosphatase. (B) Indirect method. The antigen-specific primary antibody is unlabeled. The secondary, biotin-labeled antibody binds to primary antibody. Visualization is achieved accordingly through avidin/streptavidin and peroxidase/alkaline phosphatase complexes. The indirect method increases versatility, because unlabeled primary antibodies can be used. (C) Indirect method with polymer chain detection system. Biotin and avidin/streptavidin are replaced by a labeled polymer chain, allowing for increased sensitivity and specificity. (Modified from Schacht V, Kern JS: Basics of immunohistochemistry, *J Invest Dermatol* 135:3, 2012.)

or streptavidin. Through this second layer of labeling, the staining is amplified. The development of a multiple-step detection method allows for detection of a wide range of antigens in tissues.

The indirect method uses two layers of antibodies. Progression from the one-step direct conjugate method to the multiple-step indirect method greatly increased the versatility of IHC, because a wide range of unlabeled primary antibodies could then be used.

Antibody molecules cannot be seen, even under electron microscopy, unless they are labeled or tagged for visualization. Labeling techniques include fluorescent compounds such as direct immunofluorescence or active enzymes for IHC. In IHC, enzymes are added to the tissue sections, and these enzymes bind to the biotin or avidin/streptavidin-labeled antibodies; the enzymes used are horseradish peroxidase or calf intestine alkaline phosphatase. Then chromogens are added to the sections and oxidized by horseradish peroxidase or alkaline phosphatase, leading to a color reaction. The most widely used chromogens result in red or brown IHC staining.

Polymer-Based Immunohistochemistry Methods

The traditional direct and indirect IHC methods are the most widely used, but newly developed detection systems do not rely on antibody labeling through biotin and avidin/streptavidin. Instead, multiple secondary antibodies and enzymes are linked to a polymer backbone. These new methods have the advantage of decreased background staining (higher specificity) and increased sensitivity. Double staining using different colors in one tissue section can be achieved through a combination of two immunoenzymatic systems or one immunoenzymatic system with different substrates.

In July 2015, The Joint Commission revised the laboratory requirements revision of Standards (QSA.02.10.01, EP 7 and QSA.13.06.01, EP 2) for Microbiology Polymer-Based Immunohistochemistry Methods. The first change pertains to the use of a negative control for polymer-based IHC methods. Polymer-based IHC methods allow for the visualization of target proteins through the use of antibodies conjugated to enzyme-labeled polymers. The polymer-based method is more sensitive than traditional techniques, and the polymers do not bind nonspecifically to the tissue sample. Because the absence of nonspecific binding eliminates the likelihood of false-positive results, a negative control is not necessary for this method.

Newer Molecular Testing Approaches

The FDA has cleared the FilmArray system from BioFire Diagnostics, which has set a new standard in molecular diagnostics. The BioFire system is a panel-based multiplex PCR-based assay for viral and bacterial testing. FilmArray's Respiratory and Blood Culture Identifications panels are comprehensive and when combined can test for more than a hundred pathogens. FilmArray requires 2 minutes of hands-on time and returns results in about 1 hour.

Respiratory Virus Panels

The first test of its kind, Nanosphere's (Vancouver, BC, Canada) Verigene Respiratory Pathogens FlexTest (RPFlex) is an automated, multiplex, and flexible nucleic acid test for the identification of the viruses and bacteria that most commonly cause respiratory infections.

To meet diverse testing needs, labs must choose between running expensive megapanels on all samples, offering an assortment of overlapping small and large panels, or using costly reference laboratories. RPFlex consists of one platform and one comprehensive panel.

CASE STUDY 13.1

This 34-year-old Black male was a local delivery truck driver until 2 weeks ago when he was laid off because of the SARS-CoV-2 pandemic. He has been an organist at his local church for the past 5 years.

Two weeks ago he began to feel very tired but with no other medical complaints. Ten days ago he began having difficulty breathing and visited his local emergency care clinic. His blood saturation level was low but he had no other symptoms. Two days after that emergency room visit he began to experience severe shortness of breath. He again returned to the emergency care clinic. On this visit he had a temperature of 100.5°F and a significantly decreased oxygen saturation level. The physician in attendance wanted to admit him to the hospital but he declined because he no longer had healthcare insurance.

The patient returned home, where he expired the next day.

Relevant Laboratory Data
Hemoglobin 10.0 g/dL, WBC 15 × 10^9/L, CRP elevated, oxygen saturation severely decreased.

Questions
1. Patients infected with COVID-19 can have a fever because of:
    a. Acute infection
    b. Hemoglobin deficiency
    c. Increase in lymphocytes in peripheral blood
    d. Cardiac muscle damage
2. The method for initial screening for COVID-19 is:
    a. Chemiluminescence
    b. ELISA
    c. RT-PCR
    d. Evaluation of cytokine levels

Answers to these questions can be found in Appendix A.

Critical Thinking Group Discussion Questions
1. How did SARS-CoV-2 cause the patient's death?
2. When is antibody analysis of serum not an acceptable initial method for detection of COVID-19 infection?

CASE STUDY 13.2

History and Physical Examination
A 24-year-old woman with a history of AIDS comes to the clinic for evaluation of left-sided weakness. She has been experiencing headaches and seizures, and others have observed an alteration in her mental status.

The patient's medical history is notable for an episode of *Pneumocystis jirovecii* (previously called *Pneumocystis carinii*) pneumonia, primary syphilis treated with penicillin 5 years ago, and occasional thrush. She is taking oral prophylactic medications for *Pneumocystis*. An urgent computed tomography (CT) scan of the head shows two 1-cm lesions in the right basal ganglia, enhanced with intravenous contrast media.

Laboratory Data
- CD4 cell count: 50 × 10^9/L
- Rapid plasma reagin (RPR): Positive at 1:2
- Toxoplasmosis IgG: Positive
- Toxoplasmosis IgM: Negative

Questions
1. In cases of toxoplasmosis, the diagnosis can be established by:
    a. Isolation of the organism
    b. PCR
    c. IFA
    d. All of the above
2. In cases of current toxoplasmosis infection, the earliest that *Toxoplasma* antibodies can be detected is _____ after infection.
    a. 48 hours
    b. 72 hours
    c. Within the first 2 weeks
    d. Within the first 6 months

Answers to these questions can be found in Appendix A.

Critical Thinking Group Discussion Questions
1. What is the most common cause of lesions in the brain?
2. What is the source of this infection?
3. Is this a newly acquired infection?
4. How can the patient be treated?
5. Should pregnant women be tested for this microorganism?

See instructor site for a discussion of the answers to these questions.

CASE STUDY 13.3

History and Physical Examination
A 20-year-old college junior comes to the student health office because she was exposed to rubella during a recent outbreak at the college. She was immunized as a child.

Laboratory Data
- Screening procedure for rubella—negative
- Pregnancy test—positive

Ultrasonography shows that the fetus is in the eighth week of development.

Questions
1. What constitutes proof of immunity to rubella infection?
    a. Physician-documented infection
    b. IgG antibody (1:8 dilution or greater)
    c. IgM antibody
    d. Both b and c
2. To confirm congenital rubella syndrome _____ antibody must be demonstrated in the newborn's serum.
    a. IgM
    b. IgG
    c. IgA
    d. IgE

Answers to these questions can be found in Appendix A.

Critical Thinking Group Discussion Questions
1. Is this woman susceptible to rubella infection?
2. Is the fetus at risk of a congenital defect?
3. Is there any treatment for the infection?
4. What are the immunologic manifestations of infection?

CASE STUDY 13.4

History and Physical Examination
A 35-year-old man recently received a kidney transplant. He had been feeling well until 2 weeks ago when he experienced a sore throat, fever, chills, profound malaise, and myalgia. Lymphadenopathy and splenomegaly were observed. His medications included cyclosporine.

Questions
1. In cytomegalovirus (CMV) infection, the presence of IgM antibodies to CMV can be found in:
   a. Primary CMV
   b. Reactivation of CMV
   c. Reinfection with CMV
   d. All of the above
2. Reactivation of latent CMV may:
   a. Elicit a detectable IgM response
   b. Produce a significant increase in IgG antibody to CMV
   c. Produce IgM and IgG
   d. Produce neither IgM nor IgG

Answers to these questions can be found in Appendix A.

Critical Thinking Group Discussion Questions
1. Could this patient be suffering from an infectious disease?
2. Why would this patient be susceptible to an opportunistic infection?
3. How could an infection of this type be potentially eliminated?
4. Are healthcare workers at risk for infections of this type?
5. Can congenital infections of this type occur?
6. How can this disease be diagnosed?

REVIEW QUESTIONS

1. Effective immunologic defenses against bacteria are:
   a. Interferons
   b. Lysozymes and phagocytosis
   c. Complement, antibody-dependent cell-mediated cytotoxicity, and cellular defenses
   d. Immunoglobulins and complement
2. The detection of _____ can be of diagnostic significance during the first exposure of a patient to an infectious agent.
   a. IgM
   b. IgG
   c. IgA
   d. IgD
3. Serologic procedures for the diagnosis of recent infection should include:
   a. Only an acute specimen
   b. Only a convalescent specimen
   c. Acute and convalescent specimens
   d. Acute, convalescent, and 6-month postinfection specimens
4. Viral diseases are:
   a. Affected by immune responses such as immunoglobulin, complement, and antibody-dependent cell-mediated cytotoxicity
   b. Inhibited by antibiotics, lysozymes, and phagocytosis
   c. Stimulated by production of, and in turn inhibited by, interferon
   d. Found exclusively in tropical climates
5. Toxoplasmosis is a _____ infection.
   a. Bacterial
   b. Mycotic
   c. Parasitic
   d. Viral
6. The presence of IgM antibodies to *T. gondii* in an adult is indicative of a(an):
   a. Carrier state
   b. Active infection
   c. Chronic infection
   d. Latent disease
7. Congenital toxoplasmosis can cause:
   a. Congenital heart disease
   b. Central nervous system malformation
   c. Urinary tract infections
   d. Muscular disorders
8. Antibodies to *T. gondii* are demonstrable _____ after infection.
   a. 3 to 5 days
   b. Within 10 days
   c. Within 2 weeks
   d. Within 4 weeks
9. The method of choice for detecting IgM antibodies in toxoplasmosis is:
   a. Enzyme-linked immunosorbent assay (ELISA)
   b. Indirect fluorescent antibody (IFA)
   c. Indirect hemagglutination (IHA)
   d. Complement fixation (CF)
10. The greatest risk of the manifestation of anomalies in maternal rubella is _____ of gestation.
    a. During the first month
    b. During the first trimester
    c. During the third month
    d. During the fourth or fifth month
11. Testing for _____ antibody is invaluable for the diagnosis of congenital rubella syndrome.
    a. IgM
    b. IgG
    c. IgD
    d. IgE
12. Before the licensing of rubella vaccine in the United States in 1969, epidemics occurred at _____ year intervals.
    a. 2- to 3-
    b. 5- to 7-
    c. 6- to 9-
    d. 10- to 20-
13. IgM antibodies to rubella virus reach peak levels at _____ days.
    a. 2 to 4
    b. 3 to 5
    c. 5 to 7
    d. 7 to 10
14. IgG antibodies to rubella virus increase rapidly for _____ days after the acquisition of infection.
    a. 2 to 8
    b. 3 to 10
    c. 5 to 15
    d. 7 to 21

15. Which percentage of serologically confirmed cases of maternal rubella infection occur before 11 weeks of gestation?
    a. 11%
    b. 24%
    c. 33%
    d. 90%
16. Laboratory confirmation of rubeola antibody is done by:
    a. Detection of IgM antibodies in serum
    b. Detection of measles virus RNA by nucleic acid amplification in a clinical specimen
    c. Isolation of rubella virus
    d. Either a or b
17. CMV is recognized as the cause of congenital viral infection in what percentage of all live births?
    a. 0.1% to 0.4%
    b. 0.4% to 2.5%
    c. 2.5% to 4.9%
    d. 4.9% to 9.9%
18. A reactivated CMV infection can be described as:
    a. Having a significant antibody response and viral shedding caused by a different strain of virus
    b. A condition in which a seronegative recipient is transfused with blood from an actively or a latently infected donor
    c. A condition in which a seropositive recipient is transfused with blood from a CMV antibody–positive or negative donor
    d. Either b or c
19. A reinfection with CMV can be described as:
    a. Having a significant antibody response and viral shedding caused by a different strain of virus
    b. A condition in which a seronegative recipient is transfused with blood from an actively or a latently infected donor
    c. A condition in which a seropositive recipient is transfused with blood from a CMV antibody–positive or negative donor
    d. Either b or c
20. A characteristic of CMV early antigens is:
    a. They appear 72 hours after infection or at the end of the viral replication cycle
    b. They appear within 1 hour of cellular infection
    c. They are present within 24 hours
    d. Either a or c
21. A characteristic of CMV immediate-early antigens is:
    a. They appear 72 hours after infection or at the end of the viral replication cycle
    b. They appear within 1 hour of cellular infection
    c. They are present within 24 hours
    d. Either a or c
22. The characteristic antibody response in a primary CMV infection is:
    a. IgG, but IgM response unknown
    b. Specific IgM antibody response
    c. IgG with no detectable IgM response
    d. No identifiable antibody response
23. The characteristic antibody response in a reactivation of latent CMV infection in a seropositive IgG patient is:
    a. IgG, but IgM response unknown
    b. Specific IgM antibody response
    c. IgG with no detectable IgM response
    d. No identifiable antibody response
24. A characteristic of CMV is:
    a. Primary and recurrent maternal CMV infections cannot be transmitted in utero
    b. CMV is the least common intrauterine infection
    c. Many CMV-infected newborns are asymptomatic
    d. Normal adults and children usually experience CMV infection with serious complications
25. A distinguishing characteristic of the herpes viruses is that:
    a. They are cell-associated viruses
    b. They are enveloped RNA
    c. Human beings are the only known reservoir of infection
    d. Both a and c
26. Up to _____ of infants develop antibody to HHV-6 by 10 to 11 months of age.
    a. 25%
    b. 50%
    c. 75%
    d. 95%
27. Rapid preliminary diagnosis of varicella-zoster virus can be done in the laboratory by:
    a. Direct immunofluorescence
    b. Viral isolation
    c. ELISA method
    d. Complement fixation

Streptococcal Infections

Mary Lou Turgeon

LEARNING OUTCOMES

- Describe the etiology, epidemiology, signs and symptoms, and complications of streptococcal infection.
- Discuss the immunologic manifestations and diagnostic evaluation of streptococcal infection.
- Analyze and apply laboratory data to a case study.
- Correctly answer case study–related multiple-choice questions.
- Participate in a discussion of critical thinking questions.
- Explain the principle and applications of the classic anti–streptolysin O (ASO) procedure.
- Briefly explain other methods of detection of group A streptococcus (GAS).
- Correctly answer end-of-chapter review questions.

OUTLINE

Etiology, 221
    Morphologic Characteristics, 222
    Extracellular Products, 222
Epidemiology, 223
Signs and Symptoms, 223
    Upper Respiratory Infection, 223
    Impetigo and Cellulitis, 223
    Scarlet Fever, 223
    Complications of *Streptococcus pyogenes* Infection, 224
    Immunologic Manifestations, 224
Diagnostic Evaluation, 224
    Antistreptolysin O, 224
    Deoxyribonuclease B, 224
    Specimen Pairing, 224
Streptococcal Toxic Shock Syndrome, 225
    Etiology, 225
    Immunologic Mechanisms, 225
    Epidemiology, 225
    Signs and Symptoms, 225
    Laboratory Data, 225
    Treatment, 225
    Epidemiology, 226
    Etiology, 226
    Laboratory Data, 226
    Signs and Symptoms, 226
    Future Directions, 226
Case Study 14.1, 226
Procedure: Antistreptolysin O Latex Test Kit, 227.e1
Procedure: OSOM Ultra Streptococcus A Test, 227.e1
Procedure: Group A Streptococcus Direct Test, 227.e1
Procedure: Antistreptolysin O Classic Procedure, 227.e1

KEY TERMS

anti–deoxyribonuclease B (anti–DNase B)
antistreptolysin O (ASO)
erythrogenic toxin
exogenous endotoxin
exudate
hemoglobinuria
hemolysins
necrotizing fasciitis
neonatal septicemia
osmotic lysis
poststreptococcal glomerulonephritis
purulent
serogroups
streptokinase
streptolysin O (SLO)
streptolysin S
tumor necrosis factor

ETIOLOGY

Most streptococci that contain cell wall antigens of the Lancefield group A (Table 14.1) are known as *Streptococcus pyogenes*. Members of this species are almost always beta-hemolytic streptococci. *S. pyogenes* is the most common causative agent of pharyngitis and its resultant disorder, scarlet fever, and the skin infection impetigo. The most common type of bacteria causing necrotizing fasciitis is *S. pyogenes*.

In terms of human morbidity and mortality worldwide, however, the role of *S. pyogenes* in the subsequent development of complications such as acute rheumatic fever and poststreptococcal glomerulonephritis is more important. Other *S. pyogenes*–associated infections include otitis media in children; sinusitis in adults; and osteomyelitis, septic arthritis, neonatal septicemia, and rare cases of pneumonia.

Necrotizing fasciitis (NF) is a rare infection that can destroy skin and soft tissues, including fat and the tissue covering muscles (fascia).

TABLE 14.1 Lancefield Streptococcus Classifications[a].

Lancefield Group	Examples of Bacterial Species in the Group	Comments
A	*Streptococcus pyogenes*	Strains most pathogenic for human beings can cause strep throat, rheumatic fever, scarlet fever, acute glomerulonephritis, and necrotizing fasciitis.
B	*Streptococcus mastitis* *Streptococcus agalactiae*	Strains from mastitis in cows and from normal milk, including strains from the human throat and vagina. Can cause pneumonia and meningitis in neonates and older adults, with occasional systemic bacteremia.
C	*Streptococcus equi* *Streptococcus dysgalactiae*	Strains from various lower animals, including cattle, and from the human throat. Can cause pharyngitis and other pyogenic infections similar to group A streptococci.
D	*Streptococcus faecalis* (now *Enterococcus faecalis*) Other nonenterococcal group D strains include *Streptococcus bovis* and *Streptococcus equinus*	Strains from cheese and humans. Many former group D streptococci have been reclassified and placed in the genus *Enterococcus*.
E	–	Strains from certified milk.
F	*Streptococcus anginosus* (Lancefield classification) or *Streptococcus milleri* group (European system)	Strains mainly from the human throat, associated with tonsillitis; minute hemolytic.
G	*Streptococcus canis* is an example of a GBS that is typically found in animals but does not cause infection except in newborns at birth.	Strains can cause infection in human beings (a few strains from monkeys and dogs). **Note:** This is not exclusively beta-hemolytic.
H, K, O	–	Nonpathogenic strains occasionally form normal human respiratory tracts.

[a]This is a serologic classification of hemolytic streptococci, dividing them into groups based on antigenic serocharacteristics. It is based on precipitation tests, depending on group-specific carbohydrate substances.
GBS, Group B streptococcus.

Because these tissues die rapidly, a person with NF is sometimes said to be infected with so-called flesh-eating bacteria. A highly invasive group A streptococcal infection is associated with toxic shock syndrome.

> **KEY CONCEPTS: Characteristics of Streptococcus Group A**
> - Most streptococci that contain cell wall antigens of Lancefield group A are known as *Streptococcus pyogenes*. Members of this species are almost always beta-hemolytic streptococci.
> - *S. pyogenes* is important in the development of complications such as acute rheumatic fever and poststreptococcal glomerulonephritis.
> - Strains of *S. pyogenes* that lack M protein cannot cause infection.
> - Extracellular products are important in the pathogenesis and serologic diagnosis of streptococcal disease. Antibodies produced in response to these substances indicate recent streptococcal infection.
> - Substances produced by group A streptococci presumably facilitate rapid spread through subcutaneous or deeper soft tissues.

Morphologic Characteristics

S. pyogenes is a gram-positive coccus and the serotype most commonly associated with human infection. Lancefield (see Table 14.1) divided these beta-hemolytic streptococci into **serogroups** A through O on the basis of the immunologic action of the cell wall carbohydrate (Fig. 14.1).

Structures called *fimbriae* arise near the plasma membrane and project through the cell wall and capsule. These processes contain important surface components of the streptococcus. Lipoteichoic acid on the fimbriae is important in the organism's adherence to human epithelium and the initiation of infection. The M and R antigens, which are structurally similar but immunologically distinct, are also found on the fimbriae. R antigen has no known biological role.

M protein, a cell protein found in association with the hyaluronic capsule, is a major virulence factor of *S. pyogenes*. Strains of *S. pyogenes* that lack M protein cannot cause infection. M protein inhibits

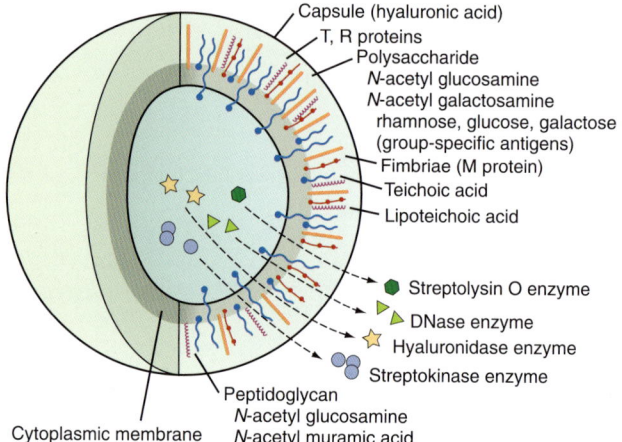

Fig. 14.1 *Streptococcus pyogenes* contains many antigenic structural components and produces several antigenic enzymes, each of which may elicit a specific antibody response from the infected host. (Adapted from Forbes BA, Sahm DF, Weissfeld AS: *Bailey and Scott's diagnostic microbiology*, ed 12, St. Louis, 2007, Mosby.)

phagocytosis, and antibody synthesized against M protein provides type-specific immunity to group A streptococci. In addition, M protein is the basis for a subclassification of group A streptococci into more than 60 M serotypes.

Extracellular Products

Extracellular products are important in the pathogenesis of disease and in the serologic diagnosis of streptococcal disease. Antibodies produced in response to these substances provide evidence of recent streptococcal infection. Two **hemolysins**, with the ability to damage human and animal erythrocytes, polymorphonuclear leukocytes (PMNs), and platelets, are produced by most group A strains as follows:
- **Streptolysin O (SLO)**, an oxygen-labile enzyme, binds to sterols in the red blood cell (RBC) membrane, causing stearic rearrangement.

This rearrangement produces submicroscopic holes in the RBC membrane and hemoglobin diffuses from the cells. SLO is antigenic; the antibody response to it is the most commonly used serologic indicator of recent streptococcal infection.
- **Streptolysin S**, an oxygen-stable enzyme, is responsible for beta (clear-appearing) hemolysis on the surface of a blood agar culture plate. Streptolysin S disrupts the selective permeability of the RBC membrane, causing **osmotic lysis**. It is not antigenic.
- Other substances produced by group A streptococci presumably facilitate rapid spread through subcutaneous or deeper soft tissues and include the following:
  - Hyaluronidase, also called *spreading factor*, breaks down hyaluronic acid found in the host's connective tissue.
  - Four immunologically distinct deoxyribonucleases (DNases A, B, C, and D) degrade DNA.
  - **Streptokinase**, an enzyme, dissolves clots by converting plasminogen to plasmin.
  - Other extracellular products that can elicit an antibody response include NADase, proteinase, esterase, and amylase.
  - **Erythrogenic toxin** is elaborated by scarlet fever–associated strains and is responsible for the characteristic rash.

EPIDEMIOLOGY

S. pyogenes is one of the most common and ubiquitous of human pathogens. It is found in the human respiratory tract and is always considered a potential pathogen. Upper respiratory infections caused by *S. pyogenes* occur most commonly in school-age children and are uncommon in children younger than 3 years. No sex or race predilection has been described.

Infection is spread by contact with large droplets produced in the upper respiratory tract. Although not as common, foodborne and milkborne epidemics do occur. Crowding enhances the spread of microorganisms.

A number of individuals, particularly school-age children, carry *S. pyogenes* without signs of illness. Carriers have positive cultures without serologic evidence of infection. If a person carries the organisms in the pharynx for prolonged periods after untreated infection, the number of organisms carried and their ability to produce M protein decline during carriage. This results in a progressive decline in the likelihood of spreading infection to others.

The incidence of a major complication of *S. pyogenes*, rheumatic fever, has decreased in the United States. It occurs primarily in the rural South and in areas of crowding and lower socioeconomic status. The incidence of rheumatic fever is 2% to 3% in epidemics and 0.1% to 1% after sporadic cases of streptococcal infection. The probability of developing rheumatic fever is age related, with younger patients more likely to develop carditis than older persons.

Rheumatic fever and resultant valvular heart disease, however, are syndromes of major importance among children in developing nations. Patients with a history of rheumatic heart disease resulting from rheumatic fever are at a significantly increased risk of developing cardiac malfunction and endocarditis later. The risk of recurrent rheumatic fever depends on factors such as the age of the patient at previous recurrences, length of time since the last recurrence, and the presence of carditis. In addition, patients who develop streptococcal glomerulonephritis are at risk of later development of renal failure.

SIGNS AND SYMPTOMS

S. pyogenes causes a wide variety of infections, most often acute pharyngitis (strep throat) and upper respiratory infection, in addition to impetigo (pyoderma). Other manifestations of infection with *S. pyogenes* include sinusitis, otitis, peritonsillar and retropharyngeal abscess, pneumonia, scarlet fever, erysipelas, cellulitis, puerperal sepsis, and gangrene. A concern still exists that group A streptococcus (GAS) may be acquiring greater virulence.

Upper Respiratory Infection

The clinical manifestations of *S. pyogenes*–associated upper respiratory infection are age dependent. In an infant or a young child, the infection is characterized by an insidious onset of rhinorrhea, coughing, fever, vomiting, and anorexia. Cervical adenopathy may also be present. Rhinorrhea is sometimes **purulent**. This syndrome is called *streptococcosis*.

The classic syndrome of streptococcal pharyngitis is seen in children older than 3 years. It begins with a sudden onset of sore throat and fever, which rapidly progress in severity. Pharyngeal erythema with purulent tonsillar **exudate** and petechiae may be observed on the palate, posterior pharynx, and tonsils. Younger children may have abdominal pain, nausea, and vomiting. Most patients, however, do not manifest the classic syndrome. It is more common for a child with *S. pyogenes* pharyngitis to have a fever, mild sore throat, and pharyngeal erythema without exudate.

Viral pharyngitis can produce many of the same symptoms and cannot be reliably differentiated from streptococcal pharyngitis on the basis of clinical examination alone.

Impetigo and Cellulitis

Impetigo is a skin infection that begins as a papule (Fig. 14.2). The lesion may itch and will eventually crust over and heal. Cellulitis caused by subcutaneous infection with group A streptococci is associated with a warm, red, tender area that may be mildly swollen. Erysipelas, a distinct cellulitis syndrome usually involves the face and may be associated with pharyngitis. This syndrome is characterized by toxicity and a high fever. If left untreated, erysipelas can be fatal.

Scarlet Fever

Scarlet fever is the result of pharyngeal infection with a strain of GAS that produces erythrogenic toxin and is responsible for the characteristic rash. The signs and symptoms of scarlet fever are those of streptococcal pharyngitis with the addition of a rash. The rash usually develops on the second day of illness and results in hyperkeratosis with subsequent peeling, similar to the rash of toxic shock syndrome.

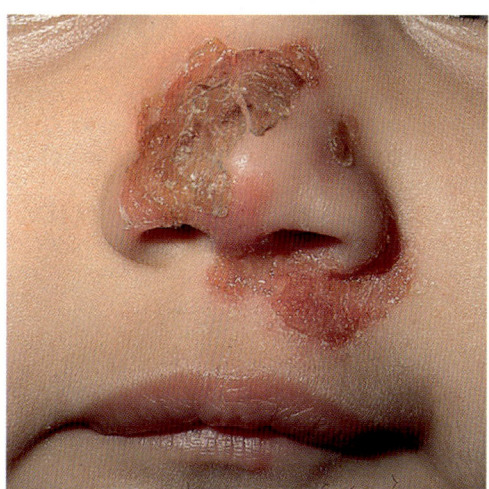

Fig. 14.2 Impetigo. Older lesions are dark and encrusted. (From Wehrle PF, Top FH: *Communicable and infectious diseases,* ed 9, St. Louis, 1981, Mosby.)

About 1 week after the onset of illness, the skin of the face begins to peel, which progresses over the next 2 weeks. Exposure to erythrogenic toxin confers specific immunity, limiting to three the number of episodes of scarlet fever in a person.

Complications of *Streptococcus pyogenes* Infection

Not all infections with *S. pyogenes* lead to complications. Acute rheumatic fever, for example, occurs only after upper respiratory tract infection. In contrast glomerulonephritis occurs after pharyngitis or skin infections (pyoderma). Acute rheumatic fever and poststreptococcal glomerulonephritis are considered nonsuppurative because the organs themselves are not directly infected and a purulent inflammatory response is not present in affected organs (e.g., heart, joints, blood, and kidneys).

The pathogenesis of this disease process has not been fully described, but an autoimmune phenomenon may be operational. It is believed that cross-reactive antibodies, originally directed against streptococcal cell membranes, bind to myosin in human heart muscle cells. Other cross-reactive antibodies bind to components of the glomerular basement membrane and form immune complexes at the affected site. These antigen–antibody complexes attract reactive host cells and enzymes that ultimately cause the cellular damage.

All M serotypes that infect the throat appear to be capable of causing rheumatic fever. Researchers have identified a few serotypes, however, that cause a much lower proportion of rheumatic fever cases than would be expected from their frequency as a cause of pharyngitis. The incidence of rheumatic fever is directly proportional to the strength of the antibody response to SLO. The prognosis of rheumatic fever is good when carditis is absent during the initial infection.

Glomerulonephritis may follow an infection of the skin or respiratory tract with one of a limited number of nephritogenic M serotypes. These serotypes are defined by antisera against the M protein, which is also associated with virulence. Why these serotypes cause glomerulonephritis is unknown.

Immunologic Manifestations

S. pyogenes is an example of a pathogen that induces the production of several different antibodies. This bacteria contains antigenic structural components and produces antigenic enzymes, each of which may elicit a specific antibody response from the infected host. In the course of an infection, the extracellular products act as antigens to which the body responds by producing specific antibodies (indications of infection).

DIAGNOSTIC EVALUATION

In addition to the traditional throat culture, rapid direct throat swab antigen tests are available. A direct molecular test for GAS is a DNA probe assay that uses nucleic acid hybridization for qualitative detection of GAS RNA.

Testing of patients with pharyngitis can demonstrate antibodies to bacterial toxins and other extracellular products. Antistreptolysin O (ASO) and anti–deoxyribonuclease B (anti–DNase B) are the standard serologic tests.

Antistreptolysin O

The ability of a patient's serum to neutralize the erythrocyte-lysing capability of SLO (ASO procedure) has been used for many years as a method for detecting previous streptococcal infections. After an infection such as pharyngitis with SLO-producing strains, most patients show a high titer of the DNase antibody ASO. The use of rapid testing has replaced the use of the classic ASO procedure archived on the Evolve website.

Most infected patients demonstrate an increased concentration of antibody against SLO. The concentration of antibody (titer) begins to rise about 7 days after the onset of infection and reaches a maximum after 4 to 6 weeks. A rise in titer in 1 to 2 weeks is of greater diagnostic significance than a single titer.

An elevated titer indicates a relatively recent infection. Peak titers are seen at the time of acute polyarthritis of acute rheumatic fever, but these titers are no longer at their peak during the carditis of acute rheumatic fever. A patient may demonstrate an elevated antibody titer for up to 1 year after infection; therefore the time of infection is not precisely determined by this technique. Low titers of ASO can be exhibited by apparently healthy persons because of the frequency of subclinical streptococcal infections, but persistently low titers rule out *S. pyogenes* infection.

Deoxyribonuclease B

DNase B is one of several extracellular enzymes produced by group A beta-hemolytic streptococci. Because DNase B is produced extensively by group A serotypes and is not produced in significant amounts by other serologic groups (C and G), anti–DNase B is a reliable streptococcal antibody test for both skin and throat infections.

The innate immune response plays a crucial role in satisfactory host resolution of bacterial infection. In response to chemotactic signals, neutrophils are early responding cells that migrate in large numbers to sites of infection. The discovery of secreted neutrophil extracellular traps (NETs) composed of DNA and histones enhanced understanding of the microbial killing capacity of these specialized leukocytes.

M1 serotype strains of the pathogen GAS are associated with invasive infections, including NF, and express a potent DNase (Sda1). A direct link between NET degradation and bacterial pathogenicity exists. NETs play a significant role in innate immunity.

The DNase B neutralization test prevents the activity of this enzyme and demonstrates recent or previous *S. pyogenes* infection. Of patients with *S. pyogenes*–related acute glomerulonephritis, 50% display a normal ASO titer but demonstrate an elevated titer to one of the other streptococcal substances (e.g., DNase). In the nephelometry method, anti-B in the serum sample will bind with DNase B in the reagent, forming complexes that result in an increase in light scatter that is interpreted by the IMMAGE Immunochemistry System.

DNase B antibody appears to be the most reliable measure of recent *S. pyogenes* skin infection. Titers of anti–DNase B are elevated in more than two-thirds of patients with recent streptococcal impetigo.

Testing for anti–DNase B also assists in the diagnosis and management of patients with acute rheumatic fever, acute glomerulonephritis, Sydenham chorea, scarlet fever, pharyngitis, and many other group A streptococcal–based illnesses. Unlike ASO, anti–DNase B is less susceptible to false positives caused by bacterial growth in the specimen, liver disease, and oxidation of the antigen.

To determine the presence of group A streptococcal infection, it is highly recommended that ASO testing be performed in conjunction with anti–DNase B, especially when the ASO titer is borderline. It has been reported in the literature that using the anti–DNase B and ASO titers together aids in the detection of streptococcal infection with a high degree of reliability. It has also been reported that in cases of skin infections, the anti–DNase B titer typically rises, whereas other antibody titers (e.g., ASO) remain low. The definition of the "reference interval" is of great importance, because results will vary with seasons, age, geographic location, and economic status of the population.

Specimen Pairing

Serologic testing should compare acute and convalescent sera collected 3 weeks apart. The ASO level becomes elevated in acute or convalescent paired specimens in 80% to 85% of patients with acute rheumatic fever.

Anti–DNase B and anti–hyaluronidase titer (AHT) levels are elevated in the remaining 15% to 20% of patients. In many cases, no acute serum specimen is available; therefore the antibody titer of the convalescent serum specimen is compared with a reference range value. False-positive ASO results may be demonstrated because of the presence of beta-lipoprotein, contamination of the serum specimen by bacterial growth products, or oxidation of ASO. These errors are not encountered with the anti–DNase B procedure, which is the serologic test of choice for acute rheumatic fever and acute glomerulonephritis after *S. pyogenes* infection.

STREPTOCOCCAL TOXIC SHOCK SYNDROME

Streptococcal toxic shock syndrome (STSS) is caused by a highly invasive group A streptococcal infection and is associated with shock and organ failure.

Etiology

The portal of entry of streptococci in STSS cannot be determined in at least 50% of cases and can only be presumed in many others. The use of tampons has been associated with acquiring the disorder. In other patients the use of nonsteroidal anti–inflammatory drugs (NSAIDs) may have masked the early symptoms or predisposed the patient to more severe streptococcal infection and shock. Usually, STSS appears after streptococci have invaded areas of injured skin (e.g., cuts, scrapes, and surgical wounds).

Immunologic Mechanisms

Pyrogenic exotoxins cause fever in human beings and animals and also help induce shock by lowering the threshold to exogenous endotoxin. Streptococcal pyrogenic exotoxins A and B induce human mononuclear cells to synthesize not only tumor necrosis factor-α (TNF-α) but also interleukin-1 beta (IL-1β) and interleukin-6 (IL-6), suggesting that TNF could mediate the fever, shock, and tissue injury observed in patients with STSS.

M protein contributes to invasiveness through its ability to impede phagocytosis of streptococci by human PMNs.

Superantigens are capable of binding to alpha and beta T-cell receptors (TCRs) and major histocompatibility complex (MHC) class II molecules. Superantigens can directly activate 1% to 2% of T cells and create high levels of cytokines in the blood. These high levels can produce shocklike symptoms.

Cytokine production by less exotic mechanisms also likely contributes to the genesis of shock and organ failure. Exotoxins such as SLO are also potent inducers of TNF-α and IL-1β. Pyrogenic exotoxin B, a proteinase precursor, has the ability to cleave pre–IL-1β to release preformed IL-1. Finally, SLO and pyrogenic exotoxin A together have additive effects in the induction of IL-1β by human mononuclear cells. Regardless of the mechanisms, induction of cytokines in vivo is likely the cause of shock, and exotoxins, cell wall components, and other substances are potent inducers of TNF and IL-1.

Epidemiology

The rates of STSS are highest in young children and older adults. More than 50% of patients have an underlying chronic illness. STSS is also associated with a substantial risk of transmission in households and healthcare institutions. Mortality after an outbreak of *S. pyogenes* that progresses to toxic shock can be as high as 70%. The illness is classified as a rare infection because it affects only about 300 people annually. STSS almost never follows a simple streptococcal throat infection.

Signs and Symptoms

The symptoms of STSS include shock; fever; blotchy rash; and a red, swollen, and painful area of infected skin. The average incubation period for STSS is 2 to 3 days, usually after minor nonpenetrating trauma.

Pain, the most common initial symptom of STSS, is abrupt and severe in onset, and usually precedes tenderness or physical findings. The pain generally involves an extremity but may also mimic peritonitis, pelvic inflammatory disease, pneumonia, acute myocardial infarction, or pericarditis.

About 20% of STSS patients have an influenza-like syndrome characterized by fever, chills, myalgia, nausea, vomiting, and diarrhea. Fever is the most common early sign, although hypothermia may be present in patients with shock.

About 80% of STSS patients have clinical signs of soft tissue infection, such as localized swelling and erythema, which in 70% of one group of patients progressed to NF or myositis and required surgical débridement, fasciotomy, or amputation. An ominous sign is the progression of soft tissue swelling to the formation of vesicles and then bullae, which appear violaceous or bluish.

Laboratory Data

The case definition of STSS includes serologic confirmation of group A streptococcal infection by a fourfold rise against SLO and DNase B. Although initial laboratory studies usually demonstrate only mild leukocytosis, the mean percentage of immature neutrophils can reach 40% to 50%. Blood cultures are positive in 60% of cases.

Renal involvement is indicated by the presence of hemoglobinuria and by serum creatinine values that are, on average, more than 2.5 times normal. Renal impairment precedes hypotension in approximately 40% to 50% of patients. Hypoalbuminemia is associated with hypocalcemia on admission and throughout the hospital course.

Treatment

STSS can be deadly and needs immediate treatment. Intravenous fluids and medications to maintain a normal blood pressure are required in acutely ill patients. Penicillin and other beta-lactam antibiotics are most efficacious against rapidly growing bacteria.

After recovery, the skin may peel as the rash heals. Surgery may be necessary to remove areas of dead skin and muscle around an infected wound.

> **KEY CONCEPTS: Group B Streptococcal Disease**
> - Group B *Streptococcus agalactiae* infections cause substantial morbidity and mortality in adults and neonates.
> - At least 30% of women asymptomatically carry this organism in the genitourinary tract, with a fatality rate ranging from 26% to 70% among men and nonpregnant women with group B streptococcus (GBS) disease.
> - GBS remains the leading cause of early-onset neonatal sepsis in the United States.
> - GBS is a gram-positive bacterium that causes invasive disease primarily in infants, pregnant or postpartum women, and older adults, with the highest incidence among young infants.
> - Culture of blood or cerebrospinal fluid, usually combined with antigen testing, including polymerase chain reaction (PCR), are the most effective methods for testing.
> - The development of a vaccine is being pursued.
>
> ### Group B Streptococcal Disease
> Group B *S. agalactiae* infections cause substantial morbidity and mortality in adults and neonates. At least 30% of women asymptomatically carry this organism in the genitourinary tract.

Epidemiology

The fatality rate ranges from 26% to 70% among men and nonpregnant women with GBS disease. Despite substantial progress in the prevention of perinatal GBS disease since the 1990s, GBS remains the leading cause of early-onset neonatal sepsis in the United States. Universal screening at 35 to 37 weeks' gestation for maternal GBS colonization and the use of intrapartum antibiotic prophylaxis has resulted in substantial reductions in the burden of early-onset GBS disease in newborns. Although early-onset GBS disease has become relatively uncommon in recent years, the rates of maternal GBS colonization (and therefore the risk for early onset GBS disease in the absence of intrapartum antibiotic prophylaxis) remain unchanged since the 1970s. GBS disease remains the leading infectious cause of morbidity and mortality in newborns in the United States.

Etiology

GBS, or *S. agalactiae*, is a gram-positive bacterium that causes invasive disease primarily in infants, pregnant or postpartum women, and older adults, with the highest incidence among young infants.

Laboratory Data

GBSs are most commonly isolated from blood, although the cerebrospinal fluid (CSF) can also be tested. Serologic identification using latex agglutination with GBS antisera is available but is not considered as effective as microbial culture and molecular methods. More rapid techniques for identifying GBS directly from enrichment broth or after subculture have been developed, including DNA probes and nucleic acid amplification tests (NAATs), such as PCR assays.

Using serology to detect colonization is ineffective; therefore culture, usually combined with antigen or, better yet, molecular methods, must be used. Standard practice is to swab a pregnant woman's tract and culture the swab. A portion of this culture can be assayed using real-time PCR.

Signs and Symptoms

The most common clinical finding is skin and soft tissue infection. Early-onset infections are acquired vertically through exposure to GBS from the vagina of a colonized woman. Neonatal infection occurs primarily when GBS ascends from the vagina to the amniotic fluid after the onset of labor or rupture of membranes, although GBS can also invade through intact membranes. Infants can also become infected with GBS during passage through the birth canal; infants who are exposed to the organism through this route can become colonized at mucous membrane sites in the gastrointestinal or respiratory tracts, but these colonized infants usually remain healthy.

Future Directions

Because of the gravity of GBS disease, especially in those who are older and those with chronic diseases, the development of a vaccine is being pursued. Determining the incidence of adult disease and groups at greatest risk helps focus prevention efforts. Intrapartum antibiotics can prevent early-onset neonatal GBS disease but have not been widely used. Women who demonstrate a GBS infection should receive an antibiotic regimen to prevent vertical transmission.

CASE STUDY 14.1

A 19-year-old woman visited the emergency department (ED) with swelling and redness of her right leg. She had fallen down while rollerblading and had a number of abrasions on the skin of her leg. She also had a body temperature of 37.8°C (100°F). The ED physician ordered a culture of her leg wound, gave her a prescription for an antibiotic, and discharged her from treatment.

The following evening, the patient collapsed onto the floor of her bedroom. Her roommate found her and called 911. On arrival, the paramedics found an unconscious woman with a blood pressure of 80/40 mm Hg and pronounced redness and swelling of her right leg. She was rushed to the ED and admitted to the intensive care unit, where she was immediately placed on intravenous fluids and medications to raise her blood pressure.

Questions

1. The patient's collapse could be due to:
   a. Dehydration
   b. Streptococcal toxic shock syndrome (STSS)
   c. Lack of sleep
   d. Swollen leg
2. What assay or assays would be the most helpful immunologic/serologic test(s)?
   a. Demonstration of streptolysin O in serum
   b. Anti–DNase B assay
   c. Throat culture for beta streptococci
   d. Both a and b

Answers to these questions can be found in Appendix A.

Critical Thinking Group Discussion Questions

1. Is there any relationship between this patient's problem with her leg and her collapse on the floor?
2. What are the symptoms of STSS?
3. What is the source of this patient's STSS?
4. Are there any immunologic/serologic manifestations of STSS?

REVIEW QUESTIONS

1. *S. pyogenes* is the most common causative agent of all the following disorders and complications *except*:
   a. Pharyngitis
   b. Gastroenteritis
   c. Scarlet fever
   d. Impetigo

2. All of the following characteristics are descriptive of M protein *except*:
   a. No known biological role
   b. Found in association with the hyaluronic capsule
   c. Inhibits phagocytosis
   d. Antibody against M protein provides type-specific immunity

3. Substances produced by *S. pyogenes* include all of the following *except*:
   a. Hyaluronidase
   b. DNases (A, B, C, D)
   c. Erythrogenic toxin
   d. Interferon

4. Laboratory diagnosis of *S. pyogenes* can be made by all of the following *except*:
   a. Culturing of throat or nasal specimens
   b. Febrile agglutinins
   c. ASO procedure
   d. Anti–DNase B

5. False ASO results may be caused by all of the following *except*:
   a. Room-temperature reagents and specimens at the time of testing
   b. The presence of beta-lipoprotein
   c. Bacterial contamination of the serum specimen
   d. Oxidation of ASO reagent caused by shaking or aeration of the reagent vial
6. Members of the *S. pyogenes* species are almost always _____ hemolytic.
   a. Alpha-
   b. Beta-
   c. Gamma-
   d. Alpha- or beta-
7. Long-term complications of *S. pyogenes* infection can include:
   a. Acute rheumatic fever
   b. Poststreptococcal glomerulonephritis
   c. Rheumatoid arthritis
   d. Both a and b
8. Particularly virulent serotypes of *S. pyogenes* produce proteolytic enzymes that cause _____ in a wound or lesion on an extremity.
   a. Necrotizing fasciitis
   b. Bone degeneration
   c. Burning and itching
   d. Severe inflammation
9. Hyaluronidase produced by group A streptococci:
   a. Degrades DNA
   b. Is called *spreading factor*
   c. Is responsible for characteristic scarlet fever rash
   d. Dissolves clots by converting plasminogen to plasmin
10. Streptokinase produced by group A streptococci:
    a. Degrades DNA
    b. Is called *spreading factor*
    c. Is responsible for characteristic scarlet fever rash
    d. Dissolves clots by converting plasminogen to plasmin
11. Erythrogenic toxin produced by group A streptococci:
    a. Degrades DNA
    b. Is called *spreading factor*
    c. Is responsible for characteristic scarlet fever rash
    d. Dissolves clots by converting plasminogen to plasmin
12. All of the following are characteristics of *S. pyogenes except*:
    a. It is an uncommon pathogen
    b. It occurs most commonly in school-age children
    c. It is spread by contact with large droplets produced in the upper respiratory tract
    d. It has been known to cause foodborne and milk-borne epidemics
13. The clinical manifestations of *S. pyogenes*–associated upper respiratory infection are:
    a. Mild and usually unnoticeable
    b. Age dependent
    c. Associated with cold sores
    d. Difficult to detect
14. The most reliable immunologic test for recent *S. pyogenes* skin infection is:
    a. ASO
    b. Anti–DNase B
    c. Anti–NADase
    d. Antibody to erythrogenic toxin
15. In the classic ASO titer, a rising titer:
    a. Suggests an increase in the severity of infection
    b. Suggests a past infection but not a current infection
    c. Is a trend toward recovery
    d. Is not of clinical significance
16. In the classic ASO titer, a declining titer:
    a. Suggests an increase in the severity of infection
    b. Suggests a past infection but not a current infection
    c. Is a trend toward recovery
    d. Is not of clinical significance
17. In the classic ASO titer, a constant (low) titer:
    a. Suggests an increase in the severity of infection
    b. Suggests a past infection but not a current infection
    c. Is a trend toward recovery
    d. Is not of clinical significance
18. If a streptococcal infection is suspected, but the ASO titer does not exceed the reference range, a(n) _____ should be performed.
    a. Repeat titer
    b. Anti–DNase B test
    c. Anti–NADase test
    d. Throat culture
19. The classic tests to demonstrate the presence of streptococcal infection are:
    a. ASO and anti-NADase
    b. ASO and anti–DNase B
    c. Anti-NADase and anti-DNase
    d. Both a and b
20. The highest reported levels of sensitivity testing for group A streptococci are in:
    a. ASO titers
    b. Direct latex agglutination tests
    c. Surface (optical) immunoassay
    d. Both a and b

15

Syphilis

LEARNING OUTCOMES

- Describe the etiology, epidemiology, and signs and symptoms of primary, secondary, latent, and late (tertiary) syphilis.
- Describe the incidence and clinical characteristics of congenital syphilis.
- Explain the immunologic manifestations and diagnostic evaluation of syphilis.
- Analyze a case study related to syphilis testing and correctly answer case study–related multiple-choice questions.
- Participate in a discussion of critical thinking questions.
- Discuss the principles and clinical applications of the rapid plasma reagin (RPR) card test and the Venereal Disease Research Laboratory (VDRL) procedure.
- Discuss the principles and clinical applications of confirmatory syphilis testing, such as the fluorescent treponemal antibody absorption (FTA) test.
- Correctly answer 80% of the end-of-chapter review questions.

OUTLINE

Etiology, 228
Epidemiology, 229
Signs and Symptoms, 230
Primary Syphilis, 230
Secondary Syphilis, 230
Latent Syphilis, 231
Late (Tertiary) Syphilis, 232
    Congenital Syphilis, 232
    Neurosyphilis, 232
Immunologic Manifestations, 233
Diagnostic Evaluation, 233
Direct Observation of Spirochetes, 233
Nontreponemal Methods, 233
    Rapid Plasma Reagin, 233
    Venereal Disease Research Laboratory Test, 234

Treponemal Methods, 234
    Chemiluminescence Immunoassays, 235
    Treponema pallidum Antibody Immunoglobulin G by Enzyme-Linked Immunosorbent Assay, 235
    Treponema pallidum Particle Agglutination, 236
    Fluorescent Treponemal Antibody Absorption, 236
Sensitivity of Representative Procedures for Syphilis, 236
Traditional Versus Reverse-Screening Algorithm Protocols, 236
Case Study 15.1, 238
Procedure: Classic Venereal Disease Research Laboratory Test – Venereal Disease Research Laboratory Qualitative Slide Test, 239.e1
Procedure: Rapid Plasma Reagin Card Test, 239.e2
Procedure: Fluorescent Treponemal Antibody Absorption Test, 239.e2

KEY TERMS

antilipoidal antibodies
antitreponemal antibodies
cardiolipin
convalescent sera
darkfield microscopy
granulomatous reactions (gummas)
morbidity
nontreponemal antibodies
rapid plasma reagin (RPR)
reagin antibodies
spirochete
Treponema pallidum antibodies
treponemes
Venereal Disease Research Laboratory (VDRL)

The disease syphilis was reported in the medical literature as early as 1495. In 1905 it was discovered that syphilis was caused by a **spirochete** type of bacteria, *Treponema pallidum* (originally called *Spirochaeta pallida*). The first diagnostic blood test for syphilis was the Wassermann test, a complement fixation test developed in 1906. This classic procedure has subsequently been replaced by a variety of methods. In the treatment of syphilis, heavy metals, such as arsenic, were replaced by penicillin in the 1940s. Penicillin continues to remain the drug of choice for the treatment of this disease.

ETIOLOGY

T. pallidum is a member of the order Spirochaetales and the family Treponemataceae (Fig. 15.1). The genus *Treponema* includes a number of species that reside in human gastrointestinal and genital tracts. *T. pallidum*, *Treponema pertenue*, and *Treponema carateum* are human pathogens responsible for significant worldwide **morbidity** (Table 15.1). Yaws, pinta, and bejel are diseases caused by bacteria closely related to *T. pallidum*. Yaws is common in the Caribbean, Latin

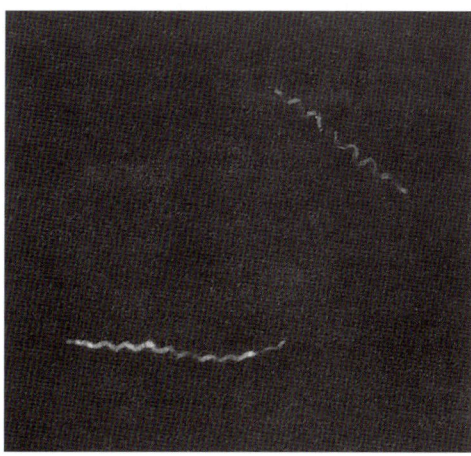

Fig. 15.1 *Treponema pallidum.* (From Bauer JD: *Clinical laboratory methods,* ed 9, St. Louis, 1982, Mosby.)

TABLE 15.1 *Treponema*-Associated Diseases

Bacteria	Associated Disease
T. pallidum	Syphilis
T. pallidum (variant)	Bejel
T. pertenue	Yaws
T. carateum	Pinta

America, Central Africa, and the Far East. Pinta is found only in Latin America, and infection is limited to the skin. Bejel is found in eastern Mediterranean countries, the Balkans, and the cooler areas of North Africa.

Direct examination of the treponemes is most often performed with darkfield microscopy. Pathogenic treponemes appear as fine, spiral (8–24 coils) organisms approximately 6 to 15 μm long. They have a trilaminar outer membrane similar to that of Gram-negative bacteria.

Pathogenic treponemes are not cultivatable with any consistency in artificial laboratory media. Outside of the host, pathogenic treponemes are extremely susceptible to a variety of physical and chemical agents. Treponemes may remain viable for up to 5 days in tissue specimens removed from diseased animals and from frozen cryoprotected specimens.

EPIDEMIOLOGY

Sexually transmitted infections (STIs) remain a major public health challenge in the United States. The surveillance report by the Centers for Disease Control and Prevention (CDC) includes data on the three STIs that physicians are required to report to the agency: chlamydia, gonorrhea, and syphilis.

Syphilis is considered to be primarily a venereal disease. It is the most common STI in the United States. The three treponematoses—yaws, pinta, and bejel—are rarely seen in the United States but are prevalent in other countries. These diseases are associated with poverty, overcrowding, and poor hygiene.

According to the latest 2022 Sexually Transmitted Infection (STI) Surveillance Report published by the Centers for Communicable Disease Control and Prevention (**http://www.CDC.gov**), surveillance provides the most current and complete data with the most alarming concerns centering around the syphilis and congenital syphilis epidemics. In 2022, 207, 255 cases of syphilis (all stages and congenital syphilis) were reported which is the greatest number of cases reported since 1950 and an increase of 17.3% since 2021. Since reaching a historic low in 2000 and 2001, the rate of primary and secondary (P&S) syphilis has increased almost every year, increasing 9.3% during 2021 to 2022. Cases of P&S syphilis are the most infectious stages of the disease, Rates of reported cases by race/Hispanic ethnicity in the United States, between 2018 to 2022 of P&S syphilis increased in most racial/Hispanic ethnicity groups. Greatest increases were among non-Hispanic American Indian/Alaska Native persons who also had the highest P&S syphilis rate in 2022.

Rates of P&S syphilis among women have increased since 2013 (Fig. 15.2). During 2021 to 2022, the national rate of P&S syphilis among women increased 19.2% with increases observed in 36 states and the District of Columbia. According to the CDC, the rate of P&S among men who have sex with women only increased between 2021 and 2022, along with the rate among women. This increase is part of a larger heterosexual syphilis epidemic in the United States.

The increase in syphilis among women has also led to a rise in congenital syphilis, syphilis in babies. In 2022, the congenital syphilis rate was 30.6% increase from 2021 and the highest rate in over 30 years. The 2022 statistics included 3,755 cases of congenital syphilis, including 282 congenital syphilis-related stillbirths and infant deaths. The national congenital syphilis rate in 2022 represents a 30.6% increase relative to 2021 and is the highest reported rate since 1991. The increases in congenital syphilis mirror sincreases in syphilis among reproductive aged women. During 2021 to 2022 the rate of P&S syphilis increased 17.2% among women aged 15–44 years.

> **KEY CONCEPTS: Facts About Syphilis**
> - Syphilis is caused by a spirochete, *T. pallidum*, usually transmitted in humans by sexual contact.
> - Untreated syphilis is a chronic disease with subacute symptomatic periods separated by asymptomatic intervals, during which the diagnosis can be made serologically. The progression of untreated syphilis is generally divided into stages.
> - In primary syphilis, the serum in about one-third of cases becomes serologically reactive after 1 week and serologically demonstrable in most cases after 3 weeks. The reagin titer increases rapidly during the first 4 weeks and then stabilizes for about 6 months.
> - Two to 8 weeks after the appearance of the primary chancre, the patient enters the stage of secondary syphilis, usually characterized by generalized illness suggestive of a viral infection. Skin lesions contain spirochetes and are highly contagious on exposed surfaces. These lesions subside spontaneously after 2 to 6 weeks, even if untreated. In this noninfectious latent stage, serologic tests for syphilis are positive.
> - The late (tertiary) stage usually occurs 3 to 10 years after primary infection; gummas can appear in about 15% of untreated syphilitic persons who eventually develop late benign syphilis. Complications include nervous system lesions, causing tabes dorsalis or cardiovascular complications. The tertiary stage is asymptomatic and determined only by serologic testing. Occasionally the lesions heal so completely that even serologic tests become nonreactive.

Syphilis remains a global problem, with an estimated 12 million people infected each year, despite the existence of effective prevention measures. The past decade has seen a pronounced resurgence of syphilis in countries of the Far East (e.g., China) and Africa. Some fundamental social problems (e.g., poverty, inadequate access to health care, and lack of education) are associated with disproportionately high levels of syphilis in certain populations.

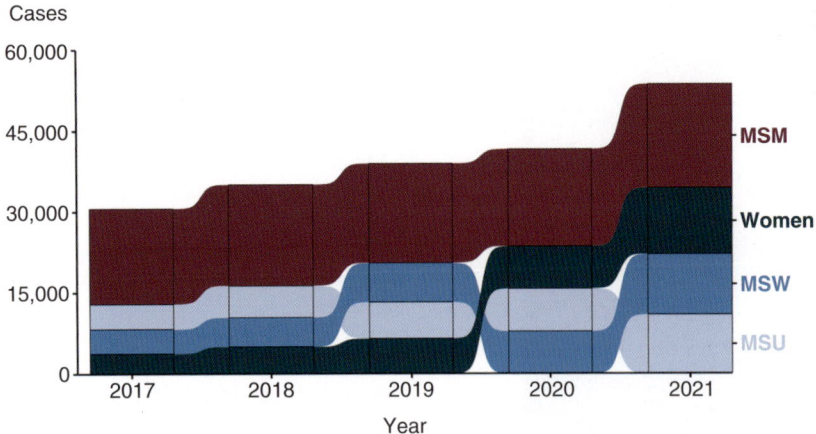

Fig. 15.2 Primary and Secondary Syphilis—Reported Cases by Sex and Sex of Sex Partners, United States, 2017–2021. Note: Over the 5-year period, 0.2% of cases were missing sex and were not included. *MSM*, Gay, bisexual, and other men who have sex with men; *MSU*, men with unknown sex of sex partners; *MSW*, men who have sex with women only. (From Sexually Transmitted Disease Surveillance 2021. https://www.cdc.gov/std/statistics/2021/data.zip [accessed May 26, 2023].)

Pathogenic treponemes are transmitted almost uniformly by direct contact. Treponemal infections of the skin or oral lesions contain many spirochetes that may be transmitted by personal, but not necessarily venereal, contact. These infections are generally acquired during childhood. In each of these diseases, infection elicits antibodies reactive in nontreponemal and treponemal methods.

Syphilis develops in 30% to 50% of the sexual partners of persons with syphilitic lesions. The risk of acquiring syphilis from a single sexual exposure to an infected partner is unknown. A high percentage of partners do seek medical treatment within 90 days of contact.

Syphilis can be acquired by kissing a person with active oral lesions. Very few cases of transfusion-acquired syphilis have been reported in recent years in the United States. During the first half of the 20th century, however, syphilis was a major bloodborne infectious disease easily transmitted through the prevailing method of direct donor-to-patient blood transfusion. The danger of syphilis transmission still exists in tropical countries in which the organization of blood banks is deficient and the use of direct blood transfusion prevails in emergency situations. Refrigerated blood storage decreases accidental transmission of the microorganism, because *T. pallidum* has a short survival period in stored blood. Spirochetes do not appear to survive in units of citrated blood at 4°C (39°F) for longer than 72 hours.

Cases have been reported of children who acquired syphilis by sharing a bed with an infected parent. In addition, syphilis may be transmitted transplacentally to the fetus. Spirochetes can be transmitted to the fetus during the last trimester of pregnancy before the mother manifests postpartum evidence of infection.

SIGNS AND SYMPTOMS

Untreated syphilis is a chronic disease with subacute symptomatic periods separated by asymptomatic intervals, during which the diagnosis can be made serologically. The progression of untreated syphilis is generally divided into stages: primary, secondary, latent (hidden), and tertiary (late) (Table 15.2).

Initially, *T. pallidum* penetrates intact mucous membranes or enters the body through tiny defects in the epithelium. On entrance, the microorganism is carried by the circulatory system to every organ of the body. Spirochetemia occurs very early in infection, even before the first lesions have appeared or blood tests become reactive. Before clinical or serologic manifestations develop, patients are said to be incubating syphilis. The incubation period usually lasts about 3 weeks but can range from 10 to 90 days.

PRIMARY SYPHILIS

At the end of the incubation period, a patient develops a characteristic primary inflammatory lesion called a *chancre* at the point of initial inoculation and multiplication of the spirochetes. The chancre begins as a papule and erodes to form a gradually enlarging ulcer, with a clean base and indurated edge (Fig. 15.3). Generally it is relatively painless. In most cases, only a single lesion is present, but multiple chancres are not rare.

Chancres are typically located around the genitalia, but in about 10% of cases, lesions may appear almost anywhere else on the body (e.g., throat, lip, and hands). In males, spirochetes are present in the lesion on the penis or discharged from deeper sites with semen. In females, infected lesions are usually located in the perineal region or on the labia, vaginal wall, or cervix. If the lesion is located inside the urethra, the only symptom may be a scanty, serous urethral discharge.

Of patients with primary syphilis of the external genitalia, 50% to 70% will subsequently develop inguinal adenopathy. Inguinal adenopathy, however, is less common with chancres involving the cervix or proximal part of the vagina because these sites are drained by the iliac nodes. Regional adenopathy may accompany primary inoculation at other sites; for example, cervical adenopathy may accompany a syphilitic lesion of the oral cavity.

The primary chancre will persist for 1 to 5 weeks and will heal completely in about 4 to 6 weeks, even without treatment. Regional adenopathy will also resolve itself.

SECONDARY SYPHILIS

Within 2 to 8 weeks (but occasionally as long as 6 months) after the appearance of the primary chancre, a patient may develop the signs and symptoms of secondary syphilis. In some patients, P&S syphilis overlap and the chancre is still obvious. Other patients never notice the primary chancre and initially have manifestations of secondary syphilis (Fig. 15.4).

TABLE 15.2 Stages of Syphilis

Phase/Stage	Features and Comments	Test
Incubating phase	The incubation period usually lasts about 3 weeks but can range from 10–90 days	Laboratory examination
Primary stage	• During the primary stage, a painless chancre develops at the site where the bacteria entered the body • A person is highly contagious during the primary stage • The chancre lasts 28–42 days and heals without treatment	Darkfield examination
Secondary stage	• This stage is characterized by a rash that appears 2–8 weeks after the chancre develops • A person is highly contagious during the secondary stage • A rash often develops all over the body, including palms of the hands and soles of the feet. The rash usually heals without scarring in 2–12 weeks • Open sores may be present on mucous membranes and may contain pus (condyloma lata) • Symptoms can include nervous system abnormalities	• RPR or VDRL • TP-PA used to confirm a syphilis infection after another method tests positive for syphilis. It can be used to detect syphilis in all stages, except during the first 3–4 weeks. This test is not done on spinal fluid • FTA-ABS test detects syphilis except during the first 3–4 weeks after exposure to syphilis bacteria. It is more difficult to perform and may be used to confirm a syphilis infection after another method tests positive for the syphilis bacteria. It can be done on a sample of blood or CSF
Latent (hidden) stage	• If untreated, an infected person will progress to the latent (hidden) stage of syphilis with no symptoms (latent period) • The latent period may be as brief as 1 year or range from 5–20 years	
Relapses of secondary syphilis	• About 20%–30% of people with syphilis have a relapse of the secondary stage of syphilis during the latent stage • A relapse means that the person had passed through the second stage, was symptom free, and then began to reexperience secondary-stage symptoms. Relapses can occur several times • When relapses no longer occur, a person is not contagious through contact • A woman in the latent stage of syphilis may still pass the disease to her unborn baby and may have a miscarriage, have a stillbirth, or give birth to a baby infected with congenital syphilis	• Nontreponemal tests are best for testing for reinfection.
Tertiary (late) stage	• Most destructive stage of syphilis • If untreated, the tertiary stage may begin as early as 1 year after infection or at any time during a person's lifetime. A person may never experience this stage of the illness • The symptoms of tertiary (late) syphilis depend on the complications that develop—gummata, large sores inside the body or on the skin, cardiovascular syphilis, or neurosyphilis	• VDRL on CSF with concurrent RPR serum • If RPR is negative and a high index of suspicion for neurosyphilis remains, FTA-ABS should be performed on serum • Some patients have nonreactive nontreponemal tests in late neurosyphilis

CSF, cerebrospinal fluid; *FTA-ABS*, fluorescent treponemal antibody absorption; *IgG*, immunoglobulin G; *IgM*, immunoglobulin M; *RPR*, rapid plasma reagin; *TP-PA*, *Treponema pallidum* particle agglutination assay; *VDRL*, Venereal Disease Research Laboratory.

The secondary stage is characterized by a generalized illness that usually begins with symptoms suggesting a viral infection: headache, sore throat, low-grade fever, and occasionally a nasal discharge. Blood tests reveal a moderate increase in leukocytes, with a relative increase in lymphocytes.

The disease progresses with the development of lymphadenopathy and lesions of the skin and mucous membranes. Approximately 75% of syphilitic patients develop generalized adenopathy. About 80% have skin lesions, which contain a large number of spirochetes and, when located on exposed surfaces, are highly contagious. Macular lesions are common and a rash invariably involves the genitalia; this rash is often prominent on the palms and soles. Patients may also develop condylomata lata, flat lesions resembling warts in moist areas of the body (e.g., around the anus or vagina). These lesions do not reflect areas of inoculation but appear to be caused by hematogenous dissemination of spirochetes.

The central nervous system (CNS) is asymptomatically involved in about one-third of patients. About 2% of cases manifest as acute syphilitic meningitis. Early CNS involvement may progress to neurosyphilis if untreated. Hepatitis and immune complex glomerulonephritis occasionally accompany secondary syphilis.

Secondary syphilis usually resolves within 2 to 6 weeks, even without therapy.

LATENT SYPHILIS

After resolution of untreated secondary syphilis, the patient enters a latent, noninfectious state in which the diagnosis can be made only by serologic methods. During the first 2 to 4 years of infection, 25% of patients will have one or more mucocutaneous relapses in which the manifestation of secondary syphilis reappears. During these relapses, patients are infectious and the

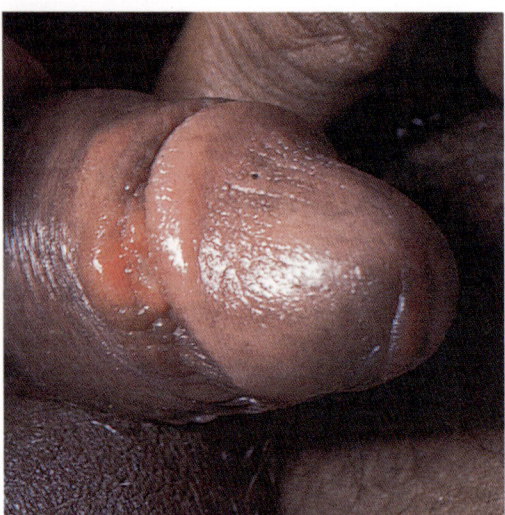

Fig. 15.3 A primary chancre of syphilis. (From Copstead-Kirkhorn LC, Banasik JL: *Pathophysiology*, ed 5, St. Louis, 2014, Elsevier.)

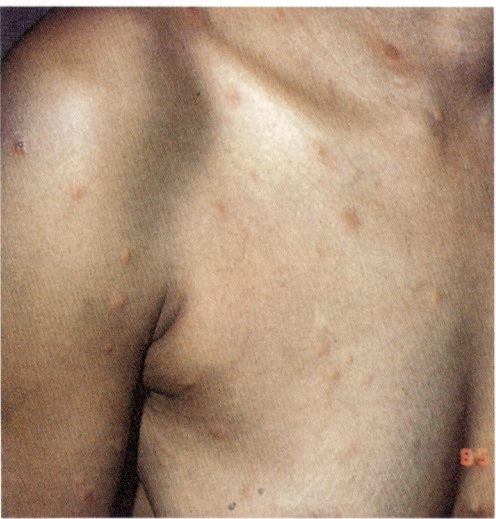

Fig. 15.4 Secondary syphilis. (From Copstead-Kirkhorn LC, Banasik JL: *Pathophysiology*, ed 5, St. Louis, 2014, Elsevier.)

underlying spirochetemia may be passed transplacentally to the fetus. Relapses are extremely rare after 4 years of latency. About one-third of patients entering latency are eventually spontaneously cured of the disease, one-third will never develop further clinical manifestations of the disease, and the remaining one-third will eventually develop late syphilis.

LATE (TERTIARY) SYPHILIS

The first manifestations of late syphilis are usually seen from 3 to 10 years after primary infection. About 15% of untreated syphilitic individuals eventually develop late benign syphilis, characterized by the presence of destructive granulomas. These granulomas, or gummas, may produce lesions resembling segments of circles that often heal with superficial scarring. The skeletal system is commonly affected, but treponemes are rarely seen.

Of untreated patients, 10% develop cardiovascular manifestations. *T. pallidum* may directly affect the aortic endothelium. Weakening of the blood vessels can occur as a syphilitic aneurysm, usually of the aortic arch.

In about 8% of untreated patients, late syphilis involves the CNS. Initially, CNS disease is asymptomatic and can be detected only by examination of cerebrospinal fluid (CSF). CSF should be examined in all patients being treated for syphilis of unknown duration or who have had syphilis for longer than 1 year.

Meningovascular syphilis usually manifests as a seizure or cerebrovascular accident (stroke). Spirochetes may also involve the brain tissues and cause general paresis, personality changes, dementia, and delusional states. Tabes dorsalis results from involvement of the posterior columns and dorsal roots of the spinal cord and is characterized by a broad-based gait. Impotence and bladder dysfunction are common in this disorder (see the section Neurosyphilis).

Congenital Syphilis

Globally, congenital syphilis is a major health problem in Africa and the Far East. The overarching global goal of the present World Health Organization (WHO) strategy is the elimination of congenital syphilis as a public health problem. This could be achieved through the reduction of prevalence of syphilis in pregnant women and by the prevention of mother-to-child transmission. The strategy rests on four pillars:

1. Ensure sustained political commitment and advocacy
2. Increase access to, and quality of, maternal and newborn health services
3. Screen and treat pregnant women and their partners
4. Establish surveillance, monitoring, and evaluation systems

Congenital syphilis is caused by maternal spirochetemia and transplacental transmission of the microorganism. Untreated syphilis during pregnancy, especially early syphilis, can lead to stillbirth, neonatal death, or infant disorders such as deafness, neurologic impairment, and bone deformities. Changes in the population incidence of P&S syphilis among women usually are followed by similar changes in the incidence of congenital syphilis.

Mother-to-infant transmission of syphilis can be prevented, or mother-to-infant transmission that has already occurred can be treated if benzathine penicillin G appropriate for the mother's stage of infection is initiated at least 30 days before delivery. For pregnant women with syphilis who deliver after 30 weeks' gestation, maternal treatment with penicillin is 98% effective at preventing congenital syphilis. A substantial percentage of congenital syphilis cases are attributable to a lack of prenatal care, but detection and treatment of maternal syphilis often occur too late to prevent congenital syphilis.

Classification of congenital syphilis is according to age at diagnosis. The early stage is seen in children younger than 2 years of age who are untreated. Symptoms of the untreated early stage can include rash, condyloma latum, bone changes, hepatosplenomegaly, jaundice, and anemia.

The late stage is seen in children older than 2 years of age who are untreated. Symptoms of the untreated late stage include eighth nerve deafness, keratitis, and Hutchinson teeth. These symptoms are called the Hutchinson triad. Other characteristics include fissuring around the mouth and anus, skeletal lesions, perforation of the palate, and collapse of nasal bones to produce a saddle-nose deformity.

Neurosyphilis

Although neurosyphilis may be asymptomatic, symptomatic forms include the following:

- Meningeal syphilis, usually less than 1 year after infection
- Meningovascular syphilis, usually 5 to 10 years after infection

- Parenchymatous syphilis

Meningeal neurosyphilis involves the brain or spinal cord. Patients can suffer from headaches and a stiff neck. Meningovascular syphilis involves inflammation of the pia mater and arachnoid space, with focal arteritis. A stroke syndrome involving the middle cerebral artery is common in young adults. Parenchymatous neurosyphilis manifests as general paresis, joint degeneration, and tabes dorsalis (demyelination of posterior columns, dorsal roots, and dorsal root ganglia). Tabes dorsalis is characterized by a gait disturbance and bladder symptoms.

IMMUNOLOGIC MANIFESTATIONS

In the treponemes, two classes of antigens have been recognized:
1. Antigens restricted to one or a few species
2. Antigens shared by many different spirochetes

Specific and nonspecific antibodies are produced in the immunocompetent host. Specific antibodies against *T. pallidum* (Treponema pallidum antibodies) and nonspecific antibodies against the protein antigen group common to pathogenic spirochetes are formed. Specific antitreponemal antibodies in early or untreated early latent syphilis are predominantly immunoglobulin M (IgM) antibodies. The early immune response to infection is rapidly followed by the appearance of immunoglobulin G (IgG) antibodies, which soon become predominant. The greatest elevation in IgG concentration is seen in secondary syphilis.

Nontreponemal antibodies, often called reagin antibodies or antilipoidal antibodies, are produced by infected patients against components of their own or other mammalian cells. Although almost always produced by patients with syphilis, these antibodies are also produced by patients with other infectious diseases. Infectious diseases in which reagin can be demonstrated include measles, chickenpox, hepatitis, infectious mononucleosis, leprosy, tuberculosis, leptospirosis, malaria, rickettsial disease, trypanosomiasis, and lymphogranuloma venereum. Reagin can also be exhibited by patients with noninfectious conditions, such as autoimmune disorders, drug addiction, old age, pregnancy, and recent immunization.

Delayed hypersensitivity immune mechanisms (see Chapter 20) also contribute to the pathophysiology of syphilis. It has been suggested that the granulomatous reactions (gummas) result from delayed hypersensitivity in the immune host. In addition, the manifestations of congenital syphilis apparently result in part from an immune inflammatory reaction. Antigen–antibody complexes have been detected in the blood of patients with secondary syphilis and are responsible for the syphilis-associated glomerulonephritis. Suppression of the various aspects of cell-mediated immunity has been noted in syphilis and may contribute to the prolonged survival of *T. pallidum*.

DIAGNOSTIC EVALUATION

> **KEY CONCEPTS: Laboratory Characteristics**
> - Classic serologic tests for syphilis measure the presence of two types of antibodies, treponemal and nontreponemal.
> - Darkfield microscopy is the test of choice for symptomatic patients with primary syphilis.
> - The widely used nontreponemal serologic test is the rapid plasma reagin (RPR) method, a flocculation method.
> - Specific treponemal serologic tests include the fluorescent treponemal antibody absorption (FTA-ABS) test and *T. pallidum* particle agglutination (TP-PA) test.

The laboratory diagnosis of syphilis depends on demonstration of microorganisms in a lesion and serologic testing (Fig. 15.5). Direct darkfield microscopy of material from a primary or secondary lesion is often unavailable and can miss up to 30% of primary cases of syphilis. Syphilis is usually diagnosed using serologic assays. Classic serologic methods measure the presence of two types of antibodies (Table 15.3) through nontreponemal methods and treponemal methods. Traditional serologic screening for syphilis initially uses nontreponemal testing with confirmation of positive results using a treponemal assay. New "reverse algorithms" are gaining in popularity. The reverse approach is to use treponemal testing initially with confirmation of reactive results using a nontreponemal assay.

Seroconversion between acute and convalescent sera is considered strong evidence of recent infection. The best evidence for infection is a significant change in two appropriately timed specimens, in which both tests are performed in the same laboratory at the same time.

DIRECT OBSERVATION OF SPIROCHETES

A method of direct observation of spirochetes is available for the examination of a patient specimen from an active syphilitic lesion. For symptomatic patients with primary syphilis, darkfield microscopy is the test of choice. A darkfield examination is also suggested for immediate results in cases of secondary syphilis, with a titer follow-up test.

NONTREPONEMAL METHODS

Nontreponemal methods determine the presence of reagin, an antibody formed against cardiolipin. An antigen composed of cardiolipin, a lipid remnant of damaged cells, cholesterol, and lecithin, is used to detect the nontreponemal reagin antibodies.

Rapid Plasma Reagin

The rapid plasma reagin (RPR) test is the most widely used nontreponemal serologic procedure, although Venereal Disease Research Laboratory (VDRL) methods may be used in some clinical and reference laboratories. Both these procedures are flocculation or agglutination tests in which soluble antigen particles coalesce to form larger particles that are visible as clumps when they are aggregated by antibody.

The RPR test, a charcoal agglutination test, can be performed on heated or unheated serum or plasma using a modified VDRL antigen suspension of choline chloride with ethylenediaminetetraacetic acid (EDTA). The RPR card test antigen also contains charcoal particles to which cardiolipin-containing antigen is bound for macroscopic reading. There are different versions of the RPR test. The original RPR method used unmeasured amounts of plasma and was used as a field procedure for screening large numbers of people. The modified RPR test uses the serum reagin test and is performed on measured volumes of unheated serum.

The RPR test measures IgM and IgG antibodies to lipoidal material released from damaged host cells and to lipoprotein-like material, and possibly cardiolipin released from the treponemes. If antibodies are present, they combine with the lipid particles of the antigen, causing them to agglutinate. The charcoal particles coagglutinate with the antibodies and show up as black clumps against the white card. If antibodies are not present, the test mixture is uniformly gray.

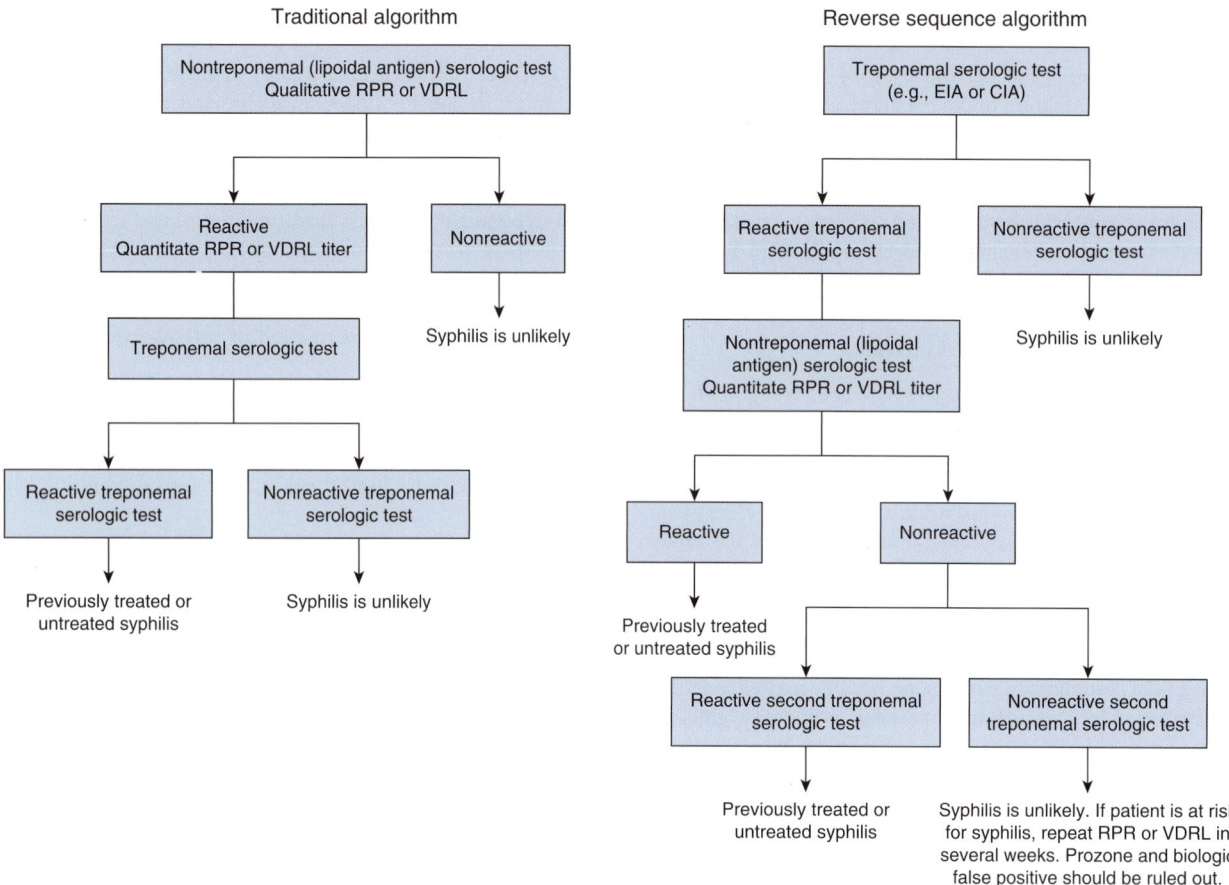

Fig. 15.5 Algorithms that can be applied to screening for syphilis with serologic tests—CDC laboratory recommendations for syphilis testing in the United States, 2024. *CIA*, chemiluminescence immunoassay; *EIA*, enzyme immunoassay; *RPR*, rapid plasma regain; *TPPA*, *Treponema pallidum* particle agglutination; *VDRL*, Venereal Disease Research Laboratory. (Papp JR, Park IU, Fakile Y, Pereira L, Pillay A, Bolan GA: CDC laboratory recommendations for syphilis testing, United States, 2024, *Recomm Rep* 73(1):1–32, 2024. (Accessed on October 15, 2024).)

Antilipoidal antibodies are antibodies that are produced not only as a consequence of syphilis and other treponemal diseases but also in response to nontreponemal diseases of an acute and chronic nature in which tissue damage occurs. Without some other evidence for the diagnosis of syphilis, a reactive nontreponemal test does not confirm *T. pallidum* infection.

The RPR test is more sensitive than the VDRL test for the detection of primary syphilis. False-positive results may occur in endemic treponematoses, herpes simplex virus (HSV) infection, HIV infection, intravenous drug use, leprosy, malaria, pregnancy, rheumatoid arthritis, and systemic lupus erythematosus (SLE).

Venereal Disease Research Laboratory Test

The VDRL test, a flocculation test, is a qualitative and quantitative screening procedure. Flocculation is a specific type of precipitation reaction that takes place over a narrow range of antigen concentrations.

Serum for testing must be heated to 56°C (133°F) for 30 minutes to inactivate complement. The test serum should be used promptly after inactivation. The antigen suspension is composed of cardiolipin, cholesterol, and lecithin. The VDRL test measures IgM and IgG antibodies to lipoidal material released from damaged host cells, to lipoprotein-like material, and possibly to cardiolipin released from the treponemes.

Without some other evidence for the diagnosis of syphilis, a reactive nontreponemal test does not confirm *T. pallidum* infection. Antilipoidal antibodies are antibodies that are not only produced as a consequence of syphilis and other treponemal diseases but also may be produced in response to nontreponemal diseases of an acute and chronic nature in which tissue damage occurs. Without some other evidence for the diagnosis of syphilis, false-positive results may occur in endemic treponematoses, HSV infection, HIV infection, intravenous drug use, leprosy, malaria, pregnancy, rheumatoid arthritis, and SLE.

VDRL with reflex testing to titer is the preferred test for CSF in suspected tertiary syphilis. A positive VDRL test result on spinal fluid is diagnostic of neurosyphilis.

TREPONEMAL METHODS

Treponemal assays detect specific IgG and/or IgM directed against *T. pallidum*. Representative assays in this category include the following:
- Chemiluminescence immunoassays (CIAs/enzyme immunoassays [EIAs])
- Enzyme-linked immunosorbent assays (ELISAs)
- *T. pallidum* antibody by microbead immunoassays (MBIAs)
- *T. pallidum* particle agglutination (TP-PA)
- Fluorescent treponemal antibody absorption (FTA-ABS)

TABLE 15.3 Tests for Syphilis Diagnosis

Test	Methodology	Comments
Direct Microscopy Observation		
Fluorescent	Fluorescent microscopy	
Darkfield	Darkfield microscopy	
Nontreponemal Assay *Quantitative*		
RPR	Charcoal particle agglutination	• CDC recommends for the screening and diagnosis of syphilis. Consider retesting in 3–12 months if patient remains in risk category • Reactive results reflex to titer and treponemal tests (e.g., TP-PA assay) for confirmation • Use to confirm reactive treponemal assay (e.g., CIAs and EIA) if using reverse algorithm testing • Preferred test for monitoring treatment response in established syphilis • RPR is being replaced by automated CIAs/EIAs
VDRL[a]	Flocculation	• Acceptable screening or monitoring test for treatment of diagnosed cases of syphilis • May use to confirm reactive treponemal test if reverse testing is used
TRUST (a modified VDRL)	Flocculation with red dye added	
Treponemal Test *Qualitative/Semiquantitative*		
CIAs/EIAs	Chemiluminescence	• Popular for point-of-care testing but cannot distinguish between active disease and old disease (treated/untreated) • CIAs/EIAs have high sensitivity but lower specificity than other methods. • Studies to compare test performance with other serologic tests are lacking • Studies evaluating performance of EIA/CIA to detect IgM antibodies in early syphilis are lacking. Confusion regarding management of patients with discrepant serology (e.g., positive EIA/CIA and a negative RPR) • All reactive EIA/CIA must be reflexively tested with a quantitative RPR
ELISAs	Enzyme-linked immunosorbent assay	• *T. pallidum* antibody IgG by ELISA is the recommended screening test in reverse-screening protocol • Abnormal results require confirmation by nontreponemal assay (e.g., RPR or VDRL)
FTA-ABS	Fluorescent antibody absorption	• Not an optimal reflex test; TP-PA is preferred
IFA	Indirect fluorescent antibody	• May assist in workup of tertiary syphilis • May be considered if suspicion of neurosyphilis remains after VDRL testing
TP-PA	Particle agglutination	• CDC recommends a confirmatory test for syphilis if initial screening (e.g., RPR or VDRL) is reactive
MBIAs	Microbead immunoassay	
MHA-TP	Microhemagglutination	• Used less commonly

[a]VDRL is the preferred test for cerebrospinal fluid (CSF). Treponemal tests (TP-PA or FTA) are *not* recommended for CSF. FTAs on CSF may be tested, but TP-PA *cannot* be tested on CSF.
CDC, Centers for Disease Control and Prevention; *CIA*, chemiluminescence immunoassay; *EIA*, enzyme immunoassay; *FTA-ABS*, fluorescent treponemal antibody absorption; *IgG*, immunoglobulin G; *IgM*, immunoglobulin M; *MBIA*, microbead immunoassay; *MHA-TP*, microhemagglutination assay for antibodies directed against *Treponema pallidum*; *RPR*, rapid plasma reagin; *TP-PA*, *Treponema pallidum* particle agglutination assay; *TRUST*, toluidine red unheated serum test; *VDRL*, Venereal Disease Research Laboratory.

Chemiluminescence Immunoassays

CIAs, EIAs, and MBIAs are becoming more popular because they can be performed at a low cost with automated equipment.

Treponema pallidum Antibody Immunoglobulin G by Enzyme-Linked Immunosorbent Assay

A negative ELISA result is seen when no specific IgG antibodies against *T. pallidum* are detected. This test should not be used to determine relapse or reinfection of syphilis because of the persistence of reactivity, likely for a lifetime. Repeat testing in 2 to 4 weeks is recommended if results are equivocal. The presence of IgG antibody in *T. pallidum* is suggestive of current or past infection.

The ELISA assay can distinguish maternally derived IgG antibodies that cross the placenta from IgM antibodies that indicate active infection in a newborn. Congenital syphilis sensitivity is approximately 80%. Hence congenital syphilis can be confirmed, but a negative IgM level does not rule out congenital syphilis. The assay is highly specific (100%) and sensitive (91%).

Treponema pallidum Particle Agglutination

TP-PA is a semiquantitative particle agglutination assay. It cannot be used to test CSF and cannot differentiate between IgM and IgG antibodies. TP-PA is useful to diagnose infection in patients whose reactive screening test is positive with atypical signs of primary, secondary, or late syphilis. TP-PA compares favorably to the FTA-ABS test but is slightly less sensitive in untreated early primary syphilis. This assay is excellent for resolving inconclusive FTA-ABS results.

Fluorescent Treponemal Antibody Absorption

FTA-ABS can be used to confirm that a positive nontreponemal test result has been caused by syphilis rather than by other biological conditions that can produce a positive serologic result. This test also can determine quantitative titers of antibody, which is useful for following response to therapy. It is not an optimal reflex test; TP-PA is preferred.

The FTA-ABS uses a killed suspension of *T. pallidum* spirochetes as the antigen. Most systems use nonviable *T. pallidum* (Nichols strain), extracted from rabbit testicular tissue, as a substrate (antigen). Sorbent, another reagent, is prepared from cultures of nonpathogenic Reiter treponemes. The sorbent that contains an antigen to the Reiter treponeme may or may not specifically absorb the reactivity that occurs in normal sera.

This procedure is performed by overlaying whole treponemes fixed to a slide with serum from patients suspected of having syphilis because of a previously positive syphilis serology. The patient's serum is first absorbed with non–*T. pallidum* treponemal antigens to reduce nonspecific crossreactivity. Fluorescein-conjugated antihuman antibody reagent is then applied as a marker for specific antitreponemal antibodies in the patient's serum.

FTA-ABS may be helpful in late neurosyphilis when the RPR is negative but there is a high clinical suspicion of syphilis. FTA tests may produce a false-positive result in a variety of disorders, such as leprosy, pregnancy, and SLE.

SENSITIVITY OF REPRESENTATIVE PROCEDURES FOR SYPHILIS

Detection of syphilis by serologic methods is related to the stage of the disease and test method (Table 15.4).

In the primary stage, about 30% of cases become serologically active after 1 week, and 90% of patients demonstrate reactivity after 3 weeks. Reagin titers increase rapidly during the first 4 weeks of infection and then remain stable for about 6 months. Patients in the secondary stage of syphilis are serologically positive.

During latent syphilis, there is a gradual return of nonreactive serologic manifestations, as seen with nontreponemal methods. About one-third of patients in the latent stage will remain seroreactive and presumably infectious. In late syphilis, treponemal tests are generally reactive and nontreponemal methods are nonreactive.

TABLE 15.4 Percentage of Positive Tests for Syphilis

Test[a]	STAGE	
	Primary	Secondary
Nontreponemal Assay		
RPR	80–86	99–100[b]
Treponemal Assays		
FTA-ABS, TP-PA, MHA-TP	84–85	100
	85–100	98–100

[a]Percentage of patients with positive serologic tests in treated or untreated primary or secondary syphilis.
[b]Treated late syphilis.
FTA-ABS, Fluorescent treponemal antibody absorption; *MHA-TP*, microhemagglutination assay for antibodies directed against *Treponema pallidum*; *RPR*, rapid plasma reagin; *TP-PA*, *Treponema pallidum* particle agglutination assay.
Adapted from Tramont E: *Treponema pallidum*. In Mandell GI, Douglas RG Jr, Bennett Jr, editors: *Principles and practice of infectious diseases*, ed 2, New York, 1985, Wiley & Sons; and LaSala PR, Smith MB: Spirochete infections. In Henry JB, editor: *Clinical diagnosis and management by laboratory methods*, ed 22, Philadelphia, 2011, WB Saunders.

TRADITIONAL VERSUS REVERSE-SCREENING ALGORITHM PROTOCOLS

The traditional protocol for serologic screening for syphilis initially uses nontreponemal testing, with confirmation of reactive results using a treponemal test. New reverse algorithms are gaining popularity due to the development of point-of-care EIA and CIA tests. Reverse algorithms initially use treponemal testing (usually EIA or CIA), with confirmation of reactive results using a nontreponemal test (Table 15.5).

The influence of automation presents a reverse protocol. Many automated protocols begin with the detection of IgM and IgG antibodies to treponemal-specific antigens for sensitive detection of primary syphilis infection. A nontreponemal assay is used to detect active disease. When a reverse protocol is used, most patient specimens are negative, with only a small percentage of specimens requiring a manual nontreponemal test. Proponents of an automated, reverse protocol cite workflow advantages and an increased detection rate of late-stage syphilis.

If discordant results are encountered, the CDC suggests confirmation of discordant results by using the TP-PA, which is necessary to rule out a false-positive result. Examples of representative discordant results are presented in Table 15.6.

TABLE 15.5 Comparison of Traditional and Reverse Syphilis Testing

Traditional[a]	Reverse
Nontreponemal Testing (Quantitative)	**Treponemal Testing (Qualitative)**
Tests: Rapid plasma reagin (RPR) with reflex to titer Venereal Disease Research Laboratory (VDRL)	*Tests:* Chemiluminescence immunoassays (CIAs; enzyme immunoassays [EIAs]) Enzyme-linked immunosorbent assays (ELISAs) *Treponema pallidum* antibody by microbead immunoassays (MBIAs) T. *pallidum* particle agglutination (TP-PA) Fluorescent treponemal antibody absorption (FTA-ABS)
Advantages • Recommended screening test for syphilis by the Centers for Disease Control and Prevention (CDC) • May use RPR to confirm reactive treponemal test results if using the reverse algorithm testing protocol • RPR tests are the preferred test for monitoring treatment response in established cases of syphilis • VDRL can be performed on serum and cerebrospinal fluid (CSF), the required specimen for diagnosing neurosyphilis • Rapid and inexpensive testing • Detects acute infection • High positive predictive value if nontreponemal testing is followed by treponemal testing for confirmation	• Increasingly used for syphilis screening with the reverse sequence algorithm (see Fig. 15.4) • Automated and low cost if high volume • Treponemal antibodies often appear earlier than nontreponemal antibodies • Treponemal immunoassays demonstrate excellent sensitivity (100%) for secondary syphilis, 92%–100% sensitivity for early latent disease, and 86.8%–98.5% sensitivity in late latent diseased seropositive primary syphilis. • Because of its high sensitivity (100%), TP-PA is preferred to adjudicate discordant results with the reverse sequence algorithm over the FTA-ABS. • TP-PA is more specific and produces fewer false-positive results than the FTA-ABS test. • No false negative caused by prozone reaction compared with traditional testing methods.
Disadvantages • Reactivity declines over time • False-negative results can occur in early and late syphilis stages • False-positive results can occur because the assay is nonspecific for *T. pallidum* infection and may signal another infection (e.g., HIV and autoimmune conditions) • Moderately high rate of false positives for initial nontreponemal tests • Reactive tests need to be reflexed to a treponemal assay for confirmation	• Treponemal antibodies usually remain detectable for life, even after treatment. • Cannot detect active versus previously treated infection. • Sensitivity of FTA-ABS in primary syphilis is poor. • FTA-ABS is less sensitive for primary syphilis than the immunoassays or TP-PA (high specificity). • Relies on confirmation with second treponemal test. Follow-up nontreponemal test with titer required for all reactive tests to detect active infection.

[a]Traditional and nontraditional test detection of active infections are equivalent.
Data from ARUP Consult, Syphilis Testing, https://www.aruplab.com; Dunseth CD, Ford BA, Krasowski MD: Traditional versus reverse syphilis algorithms: a comparison at a large academic medical center, *Pract Lab Med* 29(8):52–59, 2017; Park IU, Fakile YF Chow JM: Performance of treponemal tests for the diagnosis of syphilis, *Clin Infect Dis* 68(6):913–918, 2019; Serhir B, Labbé AC, Doualla-Bell F, et al: Improvement of reverse sequence algorithm for syphilis diagnosis using optimal treponemal screening assay signal-to-cutoff ratio, *PLOS ONE* 13(9):2018.

TABLE 15.6 Representative Discordant Serum Assay Results

Case	Treponemal Assay[a]	Nontreponemal Assay[b]	Follow-Up Assay(s)	Comments
A sexually active female patient with a recent genital lesion was suspected of having syphilis	*T. pallidum* IgG: negative	Not requested	Repeat serologic testing in 2–4 weeks to detect *T. pallidum* IgG seroconversion	Treponemal and nontreponemal assay have limited sensitivity during the acute stages of syphilis infection
A sexually active, asymptomatic male was screened for syphilis	*T. pallidum* IgG: positive	RPR: negative	TP-PA: positive	Antibodies specific to *T. pallidum* confirm exposure to the spirochete in the past This may be a latent infection or a previously treated infection A negative RPR indicates the unlikelihood of an active infection

TABLE 15.6 Representative Discordant Serum Assay Results—cont'd

Case	Treponemal Assay[a]	Nontreponemal Assay[b]	Follow-Up Assay(s)	Comments
An HIV-positive male with a 5-day history of a rash and lymphadenopathy was examined	*T. pallidum* IgG: positive	RPR: positive	RPR titer: 256	This is a case of secondary syphilis. If treatment is successful, the RPR should become negative after 2 years in cases of secondary syphilis. If titers remain elevated, the patient may have a persistent infection, or the result may be a biological false positive

[a]Chemiluminescence immunoassay (CIA), enzyme immunoassay (EIA), multiplex flow immunoassay (MFI).
[b]RPR, Venereal Disease Research Laboratory (VDRL).
IgG, Immunoglobulin G; *RPR*, rapid plasma reagin; TP-PA, *Treponema pallidum* particle agglutination.
Data from ARUP Consult, Syphilis Traditional Testing and Syphilis (Reverse Sequence) Screening, https://www.arupconsult, 2017; Theel ES, Binnicker MJ: Reverse sequence screening for syphilis, *Cl Lab News* (CLN) 40:15–19, 2014.

CASE STUDY 15.1

History and Physical Examination
A 25-year-old woman comes to an ambulatory center with pain in the right side of her pelvis and a slightly elevated temperature. She has a history of two episodes of chlamydial cervicitis and herpes simplex vulvitis.

Physical examination reveals abundant mucopurulent cervical discharge and a painless genital lesion. The patient also has some swelling of her inguinal lymph glands.

Laboratory Data
A stat pregnancy test was ordered. The result was positive.

Questions
1. Appropriate testing for a high-risk patient could include all of the following *except*:
   a. Cervical culture for gonorrhea and chlamydia
   b. Gram stain for gonorrhea
   c. Serum testing for HIV and syphilis
   d. Repeat testing every 18 months if high-risk status continues
2. Screening testing for syphilis can include:
   a. Gram stain for *T. pallidum*
   b. Rapid plasma reagin (RPR) test
   c. Treponemal microhemagglutination assay for antibodies directed against *T. pallidum* (MHA-TP)
   d. Fluorescent treponemal antibody absorption (FTA-ABS)

Answers to these questions can be found in Appendix A.

Critical Thinking Group Discussion Questions
1. What other laboratory tests would you expect to be ordered?
2. Could this patient have syphilis?
3. If syphilis is suspected, what tests should be ordered?
4. Is there risk of a congenital infection in this woman's unborn child?

REVIEW QUESTIONS

1. *Treponema pallidum (T. pallidum)* is the causative organism associated with the disease:
   a. Yaws
   b. Syphilis
   c. Pinta
   d. Bejel
2. *Treponema pallidum (T. pallidum)* variant is the causative organism associated with the disease:
   a. Yaws
   b. Syphilis
   c. Pinta
   d. Bejel
3. *Treponema pertenue (T. pertenue)* is the causative organism associated with the disease:
   a. Yaws
   b. Syphilis
   c. Pinta
   d. Bejel
4. *Treponema carateum (T. carateum)* is the causative organism associated with the disease:
   a. Yaws
   b. Syphilis
   c. Pinta
   d. Bejel

5. In the primary stage of syphilis, a clinical finding is:
   a. Diagnosis only by serologic methods
   b. Presence of gummas
   c. Development of a chancre
   d. Generalized illness followed by macular lesions in most patients
6. In the secondary stage of syphilis, a clinical finding is:
   a. Diagnosis only by serologic methods
   b. Presence of gummas
   c. Development of a chancre
   d. Generalized illness followed by macular lesions in most patients
7. In the latent stage of syphilis, a clinical finding is:
   a. Diagnosis only by serologic methods
   b. Presence of gummas
   c. Development of a chancre
   d. Generalized illness followed by macular lesions in most patients
8. In the late (tertiary) stage of syphilis, a clinical finding is:
   a. Diagnosis only by serologic methods
   b. Presence of gummas
   c. Development of a chancre
   d. Generalized illness followed by macular lesions in most patients
9. Which of the following is a term for nontreponemal antibodies produced by an infected patient against components of their own or other mammalian cells?
   a. Autoagglutinins
   b. Reagin antibodies
   c. Alloantibodies
   d. Nonsyphilis antibodies
10. The FTA-ABS test is a:
    a. Treponemal method
    b. Nontreponemal method
11. The TP-PA test is a:
    a. Treponemal method
    b. Nontreponemal method
12. The RPR test is a:
    a. Treponemal method
    b. Nontreponemal method
13. In the RPR procedure, a false-positive reaction can result from all the following *except*:
    a. Infectious mononucleosis
    b. Leprosy
    c. Rheumatoid arthritis
    d. Streptococcal pharyngitis
14. The first diagnostic blood test for syphilis was the:
    a. VDRL
    b. Wassermann
    c. RPR
    d. Colloidal gold
15. Syphilis was initially treated with:
    a. Fuller's earth
    b. Heavy metals (e.g., arsenic)
    c. Sulfonamides (e.g., triple sulfa)
    d. Antibiotics (e.g., penicillin)
16. Direct examination of the treponemes is most often performed by:
    a. Light microscopy
    b. Darkfield microscopy
    c. VDRL testing
    d. RPR testing
17. Pathogenic treponemes _____ cultivatable with consistency in artificial laboratory media.
    a. Are
    b. Are not
18. In infected blood, *T. pallidum* does not appear to survive at 4°C (39°F) for longer than:
    a. 1 day
    b. 2 days
    c. 3 days
    d. 5 days
19. The primary incubation period for syphilis (*T. pallidum*) is usually about:
    a. 1 week
    b. 2 weeks
    c. 3 weeks
    d. 4 weeks
20. The stage of syphilis that can be diagnosed only by serologic (laboratory) methods is the:
    a. Incubation phase
    b. Primary phase
    c. Secondary phase
    d. Latent phase

16

Vector-Borne Diseases

LEARNING OUTCOMES

- Describe the etiology, epidemiology, and signs and symptoms of Lyme disease.
- Analyze the immunologic manifestations and diagnostic evaluation of Lyme disease.
- Explain the principle, interpretation, and limitations of an antibody detection assay.
- Describe prevention strategies for Lyme disease.
- Summarize the etiology, epidemiology, and signs and symptoms of ehrlichiosis.
- Analyze the immunologic manifestations and diagnostic evaluation of ehrlichiosis.
- Explain the prevention of ehrlichiosis.
- Summarize the etiology, epidemiology, and signs and symptoms of Rocky Mountain spotted fever.
- Analyze the immunologic manifestations and diagnostic evaluation of Rocky Mountain spotted fever.
- Explain the prevention of Rocky Mountain spotted fever.
- Summarize the etiology, epidemiology, and signs and symptoms of babesiosis.
- Analyze the immunologic manifestations and diagnostic evaluation of babesiosis.
- Explain the prevention of babesiosis.
- Summarize the etiology, epidemiology, and signs and symptoms of malaria.
- Analyze the immunologic manifestations and diagnostic evaluation of malaria.
- Explain the treatment and prevention of malaria.
- Briefly discuss the etiology and laboratory diagnosis of chikungunya virus infection.
- Briefly discuss the etiology and laboratory diagnosis of dengue virus infection.
- Briefly discuss the etiology and laboratory diagnosis of West Nile virus infection.
- Analyze case studies related to the immune response in Lyme disease, ehrlichiosis, and babesiosis.
- Correctly answer case study–related multiple-choice questions.
- Be prepared to participate in a discussion of critical thinking questions.
- Describe the principle, limitations, and clinical applications of the rapid *Borrelia burgdorferi* antibody detection assay.
- Correctly answer 80% of the end-of-chapter review questions.

OUTLINE

Vector-borne Infectious Diseases, 241
Lyme Disease, 243
    Etiology, 243
    Epidemiology, 244
    Signs and Symptoms, 244
        Arthritis, 245
        Cutaneous Manifestations, 246
        Cardiac Manifestations, 246
        Neurologic Manifestations, 246
        Pregnancy, 246
        Immunologic Manifestations, 246
    Diagnostic Evaluation, 247
        Confirmatory Laboratory Evidence, 247
        Presumptive Laboratory Evidence, 247
        Antibody Detection Methods, 247
        Enzyme-Linked Immunosorbent Assay, 248
        Western Blot Analysis, 248
        Polymerase Chain Reaction, 248
        Cerebrospinal Fluid Analysis for Antibody Detection, 249
    Treatment and Prevention, 249
        Antibiotics, 249
        Prevention, 250

Human Ehrlichiosis, 250
    Etiology, 250
    Epidemiology, 250
    Signs and Symptoms, 250
    Diagnostic Evaluation, 250
    Treatment and Prevention, 251
Rocky Mountain Spotted Fever, 252
    Etiology, 252
    Epidemiology, 252
    Signs and Symptoms, 252
    Diagnostic Evaluation, 252
    Treatment and Prevention, 252
Babesiosis, 252
    Etiology, 252
    Epidemiology, 252
    Signs and Symptoms, 253
    Diagnostic Evaluation, 253
    Treatment and Prevention, 253
MOSQUITO VECTOR DISEASES, 253
Malaria, 253
    Etiology, 253
    Global Malaria Distribution and Statistics, 254

Characteristics of *Plasmodium* Species, 254
Epidemiology (United States), 254
Risk of Malaria, 254
The Disease Phase of Malaria in Humans, 254
Signs and Symptoms, 255
Diagnostic Laboratory Evaluation, 256
   Microscopic Examination, 256
   Molecular Testing, 256
   LAMP Assay, 258
Treatment and Prevention, 258
Chikungunya Disease, 258
Etiology, 258
Epidemiology, 258
Signs and Symptoms, 258
Diagnostic Evaluation, 258
Treatment and Prevention, 259
Dengue Virus, 259
Etiology, 259
Epidemiology, 259
Signs and Symptoms, 259

Diagnostic Evaluation, 260
Nucleic Acid Amplification Tests (NAATs), 260
   Serologic Tests, 260
   Crossreactive Flaviviruses, 260
   IgG Antibody Testing, 260
Treatment and Prevention, 262
West Nile Virus, 262
Etiology, 262
Epidemiology, 262
Signs and Symptoms, 263
Diagnostic Evaluation, 263
Treatment and Prevention, 263
Case Study 16.1, 263
Case Study 16.2, 263
Case Study 16.3, 264
Case Study 16.4, 264
Case Study 16.5, 264
Procedure: Rapid *Borrelia Burgdorferi* Antibody Detection Assay, 266.e1

KEY TERMS

anaplasmosis	chikungunya	Lyme disease
anticardiolipin	dengue fever	rickettsial
arthralgia	erythema migrans (EM)	Rocky Mountain spotted fever (RMSF)
aseptic meningitis	human ehrlichiosis	vector-borne
babesiosis	intraerythrocytic	
bacteriostatic	intraleukocytic morulae	

VECTOR-BORNE INFECTIOUS DISEASES

Microbial infectious diseases can be transmitted by infected ticks mosquitoes, or fleas (Table 16.1). The number of **vector-borne** infections is increasing globally due to climate change. Specific infected mosquitoes are carriers of genus *Plasmodium* species: *P. falciparum, P. vivax, P. malariae, P. ovale,* and *P. knowlesi.*

Tick vectors in the United States include blacklegged tick, lone star tick, American dog tick, brown dog tick, groundhog tick, Gulf Coast tick, Rocky Mountain wood tick, soft tick *Ornithodoros* spp., and western blacklegged tick.

According to the Centers for Disease Control and Prevention, some human diseases in the United States (examples discussed in more detail later) are caused by ticks that carry pathogens, including:

- **Anaplasmosis** is transmitted primarily from the blacklegged tick (*Ixodes scapularis*) in the northeastern and upper midwestern United States and the western blacklegged tick (*Ixodes pacificus*) along the Pacific Coast.
- **Babesiosis** is caused by *Babesia microti*, which is transmitted by the blacklegged tick (*I. scapularis*) and is found primarily in the northeast and upper midwestern United States.
- *Borrelia mayonii* infection has recently been described as a cause of illness in the upper midwestern United States. It has been found in blacklegged ticks (*I. scapularis*) in Minnesota and Wisconsin. *B. mayonii* is a new species and is the only species besides *B. burgdorferi* known to cause Lyme disease in North America.
- *Borrelia miyamotoi* infection has recently been described as a cause of illness in the United States. It is transmitted by the blacklegged tick (*I. scapularis*) and has a range similar to that of Lyme disease.
- **Bourbon virus** infection has been identified in a limited number of patients in the midwestern and southern United States.
- **Colorado tick fever** is caused by a virus transmitted by the Rocky Mountain wood tick (*Dermacentor andersoni*). It occurs in the Rocky Mountain states at elevations of 4000 to 10,500 feet.
- **Ehrlichiosis** is transmitted to humans by the lone star tick (*Amblyomma americanum*), found primarily in southcentral and eastern United States.
- **Heartland virus** cases have been identified in the midwestern and southern United States. Studies suggest that lone star ticks can transmit the virus.
- **Lyme disease** is transmitted by the blacklegged tick (*I. scapularis*) in the northeastern United States and upper midwestern United States, and the western blacklegged tick (*I. pacificus*) along the Pacific Coast.
- **Powassan disease** is transmitted by the blacklegged tick (*I. scapularis*) and the groundhog tick (*Ixodes cookei*). Cases have been reported primarily from northeastern states and the Great Lakes region.
- *Rickettsia parkeri* rickettsiosis is transmitted to humans by the Gulf Coast tick (*Amblyomma maculatum*).
- **Rocky Mountain spotted fever (RMSF)** is transmitted by the American dog tick (*Dermacentor variabilis*), Rocky Mountain wood tick (*D. andersoni*), and the brown dog tick (*Rhipicephalus sanguineus*) in the United States. The brown dog tick and other tick species are associated with RMSF in Central and South America.
- **STARI (Southern tick-associated rash illness)** is transmitted via bites from the lone star tick (*A. americanum*), found in the southeastern and eastern United States.
- **Tickborne relapsing fever (TBRF)** is transmitted to humans through the bite of infected soft ticks. TBRF has been reported in 15 states—Arizona, California, Colorado, Idaho, Kansas, Montana, Nevada, New Mexico, Ohio, Oklahoma, Oregon, Texas, Utah, Washington, and Wyoming—and is associated with sleeping in rustic cabins and vacation homes.

TABLE 16.1 Examples of Vector-Borne Human Diseases

Vector	Human Disease	Geographic Distribution
Ticks		
Blacklegged tick (*Ixodes scapularis*) or western blacklegged tick (*Ixodes pacificus*)	Anaplasmosis (formerly human granulocytic ehrlichiosis)	Worldwide; Europe United States: *I. scapularis* in the northeastern and upper midwestern United States *Ixodes pacificus* along the Pacific Coast
Blacklegged tick (*I. scapularis*) or Western blacklegged tick (*Ixodes pacificus*)	Lyme disease	*I. scapularis* in the northeastern and upper midwestern United States *Ixodes pacificus* along the Pacific Coast
Blacklegged tick (*I. scapularis*)	Babesiosis	United States: Primarily northeastern states, rarely Pacific states
Lone star tick (*Amblyomma Americanum*)	Human monocytic ehrlichiosis	United States: Southeast, south-central states
Lone star tick (*Amblyomma americanum*)	Heartland virus	United States: Midwestern and southern United States
Lone star tick (*Amblyomma Americanum*)	STARI (Southern tick-associated rash illness)	As of September 2022, more than 60 cases of Heartland virus disease have been reported from states in the midwest and the South Southeastern and eastern United States
Blacklegged tick (*I. scapularis*) and the groundhog tick (*Ixodes cookei*)	Powassan disease	Throughout the eastern half of the United States, primarily from northeastern states and the Great Lakes region
American dog tick (*Dermacentor variabilis*), Rocky Mountain wood tick (*Dermacentor andersoni*), and the brown dog tick (*Rhipicephalus sanguinineus*) in the United States	Rocky Mountain spotted fever (RMSF)	Found in Rocky Mountain states
Dog tick (*D. variabilis*), the wood tick (*Dermacentor andersoni*), and the lone star tick (*Amblyomma americanum*)	Tuleremia	Occurs throughout the United States
Infected soft ticks, genus, *Ornithodoros* Specific species of ticks include *O. hermsi*, *O. parkeri*, and *O. Turicata*	Tickborne relapsing fever (TBRF) TBRFs also called Soft tick relapsing fever (STRF)	Reported in 15 states: Arizona, California, Colorado, Idaho, Kansas, Montana, Nevada, New Mexico, Ohio, Oklahoma, Oregon, Texas, Utah, Washington, and Wyoming[a] Each tick species has a preferred habitat and preferred set of hosts: • *O. hermsi* tends to be found at higher altitudes (1500–8000 feet) where it is associated primarily with ground or tree squirrels and chipmunks • *O. parkeri* occurs at lower altitudes, where they inhabit caves and the burrows of ground squirrels and prairie dogs, as well as those of burrowing owls • *O. turicata* occurs in caves and ground squirrel or prairie dog burrows in the plains regions of the Southwest, feeding off these animals and occasionally burrowing owls or other burrow- or cave-dwelling animals
Rocky Mountain wood tick (*Dermacentor andersoni*)	Colorado tick fever	North and South America
Pacific coast tick (*Dermacentor occidentalis*)	364D-rickettsiosis	United States: California
Gulf Coast tick (*Amblyomma maculatum*)	*R. parkeri* (rickettsiosis), a form of spotted fever	Primarily in the southeastern United States, with focal populations in the northeastern, midwestern, and southeastern United States
Tick of unknown origin, possibly lone star tick	Bourbon virus infection	Bourbon virus is a novel RNA virus in the genus *Thogotovirus* (family *Orthomyxoviridae*) that was discovered in Bourbon County, Kansas in 2014 As of 2017, a limited number of Bourbon virus disease cases have been reported in the midwestern and southern United States
Mosquitoes		
Aedes triseriatus	California encephalitis West Nile encephalitis, West Nile fever	United States: Upper midwest, Appalachian region United States: spreading nationwide Africa, Asia
Aedes species (*Ae. Aegypti* or *Ae. albopictus*)	Chikungunya Dengue fever	Africa, Asia, Europe, the Indian and Pacific Oceans, Caribbean United States: Florida, Puerto Rico, and the US Virgin Islands Locally acquired United States: Florida, Puerto Rico, American Samoa, and the US Virgin Islands The Americas, Africa, the Middle East, Asia, and the Pacific Islands

TABLE 16.1 Examples of Vector-Borne Human Diseases—cont'd

Vector	Human Disease	Geographic Distribution
Culiseta melanura	Eastern equine encephalitis	Eastern United States
		Central and South America, Caribbean
Culex spp.	St. Louis encephalitis	Eastern United States
		Central and South America
	Western equine encephalitis	Western United States
		Central and South America
Lice, Fleas, Mites		
Human body louse; squirrel flea and louse	Epidemic typhus	United States, eastern
Rat flea, *Xenopsylla cheopis*	Murine typhus	Worldwide, where rats are abundant
Cat or dog fleas	Murine typhus–like febrile disease	Worldwide
Mites (chiggers)	Scrub typhus	South Asia to Australia, East Asia in recently disturbed habitat (e.g., forest clearings or other persisting mite foci infested with rats and other rodents)
Human body louse	Louse-borne relapsing fever	Africa
	Trench fever	Industrialized countries

[a]Most recent cases and outbreaks have occurred in rustic cabins at higher elevations (8000 ft or higher) in coniferous forests in the western United States.
From Centers for Disease Control and Prevention: Tickborne Diseases of the United States, www.cdc.gov.

- **Tularemia** is transmitted to humans by the dog tick (*D. variabilis*), the wood tick (*D. andersoni*), and the lone star tick (*A. americanum*). Tularemia occurs throughout the United States.
- **364D rickettsiosis** (*Rickettsia phillipi*, proposed) is transmitted to humans by the Pacific coast tick (*Dermacentor occidentalis*). This is a new disease that has been found in California.

Other specific emerging infectious diseases in the United States include:
- Chagas disease
- Chikungunya
- Dengue
- Leishmaniasis

Some prominent examples of the more commonly occurring vector-borne diseases in the United States that are detectable by serologic methods are presented in this chapter.

LYME DISEASE

> **KEY CONCEPTS: Lyme Disease Characteristics**
> - Lyme disease (borreliosis) is caused by the tick-borne spirochete *Borrelia burgdorferi* and is a major health hazard for human beings and domestic animals.
> - Lyme disease has been considered an emerging infectious disease because of the effect of changing environmental and socioeconomic factors (e.g., transformation of farmland into suburban woodlots favorable for deer and deer ticks).
> - The basic features of Lyme disease are similar worldwide. In at least 60% to 80% of US patients, it begins with a slowly expanding skin lesion, erythema migrans (EM), at the site of the tick bite.
> - Lyme borreliosis is a multisystem illness that primarily involves the skin, nervous system, heart, and joints. It usually begins during the summer months with EM and flulike symptoms.
> - Cellular immune responses to *B. burgdorferi* antigens begin concurrently with early clinical illness, with increased spontaneous suppressor cell and reduced natural killer (NK) cell activity. Mononuclear cell, antigen-specific responses develop during spirochetal dissemination, and humoral (antibody) immune responses soon follow.
> - *B. mayonii* is a new species and is the only species besides *B. burgdorferi* known to cause Lyme disease in North America.
> - *B. miyamotoi* infection has a range similar to that of Lyme disease.

Etiology

It was not until 1982 that Burgdorfer and Barbour isolated a previously unrecognized spirochete, now called *Borrelia burgdorferi*, from *I. scapularis* ticks. Lyme disease is a cutaneous systemic infection generally transmitted by a hard-bodied tick (Fig. 16.1) and caused by *B. burgdorferi* (Fig. 16.2), and rarely *B. mayonii*. has also been shown to cause Lyme disease in the upper midwestern United States. The complete genome of *B. burgdorferi* (strain B31) has now been sequenced.

The spirochete is transmitted by certain ixodid ticks that are part of the *Ixodes ricinus* complex. These include *I. scapularis* (formerly classified as *Ixodes dammini*) in the northeastern and midwestern United States, *Ixodes pacificus* in the western United States, *Ixodes ricinus* in Europe, and *Ixodes persulcatus* in Asia. The vector has not been identified in Australia. Ixodid ticks are also indigenous to Africa and South America. The lone star tick, *Amblyomma americanum*, does not transmit Lyme disease.

In the United States, the preferred host for larval and nymphal stages of *I. scapularis* is the white-footed mouse, *Peromyscus leucopus*. White-tailed deer, which are not involved in the life cycle of the spirochete, are the preferred host for the *I. scapularis* adult stage, and they seem to be critical to tick survival. Ixodid ticks have also been found on at least 30 types of wild animals and 49 species of birds. Illness is not known to develop in wild animals, but clinical Lyme disease does occur in domestic animals, including dogs, horses, and cattle.

Two factors influence the chance that a bitten patient will contract the disease: the likelihood that local ixodid ticks carry the Lyme spirochete and the likelihood of infection after a bite by an infected tick. The probability of infection after an ixodid tick bite in an area of endemic disease is about 3% but varies in different regions from less than 1% to as high as 5%. It has been suggested that human leukocyte antigen (HLA)-DR4 and, secondarily, HLA-DR2 may increase the risk that Lyme arthritis will become chronic and fail to respond to antibiotics.

Lyme disease spreads because of the effect of changing environmental and socioeconomic factors, such as the transformation of farmland into suburban woodlots favorable for deer and deer ticks. Although pets may represent a spirochete reservoir, it is unlikely that humans can be infected directly by them. In areas of endemic Lyme disease, however, both adult and nymphal ticks, carried into the household by dogs and cats, may infect humans.

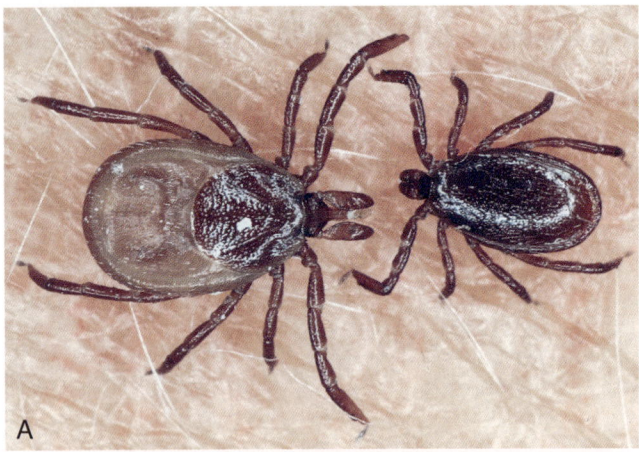

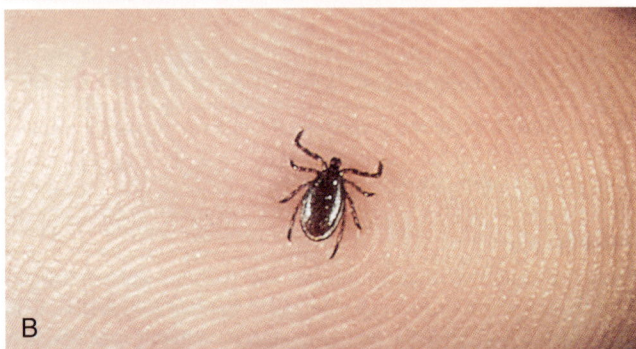

Fig. 16.1 (A and B) Deer tick. (From Habif TP: *Clinical dermatology*, ed 2, St. Louis, 1990, Mosby.)

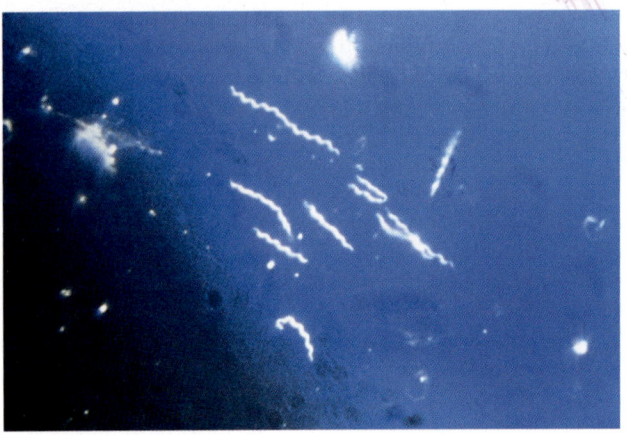

Fig. 16.2 *Borrelia burgdorferi*. Using the dark-field microscopy technique, under a magnification of 400×, this photomicrograph reveals the presence of spirochetes or corkscrew-shaped bacteria known as *Borrelia burgdorferi*, which is the pathogen responsible for causing Lyme disease. They are helical-shaped bacteria, 10–25 μm in length. (From CDC Public Health Image Library. https://phil.cdc.gov/.)

Epidemiology

Currently, Lyme disease is a global illness. Cases have been reported on all continents except Antarctica. Since its original description, Lyme disease has become the most commonly reported (95%) vector-borne illness in the United States. This infection has emerged as a major health hazard for human beings and domestic animals. The disease is concentrated heavily in the northeast and upper midwest (Fig. 16.3), but the geographic distribution of high-incidence areas of patients with Lyme disease appears to be increasing.

States with an average annual incidence of ≥10 confirmed Lyme disease cases per 100,000 population are classified as high-incidence states. States sharing a border with those states or located between high-incidence states are classified as neighboring and all of the other states are classified as low incidence.

According to the Centers for Disease Control and Prevention (CDC), over 63,000 cases of Lyme disease were reported to CDC by state health departments and the District of Columbia in 2022. This number reflects cases reported through routine national surveillance, which is only one way public health officials track diseases. Recent estimates using other methods suggest that approximately 476,000 people may be diagnosed and treated for Lyme disease each year in the United States. This number likely includes patients who are treated based on clinical suspicion but do not actually have Lyme disease.

Signs and Symptoms

In some patients, Lyme disease may be transitory and of little consequence, but in others it may become chronic and severely disabling. Accurate diagnosis is therefore essential, although better laboratory techniques are still needed.

Retrospectively the first symptom of Lyme disease was apparently recognized as early as 1908 in Sweden. Spirochetes are transmitted from the gut of the tick to human skin at the site of a bite and then migrate outwardly into the skin. This migration causes the unique expanding skin lesions, *erythema migrans (EM)*. Subsequent dissemination of spirochetes to secondary sites may cause major organ system involvement in humans. In dogs, the most common symptom is arthritis. Secondary symptoms, such as impairment of the nervous system, were described in France, Germany, and again in Sweden.

In the United States, the European rash was almost unknown until 1969, when a case of a physician bitten by a tick while hunting in Wisconsin was reported. Although a few cases were seen in Americans who had traveled to Europe, there were no further Native American cases until 1975, when physicians at the US Navy base in Groton, Connecticut, reported seeing four patients with a rash similar to that of EM. At the same time, an epidemiologist at the Connecticut State Department of Health and a rheumatologist at Yale University were notified of an unusual cluster of cases of arthritis occurring in children in Lyme, Connecticut.

The basic features of Lyme disease are similar worldwide, but there are regional variations, primarily between the illness in America and that in Europe and Asia. In at least 60% to 80% of US patients, Lyme disease begins with a slowly expanding skin lesion, EM, which occurs at the site of the tick bite. The skin lesion is commonly accompanied by flulike symptoms.

The CDC clinical case definition for Lyme disease includes the presence of EM or at least one objective, late-manifesting sign of musculoskeletal, neurologic, or cardiovascular disease and a positive serologic test for antibodies to *B. burgdorferi*. Many misdiagnosed patients actually have chronic fatigue syndrome or fibromyalgia, both of which can cause similar symptoms, such as joint stiffness or pain, fatigue, and sleep disturbance.

Lyme borreliosis is a multisystem illness that primarily involves the skin, nervous system, heart, and joints (Table 16.2). There are three stages of Lyme disease:

Stage 1 is called early localized Lyme disease. The bacteria have not yet spread throughout the body.
Stage 2 is called early disseminated Lyme disease. The bacteria have begun to spread throughout the body.
Stage 3 is called late disseminated Lyme disease.

Lyme disease usually begins during the summer months with EM and flulike symptoms and may be accompanied by right upper quadrant tenderness and a mild hepatitis (stage 1). This stage is followed

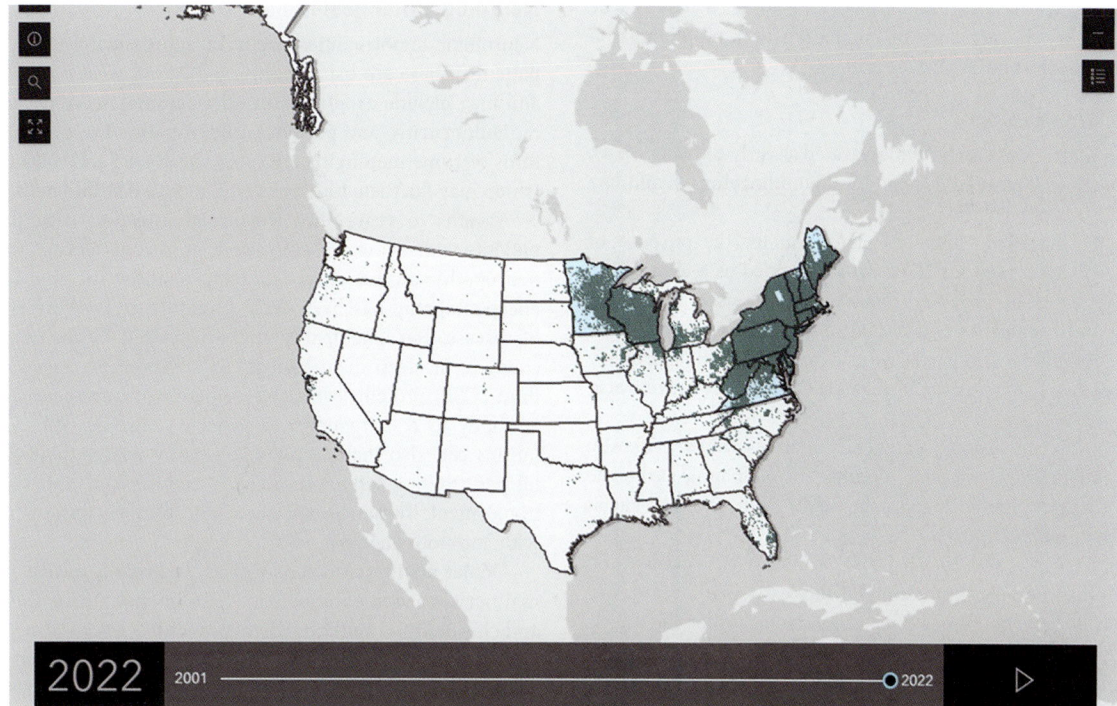

Fig. 16.3 Reported cases of Lyme disease: United States, 2022. (From Centers for Disease Control and Prevention, Atlanta.)

TABLE 16.2	Clinical Features of Lyme Disease	
Stage	Duration	Signs and Symptoms
1	4 weeks (median) after infection	• Cutaneous manifestations (erythema migrans) or other skin eruptions, flulike syndrome, fatigue. Headache and stiff neck. Muscle soreness and joint pain, swollen lymph nodes and sore throat
2	Follows a variable latent period. Early disseminated Lyme may occur several weeks or months after the blacklegged tick bite. The bacterium *B. burgdorferi* is beginning to spread throughout the body	Target organs and systems include nervous system, heart, eyes, and skin, all of which can manifest abnormalities
3	Weeks to years after infection If Lyme disease is not promptly or effectively treated in the first two stages, late disseminated (post-treatment, chronic, or neurological) Lyme occurs weeks, months or even years after the tick bite. The bacterial infection has spread throughout the body and nervous system, and many patients develop chronic Lyme arthritis as well as an increase in neurological and cardiac symptoms	Arthritis, late neurologic complications, acrodermatitis chronica atrophicans

weeks to months later by acute cardiac or neurologic disease in a minority of untreated individuals (stage 2), and then by arthritis and chronic neurologic disease (stage 3) in many untreated patients weeks to years after disease onset.

There is considerable overlap of these stages, but Lyme disease is best characterized as an illness that evolves from early to late disease without reference to an arbitrary staging system. However, a patient may have one or all of the stages, and the infection may not become symptomatic until stage 2 or 3. Most affected patients have EM and 25% manifest arthritis; neurologic manifestations and cardiac involvement are uncommon.

Arthritis

Arthralgia and myalgia are common features of early Lyme disease. Arthritis is a well-described complication of Lyme disease and characteristically occurs months to years after *Borrelia* infection. Therefore cases of Lyme arthritis occur every month of the year. Lyme arthritis and parvovirus B19 arthritis can occur in the absence of other symptoms, such as the characteristic rash. Some suspected cases of Lyme arthritis might be caused by parvovirus B19, particularly those occurring during the parvovirus B19 season.

Arthritis in patients with chronic Lyme disease may be associated with a long-standing infiltration of the joints by *B. burgdorferi* spirochetes, along with a local inflammatory response. It may not be triggered simply by the presence of circulating immunoglobulin G (IgG) antibodies against outer surface proteins.

Cutaneous Manifestations

Cutaneous manifestations can be demonstrated as early EM (Fig. 16.4), secondary lesions (disseminated lesions and lymphocytoma), and late lesions (ACA).

According to the 2020 CDC case definition for the purpose of surveillance, *Erythema migrans (EM) rash* is defined as a skin lesion (observed by a healthcare provider) that typically begins as a red macule or papule and expands over a period of days to weeks to form a large round lesion, often with partial central clearing. A single primary lesion must reach a size of ≥5 cm in diameter. Secondary lesions also may occur.

Except for the late lesions, cutaneous manifestations generally resolve spontaneously over weeks to months. The red papule at the site of the tick bite is most often located on the thigh, groin, or axilla. Facial EM is more common in children.

Several days to weeks after the onset of EM, almost 50% of untreated patients develop secondary skin lesions. A rare early manifestation of Lyme disease is *Borrelia* lymphocytoma, a violaceous, tumor-like swelling or nodule at the base of the earlobe or nipple caused by a dense lymphocytic infiltrate of the dermis. This lesion occurs at the site of a tick bite and in conjunction with other symptoms; it may be confused with lymphoma.

Acrodermatitis chronica atrophicans (ACA) is a late skin manifestation of Lyme disease more prevalent in Europe than in the United States. Lesions display bluish-red discoloration, doughy swelling, and fibrotic nodules. Eventually, striking atrophy of the skin and subcutaneous tissues follows. Polyneuropathy coexists in 30% to 45% of patients.

Cardiac Manifestations

Lyme carditis occurs in approximately 8% of untreated patients within 1 to 2 months (range, more than 1 week to 7 months) after the onset of infection and may be the initial manifestation of Lyme disease. Cardiac features of Lyme disease usually result in a fluctuating degree of atrioventricular conduction defects (first-degree, second-degree, and complete block, in addition to bundle branch and fascicular blocks) or tachyarrhythmias. Myopericarditis can occur, but symptomatic congestive heart failure is uncommon. Patients usually develop signs of lightheadedness, syncope, dyspnea, palpitations, and chest pain. Symptoms are more common in patients with more severe degrees of heart block. The carditis usually follows a self-limited and mild course, but temporary pacing may be needed in a small percentage of patients.

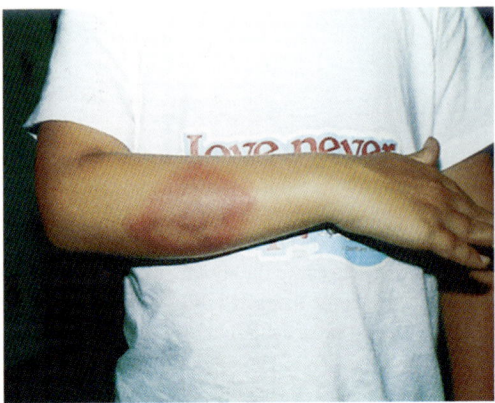

Fig. 16.4 Erythema migrans.

Neurologic Manifestations

Neurologic abnormalities occur in approximately 15% of untreated patients. These are usually observed 2 to 8 weeks after disease onset and may include aseptic meningitis, cranial nerve palsies, peripheral radiculoneuritis, and peripheral neuropathy. The predominant symptoms of Lyme meningitis are severe headache and mild neck stiffness, which may fluctuate for weeks after a post-EMEM latent period.

Months to years after the initial infection with *B. burgdorferi*, patients with Lyme disease may have chronic encephalopathy; polyneuropathy; or, less often, leukoencephalitis. The appearance of mild encephalopathy has been seen 1 month to 14 years after the onset of disease. Encephalopathy is characterized by memory loss, mood changes, or sleep disturbances. In addition, increased cerebrospinal fluid (CSF) protein levels and evidence of intrathecal production of antibody to *B. burgdorferi* may occur. Chronic neurologic manifestations can also include polyneuropathy with radicular pain or distal paresthesias, fatigue, headache, hearing loss, and verbal memory impairment. These chronic neurologic abnormalities usually improve with antibiotic therapy.

Ocular manifestations may occur in Lyme disease and include cranial nerve palsies, optic neuritis, panophthalmitis with loss of vision, and choroiditis with retinal detachment.

Any of the following signs that cannot be explained by any other etiology, alone or in combination include lymphocytic meningitis; cranial neuritis, particularly facial palsy (unilateral or bilateral); radiculoneuropathy; or, rarely, encephalomyelitis.

Pregnancy

Transplacental transmission of *B. burgdorferi* with fetal infection has been confirmed. A uniform pattern of congenital malformations has not been identified in maternal-fetal transmission of Lyme disease.

In observed cases cited, infants died shortly after birth. The mothers acquired infection during the first trimester and received inadequate or no treatment.

Immunologic Manifestations

Cellular immune responses to *B. burgdorferi* antigens begin concurrent with early clinical illness. An increase in spontaneous suppressor cell activity and reduction in NK cell activity have been noted. Mononuclear cell, antigen-specific responses develop during spirochetal dissemination, and humoral (antibody) immune responses soon follow.

Serodiagnostic tests are insensitive during the first several weeks of infection. In the United States, approximately 20% to 30% of patients with Lyme disease have positive responses, usually of the immunoglobulin M (IgM) isotype, during this period, but by convalescence 2 to 4 weeks later, about 70% to 80% have seroreactivity even after antibiotic treatment. After about 1 month, most patients with an active infection have IgG antibody responses. After antibiotic treatment, antibody titers slowly fall, but IgG and even IgM responses may persist for many years after treatment. An IgM response cannot be interpreted as a manifestation of recent infection or reinfection unless the appropriate clinical characteristics are present. Antibodies formed include cryoglobulins, immune complexes, antibodies specific for *B. burgdorferi*, and anticardiolipin antibodies. Elevated titers of IgM are noted in early disease. Immunoblot analysis demonstrates that IgM antibodies form initially against the flagellar 41-kilodalton (kDa) polypeptide but react later to additional cell wall antigens. An overlapping IgG response to these antigens develops in some individuals. These antigen-specific cellular and humoral responses are not known to eradicate infection in early disease or participate in disease pathogenesis.

Specific IgM or IgG antibodies against *B. burgdorferi* are usually not detectable in a patient's serum unless symptoms have been present for at least 2 to 4 weeks. In cases of Lyme arthritis, tests for serum antinuclear antibodies (ANAs) and rheumatoid factor (RF) and Venereal Disease Research Laboratory (VDRL) test results are generally negative. However, anti–*B. burgdorferi* antibodies of the IgG type should be present in the serum of patients with Lyme arthritis.

Outer surface protein A antibodies develop late in the course of human Lyme infection and then only in a subset of patients. A temporal association may have existed between the onset of chronic Lyme arthritis in four patients who were HLA-DR4 positive and the development of antibodies to the outer surface protein.

Persistent organisms and spirochetal antigen deposits elicit a vigorous immune reaction, as manifested by a tissue-rich plasma cell and lymphocytic exudate containing abundant T cells, predominantly of the helper subset, plus immunoglobulin D (IgD)–bearing B cells. *B. burgdorferi* antigens elicit a strong immune reaction that intensifies with chronicity of arthritis and stimulates macrophages to secrete interleukin-1 (IL-1). IL-1 is capable of stimulating synovial cells and fibroblasts to secrete collagenase and prostaglandin E2; levels of both are elevated in Lyme synovial fluid and can cause erosion of joint cartilage and bone.

> **KEY CONCEPTS: Laboratory Testing**
> - Serodiagnostic tests are insensitive during the first several weeks of *Borrelia* infection. About 20% to 30% of US patients have positive responses, usually of the IgM isotype, during this period, but by convalescence 2 to 4 weeks later about 70% to 80% have seroreactivity even after antibiotic treatment. After about 1 month, most patients with active infection have IgG antibody responses. After antibiotic treatment antibody titers fall slowly, but IgG and IgM responses may persist for years.
> - Specific IgM or IgG antibodies against *B. burgdorferi* are usually not detectable in a patient's serum unless symptoms have been present for at least 2 to 4 weeks. In Lyme arthritis, test results (antinuclear antibodies [ANAs], rheumatoid factor [RF], Venereal Disease Research Laboratory [VDRL] test) are generally negative, and anti–*B. burgdorferi* antibodies (IgG) should be present.
> - Positive serologic tests in a two-tier format include:
>   Standard two-tier test (STTT): a positive or equivocal first-tier screening assay, often an enzyme immunoassay [EIA] or immunofluorescence assay [IFA] for IgM, IgG, or a combination of immunoglobulins, followed by a concordant positive IgM or IgG immunoblot interpreted according to established criteria.
>   The most common laboratory assay for *B. burgdorferi* antibody detection is the modified two-tier test as the first-tier screen

Diagnostic Evaluation

The CDC-recommended approach to the Lyme Disease–Modified Two-Tiered Testing Algorithm (Fig. 16.5) complies with the laboratory criteria for Lyme Disease (*Borrelia burgdorferi*) 2022 Case Definition (https://ndc.services.cdc.gov/case-definitions/lyme-disease-2022).

According to the CDC laboratory evidence includes:

Confirmatory Laboratory Evidence

1. Isolation of *B. burgdorferi* sensu stricto or *B. mayonii* in culture, OR
2. Detection of *B. burgdorferi* sensu stricto or *B. mayonii* in a clinical specimen by a *B. burgdorferi* group-specific nucleic acid amplification test (NAAT) assay, OR
3. Detection of *B. burgdorferi* group-specific antigens by immunohistochemical (IHC) assay on biopsy or autopsy tissues, OR
4. Positive serologic tests[1] in a two-tier or equivalent format, including:
   a. STTT: a positive or equivocal first-tier screening assay, often an EIA or IFA for IgM, IgG, or a combination of immunoglobulins, followed by a concordant positive IgM[2] or IgG[3] immunoblot interpreted according to established criteria, OR
   b. MTTT: positive or equivocal first-tier screen, followed by a different, sequential positive or equivocal EIA in lieu of an immunoblot as a second-tier test[4].

Presumptive Laboratory Evidence

1. Positive IgG immunoblot[5], interpreted according to established criteria[3], without positive or equivocal first-tier screening assay.
   1. Currently, there are no serologic tests available for *B. mayonii* infection, but crossreactivity with *B. burgdorferi* testing may occur.
   2. IgM western blot is considered positive when at least two of the following three bands are present: 24 kDa (OspC)*, 39 kDa (BmpA), and 41 kDa (Fla). Low-incidence states should disregard IgM results for specimens collected >30 days after symptom onset. *Depending on the assay, OspC could be indicated by a band of 21, 22, 23, 24, or 25 kDa.
   3. IgG western blot is considered positive when at least 5 of the following 10 bands are present: 18 kDa, 24 kDa (OspC)*, 28 kDa, 30 kDa, 39 kDa (BmpA), 41 kDa (Fla), 45 kDa, 58 kDa (not GroEL), 66 kDa, and 93 kDa. *Depending on the assay, OspC could be indicated by a band of 21, 22, 23, 24, or 25 kDa.
   4. The MTTT algorithm should be performed using assays specifically cleared by the US Food and Drug Administration (FDA) for this purpose (Mead et al., 2019).
   5. While a single IgG western blot is adequate for surveillance purposes, a two-tier test is still recommended for clinical diagnosis.

Note that the culture of *B. burgdorferi* from specimens in Barbour-Stoenner-Kelly medium permits a definitive diagnosis. With a few exceptions, positive cultures have only been obtained early in the illness, primarily from biopsy samples of EMEM lesions, less often from plasma samples, and only occasionally from CSF samples in patients with meningitis. Later in the infection, polymerase chain reaction (PCR) testing is superior to culture for the detection of *B. burgdorferi* in joint fluid.

In the United States, the diagnosis is usually based on the recognition of the characteristic clinical findings, a history of exposure in an area in which the disease is endemic and, except in patients with EMEM, an antibody response to *B. burgdorferi*. In more than 50% of cases, physicians are comfortable making the diagnosis based on the symptoms and patient history. Testing becomes important when the telltale bull's eye rash or other symptoms characteristic of Lyme disease do not appear (Table 16.3).

Antibody Detection Methods

Assays for the detection of antibodies to *B. burgdorferi* are the most practical means for confirming infection. The CDC currently recommends a two-step process for testing blood for evidence of antibodies against the Lyme disease bacteria. Both steps can be done using the same blood sample. The first step uses an EIA or, rarely, an indirect IFA. If the first step is negative, no further

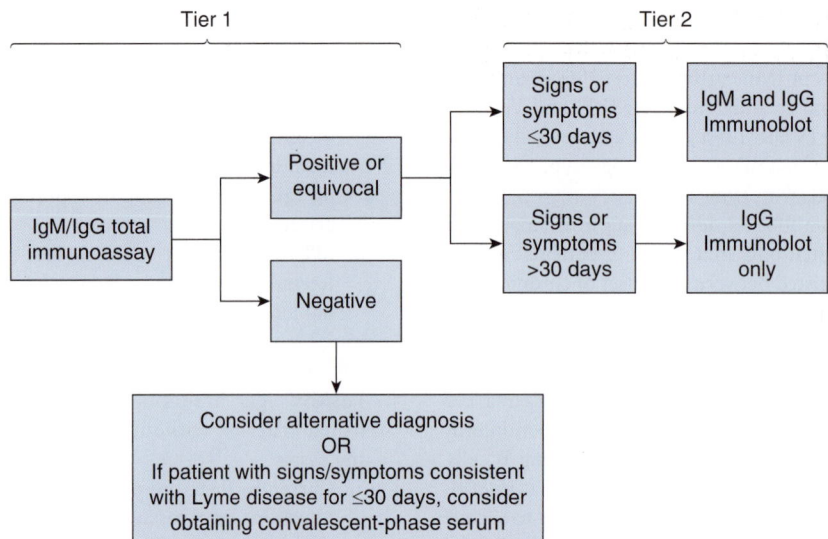

Fig. 16.5 Modified two-tiered testing algorithm (MTTT) for LD serology testing. As with STTT, a sensitive EIA is used as the first-tier test. If this is a negative and the patient has been symptomatic for >30 days, results are interpreted as negative, and no additional testing is indicated. If EIA screen is positive or equivocal, second-tier IgM- or IgG-specific EIA should be performed reflexively based on symptom duration. If second-tier EIA result is negative, the overall result is interpreted as negative. If second-tier EIA results is positive or ordered appropriately based on symptom duration, the overall results is interpreted as positive. If results of either first or second tier testing were negative and patient had symptoms for <30 days, collection of convalescent specimen should be considered. (Kenyon SM, Chan SL: A focused review on Lyme disease diagnostic testing: an update on serology algorithms, current ordering practices, and practical considerations for laboratory implementation of a new testing algorithm, Clin Biochem 117:4–9, 2023.)

testing of the specimen is recommended. If the first step is positive or indeterminate (sometimes called *equivocal*), the second step should be performed. The second step uses an immunoblot procedure, commonly a western blot test. Results are considered positive only if the EIA or IFA and the immunoblot test results are both positive.

The two steps of Lyme disease testing are designed to be done together. The CDC does not recommend skipping the first test and just doing the western blot test. Doing so will increase the frequency of false-positive results and may lead to misdiagnosis and improper treatment.

Enzyme-Linked Immunosorbent Assay

The ELISA is the standard test method; it is the most widely available and commonly performed test. The sensitivities of IFA and ELISA methods are usually low during the initial 3 weeks of infection; therefore negative results are common. The most serious disadvantages of current techniques are low sensitivity and lengthy processing time. In addition, false-positive reactions can result from crossreactivity in tests for Lyme disease. For example, tick-borne relapsing fever spirochetes, *Borrelia hermsii*, are closely related to *B. burgdorferi*. Antibodies to *B. hermsii*, an agent that coexists with the Lyme disease spirochete in portions of the western United States, strongly crossreact with *B. burgdorferi* in IFA staining and ELISA testing. Common antigens are shared among the *Borrelia* organisms and even with the treponemes. Serum from syphilitic patients reacts positively in assays for Lyme disease. Therefore serologic test results for antibodies to *B. burgdorferi* should be considered along with clinical data and epidemiologic information when a patient is evaluated for Lyme disease.

Western Blot Analysis

Western blot analysis can verify reactivity of antibody to major surface or flagellar proteins of *B. burgdorferi* (Fig. 16.6). The western blot test is helpful in determining borderline negative or weakly positive results obtained from other tests, but the values are not always reliable. This procedure is more definitive in later Lyme disease when multiple antibody bands specific for *B. burgdorferi* appear. Reported results from western blot tests for Lyme disease in its late phase indicate reactive bands for IgM levels. The 41-kDa bands are the earliest to appear but can crossreact with other spirochetes. The 18-, 23- to 25- (Osp C), 31- (Osp A), 34- (Osp B), 37-, 39-, 83-, and 93-kDa bands are the most specific but may appear later or may not appear at all.

Polymerase Chain Reaction

PCR testing can detect spirochetes in the synovial fluid around the joints or in other clinical samples. The PCR assay looks for the DNA of the organism. In the past, positive PCR assay results were taken as definitive evidence that a person had an infection, but it is possible to have antigens in the presence of nonviable organisms. This test amplifies small amounts of DNA that may remain, even when intact organisms are no longer present, an indication that the organism does or did exist. The PCR assay may miss the spirochete in the blood, allowing it to move into other tissues.

The PCR technique directly identifies the pathogen instead of measuring the host's immune response to it. It can detect DNA from as few as one to five organisms, even those that are nonviable. Different specific probes have been developed, and the PCR assay has been used to detect *B. burgdorferi* DNA in a variety of body fluids. The appeal of the PCR method lies in its rapid turnaround time (2 days vs. 6–8 weeks

TABLE 16.3	Methods of Lyme Disease Detection
Method	Comments
Isolation	Successful cultures have been obtained from ticks, skin biopsies, ear punches, CSF, blood, and synovial fluid; blood is not a reliable sample for culture. Isolation of spirochetes is highly variable
Histology	Lyme spirochetes are rarely observed in blood smears; examination of tissue is usually performed in addition to an immunologic assay, such as fluorescence microscopy. The process is labor intensive; the test is of limited value
Serology	FDA-approved IFA and EIA test systems
Molecular	DNA probe with patient DNA matched to *Borrelia* DNA

CSF, Cerebrospinal fluid; *EIA*, enzyme immunoassay; *FDA*, US Food and Drug Administration; *IFA*, indirect fluorescent antibody.

for culture) and avoidance of the difficulties associated with culture or immunohistochemistry. It has very high specificity, but the sensitivity may be as low as 70%. The PCR test may be useful in diagnosing early Lyme disease when the patient is still seronegative.

Cerebrospinal Fluid Analysis for Antibody Detection

Spinal taps are not routinely recommended; a negative tap does not rule out Lyme disease. Antibodies to *B. burgdorferi* can be detected in the CSF in only 20% of patients with late disease. Therefore spinal taps are performed only on patients with pronounced neurologic manifestations. The goal is to rule out other conditions and determine whether *B. burgdorferi* antigens are present. It is especially important to look for elevated protein levels and mononuclear cells, which would dictate the need for more aggressive therapy, and to check the opening CSF pressure, which can be elevated and contribute to headaches, especially in children.

Treatment and Prevention

Treatment decisions after a tick bite are influenced by the following factors:
- Probability that the tick is a carrier of *B. burgdorferi*
- Length of time the tick was attached
- Chance that disease will develop without the telltale rash
- Risk and severity of short- and long-term sequelae
- Accuracy of antibody tests
- Efficacy of antibiotics at various stages of the disease
- Risk of adverse reactions to the antibiotics
- Patient's level of anxiety
- Probability that the patient will comply with follow-up monitoring
- Cost of various strategies; presence of coinfections or immunodeficiencies; prior significant steroid use while infected; age and weight; gastrointestinal (GI) function; blood levels achieved

Antibiotics

It is unclear whether antimicrobial treatment after an *I. scapularis* tick bite will prevent Lyme disease. One study concluded that a single 200-mg dose of doxycycline given within 72 hours after an *I. scapularis* tick bite can prevent the development of Lyme disease.

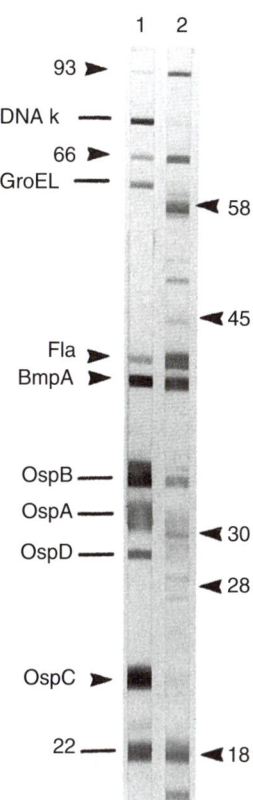

Fig. 16.6 Example of Immunoblot Calibration. *Lane 1*, Monoclonal antibodies defining selected antigens to *B. burgdorferi* B31 separated in a linear SDS-PAGE gel Marblot (MarDx Diagnostics, Carlsbad, California). *Lane 2*, Human serum (immunoglobulin G) reactive with the 10 antigens scored in recommended criteria for blot scoring; lines indicate other calibrating antibodies. Molecular masses are in kilodaltons. *Osp*, Outer surface protein. (From Detrocl B, Hamilton RG, Folds JD, editors: *Manual of molecular and clinical laboratory immunology*, ed 7, Washington, DC, 2006, American Society for Microbiology Press.)

Another study concluded that there is considerable impairment of health-related quality of life in patients with persistent symptoms despite previous antibiotic treatment for acute Lyme disease. In two clinical trials, however, treatment with intravenous (IV) and oral antibiotics for 90 days did not improve symptoms more than placebo.

Various types of antibiotics are in general use for *B. burgdorferi* treatment. The tetracyclines, including doxycycline and minocycline, are bacteriostatic unless given in high doses. If high blood levels are not attained, treatment failures in early and late disease are common because high doses of medication are difficult for patients to tolerate.

Penicillins are bactericidal. As would be expected in managing an infection with a gram-negative organism such as *B. burgdorferi*, amoxicillin has been shown to be more effective than oral penicillin V. Because of its short half-life and need for high levels, amoxicillin is usually administered along with probenecid. Because of variability, blood levels are usually measured. Third-generation agents are currently the most effective of the cephalosporins because of their very low blood level counts (0.06×10^9 for ceftriaxone), and they have been shown to be effective in penicillin and tetracycline failures. Cefuroxime axetil (Ceftin), a second-generation agent, is also effective against staphylococci and thus is useful in treating atypical EMEM, which may represent a mixed infection containing common skin pathogens in addition to *B. burgdorferi*. Because of this agent's GI side effects and high cost, cefuroxime is not used as a first-line drug.

Prevention

When hiking in the woods or mountains, picnicking at local parks, or walking in tall grass in shore areas, individuals should do the following:
- Check daily for ticks
- Wear light-colored clothing so that tick viewing is easier
- Tuck pants into socks

Note: In 2002 GlaxoSmithKline, the maker of the Lyme vaccine LYMErix, pulled the vaccine off the market. Pfizer, a pharmaceutical company, also ceased production of LYMEVAX. Currently, there is no human vaccine for the prevention of Lyme disease available and VLA15—Valneva's Lyme disease vaccine candidate—is the only Lyme disease vaccine candidate currently in advanced clinical development (Phase II).

Valneva's new vaccine works like LYMErix, but with two key differences. LYMErix only provided protection against one strain of *Borrelia* found in North America, while Valneva's vaccine protects against the six most common strains in the northern hemisphere, including those in Europe. Also, Valneva has eliminated the human protein-mimicking segment of the OspA protein and replaced it with a similar sequence from another strain as a precautionary measure.

HUMAN EHRLICHIOSIS

> **KEY CONCEPTS: Human Ehrlichiosis (Anaplasmosis)**
> - Human ehrlichiosis was first described in the United States in 1986. Tick-borne rickettsiae of the genus *Ehrlichia* cause human illness.
> - Ehrlichiosis is a general term for anaplasmosis and human monocytic ehrlichiosis (HME).
> - Anaplasmosis diagnosis is confirmed by seroconversion (fourfold rise in acute/convalescent sera titer) or a single serologic titer greater than 1:80 in patients with a history and symptoms. HME diagnosis is confirmed by seroconversion or a serologic titer greater than 1:128.

Human ehrlichiosis was first described in the United States in 1986; since then, reports of tick-borne illnesses have increased. Unlike Lyme disease, which tends to be indolent, RMSF and ehrlichiosis can be fatal and must be recognized and treated promptly.

Etiology

Tick-borne rickettsiae of the genus *Ehrlichia* have been recognized as a cause of human illness in the United States. *Ehrlichia* spp. belong to the same family as the organism that causes RMSF.

Ehrlichia chaffeensis, the etiologic agent of human monocytic ehrlichiosis (HME) in the United States, was demonstrated to cause disease in a patient from Arkansas with tick bites in 1987. Today, the CDC considers the identified agents for *Ehrlichia* disease to be *E. chaffeensis, E. ewingii*, and *E. muris eauclairensis*. The CDC identifies *Anaplasma phagocytophilum* as the agent associated with anaplasmosis (human granulocytic ehrlichiosis [HGE]). *E. ewingii* and *E. phagocytophilium* differ antigenically and genetically from *E. chaffeensis*.

Epidemiology

Although the prevalence rates are low, human ehrlichiosis is endemic in the United States. Some fatalities have been reported. Incidence rates increase with age and are higher in men than women. Human ehrlichiosis occurs most frequently in the southern Mid-Atlantic and south-central states during spring and summer.

The major vector for *E. chaffeensis* is the lone star tick, *Amblyomma americanum*. The principal reservoir for *E. chaffeensis* is the white-tailed deer, which hosts all stages of *A. americanum*. The primary tick vector for the agent of HGE is *I. scapularis* in the eastern United States and *I. pacificus* in California. *D. variabilis* represents a second tick vector in the United States. The major reservoir for infection may be the white-footed mouse in the eastern United States (Fig. 16.8). The onset of illness in spring and early summer for most cases parallels the time when *A. americanum* and *D. variabilis* ticks are most active.

Signs and Symptoms

Ehrlichiosis is a general term for HGE, now called **anaplasmosis**.

Severe and life-threatening illness is less common with anaplasmosis compared with other rickettsial diseases, such as RMSF or *E. chaffeensis* ehrlichiosis.

The syndrome of human ehrlichiosis is not typically recognized by physicians but should be considered in patients with a history of tick exposure and an acute febrile, flulike illness. Most patients are not suspected of having a rickettsial infection. Because ehrlichiosis can cause fatal infections in humans, early detection and treatment with tetracycline or chloramphenicol appear to offer the best chance for complete recovery.

Symptoms are nonspecific and include fever, chills, and headache. Fever and skin rashes are the most common physical findings. In children, fever and headache are universal. Myalgias, nausea, vomiting, and anorexia are also common.

Diagnostic Evaluation

Laboratory studies have indicated that the hematologic, hepatic, and central nervous systems are usually involved in human ehrlichiosis. Definitive diagnosis is based on inclusion in leukocytes (Fig. 16.7). *Ehrlichia* spp. undergo three developmental stages, as follows:
1. Elementary bodies enter a leukocyte by phagocytosis and multiply rapidly.
2. After 3 to 5 days, small numbers of tightly packed elementary bodies (initial bodies) are visible.
3. During the next 7 to 12 days, the initial bodies develop into morular, or mulberry, forms.

For anaplasmosis, direct observation of intraleukocytic morulae in Wright-Giemsa–stained peripheral blood or buffy coat smears is a rapid and inexpensive laboratory test. If clinical symptoms and the epidemiologic history are compatible with rickettsial infections, the following diagnostic tests should be used during the acute stage of illness and when antibiotic treatment is initiated:
- PCR test on skin biopsy of rash or eschar or an ethylenediaminetetraacetic acid (EDTA) whole-blood specimen
- Specific immunohistologic detection of rickettsiae in skin biopsy of rash or eschar

In anaplasmosis, the diagnosis is confirmed by seroconversion or by a single serologic titer higher than 1:80 in patients with a supporting history and clinical symptoms. Seroconversion is defined as a fourfold rise in the titer of paired acute and convalescent sera. Detection of IgM class antibody alone should not be interpreted as recent exposure to the rickettsial agents and should be confirmed by detection of IgG or, preferably, IgG seroconversion by parallel evaluation with a convalescent phase serum collected 4 to 6 weeks after onset of the illness.

In HME the diagnosis is confirmed by seroconversion or by a serologic titer higher than 1:128 in patients with a supporting history and clinical symptoms. Serum or CSF can be analyzed for IgM and IgG antibodies to *Ehrlichia* spp.

PCR-based detection of the *E. phagocytophila*–like agent of anaplasmosis represents the most sensitive and direct approach to diagnosis. PCR detection of *E. chaffeensis* includes the amplification of sequences with 16S ribosomal DNA (rDNA).

Treatment and Prevention

Patients with HME or anaplasmosis are treated with doxycycline. No guidelines have been established for long-term therapy. Prevention consists of reducing the risk of exposure to ticks (see earlier discussion of Lyme disease prevention).

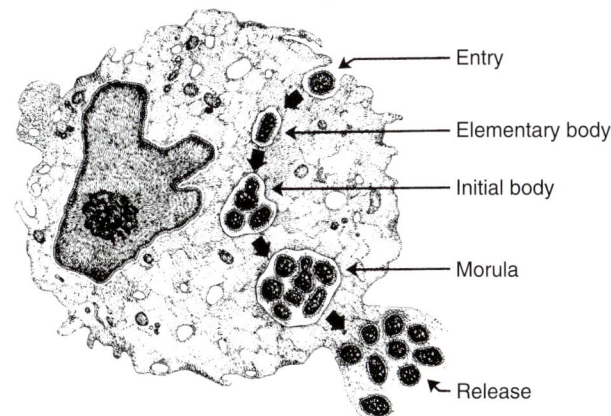

Fig. 16.7 Schematic representation of the growth cycle of ehrlichiae in an infected cell. *Elementary bodies* (EBs; individual ehrlichiae) enter the leukocyte by phagocytosis and multiply. After 3–5 days, small numbers of tightly packed EBs are observable and are called *initial bodies*. During the next 7–12 days, additional growth and replication occur, and the initial bodies develop into mature inclusions, which appear by light microscopy as mulberry (morular) forms. This *morula* is a hallmark of ehrlichial infection. (From McDade J: Ehrlichiosis: a disease of animals and human beings, *J Infect Dis.* 1990;161[4]:609–617.)

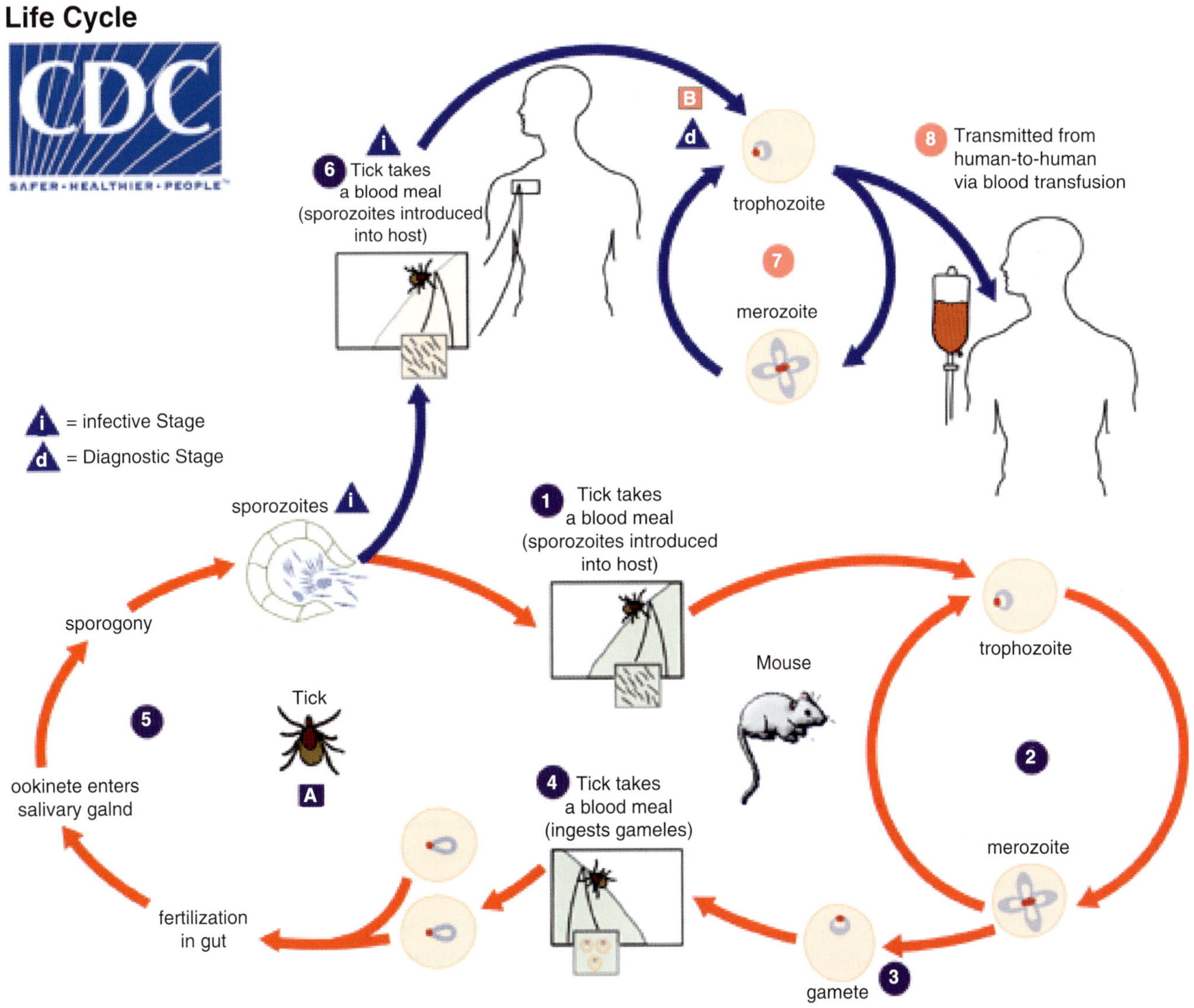

Fig. 16.8 Lifecycle of Ehrlichia. (From Centers for Disease Control and Prevention, http://www.dpd.cdc.gov/pddx.)

ROCKY MOUNTAIN SPOTTED FEVER

> **KEY CONCEPTS: Facts About Rocky Mountain Spotted Fever**
> - Since January 1, 2010, cases of Rocky Mountain spotted fever (RMSF) have been reported in a new category—spotted fever rickettsiosis (SFR).
> - The new category captures cases of RMSF, *R. parkeri* rickettsiosis, Pacific coast tick fever, and rickettsial pox.
> - The change reflects the inability to differentiate between spotted fever group *Rickettsia* species using commonly available serologic tests.

Etiology

Rocky Mountain spotted fever (RMSF) is the most severe rickettsiosis in the United States. RMSF is a rapidly progressive disease and without early administration of doxycycline can be fatal within days. This is a tick-borne disease caused by the bacterium *Rickettsia rickettsii*. This organism is a cause of potentially fatal human illness in North and South America, and is transmitted to human beings by the bite of infected tick species. In the United States, these include the American dog tick (*D. variabilis*), Rocky Mountain wood tick (*D. andersoni*), and brown dog tick (*Rhipicephalus sanguineus*).

Epidemiology

RMSF has been a nationally notifiable condition since the 1920s. In 2000, 495 cases of SFR were reported; in 2017 more than 6248 cases were reported. Cases dropped substantially in 2020 and 2021. This drop could be accounted for due to a combination of the new case definition and the COVID-19 pandemic. In the United States, SFR cases have been reported from each of the contiguous 48 states, except for Vermont and Maine. Five states (North Carolina, Oklahoma, Arkansas, Tennessee, and Missouri) account for over 60% of SFR cases. RMSF is also endemic throughout several countries in Central and South America, including Argentina, Brazil, Colombia, Costa Rica, Mexico, and Panama.

The CDC has noted that the geographic distribution of RMSF correlates with the type of tick found in that area. For example, the American dog tick is found in the eastern, central, and Pacific coastal United States; the Rocky Mountain wood tick resides in the western United States. In 2005 the brown dog tick, a vector of RMSF in Mexico, was implicated as a vector of this disease in a confined geographic area in Arizona. The cayenne tick (*Amblyomma cajennense*) is a common vector for RMSF in Central and South America, and its range extends into the United States in Texas.

Although cases of SFR can occur during any month of the year, most cases reported illness in June and July. This period coincides with the season when adult *Dermacentor* ticks are most active. Seasonal trends may vary, depending on the area of the country and tick species involved. In Arizona, the majority of SFR cases occur year-round, with peak months of illness onset in April through October. Almost all of the cases occurred within communities with large numbers of free-roaming dogs.

Signs and Symptoms

The first symptoms of RMSF typically begin 2 to 14 days after the bite of an infected tick. A tick bite is usually painless, and about 50% of those who develop RMSF do not remember being bitten. The disease typically begins as a sudden onset of fever and headache. Most patients with RMSF (90%) have some type of rash during the course of the illness. The number and combination of symptoms vary greatly from person to person. Symptoms can include fever, rash (occurs 2–5 days after fever; may be absent in some cases), headache, nausea, and vomiting.

Diagnostic Evaluation

During RMSF infection, a patient's immune system develops antibodies to *R. rickettsii*, with detectable antibody titers usually observed within 7 to 10 days of illness onset. It is important to note that antibodies are not detectable in the first week of illness in 85% of patients; a negative test during this period does not rule out RMSF as a cause of illness. As of January 1, 2020, the new case definition was updated. The key changes included raising the cutoff IFA IgG titer to >/− 1:128 from >/− 1:64 and elimination of IFA, IgM, ELISA, and latex agglutination testing methods. It also specified that specimen collection for probable cases be within 60 days of illness onset.

Treatment and Prevention

The progression of the disease varies greatly. Patients who are treated early may recover quickly on outpatient medication, whereas those who experience a more severe course may require IV antibiotics, prolonged hospitalization, or intensive care.

Doxycycline is the first-line treatment for adults and children of all ages and is most effective if started before the fifth day of symptoms. Standard duration of treatment is 7 to 14 days.

BABESIOSIS

> **KEY CONCEPTS: Babesiosis**
> - Babesiosis is a rare, severe, possibly fatal tick-borne disease caused by *Babesia*, which infects red blood cells (RBCs).
> - A less common way of acquiring the disease is by receiving an RBC transfusion from a blood donor who has a *Babesia* infection but does not have any symptoms.
> - No tests have been licensed yet for screening blood donors for *Babesia* spp.
> - Rare cases of congenital transmission (from an infected mother to her baby during pregnancy or delivery) have been reported.
> - Two rapid screening methods are used for the identification of *Babesia* organisms. The gold standard is the visualization of the intraerythrocytic organisms in thick or thin blood films.

Since January 2011, cases of babesiosis from across the United States have been formally reported to the CDC. Becoming nationally notifiable is an important step toward monitoring disease occurrence. Babesiosis is a preventable but sometimes life-threatening, tick-borne parasitic disease.

Etiology

Babesiosis is a rare, severe, and sometimes fatal tick-borne disease caused by various types of *Babesia*, a microscopic parasite that infects red blood cells (RBCs) (Fig. 16.9). The causative organism of babesiosis was first described by Babes in 1888. In New England and the eastern United States, the disease is caused by *Babesia microti*; in California, it is caused by *Babesia equi*. In Europe, the disease is caused by *Babesia divergens* and *Babesia bovis*. *Babesia canis* has been found to be responsible for several cases in Mexico and France.

Epidemiology

Babesia microti is transmitted by the tick *I. scapularis* in the northeastern United States. The larvae of the tick feed mainly on the white-footed mouse (*Peromyscus leucopus*). When larvae develop into nymphs and adults, they feed on the white-tailed deer (*Odocoileus virginianus*), but they may also choose a human host.

Babesiosis is most common in older individuals (in 2017, the median age of patients was 61 years), splenectomized patients, and immunocompromised patients.

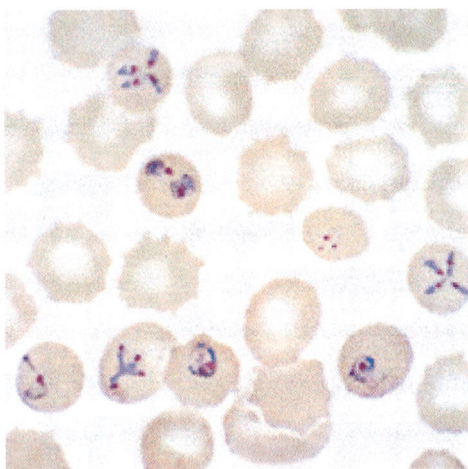

Fig. 16.9 *Babesia* in red blood cells (1000× magnification). (From Tille P: *Bailey & Scott's diagnostic microbiology,* ed 14, St. Louis, 2017, Elsevier.)

According to the CDC, for 2020, CDC received reports for a total of 1827 cases of babesiosis in the US, a 24% decrease from the total of 2418 cases for 2019
- Babesiosis was a reportable disease in 40 states and the District of Columbia (DC) in 2020; 24 (60%) of the 40 states notified CDC of at least 1 case
- Most of the reported cases (98%) were in residents of 10 states where tickborne transmission of *Babesia* parasites is well established (the Northeast and upper Midwest: Connecticut, Maine, Massachusetts, Minnesota, New Hampshire, New Jersey, New York, Rhode Island, Vermont, and Wisconsin)

Signs and Symptoms

The incubation period is approximately 7 to 21 days. The clinical presentation is variable, ranging from asymptomatic to rapidly progressive and sometimes fatal. Infections caused by *Babesia divergens* tend to be more severe (commonly fatal if not appropriately treated) than those caused by *Babesia microti* (clinical recovery usually occurs).

The disease can cause fever, fatigue, and hemolytic anemia lasting several days to several months. It may take from 1 to 8 weeks, sometimes longer, for symptoms to appear. The disease course is characterized by high fever, massive hemolysis, hemoglobinemia, and hemoglobinuria.

Diagnostic Evaluation

In symptomatic people, babesiosis usually is diagnosed by examining blood specimens under a microscope and observing *Babesia* parasites inside RBCs. Multiple smears may need to be examined to detect low levels of parasites. Two rapid screening methods are used for the identification of *Babesia* organisms. The gold standard for their identification is the visualization of the intraerythrocytic organisms in thick or thin blood films. Sometimes it is hard to distinguish *Babesia* spp. from *Plasmodium falciparum* (malaria) by blood smear examination. Also, some *Babesia* spp. (e.g., *B. microti*, *B. duncani*) appear identical; they cannot be distinguished from each other by microscopy.

Acute and convalescent antibody titers may be useful for diagnosis. A titer higher than 1:256 is considered diagnostic of acute infection. Only IgG antibody determinations are performed. PCR amplification can be used for diagnosis.

Molecular diagnosis can also be useful. In some infections with intraerythrocytic parasites, the morphologic characteristics observed on microscopic examination of blood smears do not allow an unambiguous differentiation between *Babesia* and *Plasmodium* organisms. In these cases, the diagnosis can be derived from molecular techniques such as PCR testing using the appropriate primers and single-step or the more sensitive nested PCR technique. In addition, molecular approaches are valuable for the investigation of new *Babesia* variants (or species) observed in recent human infections in the United States and Europe.

No *Babesia* test approved by the FDA is currently available for screening prospective blood donors, who may feel healthy despite being infected. Some manufacturers are working with investigators at blood centers to develop FDA-approved tests for *Babesia* for donor screening.

Treatment and Prevention

Standardized treatments for babesiosis have not been developed. However, some drugs used for the treatment of malaria have been found to be effective in some patients with babesiosis.

Antimicrobial therapy is recommended for splenectomized or immunodeficient patients, older patients, and patients with severe infections. The usual regimen consists of a combination of clindamycin and oral quinine. An alternate treatment option is oral azithromycin and oral atovaquone. Exchange transfusion has been effective for patients with a high level of parasites (>10%), severe disease, or massive hemolysis.

Prevention requires vigilance when in tick-infested areas (see earlier discussion of Lyme disease prevention).

MOSQUITO VECTOR DISEASES

> **KEY CONCEPTS: Malaria**
> - Malaria is caused by the genus *Plasmodium*: *P. falciparum, P. vivax, P. malariae, P. ovale,* and *P. knowlesi.*
> - According to the CDC, every year millions of US residents travel to countries where malaria is endemic. Travelers to sub-Saharan Africa have the greatest risk of both contracting malaria and dying from their infection.
> - *Anopheles* mosquitoes capable of transmitting malaria ("vectors") exist in the United States. There is a constant risk that malaria transmission can resume in the United States.
> - Severe manifestations of malaria are mostly restricted to young children, but it is also a major factor of morbidity in pregnancy-associated malaria.
> - The presence of malarial parasites can be detected by microscopy, which continues to be the gold standard.
> - Three main groups of antigens detected by commercially available rapid diagnostic tests (RDTs) are histidine-rich protein II (HPR-II), which is specific to *P. falciparum* antigen, parasite-specific *Plasmodium* lactate dehydrogenase (pLDH) and aldolase.
> - Prevention strategies include several drugs and a newly approved vaccine for children in Africa.

MALARIA

Etiology

Malaria is caused by any of five species of protozoan parasite of the genus *Plasmodium*:
- *P. falciparum*
- *P. vivax*
- *P. malariae*
- *P. ovale*
- *P. knowlesi*

The modern tendency is to refer to the various forms of malaria by the name of the causative parasitic agent. Malaria is a serious and potentially fatal disease transmitted through the bite of an infective female anopheline mosquito. Although rare, malaria can also be transmitted congenitally from mother to fetus or to the neonate at birth, through blood transfusion or organ transplantation, or through unsafe needle-sharing practices.

Global Malaria Distribution and Statistics

In 2020, an estimated 241 million cases of malaria occurred worldwide and 627,000 people died, mostly children in sub-Saharan Africa. According to the CDC every year, millions of US residents travel to countries where malaria is endemic. Travelers to sub-Saharan Africa have the greatest risk of both contracting malaria and dying from their infection.

Before the COVID-19 pandemic, approximately 2000 cases of mostly travel-related malaria were diagnosed in the United States each year; approximately 300 people experienced severe disease (mostly *P. falciparum*), and 5 to 10 people with malaria died yearly. Most imported cases of malaria in the United States are diagnosed during summer and early fall.

In 2023, the CDC expects summer international travel among US residents will be increasing to pre-COVID-19 pandemic levels. This may contribute to an increased number of cases of malaria in the United States.

Characteristics of *Plasmodium* Species

Plasmodium falciparum affects more than 500 million people each year. It is almost entirely confined to the tropics and subtropics. Fortunately, most cases of malarial anemia have a mild clinical outcome, but more than 1 to 2 million fatalities occur each year.

The current geographic distribution of group O individuals suggests a survival advantage if infected with *P. falciparum* to persons of group O in malaria-endemic regions. In addition, individuals with sickle cell trait are protected predominantly from *P. falciparum*.

Plasmodium vivax is a predominant species of malaria worldwide. *P. vivax* and *P. falciparum* are responsible for 80% to 95% of all malaria cases worldwide.

Plasmodium malariae occurs primarily in subtropical and temperate areas where other species of malaria are found but is seen less frequently than *P. vivax* or *P. falciparum*.

Plasmodium ovale is rather widely distributed in tropical Africa and replaces *P. vivax* in frequency on the West African coast. It has also been reported in South America and Asia.

Plasmodium knowlesi has assumed greater importance in recent years. It has been identified as the fifth human malaria species that can lead to fatal infections in endemic areas. Transmissions and infections with *P. knowlesi* are mainly observed in Macaque monkeys. *P. knowlesi* malaria occurs mainly on the island of Borneo but has been reported in travelers to South-East Asian countries such as Thailand between 2006 and 2013; only six cases have been identified in travelers to Southeast Asia with no evidence of man-to-man transmission of *P. knowlesi*. Routine parasitological diagnostics are associated with difficulties in determination of the species based only on microscopic examination. Recently, the molecular technique PCR has been increasingly used for diagnosis.

Epidemiology (United States)

Although malaria was eradicated in the United States in the early 1950s, in 2003, 10 patients in the United States without a travel history were diagnosed with malaria. One of the 10 infected patients had a probable transfusion-related source, eight cases were acquired as a result of local mosquito-borne transmission, and one had an unidentified source.

Of the seven deaths in 2003 attributed to malaria, five were caused by *P. falciparum* and a species was not identified in the other two cases.

On July 7, 2023 the first seven known cases of malaria in the United States were reported since 2003. None of the new infections were linked to international travel and appear to have been spread domestically by mosquitoes carrying the parasite that causes the disease. According to the CDC, six of the current cases were acquired in Florida and one case was in Texas. These first seven cases in 2023 were caused by *P. vivax* and responded to immediate treatment.

Risk of Malaria

Anopheles mosquitoes capable of transmitting malaria ("vectors") exist in the United States. Thus there is a constant risk that malaria transmission can resume in the United States. Several factors are making the United States increasingly vulnerable to malaria infection overall, regardless of whether they are locally acquired or imported infections. Climate change is causing a shift in weather patterns that can worsen malaria conditions.

Global warming could lead to higher mosquito migration and abundance in areas of the United States that were previously uninhabitable by *Anopheles* mosquitoes. According to the CDC, it is not clear that the recently reported 2023 cases are due to changes in climate, even though shifting weather conditions do influence the distribution of diseases like malaria.

The Disease Phase of Malaria in Humans

The life cycle of four *Plasmodium* species (Fig. 16.10) occurs in both humans and the mosquito. The disease phase in humans begins when sporozoites injected into the bloodstream of a human by an infected mosquito leave the circulatory system within 40 minutes and invade the liver cells of the human host. In the cells of the liver, all species undergo an asexual multiplication phase. This multiplication produces thousands of tiny merozoites in each infected cell. Subsequent rupture of the infected liver cells releases the merozoites into the circulation.

In the circulation, an asexual cycle takes place within the erythrocytes. This process, referred to as schizogony, results in the formation of 4 to 36 new parasites in each infected erythrocyte within 48 to 72 hours. At the end of this schizogonic cycle, the infected erythrocytes rupture, liberating merozoites, which in turn infect new erythrocytes.

During the intraerythrocytic phase of the life cycle, malaria parasites hydrolyze host proteins. Hemoglobin is processed into individual amino acids, which are used for parasite protein synthesis. Erythrocyte cytoskeletal proteins are cleaved during erythrocyte invasion and rupture. A number of plasmodial protease enzymes (cysteine, aspartic, and metalloproteases and a neutral aminopeptidase) appear to be responsible for key cleavages of host proteins. Cysteine and aspartic proteases hydrolyze hemoglobin and cleave host cytoskeletal proteins. These and additional protease enzymes likely cleave the cytoskeleton to mediate erythrocyte rupture and invasion.

Usually, after a patient has become clinically ill, gametocytes appear in circulating erythrocytes. Gametocytes circulate in the blood for some time and if ingested by an appropriate species of mosquito undergo the sexual cycle, gametogony, which develops into sporogony in the mosquito.

Proteins exported from *P. falciparum* parasites into RBCs interact with the membrane skeleton and contribute to the pathogenesis of malaria. These proteins increase RBC membrane rigidity, decrease deformability, and increase adhesiveness, which produces intravascular sequestration of infected RBCs.

CHAPTER 16 Vector-Borne Diseases

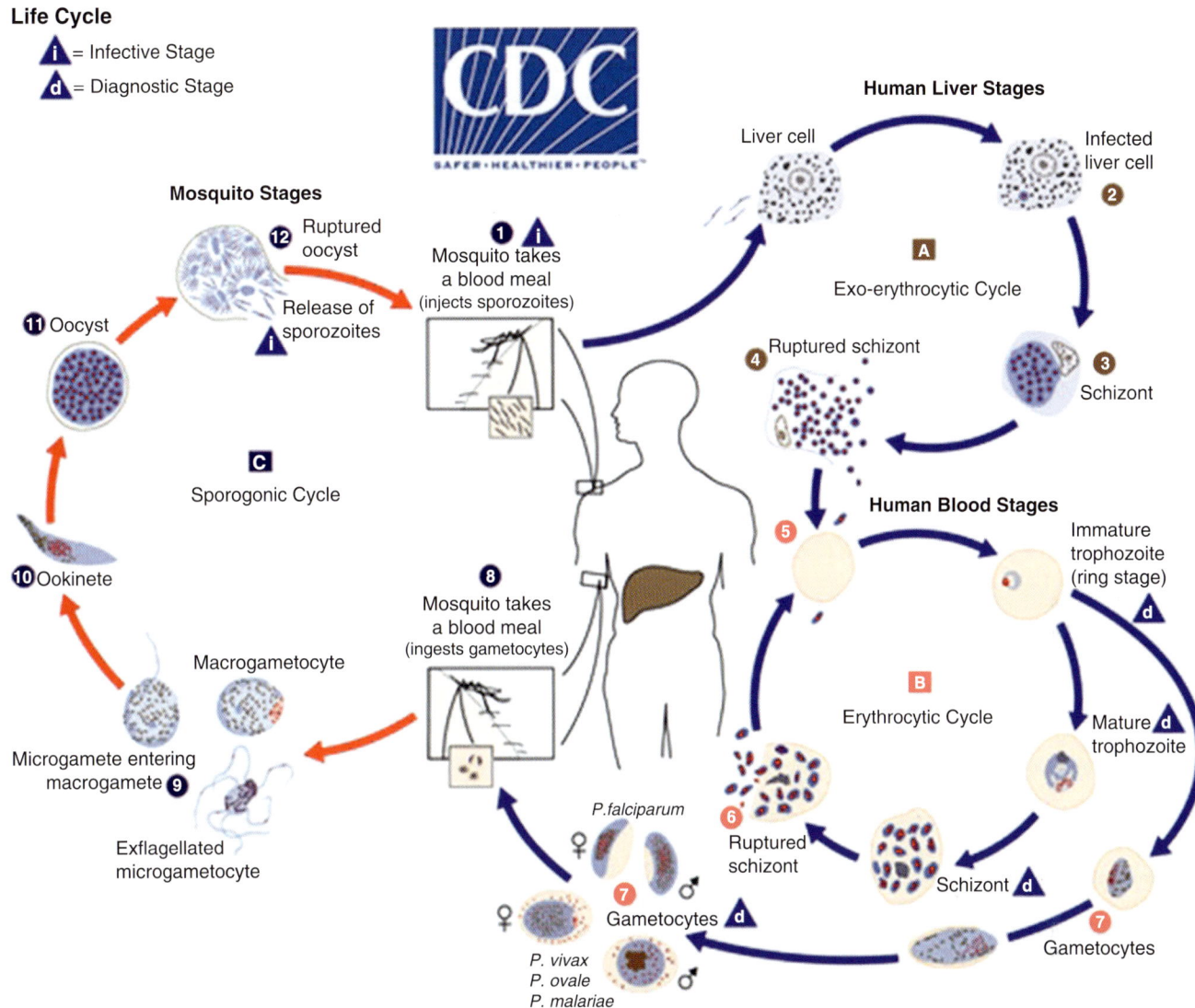

Fig. 16.10 Lifecycle of *Plasmodium* Species. The malaria parasite life cycle involves two hosts. During a blood meal, a malaria-infected female *Anopheles* mosquito inoculates sporozoites into the human host ❶ Sporozoites infect liver cells ❷ and mature into schizonts ❸, which rupture and release merozoites ❹. (Of note, in *P. vivax* and *P. ovale* a dormant stage [hypnozoites] can persist in the liver [if untreated] and cause relapses by invading the bloodstream weeks, or even years later.) After this initial replication in the liver (exo-erythrocytic schizogony Ⓐ), the parasites undergo asexual multiplication in the erythrocytes (erythrocytic schizogony Ⓑ). Merozoites infect red blood cells ❺. The ring stage trophozoites mature into schizonts, which rupture releasing merozoites ❻. Some parasites differentiate into sexual erythrocytic stages (gametocytes) ❼. Blood-stage parasites are responsible for the clinical manifestations of the disease. The gametocytes, male (microgametocytes) and female (macrogametocytes) are ingested by an *Anopheles* mosquito during a blood meal ❽. The parasites' multiplication in the mosquito is known as the sporogonic cycle Ⓒ. While in the mosquito's stomach, the microgametes penetrate the macrogametes generating zygotes ❾. The zygotes in turn become motile and elongated (ookinetes), ❿ which invade the midgut wall of the mosquito where they develop into oocysts ⓫. The oocysts grow, rupture, and release sporozoites ⓬, which make their way to the mosquito's salivary glands. Inoculation of the sporozoites ❶ into a new human host perpetuates the malaria life cycle. (From Centers for Disease Control and Prevention, Lifecycle of *Plasmodium* spp. https://www.dpd.cdc.gov/pddx/.)

Signs and Symptoms

Severe manifestations of malaria are mostly restricted to young children, but it is also a major factor of morbidity in pregnancy-associated malaria. On a global basis, infection of RBCs by protozoa is a common cause of hemolytic anemia.

Malaria should be considered a potential medical emergency and should be treated accordingly. Delay in diagnosis and treatment is a leading cause of death in malaria patients in the United States. Malaria can be suspected based on the patient's travel history, symptoms, and the physical findings at examination. However, for a definitive diagnosis to be made, laboratory tests must verify the presence of malaria parasites or their immunologic components.

There are usually no symptoms of malaria until several continuous life cycles have been completed. The simultaneous rupturing of erythrocytes liberates toxic products that characteristically produce chills followed by a fever in a few hours. A patient's temperature may rise to 104°F to 105°F. The symptoms last from 4 to 6 hours and recur at regular intervals, depending on the species of malaria.

Diagnostic Laboratory Evaluation
Microscopic Examination

The presence of malarial parasites can be detected by microscopy (Fig. 16.11), which continues to be the gold standard. The diagnosis of malaria is based on the demonstration of the parasite in a thick blood smear (refer to Turgeon ML: Clinical hematology, ed. 7. Burlington, MA: Jones & Bartlett; 2024 for the manual procedure). Many of the general morphological features are shared by all of the malarial species, but differences are usually sought to establish the species producing the illness.

All the stages seen in thin films may also be found in thick-film preparations, but the parasites appear somewhat distorted. Young trophozoites may be seen but *cannot* be distinguished from similar stages of *P. ovale* or *P. falciparum*. Gametocytes of *P. vivax*, *P. ovale*, and *P. malariae* are very similar in appearance. Schizogony does not usually take place in peripheral blood in *P. falciparum*. Young trophozoites and gametocytes are generally the only stages seen on the peripheral blood smear.

Molecular Testing

The three main groups of antigens detected by commercially available RDTs are:

1. HPR-II, which is specific to *P. falciparum* antigen. The HRP-II antigen is synthesized and released by trophozoites and immature gametocyte stages, and persists in a patient's circulating blood for up to 2 weeks following chemotherapy and the appearance of the parasite in the blood. Tests for HPR-II have low sensitivity for a concentration of <100 parasites/μL but HPR-II has a high specificity of >90%.
2. Parasite-specific pLDH is produced by asexual and sexual stages (gametocytes) of malaria parasites. pLDH can distinguish *P. falciparum* from non-*falciparum* species but cannot distinguish *P. vivax*, *P. malariae*, and *P. ovale* from each other. Tests that detect pLDH can detect a persistent positive result following chemotherapy, like the HRP-II assay.
3. Aldolase is a pan-malarial antigen.

PCR testing. Molecular testing based on a hypervariable region with the 18s rRNA gene includes PCR kits from www.clonit.it. The Clonit system malaria panel allows for the detection of the DNA target (18s rRNA gene) through a genomic amplification reaction and the identification of the different species of malaria—*P. falciparum*, *P. ovale*, *P. malariae*, and *P. vivax*. Analysis of the results is obtained using a real-time PCR analyzer (thermal cycler integrated with a system for fluorescence detection and a dedicated software).

Rapid testing. Laboratories may now use a rapid testing device, or RDT, to quickly screen for the presence of malaria. On June 13, 2007, the FDA approved the first and only RDT device for use in the United States, the BinaxNOW™ Malaria RDT (Figs. 16.12 and 16.13). The BinaxNOW™ Malaria RDT is an *in vitro* lateral flow immunochromatographic antigen-detection assay for the qualitative detection of *Plasmodium* antigens circulating in the blood of a patient with the signs and symptoms of malarial infection.

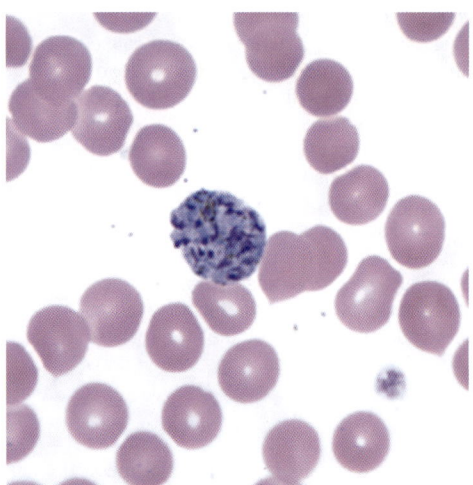

Fig. 16.11 Malaria Microscopic Examination. Blood smear from a patient with malaria; microscopic examination shows *Plasmodium falciparum* parasites. (From Centers for Disease Control and Prevention. https://www.CDC.gov.)

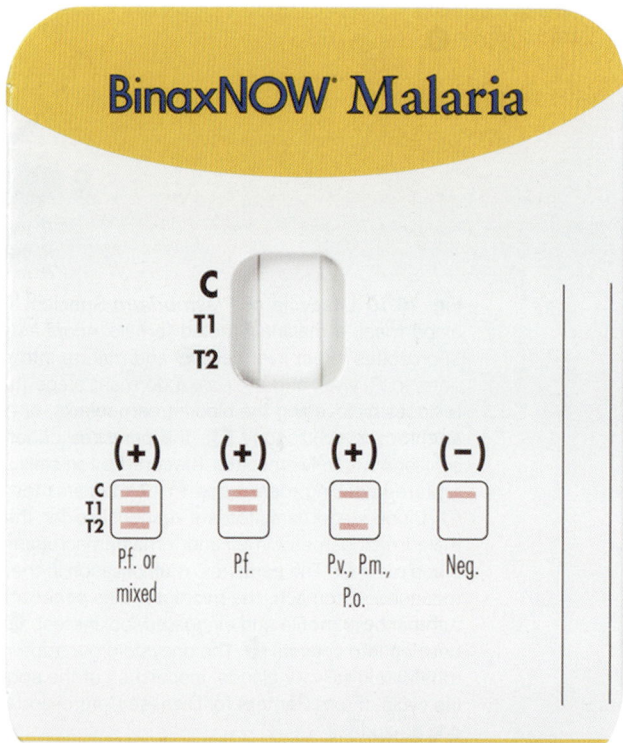

Fig. 16.12 BinaxNOW testing targets the histidine-rich protein II (HRP-II) antigen specific to *Plasmodium falciparum* (*P.f.*) and a pan-malarial antigen common to all four malaria species capable of infecting humans: *P. falciparum*, *P. vivax* (*P.v.*), *P. ovale* (*P.o.*), and *P. malariae* (*P.m.*). This picture demonstrates a positive test for *Plasmodium falciparum*. (Reproduced with permission of Abbott, © 2024. All rights reserved.)

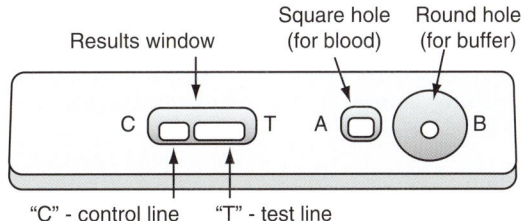

Inside the cassette is a strip made of filter paper and nitrocellulose. Typically, a drop of blood is added to the Rapid Diagnostic Test (RDT) through one hole (A; sample well), and then a number of drops of buffer usually through another hole (B; buffer well). Buffer carries the blood along the length of the RDT.

Mode of action of common malaria RDT format

1. The first step of the test procedure involves mixing the patient's blood with a lysing agent in a test strip or well. This ruptures the red blood cells, releasing more parasite protein.

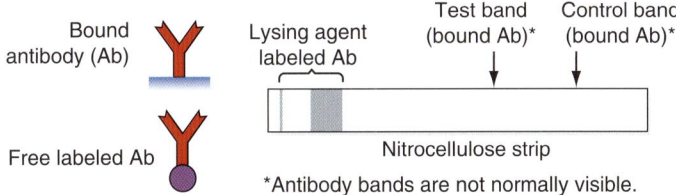

2. Dye-labeled antibody, specific for target antigen, is present on the lower end of nitrocellulose strip or in a plastic well provided with the strip. Antibody, also specific for the target antigen, is bound to the strip in a thin (test) line, and either antibody specific for the labeled antibody, or antigen, is bound at the control line.

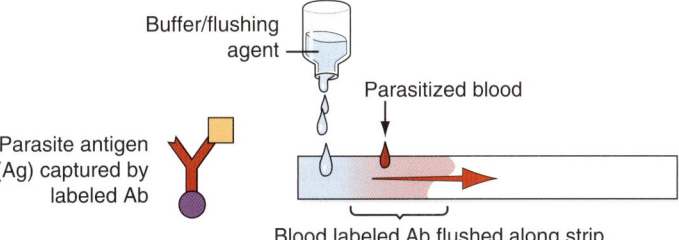

3. Blood and buffer, which have been placed on strip or in the well, are mixed with labeled antibody and are drawn up the strip across the lines of bound antibody.

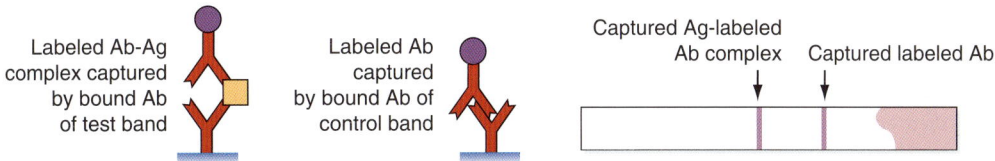

4. If antigen is present, some labeled antibody-antigen complex will be trapped and accumulate on the test line. Excess-labeled antibody is trapped and accumulates on the control line. A visible line indicates that labeled antibody has traversed the full length of the strip, past the test line, and that at least some free antibody remains conjugated to the eye, and that some of the capturing properties of the antibodies remain intact.

5. The intensity of the test band will vary with the amount of antigen present, at least at low parasite densities (antigen concentration), as this will determine the amount of dye particles, which will accumulate on the line. The control band intensity may decrease at higher parasite densities, as much of the labeled antibody will have been captured by the test band before reaching the control.

Fig. 16.13 Malaria Rapid Device Testing (RDT). (From World Health Organization. https://www.who.int/malaria/areas/diagnosis/rapid-diagnostic-tests/en/. Accessed December 21, 2017.)

The procedure is intended to aid in the rapid diagnosis of human malaria infections and in the differential diagnosis of *P. falciparum* infections from other less virulent malarial infections. The Binax test provides results in 15 minutes. It is approved for use by hospital or commercial laboratories, but not for use by individual clinicians or by patients themselves.

The test rapidly targets HRP-II and aldolase. HRP-II antigen is specific to *P. falciparum* and a pan-malarial antigen common to malaria species capable of infecting humans—*P. falciparum*, *P. vivax*, *P. ovale*, and *P. malariae*.

The Binax assay contains both the HRP-II (for *P. falciparum*) and aldolase, which is a pan-malarial antigen. It cannot separate the non-*falciparum* species from each other. This RDT is intended to aid in the rapid diagnosis of human malaria infections and in the differential diagnosis of *P. falciparum* infections from other, less virulent malarial infections.

Antimalaria antibody RDTs exist and can be used in applications such as screening donated blood; however, malaria RDTs commonly detect specific antigens produced by malaria parasites in the blood of infected patients.

Negative results must be confirmed by thin/thick smear microscopy. The use of the RDT does not eliminate the need for malaria microscopy. The RDT may not be able to detect some infections with lower numbers of malaria parasites circulating in the patient's bloodstream. Patients with negative RDT results can be followed up by microscopy, where available, to confirm the result.

Patients with positive RDT results who are not responding to initial antimalarial treatment should be evaluated for other causes of their symptoms to determine whether the treatment was appropriate and to examine parasites in the blood by microscopy to determine the possibility of drug resistance.

LAMP Assay

The CDC reported that in the summer of 2023, CDC experts and interns developed a test, known as the colorimetric loop mediated isothermal amplification (LAMP) assay, also known as the CLASS assay, for quickly detecting *Anopheles stephensi* mosquito, an invasive mosquito that can carry malaria. The new CLASS assay a portable, can be used in the field and other settings with limited resources, and can detect *A. stephensi* in as little as 30 minutes, removing major barriers.

Treatment and Prevention

There are approximately 300 cases of severe malaria in the United States each year, most of them acquired from travel to malaria-endemic countries. Severe malaria should be treated with IV antimalarial medications.

IV artesunate is the first-line drug for the treatment of severe malaria in the United States. Artesunate for Injection™, manufactured by Amivas, is approved by the FDA and is commercially available in the United States.

Prevention strategies include the following FDA-approved drugs:
- Attovaquone/proguanil (Malarone). Cannot be used in areas where chloroquine- or mefloquine-resistant *Plasmodium* species are present.
- Cloroquine. Cannot be used in areas where chloroquine- or mefloquine-resistant *Plasmodium* species are present.
- Deoxycycline.
- Mefloquine. Cannot be used in areas where mefloquine-resistant *Plasmodium* species are present.
- Primaquine. One of the most effective medications for preventing *P. vivax*. It is a good choice for travel to locations with >90% *P. vivax* present.
- Tafenoquine (Arakoda™). One of the most effective drugs for the prevention of *P. vivax* and also to prevent *P. falciparum* infection.

In 2021, one vaccine, RTS, S/AS01 AS01 (Mosquirix; GlaxoSmithKline) malaria vaccine was approved for children living in sub-Saharan Africa and other regions with moderate-to-high levels of *P. falciparum* malaria transmission. See Chapter 27 for content presentation on this new vaccine.

CHIKUNGUNYA DISEASE

> **KEY CONCEPTS: Chikungunya Virus**
> - **Chikungunya** virus is transmitted to people through mosquito bites, and most often spread to people by *Aedes aegypti* and *Aedes albopictus* mosquitoes. These are the same mosquitoes that transmit dengue virus (DENV).
> - Chikungunya virus disease became a nationally notifiable condition in 2015.
> - As of October 3, 2019, cases of chikungunya virus disease with illness onset in 2019 had been reported by 23 US states.
> - All cases in 2019 occurred in travelers returning from affected areas.
>
> A total of two chikungunya virus disease cases with illness onset in 2019 have been reported to ArboNET from US territories. To date, two locally acquired cases have been reported from Puerto Rico.

Etiology

Chikungunya virus is transmitted to people through mosquito bites. The virus is most often spread to people by *A. aegypti* and *A. albopictus* mosquitoes. These are the same mosquitoes that transmit DENV.

Epidemiology

Outbreaks of chikungunya infection have occurred in Africa, Asia, Europe, and the Indian and Pacific Oceans. Chikungunya virus disease became a nationally notifiable condition in 2015. Cases are reported to the CDC by state and local health departments using standard case definitions. A total of 69 chikungunya virus disease cases with illness onset in 2019 have been reported from 23 US states, with all reported cases occurring in travelers returning from affected areas. No locally transmitted cases have been reported from US states. A total of two chikungunya virus disease cases with illness onset in 2019 have been reported from US territories. To date, two locally acquired cases have been reported from Puerto Rico.

Signs and Symptoms

Symptoms usually begin 3 to 7 days after a person is bitten by an infected mosquito. The most common symptoms of chikungunya virus infection are fever and joint pain. Other symptoms may include headache, muscle pain, joint swelling, or rash. The symptoms are similar to those of dengue.

Diagnostic Evaluation

Chikungunya IgM and IgG antibody testing can be performed by reference laboratories. The detection method is a semiquantitative ELISA assay. In addition to testing of an acute serum specimen, parallel testing

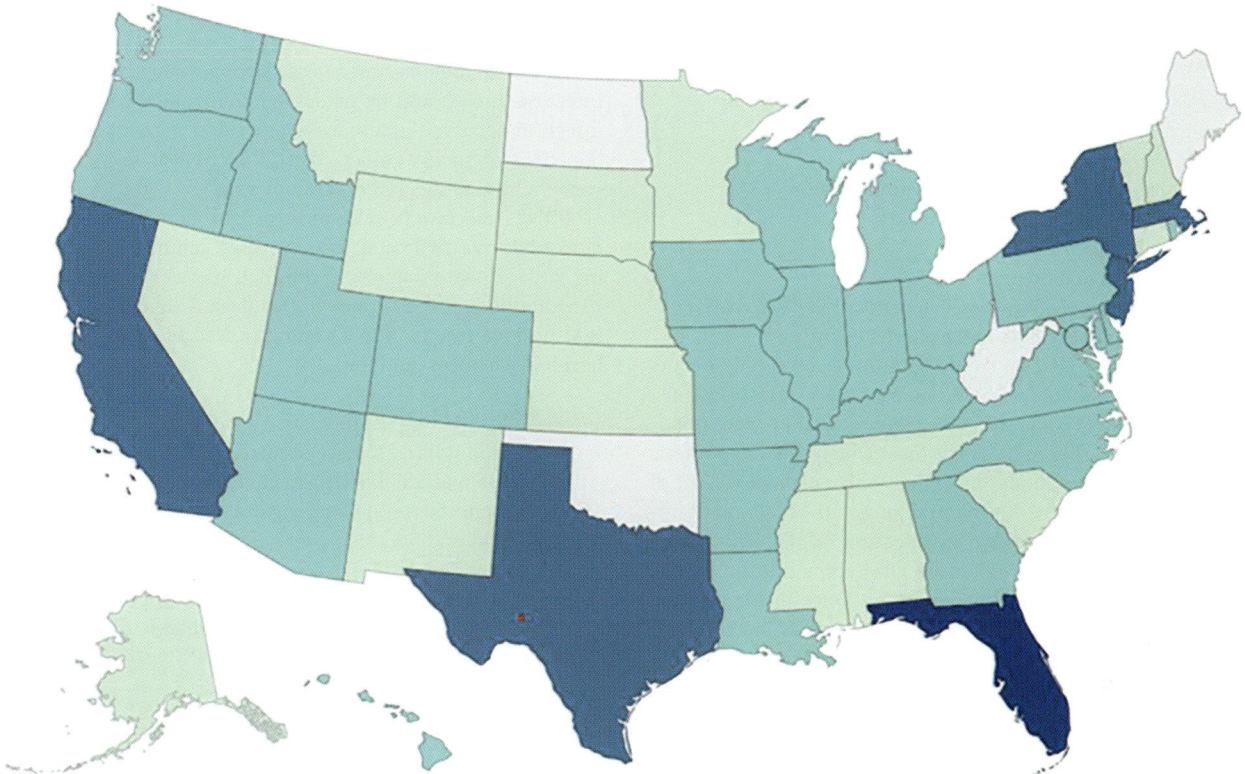

Fig. 16.14 States and territories reporting dengue cases—United States, 2024. (From Centers for Disease Control and Prevention, https://www.cdc.gov/ncidod/dvbid/westnile/Mapsactivity/surv&control11MapsAny-byState.htm.)

of an acute specimen and a convalescent specimen obtained within 30 days should be tested together.

The presence of chikungunya IgM antibody suggests a new, active infection. Detection of chikungunya IgG antibody suggests a current or past infection.

Treatment and Prevention

Treatment to relieve fever and pain is the only available medication, and there is no vaccine to prevent or medicine to treat chikungunya virus infection. Travelers can protect themselves by taking precautions to prevent mosquito bites.

DENGUE VIRUS

> **KEY CONCEPTS: Characteristics of Dengue Fever**
> - Dengue virus disease became a nationally notifiable condition in 2010.
> - Dengue hemorrhagic fever (DHF) and dengue shock syndrome (DSS) are caused by any one of four related viruses transmitted by mosquitoes.
> - Dengue is one of the most common vector-borne flaviviral infections globally.
> - According to the CDC, dengue testing is divided into confirmatory testing and testing for probable or suspected dengue infection.

Etiology

Dengue hemorrhagic fever (DHF) and dengue shock syndrome (DSS) are caused by any one of four related viruses transmitted by mosquitoes (dengue 1–4 serotypes). Dengue is transmitted between people by the mosquitoes *A. aegypti* and *A. albopictus*, which are found throughout the world.

Epidemiology

Statistics for mid-2024 identified 1059 dengue cases in patients with a travel history and 2231 locally acquired dengue cases. The highest number of cases was in the state of Florida (Fig. 16.14).

According to the CDC, dengue is one of the most common vector-borne flaviviral infections globally. In 2019 and 2020, the Pan American Health Organization reported approximately 5.5 million dengue cases from the Americas, the highest number on record.

Dengue is endemic in at least 100 countries in Asia, the Pacific, the Americas, Africa, and the Caribbean. It is endemic in the US territories of American Samoa, Puerto Rico (reported 2,190 cases), and the US Virgin Islands (reported 27 cases of Dengue fever). The risk of dengue infection in Guam and the Commonwealth of the Northern Mariana Islands is considered to be sporadic or uncertain. In the United States, nearly all dengue cases reported in the 48 continental states were acquired elsewhere by travelers or immigrants.

Signs and Symptoms

The new World Health Organization (WHO) classification for dengue severity is divided into dengue without warning signs, dengue with warning signs, and severe dengue. Symptoms of infection usually begin 4 to 7 days after the mosquito bite and typically last 3 to 10 days. The newest 2015 CDC case definition of dengue fever without warning signs is fever and two of the following: nausea, vomiting, rash, aches and pains, leukopenia, and a positive tourniquet test.

Dengue with warning signs can include any of the following:
- Abdominal pain or tenderness
- Persistent vomiting
- Clinical fluid accumulation (ascites, pleural effusion)
- Mucosal bleeding
- Lethargy, restlessness
- Liver enlargement of more than 2 cm
- Laboratory findings of an increased hematocrit, red cell mass, concurrent with a rapid decrease in the platelet count

According to the CDC, severe dengue most commonly occurs among infants and patients with secondary DENV infections (i.e., infection with a DENV type different from what they were previously infected with earlier in life). The most widely cited hypothesis for this occurrence is antibody-dependent enhancement (ADE) of disease. ADE occurs when non-neutralizing anti-DENV antibodies bind to but do not neutralize an infecting DENV. This virus-antibody complex allows for enhanced viral entry into host cells, specifically dendritic cells and macrophages. Once inside the cell, the virus replicates and generates higher virus titers in the blood than when anti-DENV antibody is not present, which results in a "cytokine storm" and ultimately leading to more severe disease.

Severe dengue must include dengue symptoms with at least one of the following criteria:
- Severe plasma leakage leading to:
  - Shock (DSS)
  - Fluid accumulation with respiratory distress
- Severe bleeding as evaluated by a clinician
- Severe organ involvement
  - Liver: aminotransferase (AST) or alanine aminotransferase (ALT) of 1000 or higher
  - CNS: impaired consciousness
  - Failure of the heart and other organs

Diagnostic Evaluation

A summary of CDC diagnostic testing is summarized in Box 16.1.

Nucleic Acid Amplification Tests (NAATs)

NAATs should be performed on serum specimens collected 7 days or less after symptom onset. Laboratory confirmation can be made from a single acute-phase serum specimen obtained early (≤7 days after fever onset) in the illness by detecting viral genomic sequences with rRT-PCR or dengue nonstructural protein 1 (NS1) antigen by immunoassay. The presence of virus by rRT-PCR or NS1 antigen in a single diagnostic specimen is considered laboratory confirmation of dengue in patients with a compatible clinical and travel history.

Serologic Tests

IgM antibody testing can identify additional infections and is an important diagnostic tool. However, interpreting the results is complicated by crossreactivity with other flaviviruses and determining the specific timing of infection can be difficult. Later in the illness (≥4 days after fever onset), IgM against DENV can be detected with MAC-ELISA. For patients presenting during the first week after fever onset, diagnostic testing should include a test for DENV (rRT-PCR or NS1) and IgM.

For patients presenting >1 week after fever onset IgM detection is most useful, although NS1 has been reported to be positive up to 12 days after fever onset. In the United States, both MAC-ELISA and rRT-PCR are approved as in vitro diagnostic tests.

IgM in a single-serum sample strongly suggests a recent DENV infection and should be presumed confirmatory for dengue if the infection occurred in a place where other potentially crossreactive flaviviruses (such as Zika, West Nile, yellow fever, and Japanese encephalitis viruses [JEV]) are not a risk.

PRNTs can resolve false-positive IgM antibody results caused by nonspecific reactivity and, in some cases, can help identify the infecting virus. However, in areas with high prevalence of DENV neutralizing antibodies, PRNT may not confirm a significant proportion of IgM-positive results. PRNT testing is available through several state health departments and the CDC.

Crossreactive Flaviviruses
- If infection is likely to have occurred in a place where other potentially crossreactive flaviviruses circulate, both molecular and serologic diagnostic testing for dengue and other flaviviruses should be performed.
- People infected with or vaccinated against other flaviviruses (such as yellow fever or Japanese encephalitis) may produce crossreactive flavivirus antibodies, yielding false-positive serologic dengue diagnostic test results.

IgG Antibody Testing

IgG detection by ELISA in a single-serum sample is not useful for diagnostic testing because it remains detectable for life after a DENV infection.

According to the CDC, dengue testing is divided into confirmatory testing and testing for probable or suspected dengue infection. Confirmatory testing for dengue consists of one of the following:
- Detection of DENV nucleic acid in serum, plasma, blood, CSF, other body fluid, or tissue by validated reverse transcriptase PCR (RT-PCR).
- Detection of DENV antigens in tissue by a validated IFA or IHC assay.
- Detection in serum or plasma of DENV NS1 antigen by a validated immunoassay.
- Cell culture isolation of DENV from a serum, plasma, or CSF specimen.
- Detection of IgM anti-DENV by validated immunoassay in a serum specimen or CSF in a person living in a dengue-endemic or nonendemic area of the United States without evidence of other flavivirus transmission (e.g., West Nile virus [WNV] and St. Louis encephalitis virus [SLEV]) or recent vaccination against a flavivirus (e.g., yellow fever virus [YFV] and JEV).
- Detection of IgM anti-DENV in a serum specimen or CSF by validated immunoassay in a traveler returning from a dengue-endemic area without ongoing transmission of another flavivirus (e.g., WNV), clinical evidence of coinfection with one of these flaviviruses, or recent vaccination against a flavivirus (e.g., YFV, JEV).
- IgM anti-DENV seroconversion by validated immunoassay in acute (i.e., collected within 5 days of illness onset) and convalescent (i.e., collected more than 5 days after illness onset) serum specimens.
- IgG anti-DENV seroconversion or at least a fourfold rise in titer by a validated immunoassay in serum specimens collected more than 2 weeks apart and confirmed by a neutralization test (e.g., plaque-reduction neutralization test), with more than a fourfold higher endpoint titer compared with other flaviviruses tested.

BOX 16.1 Summary of Centers for Disease Control and Prevention Dengue Fever Diagnostic Tests

1. **Molecular**
   - Centers for Disease Control and Prevention (CDC) DENV-1-4 rRT-PCR Multiplex and Trioplex rRT-PCR Assays
   - CDC DENV-1-4 Real-Time RT-PCR Multiplex Assay
   - Nucleic acid amplification test (NAAT) for fixed tissue specimens
   - Immunohistochemical (IHC) analysis to identify dengue virus (DENV) in tissues.

   A NAAT, like real-time reverse transcription polymerase chain reaction (rRT-PCR) or in situ hybridization, detects DENV RNA. The CDC DENV-1-4 rRT-PCR multiplex assay is a laboratory test designed to detect and serotype DENV infections. If positive, the result indicates the infecting DENV serotype. The US Food and Drug Administration (FDA) cleared this test in 2013.

2. **Dengue Virus Antigen Detection (NS1 Detection)**
   - NS1 tests detect the nonstructural protein NS1 of DENV. This protein is secreted into the blood during dengue infection. NS1 is detectable during the acute phase of DENV infections. NS1 tests can be as sensitive as molecular tests during the first 0–7 days of symptoms. After day 7, NS1 tests are not recommended.
   - Most NS1 tests have been developed for use in serum. Most of these tests use synthetically labeled antibodies to detect dengue NS1 protein. It does not provide serotype information. Knowing the serotype of the infecting virus is not necessary for patient care; however, if serotype information is needed for surveillance purposes, the sample should be tested by NAAT.
   - Combined testing with an NS1 and IgM antibody test can usually provide a diagnostic result during the first 1–7 days of illness, a second, convalescent phase specimen should be obtained and tested for IgM when both antigen and antibody tests are negative.
   - A negative NS1 test result does not rule out infection. People with negative NS1 results should be tested for the presence of dengue IgM antibodies to determine possible recent dengue exposure.
   - DENV-specific IgM and neutralizing antibodies typically develop toward the end of the first week of illness. IgM levels are variable, but generally are positive starting 4–5 days after onset of symptoms and continuing for approximately 12 weeks post symptom onset, but may persist longer.

3. **Serologic Tests**
   IgM Antibody Capture Enzyme-Linked Immunosorbent Assay (MAC-ELISA)
   - The dengue MAC-ELISA is used for the qualitative detection of DENV IgM antibodies. The MAC-ELISA is based on capturing human IgM antibodies on a microtiter plate using anti-human–IgM antibody followed by the addition of DENV antigens. The antigens used for this assay are derived from the envelope proteins of the four DENV serotypes (DENV-1–4).
   - IgM antibodies against DENV are detectable starting 4–5 days after onset of symptoms and are reliably detectable for approximately 12 weeks.
   - Combined testing with a NAAT and MAC-ELISA usually provides a diagnostic result during the first 1–7 days of illness. A convalescent-phase specimen is needed to make a diagnosis of DENV infection when results are negative on both tests from the acute specimen.
   - IgM antibody detection is not useful for DENV serotype determination.
   - Specimen types include serum and cerebrospinal fluid (CSF). Some IgM tests can be performed on plasma and whole blood but these tests have not been extensively evaluated for these specimen types.
   - Positive IgM: Patients with a positive IgM test result are classified as presumptive, recent DENV infections.
   - Negative IgM:
     - Patients with negative IgM results before day 8 of illness and absent or negative NAAT or NS1 results are considered unconfirmed cases. For these cases, a second sample should be obtained after day 7 of symptoms for additional serologic testing.
     - Patients with negative IgM results after 7 days of symptoms, and absent or negative NAAT or NS1 (DENV antigen detection) are classified as negative for recent infection.
     - Patients with a change from negative to positive IgM results in paired samples (first sample collected during the first 7 days of illness, and second sample collected after symptoms subside) are classified as current dengue infections.
   - Due to crossreaction with other flaviviruses and possible nonspecific reactivity, results may be difficult to interpret. Consequently, presumed positive, indeterminate, and equivocal, IgM antibody test results may be forwarded for confirmation by plaque-reduction neutralization testing (PRNT).

4. **Plaque-reduction Neutralization Testing (PRNT)**
   - PRNT can detect specific neutralizing antibodies against DENV and other flaviviruses. It is used to more precisely determine the cause of infection in IgM-positive patients for whom a specific diagnosis is clinically or epidemiologically important (e.g., to rule out other flaviviruses such as yellow fever).
   - PRNT measures the titer of the neutralizing antibodies in the serum of the infected person. Specimen types include serum and CSF. A fourfold rise in PRNT titers in paired acute and convalescent samples with antibodies to multiple DENV serotypes or other flaviviruses in the convalescent sample is classified as a recent flavivirus infection.
   - PRNT is a biological assay based on the principle of interaction of virus and antibody resulting in inactivation of virus such that the virus is no longer able to infect and replicate in cell culture. PRNT and microneutralization PRNT can be used when a specific serologic diagnosis is required; for example in pregnant women or cases of clinical and epidemiologic importance.
   - PRNT is used in an attempt to confirm the infecting virus in a dengue or Zika virus IgM-positive specimen and can in some cases determine the infecting DENV serotype. This testing is not routinely performed in the US territory of Puerto Rico where dengue is endemic and has circulated. However, strong consideration should be given to performing PRNT in symptomatic pregnant women with negative NAAT testing and positive IgM serology. Another situation in which PRNT testing would not likely add value is in the context of a documented dengue outbreak in an area without evidence of concurrently circulating flaviviruses.

Note: PRNT is performed at the CDC or a laboratory designated by CDC (i.e., a laboratory that has independently demonstrated proficiency to perform PRNT testing by completing a proficiency panel provided by CDC). Public health laboratories may refer IgM-positive specimens to CDC for PRNT to confirm positive, equivocal, or inconclusive IgM results.
From Centers for Disease Control and Prevention, National Center for Emerging and Zoonotic Infectious Diseases (NCEZID), Division of Vector-Borne Diseases (DVBD); https://www.cdc.gov/dengue/healthcare-providers/testing/serologic-tests.html. (Last reviewed June, 2019).

Testing for probable dengue diagnostic testing consists of one of the following:
- Detection of IgM anti-DENV by validated immunoassay in a serum specimen or CSF in a person living in a dengue-endemic or nonendemic area of the United States with evidence of other flavivirus transmissions (e.g., WNV and SLEV) or recent vaccination against a flavivirus (e.g., YFV and JEV).
- Detection of IgM αντι-DENV in a serum specimen or CSF by validated immunoassay in a traveler returning from a dengue-endemic area with ongoing transmission of another flavivirus (e.g., WNV,

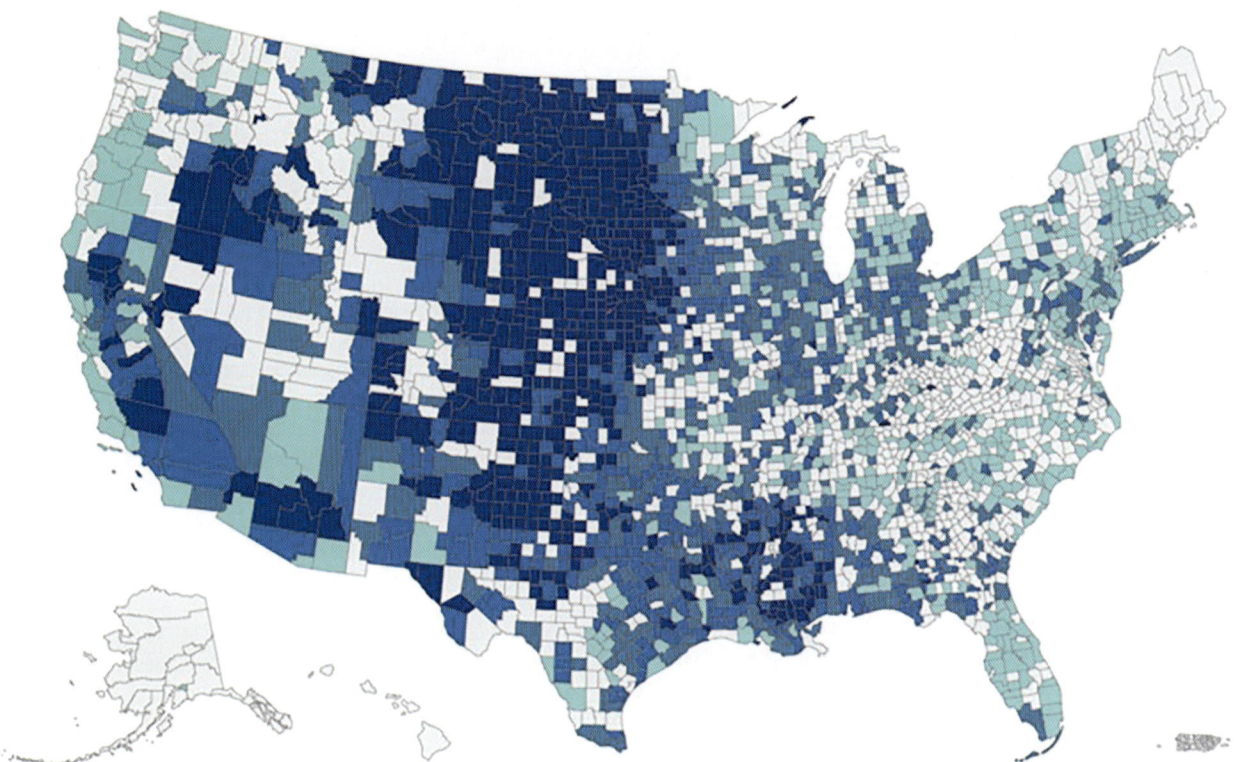

Fig. 16.15 West Nile virus human disease cases reported by state of residence, 2024. (From Centers for Disease Control and Prevention cdc.gov.)

JEV, and YFV), clinical evidence of coinfection with one of these flaviviruses, or recent vaccination against a flavivirus (e.g., YFV and JEV).

Testing for a suspected case of dengue infection includes the following:
- The absence of IgM anti-DENV by validated immunoassay in a serum or CSF specimen collected within 5 days after illness onset and in which molecular diagnostic testing was not performed in a patient with an epidemiologic linkage.

Dengue infection results in long-lasting immunity to symptomatic infection (dengue) with a specific dengue serotype. However, crossprotective (heterotypic) immunity against dengue is short lived, with estimated durations of 1 to 3 years. In dengue-endemic areas where infection pressure is high, rarely individuals have been shown to have sequential episodes of dengue with two different infecting serotypes.

Treatment and Prevention

Treatment is consistent with the classification of the dengue infection. The most effective protective measures are those that prevent mosquito bites.

According to the CDC, a new dengue vaccine is approved for use in children aged 9 to 16 years with laboratory-confirmed previous DENV infection and living in areas where dengue is endemic. Dengue vaccine is now recommended for the US territories of American Samoa, Puerto Rico, and the US Virgin Islands, and freely associated states, including the Federated States of Micronesia, the Republic of Marshall Islands, and the Republic of Palau.

The vaccine is not approved for use in US travelers who are visiting but not living in an area where dengue is common.

WEST NILE VIRUS

> **KEY CONCEPTS:** West Nile Virus
> - West Nile virus (WNV), a mosquito-borne virus present in the United States since at least 1999, causes febrile illness and encephalitis in human beings.
> - In WNV, IgM antibody is evident in most infected patients 7 to 8 days after the onset of symptoms, persisting for more than 500 days in 60% of cases. Most patients demonstrate IgG antibody 3 to 4 weeks after infection.

Etiology

West Nile virus (WNV) is a member of the JEV group of flaviviruses that cause febrile illness and encephalitis in human beings. WNV is a mosquito-borne pathogen.

Epidemiology

The virus has been in the United States since at least the summer of 1999. Data current as of August, 6, 2024 indicated 103 cases of West Nile human disease and 68 cases of neuroinvasive human cases reported by 26 states of residence (Fig. 16.15). If WNV infection is reported to the CDC from any area of a state, the entire state is shaded.

WNV is the leading cause of mosquito-borne disease in the continental United States. Cases of WNV occur during mosquito season, which starts in the summer and continues through fall.

In a very small number of cases, WNV has been spread through:
- Exposure in a laboratory setting
- Blood transfusion and organ transplant
- Mother to baby, during pregnancy, delivery, or breastfeeding

The median patient age was 62 years (range: 50–71 years), of whom 63% were male. A total of 80% of patients were hospitalized, and 66 (9%) died. The median age of patients who died from neuroinvasive disease was 70 years (range: 64–82 years).

In 2020 a total of 559 cases of neuroinvasive WNV disease were reported. The largest numbers of neuroinvasive cases were reported from California, Texas, Florida, and Illinois, which together accounted for 64% of cases nationwide.

Signs and Symptoms

WNV infection is characterized by fever, headache, fatigue, aches, and sometimes a rash. Illness can last from a few days to several weeks.

Diagnostic Evaluation

Historically, flavivirus infections have been diagnosed by serologic tests or virus isolation. IgM antibody is evident in most infected patients 7 to 8 days after the onset of symptoms. IgM antibody has been shown to persist for longer than 500 days in approximately 60% of cases. Most patients demonstrate IgG antibody in 3 to 4 weeks after infection.

Several molecular techniques are available for diagnosis. Molecular detection of WNV is used for prevention of transmission by blood transfusion and transplantation. Laboratory diagnosis of WNV infection is generally accomplished by testing of serum or CSF to detect virus-specific IgM and neutralizing antibodies.

Four FDA-approved WNV IgM ELISA kits from different manufacturers are commercially available in the United States. According to the package inserts, each of these kits is indicated for use on serum to aid in the presumptive laboratory diagnosis of WNV infection in patients with clinical symptoms of meningitis or encephalitis. The package inserts also state that all positive results obtained with any of the commercially available WNV test kits should be confirmed by additional testing at a state health department laboratory or by the CDC.

In fatal cases, nucleic acid amplification, histopathology with immunohistochemistry, and virus culture of autopsy tissues can also be useful. Only a few state laboratories or other specialized laboratories, including those at the CDC, can carry out this specialized testing.

Treatment and Prevention

No vaccine or specific medicines are available for WNV infection. Antibiotics do not treat viruses. In patients with milder disease symptoms resolve over time, although even healthy people have been sick for several weeks. In patients with more severe disease, hospitalization is usually required for supportive treatment, including IV fluids.

Prevention consists of preventing mosquito bites.

CASE STUDY 16.1

A 42-year-old executive lives in New York City. Her company annually sponsors a Memorial Day weekend golf outing at a Long Island club. In early June she noticed a solid, bright red spot on her left thigh. The spot was about 2 inches wide in the bright red area with an overall diameter of about 6 inches, including the surrounding pale area. The ensuing 11 months passed without further incident.

The following Memorial Day weekend, she was stung several times by bees. Both systemic and local reactions followed. About 1 week later, the previous year's red ring on the thigh reappeared. During this interval, she experienced fever, malaise, arthromyalgias, headache, and a stiff neck but recovered completely.

In the fall, the woman noticed insidiously progressive fatigue, malaise, memory deficits, irritability, and inattentiveness to the demands of her job. She visited a physician, but no abnormalities were noted, and she was referred to a Manhattan neurologist. The patient was eventually diagnosed as having Lyme disease.

Question

1. A major focus of Lyme disease infection is:
    a. Massachusetts to Maryland
    b. Virginia to Florida
    c. Florida to Louisiana
    d. Louisiana to North Dakota

The answer to this question can be found in Appendix A.

Critical Thinking Group Discussion Questions

1. Did the patient's residence or travel history suggest that she might have been exposed to Lyme disease?
2. Why did it take so long for the patient to develop symptoms of Lyme disease?

CASE STUDY 16.2

A 25-year-old graduate student visits his local family physician because of episodic arthromyalgias, sporadic global headaches, fatigue, irritability, and depression. Over the past several months he had become seriously dysfunctional at work and home.

His residence and travel history revealed a week-long vacation on Cape Cod the previous summer. He could not recall any tick bites or skin lesions fitting the description of EM.

A laboratory test yielded a positive result, and a 4-week course of doxycycline was initiated. Two weeks later, he noted significant improvement in symptoms, but 3 months later his previous symptoms recurred. His laboratory test was repeated, and again the result was positive. A 1-month regimen of amoxicillin and probenecid was initiated. This time, there was no improvement. No neurologic findings were apparent. His joints were painful, but no overt synovitis was present. Two months after the second course of antibiotic, his Lyme test result was still positive, and the patient was given 2 weeks of infusion therapy with ceftriaxone. His symptoms disappeared after this treatment.

Question

1. The western blot procedure is more definitive in the _____ stage of Lyme disease.
    a. Initial
    b. Early
    c. Mid
    d. Late

The answer to this question can be found in Appendix A.

Critical Thinking Group Discussion Questions

1. Why was the initial treatment regimen unsuccessful?
2. Why did the patient demonstrate a positive laboratory result?

CASE STUDY 16.3

A 45-year-old man from upstate New York visits his physician because of a worsening headache, myalgia, arthralgia, and generalized weakness. He had been in good health until about 1 week before the appointment. A fever and myalgia began after the patient removed a small tick from his left thigh while on vacation in an area in which *B. burgdorferi* was endemic. In addition, the deer tick found in the area that he visited on vacation is the vector of Lyme disease, babesiosis, and, most likely, anaplasmosis.

On physical examination, the patient had a slight fever. His thigh had a rash suggestive of erythema migrans (EM). Laboratory results included a complete blood count and liver function tests. A skin scraping was obtained to culture *B. burgdorferi*. Buffy coat smears of peripheral blood were also requested.

The patient had a slight leukopenia, normal white blood cell differential, and normal hemoglobin and hematocrit values. His liver function test results were slightly abnormal. Wright-stained buffy coat smears revealed the presence of morulae of anaplasmosis. The patient was prescribed oral doxycycline twice daily for 14 days. Nine days after initiation of treatment, the patient improved greatly. Repeat laboratory test results were all within the normal reference range. His rash had resolved.

Question
1. *B. burgdorferi* and the agent of anaplasmosis (HE) can be demonstrated by:
   a. Isolation of both organisms from a clinical specimen
   b. Latex agglutination for Lyme disease
   c. ELISA testing
   d. Indirect fluorescent antibody (IFA) testing
   The answer to this question can be found in Appendix A.

Critical Thinking Group Discussion Questions
1. Can the vector of *B. burgdorferi* and the agent of anaplasmosis be the same?
2. Is it important to determine whether one or both infections are present in the same host?
3. How can coinfection with *B. burgdorferi* and the agent of anaplasmosis be demonstrated in the laboratory?

CASE STUDY 16.4

A 73-year-old, previously healthy man had spent the summer on Martha's Vineyard. On returning to his home in Boston after Labor Day, he began to feel unusually tired and had difficulty breathing. He also reported that his urine had become dark brown several days after returning home.

On physical examination, the patient was found to be jaundiced and he had an enlarged spleen. A complete blood count, urinalysis, and blood chemistries were ordered. His total white blood cell count was normal, but he had an increased percentage of segmented neutrophils. His hemoglobin and hematocrit values and platelet count were all below the normal reference range. He had hematuria and proteinuria. His liver function test results were greatly elevated. His renal function assays were also elevated. A follow-up Wright-stained peripheral blood smear revealed numerous *Babesia microti* organisms.

The patient was treated with quinine and the antibiotics clindamycin and doxycycline. He also received two units of packed red blood cells (RBCs). Six days later, the patient was discharged from the hospital.

Question
1. If *Babesia* cannot be observed by microscopic examination of a peripheral blood smear from a patient who is ill but has no travel history to a malaria-endemic area, an acute infection with *Babesia* can be diagnosed by:
   a. Repeat blood smear examination in 4 weeks
   b. Testing acute and convalescent patient sera for a rise in the IgG antibody titer
   c. Use of a molecular technique to detect the microorganism
   d. Either b or c
   The answer to this question can be found in Appendix A.

Critical Thinking Group Discussion Questions
1. Would the patient's travel history be suggestive of malaria or another bloodborne infectious disease?
2. What is the definitive diagnosis for babesiosis?
3. What additional laboratory tests are of diagnostic value?

CASE STUDY 16.5

A 35-year-old field biologist from central Missouri tested positive for HIV. Her work required that she spend a great deal of time in the woods in the surrounding areas. Although she was in good health despite the HIV positivity, she began having back pain, fever, chills, sweats, a productive cough, and extreme tiredness before her visit to the emergency department.

She was admitted to the hospital because her laboratory results demonstrated severe leukopenia and thrombocytopenia. Her liver function tests were also extremely abnormal. Later on the day of admission, renal failure developed. The patient died the next day.

Question
1. In suspected human monocytic ehrlichiosis (HME), if a patient has a supporting history and clinical symptoms, the diagnosis can be confirmed by a serologic titer greater than:
   a. 1:32
   b. 1:64
   c. 1:128
   d. 1:256
   The answer to this question can be found in Appendix A.

Critical Thinking Group Discussion Questions
1. What was the cause of death?
2. What immunologic studies could be performed?
3. Is human monocytic ehrlichiosis a risk in the United States?

REVIEW QUESTIONS

1. Common vectors of Lyme disease include all of the following *except*:
   a. *I. pacificus*
   b. *I. scapularis*
   c. *I. ricinus*
   d. *D. variabilis*
2. The only continent without Lyme disease is:
   a. Asia
   b. Europe
   c. Africa
   d. Antarctica
3. The primary reservoir in nature for *B. burgdorferi* is the:
   a. White-tailed deer
   b. White-footed mouse
   c. Lizard
   d. Meadowlark
4. The first *B. burgdorferi* antigen to elicit an antibody response is:
   a. Outer surface protein A
   b. Outer surface protein B
   c. Flagellar 41-kDa polypeptide
   d. 60-kDa polypeptide
5. On average, the incidence of infection after an *I. scapularis* tick bite in an endemic area is:
   a. 1%
   b. 3%
   c. 5%
   d. 10%
6. Erythema migrans (EM):
   a. Occurs in all patients
   b. Harbors *B. burgdorferi* in the advancing edge
   c. Is easily distinguished from other erythemas
   d. Is more common in the winter months
7. The predominant symptoms of Lyme meningitis are:
   a. Severe headache and mild neck stiffness
   b. Aseptic meningitis and double vision
   c. Cranial nerve palsies and blurred vision
   d. Peripheral radiculoneuritis and peripheral neuropathy
8. Cardiac involvement in Lyme disease may include:
   a. Murmurs
   b. Conduction abnormalities
   c. Congestive heart failure
   d. Vasculitis
9. Ocular involvement in Lyme disease includes all of the following *except*:
   a. Cranial nerve palsies
   b. Conjunctivitis
   c. Panophthalmitis with loss of vision
   d. Chorioditis with retinal detachment
10. Pregnancy in Lyme disease:
    a. Does not result in high fetal mortality
    b. Has been associated with transplacental infection
    c. Should be terminated because of maternal risk
    d. Is not associated with congenital abnormalities
11. The most useful test for distinguishing between true-positive and false-positive serologic test results in Lyme disease is:
    a. Enzyme-linked immunosorbent assay
    b. Immunofluorescence assay
    c. Polymerase chain reaction
    d. T-cell assay
12. Lyme disease, the most common tick-borne disease in the United States, is a major health hazard for:
    a. Dogs
    b. Cheetahs
    c. Humans
    d. Both a and c
13. Lyme disease is a _____ type of infection.
    a. Bacterial
    b. Parasitic
    c. Viral
    d. Fungal
14. The first Native American patient case of what would later be called Lyme disease occurred in:
    a. Connecticut
    b. Wisconsin
    c. Florida
    d. New York
15. The median length of time for stage 1 of Lyme disease is:
    a. 3 days
    b. 1 week
    c. 4 weeks
    d. 3 months
16. Common signs and symptoms as manifestations after infection in stage 1 of Lyme disease are:
    a. Neurologic
    b. Rheumatoid
    c. Cutaneous (e.g., erythema migrans)
    d. Cardiac
17. In stage 3 of Lyme disease, the length of time after initial infection is:
    a. Hours to weeks
    b. Days to weeks
    c. Weeks to months
    d. Weeks to years
18. In stage 3 of Lyme disease, in addition to late neurologic complications, another clinical manifestation can be:
    a. Arthritis
    b. Lyme carditis
    c. Transplacental transmission
    d. Lymphocytoma
19. Unlike some procedures, the polymerase chain reaction (PCR) assay can be used to detect Lyme disease–causing organisms in:
    a. Urine
    b. Cerebrospinal fluid
    c. Synovial fluid
    d. Blood

Question 20. Antigen-detection systems for Lyme disease testing screen for _____.
   a. Antibody
   b. Microorganisms
   c. Antigenic products
   d. An infected tick

Question 21. Antigen-detection systems for Lyme disease testing do not screen for _____.
   a. Antibody
   b. Microorganisms
   c. Antigenic products
   d. An infected tick

22. Patients who have specific Lyme disease–associated manifestations may be treated with:
    a. Vaccination
    b. Interferon
    c. Antibiotics
    d. Analgesics
23. *Ehrlichia* spp. belong to the same family as the organism that causes:
    a. Lyme disease
    b. Rocky Mountain spotted fever
    c. Toxoplasmosis
    d. Infectious mononucleosis
24. One of the most common physical findings in adults with ehrlichiosis is:
    a. Hives
    b. Fever
    c. Erythema migrans
    d. Nausea
25. Definitive diagnosis of ehrlichiosis requires:
    a. A complete blood count
    b. Detection of the presence of lymphocytopenia
    c. Acute and convalescent serum antibody titers
    d. Direct microscopic observation of inclusions in leukocytes
26. In human granulocytic ehrlichiosis (anaplasmosis), the diagnosis is confirmed by seroconversion or by a single serologic titer of _____ in patients with a supporting history and clinical symptoms.
    a. 1:2
    b. 1:16
    c. 1:80
    d. 1:160
27. In the eastern United States, babesiosis is caused by:
    a. *B. microti*
    b. *B. canis*
    c. *B. bovis*
    d. *B. equi*
28. *Babesia* organisms can be found in:
    a. Peripheral blood
    b. Sputum
    c. Synovial fluid
    d. Various exudates
29. In cases of malaria, after the injection of sporozoites into a person, they multiply in the:
    a. Sporogonic cycle
    b. Exo-erythrocytic cycle
    c. Erythrocytic cycle
    d. Either a or b
30. In cases of malaria, sickle cell trait protects individuals predominantly against _____ infection.
    a. *Plasmodium falciparum*
    b. *Plasmodium vivax*
    c. *Plasmodium ovale*
    d. *Plasmodium malariae*
31. West Nile virus causes:
    a. Encephalitis
    b. Polio
    c. Measles
    d. Arthritis

17

Infectious Mononucleosis

LEARNING OUTCOMES

- Describe the etiology, epidemiology, and signs and symptoms of infectious mononucleosis.
- Explain the immunologic manifestations of infectious mononucleosis, including heterophile antibodies.
- Discuss the elements of Epstein-Barr virus (EBV) serology and the diagnostic clinical applications of the presence of each component.
- Analyze and apply laboratory data to a case study.
- Correctly answer case study–related multiple-choice questions.
- Participate in a discussion of critical thinking questions.
- Compare the serologic procedures and clinical applications of the Paul-Bunnell, Davidsohn differential, and rapid agglutination techniques.
- Correctly answer 80% of the end-of-chapter review questions.

OUTLINE

Etiology, 267
Epidemiology, 268
Transmission of Infection, 268
Pathophysiology, 268
Signs and Symptoms, 268
Laboratory Diagnostic Evaluation, 269
Immunologic Manifestations, 269
    Heterophile Antibodies, 269
    Epstein-Barr Virus Serology, 269

Viral Capsid Antigen, 270
Early Antigen, 270
Epstein-Barr Nuclear Antigen, 270
Additional Testing, 271
Case Study 17.1   History and Physical Examination, 271
Procedure: Paul-Bunnell Screening Test, 272.e1
Procedure: Davidsohn Differential Test, 272.e1
Procedure: MonoSlide Test, 272.e2

KEY TERMS

acute	carcinoma	neoplasms
asymptomatic	leukopenia	prognostic
benign	morphologic	splenomegaly S

KEY CONCEPTS: Characteristics of Epstein-Barr Virus

- Epstein-Barr virus (EBV), a human herpes DNA virus that infects B lymphocytes, is the cause of infectious mononucleosis.
- EBV is also the cause of Burkitt lymphoma (a malignant tumor of the lymphoid tissue occurring mainly in African children); nasopharyngeal carcinoma; and neoplasms of the thymus, parotid gland, and supraglottic larynx.
- EBV is widely disseminated. An estimated 95% of the world's population is exposed to EBV, making it the most ubiquitous virus known.
- In Western societies, primary exposure to EBV occurs in two waves:
  - Approximately 50% of the population is exposed to the virus before age 5 years;
  - A second wave of seroconversion occurs during late adolescence (age 15–24 years). Approximately 90% of adults older than 35 years demonstrate antibodies to the virus.

ETIOLOGY

The Epstein-Barr virus (EBV), a human herpes DNA virus that infects B lymphocytes, is the cause of infectious mononucleosis. EBV was discovered by Dr. M. Anthony Epstein and his colleague, Yvonne Barr. Subsequently, Dr. Werner Henle and Dr. Gertrude Henle screened human serum samples for antibodies to viral capsid antigens of EBV and established the relationship of EBV to several cancers (e.g., Burkitt lymphoma). EBV became the most intensively studied human cancer virus. The entire genome of one EBV strain was completely sequenced in 1964.

EBV is also the cause of Burkitt lymphoma (a malignant tumor of the lymphoid tissue occurring mainly in African children); nasopharyngeal carcinoma; and neoplasms of the thymus, parotid gland, and supraglottic larynx.

EBV is an important factor in the development of nasopharyngeal carcinoma, an epithelial cancer. Although nasopharyngeal carcinoma is rare in White North American and European individuals, it is one of the most common cancers in southern China and parts of Southeast Asia. Genetics and environmental factors appear to contribute to the elevated risk of nasopharyngeal carcinoma among the Chinese.

EPIDEMIOLOGY

EBV is widely disseminated. It is estimated that 95% of the world's population is exposed to the virus, which makes EBV the most ubiquitous virus known to humans. Clinically apparent infectious mononucleosis has an estimated frequency of 45 per 100,000 in adolescents. In immunosuppressed patients, the incidence of EBV infection ranges from 35% to 47%. As with other herpes viruses, there is a carrier state after primary infection.

The frequency of seronegative patients is almost 100% in early infancy. After primary exposure, a person is considered to be immune and generally no longer susceptible to overt reinfection.

In Western societies, primary exposure to EBV occurs in two waves:
1. Approximately 50% of the population is exposed to the virus before age 5 years;
2. A second wave of seroconversion occurs during late adolescence (age 15–24 years). Approximately 90% of adults older than 35 years demonstrate antibodies to the virus.

> **KEY CONCEPTS: Transmission of Infection**
> - Although transmitted primarily by infectious oropharyngeal secretions, under normal conditions, EBV transmission through transfusion or transplacental exposure is unlikely.
> - However blood transfusion from an immune donor to a nonimmune recipient may produce a primary infection in the recipient known as *infectious mononucleosis postperfusion syndrome*.
> - EBV is only a minor problem for immunocompetent persons but can become a major concern for immunocompromised patients.
> - A final consideration is the association with EBV that appears to be a specific finding in malignant lymphoma developing after severe immunosuppression, such as that induced by cyclosporine therapy.

TRANSMISSION OF INFECTION

The virus is transmitted primarily by close contact with infectious oropharyngeal secretions. Although EBV can reportedly be transmitted by blood transfusion and transplacental routes, under normal conditions, exposure is unlikely. However blood transfusion from an immune donor to a nonimmune recipient may produce a primary infection in the recipient known as *infectious mononucleosis postperfusion syndrome*. Infectious mononucleosis or an infectious mononucleosis–like illness after blood transfusion often may result from a concomitant cytomegalovirus (CMV) infection rather than EBV.

In addition, EBV-associated posttransplantation lymphoproliferative disorder (PTLD) develops in 1% to 10% of organ transplant recipients.

Individuals at risk include those who lack antibodies to the virus. EBV is only a minor problem for immunocompetent persons but can become a major concern for immunocompromised patients.

A final consideration is the association with EBV that appears to be a specific finding in malignant lymphoma developing after severe immunosuppression, such as that induced by cyclosporine therapy.

> **KEY CONCEPTS: Pathophysiology**
> - EBV parasitizes every cell system—signal transduction, cell cycle control, regulation of gene expression, posttranscriptional RNA processing, protein modification and stability, and DNA replication.
> - The variant lymphocytes produced in response to and seen in microscopic examination of the peripheral blood have T-cell characteristics.
> - CD8+ T cells expand dramatically with subpopulations specific for individual viral epitopes at frequencies as high as 10% of circulating CD8+ T cells.

PATHOPHYSIOLOGY

EBV parasitizes every cell system—signal transduction, cell cycle control, regulation of gene expression, posttranscriptional RNA processing, protein modification and stability, and DNA replication.

The variant lymphocytes produced in response to and seen in microscopic examination of the peripheral blood have T-cell characteristics. The mononucleosis is not from stimulation of B cells by viral infection (EBV will transform cell lines in vitro), but is from a large, effective, CD8 cytotoxic T-cell (Tc) response against the EBV-infected circulating B lymphocytes.

Virus-specific CD8+ T cells have been associated with severity of disease and expand dramatically during acute EBV infection. CD8+ T cells expand dramatically with subpopulations specific for individual viral epitopes at frequencies as high as 10% of circulating CD8+ T cells. Persistence of CD8+ T cells is important for lifelong control of EBV-associated disease. One of the habitats of the persisting viral genome in hosts with a latent infection is the B lymphocytes of the lymphoreticular system and epithelial cells of the oropharynx.

> **KEY CONCEPTS: Signs and Symptoms**
> - Infectious mononucleosis, caused by EBV, is usually an acute, benign, and self-limiting lymphoproliferative condition.
> - Infants typically have asymptomatic infection.
> - Most individuals experience seroconversion without any significant clinical signs or symptoms of disease.
> - EBV-associated neurologic syndromes include Bell palsy, Guillain-Barré syndrome, meningoencephalitis, Reye syndrome, myelitis, cranial nerve neuritis, and psychotic disorders. Respiratory paralysis caused by bulbar involvement can be fatal.

SIGNS AND SYMPTOMS

Infectious mononucleosis, caused by EBV, is usually an **acute**, **benign**, and self-limiting lymphoproliferative condition. Although EBV infects more than 95% of the world's population, most individuals experience no adverse effects.

Infants typically have **asymptomatic** infections. The timing of initial infection is a key indicator of the ensuing symptoms. Infectious mononucleosis is the typical illness experienced by adolescents newly infected with EBV.

Most individuals experience seroconversion without any significant clinical signs or symptoms of disease. Immunocompetent persons maintain EBV as a chronic latent infection. In children younger than 5 years, infection is asymptomatic or frequently characterized by mild, poorly defined signs and symptoms. Although anyone can suffer from this viral disorder, it is typically manifested in young adults.

The incubation period of infectious mononucleosis is from 10 to 50 days; once fully developed, it lasts for 1 to 4 weeks. Clinical manifestations include extreme fatigue, malaise, sore throat, fever, and cervical lymphadenopathy. Splenomegaly occurs in about 50% of cases. Jaundice is uncommon, although the most common complication is hepatitis. A smaller percentage of patients develops hepatomegaly or splenomegaly and hepatomegaly. Because abnormal liver function is more marked with EBV-induced than CMV-associated infectious mononucleosis, EBV must be considered in the differential diagnosis of hepatitis.

A significant number of patients with infectious mononucleosis do not manifest classic signs and symptoms. A low percentage of patients experience symptomatic reactivation. Reactivation of latent EBV infection has been implicated in a persistent illness referred to as *EBV-associated fatigue syndrome*.

EBV infections can result in complications involving the cardiac, ocular, respiratory, hematologic, digestive, renal, and neurologic systems. EBV-associated neurologic syndromes include Bell palsy, Guillain-Barré syndrome, meningoencephalitis, Reye syndrome, myelitis, cranial nerve neuritis, and psychotic disorders. Respiratory paralysis caused by bulbar involvement can be fatal.

> **KEY CONCEPTS: Laboratory Diagnostic Evaluation**
> - Laboratory testing is necessary to establish or confirm the diagnosis of infectious mononucleosis.
> - Lymphocytes express a variety of new antigens encoded by the virus. Infection with EBV results in:
>   - expression of viral capsid antigen (VCA),
>   - early antigen (EA), and
>   - nuclear antigen (NA), with corresponding antibody responses.
> - Assays for immunoglobulin M (IgM) and immunoglobulin G (IgG) antibodies to these EBV antigens are available.
> - EBV-specific serologic studies are beneficial for defining immune status. The time of antibody appearance may indicate the stage of the disease.

LABORATORY DIAGNOSTIC EVALUATION

Laboratory testing is necessary to establish or confirm the diagnosis of infectious mononucleosis (Table 17.1).

Hematologic studies reveal a leukocyte count ranging from 10 to 20 $\times 10^9$/L in about two-thirds of patients; about 10% of patients demonstrate leukopenia. A differential leukocyte count may initially disclose a neutrophilia, although mononuclear cells usually predominate as the disorder develops. Typical relative lymphocyte counts range from 60% to 90%, with 5% to 30% variant lymphocytes. These variant lymphocytes exhibit diverse morphologic features and persist for 1 to 2 months and as long as 4 to 6 months (Fig. 17.1).

TABLE 17.1 Classic Laboratory Findings in Acute Infectious Mononucleosis.

Assay	Result
Heterophile antibody test	Positive
Anti-VCA IgM	Elevated titer
Liver enzymes	Elevated
Leukocyte differential	Increased number of variant (atypical) lymphocytes

IgM, Immunoglobulin M; *VCA*, viral capsid antigen.

IMMUNOLOGIC MANIFESTATIONS

If the classic signs and symptoms are absent, a diagnosis of infectious mononucleosis is more difficult to make. A definitive diagnosis can be established by serologic antibody testing. The antibodies present in infectious mononucleosis are heterophile and EBV antibodies.

Heterophile Antibodies

Heterophile antibodies are composed of a broad class of antibodies. These antibodies are stimulated by one antigen and react with an entirely unrelated surface antigen present on cells from different mammalian species. Heterophile antibodies may be present in normal individuals in low concentrations (titers), but a titer of 1:56 or greater is clinically significant in patients with suspected infectious mononucleosis.

The immunoglobulin M (IgM) type of heterophile antibody usually appears during the acute phase of infectious mononucleosis, but the antigen that stimulates its production remains unknown. IgM heterophile antibody is characterized by the following features:
- Reacts with horse, ox, and sheep erythrocytes
- Absorbed by beef erythrocytes
- Not absorbed by guinea pig kidney cells
- Does not react with EBV-specific antigens

Paul and Bunnell first associated infectious mononucleosis with sheep cell agglutination and developed a test for the infectious mononucleosis heterophile. Davidsohn modified the original Paul-Bunnell test, introducing a differential adsorption aspect to remove the cross-reacting Forssman and serum sickness heterophile antibodies. Rapid agglutination slide tests are now available.

Epstein-Barr Virus Serology

Within the adult population, 10% to 20% of individuals with acute infectious mononucleosis do not produce infectious mononucleosis heterophile antibody. The pediatric population is of particular concern, because more than 50% of children younger than 4 years with infectious mononucleosis are heterophile negative. In diagnostically inconclusive cases of infectious mononucleosis, a more definitive assessment of immune status may be obtained through an EBV serologic panel. Candidates for EBV serology include those who do not exhibit classic symptoms of infectious mononucleosis, who are heterophile negative, or who are immunosuppressed.

Epstein-Barr–infected B lymphocytes express a variety of new antigens encoded by the virus. Infection with EBV results in the expression

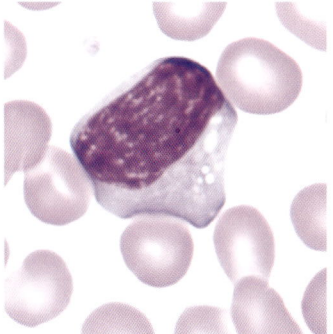

Fig. 17.1 Variant Lymphocytes Seen in Epstein-Barr Virus Infection (Mononucleosis). (From Rodak BF, Carr JH: *Clinical hematology atlas*, ed 4, St. Louis, 2013, Saunders.)

of viral capsid antigen, early antigen, and nuclear antigen, with corresponding antibody responses. Assays for IgM and IgG antibodies to these EBV antigens are available. EBV-specific serologic studies are beneficial in defining immune status, and their time of appearance may indicate the stage of disease (Fig. 17.2 and Table 17.2). This can provide important information for the diagnosis and management of EBV-associated disease. Patients with nasopharyngeal carcinoma have elevated titers of immunoglobulin A (IgA) antibodies to EBV replicative antigens, including VCA. These antibodies, which commonly precede the appearance of the tumor, serve as a prognostic indicator of remission and relapse.

Viral Capsid Antigen

VCA is produced by infected B cells and can be found in the cytoplasm. Anti-VCA IgM is usually detectable early in the course of infection but is low in concentration and disappears within 2 to 4 months. Anti-VCA IgG is usually detectable within 4 to 7 days after the onset of signs and symptoms and persists for an extended period, perhaps lifelong.

Early Antigen

EA is a complex of two components, early antigen–*diffuse* (EA-D), which is found in the nucleus and cytoplasm of the B cells, and early antigen–*restricted* (EA-R), usually found as a mass only in the cytoplasm.

Anti–EA-D of the IgG type is highly indicative of acute infection, but it is not detectable in 10% to 20% of patients with infectious mononucleosis. EA-D disappears in about 3 months; however, a rise in titer is demonstrated during reactivation of a latent EBV infection.

Anti–EA-R IgG is not usually found in young adults during the acute phase but may be seen in the serum of very young children during the acute phase. Anti–EA-R IgG appears transiently in the later, convalescent phase. In general, anti–EA-D and anti–EA-R IgG are not consistent indicators of the disease stage.

Epstein-Barr Nuclear Antigen

Epstein-Barr nuclear antigen (EBNA) is found in the nucleus of all EBV-infected cells. Although the synthesis of NA precedes EA synthesis during the infection of B cells, EBNA does not become available

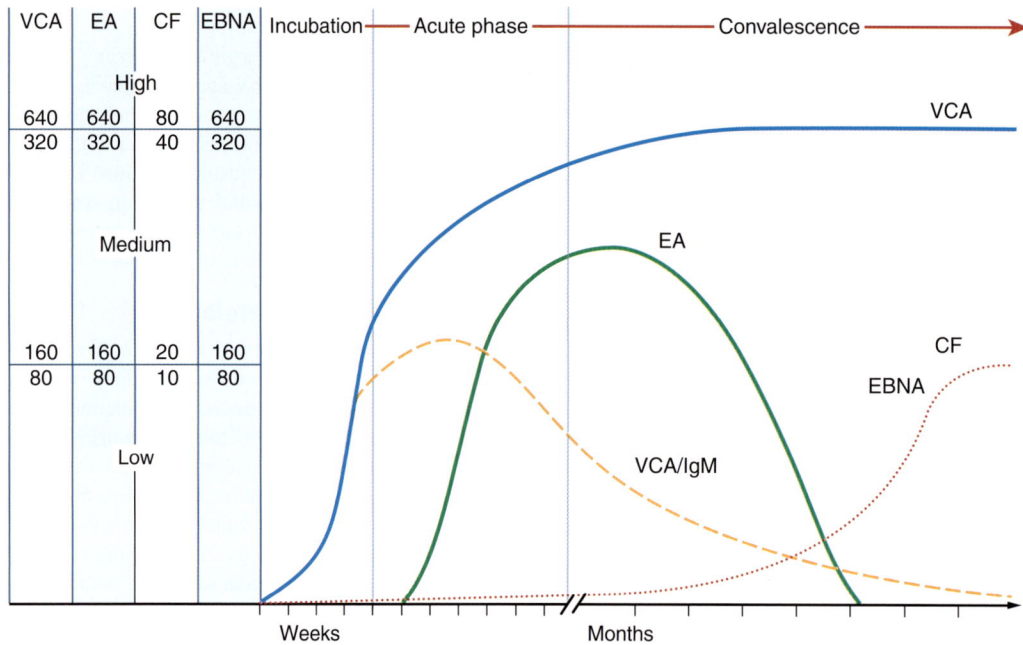

Fig. 17.2 Epstein-Barr Virus (EBV) Antibody Response During the Course of Infectious Mononucleosis. *CF*, Complement fixation test; *EA*, early antigen; *EBNA*, Epstein-Barr nuclear antigen; *IgM*, immunoglobulin M; *VCA*, viral capsid antigen. (Redrawn from Krugman S, Katz SL, Gershon AA, Wilfert CM, editors: *Infectious disease of children*, ed 9, St. Louis, 1992, Mosby Year Book.)

TABLE 17.2	Characteristic Antibody Formation in Infectious Mononucleosis.					
Parameter	VCA IgM	VCA IgG	EA-D	EA-R	EBNA IgG	Heterophile
No previous exposure	−	−	−	−	−	−
Recent (acute) infection	+	+	±	−	−	+
Past infection (convalescent) period	−	+	−	−	+	−
Reactivation of latent infection	±	+	±	±	+	±

EA-D, Early antigen–diffuse; *EA-R*, early antigen–restricted; *EBNA*, Epstein-Barr nuclear antigen; *IgG*, immunoglobulin G; *IgM*, immunoglobulin M; *VCA*, viral capsid antigen.

for antibody stimulation until after the incubation period of infectious mononucleosis, when activated T lymphocytes destroy the EBV genome–carrying B cells. As a result antibodies to EBNA are absent or barely detectable during acute infectious mononucleosis.

Anti-EBNA IgG does not appear until a patient has entered the convalescent period. EBNA antibodies are almost always present in sera containing IgG antibodies to VCA of EBV unless the patient is in the early acute phase of infectious mononucleosis. Patients with severe immunologic defects or immunosuppressive disease may not have EBNA antibodies, even if antibodies to VCA are present.

Under normal conditions, antibody titers to NA gradually increase through convalescence and reach a plateau 3 to 12 months after infection. The antibody titer remains at a moderate, measurable level indefinitely because of the persistent viral carrier state established after primary EBV infection. Most healthy individuals with previous exposure to EBV have antibody titers to EBNA that range from 1:10 to 1:160. In EBV-associated malignancies, the levels of EBNA antibody are usually high in patients with nasopharyngeal carcinoma and can range from barely detectable to very high levels in patients with Burkitt lymphoma.

Test results of antibodies to EBNA should be evaluated in relation to patient symptoms, clinical history, and antibody response patterns to VCA and EA to establish a diagnosis (Table 17.3). The antibody profile can be especially useful. For example, a patient with an infectious mononucleosis–like illness caused by reactivation of a persistent EBV infection resulting from an immunosuppressive malignancy or nonmalignant disease can demonstrate high titers of IgM and IgG VCA antibodies. If the antibody to EBNA is also elevated, however, a diagnosis of primary EBV infection can be excluded.

Additional Testing

Immunofluorescence is a common method used for EBV serology testing. Antigen substrate slides containing EBV-infected B cells are incubated with the patient's serum. The presence of specific antibody is detected by the addition of fluorescein-conjugated antihuman IgG or IgM. The disadvantages of this type of testing are that it is time-consuming, difficult to interpret, and prone to interference from other serum components (e.g., rheumatoid factor).

TABLE 17.3 Characteristic Diagnostic Profile of Epstein-Barr Virus.

Stage	Description
Susceptibility	If the patient is seronegative (lacks antibody to VCA).
Primary infection	Antibody (IgM) to VCA is present; EBNA is absent. High or rising titer of antibody (IgG) to VCA and no evidence of antibody to EBNA after at least 4 weeks of symptoms.
Reactivation	If antibody to EBNA and increased antibodies to EA are present, patient may be experiencing reactivation.
Past infection	Antibodies to VCA and EBNA are present.

EA, Early antigen; *EBNA*, Epstein-Barr nuclear antigen; *IgG*, immunoglobulin G; *IgM*, immunoglobulin M; *VCA*, viral capsid antigen.

CASE STUDY 17.1 History and Physical Examination

A female college freshman visits the infirmary complaining of extreme fatigue, frequent headaches, and a sore throat. A routine physical examination by the college physician shows that the patient had swollen lymph nodes (lymphadenopathy), redness of the throat, and a slightly enlarged spleen. A complete blood count (CBC), urinalysis (UA), and mononucleosis screening test are ordered.

Laboratory Data
CBC
- Hemoglobin and microhematocrit—within normal range
- Total leukocyte count—elevated (13.5×10^9/L)
- Leukocyte differential—elevated lymphocytes (56%)
- Many variant forms of lymphocytes (25%)

Urinalysis—normal
Mononucleosis screening test—negative

Therapy and Follow-Up
The physician prescribes bed rest and medication for the patient's headache. A follow-up appointment is scheduled for 10 days later.

Questions
1. Heterophil antibodies cannot be characterized as:
    a. Reacts with horse and sheep RBCs
    b. Absorbed by beef RBCs
    c. Not absorbed by guinea pig kidney cells
    d. Not absorbed by beef RBCs

2. The immunologic response expressed by Epstein-Barr virus (EBV)–infected lymphocytes encoded by the virus that may persist for a lifetime is:
    a. Early antigen (EA)
    b. Viral capsid antigen (VCA)
    c. Epstein-Barr nuclear antigen (EBNA)
    d. Anti-VCA IgM

Answers to these questions can be found in Appendix A.

Critical Thinking Group Discussion Questions
1. What is this patient's absolute lymphocyte count? Is this considered normal?
2. What is the most probable diagnosis of this disorder?
3. If repeat testing is performed on the patient after 10 days, could any of the results vary?
4. Discuss the antibodies that could occur in this patient's condition.
5. What type of antigens could be tested for in the blood?

The enzyme-linked immunosorbent assay (ELISA) may be used to detect antibodies to EBNA. This ELISA uses a synthetic peptide antigen to determine the relative amounts of IgM and IgG antibodies in patient serum or plasma. Its sensitivity is reportedly 98.9%, with a specificity of 99.0%.

TABLE 17.4	Agglutinins for Sheep Erythrocytes in Human Serum.	
Type of Serum	Absorbed by Guinea Pig Kidney	Absorbed by Beef Erythrocytes
Normal	Positive (+)	Negative (−)
Infectious mononucleosis	Negative (−)	Positive (+)
Serum sickness	Positive (+)	Positive (+)

REVIEW QUESTIONS

1. Epstein-Barr virus (EBV) can cause all the following *except*:
   a. Infectious mononucleosis
   b. Burkitt lymphoma
   c. Nasopharyngeal carcinoma
   d. Neoplasms of the bone marrow
2. The primary mode of EBV transmission is:
   a. Exposure to blood
   b. Exposure to oropharyngeal secretions
   c. Congenital transmission
   d. Fecal contamination of drinking water
3. An asymptomatic infection with EBV is a typical illness seen in:
   a. Infants
   b. Adolescents
   c. Adults over 30 years old
   d. Adults over 65 years old
4. IgM heterophile antibody is characterized by all of the following features *except*:
   a. Reacts with horse, ox, and sheep RBCs
   b. Absorbed by beef erythrocytes
   c. Absorbed by guinea pig kidney cells
   d. Does not react with EBV-specific antigens
5. Characteristics of EBV-infected lymphocytes include all of the following *except*:
   a. B type
   b. Expression of viral capsid antigen
   c. Expression of early antigen
   d. Expression of EBV genome
6. Which of the following stages of infectious mononucleosis infection is characterized by antibody to Epstein-Barr nuclear antigen (EBNA)?
   a. Recent (acute) infection
   b. Past infection (convalescent) period
   c. Reactivation of latent infection
   d. Both b and c
7. Which of the following stages of infectious mononucleosis infection is/(are) characterized by heterophile antibody?
   a. Recent (acute) infection
   b. Past infection (convalescent) period
   c. Reactivation of latent infection
   d. Both a and c
8. What percentage of the world's population is exposed to EBV?
   a. 25%
   b. 50%
   c. 75%
   d. 95%
9. Infectious mononucleosis postperfusion syndrome is a primary infection resulting from a blood transfusion from a(n) _____ to a(n) _____ recipient.
   a. Immune; nonimmune
   b. Nonimmune; immune
   c. Infected; nonimmune
   d. Infected; immune
10. In infectious mononucleosis, there is no:
    a. Acute state
    b. Latent state
    c. Carrier state
    d. Reactivation
11. The incubation period of infectious mononucleosis is:
    a. 2 to 4 days
    b. 10 to 15 days
    c. 10 to 50 days
    d. 51 to 90 days
12. The use of horse erythrocytes in rapid slide tests for infectious mononucleosis increases their:
    a. Cost
    b. Sensitivity
    c. Specificity
    d. Both b and c
13. EBV-infected B lymphocytes express all the following new antigens *except*:
    a. Viral capsid antigen (VCA)
    b. Early antigen (EA)
    c. Cytoplasmic antigen (CA)
    d. Nuclear antigen (NA)
14. Anti-EBNA IgG does not appear until a patient has entered the:
    a. Initial phase of infection
    b. Primary infection phase
    c. Convalescent period
    d. Reactivation of infectious stage
15. An appropriate description of the Paul-Bunnell screening test is:
    a. Distinguishes between heterophile antibodies; uses beef erythrocytes, guinea pig kidney cells, and sheep erythrocytes
    b. Detects heterophile antibodies and uses horse erythrocytes
    c. Detects heterophile antibodies and uses sheep erythrocytes
    d. Detects heterophile antibodies and uses rabbit erythrocytes
16. An appropriate description of the Davidsohn differential test is:
    a. Distinguishes between heterophile antibodies; uses beef erythrocytes, guinea pig kidney cells, and sheep erythrocytes
    b. Detects heterophile antibodies and uses horse erythrocytes
    c. Detects heterophile antibodies and uses sheep erythrocytes
    d. Detects heterophile antibodies and uses rabbit erythrocytes
17. An appropriate description of the MonoSlide agglutination test is:
    a. Distinguishes between heterophile antibodies; uses beef erythrocytes, guinea pig kidney cells, and sheep erythrocytes
    b. Detects heterophile antibodies and uses horse erythrocytes
    c. Detects heterophile antibodies and uses sheep erythrocytes
    d. Detects heterophile antibodies and uses rabbit erythrocytes
18. What is the correct sequence of the immunologic EBV response in infectious mononucleosis?
    a. VCA, VCA/IgM, EA, EBNA
    b. EA, EBNA, VCA, VCA/IgM
    c. VCA/IgM, EBNA, VCA, EA
    d. EBNA, VCA, EA, VCA/IgM

18

Viral Hepatitis

LEARNING OUTCOMES

- Identify and describe the characteristics of the various forms of primary infectious hepatitis, including laboratory assays.
- Compare the etiology, epidemiology, signs and symptoms, laboratory evaluation, and prevention of hepatitis A, acute hepatitis B, chronic hepatitis B, and hepatitis C.
- Analyze case studies related to the immune response for various forms of hepatitis.
- Correctly answer case study–related multiple-choice questions.
- Participate in a discussion of critical thinking questions.
- Describe the principle, results, and limitations of the rapid hepatitis C virus test.
- Correctly answer 80% of the end-of-chapter review questions.

OUTLINE

General Characteristics of Hepatitis, 274
    Etiology, 274
    Incidence, 274
    Signs and Symptoms, 274
    Differential Diagnosis of Hepatitis, 274
Hepatitis A, 274
    Etiology, 275
    Epidemiology, 275
    Signs and Symptoms, 275
    Immunologic Manifestations, 276
    Diagnostic Evaluation, 276
    Prevention and Treatment, 276
Hepatitis B, 278
    Etiology, 278
    Epidemiology, 278
    Signs and Symptoms, 280
        Asymptomatic Infection, 280
    Laboratory Assays, 281
        Hepatitis B Surface Antigen, 281
        Hepatitis B–Related Antigen, 284
        Hepatitis B Core Antibody, 284
        Antibodies to Hepatitis B e Antigen and Hepatitis B Surface Antigen, 285
        Hepatitis B Viral DNA, 285
    Diagnostic Evaluation, 285
        Interrelationship of Test Results, 285
    Differentiating Acute and Chronic Hepatitis and the Chronic Carrier State, 285
        Acute Infection, 285
        Chronic Infection, 286
        Carrier State, 286
    Prevention and Treatment, 287
Hepatitis D, 287
    Etiology, 287
    Epidemiology, 287
    Signs and Symptoms, 288
    Immunologic Manifestations, 288
        Coinfection with Hepatitis B Virus, 288
        Superinfection of Hepatitis B Carrier, 288
    Diagnostic Evaluation, 288
Hepatitis C, 288
    Etiology, 288
    Epidemiology, 288
    Viral Transmission, 289
        Posttransfusion Hepatitis, 289
        Parenteral and Occupational Exposure, 289
        Sexual Transmission, 289
        Other Sources, 289
        Prognosis, 289
    Signs and Symptoms, 290
    Traditional Hepatitis C Virus Testing, 290
        Polymerase Chain Reaction, 290
    Acute and Chronic Hepatitis C, 291
        Acute Hepatitis C, 291
        Chronic Hepatitis C, 291
    Treatment, 292
    Prevention, 292
Hepatitis E, 292
    Etiology, 292
    Epidemiology, 292
    Signs and Symptoms, 292
    Immunologic Manifestations, 293
    Diagnostic Evaluation, 293
    Prevention and Treatment, 293
Transfusion-Transmitted Virus, 293
    Etiology, 293
    Epidemiology, 293
    Signs and Symptoms, 293
Case Study 18.1, 293
Case Study 18.2, 294

Case Study 18.3, 294
Case Study 18.4, 294

Procedure: Rapid Hepatitis C Virus Testing, 297.e1

KEY TERMS

- anicteric
- capsid
- chronicity
- coinfection
- **Dane particles**
- fulminant disease
- hepadnavirus
- hepatitis B core antigen (HBcAg)
- hepatoma
- necrosis
- nucleocapsid protein
- prodromal
- sequelae
- viremia
- virions

GENERAL CHARACTERISTICS OF HEPATITIS

The term *hepatitis* refers to inflammation of the liver. This chapter discusses infectious hepatitis caused by various viruses.

According to the World Health Organization (WHO), 2 billion people are infected with hepatitis and almost one-third of the world's population has been infected with one of the known hepatitis viruses. In the United States acute viral hepatitis most commonly is caused by infection with hepatitis A virus (HAV), hepatitis B virus (HBV), or hepatitis C virus (HCV). These unrelated viruses are transmitted via different routes and have different epidemiologic profiles. Safe and effective vaccines have been available for hepatitis B since 1981 and for hepatitis A since 1995.

> **KEY CONCEPTS: Facts About Hepatitis Virus**
> - Viral agents of acute hepatitis can be divided into primary hepatitis viruses—A, B, C, D, E, and G—and also secondary hepatitis viruses, including Epstein-Barr virus, cytomegalovirus, herpes virus, and others. Primary hepatitis viruses account for approximately 95% of the cases of hepatitis.
> - As a clinical disease, hepatitis can occur in an acute or chronic form.

Etiology

Viral hepatitis is the most common liver disease worldwide. The viral agents of acute hepatitis can be divided into two major groups as follows:
- Primary hepatitis viruses: A, B, C, D, E, and G
- Secondary hepatitis viruses: Epstein-Barr virus (EBV), cytomegalovirus (CMV), herpes virus, and others

Incidence

Primary hepatitis viruses account for approximately 95% of the cases of hepatitis. These viruses are classified as primary hepatitis viruses because they attack primarily the liver and have little direct effect on other organ systems. The secondary viruses involve the liver secondarily in the course of systemic infection of another body system. The viruses for hepatitis types A, B, C, D, E, and GB virus C, as well as the secondary viruses (e.g., EBV and CMV), have been isolated and identified (Table 18.1).

Signs and Symptoms

As a clinical disease, hepatitis can occur in an acute or a chronic form. The signs and symptoms of hepatitis are extremely variable. It can be mild, transient, and completely asymptomatic, or it can be severe, prolonged, and ultimately fatal. Many fatalities are attributed to hepatocellular carcinoma, of which hepatitis viruses B and C are the primary causes. The course of viral hepatitis can take one of four forms: acute, fulminant acute, subclinical without jaundice, and chronic (Table 18.2).

Differential Diagnosis of Hepatitis

Identification of various types of hepatitis can be initiated with an overall screening approach (Fig. 18.1).

HEPATITIS A

> **KEY CONCEPTS: Hepatitis A Characteristics**
> - Hepatitis A virus (HAV; formerly infectious or short-incubation hepatitis) is common in underdeveloped or developing countries.
> - HAV is transmitted almost exclusively by a fecal-oral route during the early phase of acute illness because the virus is shed in feces for up to 4 weeks after infection occurs.
> - The incidence of HAV is not increased in healthcare workers or dialysis patients.

TABLE 18.1 Characteristics of Viral Hepatitis

Parameter	Type A	Type B	Type D (delta agent)	Type C	Type E	GB Virus
Molecular Composition	RNA	DNA	RNA	RNA	RNA	RNA
Antigens	HA Ag	HBsAg, HBcAg, HBeAg	Delta	HCV	HEV	GB-C
Antibodies	Anti-HAV	Anti-HBs, anti-HBc, anti-HBe	Antidelta	Anti-HCV	IgM anti-HEV IgG anti-HEV	Anti-HGV
Epidemiology	Fecal-oral	Parenteral, other	Parenteral, other	Parenteral and nonparenteral	Fecal-oral	Parenteral

Anti-HBc, Hepatitis B core antibody; *anti-HBe*, hepatitis B e antibody; *anti-HBs*, hepatitis B surface antibody; *anti-HCV*, hepatitis C antibody; *anti-HEV*, hepatitis E antibody; *anti-HGV*, hepatitis G antibody; *HA Ag*, hepatitis A antigen; *HBcAg*, hepatitis B core antigen; *HBeAg*, hepatitis B e antigen; *HBsAg*, hepatitis B surface antigen; *HCV*, hepatitis C virus; *HEV*, hepatitis E virus.
From the Centers for Disease Control and Prevention: What is viral hepatitis? https://www.cdc.gov/hepatitis.

TABLE 18.2 Forms of Hepatitis

Form	Characteristics
Acute hepatitis	Typical form with associated jaundice. Four phases: incubation, preicteric, icteric, and convalescence. Incubation period, from time of exposure and first day of symptoms, ranges from a few days to many months. Average length of time is 75 days (range: 40–180 days) in HBV infection.
Fulminant acute hepatitis	Rare form of hepatitis associated with hepatic failure.
Subclinical hepatitis without jaundice	Probably accounts for persons with demonstrable antibodies in their serum but no reported history of hepatitis.
Chronic hepatitis	Accompanied by hepatic inflammation and necrosis that lasts for at least 6 months. Occurs in about 10% of patients with HBV infection.

HBV, Hepatitis B virus.

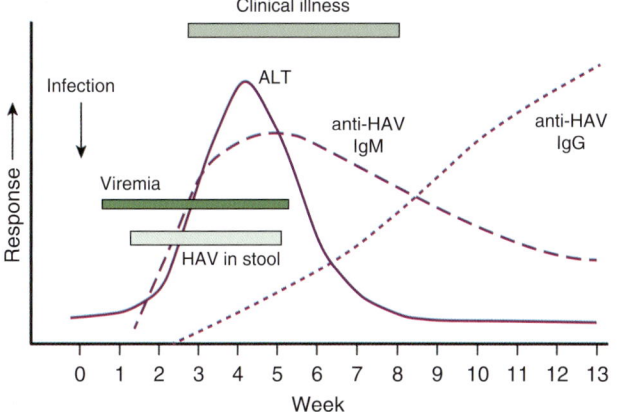

Fig. 18.1 Hepatitis Virus Screening. (From CDC.gov Serological Course of HAV infection and recovery. https://www.cdc.gov/hepatitis-a/hcp/diagnosis-testing/index.html#:~:text=Typical%20serologic%20course%20of%20HAV,persists%20to%20provide%20lifelong%20immunity. Accessed on October 16, 2024.)

Etiology

HAV is a small, RNA-containing picornavirus and the only hepatitis virus that has been successfully grown in culture (Fig. 18.2A). The structure is a simple, nonenveloped virus with a nucleocapsid designated as the hepatitis A (HA) antigen (HA Ag). Inside the capsid is a single molecule of single-strand RNA. The RNA has a positive polarity, and proteins are translated directly from the RNA. Replication of HAV appears to be limited to the cytoplasm of the hepatocyte.

The highest titers of HAV are detected in acute-phase stool samples. Human infectivity of saliva and urine from patients with acute hepatitis A does not pose a significant risk. Sexual contact has been suggested as a possible mode of transmission.

Epidemiology

HAV was formerly called *infectious hepatitis* or *short-incubation hepatitis*. In unvaccinated children, primarily in resource-limited countries, hepatitis A is primarily a disease of young children. The prevalence of infection, as measured by the presence of antibody (immunoglobulin G [IgG] anti-HAV), approaches 100% at or shortly after 5 years of age. The incidence of hepatitis A varies by age.

According to the Centers for Disease Control and Prevention (CDC), outbreaks associated with person-to-person transmission have since been reported in multiple states, resulting in substantial increases in hepatitis A peaking at 18,846 reported cases in 2019, then decreasing in 2020 and 2021. During 2022, the number of reported cases was 2265, which corresponds to 4500 estimated infections after adjusting for case underascertainment and underreporting. The number of reported cases during 2022 corresponds to a 60% decrease from 2021 but remains 1.6 times the number reported during 2015, before the hepatitis A outbreaks associated with person-to-person transmission were first reported. During 2022, 14 out of 23 states with ongoing outbreaks declared an end to their outbreaks. Disruptions to healthcare access and health department surveillance capacity during the COVID-19 pandemic may have affected the ability to detect, investigate, and report all hepatitis A cases during 2020–2022.

Persons aged 30–39 years have the highest rate of hepatitis A. Hepatitis A infection is noted for occurring in isolated outbreaks or as an epidemic, but it also may occur sporadically. It is rarely a transfusion-acquired hepatitis because of its transient nature.

Globally, HAV infection is most common in countries with poor sanitary conditions and hygienic practices and in transitional economies according to the WHO.

Susceptibility to infection is independent of gender and race. Crowded, unsanitary conditions are a definite risk factor. HAV is transmitted almost exclusively by a fecal-oral route during the early phase of acute illness; the virus is shed in feces for up to 4 weeks after infection. Large outbreaks are usually traceable to a common source, such as an infected food handler, contaminated water supply, or consumption of raw shellfish. Institutions and day care centers also are known to be favorable sources for transmission.

Improvements in socioeconomic and sanitary conditions and declining family size may be responsible for a decreasing frequency of infection, and the incidence of HAV infection is not increasing among healthcare workers or in dialysis patients. Maternal-neonatal transmission of HAV is not recognized as an epidemiologic entity. Person-to-person contact, usually among children and young adults, remains the major route of HAV infection.

The most commonly identified risk factor for hepatitis A has been international travel by unvaccinated persons. Most travel-related cases have been associated with travel to Mexico and Central or South America. As HAV transmission in the United States has decreased, cases among travelers to countries where hepatitis is endemic have accounted for an increased proportion of all cases.

Sexual contact and household contact with another person with hepatitis A have been among the most commonly identified risk factors. Street drugs are also a source of HAV infection.

Signs and Symptoms

Nonimmune adult patients infected with HAV develop clinical symptoms on average 28 days after exposure. However, hepatitis A is often a subclinical disease, and many patients are anicteric. Clinically apparent cases show elevated serum liver chemistry enzyme and bilirubin levels, with jaundice developing several days later. Viremia and fecal shedding of virus disappear at the onset of jaundice. Atypical presentations include prolonged intrahepatic cholestasis, relapsing course, and extrahepatic immune complex deposition, all of which resolve spontaneously.

Complete clinical recovery is anticipated in almost all patients. Hepatitis A rarely causes fulminant hepatitis and does not progress to chronic liver disease. Unusual clinical variants of hepatitis A include cholestatic, relapsing, and protracted hepatitis. In cholestatic hepatitis, serum bilirubin levels may be dramatically elevated (>20 mg/dL), and jaundice persists for weeks to months before resolution. In relapsing hepatitis and protracted hepatitis, complete resolution is anticipated.

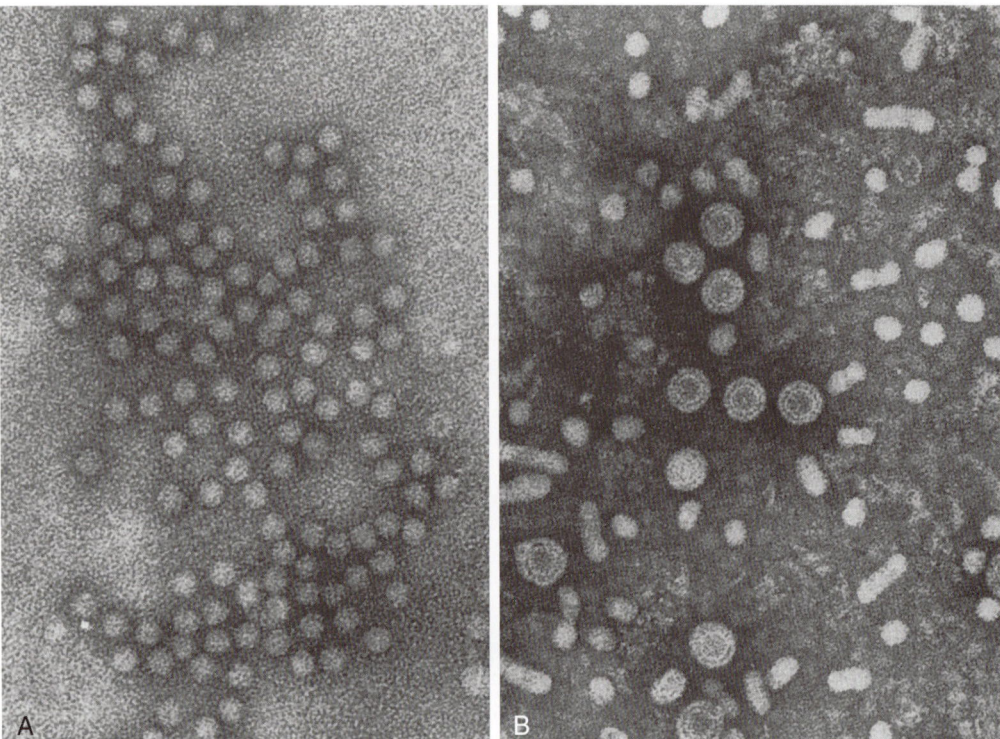

Fig. 18.2 Electron Micrographs of Hepatitis Viruses. (A) Hepatitis A virus (HAV). (B) Hepatitis B virus (HBV). Note the Dane particles. (From Katz SL, Gershon AA, Wilfert CM, Krugman S, editors: *Infectious diseases of children,* ed 9, St. Louis, 1992, Mosby.)

A chronic carrier state (persistent infection) and chronic hepatitis (chronic liver disease) do not occur as long-term sequelae of hepatitis A. Rarely, injection with HAV may cause fulminant hepatitis, with about 0.1% mortality. Fulminant hepatitis is the most likely complication of coinfection with other hepatitis viruses.

Immunologic Manifestations

Shortly after the onset of fecal shedding, an immunoglobulin M (IgM) antibody is detectable in serum, followed within a few days by the appearance of an IgG antibody. IgM anti-HAV is almost always detectable in patients with acute HAV. IgG anti-HAV, a manifestation of immunity, peaks after the acute illness and remains detectable indefinitely, perhaps lifelong.

The finding of IgM anti-HAV in a patient with acute viral hepatitis is highly diagnostic of acute HAV. Demonstration of IgG anti-HAV indicates previous infection. The presence of IgG anti-HAV protects against subsequent infection with HAV but is not protective against hepatitis B or other viruses.

Diagnostic Evaluation

Testing methods for HAV include HAV antibody, IgM, or an acute hepatitis panel A virus. If this assay is positive, a diagnosis of acute hepatitis A is confirmed.

The short period of viremia makes detection difficult. Specific IgM antibody usually appears about 4 weeks after infection and may persist for up to 4 months after the onset of clinical symptoms. The presence of IgG or total (IgM and IgG) antibody indicates past infection or immunization and associated immunity. The total assay detects IgM and IgG antibodies but does not differentiate between them. The hepatitis A antibody IgM assay is appropriate when acute HAV infection is suspected. Specific IgG antibody apparently protects an individual from symptomatic infection, but specific IgM may increase with reinfection. In the acute phase of HAV, liver chemistry levels (e.g., serum liver enzyme levels) will be elevated and may aid in establishing the diagnosis.

Molecular testing is not used routinely in the clinical laboratory for detection of HAV. This methodology is used by public health officials when investigating disease outbreaks and testing of water sources.

Prevention and Treatment

The first effective control measures to prevent enterically transmitted viral hepatitis resulted from World War II research. In 1945 the following were demonstrated: (1) infectious virus could be transmitted by contaminated drinking water; (2) treatment of the water by filtration and chlorination made it safe to drink; and (3) gamma globulin derived from convalescent-phase serum from patients with hepatitis could protect adults from clinical hepatitis. For 50 years, refining food and water preparation and establishing standards for immunoglobulin constituted the methods of HAV prevention. An individual who has had close contact with an HAV-infected person should receive passive immunization with immunoglobulin intramuscularly.

A safe, highly immunogenic, formalin-inactivated, single-dose vaccine is available to prevent HAV infection (Box 18.1). HAV vaccine should be targeted at high-risk groups (e.g., staff in childcare centers; food handlers; international travelers, including military personnel; homosexual men; and institutionalized patients).

Universal childhood vaccination may prove to be the most cost-effective method of protecting large populations, both nationally and globally. Routine childhood hepatitis A vaccination is recommended.

In May 2001, the US Food and Drug Administration (FDA) approved a new combination vaccine that protects individuals 18 years of age or older against diseases caused by HAV and HBV. The vaccine, Twinrix

BOX 18.1 Hepatitis Vaccine: Questions and Answers

Hepatitis A

Who Should Get Vaccinated Against Hepatitis A?

The Advisory Committee on Immunization Practices (ACIP) recommends hepatitis A vaccination for the following people:

- All children at age 1 year
- Travelers to countries where hepatitis A is common
- Family and caregivers of adoptees from countries where hepatitis A is common
- Men who have sexual encounters with other men
- Users of recreational drugs, whether injected or not
- People with unstable housing or experiencing homelessness
- People with chronic or long-term liver disease, including hepatitis B or hepatitis C
- People with clotting factor disorders
- People with direct contact with others who have hepatitis A
- Any person wishing to obtain immunity (protection)

How is the Hepatitis A Vaccine Given?

The hepatitis A vaccine is safe and effective and given as two shots, 6 months apart. Both shots are needed for long-term protection. The hepatitis A vaccine also comes in a combination form, containing both hepatitis A and B vaccine, that can be given to anyone 18 years of age or older. This combination vaccine is given as three shots, over 6 months. All three shots are needed for long-term protection against both hepatitis A and B.

Is the Hepatitis A Vaccine Effective?

Yes, the hepatitis A vaccine is highly effective in preventing hepatitis A virus infection. A second hepatitis A shot results in long-term protection.

Is the Hepatitis A Vaccine Safe?

Yes, the hepatitis A vaccine is safe. No serious side effects have been reported from the hepatitis A vaccine. Soreness at the injection site is the most common side effect reported. As with any medicine, there is always a small risk that a serious problem could occur after someone gets the vaccine. However, the potential risks associated with hepatitis A are much greater than the potential risks associated with the hepatitis A vaccine. Since the licensure of the first hepatitis A vaccine in 1995, millions of doses of hepatitis A vaccine have been given in the United States and worldwide.

Who Should not Receive the Hepatitis A Vaccine?

People who have ever had a serious allergic reaction to the hepatitis A vaccine or who are known to be allergic to any part of the hepatitis A vaccine should not receive the vaccine. Tell your doctor if you have any severe allergies. In addition, the vaccine is not licensed for use in infants under age 1 year.

What is Immunoglobulin?

Immunoglobulin (IG) is a substance made from human blood plasma that contains antibodies that protect against infection. IG is a shot and provides short-term protection against hepatitis A for up to 2 months, depending on the dosage given. IG is sometimes used before travel to a country where hepatitis A is common. IG is also used to prevent infection after exposure to the hepatitis A virus but must be given within 2 weeks after exposure for the best protection.

Will the Hepatitis A Vaccine Protect Me from Other Forms of Hepatitis?

No, the hepatitis A vaccine will only protect you against hepatitis A. There is a separate vaccine available for hepatitis B. There is also a combination of hepatitis A and hepatitis B vaccine that offers protection for both viruses. There is no vaccine for hepatitis C at this time.

Can Hepatitis A Vaccine Be Given to People with Compromised Immune Systems, Such as Hemodialysis Patients or People with AIDS?

Yes. The hepatitis A vaccine is inactivated (not "live"), so it can be given to people with compromised immune systems.

Is it Harmful to Have an Extra Dose of Hepatitis A Vaccine or to Repeat the Entire Hepatitis A Vaccine Series?

No, getting extra doses of hepatitis A vaccine is not harmful.

What Should be Done if the Last Dose of Hepatitis A Vaccine is Delayed?

If the second dose has been delayed (more than 6 months since the first dose was given), the second, or last dose, should be given as soon as possible. The first dose does not need to be given again.

Hepatitis B

Who Should Get Vaccinated Against Hepatitis B?

Hepatitis B vaccination is recommended for:

- All infants
- All children and adolescents younger than 19 years of age who have not been vaccinated
- People at risk for infection by sexual exposure
- People whose sex partners have hepatitis B
  - Sexually active people who are not in a long-term, mutually monogamous relationship (for example, people with more than one sex partner during the previous 6 months)
  - People seeking evaluation or treatment for a sexually transmitted infection
  - Men who have sex with men
- People at risk for infection by exposure to blood
  - People who inject drugs
  - People who live with a person who has hepatitis B
  - Residents and staff of facilities for developmentally disabled people
  - Healthcare and public safety workers at risk for exposure to blood or blood-contaminated body fluids on the job
  - Hemodialysis patients and predialysis, peritoneal dialysis, and home dialysis patients
  - People with diabetes aged 19 to 59 years; people with diabetes aged 60 or older should ask their healthcare professional.
- International travelers to countries where hepatitis B is common
- People with hepatitis C virus infection
- People with chronic liver disease
- People with human immunodeficiency virus (HIV) infection
- People who are in jail or prison
- All other people seeking protection from hepatitis B virus infection

Is the Hepatitis B Vaccine Recommended Before International Travel?

The risk of hepatitis B virus infection in international travelers is generally low, although people traveling to certain countries are at an increased risk. Travelers to countries where hepatitis B is common should get the hepatitis B vaccine.

Is the Hepatitis B Vaccine Safe?

Yes, the hepatitis B vaccine is safe. Soreness at the injection site is the most common side effect reported. As with any medicine, there are very small risks that a serious problem could occur after getting the vaccine. The safety of vaccines is always being monitored. For more information, visit the Centers for Disease Control and Prevention (CDC) vaccine safety site.

Continued

BOX 18.1 Hepatitis Vaccine: Questions and Answers—cont'd

Is it Harmful to have an Extra dose of Hepatitis B Vaccine or to Repeat the Entire Hepatitis B Vaccine Series?
No, getting extra doses of hepatitis B vaccine is not harmful.

What Should be done if Hepatitis B Vaccine Series was not Completed?
Talk to your doctor to resume the vaccine series as soon as possible. The series does not need to be restarted. If the series is interrupted, the next dose should be given as soon as possible.

Who Should not Receive the Hepatitis B Vaccine?
Anyone who has had a serious allergic reaction to a prior dose of hepatitis B vaccine, to any part of the vaccine, or yeast should not get the hepatitis B vaccine. When hepatitis B vaccine is given as part of a combination vaccine, possible reasons for not getting the other vaccine(s) should be checked.

Are Booster Doses of the Hepatitis B Vaccine Necessary?
It depends. A "booster" dose of hepatitis B vaccine is a dose that increases or extends the effectiveness of the vaccine. Booster doses are not recommended for most healthy people. Booster doses are recommended only in certain circumstances, and the need for booster doses is determined by a certain blood test that looks for hepatitis B surface antibody (anti-HBs).

Are there Reasons to get Tested for Hepatitis B Immunity?
There are many different reasons for a person to get a blood test that looks for hepatitis B immunity through the presence of surface antibody (anti-HBs). The test is especially important for people who may or have been exposed to the blood of a person infected with the hepatitis B virus. This includes:
- Infants born to mothers with hepatitis B
- Healthcare providers
- Hemodialysis patients
- Sex partners of someone with hepatitis B
- Any other people who have an ongoing risk of exposure to the blood of an infected person

The test can help determine if the person needs another dose of the hepatitis B vaccine in order to help give them further protection against infection.

Is there a vaccine that will protect me from both hepatitis A and hepatitis B?
Yes, there is a combination vaccine approved for adults that protects people from both hepatitis A and hepatitis B. The combined hepatitis A and B vaccine is usually given as three separate doses over a 6-month period.

Can I get the hepatitis B vaccine at the same time as other vaccines?
Yes. Getting two different vaccines at the same time has not been shown to be harmful.

From the Centers for Disease Control and Prevention (CDC): Viral hepatitis. https://www.cdc.gov/hepatitis.

(GlaxoSmithKline Beecham, Philadelphia, Pennsylvania), combines two already approved vaccines, Havrix (hepatitis A vaccine, inactivated) and Engerix-B (hepatitis B vaccine, recombinant) so that those at high risk for exposure to both viruses can be immunized against both at the same time. Areas with a high rate of both HAV and HBV include Africa, parts of South America, most of the Middle East, and South and Southeast Asia. Clinical trials of Twinrix, given in a three-dose series at ages 0, 1, and 6 months, have shown that the combination vaccine is as safe and effective as the already licensed, separate HAV and HBV vaccines.

HEPATITIS B

> **KEY CONCEPTS: Facts About Hepatitis B**
> - Reported cases of acute hepatitis B have decreased dramatically in the United States in the past 15 years.
> - HBV is largely spread parenterally through blood transfusion, needlestick accidents, and contaminated needles, although the virus can be transmitted in the absence of obvious parenteral exposure.
> - Serologic markers for HBV infection include hepatitis B surface antigen (HBsAg), hepatitis B e antigen (HBeAg), hepatitis B core antibody (anti-HBc), hepatitis B e antibody (anti-HBe), hepatitis B surface antibody (anti-HBs), and DNA analysis.
> - Hepatitis D virus (HDV; initially the delta agent) superinfects some patients already infected with HBV.

Etiology

HBV is the classic example of a virus acquired through blood transfusion before the development of laboratory screening procedures and vaccination. HBV serves as a model for viral infections transmitted by blood (Fig. 18.2B).

Hepatitis B surface antigen (HBsAg) was discovered in 1966. This discovery, and its subsequent association with HBV, led to the biochemical and epidemiologic characterization of HBV infection.

Hepatitis B is a complex DNA virus that belongs to the family Hepadnaviridae; a member of this family is known as a **hepadnavirus**. Eight different HBV genotypes with differences in clinical outcomes have been identified. Viral proteins of importance include the following:

1. The envelope protein: HBsAg
2. A structural nucleocapsid core protein: **hepatitis B core antigen (HBcAg)**
3. A soluble **nucleocapsid protein**: hepatitis B e antigen (HBeAg)

The unique structure of the DNA of HBV is one of the distinguishing characteristics of a hepadnavirus. The DNA is circular and double stranded, but one of the strands is incomplete, leaving a single-strand or gap region that accounts for 10% to 50% of the total length of the molecule. The other DNA strand is nicked (3′ and 5′ ends are not joined). The entire DNA molecule is small, and all the genetic information for producing both HBsAg and HBcAg is on the complete strand.

HBV relies on a retroviral replication strategy (reverse transcription from RNA to DNA). The steps in viral replication are described in Fig. 18.3.

Epidemiology

Since the first hepatitis B vaccine became available in 1969, the greatest decline in the number of HBV infections has occurred in children and adolescents. The number of reported acute hepatitis B cases has declined from 2015 to 2022 in the United States (Fig. 18.4). However, many HBV infections are either asymptomatic or never reported.

CHAPTER 18 Viral Hepatitis

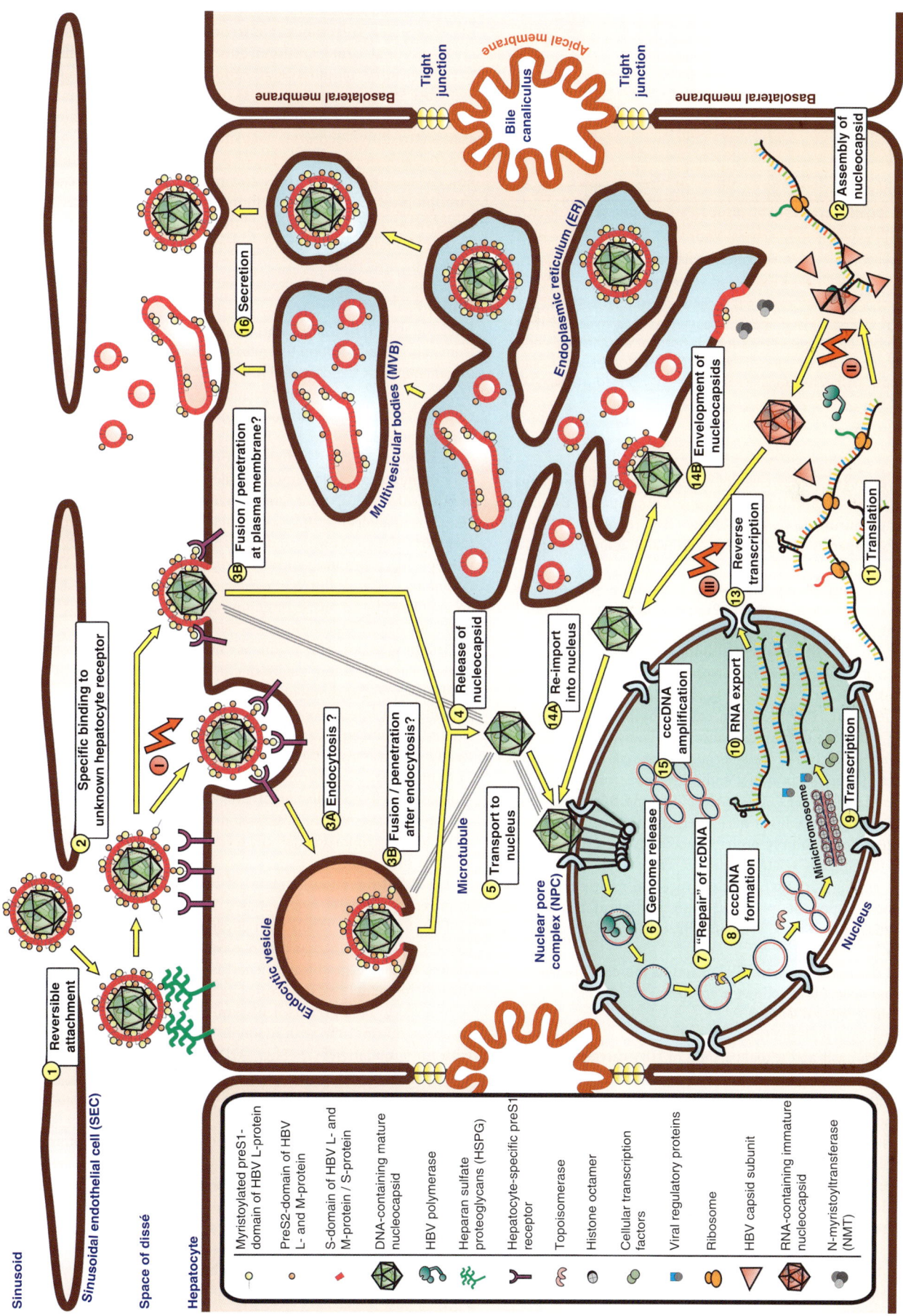

Fig. 18.3 The Replication Cycle of the Hepatitis B Virus (HBV). (From Urban S, Schulze A, Dandri M: The replication cycle of hepatitis B virus, *J Hepatol.* 52[2]:282–284, 2010. © 2009 European Association for the Study of the Liver.)

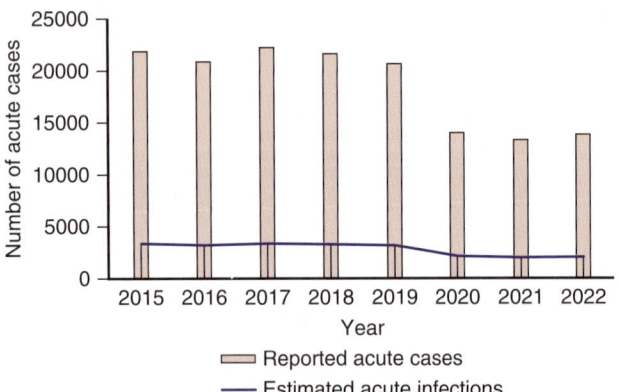

Fig. 18.4 Number of acute hepatitis B cases – United States, 2015–2022. The number of estimated viral hepatitis cases was determined by multiplying the number of reported cases by a factor that adjusted for underascertainment and underreporting. (From the Centers for Disease Control and Prevention [CDC]: Viral Hepatitis Surveillance – United States: 2022 Surveillance.)

The CDC reported 16,729 cases of newly reported chronic hepatitis B during 2022. In addition, there were 1797 hepatitis B-related deaths reported during 2022. In 2022 the CDC reported 2126 new cases of acute hepatitis B and 13,800 estimated acute hepatitis B infections.

Although the rate of reported acute hepatitis B was the lowest among Asian/Pacific Islander (API) persons, the rate of newly reported chronic hepatitis B was highest among this group during 2020. The death rate of hepatitis B among Asian/Pacific Islander persons was nearly nine-times the death rate among non-Hispanic White persons.

The incidence of HBV infection caused by blood transfusion is increasingly rare in developed countries. Transfusion-acquired HBV has been severely reduced because high-risk donor groups (e.g., paid donors, prison inmates, and military recruits) have been eliminated as major sources of donated blood and because specific serologic screening procedures have been instituted. This shift to an all-volunteer donor supply probably accounts for a 50% to 60% reduction of transfusion-related hepatitis. The overall incidence of HBV is high among patients who have received multiple transfusions or blood components prepared from multiple-donor plasma pools, hemodialysis patients, drug addicts, and medical personnel (see Table 18.1).

Persons at risk of exposure to HBV, including those mentioned earlier, include members of the following groups:
- Heterosexual men and women
- Homosexual men with multiple partners
- Household contacts and sexual partners of HBV carriers
- Infants born to HBV-infected mothers
- Patients and staff in custodial institutions for developmentally disabled persons
- Recipients of certain plasma-derived products, including patients with congenital coagulation defects
- Healthcare and public safety workers who may be in contact with infected blood
- Persons born in HBV-endemic areas and their children

HBV does not seem capable of penetrating the skin or mucous membranes; therefore some break in these barriers is required for disease transmission. Transmission of HBV occurs via percutaneous or permucosal routes, and infective blood or body fluids can be introduced at birth, through sexual contact, or by contaminated needles. Infection can also occur in settings of continuous close personal contact. About 50% of patients with acute HBV have a history of parenteral exposure. Unapparent parenteral exposure involves intimate or sexual contact with an infectious individual. Transmission between siblings and other household contacts readily occurs via transmission from skin lesions such as eczema or impetigo, sharing of potentially blood-contaminated objects such as toothbrushes and razor blades, and occasionally through bites. HBV has been found in saliva, semen, breast milk, tears, sweat, and other biological fluids of HBV carriers. Urine and wound exudate are capable of harboring HBV. Stool is not considered to be infectious.

Signs and Symptoms

Infection with HBV causes a broad spectrum of liver disease, ranging from subclinical infection to acute, self-limited hepatitis and fatal fulminant hepatitis. Exposure to HBV, particularly when it occurs early in life, may also cause an asymptomatic carrier state that can progress to chronic active hepatitis, cirrhosis of the liver, and eventually hepatocellular carcinoma.

A number of factors, including the dose of the agent and an individual's immunologic host response ability, influence the clinical course of HBV infection. Extrahepatic manifestations, reflecting an immune complex–mediated, serum sickness–like syndrome, are seen in fewer than 10% of patients with acute hepatitis B and include rash, glomerulonephritis, vasculitis, arthritis, and angioneurotic edema. Manifestations such as vasculitis, glomerulonephritis, arthritis, and dermatitis are mediated by circulating immune complex deposition (HBV antigen–antibody) in blood vessels.

The progression of liver disease in HBV infection is fostered by active virus replication, manifested by the presence of an HBV DNA level above a threshold of approximately 1000 to 10,000 IU/mL. Patients with lower levels and normal liver enzyme levels are considered to be inactive carriers, with a low risk of clinical progression. Rarely, reactivation in these patients can occur spontaneously or with immunosuppression. Perinatal infection can result in high HBV level replication without substantial liver injury in the early decades of life; however, the risk of progression to cirrhosis and hepatocellular carcinoma is proportional to the level of HBV DNA maintained persistently over time.

Persistent infection is the usual consequence of HBV infection acquired at an early age, signaled by the prolonged presence of HBsAg. Some individuals with chronic HBV infection are asymptomatic carriers, whereas others have clinical, laboratory, and histologic evidence of chronic hepatitis that may be associated with the development of postnecrotic cirrhosis. Persistent HBV infection is believed to be a precursor of primary hepatocellular carcinoma. In about 5% to 10% of individuals with HBV, especially patients with immunodeficiencies (e.g., AIDS), the disease will progress to a chronic state.

Asymptomatic Infection

The most common clinical response to HBV is an asymptomatic or a subclinical infection. In patients developing clinical symptoms of transfusion-associated HBV, jaundice and abnormal liver serum enzyme can be manifested from a few weeks to up to 6 months after a single transfusion episode, with an average of 90 days. However, in patients with a classic serologic response associated with HBV the diagnosis is rarely in doubt, even in the absence of significant symptoms. Diagnosis is more difficult in asymptomatic patients with negative HBV serology who develop a mild elevation of alanine transaminase

(ALT) levels a few weeks after a transfusion. Elevated enzyme levels may persist for 1 or 2 weeks.

Laboratory Assays

Laboratory diagnosis (Fig. 18.5) and monitoring of acute and chronic HBV infections involve the use of several of the following tests (Tables 18.3 and 18.4):

1. Hepatitis B surface antigen (HBsAg)
2. Hepatitis B e antigen (HBeAg)
3. Hepatitis B core antibody, total or IgM (anti-HBc)
4. Hepatitis B e antibody (anti-HBe)
5. Hepatitis B surface antibody (anti-HBs)
6. Hepatitis B viral DNA by polymerase chain reaction (PCR; qualitative and quantitative)

Serum testing procedures may be performed by qualitative chemiluminescent immunoassay (CIA), qualitative enzyme immunoassay (EIA), quantitative PCR, or genotype sequencing. Immunohistochemistry may be used to detect HBsAg in liver tissue samples.

Hepatitis B Surface Antigen

Serum HBsAg is a marker of HBV infection. Antibodies against HBsAg signify recovery. The initial detectable marker found in serum during the incubation period of HBV infection is HBsAg. HBsAg usually becomes detectable 2 weeks to 2 months before clinical symptoms and as soon as 2 weeks after infection. This marker is usually present for 2 to 3 months. The HBsAg screening procedure was developed to detect the presence of the major coat protein of the virus (HBsAg) in serum and is considered to be the most reliable method for preventing the transmission of HBV through blood. The presence of HBsAg indicates active HBV infection, acute or chronic.

The titer of HBsAg rises and generally peaks at or shortly after the onset of elevated liver serum enzyme levels (e.g., ALT or serum glutamate-pyruvate transaminase [SGPT]). Clinical improvement of the patient's condition and a decrease in serum enzyme concentrations are paralleled by a fall in the titer of HBsAg. There is variability in the duration of HBsAg positivity and in the relationship between clinical recovery and the disappearance of HBsAg (Fig. 18.6). Approximately 5% of positive HBsAg values are false-positive results.

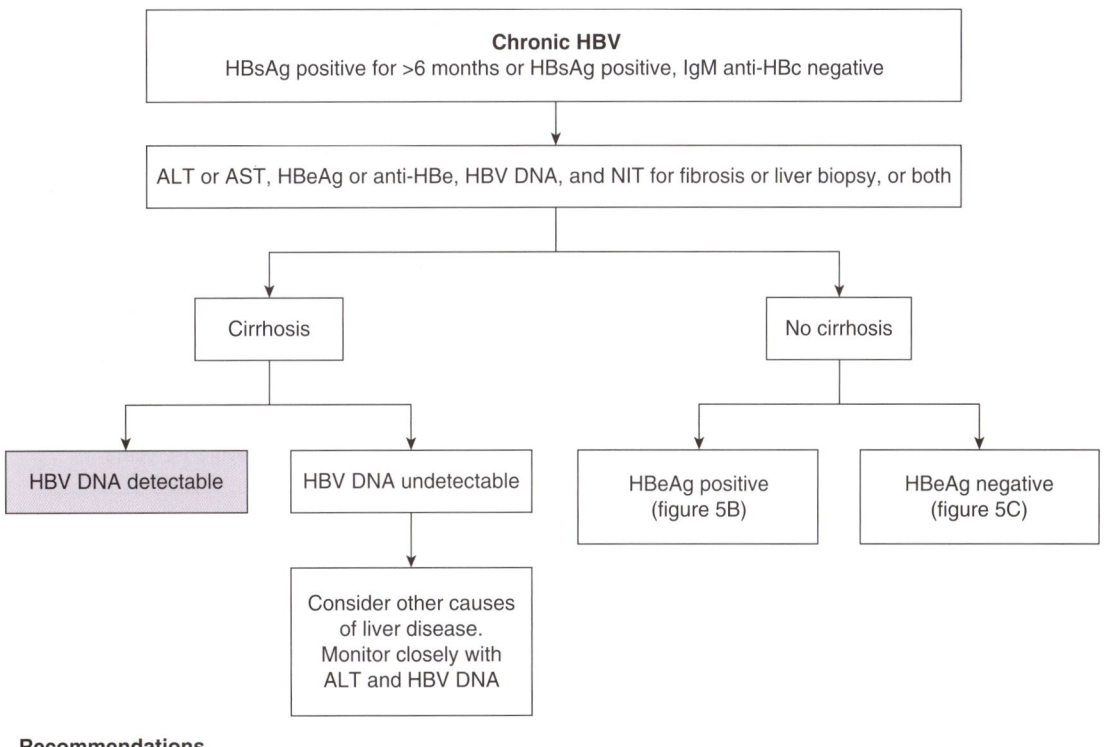

Fig. 18.5 Monitoring and decisions on treatment for patients with chronic HBV infection in relation to presence of cirrhosis and HBeAg status. (A) For patients with cirrhosis, most guidelines, recommend treatment for patients with decompensated or compensated cirrhosis if HBV DNA is detectable regardless of HBeAg status and ALT levels.

Continued

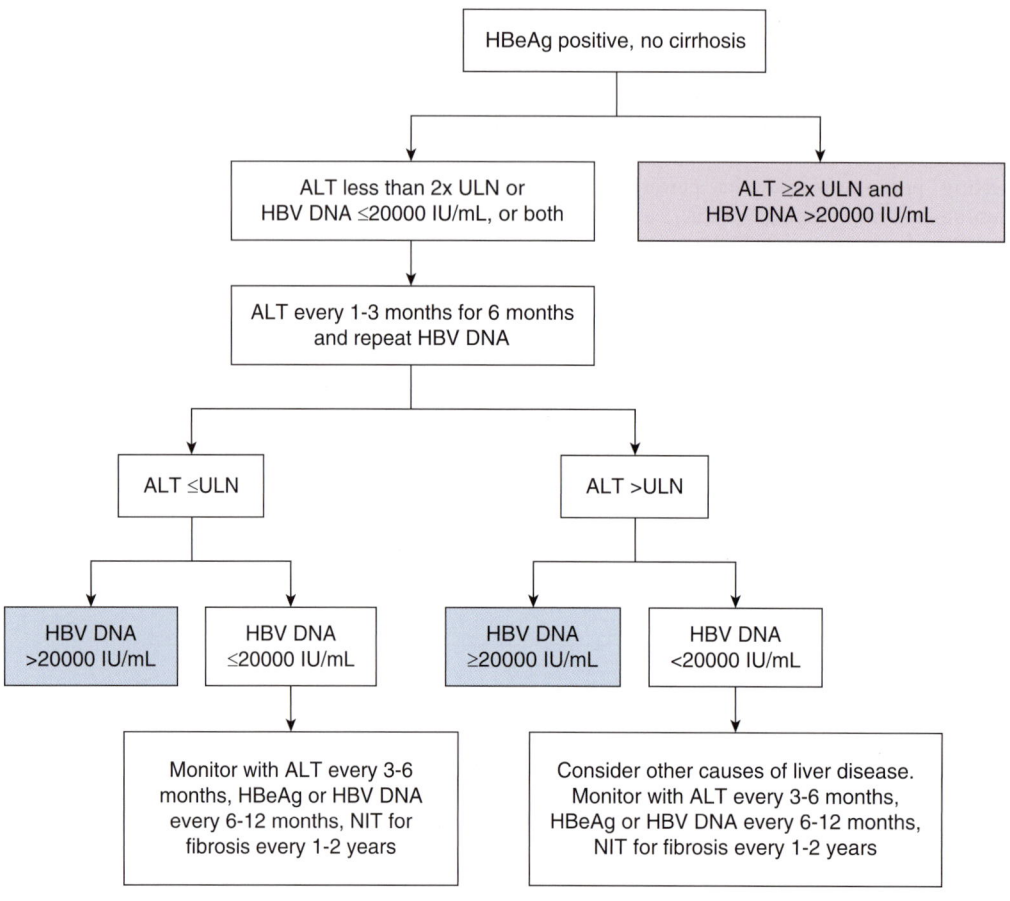

Fig. 18.5 cont'd (B) For HBeAg-positive patients without cirrhosis, all guidelines recommend treatment for patients with ALT ≥2 × ULN and HBV DNA >20 000 IU/mL; ALT >ULN and HBV DNA ≥2000 IU/mL with at least moderate inflammation (Metavir activity grade 2–3, range 0–3) or fibrosis (Metavir fibrosis stage ≥2, range 0–4), or both; and ALT ≤ULN and HBV DNA >20 000 IU/mL who are older than 30 years or 40 years.

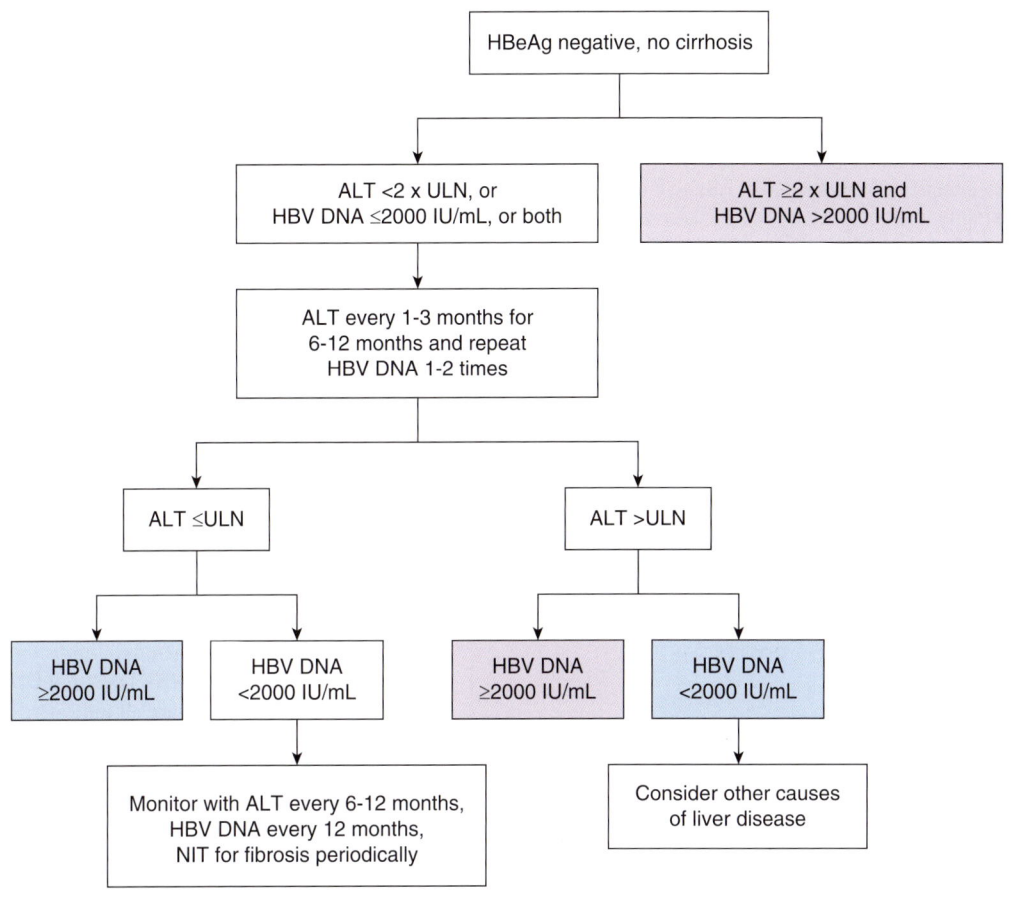

Fig. 18.5 cont'd (C) For HBeAg-negative patients without cirrhosis, all guidelines recommend treatment for patients with ALT ≥2 × ULN and HBV DNA >2000 IU/mL; and HBV DNA ≥2000 IU/mL and at least moderate inflammation or fibrosis, or both, regardless of ALT. For patients with HBV DNA <2000 IU/mL, treatment is recommended only if ALT is persistently >ULN or there is at least moderate inflammation or fibrosis, or both, and other causes of liver disease have been excluded. Patients who do not meet treatment indications should be regularly tested for ALT, HBV DNA, and liver fibrosis. Frequency of monitoring, particularly testing for HBV DNA and liver fibrosis, might vary depending on availability of resources. NIT can be used in place of liver histology to assess stage of liver fibrosis. Patients with cirrhosis and those with increased risk for HCC should undergo surveillance with ultrasonography with or without AFP every 6 months. *AFP*, Alphafetoprotein; *ALT*, alanine aminotransferase; *HBeAg*, hepatitis B e-antigen; *HBsAg*, hepatitis B surface antigen; *HBV*, hepatitis B virus; *HCC*, hepatocellular carcinoma; *NIT*, noninvasive tests; *ULN*, upper limit of normal. (From Jeng W-J, Papatheodoridis GV, Lok ASF: Hepatitis B, *Lancet* 401(10381):1039–1052, 2023.)

TABLE 18.3 Serologic Markers for Hepatitis B Virus Infection

Marker	Early (Asymptomatic)	Acute or Chronic	Low-Level Carrier	Immediate Recovery	Long After Infection	Immunized with HBsAg
HBsAg	+	+	−	−	−	−
Anti-HBs	−	±	−	−	±	+
Anti-HBc	−	+	+	+	±	−
Anti-HBc (IgM)	−	+	−	+	−	−

−, Negative; +, positive; ±, questionable.
Hepatitis B surface antigen (*HBsAg*): A protein on the surface of the hepatitis B virus (HBV); it can be detected in high levels in serum during acute or chronic HBV infection. The presence of HBsAg indicates that the person is infectious. The body normally produces antibodies to HBsAg as part of the normal immune response to infection. HBsAg is the antigen used to make hepatitis B vaccine.
Hepatitis B surface antibody (*anti-HBs*): The presence of anti-HBs is generally interpreted as indicating recovery and immunity from HBV infection. Anti-HBs also develop in a person who has been successfully vaccinated against hepatitis B.
Total hepatitis B core antibody (*anti-HBc*): Appears at the onset of symptoms in acute hepatitis B and persists for life. The presence of anti-HBc indicates previous or ongoing infection with HBV in an undefined time frame.
Immunoglobulin M (*IgM*) antibody to hepatitis B core antigen *anti-HBc (IgM)*: Positivity indicates recent infection with HBV (6 months or less). Its presence indicates acute infection.
Adapted from Hoofnagle JH: Type A and type B hepatitis, *Lab Med.* 14(11):713, 1983.

TABLE 18.4 Interpretation of Hepatitis B Panel

Tests	Results	Interpretation
HBsAg	Negative	Susceptible
Anti-HBc	Negative	
Anti-HBs	Negative	
HBsAg	Negative	Immune because of natural infection
Anti-HBc	Positive	
Anti-HBs	Positive	
HBsAg	Negative	Immune because of hepatitis B vaccination
Anti-HBc	Negative	
Anti-HBs	Positive	
HBsAg	Positive	Acutely infected
Anti-HBc	Positive	
IgM Anti-HBc	Positive	
Anti-HBs	Negative	
HBsAg	Positive	Chronically infected
Anti-HBc	Positive	
IgM Anti-HBc	Negative	
Anti-HBs	Negative	
HBsAg	Negative	Interpretation unclear; four possibilities[a]
Anti-HBc	Positive	
Anti-HBs	Negative	

[a]Interpretation unclear; four possibilities:
1. Resolved infection (most common)
2. False-positive anti-HBc, thus susceptible
3. "Low-level" chronic infection
4. Resolving acute infection

Anti-HBc, Hepatitis B core antibody; *Anti-HBs*, hepatitis B surface antibody; *HBsAg*, hepatitis B surface antigen; *IgM*, immunoglobulin M.
Adapted from https://www.medscape.org.

Among persons infected with HBV with detectable HBsAg in their serum, not all the HBsAg represents complete **Dane particles**. HBsAg-positive serum also contains two other viruslike structures, which are incomplete spherical and tubular forms consisting entirely of HBsAg and devoid of HBcAg, DNA, or DNA polymerase. The incomplete HBsAg particles can be present in serum in extremely high concentrations and form the bulk of the circulating HBsAg.

Hepatitis B–Related Antigen

A hepatitis B–related antigen, HBeAg, is found in the serum of some HBsAg-positive patients. HBV DNA and DNA polymerase will appear along with HBeAg. These are all indicative of active viral replication. HBeAg is rarely found in the absence of HBsAg. HBeAg appears to be associated with the HBV core; however, the relationship between HBeAg and the structure of HBV is unclear. HBeAg appears to be a reliable marker for the presence of high levels of virus and a high degree of infectivity.

One of the primary reasons this test is ordered is to monitor a patient's response to HBV therapy.

Hepatitis B Core Antibody

During the course of most HBV infections, HBsAg forms immune complexes with the antibodies produced as part of the recovery process. Because the HBsAg contained in these complexes is usually undetectable, HBsAg disappears from the serum of up to 50% of symptomatic patients. During this phase, an indicator of a recent hepatitis B infection is anti-HBc, the antibody to the core antigen. The time between the disappearance of detectable HBsAg and the appearance of detectable antibody to HBsAg (anti-HBs) is called the *anticore window* or *hidden antigen phase* of HBV infection. This window phase may last for a few weeks, several months, or 1 year, during which anti-HBc may be the only serologic marker. Anti-HBc is found in 3% to 5% of individuals. Of 100 anti-HBc–positive persons, 97 will have anti-HBs, 2 will have HBsAg, and 1 may have only anti-HBc.

Testing for antibody to the core of the virus (anti-HBc) may provide an additional advantage and lead to the identification of a person recently recovered from an HBV infection who may still be infectious. EIA or microparticle EIA is the method of choice.

An anti-HBc test is the Corzyme test (Abbott Laboratories, Abbott Park, Illinois) EIA. The most recent assay to be developed is the test for anti-HBc IgM. This is considered a reliable marker during the window period, diagnostic of acute infection, when most other markers may be absent. The IgM anti-HBc titer rises rapidly in the acute phase and becomes negative in most patients in 3 to 9 months, although it may persist for many years.

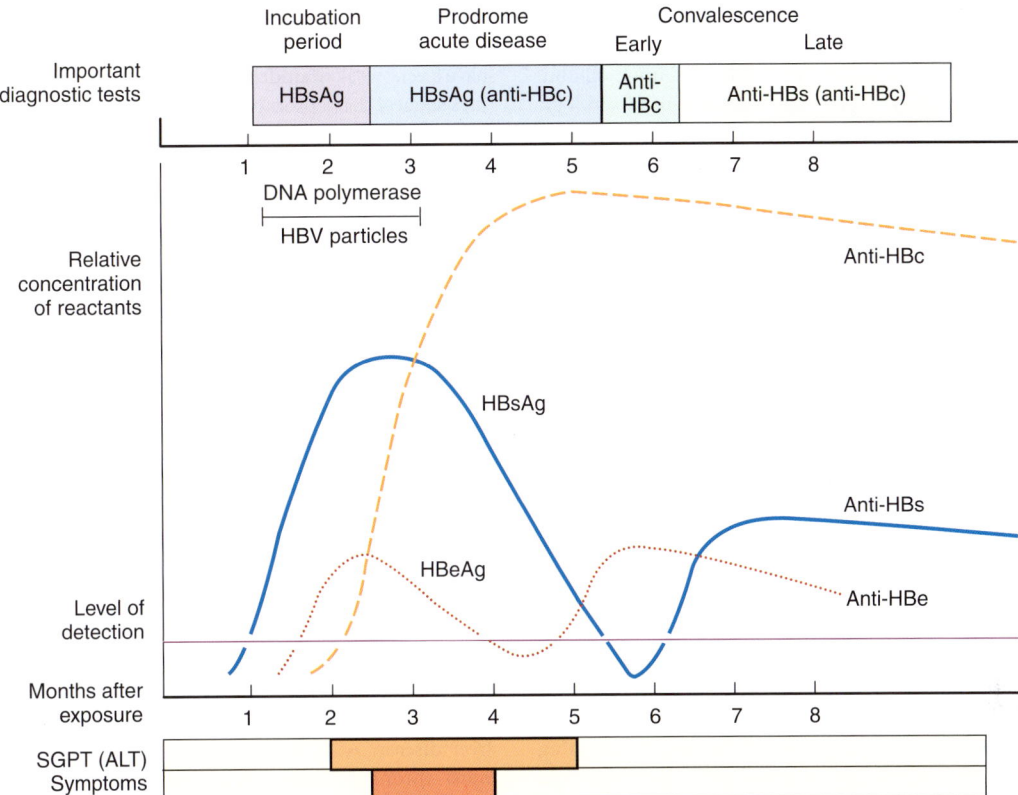

Fig. 18.6 Serologic and Clinical Patterns Observed During Acute Hepatitis B Viral Infection. *Anti-HBc*, Hepatitis B core antibody; *anti-HBs*, hepatitis B surface antibodies; *anti-HBe*, hepatitis B e antibody; *HBeAg*, hepatitis B e antigen; *HBsAg*, hepatitis B surface antigen; *SGPT (ALT)*, serum glutamate-pyruvate transaminase (alanine aminotransferase). (Adapted from Hollinger FB, Dreesman GR, Rose RN, Friedman H, editors: *Manual of clinical immunology*, ed 2, Washington, DC, 1980, American Society for Microbiology.)

Antibodies to Hepatitis B e Antigen and Hepatitis B Surface Antigen

HBeAg is a serum marker of active viral replication. Antibodies to HBeAg (anti-HBe) and HBsAg (anti-HBs) develop during convalescence and recovery from HBV infection. The development of anti-HBe in a case of acute hepatitis is the first serologic evidence of the convalescent phase. Antibody to HBsAg (anti-HBs), unlike anti-HBc and anti-HBe, does not arise during the acute disease; it is manifested during convalescence. Anti-HBs is a serologic marker of recovery and immunity, and is probably the major protective antibody in this disease. Thus hepatitis B immune globulin (HBIG) is so named because it contains high levels of anti-HBs.

Hepatitis B Viral DNA

Current tests for the assessment of HBV infections are the qualitative and quantitative measures of HBV DNA by molecular methods (e.g., PCR). In the qualitative assay, a highly conserved region of the surface gene of HBV is detected at a level as low as 1.5×10^4 copies of the viral genome per milliliter. This assay may be of value in confirming HBV infection in patients with questionable results. A less sensitive quantitative assay that uses an RNA probe is available for monitoring therapeutic responsiveness in chronically infected patients.

Diagnostic Evaluation

Appropriate diagnostic procedures should be ordered, depending on clinical factors such as patient history, signs and symptoms being evaluated, and cases involving donated blood. The various components of HBV infection can be measured by a laboratory assay.

Interrelationship of Test Results

If HBsAg is negative and anti-HBc is positive, the anti-HBs will confirm previous HBV infection or immunity. The presence of anti-HBc IgM in the absence of HBsAg in the serum indicates a recent HBV infection. An absence of IgM anti-HBc in the presence of HBsAg and HBeAg suggests high infectivity in chronic HBV disease; the presence of anti-HBe in this situation indicates low infectivity.

A vaccine-type response includes test results negative for anti-HBc and positive for anti-HBs. In the evaluation of individuals before vaccination, positive results for both anti-HBc and anti-HBs should be required as proof of immunity, especially if the result for anti-HBs displays a low positive reaction. Because there is a positive relationship between the amount of HBsAg present and a positive reaction for HBeAg, testing for HBeAg is usually not necessary, except in pregnant women. A positive HBsAg value during pregnancy results in an 80% to 90% risk of infection in the newborn in the absence of prophylaxis.

Differentiating Acute and Chronic Hepatitis and the Chronic Carrier State

Acute Infection

In an HBsAg-positive individual, the differential diagnosis should include acute hepatitis B, reactivation of chronic HBV infection, HBeAg seroconversion to anti-HBe flare, superinfection by other hepatitis viruses, and liver injury resulting from other causes (e.g., drug-induced, alcoholic, or ischemic hepatitis). Accurate diagnosis requires testing for serologic markers and sequential studies.

The first antibody to appear during an acute HBV infection is antibody to hepatitis B core antigen (anti-HBc). Anti-HBc becomes measurable shortly after HBsAg is detected and reaches peak levels within several weeks of the onset of infection. It persists long after the disappearance of HBsAg. Initially, the predominant immunoglobulin class of anti-HBc is IgM. Early after the development of serologic tests for HBV markers, when tests for anti-HBs were less sensitive than current assays, a window period between the loss of HBsAg and the appearance of anti-HBs was recognized. During this infrequently encountered window, or when levels of HBsAg do not reach detection thresholds, the detection of IgM anti-HBc is the sole marker of acute HBV infection. Over several weeks to months, the titer of IgM anti-HBc falls, tending to become undetectable after 6 months. Total anti-HBc reactivity declines at a considerably slower rate; the predominant immunoglobulin form of anti-HBc during the late recovery phase is IgG. This IgG anti-HBc persists in slowly declining titers for many years to decades after acute infection.

Within a few days to 1 or 2 weeks of the appearance of HBsAg, HBeAg also becomes detectable in the circulation of acutely infected individuals. HBeAg, a nonstructural nucleocapsid protein, is a marker of HBV replication; its presence is correlated with the presence of complete HBV particles and HBV DNA in the circulation. In acute HBV infection, patients are most infectious during the period in which HBeAg can be detected. In self-limited HBV infection, HBeAg disappears before HBsAg disappears. With the disappearance of HBeAg, its corresponding antibody, anti-HBe, becomes detectable and persists for a prolonged period.

HBV DNA, and possibly HBV virions, may persist in circulating immune complexes. The viral genome can remain in an active form in peripheral blood mononuclear cells for more than 5 years after complete clinical and serologic recovery from acute viral hepatitis B.

Chronic Infection

Recent statistics have indicated that 800,000 to 1.4 million persons are living with chronic hepatitis B infection; 3000 patients die annually as the result of chronic liver disease associated with hepatitis B.

Progression from acute to chronic HBV is influenced by a patient's age at acquisition of the virus. Clinical expression of HBV infection is high in Asia but low in Western countries. In the Far East, where HBV infection is acquired perinatally, the immune system does not recognize the difference between the virus and the host. Consequently a high level of immunologic tolerance emerges. The cellular immune responses to hepatocyte membrane HBV protein associated with acute hepatitis do not occur, and chronic, usually lifelong, infection is established in more than 90% of infected patients. In Western countries, most acute HBV infections occur during adolescence and early adulthood. These segments of immunocompetent, HBV-infected patients produce a strong cellular immune response to foreign HBV proteins expressed by hepatocytes, with resulting clinically apparent acute hepatitis. All but about 1% of infected patients clear the HBV infection.

HBV can lead to chronic infection, and patients with HBV have been shown to have the viral DNA actually incorporated into the DNA of their liver cells. This integration may be an important factor in the eventual development of liver cell cancer—hepatocellular carcinoma, a well-known long-term outcome of chronic HBV infection.

The hepatitis B virus is not directly cytopathic, and the hepatocellular necrosis results from the host's immune response to the viral antigens of the replicating virus present in infected hepatocytes. Cytotoxic T cells recognize histocompatibility and HBcAg receptors on the liver cell membrane surface. Attachment of T cells to the receptors, together with natural killer (NK) cells, results in hepatocellular necrosis; in the setting of an effective immune response, HBV replication ceases.

Studies of peripheral blood mononuclear cells have revealed that patients with acute HBV produce vigorous T-cell responses against multiple HBV antigenic determinants located on the viral core, envelope, and polymerase proteins, whereas patients with chronic infection have a very weak or undetectable cellular immune response. These findings suggest that a prompt, vigorous, and broad-based cellular immune response results in clearance of the virus from the liver, whereas a qualitatively or quantitatively less efficient or restricted immune response may permit the persistence of virus and the development of ongoing, immunologically mediated liver cell injury. In addition to a patient's immune response, viral factors (HBV genome) may also be important in determining the course of HBV infection.

Chronic HBV occurs in two phases, a more infectious replicative phase (high levels of circulating virions, HBV DNA, HBeAg) and a minimally infectious nonreplicative phase (few virions, circulating spherical and tubular forms of HBsAg, undetectable HBV DNA and HBeAg, but circulating anti-HBe and integrated HBV DNA in hepatocytes). In patients with chronic HBV infection, HBsAg remains detectable for more than 6 months and, in rare cases, HBsAg persists for decades. Spontaneous HBsAg clearance in chronic infection is unusual. Clearance of the virus results in complete clinical and histologic recovery, ultimately leaving the patient with a serologic pattern characterized by hepatitis B core antibody (IgG anti-HBc) and anti-HBs, with the latter conferring immunity.

Asymptomatic individuals in whom test results for HBsAg remain positive are labeled *HBsAg carriers*. Other chronically infected HBsAg-positive individuals may have clinical or laboratory evidence of chronic liver disease. Anti-HBc is present in all chronic HBV infections. In most chronically infected patients, IgM anti-HBc is a minor fraction of total anti-HBc reactivity. In all patients with HBV infection, HBeAg can be detected during the early phase of infection, but in contrast to the situation with acute self-limited HBV infection, HBeAg may remain detectable in chronically infected individuals for many months to years. In these patients, HBV DNA is also readily detected in the circulation. The presence of circulating HBV DNA is highly correlated with the presence of whole-virus replication, and thus with the potential infectivity of the patient. HBV DNA is also detectable in the hepatocytes of individuals with chronic HBV infection. For a variable but generally prolonged period, this hepatic HBV DNA is present in a free, episomal replicating form. In some patients, HBV DNA becomes integrated into the genome of the host hepatocyte. Viral replication may diminish spontaneously over time or after treatment, signaled by the decline or disappearance of serum HBV DNA, loss of HBeAg, and appearance of anti-HBe in the circulation, as detected by commercial assays. Research has suggested that both anti-HBe and anti-HBs may be present early in chronic hepatitis B complexed to HBeAg and HBsAg.

In 10% to 40% of patients with chronic HBV infection, anti-HBs is detected concurrently with HBsAg. The presence of anti-HBs does not signal reduced infectivity or imminent clearance of HBsAg.

Carrier State

There are an estimated 400 to 500 million HBV carriers worldwide. In the United States 50,000 to 100,000 people still acquire HBV infection each year, even though a highly effective vaccine is available. Immunocompromised patients, including those with HIV infection, are at increased risk for chronic HBV infection. Age at the time of acquisition of HBV infection is a major determinant of chronicity, as reflected by the development of the HBsAg carrier state. As many as 90% of infected neonates become carriers. The rate falls progressively with increasing age at the time of infection, so that only 1% to 10% of newly infected adults fail to clear HBsAg. Another important risk factor for chronicity is the presence of intrinsic or iatrogenic immunosuppression. Immunosuppressed individuals are at increased risk of becoming carriers after HBV infection and gender is a determinant of chronicity. Women are more likely than men to clear HBsAg; therefore men predominate in all populations of HBsAg carriers.

The worldwide prevalence of the HBsAg carrier state varies widely. In the United States, as in many Western nations, carriers account for approximately 0.2% of the general population. However, among certain groups (e.g., homosexual men and intravenous [IV] drug abusers) in the general population, carrier rates 4 to 10 times greater have been identified. Carrier rates as high as 25% have been recognized among Alaskan natives in some Alaskan villages.

Perinatal transmission continues to occur. This rate should be reduced significantly by the implementation of routine screening of all pregnant women for HBsAg, followed by vaccination of their newborns. Hepatitis B vaccination is gradually being incorporated into routine infant immunization programs. A newer multivalent, triple-antigen HBV vaccine should have wide practical application.

Carriers can be divided into two categories based on differing infectivity, depending on the presence in their serum of another antigen, HBeAg, or its antibody (anti-HBe). The types of carrier states include the following:

- The more commonly identified carriers have anti-HBe in their serum and are at a later stage of infection.
- Anti-HBe carriers are less infectious but may transmit infection through blood transfusion.
- HBsAg-positive carriers will become anti-HBe–positive carriers at a rate of about 5% to 10% per year.
- All HBsAg-positive individuals must be excluded from giving blood for transfusion.
- About one in four carriers has HBeAg in their serum. It is likely that these individuals have recently become carriers and that their blood is highly infectious.
- Patients with HBeAg-negative chronic HBV infection, in which precore or core promoter gene mutations preclude or reduce the synthesis of HBeAg, account for an increasing proportion of cases. These patients tend to have progressive liver injury, fluctuating liver enzyme activity, and lower levels of HBV DNA than patients with HBeAg-reactive HBV infection.

Prevention and Treatment

Routine hepatitis B vaccination of children and at-risk adults has significantly prevented HBV infection.

The most important factors in preventing transfusion-acquired HBV are donor interviewing, screening of donor blood, use of hepatitis-free products when possible, and appropriate use of blood and blood components. In addition, the avoidance of high-risk blood components (e.g., untreated factor VIII prepared from multiple-donor pools) reduces the incidence of HBV.

Elimination of high-risk donors has accounted for at least a 50% reduction in the incidence of hepatitis; routine testing of donated blood for HBsAg has further reduced the incidence by another 20% to 30%. Testing for anti-HBc will detect almost 100% of HBsAg-positive persons, the rare asymptomatic donor in the core window, and the large number of donors who have had subclinical hepatitis B infections and are now immune.

The use of recombinant vaccine against hepatitis B, licensed in 1982, is warranted for high-risk persons, including medical personnel (see Box 18.1). HBV vaccine is administered in three doses over 7 months and is about 80% to 95% effective. The vaccine is now included in the childhood vaccination schedule. Hepatitis B vaccine is also a vaccine against cancer (hepatocellular carcinoma). Vaccination offers a new approach to preventing transfusion-acquired HBV and the dependent HDV in patients who are likely to need ongoing transfusion therapy, such as nonimmune patients with hemophilia, sickle cell anemia, or aplastic anemia.

In cases of accidental needlestick exposure or exposure of mucous membranes or open cuts to HBsAg-positive blood, HBIG should be administered within 24 hours of exposure and again 25 to 30 days later to nonimmunized patients. Infants born to mothers with acute hepatitis B in the third trimester, or with HBsAg at delivery, should be given HBIG as soon as possible and no later than 24 hours after birth. Persons who are HBsAg-positive or who have anti-HBs need not be given HBIG unless the HBV titer is shown to be low or unknown.

Seven drugs have been licensed in the United States for the treatment of HBV infection. Treatment for a duration of about 1 year usually results in the reduction of serum HBV DNA levels and a serum level of HBV DNA that is undetectable by PCR assay. Therapeutic agents interfere with the HBV life cycle. Acylated preS1-peptides have been shown to bind the HBV receptor and block viral entry in vivo. Dihydroarylpyrimidines interfere with nucleocapsid assembly and induce core protein degradation. Polymerase inhibitors suppress reverse transcription and synthesis of the DNA-plus strand. The preS1-derived lipopeptides and the dihydroarylpyrimidines are presently in preclinical development. Nucleoside and nucleotide analogs (lamivudine, adefovir, entecavir, telbivudine, and tenofovir) and interferon-alpha (IFN-α) and peginterferon-alpha (PEG-IFN-α) are currently approved therapeutic treatments. IFN-α inhibits HBV both through immune modulatory effects and directly by reducing steady-state levels of HBV transcripts.

Liver transplantation is also used for some severe cases of liver disease caused by HBV, although the new organ usually becomes infected with HBV.

HEPATITIS D

Etiology

HDV was first described in 1977 as a pathogen that superinfects some patients already infected with HBV (see Table 18.1). Persons with acute or chronic HBV infection, as demonstrated by serum HBsAg, can be infected with HDV. HBV is required to supply envelope proteins for its assembly into mature virions.

The natural reservoir for HDV is a negative-strand RNA virus. The HDV is a replication-defective or incomplete RNA virus that by itself is unable to cause infection. HDV consists of a single-strand, circular RNA coated in HBsAg. HDV is interesting because it can force the host's RNA polymerase to transcribe the HDV RNA genome. Multiple genotypes (1–8) are distributed by geography, except for genotype 1, which is worldwide.

Epidemiology

Hepatitis D was originally described in Italy and appears to be most common in southern European countries. It also appears to be endemic among Indian tribes living in the Amazon basin. In the United States, Northern Europe, and Asia, infection is uncommon. In the United States hepatitis D is seen predominantly in IV drug users and their sexual partners, but it has been reported in homosexual men and men with hemophilia. According to the CDC, there are approximately 70,000 people with chronic HDV infection in the United States.

Hepatitis D is a severe and rapidly progressive liver disease for which no therapy has proven effective. Patients with this form of hepatitis are significantly more likely to have cirrhosis and liver failure and to require liver transplantation than patients with HBV infection alone. Chronic HDV infection is responsible for more than 1000 deaths per year in the United States. The mortality rate can be up to 20% of infected patients.

HDV is spread chiefly by direct contact of HBsAg carriers with HDV- or HBV-infected individuals. Family members and intimate contacts of infected individuals are at greatest risk. IV drug users and intranasal cocaine users, organ recipients, and hemodialysis patients are high-risk groups. Sexual transmission is uncommon, except in some countries (e.g., Taiwan). Maternal-neonatal transmission is rare.

Hepatitis D can be acquired either as a coprimary infection (coinfection) with HBV (e.g., after inoculation with blood or secretions containing both agents) or as a superinfection in patients with established HBV infection (HBsAg carriers or patients with chronic hepatitis B). A superinfection can make an HBV infection worse by transforming a mild infection into a persistent infection in 80% of patients. In contrast, coinfection rarely leads to a chronic condition. Although HDV is dependent on HBV for its expression and pathogenicity, replication of HDV appears to be independent of the presence of its associated hepadnavirus.

Signs and Symptoms

Hepatitis D infection may be benign and brief, but fulminant hepatitis and chronic hepatitis have been attributed with increasing frequency to HDV. Chronic HDV infection is associated with increased hepatic damage and a more severe clinical course than is expected from chronic HBV infection alone. The occurrence of sequential attacks of HBV in the same patient is probably attributable in most cases to HDV infection superimposed on a previous acute HBV infection.

HDV infection with an HDV agent can occur in several conditions; the symptoms are typical of acute or chronic hepatitis, as follows:
- Acute hepatitis D with concurrent acute hepatitis B (coinfection)
- Acute hepatitis D in a chronic HBsAg carrier
- Chronic hepatitis D in a chronic HBsAg carrier

Immunologic Manifestations

The HDV probably partially suppresses HBV replication. Hepatitis D infection is diagnosed by the appearance of HDV antigen in serum or the development of IgM or IgG HDV antibodies that appear sequentially in a time frame similar to that described for hepatitis A or B antibodies. HBsAg will also be present.

Coinfection with Hepatitis B Virus

In patients with acute, self-limited HDV coinfection with HBV, various serologic responses indicative of HDV infection have been identified. Serum HDV RNA and HDV antigen (HDAg) may be detected early, concurrently with the detection of HBsAg. HDAg disappears as HBsAg disappears, and seroconversion to anti–hepatitis D (anti-HD; initially IgM and later IgG) follows. The IgM reactivity usually appears several days to a few weeks after the onset of illness, whereas IgG anti-HD appears in the convalescent phase. In about 60% of coinfections HDAg is not detected by anti-HD, but patients can manifest both IgM and IgG antibodies. IgM anti-HD in self-limited coinfections is usually transient. IgG anti-HD also often disappears but occasionally persists in declining titer for many months and may remain detectable as long as 1 to 2 years after the disappearance of HBsAg. In a small number of patients, the early appearance of isolated IgM anti-HD, or its appearance during convalescence of isolated IgG anti-HD, may be the only detectable marker of HDV infection.

Superinfection of Hepatitis B Carrier

HDV superinfection of HBV (HBsAg) carriers causes the appearance of HDAg and HDV RNA, a simultaneous reduction in HBV replication, and a consequent diminution in the titer of circulating HBsAg. Termination of the HBsAg carrier state appears to occur infrequently after HDV inhibition of HBV replication. Often, HDV infection becomes chronic and HDAg and HDV RNA may remain detectable at low levels in the serum; in persistent HDV infection, large quantities of HDAg can be detected in hepatocytes. High titers of IgM and IgG anti-HD are maintained in persistent infection, reflecting progressive, HDV-induced, chronic liver disease.

Diagnostic Evaluation

The HDV appears in the circulating blood as a particle with a core of delta antigen and a surface component of HBsAg. A person with hepatitis D will have detectable antigen in the liver and antibody in the serum. Test methodologies for HDV IgM antibody use EIA, and HDV antigen is detected by qualitative enzyme-linked immunosorbent assay (ELISA).

Screening for total HDV antibodies in serum is important in the identification of a subpopulation of apparently healthy HBsAg carriers whose risk of serious liver damage is fourfold higher than that of anti-HDV–negative carriers. The combined presence of total anti-HDV antibody and abnormal liver chemistry test results in a symptom-free carrier suggests parenchymal damage and is considered an indication for liver biopsy. Hepatic lesions in anti-HDV–positive carriers often consist of chronic active hepatitis or advanced cirrhosis. A positive test result for IgM anti-HDV increases the likelihood of occult active HBV infection.

HEPATITIS C

> **KEY CONCEPTS: Hepatitis C Facts**
> - Hepatitis C virus (HCV) is prevalent in the United States and Western Europe, and resembles HBV in terms of transmission characteristics.
> - Healthcare workers should prevent needlestick injuries.

Etiology

HCV is an enveloped flavivirus. It is a small, single-strand RNA virus. After binding to the cell surface, HCV particles enter the cell by receptor-mediated endocytosis. Because the virus mutates rapidly, changes in the envelope protein may help it evade the immune system.

There are at least six major HCV genotypes and more than 50 subtypes of HCV. The different genotypes have different geographic distributions. Genotype 1 represents most infections in North and South America and Europe. Genotypes 1a and 1b are the most common genotypes in the United States. The HCV genotype does not appear to play a role in the severity of disease. Knowing the genotype of HCV is useful to physicians when making recommendations and counseling patients regarding therapy. Patients with genotypes 2 and 3 have a more favorable prognosis and are more likely to respond to treatment.

Epidemiology

Worldwide an estimated 180 million people are infected with HCV. In the United States an estimated 5 to 7 million persons, or 1.6% to 1.8% of the total population, suffer from HCV infection. Annually approximately 12,000 patients die in the United States as the result of chronic liver disease associated with HCV. HCV infection is a leading cause of chronic hepatitis, cirrhosis, and liver cancer. This virus is the primary indication for liver transplantation in Western countries.

In the past, hepatitis C was considered a disease limited to transfusion recipients. HCV is now recognized in many other epidemiologic settings (see Table 18.1) and as a major cause of chronic hepatitis worldwide, particularly in adults in the United States born between 1945 and 1965 with or without symptoms. This cohort is affected because of a confluence of risk factors, including contaminated blood transfusions and expanded use of illicit IV drugs, and represents about three-fourths of cases of chronic HCV infection in the United States.

In the United States, the national rate of acute cases of hepatitis C has demonstrated an increase from 2015 to 2022 and a slight decrease between 2021 and 2022, according to the CDC (Fig. 18.7). The number of reported cases in 2022 was 4848 but the CDC estimated that there were 67,400 cases in 2022. According to the US Department of Health and Human Services, more than 3 million people in the United States are living with chronic hepatitis C, and most do not feel ill or know they are infected.

Viral Transmission

HCV is spread primarily by percutaneous contact with infected blood or blood products. Currently, injectable drug abuse is the most common risk factor. Workers with needlestick injuries, infants born to HCV-infected mothers, individuals with multiple sexual partners, and recipients of unscreened donor blood are also at risk for contracting HCV.

Although most hepatitis C patients are injectable drug users, many patients acquire HCV without any known exposure to blood or drug use. Sporadic or community-acquired infections without a known source occur in about 10% of acute hepatitis C cases and 30% of chronic cases.

Posttransfusion Hepatitis

The incubation time for posttransfusion hepatitis C is 2 to 12 weeks, with a range of 2 to 26 weeks. After the introduction of nucleic acid testing (NAT) in the screening of blood donors, the rate of posttransfusion hepatitis C plummeted. Before NAT, the transfusion of infected blood or blood components (e.g., factor VIII or IX) constituted a clear route of HCV transmission. Another reason the incidence of posttransfusion hepatitis C declined in the 1980s was the effort to replace the pool of high-risk, paid donors. In addition, dialysis patients now require fewer blood transfusions because recombinant erythropoietin (EPO) is used to stimulate the patient's own bone marrow to produce red blood cells.

Parenteral and Occupational Exposure

Illegal IV drug use continues to be the most commonly identified risk factor for HCV infection. Accidental needlestick injuries also are a clearly documented route of hepatitis transmission. The Occupational Safety and Health Administration (OSHA) has estimated that the general risk to healthcare workers of occupational transmission of HCV is 20- to 40 times higher than the risk of contracting HIV. The CDC has more conservatively estimated that the average risk of HCV transmission after a needlestick injury is six times greater than the risk of HIV transmission. Because of these grim statistics, occupationally acquired HCV infection is a growing concern for healthcare providers.

A person with a high level of circulating HCV may be capable of transmitting the virus by exposing others percutaneously or mucosally to small amounts of blood or other body fluids. A person with a low level of circulating HCV may be capable of transmitting the virus only by exposing others percutaneously to a large volume of blood. The threshold concentration of virus needed to transmit or cause infection is uncertain.

Sexual Transmission

Sexual transmission is believed to occur but is uncommon. Spouses of patients with HCV viremia and chronic liver disease have an increased risk of acquiring HCV proportional to the duration of the marriage.

Other Sources

Mother-to-infant transmission has been documented. HCV is vertically transmitted from mother to infant, and the risk of transmission is correlated with the level of HCV RNA in the mother. Personal contact is thought to be a route of infection but has not been conclusively demonstrated; the actual risk for such transmission is unknown.

Between 25% and 50% of sporadic community-acquired cases of hepatitis in the United States are of the HCV type and are unrelated to parenteral exposure. Some of these cases are believed to result from heterosexual transmission, but in approximately 40% the route of infection cannot be identified. Therefore transmission can occur by unapparent and apparent parenteral routes; this form of hepatitis cannot be distinguished from other types of viral hepatitis solely by its epidemiologic characteristics.

In addition, liver disease can occur in the recipients of organs from donors with antibodies to HCV. Almost all the recipients of organs from anti-HCV–positive donors become infected with HCV. The current tests for anti-HCV antibodies may underestimate the incidence of transmission and the prevalence of HCV infection in immunosuppressed organ recipients. If the medical condition of the potential recipient is so serious that other options no longer exist, however, the use of an organ from an anti-HCV–seropositive donor should be considered.

Prognosis

Several strains of HCV exist. The genotype of HCV influences the clinical course of HCV infection, in addition to the response to IFN and newer treatments. Six major genotypes with multiple subtypes (e.g., 1a, 1b, and 1c) exist. Genotype is an important predictor of virologic response to HCV treatment:

- Type 1 is the predominant genotype in the United States and more difficult to treat.
- Types 2 and 3 are less aggressive and easier to treat.

It is believed that about 50% of patients with acute hepatitis C will continue to have elevated serum liver enzyme levels more than 6

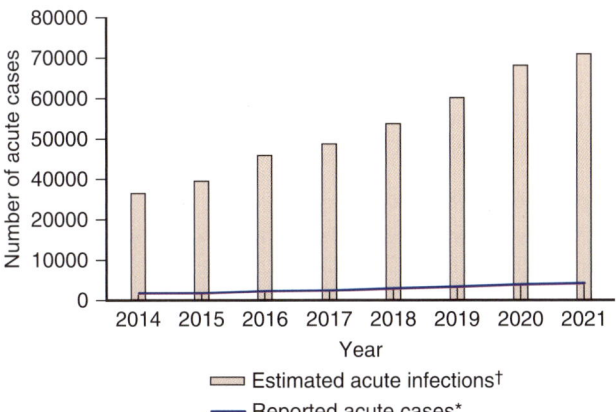

Fig. 18.7 Actual number and estimated number of acute hepatitis C cases submitted to the Centers for Disease Control and Prevention (CDC) by states, and estimated number of acute hepatitis cases – United States, 2014–2021. The number of estimated viral hepatitis cases was determined by multiplying the number of reported cases by a factor that adjusted for underascertainment and underreporting. (From the Centers for Disease Control and Prevention [CDC]: Viral Hepatitis Surveillance – United States: 2017 Surveillance. https://www.cdc.gov/hepatitis/statistics/2021surveillance/hepatitis-c/figure-3.1.htm Accessed on October 16, 2024.)

months after the onset of illness. These patients usually have persistent HCV RNA detected in their serum and evidence of chronic hepatitis on liver biopsy. Viremia, as detected by HCV RNA assay, may persist for months to years in patients in whom serum liver enzyme levels return to normal, and liver biopsy may reveal chronic hepatitis.

Chronic hepatitis C appears to be a slowly progressive, often silent disease. In addition, HCV may be associated with hepatocellular carcinoma predominantly, if not exclusively, in the setting of cirrhosis.

Signs and Symptoms

Although the clinical characteristics of the acute disease of both types of hepatitis C are basically indistinguishable, the chronic consequences are very different. The signs and symptoms of hepatitis C are extremely variable. It can be mild, transient, and completely asymptomatic, or it can be severe, prolonged, and ultimately fatal.

Hepatitis C more closely resembles HBV than HAV in regard to its transmission and clinical features. Hepatitis C, as with HBV, can be acute and ranges from mild anicteric illness to *fulminant disease*. A fulminant course with a rapidly fatal outcome is rare. Usually the patient is only mildly symptomatic and nonicteric; less than 25% of patients develop jaundice. Transfusion-associated hepatitis C has a typical incubation time of 2 to 12 weeks, with a range of 2 to 26 weeks.

Hepatitis C is characterized by serum liver enzyme levels in the range of 200 to 800 U/L and marked fluctuations, with intervening periods of normalcy. Mean serum liver enzyme and bilirubin levels of patients with hepatitis C, however, are significantly lower than those of patients with HBV; the extensive overlap of the ranges of elevation precludes the identification of the type of viral hepatitis by the use of these assays.

The diagnosis of hepatitis C has a guarded prognosis. Although hepatitis C was initially thought to be a relatively benign disease, there is increasing evidence of progression to cirrhosis in about 20% of patients, liver failure, and even *hepatoma*. The hepatic damage is caused by the cytopathic effect of the virus and the inflammatory changes secondary to immune activation. Up to 60% of patients with posttransfusion hepatitis C develop chronic liver disease based on biopsy analysis, and up to 20% of these patients develop cirrhosis.

Posttransfusion hepatitis C affects men and women equally, but a reported 75% of patients who develop chronic hepatitis are men. Patients with parenterally acquired (nontransfusion) hepatitis C, including those who have no identifiable source, have the same clinical characteristics and develop chronic liver disease with the same frequency.

Extrahepatic immunologic abnormalities have been shown to occur commonly in patients with chronic HCV infection. HCV infection has been linked to a number of extrahepatic conditions, including Sjögren syndrome, cryoglobulinemia, urticaria, erythema nodosum, vasculitis, glomerulonephritis, and peripheral neuropathy. HCV apparently causes the cases of mixed cryoglobulinemia previously mentioned.

Immunologic failure results in chronic infection, persistent stimulation of the immune system, and subsequent production of circulating immune complexes, of which almost one-third become insoluble when exposed to low temperatures and which are associated with the clinical picture of cryoglobulinemia. Many epidemiologic studies have demonstrated an association between HCV infection and an increased incidence of B-cell non-Hodgkin lymphoma (NHL), ranging from 20% to 30% to almost twice that of HCV-negative control subjects.

Traditional Hepatitis C Virus Testing

HCV testing follows a flow chart protocol (Fig. 18.8). Based on a patient's symptoms or whether they are in a high-risk cohort, testing

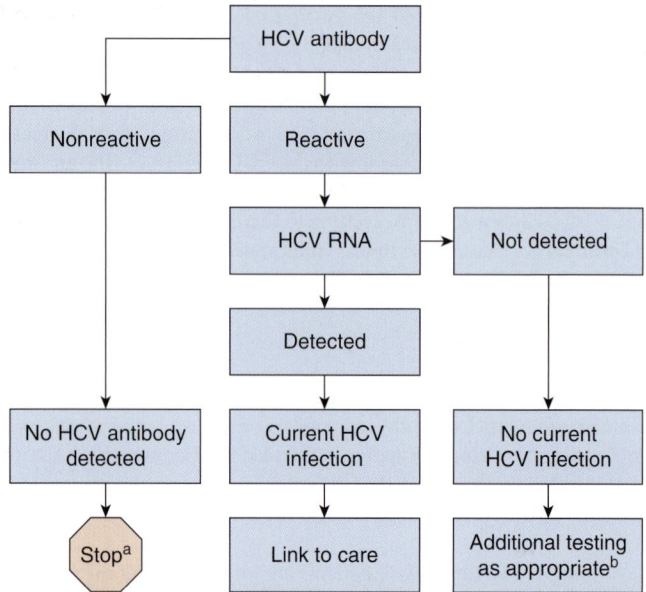

Fig. 18.8 CDC-Recommended Testing Sequence for Identifying Current HCV Infection. (Centers for Disease Control and Prevention (CDC): Testing for HCV infection: an update of guidance for clinicians and laboratorians, *MMWR Morb Mortal Wkly Rep* 62(18):362–365, 2013.)

[a]For persons who might have been exposed to HCV within the past 6 months, testing for HCV RNA or follow-up testing for HCV antibody should be performed. For persons who are immunocompromised, testing for HCV RNA should be performed.

[b]To differentiate past, resolved HCV infection from biologic false positivity for HCV antibody, testing with another HCV-antibody assay can be considered. Repeat HCV-RNA testing if the person tested is suspected to have had HCV exposure within the past 6 months or has clinical evidence of HCV disease, or if there is concern regarding the handling or storage of the test specimen.

begins with CIA or third-generation ELISA. Point-of-care testing (POCT) rapid tests for anti-HCV antibody use the same viral antigens as do third-generation ELISAs (Table 18.5).

ELISAs have high specificity in the testing of at-risk populations, but they have a low positive predictive value when used for screening the general population. If a patient's result is positive or reactive, an HCV by quantitative PCR should be ordered.

Polymerase Chain Reaction

The PCR amplification technique can detect low levels of HCV RNA in serum. Testing for HCV RNA is a reliable way of demonstrating that hepatitis C infection is present, and it is the most specific test for infection.

A negative HCV result by quantitative PCR indicates that the patient is not currently infected. However, a patient may have been previously infected and recovered. Test results may reflect a false-positive anti-HCV screening assay.

A positive result indicates that a patient is currently infected. Acutely symptomatic patients should be retested in 3 to 6 months to assess for resolution of infection. If a patient has minimal or no symptoms, they are considered to have chronic HCV.

The best method to confirm a diagnosis of hepatitis C is to test for HCV RNA using a PCR assay. In addition, HCV RNA testing is of value when EIA tests for anti-HCV are unreliable (e.g., immunocompromised

TABLE 18.5	Interpretation of Results of Tests for Hepatitis C Virus (HCV) Infection and Further Actions	
Test Outcome	Interpretation	Further Actions
HCV antibody nonreactive	No HCV antibody detected	Sample can be reported as nonreactive for HCV antibody. No further action required. If recent exposure in person tested is suspected, test for HCV RNA.[a]
HCV antibody reactive	Presumptive HCV infection	A repeatedly reactive result is consistent with current HCV infection, or past HCV infection that has resolved, or biological false positivity for HCV antibody. Test for HCV RNA to identify current infection.
HCV antibody reactive, HCV RNA detected	Current HCV infection	Provide person tested with appropriate counseling and link person tested to care and treatment.[b]
HCV antibody reactive, HCV RNA not detected	No current HCV infection	No further action required in most cases. If distinction between true positivity and biological false positivity for HCV antibody is desired, and if sample is repeatedly reactive in the initial test, test with another HCV antibody assay. In certain situations,[c] follow-up with HCV RNA testing and appropriate counseling.

[a] If HCV RNA testing is not feasible and the person tested is not immunocompromised, carry out follow-up testing for HCV antibody to demonstrate seroconversion. If the person tested is immunocompromised, consider testing for HCV RNA.
[b] It is recommended before antiviral therapy is initiated to retest for HCV RNA in a subsequent blood sample to confirm HCV RNA positivity.
[c] If the person tested is suspected of having HCV exposure within the past 6 months or has clinical evidence of HCV disease, or if there is concern regarding the handling or storage of the test specimen.
From the Centers for Disease Control and Prevention: Testing for HCV infection: An update of guidance for clinicians and laboratorians, *MMWR* 62(18):000, 2013, pp. 362–365.

patients may not produce sufficiently high antibody titer for detection with EIA). Immunosuppressed or immunocompromised patients pose diagnostic problems because of their inability to produce anti-HCV. HCV RNA testing may be required for the following:
- Immunosuppressed patients (e.g., recipients of a solid-organ transplant)
- Patients undergoing dialysis because of chronic renal failure
- Patients taking corticosteroids
- Patients experiencing agammaglobulinemia

Patients exhibiting anti-HCV who have another form of liver disease (e.g., alcoholism and autoimmune disorder) can be difficult to diagnose. In these situations, the anti-HCV may represent a false-positive reaction, previous HCV infection, or mild hepatitis C occurring concurrently with another hepatic abnormality. In these cases, HCV RNA testing can help confirm that hepatitis C is contributing to the liver problem.

Patients with minimal or no symptoms who test positive for HCV by quantitative PCR, who then are diagnosed with chronic HCV, should be tested for genotype 1. HCV genotyping guides selection of the most appropriate antiviral regimen.

If a patient does not demonstrate genotype 1, a treatment decision is made. Subsequently, treatment is monitored and the end of treatment is monitored by HCV by quantitative PCR. If a patient demonstrates genotype 1, assays for interleukin-28B (IL-28B)–associated variants and two single-nucleotide polymorphisms (SNPs) should be ordered. Determination of genotype assists with the selection of the most appropriate antiviral regimen. IL-28B genotyping predicts the response to PEG-IFN-α and ribavirin (RBV) therapy for patients with chronic genotype 1 HCV. Patients with HCV genotype 1 tend to have more advanced disease and an associated lower response to therapy.

Acute and Chronic Hepatitis C
Acute Hepatitis C
The coordinated activities of CD4+ T cells and cytotoxic CD8+ T cells, primed in the context of human leukocyte antigen (HLA) class II and I alleles, respectively, on antigen-presenting cells, are critically important for the control of acute HCV infections. The signs and symptoms of acute hepatitis C infection usually include jaundice, fatigue, and nausea. Laboratory manifestations include a significant increase in serum liver enzyme levels (usually more than tenfold) and the presence or de novo development of anti-HCV.

Demonstration of HCV antibodies can be problematic because anti-HCV is not always present in patients with symptoms. In 30% to 40% of patients, anti-HCV is not detected until 2 to 8 weeks after the onset of symptoms. Acute hepatitis C can also be diagnosed by testing for HCV RNA, apparently the earliest detectable marker of acute HCV infection, preceding the appearance of anti-HCV by several weeks. The current ELISA for antibodies to recombinant HCV antigens becomes positive earlier and is more sensitive than preceding ELISAs. Another approach is to repeat the anti-HCV testing 1 month after the onset of illness.

Hepatitis C viremia may persist despite the normalization of serum ALT levels. Intracytoplasmic HCV antigen has been found in the hepatocytes of acutely infected chimpanzees and, by analogy, is presumed to be present in acute hepatitis C in human beings. HCV antigens were not detected in hepatocyte nuclei, Kupffer or sinusoidal lining cells, bile duct epithelium, or blood vessels.

Chronic Hepatitis C
Chronic hepatitis C varies greatly in its course and outcome. At one end of the spectrum are asymptomatic patients who generally have a favorable prognosis; at the other end are patients with severe hepatitis C who have symptoms, HCV RNA in their serum, and elevated serum liver enzyme levels. These patients typically develop cirrhosis and end-stage liver disease.

Episodic fluctuations in serum liver enzyme levels appear to be a feature of chronic hepatitis C. This pattern, presumably reflecting waves of hepatocellular inflammation and necrosis, may last for months to years. Such episodes of disease activity may be related to the emergence of so-called HCV neutralization escape mutants, but other poorly defined mechanisms also may play a role. HCV RNA is detected in the serum by PCR in almost all patients with chronic hepatitis C. HCV replication may be increased in advanced liver disease and may contribute to the progression of disease.

At least 20% of patients with chronic hepatitis C develop cirrhosis, a process that takes 10 to 20 years. After 20 to 40 years, a smaller percentage of patients with chronic disease develop liver cancer. Liver failure from chronic hepatitis C is one of the most common reasons for liver transplantation in the United States.

Chronic hepatitis C is diagnosed when anti-HCV is present and serum liver enzyme levels remain elevated for more than 6 months. Testing for HCV RNA by PCR assay confirms the diagnosis and documents that viremia is present. Most patients with chronic infection will have the viral genome detectable in serum by PCR.

Approximately one-third of those infected with HCV manifest anti-HCV antibodies within several weeks; others may take months or, less often, as long as 1 year to express antibodies. The current test antigen represents only 12% of the encoding capacity of the virus.

A reactive test implies infection with HCV but not infectivity or immunity.

Treatment

The main goal of treatment of chronic hepatitis C is to eliminate detectable viral RNA from the blood. Lack of detectable HCV RNA from the blood 6 months after the completion of therapy is known as a *sustained response* and has a very favorable prognosis that may be equivalent to a cure. Other, more subtle benefits of treatment may include slowing the progression of fibrosis in patients who do not achieve a sustained response.

The standard of care for HCV treatment since the early 1990s had been interferon, which aimed to boost the immune system rather than attacking the HCV directly.

Direct-acting antivirals (DAAs) are a newer class of drug that achieves cure rates of up to 99%. Compared with older-generation drugs, DAAs have far fewer side effects and can even treat advanced liver disease. Some newer combination DAAs can even treat all six major genetic strains (genotypes) of HCV.

In 2019 the following DAAs (alone or in combination with another drug) were approved by the FDA (https://www.fda.gov) for the treatment of chronic hepatitis C infection:

- Daklinza (daclatasvir): approved for HCV genotype 3
- Epclusa (sofosbuvir/velpatasvir): approved for all HCV genotypes (1–6)
- Harvoni (sofosbuvir, ledipasvir): approved for HCV genotype 1
- Mavyret (glecapravir, pibrentasvir): approved for all HCV genotypes (1–6)
- Sovaldi (sofosbuvir): approved for HCV genotypes 1, 2, 3, and 4
- Vosevi (sofosbuvir, velpatasvir, voxilaprevir): approved for all HCV genotypes (1–6)
- Zepatier (grazoprevir + elbasvir): approved for HCV genotypes 1, 4, and 6

In April, 2019, the FDA approved the use of glecaprevir/pibrentasvir (Mavyret) tablets to treat all six genotypes of HCV in children aged 12 to 17 years. This drug had been approved in 2017 only to treat HCV in adults.

Therapeutic vaccines are also being developed to enhance the immune response against the HCV.

Prevention

Precautionary practices among healthcare workers to prevent needlestick injuries should be promoted. Investigations have shown that removal of blood from donors with anti-HBcAg from the blood supply and use of third-generation anti-HCV testing can reduce the incidence of posttransfusion hepatitis C.

Vaccines and immunoglobulin products do not exist for the prevention or treatment of hepatitis C. Development of preventive strategies appears unlikely in the near future because these products would require antibodies to all the genotypes and variants of hepatitis C; however, some type of vaccine may eventually be developed.

HEPATITIS E

> **KEY CONCEPTS: Things to Know About Hepatitis E**
> - Hepatitis E virus (HEV) is transmitted by the fecal-oral route and usually is caused by poor sanitation.
> - No form of chronic liver disease has been attributable to HEV infection.
> - Although most acute infections are self-limited and mild, about 10% to 20% of HEV infections in pregnant women result in fulminant hepatitis, especially in the third trimester of pregnancy.

Etiology

The agent that causes hepatitis E is the hepatitis E virus (HEV).

Epidemiology

Only a few cases of hepatitis E have been reported, with none originating in the United States. All have been in travelers returning from the Indian subcontinent, northern Africa, the Far East, portions of Russia and Mexico.

HEV is transmitted by the fecal-oral route. Infection is usually the result of poor sanitation conditions. HEV is responsible for large, water-borne outbreaks of hepatitis in the developing world and is the most common cause of sporadic hepatitis in young adults in developing nations. Clinically apparent disease typically is found in patients 15 to 40 years old.

The HEV infection rate among household contacts of infected patients appears to be low. The seroprevalence of HEV in blood donors is approximately 2%.

Viruslike particles have been observed in stools from patients with HEV infection. In addition, serologic tests (IgM and IgG anti-HEV) have been developed now that the HEV genome has been cloned and sequenced.

Signs and Symptoms

The incubation period of HEV ranges from 2 to 9 weeks, with an average of 6 weeks. The symptoms of HEV infection are similar to those of other forms of viral hepatitis. HEV particles may appear in feces, inconstantly, during prodromal symptoms of hepatitis E. Fecal HEV shedding occurs predominantly during the first week after the onset of jaundice and has not been identified in stool samples obtained at 8 to 15 days. Viremia may occur during the period of fecal HEV shedding.

No form of chronic liver disease has been attributable to infection by HEV. Although most acute infections are self-limited and mild, 10%

to 20% of HEV infections in pregnant women result in fulminant hepatitis, especially in the third trimester of pregnancy.

Immunologic Manifestations
A short-lived IgM anti-HEV has been found in acute-phase sera. IgG anti-HEV appears and replaces IgM anti-HEV about 2 to 4 weeks after symptoms subside. The duration of detectable IgG anti-HEV remains uncertain.

Diagnostic Evaluation
Specific serologic tests for IgM and IgG anti-HEV are available. HEV can be diagnosed by performing immunoelectron microscopy on a stool specimen. Liver serum enzyme levels, if elevated, are indicative of the acute phase of the infection.

Prevention and Treatment
Standard gamma globulin preparations have not been shown to be effective in the prevention of viral E hepatitis. No effective vaccine has been developed. Treatment of HEV is usually supportive care.

TRANSFUSION-TRANSMITTED VIRUS

> **KEY CONCEPTS: Facts About Transfusion-Transmitted Virus**
> - Transfusion-transmitted virus (TTV) is a recent addition to the infectious hepatitis family.
> - The most remarkable feature of TTV is the extraordinarily high prevalence of chronic viremia in apparently healthy people, almost 100% in some countries.
> - As with HGV, the pathogenicity of TTV has not been proven.

Etiology
A more recent addition to the infectious hepatitis family is the transfusion-transmitted virus (TTV). TTV is a nonenveloped, single-strand DNA virus with 3739 nucleotides. Two genetic groups have been identified, differing by 30% in nucleotide sequences. It was discovered in 1997 through cloning and DNA sequence analysis by Japanese scientists. This novel, single-strand linear DNA virus has been designated the TT virus, or TTV, after the initials of the first patient (TT) from whom the virus was isolated.

The most remarkable feature of TTV is the extraordinarily high prevalence of chronic viremia in apparently healthy people, up to almost 100% in some countries.

Epidemiology
TTV has been associated with posttransfusion hepatitis of unknown etiology (non–A-G). The prevalence in the global population, particularly, the United States, United Kingdom, Japan, Germany, and Thailand, can reach 100% in healthy people.

There is evidence that TTV may be transmitted not only by parenteral exposure to blood but also by the fecal-oral route and from mother to child.

Signs and Symptoms
Although similar to HGV, TTV may be an example of a human virus with no clear disease association. This hypothesis is supported by the fact that the high prevalence of active TTV infection in the general population, both in the United Kingdom and Japan, is not comparable to the rate of significant liver damage.

As with HGV, the pathogenicity of TTV has not been proven.

CASE STUDY 18.1

History and Physical Examination
Several workers at a local fast food restaurant call in sick and report to the local ambulatory clinic for treatment. All of them complain of extreme fatigue. In addition, another 26-year-old food handler, who returned from visiting his relatives in Costa Rica a month ago, is sick. Within the past 1 or 2 weeks, he has had no energy and "just doesn't feel well." When he recently visited a physician at a local ambulatory clinic, he was slightly jaundiced.

Laboratory Data
Food handler's test results—Complete blood count, normal
Serum bilirubin level—Slightly elevated
  All of the other workers in the restaurant were asymptomatic and were not tested.

Questions
1. What is the most likely source route of hepatitis infection in this patient?
   a. Fecal-oral
   b. Parenteral
   c. Maternal-neonatal transmission
   d. Blood transfusion
2. Prevention and prophylaxis of hepatitis A consists of all of the following *except*:
   a. Handwashing
   b. Vaccination for hepatitis A virus
   c. Immunoglobulin injection if travel to or residence in an endemic area for more than 3 months
   d. Avoiding domestic and international travel

Answers to these questions can be found in Appendix A.

Critical Thinking Group Discussion Questions
1. What types of additional laboratory tests could be of value in determining the food handler's source of illness?
2. What are the immunologic manifestations?
3. What is the prognosis of this disease?
4. What are the methods of prevention and prophylaxis?
5. Because of this patient's occupation, could particular infectious diseases be of concern?

CASE STUDY 18.2

History and Physical Examination
A 30-year-old phlebotomist presents with fever, persistent fatigue, and joint pain. She reports that a needle in a plastic garbage bag nicked her finger about 2 months ago. Her physical examination is within normal limits.

Laboratory Data
The patient's laboratory data reveal elevated liver serum enzyme levels and total bilirubin levels. Additional laboratory data include a positive HBsAg and positive IgM anti-HBc. Her IgM, anti-HAV, and anti-HCV tests are negative.

Questions
1. The serologic marker of a low-level hepatitis B (HBV) carrier is:
   a. HBsAg
   b. Anti-HBs
   c. Anti-HBe
   d. Anti-HBc (IgM)
2. During the "window phase" of HBV infection, only _____ may be detectable as a marker.
   a. Anti-HBc
   b. Anti-HBe
   c. Anti-HBs
   d. HBsAg

Answers to these questions can be found in Appendix A.

Critical Thinking Group Discussion Questions
1. Does this patient have a form of infectious hepatitis? If so, what type?
2. Can any further tests be done to confirm the diagnosis?
3. What is the patient's prognosis?

CASE STUDY 18.3

History and Physical Examination
A 75-year-old woman has an 18-month history of right-sided abdominal pain and progressive fatigue. Her other medical problems include insulin-dependent diabetes mellitus and hypertension.

She reports no history of blood transfusion, IV drug use, or excessive alcohol use. She has no family history of liver disease. Her physical examination shows no cutaneous stigmata of chronic liver disease, hepatosplenomegaly, or ascites. Her daily medications include Humulin U-100 insulin and a drug for her high blood pressure.

Laboratory Data
Her abnormal laboratory values include elevated liver serum enzyme levels (ALT) and total bilirubin. She also exhibits hypergammaglobulinemia. Other relevant findings include negative HBsAg, positive anti-HCV antibody, and positive HCV RNA (by PCR).

Questions
1. Risk factors for hepatitis C virus (HCV) do not include:
   a. Illegal IV drug use
   b. Occupational exposure
   c. Multiple sexual partners
   d. A person's age
2. The most specific assay for detection of HCV infection is:
   a. Enzyme immunoassay (EIA)
   b. Western blot
   c. HCV RNA
   d. Southern blot

Answers to these questions can be found in Appendix A.

Critical Thinking Group Discussion Questions
1. Does this patient have a form of infectious hepatitis? If so, what type?
2. Can any further tests be done to confirm the diagnosis?
3. What is the patient's prognosis?

CASE STUDY 18.4

History and Physical Examination
A 45-year-old, previously healthy medical technologist visits her primary care physician because of increasing fatigue and loss of appetite. She has had a monogamous sexual relationship with her husband for 25 years.

Laboratory Data
After an initial workup for chronic fatigue, including a risk factor history that revealed several needlesticks on the job, the patient is found to be anti-HCV positive by EIA and to have an abnormal liver chemistry profile.

Questions
1. What risk factor for HCV does this patient have?
   a. Recent vaccination
   b. Monogamous sexual relationship
   c. Accidental needlestick (occupational)
   d. Advancing age
2. What percentage of HCV-infected individuals do not have the virus circulating in their blood?
   a. 5%
   b. 10%
   c. 15%
   d. 25%

Answers to these questions can be found in Appendix A.

Critical Thinking Group Discussion Questions
1. What is the probable source of the HCV infection?
2. What steps should be taken after exposure?
3. What behavioral changes are necessary now that the patient knows that she has HCV infection?

REVIEW QUESTIONS

1. An appropriate description of acute hepatitis is:
   a. A rare form associated with hepatic failure
   b. A typical form of hepatitis with associated jaundice
   c. Probably accounts for persons with serum antibodies but no history of hepatitis
   d. Accompanied by hepatic inflammation and necrosis
2. An appropriate description of fulminant acute hepatitis is:
   a. A rare form associated with hepatic failure
   b. A typical form of hepatitis with associated jaundice
   c. Probably accounts for persons with serum antibodies but no history of hepatitis
   d. Accompanied by hepatic inflammation and necrosis
3. An appropriate description of subclinical hepatitis without jaundice is:
   a. A rare form associated with hepatic failure
   b. A typical form of hepatitis
   c. Probably accounts for persons with serum antibodies but no history of hepatitis
   d. Accompanied by hepatic inflammation and necrosis
4. An appropriate description of chronic hepatitis is:
   a. A rare form associated with hepatic failure
   b. A typical form of hepatitis with associated jaundice
   c. Probably accounts for persons with serum antibodies but no history of hepatitis
   d. Accompanied by hepatic inflammation and necrosis
5. A representative characteristic of hepatitis A is:
   a. Intact virus is the Dane particle
   b. Transmission by both parenteral and nonparenteral routes
   c. Requires HBV as a helper
   d. Most common form of hepatitis
6. A representative characteristic of hepatitis B is:
   a. Intact virus is the Dane particle
   b. Transmission by both parenteral and nonparenteral routes
   c. Requires HBV as a helper
   d. Most common form of hepatitis
7. A representative characteristic of hepatitis D is:
   a. Intact virus is the Dane particle
   b. Transmission by both parenteral and nonparenteral routes
   c. Requires HBV as a helper
   d. Most common form of hepatitis
8. A representative characteristic of hepatitis C is:
   a. Intact virus is the Dane particle
   b. Transmission by both parenteral and nonparenteral routes
   c. Requires HBV as a helper
   d. Most common form of hepatitis
9. An associated characteristic of hepatitis A is:
   a. Should receive immunoglobulin intramuscularly after exposure
   b. Defective or incomplete RNA virus
   c. Has an epidemiology similar to that of HAV
   d. Originally called *Australia antigen*
10. An associated characteristic of hepatitis B is:
    a. Should receive immunoglobulin intramuscularly after exposure
    b. Defective or incomplete RNA virus
    c. Has an epidemiology similar to that of HAV
    d. Originally called *Australia antigen*
11. An associated characteristic of delta agent is:
    a. Should receive immunoglobulin intramuscularly after exposure
    b. Defective or incomplete RNA virus
    c. Has an epidemiology similar to that of HAV
    d. Originally called *Australia antigen*
12. An associated characteristic of hepatitis C is:
    a. Should receive immunoglobulin intramuscularly after exposure
    b. Defective or incomplete RNA virus
    c. Has an epidemiology similar to that of HAV
    d. Originally called *Australia antigen*
13. What three hepatitis B virus (HBV) markers are detectable in serum during the first two months after infection?
    a. HBsAg, HBeAg, anti-HBc
    b. HBeAg, anti-HBe, anti-HBs
    c. Anti-HBc, anti-HBs, anti-HBe
    d. HBsAg, anti-HBs, anti-HBe
14. HBsAg is:
    a. An indicator of recent HBV infection; may be the only serologic marker during the window phase
    b. Found in the serum of some patients who are ABsAg positive; marker for level of virus infectivity
    c. A serologic marker of recovery and immunity
    d. Initially detectable marker found in serum during the incubation period of HBV infection
15. HBeAg is:
    a. An indicator of recent HBV infection; may be the only serologic marker during the window phase
    b. Found in the serum of some patients who are ABsAg positive; marker for level of virus infectivity
    c. A serologic marker of recovery and immunity
    d. Initially detectable marker found in serum during the incubation period of HBV infection
16. Anti-HBc is:
    a. An indicator of recent HBV infection; may be the only serologic marker during the window phase
    b. Found in the serum of some patients who are ABsAg positive; marker for level of virus infectivity
    c. A serologic marker of recovery and immunity
    d. In the case of acute hepatitis, the first serologic evidence of the convalescent phase
17. Anti-HBe is:
    a. An indicator of recent HBV infection; may be the only serologic marker during the window phase
    b. Found in the serum of some patients who are ABsAg positive; marker for level of virus infectivity
    c. A serologic marker of recovery and immunity
    d. In the case of acute hepatitis, the first serologic evidence of the convalescent phase
18. Anti-HBs is:
    a. An indicator of recent HBV infection; may be the only serologic marker during the window phase
    b. Found in the serum of some patients who are HBsAg-positive; marker for level of virus infectivity
    c. A serologic marker of recovery and immunity
    d. Initially detectable marker found in serum during the incubation period of HBV infection
19. Of patients in the United States with chronic hepatitis B, _____ of them acquired the virus in childhood.
    a. Less than 20%
    b. 20% to 30%
    c. 30% to 40%
    d. More than 40%

20. The rate of posttransfusion hepatitis C decreased to _____ after the introduction of serologic testing in the screening of blood donors.
    a. Less than 1%
    b. 5%
    c. 10%
    d. 15%
21. The average incubation time for hepatitis A is:
    a. 5 days
    b. 28 days
    c. 50 days
    d. 75 days
22. The average incubation time for hepatitis B is:
    a. 5 days
    b. 25 days
    c. 50 days
    d. 90 days
23. The average incubation time for posttransfusion hepatitis C is _____ weeks.
    a. 2–12
    b. 2–26
    c. 4–12
    d. 6–26
24. Which form of hepatitis does *not* have a chronic form of the disease?
    a. Hepatitis A
    b. Hepatitis B
    c. Hepatitis C
25. Another name for hepatitis B infection is:
    a. Infectious hepatitis
    b. Long-incubation hepatitis
    c. Australia antigen
    d. Dane particle
26. The most common clinical response to hepatitis B virus is:
    a. Jaundice within 75 days
    b. Asymptomatic infection
    c. Subclinical infection
    d. Both b and c
27. The first laboratory screening test of donor blood was for the detection of:
    a. HBc
    b. HBsAg
    c. HBe
    d. Anti-HBe
28. Which surface marker is a reliable marker for the presence of high levels of hepatitis B virus (HBV) and a high degree of infectivity?
    a. HBeAg
    b. HBsAg
    c. HBcAg
    d. Anti-HBsAg
29. The only serologic marker during the anticore window period of hepatitis B (the time between disappearance of detectable HBsAg and appearance of detectable anti-HBs) may be:
    a. Anti-HBs
    b. Anti-HBc
    c. Anti-HBe
    d. HBsAg
30. Which of the following is a characteristic of the delta agent?
    a. Is a DNA virus
    b. Usually replicates only in HBV-infected hosts
    c. Infects patients who are HBcAg positive
    d. Is commonly found in the United States
31. Which of the following viruses is rarely implicated in transfusion-associated hepatitis?
    a. Hepatitis A
    b. Hepatitis B
    c. Hepatitis C
    d. Cytomegalovirus
32. In healthcare workers, the risk of contracting hepatitis C is _____ the risk of contracting AIDS.
    a. Lower than
    b. Higher than
    c. The same as
    d. Not something to worry about compared with
33. The specific diagnostic test for hepatitis C is:
    a. Absence of anti-HAV and anti-HBsAg
    b. Increase in liver serum enzyme levels
    c. Detection of non-A, non-B antibodies
    d. Anti-HCV
34. The earliest detectable serologic marker of acute hepatitis C is:
    a. Anti-HCV
    b. Anti-HBc and liver serum enzyme abnormalities
    c. HCV RNA
    d. Anti-HBs and anti-HBc
35. Primary hepatitis viruses are given this name because they primarily attack:
    a. A variety of body systems
    b. The liver
    c. The skin
    d. The nervous system
36. Hepatitis A has all the following characteristics *except*:
    a. DNA virus
    b. Short-incubation hepatitis
    c. Crowded, unsanitary conditions as a risk factor
    d. Rare occurrence of transfusion acquisition
37. The Australia antigen is now called:
    a. Dane particle
    b. Long-incubation hepatitis
    c. Hepatitis B surface antigen (HBsAg)
    d. Hepatitis B core antigen (HBcAg)
38. The serologic marker HBsAg for hepatitis B virus (HBV) infection in early (asymptomatic) infection is:
    a. Positive
    b. Negative
    c. Questionable (±)
39. The serologic marker HBsAg for hepatitis B virus (HBV) infection in the acute or chronic stage is:
    a. Positive
    b. Negative
    c. Questionable (±)
40. The serologic marker anti-HBc for hepatitis B virus (HBV) infection in the acute or chronic stage is:
    a. Positive
    b. Negative
    c. Questionable (±)

41. The serologic marker anti-HBc for hepatitis B virus (HBV) infection in a low-level carrier state is:
    a. Positive
    b. Negative
    c. Questionable (±)
42. The serologic marker anti-HBc for immunity with HBsAg is:
    a. Positive
    b. Negative
    c. Questionable (±)
43. The serologic marker anti-HBc (IgM) for immunity with HBsAg is:
    a. Positive
    b. Negative
    c. Questionable (±)
44. Which category has the highest risk for acute hepatitis C?
    a. Low socioeconomic status
    b. Dialysis
    c. Transfusion
    d. Illegal drug use
45. Which category has the lowest incidence of acute hepatitis C?
    a. Sexual, household
    b. Dialysis
    c. Drug abuse
    d. Community acquired without any known risk factors
46. The mode of transmission of hepatitis A is:
    a. Fecal-oral
    b. Parenteral
    c. Nonparenteral
    d. Unknown
47. The mode of transmission of hepatitis B is:
    a. Fecal-oral
    b. Parenteral
    c. Nonparenteral
    d. Unknown
48. The mode of transmission of hepatitis C is:
    a. Fecal-oral
    b. Parenteral
    c. Nonparenteral
    d. Unknown
49. The mode of transmission of hepatitis E is:
    a. Fecal-oral
    b. Parenteral
    c. Nonparenteral
    d. Unknown
50. What form of immunity is anticipated to provide long-term immune protection after a series of HBV vaccinations is administered to an immunocompetent person?
    a. Active
    b. Passive
    c. Adaptive
    d. Innate
51. What is the anticipated serological response in an immunocompetent person who has been properly vaccinated
    a. HBsAg (neg), anti-HBcAg (neg), anti-HBs (pos)
    b. HBsAg (pos), HBcAg (pos), anti-HBs (neg)
    c. HBsAg (neg), anti-HBcAg (pos), anti-HBs (pos)
    d. HBsAg (neg), anti-HBcAg (pos), anti-HBs (pos)

PART IV

Immune Disorders

Chapter 19: Primary and Acquired Immunodeficiency Syndromes, 300

Chapter 20: Hypersensitivity Reactions, 337

Chapter 21: Plasma Cell Neoplasms and Other Diseases With Paraproteins, 353

Chapter 22: Tolerance, Autoimmunity, and Autoimmune Disorders, 369

Chapter 23: Systemic Lupus Erythematosus, 396

Chapter 24: Rheumatoid Arthritis, 414

19

Primary and Acquired Immunodeficiency Syndromes

LEARNING OUTCOMES

- Compare the major characteristics of primary immunodeficiency disorders (PIDs) versus secondary immunodeficiencies.
- Describe general laboratory evaluation of PIDs.
- Compare the etiology, signs and symptoms, and immunologic manifestations of these PIDs:
  - DiGeorge syndrome
  - Severe combined immunodeficiency (SCID)
  - Chronic mucocutaneous candidiasis
  - Bruton X-linked agammaglobulinemia
  - Common variable immunodeficiency
  - Immunodeficiency with elevated immunoglobulin M (hyper-IgM)
  - Selective immunoglobulin A deficiency
  - X-linked lymphoproliferative disease (XLP) syndromes 1 and 2 (Duncan disease)
    - Compare the etiology, signs and symptoms, and immunologic manifestations of the combined cellular immunodeficiency disorder—hereditary ataxia-telangiectasis.
    - Compare the etiology, signs and symptoms, and immunologic manifestations of the partially combined immunodeficiency disorder—Wiskott-Aldrich syndrome (WAS).
- Compare the etiology, signs and symptoms, and immunologic manifestations of an example of other primary immune disorders—hyper-E syndrome (Job syndrome)
- Describe the etiology and viral characteristics of the human immunodeficiency virus type 1 (HIV-1).
- Explain the epidemiology, including modes of transmission, and prevention of HIV-1.
- Discuss the signs and symptoms of various stages and the classification of HIV infection.
- Describe the immunologic manifestations and cellular abnormalities of HIV-1 infection.
- Explain the serologic markers and diagnostic evaluation of HIV.
- Compare the features of fourth-generation HIV testing with other generations of testing.
- Analyze a representative HIV-1 case study.
- Correctly answer case study–related multiple-choice questions.
- Participate in a discussion of critical thinking questions.
- Describe the principles of various rapid HIV assays, GS HIV combo antigen/antibody enzyme immunoassay (EIA), and simulation of HIV-1 detection.
- Correctly answer the end-of-chapter review questions.

OUTLINE

Primary Immunodeficiency Disorders, 302
Characteristics of Primary Immunodeficiency Disorders, 304
General Laboratory Evaluation, 304
    Newborn Screening, 304
T-Cell Immunodeficiency Disorders, 306
Digeorge Syndrome, 307
    Etiology, 307
    Signs and Symptoms, 307
    Immunologic Manifestations, 307
Severe Combined Immunodeficiency (SCID), 307
    Etiology, 307
    Signs and Symptoms, 308
    Immunologic Manifestations, 308
        Newborn Screening Test for SCID: T-Cell Receptor Excision Circles, 308
Chronic Mucocutaneous Candidiasis, 308
    Etiology, 308
    Signs and Symptoms, 308
    Immunologic Manifestations, 309
        T-Cell Activation Defects, 309
        B-Cell and Antibody Deficiency Disorders, 309

Bruton X-Linked Agammaglobulinemia (XLA), 309
    Etiology, 309
    Signs and Symptoms, 309
    Immunologic Manifestations, 310
Common Variable Immunodeficiency, 310
    Etiology, 310
    Epidemiology, 310
    Signs and Symptoms, 310
    Immunologic Manifestations, 310
    Prognosis, 311
Transient Hypogammaglobulinemia of Infancy, 311
Immunodeficiency With Elevated Immunoglobulin M (Hyper-IgM), 311
    Etiology, 311
    Signs and Symptoms, 311
    Immunologic Manifestations, 311
        Immunoglobulin Subclass Deficiencies, 311
Selective Immunoglobulin A Deficiency, 311
    Etiology, 311
    Signs and Symptoms, 311
    Immunologic Manifestations, 311

Hyper-E Syndrome (HIES), 311
    Etiology, 311
    Signs and Symptoms, 311
X-Linked Lymphoproliferative Disease (XLP) Syndromes 1 and 2 (Duncan Disease), 312
    Etiology, 312
    Signs and Symptoms, 312
    Immunologic Manifestations, 312
    Treatment, 312
Combined Cellular Immunodeficiency Disorders, 312
    Hereditary Ataxia-Telangiectasia (Louis Bar Syndrome), 312
        Etiology, 312
        Signs and Symptoms, 312
        Immunologic Manifestations, 312
Partial Combined Immune Deficiency Disorders, 312
    Wiskott-Aldrich Syndrome, 312
        Etiology, 312
        Signs and Symptoms, 312
        Immunologic Manifestations, 312
        Autoimmune Disorders in Wiskott-Aldrich Syndrome, 313
        Malignancies in Wiskott-Aldrich Syndrome, 313
        Vaccination, 313
        Stem Cell Transplantation and Gene Therapy, 313
Other Primary Immune Disorders, 313
Acquired (Secondary) Immunodeficiency Disorders, 313
Acquired Immunodeficiency Syndrome, 313
    Etiology, 313
    Viral Characteristics, 314
        Viral Structure, 314
        Viral Replication, 315
    Epidemiology, 316
        Global Data, 316
    Infectious Patterns, 317
        HIV-1, 317
        HIV-2, 318
    Modes of Transmission, 318
    Signs and Symptoms, 318
    Opportunistic Infections, 319
        Kaposi Sarcoma, 320
        Cryptosporidiosis, 320
    Disease Progression, 321
    Immunologic Manifestations, 321
        Cellular Abnormalities, 321
        Immune System Alterations, 321
    Serologic Markers, 322
        Detection of Core Antigen, 322
        Antibodies to HIV-1, 322
    Diagnostic Evaluation and Monitoring, 322
    Testing Methods, 322
    HIV-1 Antibody Assays, 322
    HIV Antigen and Genome Testing, 324
        Enzyme Immunoassay: p24 Antigen, 324
        Polymerase Chain Reaction, 324
    Alternative Screening for HIV, 324
        Western Blot, 325
        Quantitative RNA Assay, 326
    Fourth-Generation Testing, 326
    Pediatric Testing, 326
    Rapid Testing, 326
    Tests for Therapeutic Monitoring, 326
        Viral Load Testing, 326
        CD4+ T-Lymphocyte Testing, 326
Prevention, 326
    Reducing Viral Transmission, 326
    Vaccines, 326
Treatment, 326
    Drug Therapy, 327
    Actions of Mechanistic Classes of Antiretroviral Drugs, 328
        Nucleoside Reverse Transcriptase Inhibitors, 328
        Nonnucleoside Reverse Transcriptase Inhibitors, 328
        Protease Inhibitors, 328
        Fusion Inhibitors, 328
        Entry Inhibitors (CCR5 Antagonist), 328
        Integrase Strand Transfer Inhibitors, 328
    Investigational Drugs, 331
        HIV Drug Resistance, 331
Preexposure and Postexposure Prophylaxis, 332
    Preexposure Prophylaxis, 332
    Postexposure Prophylaxis, 332
Case Study 19.1, 333
Case Study 19.2, 333
Case Study 19.3, 334
Procedure: Rapid HIV Antibody Test, 336.e1
Procedure: GS HIV Combo AG/AB EIA, 336.e1
Procedure: Simulation of HIV-1 Detection, 336.e1

KEY TERMS

acquired immunodeficiency disorders
acquired immunodeficiency syndrome (AIDS)
antiretroviral therapy (ART)
bare lymphocyte syndrome
cytochrome P-450
dysplastic
envelope protein
gag region
highly active antiretroviral therapy (HAART)
human immunodeficiency virus (HIV)
long terminal redundancies (LTRs)
Phase I trials
Phase IV trials
primary immunodeficiency disorders (PIDs)
protease
protease inhibitors (PIs)
proviral genome
retrovirus
reverse transcriptase
single-nucleotide polymorphism (SNP)
specific oligomer primers
structural protein
transcriptase
viral core protein

Primary immunodeficiency disorders (PIDs) were previously described as disorders caused by one or more defects of the immune system that resulted in an increased susceptibility to microbial infections. Today, the PIDs are defined in more complex terms. There are now more than 320 single-gene inborn errors of immunity underlying phenotypes as diverse as infection, allergy, autoimmunity, and autoinflammation.

According to the National Institute of Allergy and Infectious Diseases, there are more than 200 different forms of PIDs affecting approximately 500,000 people in the United States (Box 19.1A). These rare genetic diseases may be chronic, debilitating, and costly. PIDs are now recognized as a more complicated group of heterogeneous immune disorders characterized by various combinations of repeated infections, autoimmunity, lymphoproliferation, atopy, malignancy, and a granulomatous process (Fig. 19.1).

The types of repeated infections are based on the type of cellular defect in the PID. For example, bacterial infections are typically manifested in B-cell defects, whereas viral, fungal, and bacterial infections may be manifested in T-cell or B-cell defects (Box 19.1B).

> **KEY CONCEPTS: Origin and Effects of Primary Immunodeficiency Disorders**
> - Primary immune deficiency disorders (PIDs) are a group chronic disorders in which a genetic error related to the body's immune system is missing or functions improperly.
> - These unusual autosomal or X-linked hereditary disorders of the innate or adaptive immune system are usually monogenic disorders.
> - Gene mutations have been identified that cause impairment in the differentiation and/or function of immune cells with different degrees of severity and may produce associated anatomic abnormalities.
> - Disorders of immunologic origin include hematologic progenitor cells, T cells, B cells, antibody-production disorders, phagocytic abnormalities, and complement alterations.
> - Some PIDs are specific to a single type of blood cell, but others can involve one or more components of the immune system.
> - Identification of gene defects in PIDs complicated by autoimmune disorders has expanded understanding of central and peripheral tolerance.
> - Laboratory evaluation of patients with a suspected immunodeficiency varies for infants and children compared with older children and adults.

PRIMARY IMMUNODEFICIENCY DISORDERS

Immunologic disorders can be divided into primary, secondary, and other types of disorders mediated through immune mechanisms. Most primary immune disorders are caused by an inherited dysfunction of the immune system caused by a genetic irregularity, but secondary immune disorders are the result of other underlying causes (Box 19.2).

Primary immunodeficiency disorders (PIDs), also called *inborn errors of immunity*, are a group of uncommon, chronic disorders. They are classified according to the immunologic mechanisms and clinical presentations that result from the underlying defects and functional consequences of mutations upon their gene products.

Innate immune disorders result from impaired antigen-independent pathways and include defects in natural killer (NK) cell cytotoxicity, toll-like receptor (TLR) activation, phagocytosis, macrophage activation, and complement defects. Adaptive immune defects predominantly affect antigen-driven processes. These defects include humoral immune deficiencies (due to impaired production of antibody by B cells) and combined immunodeficiencies (with impairments in both T and B cells). The autosomal or X-linked hereditary disorders of the innate or adaptive immune system are usually monogenic disorders affecting host defenses. Different gene mutations have been identified that cause impairment in the differentiation and/or function of immune cells with different degrees of severity and may produce associated anatomic abnormalities.

> **BOX 19.1A Examples of Primary Immune Deficiency Diseases Under Study**
>
> Autoimmune lymphoproliferative syndrome (ALPS)
> APS-1 (APECED) Autoimmune polyglandular syndrome type 1
> CARD9 and other syndromes of susceptibility to candidiasis
> Chronic granulomatous disease (CGD)
> Common variable immunodeficiency (CVID)
> Congenital neutropenia syndromes
> CTLA4 deficiency
> DOCK8 deficiency
> Glycosylation disorders with immunodeficiency
> Hyper-immunoglobulin E syndromes (HIES)
> Hyperimmunoglobulin M syndromes
> Leukocyte adhesion deficiency (LAD)
> PI3 kinase disease
> PLCG2-associated antibody deficiency and immune dysregulation (PLAID)
> Severe combined immunodeficiency (SCID)
> STAT3 dominant-negative disease
> X-linked agammaglobulinemia (XLA)
> X-linked lymphoproliferative disease (XLP)

From NIH National Institute of Allergy and Infectious Diseases Types of Primary Immune Deficiency Diseases www.niaid.nih.gov. Accessed August 13, 2023.

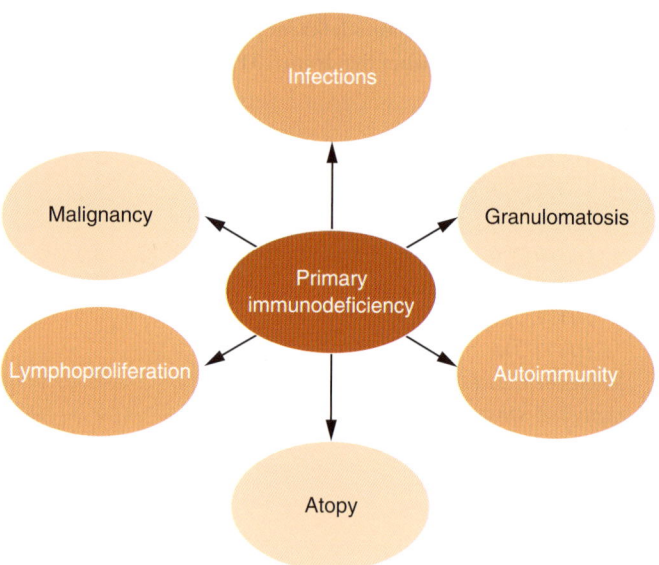

Fig. 19.1 Features of Primary Immunodeficiencies. (From Raje N, Dinakar C: Overview of immunodeficiency disorders in primary immunodeficiency disorders, *Immunol Allergy Clin North Am* 35[4]:600, 2015.)

Primary (congenital) and secondary (acquired disease or therapy produced) immune deficiency disorders encompass all major components of the immune system. A breakdown in any part of the immune mechanism can lead to a disorder. Disorders of immunologic origin include hematologic progenitor cells, T cells, B cells, antibody-production disorders, phagocytic abnormalities, and complement alterations (Table 19.1 and Fig. 19.2).

Some PIDs are specific to a single type of blood cell, but others can involve one or more components of the immune system. The most common T-cell deficiency disorders are associated with a concurrent B-cell abnormality.

BOX 19.1B Examples of Types of Cells in Primary Immune Deficiencies

Cellular Immunodeficiencies
T Cells
- DiGeorge syndrome
- Severe combined immune deficiency
- Chronic mucocutaneous candidiasis
- T-cell activation defects

T Cells and Partially Combined Immunodeficiency Disorders
- Ataxia-telangiectasia
- Wiskott-Aldrich syndrome
- Nezelof syndrome

B-Cell and Antibody Deficiencies
- Bruton X-linked agammaglobulinemia
- Common variable immunodeficiency
- Immunoglobulin subclass deficiencies
  - Selective IgA deficiency
  - Hyper-IgM
  - Transient hypogammaglobulinemia
- X-linked lymphoproliferative disease

Innate Immune Disorders
- Chronic granulomatous disease
- Leukocyte adhesion deficiency
- Hyper-IgE syndrome
- Complement deficiencies
- NEMO deficiency syndrome

Adapted from Blaese RM, editor: *Immune Deficiency Foundation patient and family handbook for primary immunodeficiency diseases,* ed 5, Towson, Maryland, 2013, Immune Deficiency Foundation.

BOX 19.2 Categories of Primary Immunodeficiencies

Predominantly Antibody Deficiencies
Disorders include hypogammaglobulinemia, Bruton X-linked agammaglobulinemia, common variable immunodeficiency phenotypes, and selective IgA deficiency.

T-Cell Immunodeficiencies or Combined Immunodeficiencies
Disorders include severe combined immunodeficiencies (SCIDs) defined by CD3 T-cell lymphopenia, combined immunodeficiencies.

Combined Immunodeficiency Disorders (CIDs) with Syndromic Immunodeficiencies
Disorders include congenital thrombocytopenia (Wiskott-Aldrich syndrome), ataxia-telangiectasia, and hyper-IgE syndromes.

Complement Defects
Disorders include disseminated neisserial infections, recurrent pyogenic infections, systemic lupus erythematosus (SLE)–like syndrome, and atypical hemolytic syndrome. Early complement defect C1q, C1r, C1s, C4, and C2 deficiency present with SLE. C3, factor I, H deficiency, and CD46 deficiency can present with infection, glomerulonephritis, and atypical hemolytic-uremic syndrome. Late complement C5–C9, factor D, and properdin deficiency are caused by infections with neisserial species.

Congenital Defects of Phagocyte Number, Function, or Both
Disorders include neutropenia, chronic granulomatous disease; chronic myelomonocytic leukemia; motility defects leukocyte adhesion deficiency (LAD) 1, 2, or 3; respiratory burst defects chronic granulomatous (CGD), mendelian susceptibility to mycobacterial disease.

Defects of Intrinsic and Innate Immunity
Disorders include chronic mucocutaneous candidiasis (CMC), mendelian susceptibility to mycobacterial disease (MSMD).

Diseases of Immune Dysregulation
Disorders include hemophagocytic lymphohistiocytosis, autoimmune lymphoproliferative syndrome (ALPS), autoimmune polyendocrinopathy syndrome (APS), familial hemophagocytic lymphohistiocytosis (FHL), (hepato)splenomegalia ([H]SM), inflammatory bowel disease (IBD), SLE.

Autoinflammatory Disorders
Disorders affecting the inflammation include cryopyrin-associated periodic syndrome (CAPS), familial chilblain lupus (FCL), hemophagocytic lymphohistiocytosis (HLH), hepatosplenomegaly (HSM), intracranial calcifications (ICC), SLE.

Phenocopies of Primary Immunodeficiencies
These disorders behave and present like primary immunodeficiency diseases, but they are acquired secondary to the occurrence of autoantibodies or somatic mutations. Examples of disorders include autoimmune lymphoproliferative syndrome due to a somatic FAS mutation (ALPS-sFAS), combined immunodeficiency (CID), chronic mucocutaneous candidiasis (CMC), mendelian susceptibility to mycobacterial disease (MSMD), and pure red cell aplasia (PRCA).

Adapted from Bousfiha A, Jeddane L, Picard C et al: The 2017 IUIS phenotypic classification for primary immunodeficiencies, *J Clin Immunol* 38(1):129–143, 2018; Al-Herz W, Bousfiha A, Casanova JL, et al: Primary immunodeficiency diseases: an update on the classification from the international union of immunological societies expert committee for primary immunodeficiency, *Front Immunol* 5:162, 2014.

TABLE 19.1 T-Cell and B-Cell Disorders

T-Cell Disorders	B-Cell Disorders
Congenital	
Thymic hypoplasia (DiGeorge syndrome)	Bruton agammaglobulinemia
Acquired	
Acquired immunodeficiency syndrome	Autoimmune disorders
Hodgkin disease	Multiple myeloma
Chronic lymphocytic leukemia	
Systemic lupus erythematosus	

Commonly reported specific primary immune deficiency disorders in order of approximate incidence, are:
- Common variable immune deficiency
- IgG subclass deficiency
- Selective IgA deficiency
- X-linked agammaglobulinemia
  Less common disorders include:
- Severe combined immune deficiency
- Chronic granulomatous disease
- Hyper-IgM
- DiGeorge syndrome

PART IV Immune Disorders

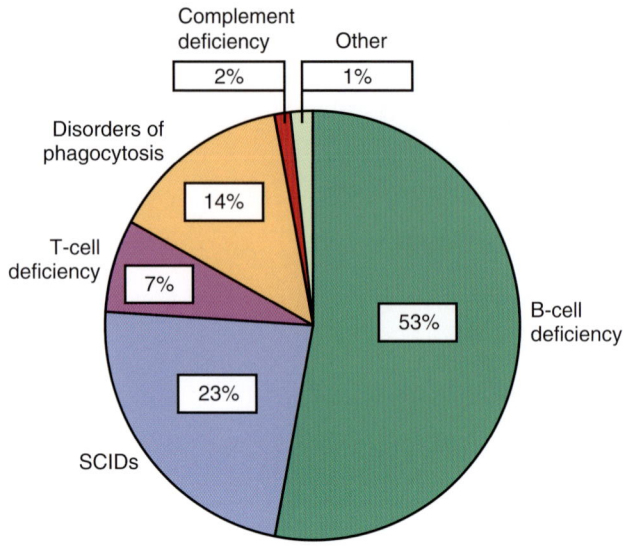

Fig. 19.2 Distribution of Immunodeficiency Disorders. *SCIDs,* Severe combined immunodeficiency disorders.

- Wiskott-Aldrich syndrome (WAS)
- Ataxia-telangiectasia
- Complement disorders

Another category (diseases mediated through immune mechanisms) exists. Autoimmunity (see Chapter 22) and PID are frequently associated. This relationship highlights the relationship between various elements of the immune system and the selection and regulatory mechanisms that maintain self-tolerance (Table 19.2 and Fig. 19.3).

CHARACTERISTICS OF PRIMARY IMMUNODEFICIENCY DISORDERS

Infants and children with recurrent upper and lower respiratory tract infections and/or diarrhea, abscesses, sepsis, or meningitis should be evaluated for immune deficiency. Before proceeding with laboratory testing, primary care providers need to rule out the following:

- Anatomic or physical causes (e.g., foreign bodies and indwelling catheters)
- Cancer
- Connective tissue disease
- Diabetes
- Renal disease

GENERAL LABORATORY EVALUATION

Newborn Screening

Currently, over 380 PIDs have been described and they are estimated to occur in as many as 1 in 1200 live births. Delay in diagnosis and treatment of PIDs leads to significant morbidity and sometimes early death from infections; affected infants may die of infections without recognition that they had an immune system defect. The overall goal of newborn screening (NBS) is to detect treatable disorders that can threaten life or long-term health before a disorder becomes symptomatic (e.g., repeated infections). Thus early identification via NBS prior to the onset of infections should improve detection and reduce the morbidity and mortality associated with these disorders. Early treatment of these rare disorders may significantly reduce mortality and morbidity in affected patients.

TABLE 19.2 Examples of the Relationship of Primary Immunodeficiencies to Autoimmune Inflammatory Conditions

Primary Immunodeficiency	Genetic Defect	Mechanisms	Autoimmune Features
Complement deficiencies	C11, C1r, C1s, C4, C2	Defective clearance of apoptotic bodies Impaired clearance of immune complexes	Systemic lupus erythematosus (SLE), Antineutrophil cytoplasmic antibody (ANCA) vasculitis
Hyper-IgM syndrome	CD40L/CD40	Defective peripheral tolerance Reduced regulatory T cells (T_{reg}) Elevated B-cell–activating factor (BAFF) levels	Autoimmune hemolytic anemia (AIHA), chronic neutropenia, immune thrombocytopenia (ITP), polyarthritis, inflammatory bowel disease (IBD), biliary tract/liver disease, thyroiditis
Common variable immunodeficiency (CVID)	Unknown in majority of cases	Mechanisms unclear	Autoimmune cytopenias, enteropathy, granulomatous lymphocytic interstitial lung disease (GLILD), hepatitis, rheumatologic diseases
Chronic granulomatous disease (CGD)	Gp91 phox p22 phox p47 phox p67 phox p40 phox	Ineffective clearance of antigens, leading to chronic stimulation Enhanced type 1 interferon (IFN-1) signature Defective induction of regulatory T cells (T_{reg}) cells	Colitis, discoid lupus, carriers with rheumatologic disease
Wiskott-Aldrich syndrome (WAS)	WASp	Intrinsic signaling abnormality in B cells Reduction in T_{reg} numbers and function	Thrombocytopenia, AIHA, neutropenia, IBD, arthritis, vasculitis, renal disease
Hyper-IgE syndrome	STAT3 DOCK8	Altered T_{reg} and cytokine signaling Decreased number and function of T_{regs} Autoreactive B cells	Cytopenias, organ-specific autoimmunity (lung, gastrointestinal, hepatic, and/or endocrine), enteropathy, type 1 diabetes mellitus, lymphadenopathy, SLE

Adapted from Raje N, Dinakar C. Overview of immunodeficiency disorders in autoimmune disease in primary immunodeficiency. *Immunol Allergy Clin North Am* 35(4):599-623, 2015.

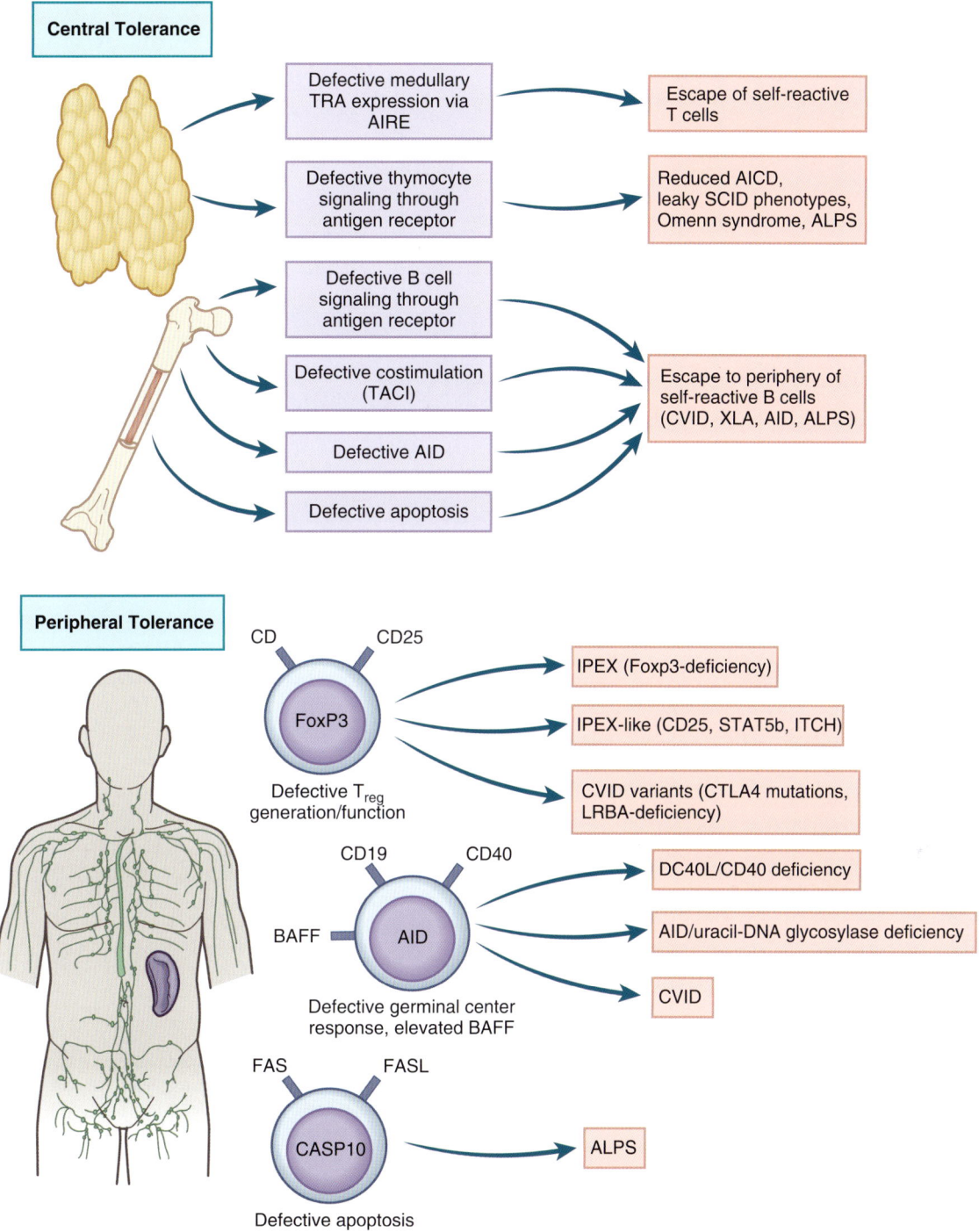

Fig. 19.3 Mechanisms of autoimmunity in primary immunodeficiency disorders (PIDs) and some of the major mechanisms through which loss of self-tolerance and autoimmunity occur in PID syndromes. *AID*, Activation-induced cytidine deaminase; *AICD*, active induced cell death; *AIRE*, autoimmune regulator; *ALPS*, autoimmune lymphoproliferative syndrome; *BAFF*, B-cell–activating factor; *CVID*, common variable immunodeficiency; *FASL*, FAS ligand; *LRBA*, lipopolysaccharide-responsive and beige-like anchor protein; *SCID*, severe combined immunodeficiency disorders; *TRA*, tissue-restricted antigen; *XLA*, X-linked agammaglobulinemia. (From Saifi M, Wysocki CA: Autoimmune disease in primary immunodeficiency: At the crossroads of anti-infective immunity and self-tolerance, *Immunol Allergy Clin North Am* 35[4]:731–52. 2015.)

Severe combined immunodeficiency (SCID) is included in NBS because of the recent emergence of an effective assay for T-cell receptor excision circles (TRECs), a biomarker for normal T-cell development. TRECs are found in every healthy newborn's blood. NBS for SCID is carried out in some states.

Preliminary laboratory assessment can include examination of a peripheral blood smear, the erythrocyte sedimentation rate (ESR), and C-reactive protein (CRP). Laboratory evaluation of patients with a suspected immunodeficiency is different for infants and children than for older children and adults.

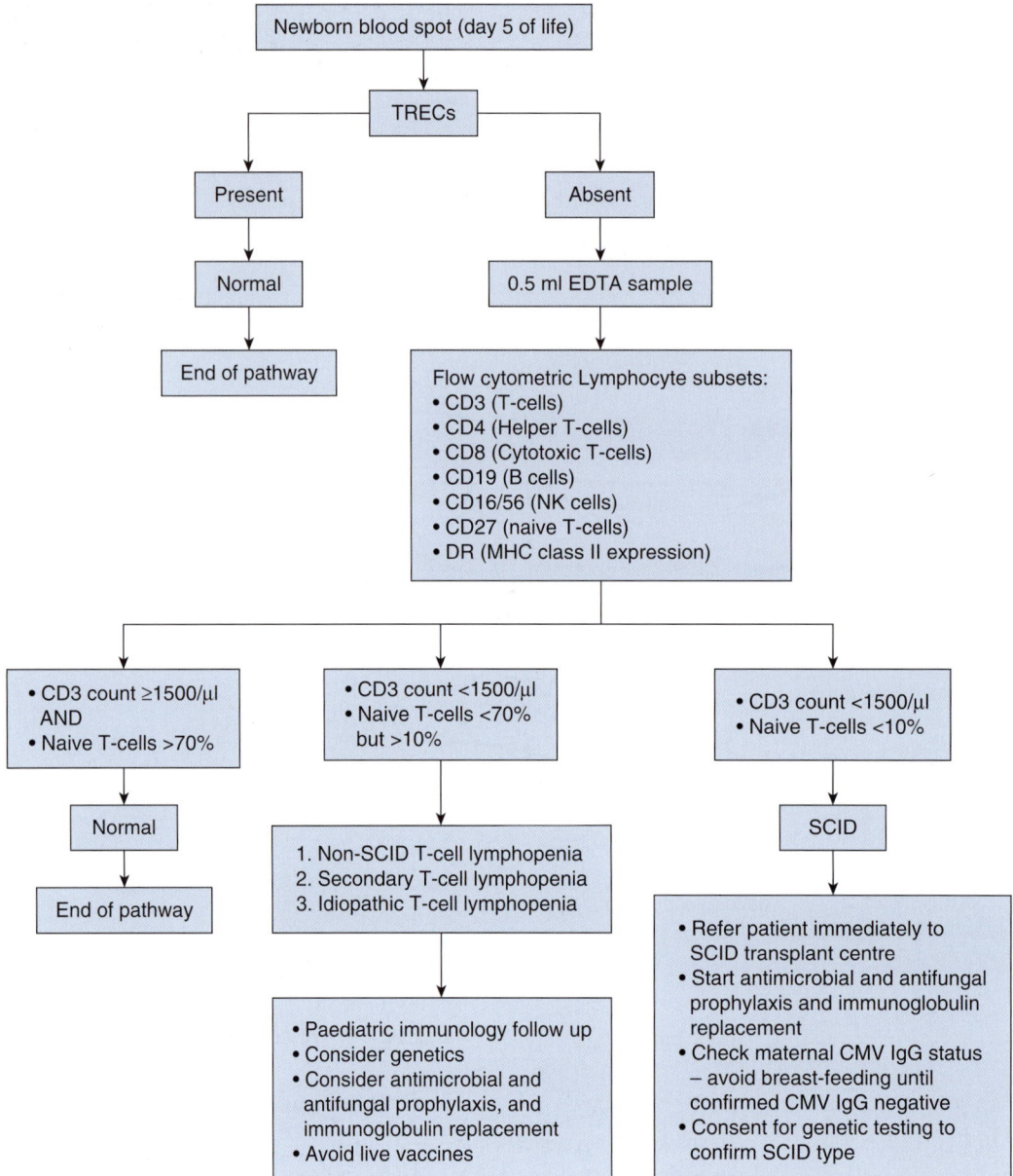

Fig. 19.4 Clinical pathway for SCID newborn screening in the UK. *CMV*, Cytomegalovirus; *SCID*, severe combined immune deficiency; *TRECs*, T-cell receptor excision circles. (Torpiano P, Buckland M, Gilmour K: Symposium: immunity and infection. Investigating suspected immune deficiency in children, *Paediatr Child Health* 32(6):213–219, 2022.)

Specific laboratory testing for the evaluation of immune deficiency in chronic infections in infants and children can follow various paths, depending on the presenting symptoms (Fig. 19.4). The evaluation of chronic infections in older children and adults is presented in Fig. 19.4. The algorithm for testing adults has variations from the evaluation of infants and young children. Among the important laboratory assessments, the absolute lymphocyte count can be critical (Box 19.3).

BOX 19.3 Determination of Absolute Lymphocyte Count

1. Absolute number of lymphocytes = Total leukocyte count × percentage (%) of lymphocytes
2. Total leukocyte count = 25×10^9/L
3. Relative percentage (%) of lymphocytes = 76%
4. Absolute number = 19×10^9/L

T-CELL IMMUNODEFICIENCY DISORDERS

Infants and children who are 18 months old or older and suffer from chronic respiratory infections, severe viral infections, or *Candida* or other fungal infections should be screened for the human immunodeficiency virus (HIV). If HIV screening result is positive, an HIV workup should be conducted (see discussion of acquired immunodeficiency syndrome [AIDS] later in the chapter). If the HIV screening result is negative, a further T-cell disorder evaluation should be conducted. Specific testing includes:

- CD4+ T-cell recent thymic emigrants (RTEs)
- Lymphocyte subset panel
- Lymphocyte antigen and mitogen (LAM) proliferation panel

DIGEORGE SYNDROME

Etiology

DiGeorge syndrome, also called *22q11.2 deletion syndrome*, is a disorder resulting from a heterogeneous mutation in *TBX1* (chromosome 22q11.2 deletion).

The T-cell defect is a congenital anomaly, with a contiguous gene defect found in 90% of patients that results in faulty embryogenesis of the endodermal derivation of the third and fourth pharyngeal pouches; this results in aplasia of the parathyroid and thymus glands. At autopsy, parathyroid and vestigial thymus glands may be found in ectopic locations.

A newborn may exhibit various facial and vascular anomalies, collectively referred to as *pharyngeal pouch syndrome*. In addition to the established embryonic cause of DiGeorge syndrome, a nutrient (zinc) deficiency in utero has been suggested as a cause of this process.

Signs and Symptoms

DiGeorge syndrome is present at birth. Initial manifestations can include hypocalcemic tetany, unusual facies, and congenital heart defects. An increased susceptibility to viral, fungal, and disseminated bacterial infections (e.g., acid-fast bacilli, *Listeria monocytogenes*, and *Pneumocystis jirovecii* [formerly known as *P. carinii*]) result from the defect of T cells normally controlled by cell-mediated immunity. Infants usually die of sepsis during the first year of life.

Immunologic Manifestations

Peripheral lymphoid tissue appears to be normal except for the depletion of T cells in thymus-dependent zones, such as the subcortical region of the lymph nodes and perifollicular and periarteriolar lymphoid sheaths of the spleen. Lymph node paracortical areas and thymus-dependent regions of the spleen show variable degrees of depletion.

Thymic aplasia results in impaired T-cell maturation and function. B cells (CD19, HLA-DR) and NK cells (CD16, CD56) are normal, but T cells (CD2, CD3) are usually decreased, with an elevated CD4:CD8 ratio.

In the circulating blood lymphopenia is generally present, although in some cases the concentration of lymphocytes is normal. An abnormally high CD4+ to CD8+ ratio is present because of a decrease in CD8+ cells. Most patients with DiGeorge syndrome have a decreased percentage of cells expressing the CD3+ (mature T-cell) antigen. Because patients do demonstrate lymphocytes capable of differentiating to the more mature surface markers, such as CD4+, a small rudimentary thymus is believed to be present in these patients.

Lymphocytic responsiveness to antigenic and mitogenic (LAM) stimulation is typically low, but the result reflects the degree of thymic deficiency. Cell-mediated immune reactions, such as delayed-hypersensitivity and skin allograft rejections, are absent or feeble. In addition to a low T-cell count and a low LAM assay result, abnormal results in CD4+ T-cell RTEs are expressed by patients suffering from DiGeorge syndrome.

Serum immunoglobulin (Ig) antibody concentrations are near normal. Levels of IgA may be diminished, and those of IgE may be elevated. Antibody response to primary antigenic stimulation may be unimpaired.

The definitive diagnostic assay is the demonstration of 22q11.2 deletion using the chromosome fluorescence in situ hybridization (FISH) technique.

SEVERE COMBINED IMMUNODEFICIENCY (SCID)

Etiology

SCID is a group of rare, life-threatening disorders caused by mutations in different genes involved in the development and function of T and B cells. SCID has multiple genetic causes, including mutations in the gamma chain of the interleukin-2 (IL-2) receptor and the purine degradation enzymes adenosine deaminase (ADA) and nucleoside phosphorylase. Mutations in the IL-2 receptor complex, a hematopoietic growth factor, have been shown to cause X-linked SCID in humans. Two modes of inheritance are known: autosomal-recessive and X-linked recessive (Table 19.3). X-linked–recessive SCID is thought to be the most common form in the United States, which accounts for the 3:1 male-to-female ratio with the disorder.

Of patients with autosomal SCID, 50% have a concomitant deficiency of ADA, an aminohydrolase that converts adenosine to inosine. Analysis by complementary (copy) DNA (cDNA) probe has revealed that the deficiency results from a hereditable point mutation in the

TABLE 19.3 Identified Forms of Severe Combined Immunodeficiency Based on Combined Immunodeficiencies

Gene	Circulating T Cells	Circulating B Cells	Natural Killer (NK) Cells	Genetics?
IL2RG	Markedly decreased	Normal or increased	Markedly decreased	XL
JAK3	Markedly decreased	Normal or increased	Markedly decreased	AR
IL7RA	Markedly decreased	Normal or increased	Normal	AR
PTPRC	Markedly decreased	Normal	N/A	AR
CD3D	Markedly decreased	Normal	Normal	AR
CD3E	Markedly decreased	Normal	Normal	AR
CD3Z	Markedly decreased	Normal	Normal	AR
CORO1A	Markedly decreased	Normal	N/A	AR
RAG1	Markedly decreased	Markedly decreased	N/A	AR
RAG2	Markedly decreased	Markedly decreased	N/A	AR
ARTEMIS	Markedly decreased	Markedly decreased	N/A	AR
PRKDC	Markedly decreased	Markedly decreased	N/A	AR
AK2	Markedly decreased	Decreased or normal	N/A	AR
ADA	Absent from birth (null mutations) or progressive decrease	Absent from birth or progressive decrease	Decreased	AR

AR, Autosomal-recessive inheritance; *N/A*, not applicable; *XL*, X-linked inheritance.
Modified from the International Union of Immunologic Societies Expert Committee for Primary Immunodeficiency, 2013; Al-Herz W, Bousfiha A, Casanova J, et al: Primary immunodeficiency diseases: an update on the classification from the International Union of Immunologic Societies Expert Committee for Primary Immunodeficiency, *Front Immunol* 5:162–180, 2014.

ADA gene. Another variant with a severe deficiency in T-cell immunity but normal B-cell concentrations is associated with purine nucleotide phosphorylase deficiency.

There are two main forms of defective expression of major histocompatibility complex (MHC) antigens. In a less common form of SCID, MHC class II deficiency, bare lymphocyte syndrome, is caused by defective transcription of human leukocyte antigen (HLA) class II genes; B cells (CD19) and T cells (CD2, CD3) are present in normal numbers, but HLA-DR is absent. The CD4+ cells are usually CD45RA+. In another form of defective expression, MHC class I antigen deficiency plus the absence of class II antigens is present.

Signs and Symptoms

Infants with SCID appear healthy at birth but are highly susceptible to severe infections. SCID leads to life-threatening infections unless the immune system can be restored through a bone marrow transplant, enzyme replacement, or gene therapy. Severe infections can be fatal within the first 2 years of life without treatment.

No important differences in signs and symptoms exist between the two major genetic types of SCID. Initial manifestations of SCID are repeated, debilitating infections beginning within the first 6 months of life. These are dominated by bacterial, viral, and fungal infections of the respiratory and intestinal systems and skin. Infants with SCID usually die within 3 years of birth from lung abscesses, *Pneumocystis* pneumonitis, or a common viral disorder such as chickenpox or measles.

Approximately 10% to 15% of patients have delayed- or late (adult)-onset combined immunodeficiency, a milder form of the disease, as more than 12 types of SCID have been identified. If flow cytometry studies show that CD19+ and CD20+ are at least present and in normal quantities, this would point more toward common variable immunodeficiency (CVID) because this defect in this disease lies in the maturation of B cells into plasma cells, not in the production of cells.

Immunologic Manifestations

SCID disorders are characterized by a lack of protective T-, B-, and sometimes NK-cell responses to infections.

The thymus and other lymphoid organs are severely hypoplastic. The bone marrow is devoid of lymphoblasts, lymphocytes, and plasma cells. Lymphocytes are also absent from lymphoid tissues such as the spleen, tonsils, appendix, and intestinal tract.

SCID is characterized by blocking T-lymphocyte differentiation or function and can be associated with abnormal development of other types of lymphocytes (B cells and NK cells). In ADA deficiency, both B cells (CD19, HLA-DR) and T cells (CD2, CD3) are decreased in the peripheral blood.

Moderate lymphocytopenia is detectable early in infancy. T-cell functions are decreased. The circulating blood contains no CD4+, CD8+, or CD3+ cells. In addition to a low T-cell count and a low LAM assay result, abnormal results of CD4+ T-cell RTEs are expressed by patients suffering SCID. T-cell lymphopenia in SCID is defined by a CD3+ T-cell count below 300/μL.

The percentage of B cells is usually normal. Patients with the X-linked form of SCID usually appear similar to those with the autosomal-recessive form, except they tend to have an increased percentage of B cells. However, the defect affects both B lineage cells and T lineage cells. Variable hypogammaglobulinemia with decreased serum immunoglobulin M (IgM) and immunoglobulin A (IgA) levels and poor-to-absent antibody production are representative features.

In other forms of SCID, the lymphopenia is not as severe, but the lymphocyte count is usually less than 1000/μL, even though B cells (CD19, HLA-DR) may be normal or increased. In contrast to thymic aplasia, any T cells present may have an immature phenotype.

Leaky SCID, which is less severe and/or delayed in onset compared with typical SCID, is defined as age-adjusted relative CD3+ T-cell lymphopenia (age <2 years, <1000 cells/μL; age 2–4 years, <800 cells/μL; age >4 years, <600 cells/μL) and proliferation to mitogens <30% of normal. SCID is a very rare disease and more than 90% of cases are the X-linked form. The leaky SCID form is extremely rare and would have been diagnosed in infancy with life-threatening infections. Omenn syndrome is an inherited disorder of the immune system (immunodeficiency) and is one of several forms of SCID, a group of disorders that cause individuals to have virtually no immune protection from bacteria, viruses, and fungi. Omenn syndrome is characterized by a combination of SCID and severe allergy symptoms. The life expectancy for any type of untreated SCID is about 2 years.

A SCID genetic panel for the sequencing and deletion or duplication of 19 frequent genes can be performed using FISH technology.

Newborn Screening Test for SCID: T-Cell Receptor Excision Circles

Unlike individual clinical tests carried out because of suspicion for a disease by either genetic or clinical information, a screening test looks for serious conditions in infants. Population-based NBS is different from testing with a known or suspected case of immune deficiency. Screening tests on a large scale use blood from a heel stick that is spotted onto filter paper and dried. Dried blood spots (DBS) can be tested using automated polymerase chain reaction (PCR) systems.

TRECs are circular DNA molecules formed within T cells developing in the thymus. TREC DNA circles are measured by PCR. Normal infant blood samples have one TREC per 10 T cells, reflecting the high rate of new T-cell generation early in life. Infants with SCID lack TREC altogether. When PCR indicates low or absent TRECs, follow-up testing includes assays of the total lymphocyte count; analysis of subsets of T, B, and NK cells; and evaluation of naïve and memory T cells by flow cytometry.

In addition to traditional SCID, other immunologic conditions in which low T-cell numbers can be flagged by TREC testing include leaky SCID or Omenn syndrome due to mutations in typical SCID genes that do not completely abolish gene function, and variant SCID, with persistently low T cells but no defect in a known SCID gene.

Not all T-cell deficiency diseases are detected by the TREC test. Diseases in which T cells develop in the thymus to the point of production of the DNA circles but with impaired function are missed. Newborns with Zap70 deficiency, MHC class II deficiency, and nuclear factor kappa B (NF-κB) essential modulator (NEMO) deficiency have expressed normal TRECs.

Screening for dysfunctional B cells is a goal for continued advances in molecular and genomic technology. This testing could be for B-cell kappa chain excision circles.

CHRONIC MUCOCUTANEOUS CANDIDIASIS

Etiology

Chronic mucocutaneous candidiasis (CMC) results from a primary defect in cell-mediated immunity. T cells specifically fail to recognize only the *Candida* (fungus) antigen.

Signs and Symptoms

CMC is usually hereditary and presents soon after birth with persistent oral *Candida* infections (thrush). The characteristic manifestation is *Candida* infection of the mucous membranes, scalp, skin, and nails.

Endocrine abnormalities, often polyendocrinopathies, are frequently associated with fungal manifestations. Sudden death from adrenal insufficiency has been reported in patients with CMC. These infections respond to anti-*Candida* treatment but recur when the treatment stops.

Immunologic Manifestations

Patients demonstrate normal skin reactions to testing with all antigens except *Candida*.

One hereditary form of CMC is APECED syndrome (autoimmune polyendocrinopathy-candidiasis-ectodermal dysplasia), which is associated with multiple endocrine problems, such as hypothyroidism, diabetes, or Addison disease, due to a gene defect on chromosome 21. This CMC disorder is partly caused by autoantibodies or mutations in very uncommon genes such as interleukin-17. Several other forms of CMC are caused by mutations in the gene signal transducer and activator of transcription 1 (STAT1).

An effective laboratory screening test for patients with a decreased response to *Candida* is a TLR function assay. TLRs enable innate immunity to prevent infection and function as recognition factors for microbes and viruses. A TLR assay assists in the diagnosis of innate immunodeficiencies when genetic defects of the innate immune system are suspected in patients who have no detectable abnormalities in antibody function, complement activity, neutrophil function, or cell-mediated immunity. TLRs induce appropriate cytokine pathways by stimulating interferons, tumor necrosis factor-alpha (TNF-α), IL-1β, and IL-6. There are suspected genetic associations with IRAK4, MYD88, and TLR3.

T-Cell Activation Defects

Some patients with defective activation of T cells have experienced the following:
- Defective surface expression of the CD3-TCR complex caused by a mutation in the gene encoding the CD3γ subunit
- Defective signal transduction from the TCR to intracellular metabolic pathways
- Pretranslational defect in IL-2 or other cytokine production

B-Cell and Antibody Deficiency Disorders

Because the primary function of B cells is to produce antibody, the major clinical manifestation of a B-cell deficiency is an increased susceptibility to severe bacterial infections. Selective IgA deficiency is the most common B-cell disorder, affecting 1 in 400 to 800 persons. Because IgA is the primary Ig in secretions, a deficiency contributes to pulmonary infections, gastrointestinal (GI) disorders, and allergic respiratory disorders.

Most cases (50% of reported cases are associated with Ig deficiencies) are autoimmune in nature, including rheumatoid arthritis (RA), systemic lupus erythematosus (SLE), thyroiditis, and pernicious anemia. Immunophenotyping is generally not useful in characterizing selective IgA deficiency, IgG subclass deficiencies, the hyper-IgM syndrome, or hyperimmunoglobulin E syndrome (Job syndrome).

Infants and children who are 18 months old or older and suffer from recurrent respiratory infections, with or without diarrhea, should be evaluated using the following laboratory protocols:
- Quantitative Ig levels: IgM, IgG, IgA
- Lymphocyte subset panels (Table 19.4), including congenital immunodeficiencies
- Response to polyvalent pneumococcal vaccine
- Immune response to diphtheria and tetanus (DT) vaccine
- Sweat chloride testing at an accredited cystic fibrosis center

TABLE 19.4 Lymphocyte Subset Reference Ranges in Adolescents and Adults[a]

	Adolescent (%)	Adults (%)
CD3:	49–83	65–88
CD4:	27–53	26–62
CD8:	16–40	14–44
CD19+ B cells:	8–31	2–27
CD16+CD56+ NK cells:	3–30	2–27
CD4:CD8 ratio	0.7–2.6	0.6–4.4

[a]adolescent age range 12–18, adult age range: 21–67
Note: Gender based analysis of relative percentages of lymphocyte subsets showed no significant differences between adult and adolescent males and females.
Adapted from Valiathan R, Deeb K, Diamante M, Ashman M, Sachdeva N, Asthana D. Reference ranges of lymphocyte subsets in healthy adults and adolescents with special mention of T cell maturation subsets in adults of South Florida. Immunobiology. 2014 Jul;219(7):487–96. http://doi.org/10.1016/j.imbio.2014.02.010. Epub 2014 Mar 2. PMID: 24661720.

Specific antibody deficiency (SAD) is also known as *selective polysaccharide antibody deficiency of B cells*, and it exhibits an insufficient antibody response to polysaccharide antigens. Evaluation of response to the 23-valent pneumococcal polysaccharide vaccine is the current gold standard. Failure of polysaccharide response may be observed as a component of a more global PID or multiple secondary immunodeficient states (Box 19.4).

BRUTON X-LINKED AGAMMAGLOBULINEMIA (XLA)

Etiology

Bruton X-linked agammaglobulinemia is a classic example of an X-linked agammaglobulinemia, in which a disease-causing variant in the gene coding for Bruton tyrosine kinase (BTK) leads to the arrest of B-cell development at the pre–B-cell stage. X-linked hypogammaglobulinemia can be distinguished from transient hypogammaglobulinemia of infancy by the absence of B cells. Transient hypogammaglobulinemia of infancy results from delayed capacity for Ig synthesis and spontaneously resolves with age.

Signs and Symptoms

X-linked agammaglobulinemia occurs primarily in young boys, but scattered cases have been identified in girls. Manifestations begin in the first or second year of life. Hypersusceptibility to infection does not develop until 9 to 12 months after birth because of passive protection by residual maternal immunoglobulin. Thereafter patients repeatedly acquire infections with high-grade extracellular pyogenic organisms, such as streptococci. This disorder is characterized by sinopulmonary and central nervous system (CNS) infectious episodes and severe septicemia, but patients are not abnormally susceptible to common viral infections (excluding fulminant hepatitis), enterococci, or most gram-negative organisms. Chronic fungal infections are not usually present.

An autoimmune phenomenon, especially a juvenile RA type of disease, has also been associated with X-linked agammaglobulinemia. In addition, patients are highly vulnerable to a malignant form of dermatomyositis that eventually involves destructive T-cell infiltration surrounding the small vessels of the CNS. In addition to infections and connective tissue disorders, agammaglobulinemic patients have hemolytic anemia, drug eruptions, atopic eczema, allergic rhinitis, and asthma.

BOX 19.4 Causes of Secondary Immunodeficiencies

Infections
- Acquired immunodeficiency syndrome (AIDS)
- Cytomegalovirus (CMV)
- Epstein-Barr virus (EBV)

Surgical Procedures and Trauma
- Splenectomy
- Anesthesia
- Post–stem cell transplantation
- Burns

Nutrition
- Malnutrition
- Zinc deficiency
- Vitamin/other mineral deficiencies

Hereditary Disorders
- Chromosomal disorders
- Sickle cell disease

Hematologic Lymphoproliferative Disorders
- Hodgkin disease and lymphoma
- Leukemia, myeloma, macroglobulinemia
- Agranulocytosis and aplastic anemia

Other Systemic Processes and Metabolic Disorders
- Nephrotic syndrome
- Protein-losing enteropathy
- Diabetes mellitus
- Malnutrition
- Hepatic disease
- Uremia
- Age: Prematurity, infancy, elderly

Treatment Agents
- Antimetabolites
- Corticosteroids
- Radiation

Adapted from Stiehm RE, Ochs HD, Winkelstein JA: *Immunodeficiency disorders in infants and children*, ed 5, Philadelphia, 2004, Saunders.

Immunologic Manifestations

The diagnosis of X-linked agammaglobulinemia is suspected if serum concentrations of IgG, IgA, and IgM are notably below the appropriate level for the patient's age. Tests for natural antibodies to blood group substances and for antibodies to antigens given during standard courses of immunization (e.g., diphtheria) are useful in distinguishing this disorder from transient hypogammaglobulinemia of infancy (discussed later).

T cells (CD2, CD3) are normal or increased in number, and the CD4:CD8 ratio is normal or decreased. Most of the CD4 cells express the CD45RA antigen characteristic of naïve rather than memory cells. B cells (CD19, HLA-DR) are severely decreased or absent from bone marrow and lymphoid tissues. A deficiency or absence of peripheral B lymphocytes is usually noted. If present, B cells are unresponsive to T cells and incapable of antibody synthesis or secretion. Surface immunoglobulins are absent. However, patients have normal numbers of CD3+ and CD8+ cells, and many have normal CD4+ cells. Male children have normal T-cell function; therefore homograft rejection mechanisms are intact and delayed-hypersensitivity reactions for both tuberculin and skin contact types can be elicited.

COMMON VARIABLE IMMUNODEFICIENCY

Etiology

CVID is a primary immune deficiency disease characterized by low levels of protective antibodies and an increased risk of infections. The name *common variable immunodeficiency* describes a very heterogeneous group of disorders with defective antibody formation. CVID is the most common clinically relevant PID and genetic causes of CVID are largely unknown. Implicated genes include inducible costimulatory (ICOS) and a few other proteins in B cells. These appear to be causes of autosomal-recessive CVID. Mutations in a cell receptor (TACI) that is needed for normal growth and regulation of B cells have been found in about 8% of patients with CVID. A causative role of TACI mutations in this immune defect is not yet clear because some of these mutations can be found in people with normal immunoglobulins.

Findings of rare alleles or deletions of MHC class III genes in patients with IgA deficiency of CVID have suggested that the susceptible gene(s) is (are) on chromosome 6.

Epidemiology

The incidence of CVID is estimated at 1 per 25,000 individuals. A familial inheritance of CVID is rare. CVID is a relatively frequent form of primary acquired agammaglobulinemia, occurring equally in males and females. Twenty percent of patients with CVID have associated autoimmunity, with autoimmune cytopenias being the most common. Classic RA occurs in about 2% to 3% of CVID patients. However, polyarthritis, a distinct form of RA, occurs in 10% to 30% of CVID patients. Mutations in the *TACI* gene may be found in 8% to 10% of CVID patients and appear to increase patient predisposition to autoimmunity.

Signs and Symptoms

CVID usually manifests in the third or fourth decade of life. About 20% of patients are symptomatic or diagnosed in childhood, but usually not until the age of 4 years. Although the disease usually is diagnosed in adults, it also can occur in children. CVID also is known as hypogammaglobulinemia, adult-onset agammaglobulinemia, late-onset hypogammaglobulinemia, and acquired agammaglobulinemia.

Signs and symptoms include frequent sinopulmonary infections, diarrhea, endocrine and autoimmune disorders, and malabsorption (e.g., of vitamin B_{12}). Intestinal giardiasis is also prevalent.

Immunologic Manifestations

CVID is largely a diagnosis of exclusion. It is characterized by low levels of Ig isotypes (IgM, IgG, IgA) with a poor or absent antibody response to immunization (vaccination). An IgG level less than 4.5 to 5 g/L is suggestive of CVID. However, the total IgG level may be normal while a subclass (usually IgG2 or IgG3) is deficient. Both IgA and IgM may be detectable, but IgM levels may be elevated.

Both a decreased concentration of immunoglobulins and the near absence of serum and secretory IgA are thought to represent the most common and well-defined type of PID. The pattern of inheritance suggests that an autosomal function of antibodies is usually compromised.

Cellular immunity and Ig production are impaired by the interaction between helper and suppressor T-cell subsets. The primary defect in Ig synthesis may be caused by the absence or dysfunction of CD4+

cells or by increased CD8+ suppressor cell activity. The CD4:CD8 ratio may be normal or decreased. Lymph nodes lack plasma cells but may show striking follicular hyperplasia. T-cell and B-cell immunodeficiency profile testing can be conducted. T-cell testing at minimum should include CD3, CD4, CD8, CD19, CD45RA, CD45RO, NK cell, and the CD4:CD8 ratio. A B-cell memory and naïve panel can be used as an alternate criterion to low antibody response to vaccines. Further testing can include the evaluation of prevaccination and postvaccination IgG titers. Responses to pneumococcus, diphtheria, tetanus, and *Haemophilus* are commonly used, but there are limitations, such as remaining residual antibody from childhood immunization.

Flow cytometry studies that show that CD19+ and CD20+ are at least present, and in normal quantities point more toward CVID because the defect in this disease lies in the maturation of B cells into plasma cells, not in the production of cells. The number of B cells is typically normal or mildly depressed. Despite a normal number of circulating Ig-bearing B lymphocytes and the presence of lymphoid cortical follicles, blood lymphocytes do not differentiate into Ig-producing cells. B cells (CD19, HLA-DR) and T cells (CD2, CD3) are usually normal in number, although B cells may be decreased when CVID occurs concurrently with SLE. In most patients the defect appears to be intrinsic to the B cell.

Prognosis

Patients with CVID are at an increased risk of developing a malignancy, particularly lymphoma or stomach cancer, compared with the general population. This propensity for developing a malignancy requires ruling out a malignancy as the cause of splenomegaly, if present on physical examination.

TRANSIENT HYPOGAMMAGLOBULINEMIA OF INFANCY

Unlike patients with Bruton X-linked agammaglobulinemia or CVID, patients with transient hypogammaglobulinemia of infancy can synthesize antibodies to A and B erythrocyte antigens, if they lack the antigen(s), and to DT toxoids. Antibody production usually occurs by 6 to 11 months of age. This antibody production occurs before Ig levels become normal.

IMMUNODEFICIENCY WITH ELEVATED IMMUNOGLOBULIN M (HYPER-IgM)

Etiology

A sex-linked mode of inheritance has been noted in some pedigrees. The abnormal gene in the X-linked type has been localized to Xq24 to Xq27. However, more than one genetic cause is suspected.

Signs and Symptoms

Patients with hyper-IgM defect become symptomatic during the first or second year of life, with recurrent pyogenic infections including otitis media, sinusitis, pneumonia, and tonsillitis. Hemolytic anemia and thrombocytopenia have been observed. Transient, persistent, or cyclic neutropenia is a common feature.

Immunologic Manifestations

Hyper-IgM disorder is characterized by extremely low concentrations of IgG and IgA and, most frequently, greatly elevated concentrations of polyclonal IgM. Normal or slightly reduced numbers of IgM and IgD B lymphocytes have been observed.

Immunoglobulin Subclass Deficiencies

Some patients have deficiencies of one or more subclasses of IgG despite a normal total IgG serum concentration. Most of those with absent or very low concentrations of IgG2 have been patients with selective IgA deficiency.

SELECTIVE IMMUNOGLOBULIN A DEFICIENCY

Etiology

An isolated absence mode is often seen in pedigrees of individuals with CVID. IgA deficiency has been noted to evolve into CVID, and rare alleles and deletions of MHC class III genes in both conditions suggest a common basis.

Signs and Symptoms

IgA deficiency is typically associated with poor health. Infections occur predominantly in the respiratory, GI, and urogenital tracts. There is no clear evidence that patients have any increased susceptibility to viral agents. IgA deficiency has been noted in patients treated with phenytoin, sulfasalazine, penicillamine, and gold, suggesting that environmental factors may lead to expression of the defect.

Immunologic Manifestations

As many as 44% of patients with selective IgA deficiency demonstrate antibodies to IgA. Severe or fatal anaphylactic reactions after intravenous (IV) administration of blood products containing IgA and anti-IgA antibodies (particularly IgE anti-IgA antibodies) have occurred.

HYPER-E SYNDROME (HIES)

Many different syndromes are known to lead to high levels of an antibody called immunoglobulin E (IgE). Collectively, these conditions are called hyper-IgE syndrome (HIES), autosomal-dominant hyper-IgE syndrome (AD-HIES), or Job syndrome. Other medical conditions, such as severe eczema, can produce extremely high IgE levels that are not caused by a syndrome.

Etiology

Hyperimmunoglobulinemia E (hyper-E) syndrome has an autosomal-dominant pattern of inheritance. Each set of a variety of mutations causes a specific syndrome, including autosomal-dominant CARD11 deficiency, DOCK8 deficiency, IL-6R deficiency, IL-6ST deficiency, PGM3 deficiency, and STAT3 dominant-negative disease (STAT3DN).

In 2007, National Institutes of Health investigators identified the role of STAT3 in this disease. STAT3DN is the result of mutations in the gene that encodes the signaling protein, STAT3. This protein is involved in many different activities of the body. STAT3DN affects not only the immune system but also facial appearance, bones, lungs, skin, and arteries.

Signs and Symptoms

Hyper-E syndrome is a relatively rare PID characterized by recurrent severe staphylococcal abscesses.

From infancy, patients suffer from repeated staphylococcal abscesses involving the skin, lungs, joints, and other sites. Persistent pneumatoceles—thin-walled, air-filled cysts that develop within the lung parenchyma—develop as a result of recurrent pneumonias. Pruritic dermatitis also occurs.

Treatment for PIDs depends upon the part(s) of the immune system affected and can include hematopoietic cell transplantation (HCT), gene therapy (for X-linked ADA SCID and Artemis-deficient SCID), enzyme replacement therapy (for ADA-deficient SCID), immunoglobulin replacement therapy, and antimicrobial therapy to prevent or limit infections.

X-LINKED LYMPHOPROLIFERATIVE DISEASE (XLP) SYNDROMES 1 AND 2 (DUNCAN DISEASE)

Etiology

X-linked lymphoproliferative disease is associated with a defect on the X chromosome. There are two forms of this disorder: XLP1, due to defects in the *SH2DIA* gene, and XLP2, due to defects in the *XIAP* gene.

Signs and Symptoms

Some patients are initially misdiagnosed with CVID. XLP is characterized by an inadequate immune reaction to Epstein-Barr virus (EBV) and a lifelong vulnerability to EBV infection, which can lead to severe and fatal infectious mononucleosis, lymphomas, combined immunodeficiency, and, less commonly, aplastic anemia or vasculitis. Infected patients are apparently healthy until they experience infectious mononucleosis (see Chapter 17). Approximately two-thirds of patients die of overwhelming EBV-induced B-cell proliferation during mononucleosis, called *hemophagocytic syndrome*. Most patients who survive the primary infection develop hypogammaglobulinemia and/or B-cell lymphomas.

Immunologic Manifestations

A marked impairment in the production of antibodies to the EBV nucleus has been noted in affected patients. In contrast, titers of antibodies to the viral capsid antigen range from zero to extremely elevated.

Antibody-dependent, cell-mediated cytotoxicity against EBV-infected cells has been low in many patients. NK-cell function is also depressed. There is also a deficiency in long-lived T-cell immunity to EBV.

Treatment

Early recognition is crucial because the disease can be cured by bone marrow or cord blood transplantation. Early screening of infant boys in families with children suffering from XLP is critical so that they can undergo transplantation before contracting an EBV infection.

COMBINED CELLULAR IMMUNODEFICIENCY DISORDERS

Hereditary Ataxia-Telangiectasia (Louis Bar Syndrome)
Etiology

Hereditary ataxia-telangiectasia is an autosomal-recessive disorder that apparently results from the coexistence of a T-cell deficiency with a defect in DNA repair; this leads to extreme, nonrandom chromosomal instability. The sites of chromosomal breakage involve chromosomes 7 and 14 in more than 50% of patients.

The disorder is characterized by ataxia-telangiectasia mutated (ATM), a serine/threonine protein kinase that is recruited and activated by DNA double-strand breaks. ATM phosphorylates several key proteins that initiate activation of the DNA damage checkpoint, leading to cell cycle arrest, DNA repair, or apoptosis. Several of these targets, including p53, CHK2, BRCA1, NBS1, and H2AX, are tumor suppressors.

Signs and Symptoms

Ataxia-telangiectasia is characterized by ataxia and choreoathetosis in infancy. Multiple telangiectases appear on exposed oculocutaneous surfaces during childhood. A high incidence of malignancy (e.g., lymphoma) is also seen. Children with this disorder eventually die of respiratory insufficiency and sepsis.

Immunologic Manifestations

The thymus is hypoplastic or dysplastic, and the thymus-dependent zones of the lymph nodes are void of cells. About 80% of patients lack serum and secretory IgA, and some develop IgG antibodies to injections of IgA. The signs and symptoms of the disease appear to result from a concomitant T-cell deficiency, deficiency of DNA repair, and disordered IgG synthesis.

Often IgA, IgE, and IgG subclasses are decreased; IgM monomers are increased; but IgM antibodies are variably decreased.

PARTIAL COMBINED IMMUNE DEFICIENCY DISORDERS

Wiskott-Aldrich Syndrome
Etiology

WAS is unique among primary immunodeficiency diseases. In addition to being susceptible to infections, patients have problems with abnormal bleeding. The bleeding problems are the result of unusually small, dysfunctional platelets.

In 1994 the X-linked gene that is defective in patients with WAS was discovered. The gene is located on the short arm of the X chromosome, so the disease is inherited in an X-linked–recessive fashion. This is a clinical disorder in boys.

The primary defect in this uncommon X-linked–recessive pediatric disease is caused by a mutation of the gene encoding Wiskott-Aldrich syndrome protein (WASp), which plays a critical role in actin polymerization in blood cells. The mutated gene is expressed uniquely in hematopoietic cells. The effects of WAS gene mutation on this process are of interest, particularly because the actin cytoskeleton has a prominent role in the basic mechanisms of cell adhesion and migration.

Signs and Symptoms

The immune problems typically begin to manifest themselves in toddlers and older boys when patients begin to develop frequent infections. Evaluation of the immune system typically shows that patients are not able to make good antibody responses to certain types of vaccines, particularly those that contain polysaccharides or complex sugars, such as the vaccine against *Streptococcus pneumoniae* (Pneumovax). IgE levels are usually elevated, and T-lymphocyte function is often abnormal.

A definitive diagnosis of WAS can be made by sequencing the WAS gene to identify a mutation and studying the patient's blood cells to determine whether the WASp is expressed at normal levels. These tests are carried out in a few specialized laboratories and require blood or other tissue.

WAS is characterized by the triad of:
1. Thrombocytopenic purpura
2. Increased susceptibility to bacterial, viral, and fungal infections
3. Eczema of the skin, or atopic dermatitis

Affected boys rarely survive beyond 10 years of age. Thrombocytopenia and bleeding are common. Platelets are small and dysfunctional with an intrinsic defect. Patients usually die of sepsis, hemorrhage, or malignancy.

Immunologic Manifestations

There is a progressive decrease in an abnormal lymphocyte response to anti-CD3. The lymph nodes and spleen of WAS patients show relative depletion of lymphocytes from T-cell areas. Depletion of the splenic and circulating marginal zone B cells is characteristic and may explain the defective antibody responses, particularly to polysaccharide antigens. Although there are normal numbers of B cells, there is a decreased level of IgM, with antibody to polysaccharides particularly decreased. Oftentimes increased IgA and IgE levels are present.

Autoimmune Disorders in Wiskott-Aldrich Syndrome

Clinical problems caused by autoimmunity are common in WAS and affect almost half of all patients. Among the most common autoimmune manifestations are hemolytic anemia and idiopathic thrombocytopenic purpura caused by self-reactive antibodies generated inappropriately by the patient's immune system.

Another common autoimmune disorder in WAS is vasculitis, which typically causes fever and skin rash on the extremities. Occasionally vasculitis may affect the muscles, heart, brain, or other internal organs, with a range of symptoms.

Malignancies in Wiskott-Aldrich Syndrome

Patients with WAS have an increased risk of malignancies compared with normal individuals. Malignancies can occur in young children but are more frequent as a patient ages. It is estimated that 15% to 20% of WAS patients will eventually develop malignancies. Lymphomas or leukemias that arise from B lymphocytes are the most common, with non-Hodgkin lymphoma making up the majority of cases.

Vaccination

Vaccination to prevent infections is often not effective in WAS because patients do not make normal protective antibody responses to vaccines. (See Chapter 27 for a full discussion of vaccination in WAS and other conditions.)

Stem Cell Transplantation and Gene Therapy

Until recently, the only permanent cure for WAS was transplantation of stem cells from bone marrow, peripheral blood, or cord blood. Patients with WAS have some residual T-lymphocyte and NK-cell function despite having an immune deficiency. This has the potential to cause rejection of transplanted donor cells or graft-versus-host disease (GVHD) (see Chapter 25).

Gene therapy is a technique in which a normal copy of the WAS gene is inserted into the patient's own bone marrow cells using a virus. This allows blood cells from the bone marrow to make normal WAS protein. There is no risk for GVHD. The major risk of gene therapy is that the virus may insert a copy of its DNA into one of the patient's chromosomes and cause abnormal outcomes, such as leukemia. Gene therapy has been used to successfully treat a small number of patients with WAS to correct bleeding problems and immune deficiency. A number of problems remain to be solved before it becomes more broadly applicable.

OTHER PRIMARY IMMUNE DISORDERS

Patients in the other primary immune disorders group of PIDs (Table 19.5) suffer from delayed separation of the umbilical cord, abscesses, and recurrent respiratory infections, with or without diarrhea. The laboratory protocol consists of:
- Ig concentration assay for IgM, IgG, and IgA
- Complement activity enzyme immunoassay (CH50) and complement activity alternate pathway (AH50)
- Complete blood count (CBC) with leukocyte differential
- Neutrophil oxidative burst assay (DHR)
- Leukocyte adhesion deficiency (LAD) panel
- Myeloperoxidase stain
- Lymphocyte subset panel for congenital immunodeficiencies

Additional information regarding PIDs can be found in various chapters, including:
- Complement deficiency (see Chapter 2)
- Chronic granulomatous disease (CGD) (see Chapter 4)
- Leukocyte adhesion deficiency type 1 and type 2 (see Chapter 4)
- Absence of myeloperoxidase (see Chapter 4)
- Autoimmune neutropenia or thrombocytopenia (see Chapter 4)

ACQUIRED (SECONDARY) IMMUNODEFICIENCY DISORDERS

A secondary immune deficiency can result from a disease process that causes a defect in normal immune function, which leads to a temporary or permanent impairment of one or multiple components of immunity in the host (Box 19.5). Patients with secondary immunodeficiencies, which are much more common than primary deficiencies, have an increased susceptibility to infections.

In addition to acquired immunodeficiency disorders, immunosuppressive agents and burns are major causes of secondary immunodeficiencies. In varying degrees, immunosuppressive agents have been demonstrated to affect every component of the immune response. In burn patients, septicemia is a common complication in those who survive the initial period of hemodynamic shock. The mechanism that seems most critical in thermal injury is disruption of the skin, but interference with phagocytosis and deficiencies of serum Ig and complement levels have also been observed.

> **KEY CONCEPTS: HIV Facts**
> - HIV-1 is the predominant virus responsible for AIDS. In addition to the original HIV-1, a second AIDS-causing virus, HIV-2, was identified in 1985.
> - The human immunodeficiency virus is composed of structural proteins and glycoproteins that occupy the core and envelope regions of the particle.
> - Retroviruses contain a single, positive-strand RNA with the genetic information of the virus and a special enzyme, reverse transcriptase, in their core.
> - Reverse transcriptase enables the virus to convert viral RNA into DNA.

ACQUIRED IMMUNODEFICIENCY SYNDROME

Acquired immunodeficiency syndrome (AIDS) is the best-known acquired immune deficiency. Patients with AIDS exhibit some of the most severe manifestations of cell-mediated immunity.

Etiology

The human immunodeficiency virus (HIV) is the predominant virus responsible for AIDS.

In 1983 researchers at the Pasteur Institute in Paris isolated a retrovirus, termed *lymphadenopathy-associated virus* (LAV), from a homosexual man with lymphadenopathy. Concurrently an American research team headed by Dr. Robert Gallo isolated the same class of virus, which they labeled *human T-lymphotropic retrovirus* (HTLV) type III. In 1984 the Gallo team was able to demonstrate conclusively through virologic and epidemiologic evidence that HTLV-III was the cause of AIDS. When it was demonstrated that LAV and HTLV-III were the same virus, an international commission changed both names of the virus to HIV to eliminate confusion caused by the two names and to acknowledge that the virus is the cause of AIDS.

TABLE 19.5 Examples of Other Primary Cellular Immunodeficiencies

Disorder	Genetic Defect	Characteristics	Comments
Nezelof syndrome Cellular immunodeficiency with immunoglobulins	Chromosome 14q13.1 defect	Lymphocyte responses to mitogens, antigens, and allogeneic cells are profoundly depressed but not totally absent. Serum levels of most of the five Ig classes are normal or increased. Antibody-forming capacity has been reported as normal in one-third of cases	Likely to be confused with AIDS in the pediatric age group
Cartilage hair hypoplasia (CHH)	Mutations in RMRP (RNase MRP RNA) involved in processing of mitochondrial RNA and cell cycle control	Normal T cells. Normal or reduced B cells. Antibodies variably decreased	Particularly common in Amish because of close intermarriage
Hoyeraal-Hreidarsson syndrome (dyskeratosis congenita)	Mutations in dyskerin (DKC1)	Decreased number and function of natural killer (NK) cells. Pancytopenia	A progressive loss of cellular and humoral immunity
NEMO syndrome	Mutations in the X-linked NEMO gene. There is at least one additional genetic cause of a NEMO-like syndrome with defects in a similar pathway. Although this form can affect both males and females, it is extremely rare.	B cells, T cells, neutrophils, macrophages, and dendritic cells all respond poorly to bacterial and fungal invasion	NEMO stands for the "NF-kappa B essential modulator" and is also known as the inhibitor of kappa B kinase gamma (IKKγ). The modulator protein is required for the activation of the nuclear factor kappa B (NF-κB) family of transcription factors, which regulate gene expression and the development of a number of organ systems, including the immune system. In NEMO syndrome, the NEMO protein retains partial activity. An embryo develops, but many organ systems fail to develop normally, including the immune system. A complete absence of NEMO activity is not compatible with life
Defects of Vitamin B$_{12}$ and Folate Metabolism			
TCN2 deficiency	Mutation in TCN2; encodes transcobalamin, a transporter of cobalamin into blood cells	Normal T cells. Variable B cells. Antibody decreased	Megaloblastic anemia, pancytopenia
SLC46A1 deficiency	Mutation in SLC46A1, a proton-coupled folate transporter	Variable numbers of T cells and activation profile. B cells variable. Antibody decreased	Megaloblastic anemia
MTHFD1 deficiency	Mutations in MTHFD1; essential for processing of single-carbon folate derivatives	Low T cells. Low B cells. Antibody decreased	Megaloblastic anemia, neutropenia

Adapted from Blaese RM, editor: *Immune Deficiency Foundation patient and family handbook for primary immunodeficiency diseases,* ed 5, Towson, Maryland, 2013, Immune Deficiency Foundation. Copyright 2013 by Immune Deficiency Foundation, USA.

BOX 19.5 Examples of Primary Immunodeficiencies and Secondary Immunodeficient States That May Be Associated With Impaired Vaccine Response

Primary
Wiskott-Aldrich syndrome
DiGeorge syndrome
Hyperimmunoglobulin E (Job) syndrome
Common variable immune deficiency
Selective immunoglobulin A deficiency

Acquired
Human immunodeficiency virus (HIV) infection
Immunosuppression
Malnutrition
Splenectomy

Modified from Wall L, Dootroades VR, Sorensen RU: Specific antibody deficiencies in primary immunodeficiency disorders, *Immunol Allergy Clin North Am* 35(4):660, 2015.

Viral Characteristics

Viral Structure

HIV is a member of the family Retroviridae, a type D retrovirus that belongs to the lentivirus subfamily. Included in this family are oncoviruses (e.g., HTLV-I and HTLV-II), which primarily induce proliferation of infected cells and formation of tumors. Since the discovery of this virus, much has been learned about the impact of HIV on human cells. Two distinct HIV viruses, types 1 and 2 (HIV-1 and HIV-2), cause AIDS. HIV-1 is divided into nine subtypes: group M (subtypes A–H), group N, and group O. HIV-2 is divided into two subtypes: groups A and B.

The HIV-1 virus (Fig. 19.5) is composed of a lipid membrane, structural proteins, and glycoproteins that protrude. The viral genome consists of three important structural components: *pol*, *gag*, and *env*. These gene components code for various products (Table 19.6). Long terminal redundancies (LTRs) border these three components. HIV-2 has a different envelope and slightly different core proteins.

Cells infected with HIV can be examined with an electron microscope. The virus may appear as buds of the cell membrane particles. The virion has a double-membrane envelope and an electron-dense laminar crescent or semicircular cores. An intermediate, less electron-dense layer lies between the envelope and core. In a mature, free extracellular virion, the core appears as a bar-shaped nucleoid structure in cross-section. This structure appears circular and is frequently located eccentrically. It is composed of structural proteins and glycoproteins that occupy the core and envelope regions of the particle. The virion consists of knoblike structures composed of a protein called *glycoprotein (gp) 120*, which is anchored to another protein called *gp41*. Each knob includes three sets of these protein molecules. The core of the virus includes a major structural protein called *p25* or *p24* encoded by the *gag* gene. After human exposure, these and other viral components may induce an antibody response important in serodiagnosis (Table 19.7).

Retroviruses contain a single, positive-strand RNA with the genetic information of the virus and a special enzyme called **reverse transcriptase** in their core. Reverse transcriptase enables the virus to convert viral RNA into DNA. This reverses the normal process of transcription in which DNA is converted to RNA—thus the term **retrovirus**.

The genomes of all known retroviruses are organized in a similar way. In the provirus, which is formed when cDNA synthesis is completed from the retroviral RNA template, **viral core protein**, **envelope protein**, and reverse transcriptase are encoded by the *gag*, *env*, and *pol* genes, respectively, whereas viral gene expression is regulated by *tat*, *trs*, *sor*, and *3′ orf* gene products. The *gag* gene encodes a polyprotein found at high levels in infected cells and is subsequently cleaved to form p17 and p24, both of which are associated with viral particles. The *pol* gene encodes for reverse transcriptase, endonuclease, and **protease** activities. The *sor* gene stands for **s**mall **o**pen-**r**eading frame. The *sor* gene product is a protein that induces antibody production in the natural course of infection. The *tat* gene also represents a small open-reading frame; the protein product has not been identified to date.

The *env* gene encodes for a polyprotein that contains numerous glycosylation sites. The glycoprotein gp160 is found on infected cells but is deficient on viral particles; however, gp160 gives rise to two glycoproteins, gp120 and gp41, which are associated with the viral envelope. The encoding genes and gene products, or antigens, of the AIDS virus may induce an antibody response after human exposure (Table 19.8).

LTRs, which exist at each end of the **proviral genome**, play an important role in the control of viral gene expression and the integration of the provirus into the DNA of the hosts. Although a structural similarity exists between the genomes of HIV-1 and HIV-2 (HTLV-IV), the nucleotide sequence homology is limited. There is a nucleotide sequence homology of only 60% between the *gag* genes and 30% to 40% between the remainder of the genes of HIV-1 and HIV-2.

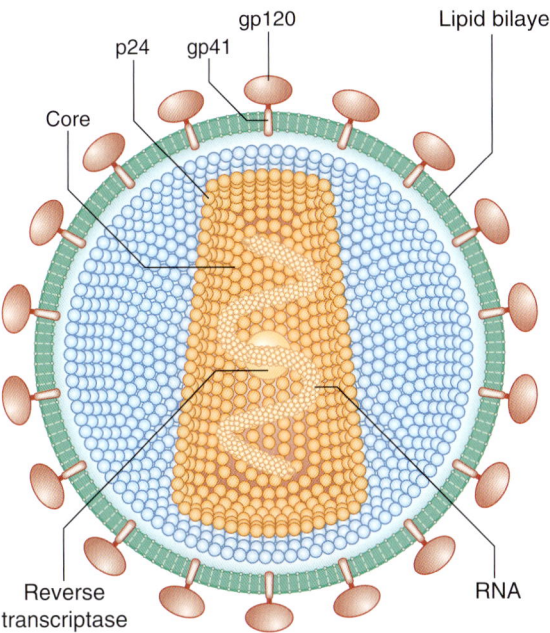

Fig. 19.5 The Human Immunodeficiency Virus. The virus's envelope is made up of glycoproteins (gps) of 120 kDa and 41 kDa. The main core protein is p19. As a ribonucleic acid *(RNA)* virus, it relies on *reverse transcriptase* to produce complementary DNA for transcription and translation. (From Peakman M, Vergani D: *Basic and clinical immunology*, ed 2, London, 2009, Churchill Livingstone.)

> **KEY CONCEPTS: HIV Characteristics**
> - HIV has a marked preference for the CD4+ subset of lymphocytes. Macrophages, as many as 40% of the peripheral blood monocytes, and cells in the lymph nodes, skin, and other organs also express measurable amounts of CD4 and can be infected by HIV.
> - In addition, about 5% of B lymphocytes may express CD4 and be susceptible to HIV infection.

Viral Replication

Retroviruses carry a single, positive-strand RNA and use reverse transcriptase to convert viral RNA into DNA. The HIV viral replication process begins when the gp120 protein on the viral envelope binds to the protein receptor CD4 located on the surface of a target cell (Fig. 19.6). HIV-1 has a marked preference for the CD4+ subset of T

TABLE 19.6 Viral Genome Components

Component	Product
Pol	Produces DNA polymerase
	Produces endonuclease
Gag	Codes for p24 and for proteins such as p17, p9, and p7
Env	Codes for two glycoproteins, gp41 and gp120

TABLE 19.7 HIV Proteins of Serodiagnostic Importance

Virus	Protein	Location	Gene
HIV-1	gp41	Envelope (transmembrane protein)	env
	gp160/120	Envelope (external protein)	env
	p24	Core (major structural protein)	gag
HIV-2	gp34	Envelope (transmembrane protein)	env
	gp140	Envelope (external protein)	env
	p26	Core (major structural protein)	gag

lymphocytes. In addition to T lymphocytes, macrophages; peripheral blood monocytes; and cells in the lymph nodes, skin, and other organs also express measurable amounts of CD4 and can be infected by HIV-1. About 5% of B lymphocytes may express CD4 and may be susceptible to HIV-1 infection. Macrophages may play an important role in spreading HIV infection in the body, both to other cells and to the target organs of HIV. Monocyte-macrophages enable HIV-1 to enter the immune-protected domain of the CNS, including the brain and spinal cord.

Fusion of the virus to the membrane of a host cell enables the viral RNA and reverse transcriptase to invade the cytoplasm of the cell. However, CD4 receptors are not sufficient for HIV envelope fusion with the T4 cell membrane or for HIV penetration or entry into the interior of the cell. Chemokine coreceptors to CD4, which HIV uses to enter a host cell after binding to it, have been identified. Beta chemokine receptors are cell surface proteins that bind small peptides. They are classified into three groups, depending on the location of the amino acid cysteine (C) in the peptide. These receptors are identified by the individual chemokine(s) that bind(s) to them. In essence, the reference to a specific chemokine also identifies its receptor. Although some cells do not produce detectable amounts of CD4, they contain low levels of messenger RNA (mRNA) encoding the CD4 protein, which indicates that they do produce some CD4. Because these cells can be infected by HIV in culture, the expression of only minimal CD4 or an alternative receptor molecule may be sufficient for HIV infection to occur. These cell types include certain brain cells, neuroglial cells, a variety of malignant brain tumor cells, and cells derived from bowel cancers. Cells of the GI system do not produce appreciable amounts of CD4, although chromaffin cells sometimes appear to be infected by HIV in vivo.

Immunologic activation of CD4+ cells latently infected with HIV induces the production of multiple viral particles, leading to cell death. The extensive destruction of cells leads to the gradual depletion of CD4+ lymphocytes. Progressive defects in the immune system include severe B-cell failure, defects in monocyte function, and defects in granulocyte function.

Epidemiology

HIV causes a chronic infection that leads to a progressive disease. Without treatment, most persons with HIV develop AIDS, which results in substantial morbidity and premature death.

Global Data

Statistics from the World Health Organization (WHO) report UNAIDS/WHO estimates demonstrate that, globally, 39.9 million (36.1–44.6 million) individuals were living with HIV at the end of 2023 (Table 19.9).

TABLE 19.8 Encoding Genes and Antigens of the AIDS Virus

Encoding Gene	Antigen
Gag	p55
Gag	p24
Gag	p17
Pol	p66
Pol	p51
Sor	p24
Env	gp160
Env	gp120
Env	gp41
3′ orf	p27

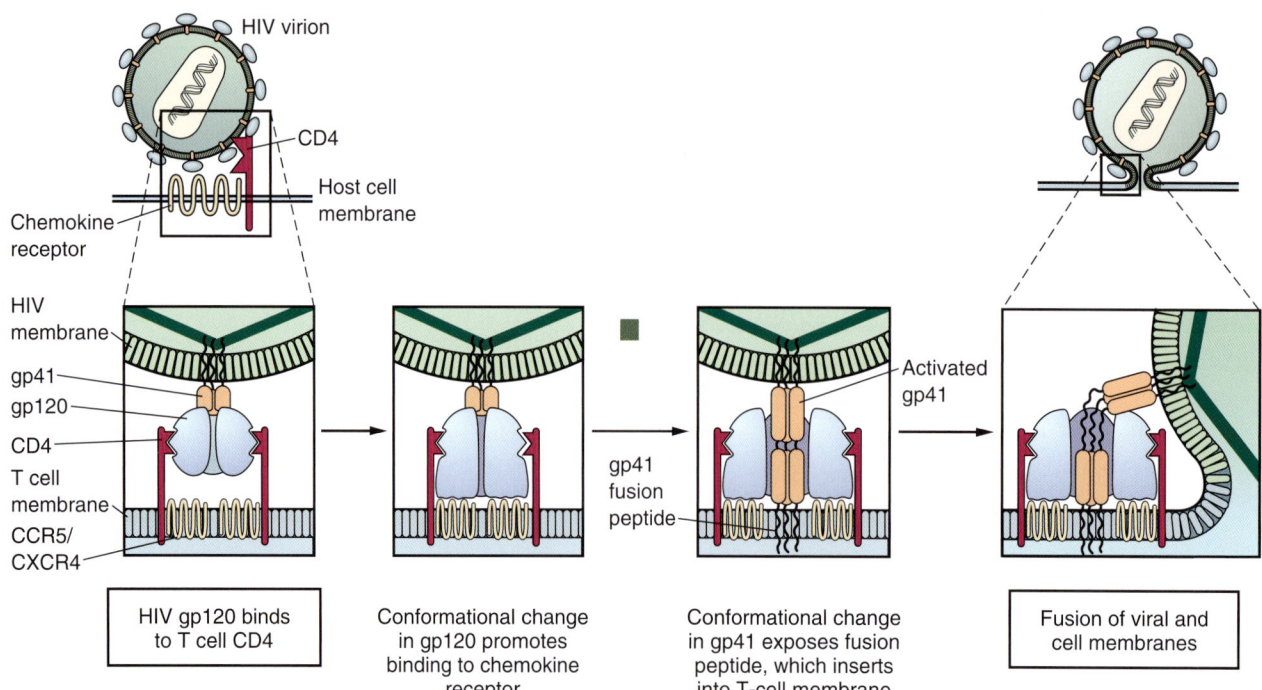

Fig. 19.6 Mechanisms of HIV Entry Into a Cell. In the model depicted, sequential conformational changes in gp120 and gp41 promote fusion of the HIV-1 and host cell membranes. The fusion peptide of activated gp41 contains hydrophobic amino acid residues that promote insertion into the lipid bilayer of the host cell's plasma membrane. (Adapted from Abbas AK, Lichtman AH, Pillai S: *Cellular and molecular immunology*, ed 6, Philadelphia, 2007, Saunders.)

TABLE 19.9 HIV Global Statistics (Regional Data—2021)

Region	HIV PREVALENCE AND INCIDENCE BY REGION	
	Total Number of People Living with HIV in 2023	Patients with HIV Accessing HIV Antiretroviral Treatment in 2023
African region	26.0 million (23.6–28.8 million)	65%–95%
Region of the Americas	4.0 million (3.5–4.5 million)	55%–85%
South-East Asian region	4.0 million (3.5–4.8 million)	60%–96%
European region	3.1 million (2.8–3.4 million)	49%–71%
Eastern Mediterranean region	530,000 (440,000–700,000)	28%–52%
Western Pacific region	2.3 million (2.2–2.4 million)	63%–83%

Modified from UNAIDS/WHO estimates, 2024. WHO regional data 2023. https://cdn.who.int/. Accessed August 16, 2024.

According to WHO, HIV-related mortality in 2023 was 630,000 [500,000–820,000] people who died from HIV-related causes globally. Since 2010, HIV-related deaths have been reduced by 51%, from 1.3 million (1.0 million–1.7 million). The global HIV epidemic claimed 69% fewer lives in 2023 since the peak in 2004. An estimated 76,000 [53,000–110,000] children died from HIV-related causes in 2023. in addition, – 560,000 [430,000–730,000] adults died from HIV-related causes in 2023.

WHO estimates that HIV continues to be a major global public health issue, claiming 42.3 million (35.7–51.1 million) lives so far.

US data. According to the latest estimates from the Centers for Disease Control and Prevention (CDC), it is estimated that 1.2 million persons in the United States were living with diagnosed and undiagnosed HIV at the end of 2022.

The new HIV incidence estimates show that national prevention efforts are continuing to move in the right direction overall, although substantial disparities exist. The estimated number of new HIV infections in 2022 (31,800) decreased 12% compared with 2018 (36,200), driven by a 30% decrease among young people aged 13–24 years. Increases in preexposure prophylaxis prescriptions, viral suppression and HIV testing likely contributed to the decline.

Data also show significant declines geographically, with estimated new HIV infections decreasing 16% in the Southern United States in 2022 compared with 2018. There were no increases in HIV incidence for any populations in 2022 compared with 2018.

The CDC estimates that a gaps remain particularly troublesome among disproportionately affected populations such as Black/African American and Hispanic/Latino.

Among women overall, in 2022, 47% (2800) of estimated new HIV infections were among Black women. New HIV infections attributed to male-to-male sexual contact (MMSC) accounted for 67% (21,400) of estimated new infections. New HIV infections among gay, bisexual, and other men who have sex with men (MSM) were about 16% lower among Black men in 2022 (7400) compared with 2018 (8800) and 20% lower among White men in 2022 (4400) compared with 2018 (5500). Although the number of new HIV infections remained about the same among Hispanic/Latino MSM (8200 in 2018 and 8300 in 2022), due to the declines among other groups, Hispanic/Latino men accounted for 39% of estimated new HIV infections among gay, bisexual, and other MSM in 2022.

Infectious Patterns

HIV-1 and HIV-2 are distinct but related retroviruses that originated from two different primate species. Globally the vast majority of infections are HIV-1, but HIV-2 is prevalent in West Africa. Transmission modes for both strains are the same, and infection with either strain can lead to the development of AIDS. HIV-2 is considered less infectious than HIV-1, and the treatment strategies are different.

AIDS is present worldwide. In some countries and regions (e.g., sub-Saharan Africa, Thailand, India), more than 90% of HIV-1 infections are acquired through heterosexual transmission, in contrast to 10% or less in the United States and Western Europe.

Within the two major HIV types, there is significant variation. Some HIV-1 variants share 50% homology in their envelope genes with the sequences of more common prototype strains. Despite some degree of immunologic crossreactivity between types and subtypes of HIV, reliable detection of antibodies derived from the more divergent strains may only be achieved by incorporating type-specific protein sequences into the assay design.

HIV-1

HIV-1 is responsible for the main AIDS epidemic. By analyzing genome sequences of representative strains, HIV-1 has been divided into three groups:
1. Group M (for major), including at least 10 subtypes (A–J)
2. Group O (for outlier)
3. Group N (for non-M, non-O)

Group M. About 90% of HIV-1 infections are classified as group M and they are distributed worldwide. Within the HIV-M group, there is a further division into at least 10 subtypes or groups of genetically related virus. Historically the distribution of subtypes followed the geographic patterns listed here:
- Subtype A: Central and East Africa and also the East European countries formerly part of the Soviet Union
- Subtype B: West and Central Europe, the Americas, Australia, South America, and several Southeast Asian countries (Thailand and Japan), in addition to northern Africa and the Middle East
- Subtype C: Sub-Saharan Africa, India, and Brazil
- Subtype D: North Africa and the Middle East
- Subtype F: South and Southeast Asia
- Subtype G: West and Central Africa
- Subtypes H, I, J, and K: Africa and the Middle East

Additionally, different subtypes can combine genetic material to form a hybrid virus, known as a *circulating recombinant form* (CRF), of which at least 20 subtypes have been identified.

Earlier in the HIV pandemic, dominant groups of genetically similar types and common routes of transmission were identified in specific geographic areas; for example in southern Africa, subtype B infection was linked to homosexual transmission and subtype C to heterosexual transmission. But assumptions can no longer be made concerning transmission patterns for particular genetically related groups of virus. Whereas heterosexual transmission drives most subtype A HIV-1 infections in sub-Saharan Africa, injection drug use is strongly linked to subtype A infection in Eastern Europe.

Subtype B is the most common form of HIV-1 found in the UK across all routes of transmission, but researchers concluded that 27% of HIV diagnoses in the UK were nonsubtype B and occurred mainly through heterosexual contact. Onward transmission has resulted in some nonsubtype B infections being identified among gay and bisexual men.

In southern Brazil, a study of mother-to-child transmission among women with either subtype C, which is the predominant subtype in that area, or subtype B found that subtype did not increase the risk of vertical transmission.

Group O. Group O infections are endemic to several west central African countries and represent 1% to 5% of all HIV-1 infection in those areas.

Group N. Group N has only been identified in a small number of individuals in Cameroon.

Superinfection. Cases of HIV superinfection have been definitively established, but there is limited evidence about their frequency. Some cases have been associated with CD4+ cell decline or transmitted drug resistance, but superinfection does not appear to have a widespread compromising effect on the health of people with HIV infection.

HIV-2

HIV-2 is endemic in parts of West Africa. HIV-2 strains have been classified into at least five subtypes (A–E). Epidemiologic data have indicated that the prevalence of HIV-2 infections in the US population is extremely low.

A persistent lower viral load is one reason for a lower incidence rate and transmission risk in HIV-2 infection than is found in HIV-1. The virulence of HIV-2 is considerably less than that of HIV-1, resulting in lower HIV-2 transmission rates, a slower course of infection, and delayed progression to AIDS. In the later stages of AIDS, HIV-2 infectiousness does increase but for a shorter duration than is seen with HIV-1 infection.

In general, after HIV-2 seroconversion the viral load tends to remain low for a longer period than is typically found in HIV-1 infection. Approximately 5% to 15% of people infected with HIV-1 are considered long-term nonprogressors versus 86% to 95% of people infected with HIV-2.

> **KEY CONCEPTS: HIV Transmission**
> - Transmission of HIV is believed to be restricted to intimate contact with body fluids from an infected person.
> - Casual contact with infected persons has not been documented as a mode of transmission.

Modes of Transmission

The primary mode of transmission of HIV-2 is via heterosexual contact. The period between infection and disease may be longer and milder for persons with HIV-2 than for those with HIV-1. HIV-2 appears to be less harmful (cytopathic) to the cells of the immune system, and it reproduces more slowly than HIV-1. Compared with persons infected with HIV-1, those with HIV-2 are less infectious early in the disease course. As the disease advances, HIV-2 infectivity seems to increase compared with HIV-1, but the duration of this increased infectivity is shorter.

HIV has been isolated from blood, semen, vaginal secretions, saliva, tears, breast milk, cerebrospinal fluid (CSF), amniotic fluid, and urine. Only blood, semen, vaginal secretions, and breast milk have been implicated in the transmission of HIV to date. HIV has been found in saliva and tears in very low quantities from some AIDS patients. It is important to understand that finding a small amount of HIV in a body fluid does not necessarily mean that HIV can be transmitted by that body fluid. HIV has not been recovered from the sweat of HIV-infected persons. Contact with saliva, tears, or sweat has never been shown to result in transmission of HIV.

HIV can be transmitted as the virus itself or as a cell associated with HIV. The virus is held within leukocytes and carried in fluid (e.g., blood, semen) to the body of another person. Transmission of HIV is believed to be restricted to intimate contact with body fluids from an infected person; casual contact with infected persons has not been documented as a mode of transmission. The risk of HIV infection to children born to women with HIV is 20% to 30%. HIV-2 seems to be less transmissible from an infected woman to her fetus or newborn.

Viral transmission of HIV-1 can be cervicovaginal, penile, rectal, oral, percutaneous, IV, in utero, or from breastfeeding after birth. More than 80% of adults infected with HIV-1 became infected through the exposure of mucosal surfaces to the virus; most of the remaining 20% were infected by a percutaneous or IV route.

Healthcare workers have been infected with HIV after being stuck with needles containing HIV-infected blood or, less frequently, after infected blood enters a worker's open cut or a mucous membrane (e.g., eyes, and inside of nose). Viral transmission can result from contact with inanimate objects, such as work surfaces or equipment recently contaminated with infected blood or certain body fluids, if the virus is transferred to broken skin or mucous membranes by hand contact.

> **KEY CONCEPTS: Stages of HIV Infection**
> - The early phase of HIV-1 infection (stage 0) may last months to years after initial infection.
> - Typically, patients in the early stages of HIV-1 infection are completely asymptomatic or show mild, chronic lymphadenopathy.
> - HIV-1 causes a predictable progressive derangement of immune function; AIDS is one late manifestation of that process.
> - Two to 10 years after HIV infection, replication of the virus can flare again, and the infection enters its final stage.
> - An average of 8 or 9 years may pass before AIDS is fully developed.
> - The virus behaves differently, depending on the host cell and its level of mitotic activity.
> - The end stage of AIDS is characterized by neoplasms and opportunistic infections.

Signs and Symptoms

Infection with HIV produces a chronic infection with symptoms that range from asymptomatic to the end-stage complications of AIDS.

Typically patients in the early stages of HIV infection are completely asymptomatic or show mild chronic lymphadenopathy. The early phase may last from many months to many years after viral exposure. Although the course of HIV-1 infection may vary somewhat in individual patients, a common pattern of development has been recognized. The newly revised HIV classification system provides uniform and simple criteria for categorizing conditions.

The CDC has a newly revised classification system (2014) to define stages of HIV-related illness (Box 19.6). The stages of HIV infection

> **BOX 19.6 Condensed Summary of Revised Surveillance Case Definition for HIV Infection—United States, 2014**
>
> **Stage 0**
> The definition of stage 0 reduces confusion between acute HIV infection (part of stage 0), when CD4+ T-lymphocyte counts can be transiently depressed, and stage 3 (AIDS), an advanced stage of HIV infection when CD4+ T-lymphocyte values are usually persistently depressed.
>
> Within 2 to 4 weeks of exposure to the virus, many patients develop flulike symptoms. Symptoms can include fever, swollen glands, sore throat, rash, muscle and joint aches and pains, and headache. This is called *acute retroviral syndrome (ARS)*, and it is a natural response to the HIV infection. During this early period of infection, large amounts of virus are produced by the immune system. Even if HIV cannot be detected in the blood (viremia), it infects lymphatic tissues in large quantities, including the tonsils and lymph nodes throughout the body. The absence of viremia generally lasts until the end stage of the disease.
>
> During this period of viral replication, the CD4+ T-lymphocyte count falls rapidly. A patient's immune response will begin to bring the level of virus in the body down to a level called a *viral set point*, a relatively stable level of virus in an infected patient's body. At this point, the CD4+ T-lymphocyte count begins to rise, but it may not return to preinfection levels.
>
> The criteria for stage 0 consist of a sequence of discordant test results indicative of early HIV infection in which a negative or indeterminate result occurs within 180 days of a positive result. The criteria for stage 0 supersede and are independent of the criteria used for other stages. Stage 0 can be established as follows:
>
> 1. Based on testing history (previous negative/indeterminate test results): A negative or indeterminate HIV test result (antibody, combination antigen/antibody, or nucleic acid test) that occurs within 180 days before the first confirmed positive HIV test result of any type. The first positive test result could be any time before the positive supplemental test result that confirms it.
> 2. Based on a testing algorithm: A sequence of tests performed as part of a laboratory testing algorithm that demonstrates the presence of HIV-specific viral markers such as p24 antigen or nucleic acid (RNA or DNA) 0 to 180 days before or after an antibody test that had a negative or indeterminate result.
> 3. A confirmed case of HIV infection is not in stage 0 if the negative or indeterminate HIV test result used as the criterion for it being a recent infection was preceded more than 60 days by evidence of HIV infection, such as a confirmed positive HIV test result; a clinical (physician-documented) diagnosis of HIV infection for which the surveillance staff have not found sufficient laboratory evidence; a CD4+ T-lymphocyte test result indicative of stage 3; or an opportunistic illness indicative of stage 3.
>
> **Progression of Stage After Initial Diagnosis in Stage 0**
> Although the stage at diagnosis does not change, if more than 180 days have elapsed after the stage was 0 at diagnosis, the stage at the later date is classified as 1, 2, 3, or unknown, depending on the CD4+ T-lymphocyte test results or whether an opportunistic illness had been diagnosed more than 180 days after diagnosis of the HIV infection.
>
> After stage 0, a prolonged period of clinical latency (range, 7–11 years; median, 10 years) can be observed. During the period of clinical latency, the patient is usually asymptomatic. Differences in the infecting virus, the host's genetic makeup, and environmental factors (e.g., concomitant infection) have been suggested as causes of the variable duration of clinical latency in persons not receiving antiretroviral therapy (ART). There are now several recommended regimens for ART-naïve patients: four integrase strand transfer inhibitor (INSTI)–based regimens and one ritonavir-boosted protease inhibitor (PI/r)–based regimen. Prophylaxis for pneumonia caused by *Pneumocystis jirovecii* (previously called *P. carinii*) has increased AIDS-free time in HIV-1–infected persons.
>
> During this next stage of HIV infection, the virus reproduces at very low levels, but it is still active. "Latency" means a period where a virus is living or developing in a patient without producing symptoms. During the clinical latency stage, patients who are infected with HIV experience no symptoms or only mild ones.
>
> If treated at this stage, patients may live with clinical latency for several decades. Without treatment, clinical latency can last for an average of 10 years. There are individual differences in disease progression.
>
> **Diagnosis of AIDS**
> If a patient's CD4+ lymphocyte count falls below 200 cells/mm^3, the patient is considered to be suffering from AIDS and is vulnerable to opportunistic infections. A patient is considered to have progressed to AIDS if one or more opportunistic infections develop, regardless of the CD4+ T-cell count. Without treatment or an effective response to ART, HIV advances in stages with an average survival time of about 3 years. If an opportunistic infection develops, life expectancy without treatment falls to about 1 year. If a patient is taking ART and maintains a low viral load, a patient most likely will never progress to AIDS and may enjoy a near-normal life span.

Modified from Revised surveillance case definition for HIV infection—United States, *MMWR* 63(RR03):1–10, 2014.

defined in this document are for surveillance staging of disease and might not be appropriate for patient care, clinical research, or other purposes. The stage characterizes the status of HIV disease at a particular point in time. Of primary interest to surveillance is the stage at initial diagnosis, but the stage can change in either direction after diagnosis.

A confirmed case that meets the criteria for diagnosis of HIV infection can be classified in one of five HIV infection stages: 0, 1, 2, 3, or unknown. An early HIV infection is inferred from a negative or indeterminate HIV test result within 6 months of a confirmed positive result, and these criteria supersede and are independent of the criteria used for later stages.

Stages 1, 2, and 3 are based on the CD4+ T-lymphocyte count. If the CD4+ count is missing or unknown, the CD4+ T-lymphocyte percentage of total lymphocytes can be used to assign the stage. Cases with no information on CD4+ T-lymphocyte count or percentage are classified as stage unknown. If a stage 3–defining opportunistic illness has been diagnosed, then the stage is 3 regardless of CD4 T-lymphocyte test results, unless the criteria described later for stage 0 are met. CD4+ T-lymphocyte counts or percentages at the time of diagnosis allow classification of cases by stage at diagnosis. Subsequent CD4+ T-lymphocyte counts or percentages help monitor disease progression and whether the person is receiving ongoing care.

Opportunistic Infections

Since AIDS was first recognized in the early 1980s, remarkable progress has been made in improving the quality and duration of life for HIV-infected persons in the industrialized world. During the first decade of the epidemic, this progress resulted from improved recognition of opportunistic disease processes, improved therapy for acute and chronic complications, and introduction of chemoprophylaxis against key opportunistic pathogens. The second decade of the epidemic witnessed extraordinary progress in developing **highly active antiretroviral therapy (HAART)**, in addition to continuing progress in preventing and treating opportunistic infections. HAART has reduced the incidence of opportunistic infections and extended life. In

TABLE 19.10 Stages of HIV Infection

The HIV infection stage[a] is based on the age-specific CD4+ T-lymphocyte count or the CD4+ T-lymphocyte percentage of total lymphocytes.

Stage	AGE ON DATE OF CD4+ T-LYMPHOCYTE TEST					
	<1 year		1–5 years		6 years	
	Cells/µL	%	Cells/µL	%	Cells/µL	%
1	1500	34	1000	30	500	26
2	750–1499	26–33	500–999	22–29	200–499	14–25
3	<750	<26	<500	<22	<200	<14

[a]The stage is based primarily on the CD4+ T-lymphocyte count; the CD4+ T-lymphocyte count takes precedence over the CD4+ T-lymphocyte percentage, and the percentage is considered only if the count is missing. There are three situations in which the stage is not based on this table: (1) if the criteria for stage 0 are met, the stage is 0 regardless of criteria for other stages (CD4 T-lymphocyte test results and opportunistic illness diagnoses); (2) if the criteria for stage 0 are not met and a stage 3–defining opportunistic illness has been diagnosed, then the stage is 3, regardless of the CD4 T-lymphocyte test results; and (3) if the criteria for stage 0 are not met and information on the criteria for other stages is missing, the stage is classified as unknown.

BOX 19.7 Opportunistic Infections in Immunosuppressed and Immunodeficient Patients

1. Oral or esophageal candidiasis
2. Cytomegalovirus
3. *Pneumocystis jirovecii (P. carinii)*
4. Herpes simplex
5. *Entamoeba histolytica*
6. *Giardia lamblia*
7. Herpes zoster
8. Atypical acid-fast bacilli
9. *Shigella*
10. *Campylobacter*
11. *Cryptococcus neoformans*
12. Adenovirus
13. Hepatitis
14. *Chlamydia*
15. *Salmonella*
16. Syphilis
17. Anal candidiasis
18. *Dientamoeba fragilis*
19. *Blastocystis hominis*
20. *Toxoplasma gondii*

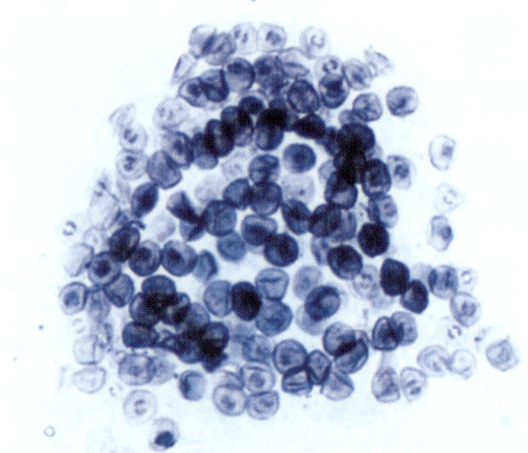

Fig. 19.7 *Pneumocystis jirovecii (P. carinii)* from a tracheobronchial aspirate (methenamine silver). (From Zeibig E: *Clinical parasitology*, ed 2, Philadelphia, 2013, Elsevier.)

addition prophylaxis against specific opportunistic infections continues to provide survival benefits even among patients receiving HAART.

The absolute number of CD4+ T lymphocytes continues to diminish as the disease progresses (Table 19.10). When the number of cells reaches a critically low level (<50 to 100×10^9/L), the risk of opportunistic infection increases. The period of susceptibility to opportunistic processes continues to be accurately indicated by CD4+ T-lymphocyte counts for patients receiving HAART.

The end stage of AIDS is characterized by the occurrence of neoplasms and opportunistic infections (Box 19.7). The most common opportunistic infections are *P. jirovecii (P. carinii)* (Fig. 19.7), cytomegalovirus (CMV), *Mycobacterium avium-intracellulare*, *Cryptococcus*, *Toxoplasma*, *Mycobacterium tuberculosis*, herpes simplex, and *Legionella*. *Histoplasma capsulatum* is being recognized with increasing frequency.

Kaposi Sarcoma

The most frequent malignancy observed is an aggressive, invasive variant of Kaposi sarcoma (KS), discovered in many cases on autopsy. Malignant B-cell lymphomas are increasingly recognized in patients with or at high risk for AIDS.

KS was first described in 1872 by the dermatologist Moritz Kaposi. Since then, until the AIDS epidemic, KS remained a rare tumor. Classic KS usually occurs in males. The tumor typically presents with one or more asymptomatic red, purple, or brown patches; plaque; or nodular skin lesions. The disease is often limited to single or multiple lesions, usually localized to one or both lower extremities, especially involving the ankle and soles. Classic KS most often has a relatively benign, indolent course for 10 to 15 years or longer, with slow enlargement of the original tumors and gradual development of additional lesions. Up to one-third of patients with classic KS develop a second primary malignancy, usually non-Hodgkin lymphoma. An increased incidence of Hodgkin disease occurs in HIV-infected homosexual men.

Cryptosporidiosis

Cryptosporidiosis is a disease caused by the parasite *Cryptosporidium parvum*. As late as 1976, this parasite was not thought to cause disease in human beings. In 1993 more than 400,000 people in Milwaukee, Wisconsin, became ill after drinking water contaminated with the parasite. Cryptosporidiosis can be chronic and severe in immunocompromised persons. The watery diarrhea can be prolonged and debilitating, and may be fatal.

Persons at risk of severe cryptosporidiosis include AIDS, cancer, or organ marrow transplant patients taking drugs that weaken the immune system, and persons born with genetically weakened immune systems.

Disease Progression

Although a large enough dose of the right strain of HIV-1 can cause AIDS on its own, cofactors can influence the progression of disease development. Debilitated patients weakened by a preexisting medical condition before HIV-1 infection may progress toward AIDS more quickly than others. Stimulation of the immune system in response to later infections can also hasten disease progression. Other pathogenic microorganisms, such as a herpes virus called *human B lymphotropic virus* (human herpes virus 6 [HHV-6]), can interact with HIV in a way that may increase the severity of HIV infection. HHV-6 is usually easily controlled by the immune system. If HIV compromises the immune system, however, HHV-6 may replicate more freely and become a health threat. The main host of HHV-6 is the B cell, but this virus can also infect CD4+ cells. If these T cells are simultaneously infected by HIV, HHV-6 can stimulate the virus, which further impairs the immune system and promotes disease progression.

The progressive decline of CD4+ cells leads to a general decline in immune function and is the primary factor in determining the clinical progression of AIDS. Plasma HIV-1 RNA is a strong CD4+ T-cell–independent predictor of a rapid progression to AIDS after HIV-1 seroconversion.

Infection with HIV is presently considered to lead to death. When the clinically apparent disease develops, untreated patients usually die within 2 years; some exposed or HIV-1–infected patients never develop AIDS. The current hope is that an AIDS-free generation is on the horizon as a result of prevention strategies (e.g., safe sex and preexposure prophylaxis).

Although scientists have known since 1986 that CD8 T cells, when stimulated, could release molecules capable of suppressing HIV, the identity of these substances eluded researchers for more than a decade. Studies have suggested that three large proteins, identified as alpha-defensins 1, 2, and 3, could be major contributors to the CD8 antiviral factor that protects some patients against AIDS. In another study, scientists at the National Institutes of Health (NIH) have linked HIV resistance to a different molecule secreted by CD8 T cells, called *perforin*. More studies related to each category of molecules are needed before either of these theories can be confirmed.

Another study at the National Institute of Allergy and Infectious Diseases has examined variations in a gene called *RANTES* (*r*egulated on *a*ctivation, *n*ormal *T* cells *e*xpressed, and presumably *s*ecreted) in HIV-infected and HIV-resistant individuals. This study searched for changes in a single-nucleotide polymorphism (SNP). The results showed that one such SNP appears more often in HIV-positive than in HIV-negative persons. In addition, this particular alteration increases the activity of the *RANTES* gene and is associated with up to twice the risk of HIV infection. However, HIV-infected patients with this SNP take about 40% longer to develop AIDS.

a receptor site for the virus. Immunologic activation (e.g., participation in an immune response to HIV-1 or viruses in other cells) of CD4+ cells latently infected with HIV-1 induces the production of multiple viral particles, leading to cell death. The extensive destruction of T cells leads to gradual depletion of the CD4+ lymphocytes. The major phenotypic cell populations affected by AIDS are CD4+ and CD8+ subsets of T lymphocytes. Normally the CD4+ to CD8+ ratio is 2:1 in heterosexual individuals and 1.5:1 in homosexual individuals. A reversal of these subsets is evident in, but not diagnostic of, AIDS. In patients with AIDS, the ratio is less than 0.5:1. It is important to note that this results from a marked decrease in the absolute number of circulating CD4+ cells, rather than from an absolute increase in suppressor or CD8+ cells. This abnormality exists in the lymph nodes and circulating T cells. A diminished CD4+:CD8+ ratio (altered lymphocyte subpopulation) can also be seen in individuals with other disorders, such as cutaneous T-cell lymphoma, SLE, and acute viral infections. The ratio, however, reverts back to normal after recovery from a viral infection in non-AIDS patients.

A decreased lymphocyte proliferative response to soluble antigens and mitogens exists in AIDS. Functional testing reveals a diminished response to pokeweed mitogen. This disease also demonstrates defective NK-cell activity.

Immune System Alterations

The HIV virus is fragile and, as the virus particle leaves its host cell, a molecule called *glycoprotein 120 (gp120)* frequently breaks off the outer coat of the virus. Gp120 can bind to the CD4 molecules of uninfected cells and, when that complex is recognized by the immune system, these cells can be destroyed. The lysis of infected cells and gp120-bound uninfected cells leads to gradual depletion of the CD4+ lymphocytes. Defects in immunity are related to this T-cell depletion. Progressive defects in the immune system also include a severe B-cell failure and defects in monocyte and granulocyte function.

Although HIV-1 destroys CD4+ cells directly and hampers the immune system, this process does not cause the severe immunodeficiency seen in AIDS. The severe deficiency can be explained only if the cells are also destroyed by other means. Several indirect mechanisms have been suggested. Infection by HIV can cause infected and uninfected cells to fuse into giant cells called *syncytia*, which are nonfunctional. Autoimmune responses, in which the immune system attacks the body's own tissues, may also be at work. In addition, HIV-infected cells may send out protein signals that weaken or destroy other cells of the immune system. It is possible that the binding of HIV to a target cell triggers the release of the enzyme protease. Proteases digest proteins; if released in abnormal quantities they might weaken lymphocytes and other cells, and decrease cell survival. The decline in T cells and subsequent alteration of the immune mechanism are the underlying factors in the progression of HIV infection.

> **KEY CONCEPTS**
> - Immunologic activities associated with HIV-1 infection include the production of different types of antibodies against HIV-1.
> - Some antibodies neutralize HIV-1 but others prevent it from binding to cells, and still others stimulate cytotoxic cells to attack HIV-infected cells.
> - A window period of seronegativity exists from the time of initial infection to 6 or 12 weeks or longer.

Immunologic Manifestations
Cellular Abnormalities

The HIV-1 virus has a marked preference for the CD4+ subset of lymphocytes because the CD4 surface marker protein on these cells serves as

> **KEY CONCEPTS: Laboratory Methods in HIV/AIDS**
> - Using enzyme immunoassay (EIA) methods based on defined HIV-1 proteins produced by recombinant DNA methods, antibodies specific for gp41 are detectable for weeks or months before assays are specific for p19.
> - The appearance of antibodies specific for p24 precedes that of anti-gp41 in Western blot (WB) serum specimens.
> - Laboratory evaluation of HIV-infected patients consists of assessment of cellular and humoral components.
> - Screening of blood donors and patients is usually by serologic methods.
> - In patients with signs and symptoms of AIDS, both the assessment of cellular concentrations and function, and the diagnosis and treatment of opportunistic infections, become important.
> - Antibodies to HIV-1 are usually detected by EIA.

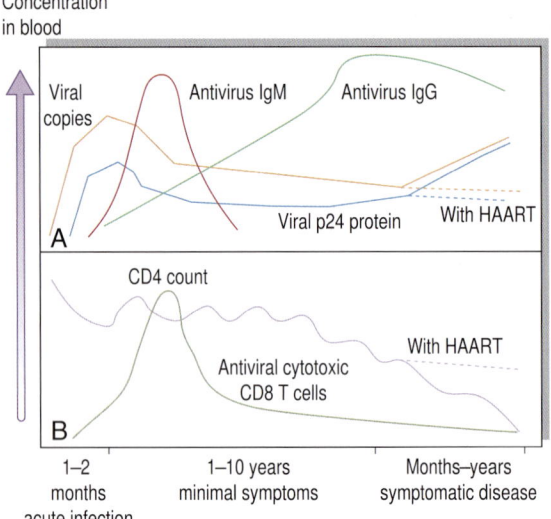

Fig. 19.8 Pattern of virus replication and immune responses in acute, chronic, and late stages of HIV infection. (A) The graph shows the acute rise in concentration of viral ribonucleic acid (RNA) and p24 protein in the blood followed by a stabilization of levels, presumably as a result of the actions of cytotoxic CD8 cells and other elements of the immune response. Antibody levels (IgM then IgG) rise acutely and, in the case of IgG, remain high throughout the disease. (B) The graph shows the early and catastrophic loss of CD4+ cells in the circulation. The loss stabilizes in association with the antiviral CD8 response emerging, but both decline during the asymptomatic period until the CD4+ count reaches 2–400 cells/μL of blood. At this point, AIDS-defining illnesses are seen, unless highly active antiretroviral therapy *(HAART)* is commenced, in which case an amelioration of viral load and CD4 cell numbers are seen. (From Peakman M, Vergani D: *Basic and clinical immunology*, ed 2, London, 2009, Churchill Livingstone.)

Serologic Markers
Detection of Core Antigen
After initial infection, the body mounts a vigorous immune response against the viremia (Fig. 19.8). The first signal of an immune response to HIV-1 infection is the appearance of acute-phase reactants, including α_1-antitrypsin and serum amyloid in plasma 3 to 5 days after transmission. This is followed by a steep rise in the HIV-1 viral load (ramp-up viremia) that coincides with a large burst of inflammatory cytokines led by interferon-α and IL-15, and by a burst of plasma microparticles derived from infected and activated CD4 T cells undergoing apoptosis.

Increased production of core antigen is believed to be associated with a burst of viral replication and host cell lysis. A sudden decrease in anti-p24 is considered to be a grave prognostic sign in HIV-1–infected patients.

Antibodies to HIV-1
Immunologic activities include the production of different types of antibodies against HIV. Some antibodies neutralize the virus, others prevent it from binding to cells, and still others stimulate cytotoxic cells to attack HIV-infected cells.

The time and sequence vary for the appearance and disappearance of antibodies specific for the serologically important antigens of HIV-1 during the course of infection. A window period of seronegativity exists from the time of initial infection to 6 or 12 weeks or longer thereafter.

Antibodies specific for gp41 are detectable for weeks or months before assays are specific for p19.

The appearance of antibodies specific for p24 has been shown to precede that of anti-gp41 in serum specimens undergoing WB analysis. This discrepancy in the sequence of antibody appearance is believed to be caused by the greater sensitivity of WB compared with viral lysate–based EIAs used for the detection of anti-p19.

The gp41 antibodies persist throughout the course of infection. Antibodies specific for p24 not only rise to detectable levels after gp41, but also can disappear unpredictably and abruptly. The disappearance of antibody directed against p24 occurs concomitantly with an increase in the concentration of core antigen in the serum. This parallel activity may result from the sequestration of antibody in immune complexes.

Specific intrathecal synthesis of HIV antibody should be assessed simultaneously with an assay for total CSF IgM and for the intrathecal synthesis of total IgG, in addition to IgG specific for an appropriate control organism (e.g., adenovirus). In progressive encephalopathy related to AIDS, an increase in HIV antibody may suggest intrathecal rather than extrathecal synthesis.

Diagnostic Evaluation and Monitoring
Multitest algorithms lead the way and now include antibody immunoassays formerly used only as initial tests or can include nucleic acid tests (NATs). Some new multitest algorithms lead to a conclusion that laboratories might classify as a "presumptive positive" result. Persons with a presumptive positive test result are expected to receive subsequent tests, such as a quantitative viral load, to confirm their HIV diagnosis.

Infection with HIV is established by detecting antibodies to the virus, viral antigens, or viral RNA-DNA or by the gold standard, viral culture. The preferred screening is by fourth-generation HIV antigen/antibody (HIV-1/2).

Both leukopenia and lymphocytopenia can exist in the AIDS patient. Total leukocyte and absolute lymphocyte concentrations need to be periodically assessed. The common denominator of AIDS is a deficiency of a specific subset of thymus-derived (CD4+) lymphocytes. Enumeration of lymphocyte subsets is usually performed by flow cytometry (see Chapter 11).

Additional testing includes viral load assay and resistance testing, an in vitro method to measure the resistance of HIV to antiretroviral agents. Resistance testing can aid in antiretroviral drug selection but has limitations.

Testing Methods
Since 2014, the CDC has recommended the use of a fourth-generation antigen–antibody test to screen for HIV-1 p24 antigen and antibodies to HIV-1 (groups M and O). Repeatedly reactive HIV-1 and HIV-2 results should be confirmed with an HIV-1/HIV-2 antibody differentiation test, as should positive results for third- or fourth-generation testing performed at a client site. Negative or indeterminate results for HIV-1 or HIV-2 antibody differentiation should be confirmed with a quantitative PCR.

Testing assays for HIV (Table 19.11) are categorized into the following three main types:
- Detection of HIV antibodies
- Detection of antigens, particularly p24
- Detection or quantification of viral nucleic acids

HIV-1 Antibody Assays
Detection of HIV antibodies by EIA (Tables 19.12 and 19.13) was the first technology developed for HIV diagnosis in 1985. Today, diagnostic testing using an algorithm (Fig. 19.9) begins in adults with fourth-generation antigen–antibody testing with reflex testing to confirm. Confirmation of repeatedly reactive results is confirmed by HIV-1/2 antibody differentiation immunoassay. If both HIV-1 and HIV-2 are positive, HIV RNA detection by nucleic acid amplification testing

TABLE 19.11 HIV Assays and Their Characteristics

Assay	Format	Target Molecule	Comments
Lymphocyte CD4 absolute count	Flow cytometry	CD4+	
HIV antigen assay for serum and plasma	Enzyme immunoassay (EIA)	HIV p24 antigen	
HIV types 1 and 2 (HIV-1, HIV-2) antibody detection in serum or plasma	EIA (first- and second-generation tests)	Recombinant HIV-1 *env* and *gag* and HIV-2 env proteins *or* purified, inactivated HIV-1 virus propagated in T-lymphocyte culture	If reactive, confirm with molecular testing (Western blot)
Detection of HIV-1 groups M and O	EIA (third generation)	Purified, inactivated HIV-1 viral lysate proteins, envelope proteins, and HIV-1 group O transmembrane protein *or* purified gp160 and p24 recombinant proteins from HIV-1, HIV-2 transmembrane gp36, and synthetic epitope of HIV-1 group O	
Enzyme-linked fluorescence p24 *or* EIA p24	EIA (fourth generation)	HIV-1 gp160, p24 antigen, and peptides representing regions of gp41 from HIV-1 group O and gp36 from HIV-2 *or* HIV-1 antigens p31 and gp41, HIV-2 p36 recombinant protein, HIV-1 group O gp41, and anti-p24 monoclonal antibodies	
HIV antibody detection in serum or plasma	Western blot	Purified and inactivated HIV-1 strain LAV grown in CEM cell line *or* purified and inactivated HIV-1 propagated in H9/HTLV-IIIB T-lymphocyte cell line	
HIV viral load assays	PCR	Reverse transcriptase PCR *or* nucleic acid sequence–based amplification *or* signal amplification, branched chain DNA	
Rapid testing	Rapid immunoassay	Uses recombinant proteins representing regions of HIV-1 envelope proteins *or* uses synthetic HIV structural proteins Rapid test rapid enzyme immunoassay to be used as a diagnostic aid for the detection and differentiation of HIV-1 and HIV-2 antibodies in human serum or plasma	
Molecular Testing			
HIV-1 RNA	Quantitative real-time PCR		Aids in assessing viral response to antiretroviral treatment
HIV-1 RNA	Quantitative bDNA	Quantitative branched chain DNA	Aids in assessing viral response to antiretroviral treatment
HIV-1 DNA	Qualitative PCR		Detects HIV-1 proviral DNA in infants <48 hours old; repeat testing at 1–2 months and 3–6 months of age
HIV-2 antibody		Qualitative enzyme immunoassay, qualitative immunoblot	Screen for HIV-2 infection in a patient with an epidemiologic link to Africa
HIV-1 genotyping	Reverse transcription PCR/nucleic acid sequencing		Detect changes in the viral genome associated with drug resistance Use in conjunction with CD4 measurement to monitor treatment efficacy
HIV-2 antibody confirmation	Qualitative immunoblot		Confirm positive screening results
HIV-1 antibody	Qualitative chemiluminescent immunoassay		

PCR, Polymerase chain reaction.
Adapted from Zetola N, Klausner JD: HIV testing: an update, *MLO Med Lab Obs* 38:58–62, 2006.

TABLE 19.12 Causes of False-Positive and False-Negative HIV Enzyme Immunoassay Results

False-Positive Result	False-Negative Result
Positive RPR (syphilis serology) test	Laboratory glove starch
Hematologic malignant disorder	Window period before seroconversion
DNA viral infections	Immunosuppressive therapy
Autoimmune disorders	Malignancies
Alcoholic hepatitis	Bone marrow transplantation
Vaccinations (e.g., hepatitis B and influenza)	Kits that mainly detect antibodies to p24
Chronic renal failure	
Renal transplantation	

RPR, Rapid plasma reagin.
Adapted from Specialty Laboratories, Santa Monica, California.

TABLE 19.13 HIV-1 and HIV-2 Antibody Differentiation Immunoassay Results in Adults

Assay Results	Additional Testing	Conclusion
HIV-1 (+) positive HIV-2 (−) negative		HIV-1 infection
HIV-1 (indeterminant) HIV-2 (−) negative	Quantitative PCR for HIV-1	Positive acute HIV-1 infection Negative for HIV-1
HIV-1 (−) negative HIV-2 (−) negative	Quantitative PCR for HIV-1	Positive acute HIV-1 infection Negative for HIV-1
HIV-1 (−) negative HIV-2 (+) positive		HIV-2 infection
HIV-1 (+) positive HIV-2 (+) positive		Cannot differentia amplification testing HIV-1 from HIV-2 Recommend consider HIV-2 nucleic acid amplification testing (NAAT)

The Centers for Disease Control and Prevention (CDC) and the Association of Public Health Laboratories (APHL) Technical Update for HIV Nucleic Acid Tests Approved for Diagnostic Purposes https://www.cdc.gov/hiv/guidelines/recommendations/technical-update-for-hiv.html. Accessed September 25, 2024.

(NAAT) can be used to differentiate HIV-2. Alternative screening using the third- or fourth-generation algorithm reflexes to the WB. Third-generation serologic assays have demonstrated that seroconversion typically occurs 3 to 12 weeks after infection, but significant delays can occur in some individuals.

HIV Antigen and Genome Testing

Enzyme Immunoassay: p24 Antigen

The EIA for the HIV-1 antigen detects primarily uncomplexed p24 antigen. This procedure is applicable to blood or CSF testing as evidence of an active infection and can be diagnostic before seroconversion, can predict a patient's prognosis, and is useful for monitoring response to therapy. Disadvantages of the procedure include poor sensitivity, inability to detect in patients with a high titer of p24 antibody, and failure of the method to detect HIV-2 antigen. Antibodies to p24 antigen are a better predictive marker of progression than p24 antigen.

Polymerase Chain Reaction

PCR allows for direct detection of HIV-1 by DNA amplification. This ultrasensitive PCR technique has revolutionized HIV-1 detection. In addition to confirmatory testing, DNA amplification can be used for the diagnosis of very early, postexposure HIV infection in the window period before production of antibodies.

The goal of direct detection of active virus in patient specimens by an ultrasensitive method is to detect less than 100 molecules of viral nucleic acid in the peripheral blood cells isolated from 1 mL of blood. This number is the assay target because as few as 1 in 10,000 lymphocytes express viral RNA in HIV-1–infected individuals. Therefore of approximately 10^6 lymphocytes per milliliter of blood, about 100 contain viral nucleic acid, corresponding to 100 to 150 copies of HIV-1 DNA. The presence of HIV-1 DNA in lymphocytes of antibody-positive, asymptomatic patients can be used to confirm exposure to the virus. The presence of viral RNA might be a sensitive indicator of viral replication and possibly of further disease progression.

The basis of PCR is the amplification of minute amounts of viral nucleic acid in lymphocyte DNA. In HIV-1–infected cells, the DNA template is a provirus that exists as integrated or episomal DNA. After amplification, isotope or nonisotope methods can detect the amplified product. The most effective means of target amplification is PCR. A pair of *specific oligomer primers* initiates DNA synthesis in combination with heat-stable Taq I DNA polymerase. After this first round of primer extension, the material is heated to denature the product from its template and cooled to 37°C (98.6°F) to permit annealing of the primer molecules to the original template DNA and to the newly synthesized DNA fragments. Primer extension is then resumed. By repetition of these cycles of denaturation, annealing, and extension, the original DNA can be increased exponentially.

Viral RNA can also be specifically amplified with some additional steps. The *gag region* is probably the best choice of a sequence for amplification. Detection of viral RNA and DNA in clinical specimens might prove to be a better indicator of biologically active virus than DNA detection alone. The presence of both provirus and viral RNA *transcriptase* would be a strong indication of viral replication. Quantitation of HIV RNA in plasma is useful for determining free viral load, assessing the efficacy of antiviral therapy, and predicting progression and clinical outcome in AIDS patients.

Alternative Screening for HIV

An alternative screening protocol uses third- or fourth-generation testing reflexing to Western blot (WB). Testing can follow one of three different combinations of assays:

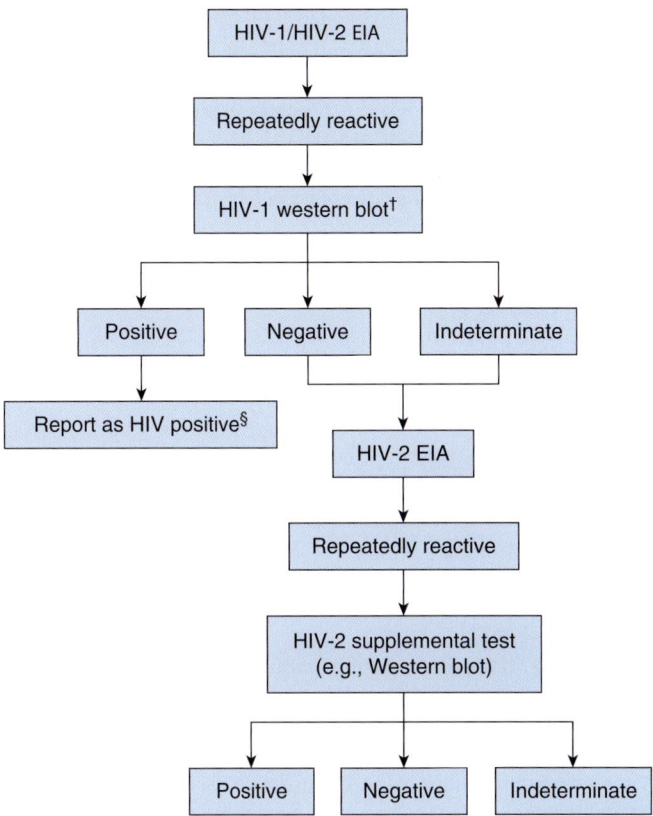

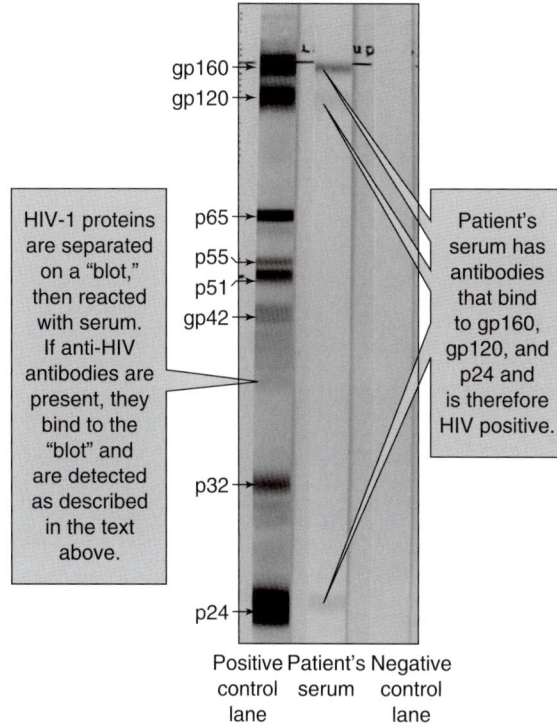

Fig. 19.10 Western Blot to Confirm HIV-Positive Status. (From Nairn R, Helbert M: *Immunology for medical students*, ed 2, Philadelphia, 2007, Mosby.)

†An immunofluorescence assay (IFA) for HIV-1 antibodies has recently been licensed by the Food and Drug Administration and can be used instead of Western blot. Positive and negative IFA results should be interpreted in the same manner as similar results from Western blot tests. An intermediate IFA should first be tested by HIV-1 Western blot then as indicated by the Western blot results.
§Perform HIV-2 EIA only if there is an identified risk factor for HIV-2 infection.

Fig. 19.9 Centers for Disease Control/Food and Drug Administration testing algorithm for use with combination HIV-1/HIV-2* enzyme immunoassays (EIAs). (Centers for Disease Controls: Testing for antibodies to human immunodeficiency virus type 2 in the United States, *MMWR Recommen Rep* 41(RR12):1–9, 1992.)

1. HIV-1 and HIV-2 antibody assay using CIA + reflex HIV-1 antibody confirmation by WB
2. HIV-1 antibody assay using CIA + reflex HIV-1 antibody confirmation by WB
3. HIV antigen/antibody (HIV-1/O/2) by enzyme-linked immunosorbent assay (ELISA) + reflex to HIV-1 antibody confirmation by WB

Western Blot

Before an HIV result is considered positive, the results can be confirmed by WB analysis to confirm HIV-1 seropositivity (Fig. 19.10).

The WB assay is based on the recognition of the major HIV proteins (p24, gp41, gp120/160) by fractionating them according to their weight by electrophoresis and then visualizing their binding with specific antibodies over nitrocellulose sheets. A positive result is indicated by the presence of any two of the following bands: p24, gp41, and gp120/160. A test result that is positive for bands gp41 and/or p24, in conjunction with a positive EIA test result, is regarded as a confirmatory test. A negative result demonstrates the absence of bands. Indeterminate results can be found in 10% to 20% of EIA-positive tests. In general, the presence of a band at p24, p31, or p55, although still classified as indeterminate, is more indicative of true infection compared with other band patterns.

The WB appears to work best with samples that contain high levels of antibody. Antibody specificities against known viral components (generally, the core component p24 and envelope component gp41) are considered true-positive results, whereas antibodies specific against nonviral cellular contaminants are nonspecific, false-positive results.

The WB technique is time-consuming and expensive. It is also open to considerable interpretation and has many sources of error. Variables in the test include the following:
- The technical skill and experience of the technologist performing the procedure
- Characteristics of the technical methodology
- General sensitivity of the WB in detecting antibodies specific for various HIV-1 antigens (especially during the window period of seronegativity)
- Frequent lack of specificity because of contamination of the viral reference preparation by histocompatibility and other antigens that electrophoretically migrate with p24 and gp41
- Variation in band reactivity patterns in sera from an individual over the course of HIV-1 infection

Indeterminate test results account for 4% to 20% of WB assays, with positive bands for HIV-1 proteins. Indeterminate WB results can be caused by the following:
- Serologic tests in the process of seroconversion; anti-p24 is usually the first antibody to appear
- End-stage HIV infection, usually with loss of core antibody
- Crossreacting nonspecific antibodies, as seen with collagen vascular disease, autoimmune diseases, lymphoma, liver disease, injection drug use, multiple sclerosis, parity, or recent immunization
- Infection with O strain or HIV-2
- Recipients of HIV vaccine
- Perinatally exposed infants who are seroconverting (losing maternal antibody)
- Technical or clerical error

In addition, nonspecific reactions producing indeterminate results in uninfected persons have occurred more frequently in pregnant women or mothers than in persons in other groups characterized by low HIV seroprevalence. The incidence of indeterminate WB results is relatively low. Indeterminant WB results need to be followed up with HIV-1 NAAT testing. If HIV-1 NAAT testing is positive, a patient is suffering from acute HIV-1 infection. If HIV-1 NAAT testing is negative, the patient is considered to be negative for HIV-1, but a primary care provider may consider HIV-2 testing if clinically indicated.

The most important factor in evaluating indeterminate results is risk assessment. Patients in low-risk categories with indeterminate test results are almost never infected with HIV-1 or HIV-2. Repeat testing usually continues to show indeterminate results, and the cause of this pattern is seldom established. Follow-up serology testing at 3 months is recommended to verify the previous results. Patients with indeterminate test results who are in the process of seroconversion usually have positive WB test results within 1 month; repeat tests at 1, 2, and 6 months are generally advocated, with appropriate precautions to prevent viral transmission in the interim.

False-positive WB results, especially those with a majority of bands, are extremely uncommon.

Quantitative RNA Assay
Recently the US Food and Drug Administration (FDA) approved a quantitative RNA assay for the confirmation of HIV infection.

Fourth-Generation Testing
Previously most tests used in the diagnostic setting detected only HIV antibodies. Fourth-generation assays detect HIV-1 p24 antigen up to 20 days earlier than WB and 5 to 7 days earlier than third-generation EIAs. Levels of p24 antigen increase early after initial infection. More specific or supplemental tests for HIV-1 and HIV-2 (e.g., NAAT, WB, or immunofluorescence) must be performed to verify the presence of HIV-1 p24 antigen or antibodies to HIV-1 or HIV-2.

Fourth-generation assays allow for the differentiation between acute infection (p24 only, no HIV-1 antibody) and established infections (both p24 antigen and HIV-1 antibody). The gold standard for acute infection screening is NAAT. HIV-1 RNA can identify HIV infection as early as 5 days after exposure.

In 2010 the FDA approved the first fourth-generation immunoassay that detects both antigen and antibodies to HIV (ARCHITECT HIV Ag/Ab Combo Assay, Abbott Laboratories, Abbott Park, Illinois). This test is a chemiluminescent microparticle immunoassay. The ARCHITECT HIV Ag/Ab Combo Assay was the first diagnostic test approved by the FDA for use in children as young as 2 years of age and pregnant women.

Other fourth-generation assays (e.g., GS HIV Combo Ag/Ab EIA, Bio-Rad Laboratories, Hercules, California) use EIA methodology (see the procedure later in this chapter). These methods simultaneously test for HIV p24 antigen and antibodies to HIV-1 (groups M and O) and HIV-2 in human serum or plasma.

Pediatric Testing
Infants born to mothers who are HIV positive need to be screened for HIV. Two testing protocols can be used:
Protocol 1: Use a qualitative PCR HIV-1 assay. Do not use cord blood. If negative or indeterminate, repeat the assay at 1 to 2 months and 3 to 6 months of age.
Protocol 2: Use a quantitative PCR HIV-1 assay. This is a more sensitive assay. Do not use cord blood. If negative or indeterminate, repeat the assay at 1 to 2 months and 3 to 6 months of age.

Rapid Testing
Routine HIV testing of whole blood in the emergency department has been shown to find unidentified cases. Currently confirmation of rapid point-of-care testing (POCT), if positive, should reflex to a fourth-generation antigen–antibody test (HIV-1, HIV-2). A disadvantage of rapid tests includes lower sensitivity than third- and fourth-generation EIAs. The sensitivity of the currently available rapid tests is similar to that of second-generation EIAs.

Many rapid POCT assays have FDA approval. Approved rapid assays differ in HIV specificity and methodology (Box 19.8). Currently approved assays include:
- Alere Determine HIV-1/2 Ag/Ab Combo
- Clearview Complete HIV 1/2
- HIV 1/2 STAT-PAK
- INSTI HIV-1/HIV-2
- Multispot HIV-1/HIV-2
- OraQuick ADVANCE Rapid HIV-1/2 Antibody Test
- Reveal G3 Rapid HIV-1 Antibody Testing Procedure
- Unigold Recombigen

Tests for Therapeutic Monitoring
Viral Load Testing
Testing of the viral load should be performed as soon as the patient treatment begins. Subsequent viral load testing can be used as a marker for HIV viremia and should be carried out every 3 to 6 months for patients undergoing treatment. New guidelines recommend viral load testing every 2 to 8 weeks after the initiation of HAART to determine early response to therapy. Fully automated assays have a fast turnaround time. Fully automated assays and real-time PCR are noted to have a lower rate of false-negative results compared with nucleic acid sequence-based amplification.

CD4+ T-Lymphocyte Testing
Monitoring of CD4+ T lymphocytes measures immune function. This information guides the initiation of antiretroviral therapy (ART) and monitors a patient's response to ART. CD4+ T-lymphocyte counts are expressed as absolute counts or as a percentage of the total population of CD4 to CD8 as a ratio. Flow cytometry, in conjunction with fluorescence-activated cell sorting (FACS; see Chapter 11) (Fig. 19.11) is considered the gold standard in CD4+ T-lymphocyte counting.

PREVENTION
Reducing Viral Transmission
WHO estimates that 1.2 million people in the United States are living with HIV infection. One in five (20%) of those people are unaware of their infection. Approximately 50,000 Americans become infected with HIV each year. The CDC has issued new testing recommendations, making HIV screening a routine part of medical care for all patients from 13 to 64 years of age. CDC officials hope that these revised guidelines will increase early HIV diagnosis so that individuals can access treatment, know their healthcare status, and prevent transmission to others.

Healthcare personnel should assume that the blood and other body fluids from all patients are potentially infectious (i.e., use Standard Precautions; see Chapter 5).

Vaccines
The development of an effective HIV vaccine is anticipated within the next decade. Limited success has been achieved with vaccines in clinical trials. Vaccines are discussed more fully in Chapter 27.

TREATMENT
Despite declines in morbidity and mortality with combination ART, its effectiveness is limited by adverse events, problems with patient

BOX 19.8 US Food and Drug Administration (FDA)–Approved Rapid Point-of-Care HIV Assays

Alere Determine HIV-1/2 Ag/Ab Combo
This assay is a qualitative immunoassay for the simultaneous detection of HIV-1 p24 antigen (Ag) and antibodies (Ab) to HIV-1 and HIV-2. It may distinguish acute HIV-1 infection from established HIV-1 infection when the specimen is positive for HIV-1 p24 antigen and negative for anti–HIV-1 and anti–HIV-2 antibodies. The assay is not intended for newborn screening or for use with cord blood specimens, specimens from individuals younger than 12 years of age, or for screening purposes.

Clearview Complete HIV 1/2
This assay uses a unique combination of a specific antibody-binding protein, which is conjugated to colloidal gold dye particles, and HIV-1/2 antigens, which are bound to the solid-phase membrane. The buffer facilitates the lateral flow of the specimen and test reagents and promotes the binding of the antibodies to the antigen. The specimen/buffer mixture migrates along the test strip by capillary action, reconstituting the conjugate. If present, the antibodies bind to the colloidal gold–conjugated antibody-binding protein. In a reactive sample, the dye conjugated–immune complex migrates on the nitrocellulose membrane and is captured by the antigens immobilized in the test area, producing a pink/purple line.

HIV-1/2 STAT-PAK
This assay uses a unique combination of a specific antibody-binding protein, which is conjugated to colloidal gold dye particles, and HIV-1/2 antigens, which are bound to the solid-phase membrane. A lateral flow of the specimen and test reagents promotes the binding of the antibodies to the antigen. If present, the antibodies bind to the colloidal gold–conjugated antibody-binding protein. In a reactive sample, the dye conjugated–immune complex migrates on the nitrocellulose membrane and is captured by the antigens immobilized in the test platform.

INSTI HIV-1/HIV-2
The anti–HIV-1 IgM enzyme-linked immunosorbent assay (ELISA) determines gp41 recombinant protein affinity to IgM. The antigen is spotted onto nitrocellulose (NC) membranes. Seroconversion panel samples with different levels of HIV IgM antibody are used as primary antibodies. Mouse monoclonal antihuman IgM, horseradish peroxidase–labeled rabbit polyclonal anti-mouse IgG, and chemiluminescence reagent are used as a secondary antibody, conjugate antibody, and a developer reagent, respectively.

Multispot HIV-1/HIV-2
This assay is based on the principle of immunoconcentration. The Multispot HIV-1/HIV-2 Cartridge contains a removable specimen prefilter, the reaction membrane, and an absorbent pad. All of the liquids added to the cartridge are absorbed by the pad and contained within the cartridge.

Microscopic particles are separately coated with the antigens that represent portions of the transmembrane proteins HIV-1 and HIV-2, respectively. The microparticles are immobilized on the reaction membrane of the cartridge and form the test spots. If antibodies against HIV-1 and/or HIV-2 are present in the specimen, they bind to the antigens on the microparticles in the specific spots on the cartridge membrane. The conjugate, which contains alkaline phosphatase–labeled goat antihuman IgG (H + L chain specific), is then added to the cartridge. The conjugate binds to the human antibody–antigen complexes that are immobilized in the spots on the cartridge membrane. After a development reagent is added to the cartridge, a purple color develops on the test platform in proportion to the amount of antibodies against HIV-1 and/or HIV-2 that have been bound to the antigen-coated microparticles and been detected by the conjugate.

OraQuick ADVANCE Rapid HIV-1/2 Antibody Test
This assay is a rapid test for the detection of HIV-1 and HIV-2 antibodies. The test uses protein A–colloidal gold, which allows for the visual detection of HIV antibodies, or second-generation enzyme immunoassay (EIA) so-called sandwich technology, with HIV-1 gp41 and HIV-2 gp36 synthetic antigen.

Reveal G3 Rapid HIV-1 Antibody Testing Procedure
This assay is composed of a single-use test cartridge containing an immunoreactive test membrane. The immunoreactive test membrane is composed of a combination of synthetic peptides corresponding to conserved regions of HIV structural proteins coated onto a membrane matrix, which functions to capture anti–HIV-1 antibodies present in human serum or plasma when a drop of the specimen is applied. Captured anti–HIV-1 antibodies are visualized through a reaction with the MedMira InstantGold Cap (which contains a proprietary protein A–colloidal gold conjugate). A reactive test result occurs only when the protein A portion of the conjugate binds to the captured antibodies, producing a distinctive red dot in the test zone.

Unigold Recombigen
This is a rapid immunoassay based on the immunochromatographic sandwich principle and is intended to detect antibodies to HIV-1. The test uses genetically engineered recombinant proteins representing the immunodominant regions of the envelope proteins of HIV-1. The recombinant proteins are immobilized at the test region of the nitrocellulose strip. These proteins are also linked to colloidal gold and impregnated below the test region of the device. If antibodies to HIV-1 are present in the sample, they combine with an HIV-1 antigen/colloidal gold reagent, and this complex binds to the immobilized antigens in the test region of the device, forming a visible pink/red band.

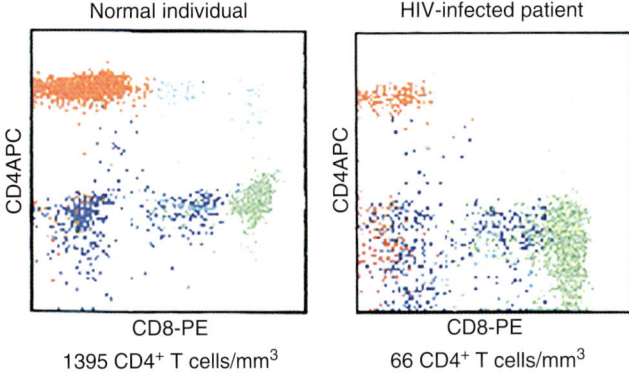

Fig. 19.11 Flow Cytometry. (From Abbas AK, Lichtman AH: *Basic immunology: functions and disorders of the immune system*, updated edition, ed 3, Philadelphia, 2011, Saunders.)

adherence, and resistance of HIV. Episodic ART, guided by the CD4+ T-lymphocyte count, significantly increases the risk of opportunistic disease or death from any cause compared with continuous ART as a consequence of lowering the CD4+ T-lymphocyte cell count and increasing the viral load. However, episodic ART does not reduce the risk of adverse events associated with ART.

Drug Therapy
Before therapy is started, the initial characteristics of a patient need to be evaluated. These characteristics include:
- Pretreatment HIV RNA level (viral load)
- Pretreatment CD4+ cell count
- HIV genotypic drug-resistance testing results
- HLA-B*5701 status

The National Institute of Allergy and Infectious Diseases endorses the initiation of ART in HIV-positive adults with a CD4+ T-lymphocyte count of more than 500 cells/mm³. This provided net benefits over starting such therapy in patients after the CD4+ T-lymphocyte count had declined to 350 cells/mm³.

Patients receiving immediate therapy were more than 70% less likely to develop an AIDS-related illness and 40% less likely to develop a severe non–AIDS-related illness, such as myocardial infarction.

More than 25 antiretroviral drugs in different mechanistic classes are FDA approved for the treatment of HIV infection (Fig. 19.12 and Table 19.14). These classes include:

- Nucleoside/nucleotide reverse transcriptase inhibitors (NRTIs)
- Nonnucleoside reverse transcriptase inhibitors (NNRTIs)
- Protease inhibitors (PIs)
- A fusion inhibitor (FI)
- A CCR5 antagonist (entry inhibitor)
- Integrase strand transfer inhibitors (INSTIs)

In addition, a pharmacokinetic enhancer or booster (CYP3A inhibitor) is used solely to improve the pharmacokinetic profiles of some drugs included in an HIV regimen. One FDA-approved drug in this category was approved in 2014. The FDA-approved use of a pharmacokinetic as an enhancer of atazanavir or darunavir in combination with other antiretroviral agents in the treatment of HIV-1 infection.

An initial antiretroviral regimen for a treatment-naïve patient generally consists of two NRTIs such as abacavir plus lamivudine or tenofovir disoproxil fumarate plus emtricitabine, plus a drug from one of three drug classes: INSTIs, NNRTIs, or a PI with a pharmacokinetic. This strategy for initial treatment has resulted in HIV RNA decreases and CD4+ T-lymphocyte cell increases in most patients.

Multiclass combination drugs are composed of components of two or more antiretroviral drugs from one or more drug classes.

Actions of Mechanistic Classes of Antiretroviral Drugs
Nucleoside Reverse Transcriptase Inhibitors

NRTIs act as HIV entry inhibitors, and these drugs block HIV's ability to infect healthy CD4+ cells. NRTIs block an enzyme of HIV, reverse transcriptase, that allows HIV to infect human cells, particularly CD4+ cells or T lymphocytes. Reverse transcriptase converts HIV genetic material, which is RNA, into human genetic material, which is DNA. The humanlike DNA of HIV then becomes part of the infected person's own cells, allowing the cell to produce RNA copies of the HIV that can then go on to infect healthy cells. Blocking reverse transcriptase prevents HIV from infecting human cells.

The original NRTI was zidovudine (AZT), approved in 1987. Zidovudine competes with one of the available DNA building blocks called *deoxythymidine 5′-triphosphate*. By replacing deoxythymidine 5′-triphosphate in the newly developing HIV DNA, zidovudine is able to stop reverse transcriptase from completing its job. This prevents the HIV DNA strand from being formed and halts the HIV life cycle.

Since zidovudine was approved, additional NRTIs have been approved. In 2001 the first nucleotide analog, tenofovir, was approved for HIV treatment. It blocks HIV replication in a manner similar to that of the nucleoside analogs. NRTIs are potent in combination with other drugs. If used alone, however, resistance to HIV will develop. Some of the drugs in this class can penetrate the blood–brain barrier.

A newer, recently approved drug, etravirine (ETR), was developed specifically to be an option for patients who have developed resistance to the earlier drugs in the class. Typically, two NRTIs and ETR are primarily being used as part of the regimens for patients with a history of different types of treatment to which they have developed resistance.

Nonnucleoside Reverse Transcriptase Inhibitors

Like NRTIs, NNRTIs block the reverse transcriptase enzyme, preventing uninfected cells from becoming infected. NNRTIs such as efavirenz and nevirapine target a key viral enzyme, reverse transcriptase, inhibiting its function by binding to a pocket near the enzyme's catalytic site. This disrupts one of the early steps in the HIV life cycle, called *reverse transcription*. However, NNRTI resistance can develop when HIV acquires one or more mutations that alter the binding pocket.

During normal reverse transcription, HIV's reverse transcriptase enzyme converts HIV's RNA into DNA. It does this by recoding the RNA building blocks into complementary DNA building blocks. As the HIV life cycle proceeds, the newly formed DNA is used to make more copies of HIV virus.

NNRTIs may interact with other cytochrome P-450–processed drugs (e.g., PIs). NNRTIs have a mixed ability to penetrate the blood–brain barrier.

Protease Inhibitors

Protease inhibitors (PIs) block the action of an HIV enzyme, protease, a protein that HIV requires to make more copies of itself within HIV-infected human cells. Thus blocking protease prevents HIV in already-infected cells from producing HIV that can infect other healthy cells.

The first drugs in this class for the treatment of HIV were approved in 1996. PIs are very potent and may interact with other drugs using cytochrome P-450 metabolic pathways, but poor drug absorption may affect potency.

Fusion Inhibitors

Currently there is only one drug, enfuvirtide (T-20), in this class. T-20, approved in 2003, blocks HIV from entering the CD4+ cells of the immune system. The drug T-20 is an example of an FI that blocks a different event rather than entry inhibition in viral invasion. An FI blocks the fusion of HIV with the host cell membrane.

Entry Inhibitors (CCR5 Antagonist)

The CCR5 antagonist, approved in 2007, is in a newer class of drugs and is the first to actually target the cell. Entry inhibitors block proteins on the CD4+ cells that HIV requires to enter the cells.

This approach involves preventing HIV from invading the human cells in which it replicates, a concept termed *entry inhibition*. To gain entry into host cells, HIV binds to the cell's CD4 receptor in tandem with a coreceptor, usually CXCR5 or CXCR4. This process allows HIV to fuse with the cell membrane and inject its genes inside the cell. Patients with certain mutations in CCR5 are resistant to HIV infection, so drugs that block this receptor might prevent the virus from invading cells.

Integrase Strand Transfer Inhibitors

The INSTI class of drugs blocks the enzyme integrase, which is required by HIV to manufacture more HIV. The drugs in this class prevent HIV DNA from entering human DNA.

The first available drug in this class was FDA approved in 2007. It represented a new drug in a new class that appeared to be very potent at suppressing HIV in all patients who have never been on this drug or other integrase inhibitors.

It was initially approved for treatment-experienced patients with drug-resistant virus. It is also now approved for those starting therapy for the first time.

When used with other anti-HIV medicines, a drug in this class may have two functions:

- To reduce the amount of HIV in the blood (the viral load)
- To increase the number of white blood cells called CD4+ (T) cells

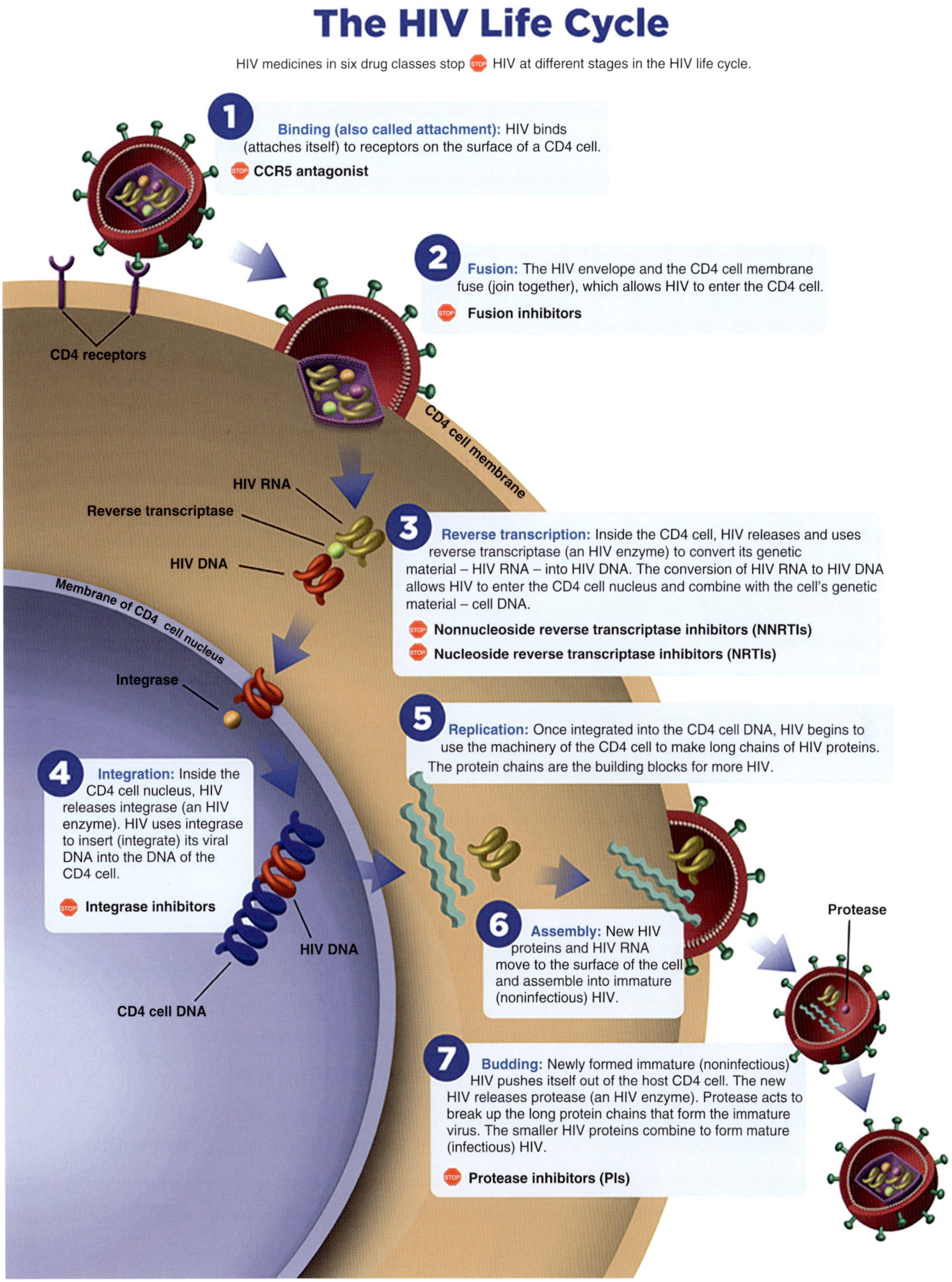

CHAPTER 19 Primary and Acquired Immunodeficiency Syndromes

The HIV Life Cycle

HIV medicines in six drug classes stop 🛑 HIV at different stages in the HIV life cycle.

1 **Binding (also called attachment):** HIV binds (attaches itself) to receptors on the surface of a CD4 cell.
🛑 **CCR5 antagonist**

2 **Fusion:** The HIV envelope and the CD4 cell membrane fuse (join together), which allows HIV to enter the CD4 cell.
🛑 **Fusion inhibitors**

CD4 receptors

CD4 cell membrane

HIV RNA
Reverse transcriptase
HIV DNA

3 **Reverse transcription:** Inside the CD4 cell, HIV releases and uses reverse transcriptase (an HIV enzyme) to convert its genetic material – HIV RNA – into HIV DNA. The conversion of HIV RNA to HIV DNA allows HIV to enter the CD4 cell nucleus and combine with the cell's genetic material – cell DNA.
🛑 **Nonnucleoside reverse transcriptase inhibitors (NNRTIs)**
🛑 **Nucleoside reverse transcriptase inhibitors (NRTIs)**

Membrane of CD4 cell nucleus

Integrase

4 **Integration:** Inside the CD4 cell nucleus, HIV releases integrase (an HIV enzyme). HIV uses integrase to insert (integrate) its viral DNA into the DNA of the CD4 cell.
🛑 **Integrase inhibitors**

HIV DNA
CD4 cell DNA

5 **Replication:** Once integrated into the CD4 cell DNA, HIV begins to use the machinery of the CD4 cell to make long chains of HIV proteins. The protein chains are the building blocks for more HIV.

6 **Assembly:** New HIV proteins and HIV RNA move to the surface of the cell and assemble into immature (noninfectious) HIV.

Protease

7 **Budding:** Newly formed immature (noninfectious) HIV pushes itself out of the host CD4 cell. The new HIV releases protease (an HIV enzyme). Protease acts to break up the long protein chains that form the immature virus. The smaller HIV proteins combine to form mature (infectious) HIV.
🛑 **Protease inhibitors (PIs)**

Fig. 19.12 Steps in the HIV Replication Cycle. The seven stages of the HIV life cycle are (1) binding, (2) fusion, (3) reverse transcription, (4) integration, (5) replication, (6) assembly, and (7) budding. (Courtesy National Institute of Allergy and Infectious Diseases, National Institutes of Health, Bethesda, MD.)

TABLE 19.14 US Food and Drug Administration–Approved HIV Medicines (last reviewed March 23, 2023)

Generic Name (Other Names and Acronyms)	Brand Name	FDA Approval Date
Nucleoside Reverse Transcriptase Inhibitors (NRTIs)		
NRTIs block reverse transcriptase, an enzyme HIV needs to make copies of itself		
Abacavir (abacavir sulfate, ABC)	Ziagen	December 17, 1998
Emtricitabine (FTC)	Emtriva	July 2, 2003
Lamivudine (3TC)	Epivir	November 17, 1995
Tenofovir disoproxil fumarate (tenofovir DF, TDF)	Viread	October 26, 2001
Zidovudine (azidothymidine, AZT, ZDV)	Retrovir	March 19, 1987
Nonnucleoside Reverse Transcriptase Inhibitors (NNRTIs)		
NNRTIs bind to and later alter reverse transcriptase, an enzyme HIV needs to make copies of itself.		
Doravirine	Pifeltro	August 30, 2018
Efavirenz (EFV)	Sustiva	September 17, 1998
Etravirine (ETR)	Intelence	January 18, 2008
Nevirapine (extended release nevirapine, NVP)	Viramune	June 21, 1996
	Viramune XR (extended release)	March 25, 2011
Rilpivirine (rilpivirine hydrochloride, RPV)	Edurant	May 20, 2011
Protease Inhibitors (PIs)		
PIs block HIV protease, an enzyme HIV needs to make copies of itself.		
Atazanavir (atazanavir sulfate, ATV)	Reyataz	June 20, 2003
Darunavir (darunavir ethanolate, DRV)	Prezista	June 23, 2006
Fosamprenavir (fosamprenavir calcium, FOS-APV, FPV)	Lexiva	October 20, 2003
Ritonavir (RTV)	Norvir	March 1, 1996
Tipranavir (TPV)	Aptivus	June 22, 2005
Fusion Inhibitors		
Fusion inhibitors block HIV from entering the CD4 T lymphocyte (CD4 cells) of the immune system		
Enfuvirtide (T-20)	Fuzeon	March 13, 2003
CCR5 Antagonists		
CCR5 antagonists block CCR5 coreceptors on the surface of certain immune cells that HIV needs to enter the cells.		
Maraviroc (MVC)	Selzentry	August 6, 2007
Integrase Strand Transfer Inhibitors (INSTIs)		
Integrase inhibitors block HIV integrase, an enzyme HIV needs to make copies of itself.		
Cabotegravir	Vocabria	January 22, 2021
Dolutegravir (DTG)	Tivicay	August 13, 2013
Raltegravir (raltegravir potassium, RAL)	Isentress	October 12, 2007
Attachment Inhibitors		
Attachment inhibitors bind to the gp120 protein on the outer surface of HIV, preventing HIV from entering CD4 cells.		
Fostemsavir	Rukobia	July 2, 2020
Post-Attachment Inhibitors		
Post-attachment inhibitors block CD4 receptors on the surface of certain immune cells that HIV needs to enter the cells.		
Ibalizumab-Uiyk	Trogarzo	March 6, 2018
Capsid Inhibitors		
Capsid inhibitors interfere with the HIV capsid, a protein shell that protects HIV's genetic material and enzymes needed for replication.		
Lenacapavir	Sunlenca	December 22, 2022
Pharmacokinetic Enhancers		
Cobicistat (COBI)	Tybost	September 24, 2014
Combination HIV Medicines		
Combination HIV medicines contain two or more HIV medicines from one or more drug classes.		
Abacavir and lamivudine	Epzicom	August 2, 2004
Abacavir, dolutegravir, and lamivudine	Triumeq	August 22, 2014
Abacavir, lamivudine, and zidovudine	Trizivir	November 14, 2000

TABLE 19.14 US Food and Drug Administration–Approved HIV Medicines (last reviewed March 23, 2023)—cont'd

Generic Name (Other Names and Acronyms)	Brand Name	FDA Approval Date
Atazanavir and cobicistat (atazanavir sulfate/cobicistat, ATV/COBI)	Evotaz	January 29, 2015
Bictegravir, emtricitabine, and tenofovir alafenamide	Biktarvy	February 7, 2018
Carbotegradevir and rilpivirine	Carbenuva	January 22, 2021
Darunavir and cobicistat	Prezcobix	January 29, 2015
Darunavir, cobicistatk, emtricitabine, and tenofovir tenoalafinide	Symtuza	July 17, 2018
Dolutegravir and lamivudine	Dovato	April 8, 2019
Dolutegravir and rilpiviridine	Juluca	November 21, 2017
Doravirine, lamivudine, and tenofovir disoproxil fumarate	Delstrigo	August 30, 2018
Efavirenz, emtricitabine, and tenofovir disoproxil fumarate	Atripla	July 12, 2006
Efavirenz, lamivudine, and tenofovir disoproxil fumarate	Simifi Lo	February 5, 2018
Elvitegravir, cobicistat, emtricitabine, and tenofovir alafenamide fumarate	Genvoya	November 5, 2015
Elvitegravir, cobicistat, emtricitabine, and tenofovir disoproxil fumarate	Stribild	August 27, 2012
Emtricitabine, rilpivirine, and tenofovir disoproxil fumarate	Complera	August 10, 2011
Emtricitabine, rilpivirine, and tenofovir alafenamide	Odefsey	March 1, 2016
Emtricitabine and tenofovir alafenamide	Descovy	April 4, 2016
Emtricitabine and tenofovir disoproxil fumarate	Truvada	August 2, 2004
Lamivudine and zidovudine	Combivir	September 27, 1997
Lamivudine and tenofovir disoproxil fumarate	Cimduo	February 28, 2018
Lopinavir and ritonavir	Kaletra	September 15, 2000

From https://fda.gov.

Investigational Drugs

An investigational drug is one that is under study and has not yet been approved by the FDA for sale in the United States. Medical research studies are required to evaluate the safety and effectiveness of an investigational drug. These research studies can be referred to as *clinical trials*.

New drugs are needed because resistant mutations that protect HIV against existing classes of antiretroviral drugs would be unlikely also to confer resistance to novel agents. Drug discovery and FDA approval currently take an average of 12 to 15 years, and it costs about $400 million for a drug to go from the research laboratory to a pharmacy in the United States.

Once an investigational drug has been proven safe and effective in clinical trials, the FDA may approve the drug for sale in the United States. Before FDA approval, clinical trials are conducted in three phases. Each phase has a different purpose and helps researchers answer different questions.

Phase I trials take about 1 year and include 20 to 80 healthy volunteers for the first time. The purpose is to evaluate the drug's safety and efficacy and to identify side effects.

Phase II trials last about 2 years and expand the number of volunteers to 100 to 300 persons with the disease to assess the effectiveness of a drug, to observe for adverse side reactions, and to further evaluate the drug's safety.

Phase III of a clinical trial lasts about 3 years and expands the number of patients with a specific disease to 1000 to 3000 to confirm its effectiveness, monitor side effects, compare it with standard or equivalent treatments, and collect information that will allow the investigational drug to be used safely.

Since the FDA Regulatory Modernization Act of 1997, the FDA review process has been streamlined to hasten approval of new therapies to treat severe diseases. Phases I and II have been allowed to be combined to shorten the approval process. It now takes about 18 months for a drug to go through the review process for approval by the FDA.

Some drugs go through the FDA's accelerated approval process and are approved before a Phase III clinical trial is complete. After a drug is approved by the FDA and made available to the public, researchers track its safety in Phase IV trials to seek more information about the drug's risks, benefits, and optimal use.

It is a long and expensive road to achieving an FDA-approved drug. Only about one in five medicines that enters a clinical trial is ultimately approved. Some drugs are withdrawn by the research company at various stages of development for various reasons.

HIV Drug Resistance

Antiviral drug resistance is defined as the reduction in the susceptibility of mutated viruses to specific antiviral drugs. The origins of drug resistance are diverse, but drug resistance is associated with the high mutation rate in the HIV genome, which is one of the key biological characteristics of the virus. Genomic mutation is determined by the following:

- The number of mistakes per genome per replication cycle. This is extremely high in HIV because reverse transcriptase has no so-called proofreading ability.
- The number of viral replication cycles per unit of time. This is reflected in an infected patient's viral load.

The relationship between resistance mutations and response to therapy is complex. Each resistance mutation is characterized by the level of associated phenotypic resistance and the specificity of the resistance mutation to one or more drugs.

A patient's response to therapy depends on a number of factors, including patient compliance, percentage of resistant virus population, dosing, and drug pharmacology issues. Genotypic or phenotypic assays can be used to assess HIV drug resistance.

Standard genotypic drug-resistance testing in antiretroviral-naïve persons involves testing for mutations in the RT and PR genes. Genotypic assays use sequenced regions of the *pol* gene of the HIV genome, the target site of most antiretroviral drugs. Enzymes coded for in those regions—reverse transcriptase, protease, and integrase—are key to HIV replication. Mutation in these regions can produce enzymes that are not susceptible to antiretroviral drug inhibition.

> **BOX 19.9 Preexposure and Postexposure HIV Prophylaxis**
>
> **Preexposure Prophylaxis (PrEP)**
> 1. PrEP is a new HIV prevention method in which people who do not have HIV infection take a pill daily to reduce their risk of becoming infected.
> 2. Only people who are HIV negative should use PrEP. An HIV test is required before starting PrEP and then every 3 months while taking PrEP.
> 3. PrEP can only be prescribed by a healthcare provider and must be taken as directed to be effective.
>
> **Postexposure Prophylaxis (PEP)**
> Step 1. PEP involves taking anti-HIV drugs as soon as possible after being exposed.
> Step 2. To be effective, PEP must begin within 72 hours after exposure, before the virus has time to rapidly replicate in the body.
> Step 3. PEP consists of two or three antiretroviral medications taken for 28 days.

From US Department of Health and Human Services (;AIDS.gov. https://aids.gov).

Genotypic and phenotypic resistance assays are used to assist selection of treatment strategies. Standard assays provide information on resistance to NRTIs, NNRTIs, and PIs. Although transmission of INSTI-resistant virus has rarely been reported, as the use of INSTIs increases, the potential for transmission of INSTI-resistant virus may also increase. When INSTI resistance is suspected, primary care providers can supplement standard baseline genotypic resistance testing with genotypic testing for resistance to this class of drugs.

Computer algorithms are now able to compare genotypic data from native HIV-1 RNA with a large database of corresponding phenotypes and genotypes to generate a virtual phenotype. A virtual phenotype offers the advantage of producing output that incorporates clinical cutoffs based on viral responses for the 14 most common forms of combination ART.

Resistance testing is necessary to determine the efficacy of drugs that act by blocking HIV entry through coreceptor activation. Tropism or coreceptor testing, like resistance testing, can be done by genotype and phenotype testing. Phenotypic testing requires amplification of the *env* sequence and the creation of viral pseudotypes. After viral material is inoculated onto CD4-, CCR5-, and CXCR4-expressing T cells, gene activity is monitored. The oldest genotypic tropism assay interrogates the coding region of the gp160 HIV-1 envelope protein and is 100% sensitive for detecting certain variants. Charges on amino acids are sought for classification. Currently phenotype testing is preferred in the United States.

PREEXPOSURE AND POSTEXPOSURE PROPHYLAXIS

Preexposure Prophylaxis

Preexposure prophylaxis (PrEP) (Box 19.9) is a newly approved method to prevent or control the spread of HIV infection. This method is for patients who are HIV negative but are at high risk of contracting an infection due to sexual practices or injection drug use. The daily medication is a pill that contains two antiretroviral drugs: tenofovir and emtricitabine. These medicines can work to keep the virus from taking hold in the body.

The CDC recommends that PrEP be considered for patients who are HIV negative and at substantial risk for HIV infection. This includes anyone who:

- Is in an ongoing relationship with an HIV-infected partner
- Is not in a *mutually monogamous* relationship with a partner who recently tested HIV negative and is a gay or bisexual man who has had sex without a condom or been diagnosed with a sexually transmitted infection within the past 6 months
- Is a heterosexual man or woman who does not regularly use condoms when having sex with partners known to be at risk for HIV (e.g., injection drug users or bisexual male partners of unknown HIV status)
- Has, within the past 6 months, injected illicit drugs and shared equipment or been in a treatment program for injection drug use

For heterosexual couples of whom one partner has HIV and the other does not, PrEP is one of several options to protect the uninfected partner during conception and pregnancy.

Patients who use PrEP must be able to take the drug every day and to return to their healthcare provider every 3 months for repeat HIV testing, prescription refills, and follow-up. PrEP is a powerful HIV prevention tool, but no prevention strategy is 100% effective.

Postexposure Prophylaxis

If healthcare workers are potentially exposed to HIV occupationally, postexposure prophylaxis (PEP) is needed. PEP is used for anyone who may have been exposed to HIV during a single high-risk event. The risk of getting HIV infection in these ways is extremely low–less than 1 in 100 for all exposures.

Healthcare workers are evaluated for PEP if they are exposed after:
- Getting cut or stuck with a needle that was used to draw blood from a person who may have HIV infection
- Getting blood or other body fluids that may have lots of HIV in their eyes or mouth
- Getting blood or other body fluids that may have lots of HIV on their skin when it is chapped, scraped, or affected by certain rashes

PEP can also be used to treat people who may have been exposed to HIV during a single high-risk event unrelated to work (e.g., during episodes of unprotected sex, needle-sharing injection drug use, or sexual assault).

PEP is not intended for long-term use. It is not a substitute for regular use of other proven HIV prevention methods, such as PrEP, correct and consistent condom use, or use of sterile injection equipment. Because PEP is not 100% effective, continued use of condoms with sex partners while taking PEP is necessary, and patients should not share injection equipment with others.

If a person has repeated exposures, HIV PEP involves taking anti-HIV medications as soon as possible (within 3 days) after being exposed to HIV to try to reduce the chance of becoming HIV positive. PEP consists of two to three antiretroviral medications and must be taken for 28 days.

PEP is safe but may cause side effects (e.g., nausea) in some people. These side effects can be treated and are not life-threatening. PEP is not 100% effective; it does not guarantee that someone exposed to HIV will not become infected; prompt treatment can reduce the subsequent risk of HIV infection by more than 80%. Optimal treatment should begin within 1 to 2 hours after exposure.

CASE STUDY 19.1

Mary is a freshman in college. She began to feel ill with diarrhea and a cough. She tried to ignore the symptoms but woke up the next morning with a severe headache and a painful stiff neck. The patient has a history of *Neisseria meningitidis* serogroup Y. She had one sibling who suffered from a meningococcal meningitis 1 year ago.

Her primary care physician admitted her to the hospital for diagnosis and treatment. Mary was started on intravenous ceftriaxone, and a sterile spinal tap was performed.

Laboratory testing included a complete blood count (CBC), blood culture ×3, and spinal fluid cell count and culture. Subsequently, the spinal fluid cell count showed 25 white blood cells (WBCs)/μL with 85% polymorphonuclear leukocytes. The blood and spinal fluid cultures grew out *Neisseria meningitidis* serotype C.

Mary responded well to the ceftriaxone and her symptoms improved steadily over the next 72 hours. She was subsequently released from the hospital. Although Mary was treated with and responded well to ceftriaxone, she may need to start a steroid (e.g., dexamethasone) to assist in diminishing the inflammation brought about by bacterial cell death. An investigation to determine if Mary has any evidence of adrenal hemorrhage should be considered. She has a low platelet count that needs to be continually monitored.

Questions
1. Based on Mary's history, what kind of immunodeficiency do you expect?
   a. Innate immunodeficiency
   b. Adaptive immunodeficiency
   c. Secondary immunodeficiency
   d. Acquired immunodeficiency
2. Which laboratory assays would be most helpful in establishing a diagnosis?
   a. Total and absolute neutrophil count
   b. Immunoelectrophoresis and total protein assay
   c. CH50 and AH50 assays
   d. EBV and CMV viral titers

Answers to these questions can be found in Appendix A.

Critical Thinking Group Discussion Questions
1. What is the significance of Mary's history?
2. How would you expect this patient to respond to relevant vaccinations?

CASE STUDY 19.2

Mr. J.J. Smith, aged 68 years, had retired to Florida and was meeting with his new primary care provider for the first time. His medical history indicated that he had suffered from recurrent upper and lower respiratory and gastrointestinal infections throughout his life. As a child, he was frequently diagnosed with ear and throat infections, and had intermittent diarrhea. Subsequently, he had been hospitalized several times since childhood for pneumonia and gastrointestinal infections.

After a 1-week vacation in Arizona the previous year he was hospitalized with severe diarrhea and was diagnosed with a *Giardia lamblia* infection.

In his medical history, Mr. Smith stated that he received a yearly flu vaccination and had received two different types of pneumococcal vaccinations. Because of his history of childhood and recent infectious diseases and his past vaccinations, Mr. Smith's physician ordered titers to investigate his pneumococcal vaccination antibody status.

Mr. Smith's physical examination revealed an enlarged spleen (splenomegaly).

Laboratory Data
CBC Results
RBC—4.8×10^6/μL
WBC—4500/μL
Segs—56%
Bands—4%
Lymphs—31%
Monos—8%
Eos—1%
Basos—0%
PLT—149×10^3/μL
Hg—11.8g/dL
Antibodies to pneumococcal vaccine—negative

Questions
1. Based on Mr. Smith's laboratory results, there should be a suspicion of:
   a. Malnutrition
   b. Malignancy
   c. Primary immunodeficiency
   d. Secondary immunodeficiency
2. Based on Mr. Smith's lack of pneumococcal antibodies after vaccination, the next applicable laboratory assay to order would be:
   a. Metabolic panel
   b. Bence Jones protein
   c. Serum protein electrophoresis
   d. Sweat chloride

Answers to these questions can be found in Appendix A.

Critical Thinking Group Discussion Questions
1. What are some of the common disorders affecting lymphocytes and the adaptive immune response (present clinically with increased susceptibility to infections in early life)?
2. Based on Mr. Smith's lack of a pneumococcal antibody response to vaccination, what is the most probable cause of his failure to respond?

CASE STUDY 19.3

History and Physical Examination

A 40-year-old man with a history of intravenous drug use came to the emergency department because of a rash and fever. In addition the patient complained of a several-day history of malaise, fatigue, fever, headache, and a sore throat.

Physical examination revealed a moderately ill–appearing man with a temperature of 38.8°C (102°F). He had a blanching, erythematous maculopapular rash over the trunk, back, and upper and lower extremities. In addition his throat showed enlarged tonsils and broad-based ulcerations on the buccal mucosa.

He had a history of an episode of endocarditis 2 years ago. At that time, an HIV serology test was performed. It was negative.

Laboratory Data

A complete blood count (CBC) and liver function tests were ordered. The results showed that the patient was anemic (hematocrit, 38%). He also had a severely decreased total leukocyte count and a severely decreased absolute lymphocyte count. Some of his liver function test results were abnormal.

Questions

1. If acute EBV or HIV is suggested clinically, a difference between the two would be that the HIV patient would have _____.
   a. Atypical lymphocytes present on a peripheral blood film
   b. Atypical lymphocytes absent on a peripheral blood film
   c. Absence of mucosal ulcerations
   d. A positive screening test for infectious mononucleosis
2. The WB assay can recognize ___ major HIV proteins.
   a. p24
   b. gp41
   c. gp120/160
   d. All of the above

Answers to these questions can be found in Appendix A.

Critical Thinking Group Discussion Questions

1. What is a likely diagnosis of this patient's condition?
2. What is the natural history of this disease?
3. What immunologic laboratory tests might be of value in establishing a diagnosis for this patient?

REVIEW QUESTIONS

1. Thymic hypoplasia is a(n):
   a. Congenital T-cell disorder
   b. Congenital B-cell disorder
   c. Acquired T-cell disorder
   d. Acquired B-cell disorder
2. AIDS is a(n):
   a. Congenital T-cell disorder
   b. Congenital B-cell disorder
   c. Acquired T-cell disorder
   d. Acquired B-cell disorder
3. Chronic lymphocytic leukemia is a(n):
   a. Congenital T-cell disorder
   b. Congenital B-cell disorder
   c. Acquired T-cell disorder
   d. Acquired B-cell disorder
4. Systemic lupus erythematosus is a(n):
   a. Congenital T-cell disorder
   b. Congenital B-cell disorder
   c. Acquired T-cell disorder
   d. Acquired B-cell disorder
5. Multiple myeloma is a(n):
   a. Congenital T-cell disorder
   b. Congenital B-cell disorder
   c. Acquired T-cell disorder
   d. Acquired B-cell disorder
6. Bruton agammaglobulinemia is a(n):
   a. Congenital T-cell disorder
   b. Congenital B-cell disorder
   c. Acquired T-cell disorder
   d. Acquired B-cell disorder
7. Most diseases associated with a primary defect are _____ disorders.
   a. T cell
   b. B cell
   c. Complement
   d. Phagocytic
8. Severe combined immunodeficiency is caused by:
   a. T-cell depletion
   b. B-cell depletion
   c. Inappropriate development of stem cells
   d. Phagocytic dysfunction
9. DiGeorge syndrome is caused by:
   a. Faulty embryogenesis
   b. Deficiency of calcium in utero
   c. Inappropriate stem cell development
   d. Autosomal-recessive disorder
10. The major clinical manifestation of a B-cell deficiency is:
    a. Impaired phagocytosis
    b. Diminished complement levels
    c. Increased susceptibility to respiratory infections
    d. Increased susceptibility to parasitic infections
11. Bruton agammaglobulinemia is a(n):
    a. Acquired disorder
    b. Autosomal genetic disorder
    c. Sex-linked genetic disorder
    d. Disorder occurring primarily in girls
12. Which of the following disorders does *not* result in a secondary immunodeficiency?
    a. Sickle cell disease
    b. Uremia
    c. AIDS
    d. Poison ivy hypersensitivity
13. In the initial evaluation of all suspected immunodeficiencies, an initial laboratory assessment of chronic infections in infants and children would be assessing:
    a. Antibody response to diphtheria-tetanus (DT) vaccination
    b. Erythrocyte sedimentation rate
    c. Absolute neutrophil count
    d. Total lymphocyte count

14. In the initial evaluation of an antibody immune deficiency, a quick laboratory procedure would be:
    a. Screening for anti-A and anti-B isoagglutinins
    b. Erythrocyte sedimentation rate
    c. Absolute neutrophil count
    d. Absolute lymphocyte count
15. In the initial evaluation of an adult with a suspected immunodeficiency, a quick laboratory procedure would be:
    a. Antibody response to vaccination
    b. Erythrocyte sedimentation rate (ESR) and complete blood count (CBC), including a platelet count
    c. Absolute neutrophil count
    d. Absolute lymphocyte count
16. In the initial evaluation of a phagocytic cell deficiency, an appropriate laboratory procedure would be:
    a. Antibody response to vaccination
    b. Erythrocyte sedimentation rate
    c. Absolute neutrophil count
    d. Absolute lymphocyte count
17. Calculate the absolute lymphocyte count when the following conditions exist:
    a. Total leukocyte count = 20×10^9/L
    b. Relative percentage of lymphocytes = 50%
    c. 5×10^9/L
    d. 10×10^9/L
    e. 15×10^9/L
    f. 20×10^9/L
18. A congenital B-cell disorder is:
    a. Chronic lymphocytic leukemia
    b. Bruton agammaglobulinemia
    c. Autoimmune disorder
    d. Leukocyte adhesions deficiency
19. An acquired B-cell disorder is:
    a. Chronic lymphocytic leukemia
    b. Bruton agammaglobulinemia
    c. Autoimmune disorder
    d. Leukocyte adhesions deficiency

20–23. Identify the distribution of immunodeficiencies shown in the illustration.

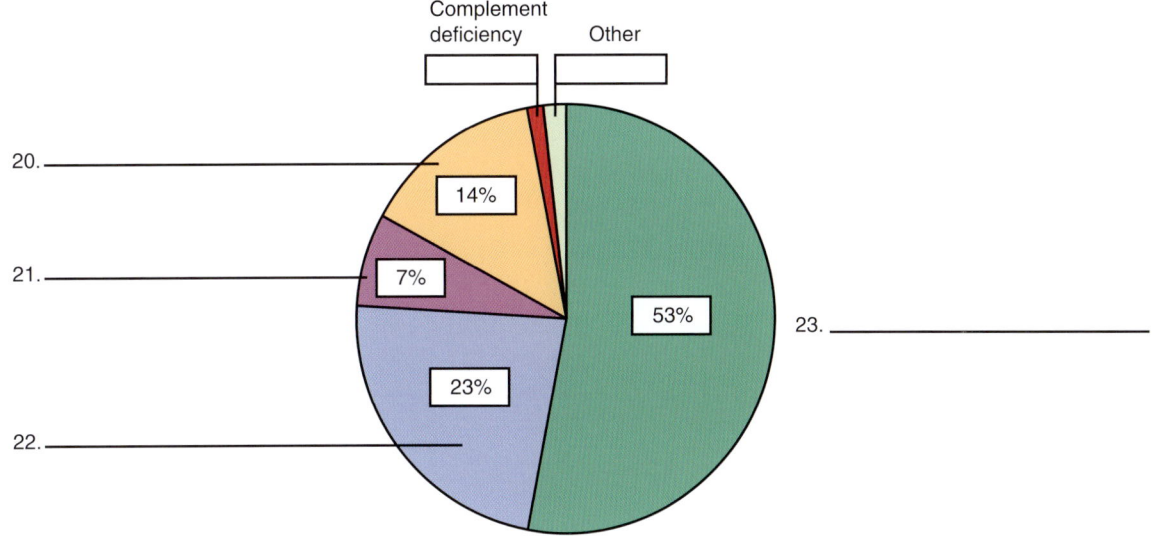

20. _____
21. _____
22. _____
23. _____
    a. T-cell disorder
    b. B-cell disorder
    c. Severe combined immunodeficiencies (SCIDs)
    d. Disorders of phagocytosis
24. A characteristic of a selective IgA deficiency is:
    a. Decreased allergic reactions
    b. Increased secretory component of IgA in saliva
    c. Increased incidence of autoimmune disease
    d. Decreased incidence of autoimmune disease
25. A characteristic of Bruton agammaglobulinemia is:
    a. Decreased presence of immunoglobulins
    b. Normal concentration of B lymphocytes
    c. Decreased risk of pyrogenic infections
    d. Increased resistance to bacterial infections
26. The most common humoral immune deficiency disorder is:
    a. DiGeorge syndrome
    b. Bruton agammaglobulinemia
    c. Selective IgA deficiency disorder
    d. Wiskott-Aldrich syndrome
27. One of the issues in the characterized triad of patients suffering from Wiscott-Aldrich syndrome include:
    a. Thrombocytopenic purpura
    b. Hemolytic anemia
    c. Vasculitis
    d. Thrombosis
28. A defect of C1q, C1r, C1s, C4, and C2 deficiency can be found in patients suffering from:
    a. Systemic lupus erythematosus (SLE)
    b. Infections and glomerulonephritis
    c. Atypical hemolytic-uremic syndrome
    d. Infections caused by neisserial species of bacteria

29. The major structural protein (core) of the human immunodeficiency virus type 1 (HIV-1) encoded by the *gag* gene is:
    a. gp41
    b. p24
    c. gp120
    d. Both a and c
30. The HIV infectious process begins when the protein on the viral envelope binds to the protein receptor _____ on the surface of a target cell:
    a. CD8
    b. CD4
    c. p24
    d. p26
31. The human immunodeficiency virus (HIV) attaches itself to receptor sites by means of:
    a. p24
    b. p31
    c. gp120
    d. gp160
32. In an established HIV infection, a patient will demonstrate:
    a. p24 antigen
    b. HIV-1 antibody
    c. p25 antigen
    d. Both a and b
33. Fourth-generation HIV testing is capable of detecting _____ in the period of initial infection:
    a. HIV-1 p24 antigen
    b. HIV-1 gp41 antigen
    c. HIV-1 gp120 antigen
    d. HIV-1 gp160 antigen
34. The most frequent malignancy observed in AIDS patients is:
    a. *Pneumocystis jirovecii*
    b. Kaposi sarcoma
    c. Toxoplasmosis
    d. Non-Hodgkin lymphoma

20

Hypersensitivity Reactions

LEARNING OUTCOMES

- Define the terms hypersensitivity, allergy, sensitization, and immunization.
- Identify and explain the three categories of antigens.
- Compare the basic differences among and give examples of types I, II, III, and IV hypersensitivity reactions.
- Discuss the acquisition and consequences of various types of latex sensitivity.
- Describe the etiology, immunologic activity, signs and symptoms, laboratory evaluation, and treatment of type I hypersensitivity reactions.
- Discuss examples of type II hypersensitivity reactions, including laboratory evaluation.
- Describe the mechanism of tissue injury, clinical manifestations, and laboratory testing for type III hypersensitivity reactions.
- Describe the characteristics and laboratory evaluation of type IV hypersensitivity reactions.
- Analyze case studies related to hypersensitivity reactions and answer case study–related multiple-choice questions.
- Participate in a discussion of critical thinking questions.
- Describe the principle, clinical applications, or sources of error of a food allergy test and the direct antiglobulin test.
- Correctly answer 80% of end-of-chapter review questions.

OUTLINE

What is Hypersensitivity?, 338
What is an Allergy?, 338
Types of Antigens and Reactions, 338
    Latex Allergies, 338
    Environmental Substances, 338
    Infectious Agents, 338
    Self-Antigens, 338
    Food Allergies, 338
Types of Hypersensitivity Reactions, 339
    Type I Anaphylactic Reactions, 340
        Etiology, 340
        Immunologic Activity, 340
        Signs and Symptoms, 341
        Testing for Type I Hypersensitivity Reactions, 341
        Skin Testing Protocols, 341
        Laboratory Evaluation of Allergic Reactions, 342
        Treatment, 343
    Type II Cytotoxic Reactions, 343
        Examples of Antibody-Dependent, Complement-Mediated Cytotoxic Reactions, 344

    Diagnostic Evaluation, 346
    Type III Immune Complex Reactions, 346
        Mechanism of Tissue Injury, 346
        Clinical Manifestations, 347
        Testing for Type III Hypersensitivity Reactions, 347
        Treatment, 347
    Type IV Cell-Mediated Reactions, 347
        Characteristics, 348
        Latex Sensitivity, 348
        Testing for Delayed Hypersensitivity, 348
        Treatment, 348
Comparison of Types of Hypersensitivity, 348
Case Study 20.1, 350
Case Study 20.2, 350
Case Study 20.3, 350
Case Study 20.4, 351
Case Study 20.5, 351
Procedure: Rapid Test for Food Allergy, 352.e1
Procedure: Direct Antiglobulin Test, 352.e1

KEY TERMS

allergens
allergy
allergy march
alloimmunization
anaphylactic reactions
Arthus reaction
atopy

autoantigens
delayed hypersensitivity
desensitization
direct antiglobulin test (DAT)
downregulation
hemolytic reactions
histocompatibility

hypersensitivity
immediate hypersensitivity
immunization
rhinitis
urticaria
vasodilation

> **KEY CONCEPTS: Hypersensitivity Facts**
> - The term *immunization*, or *sensitization*, is used to describe an immunologic reaction dependent on the response of the host to a subsequent exposure of antigen.
> - Hypersensitivity has traditionally been classified as immediate and delayed based on the time after exposure to an offending antigen.

WHAT IS HYPERSENSITIVITY?

Hypersensitivity can be defined as a normal but exaggerated or uncontrolled immune response to an antigen that can produce inflammation, cell destruction, or tissue injury. It has traditionally been classified on the basis of time after exposure to an offending antigen. When this criterion is used, the terms immediate hypersensitivity and delayed hypersensitivity are appropriate. Immediate hypersensitivity is antibody mediated; delayed hypersensitivity is cell mediated.

The term immunization, or *sensitization*, describes an immunologic reaction dependent on the host's response to a subsequent exposure to antigen. Small quantities of the antigen may favor sensitization by restricting the quantity of antibody formed. An unusual reaction, such as an allergic or hypersensitive reaction that follows a second exposure to the antigen, reveals the existence of the sensitization.

WHAT IS AN ALLERGY?

Our basic understanding of allergy has evolved from the discovery in 1967 of a previously unknown antibody, immunoglobulin E (IgE). The most significant property of IgE antibodies is that they can be specific for hundreds of different allergens. Common allergens include animal dander, pollens, foods, molds, dust, metals, drugs, and insect stings.

The term allergy originally meant any altered reaction to external substances. A related term, atopy, refers to immediate hypersensitivity mediated by IgE antibodies. The terms *allergy* and *atopy* are now often used interchangeably. Atopic allergies include hay fever, asthma, food allergies (FAs), and latex sensitivity.

Allergies are very common and are increasing in prevalence in the United States, Western Europe, and Australia. Allergies also occur in families, although not necessarily the same allergy.

TYPES OF ANTIGENS AND REACTIONS

Antigens that trigger allergic reactions are called allergens. These low-molecular-weight substances can enter the body by being inhaled, eaten, or administered as drugs.

Hypersensitivity reactions can occur in response to different types of antigens, including environmental substances, infectious agents, food, and self-antigens.

Latex Allergies

Less than 1% of the general US population has latex sensitivity. Although latex allergy is rare, the condition is more common in certain high-risk groups. The highest risk of latex allergy is in three out of five children with spina bifida. Children who have frequent medical treatments or lengthy surgeries are also at high risk.

Latex is a protein found in the sap of the Brazilian rubber tree. Use of the term *latex* refers to "natural rubber products" made from that sap. Latex is found in many everyday products, such as disposable gloves, condoms, and diaphragms. Direct contact with latex or airborne latex fibers can produce an allergic reaction. Synthetic latex does not cause an allergic reaction.

There are three types of reactions to natural rubber latex:
1. IgE-mediated allergic reactions (type I hypersensitivity)
2. Cell-mediated contact dermatitis (type IV hypersensitivity)
3. Irritant dermatitis

Irritant contact dermatitis appears as swelling, redness, and itching after contact with latex products. This is a common reaction to natural rubber latex, but it is not an allergy. Irritant contact dermatitis breaks out where latex has touched the skin. It appears 12 to 24 hours after an incident such as frequent hand washing with inadequate drying of the hands or the use of hand sanitizers. Wearing powdered latex gloves can result in an irritant contact dermatitis.

In those with allergies, contact dermatitis can be a warning sign that latex allergy may develop. Four out of five people who develop a type I hypersensitivity, IgE-mediated latex allergy, will experience contact dermatitis first.

Environmental Substances

Environmental substances in the form of small molecules can trigger several types of hypersensitivity reactions. Dust can enter the respiratory tract, mimicking parasites, and stimulate an antibody response. An immediate hypersensitivity reaction associated with IgE, such as rhinitis or asthma, can result. If dust stimulates immunoglobulin G (IgG) antibody production, it can trigger a different type of hypersensitivity reaction, such as farmer's lung. If small molecules diffuse into the skin and act as haptens, a delayed hypersensitivity reaction, such as contact dermatitis, will result.

Drugs administered orally, by injection, or on the skin can provoke a hypersensitivity reaction mediated by IgE, IgG, or T lymphocytes.

Metals (particularly nickel) and chemicals can also cause type I hypersensitivity reactions. Low–molecular-weight chemicals usually act as a hapten by binding to body proteins or major histocompatibility complex (MHC) molecules. The complex of antigen and MHC molecules is then recognized by specific T cells, which initiate the reaction.

Infectious Agents

Not all infectious agents are capable of causing hypersensitivity reactions. The influenza virus can cause hypersensitivity that results in damage to epithelial cells in the respiratory tract. Sometimes, an exaggerated immune response occurs. Influenza virus, for example, can trigger high levels of cytokine secretion or what is called a *cytokine storm*. In comparison, streptococci can cause a hypersensitivity reaction termed *immune complex disease*.

Self-Antigens

Very small immune responses to self-antigens are normal and occur in most people. When these become an exaggerated response, however, or when tolerance to other antigens breaks down, hypersensitivity reactions can occur.

Food Allergies

According to the National Institute of Allergy and Infectious Diseases (NIAID), FA is an important public health problem that affects adults and children and may be increasing in prevalence. The prevalence of FA in Europe and North America has been reported to range from 6% to 8% in children up to the age of 3 years. A recent US study has estimated that 5% of children under 5 years of age and 4% of teens and adults have FAs.

Most FAs are type I IgE-mediated reactions. Ninety percent of IgE-mediated allergies are caused by cow's milk, soy, chicken eggs, peanuts, tree nuts, wheat, fish, and crustaceans. In comparison, non-IgE-mediated reactions (also called *cell-mediated reactions*) are also common to soy, wheat, rice, oats, and cow's milk. Wheat, milk, egg, and soy allergies usually disappear gradually with age. It is important to distinguish between food intolerance and FA because they are not the same condition.

Some foods have proteins that are like those in the rubber tree sap. These latex-reactive foods have been responsible for anaphylactic reactions in latex-sensitive persons. Nuts and fruits, such as bananas, chestnuts, kiwi, avocados, and tomatoes, show cross-reactivity, perhaps because of a similarity to a latex protein component. Many other foods, including figs, apples, carrots, celery, melons, potatoes, papayas, and pitted fruits (e.g., cherries, peaches), have caused progressive symptoms, beginning with oral itching. Persons with a history of reactions to these foods are at increased risk of developing latex allergy, and those who are sensitive to latex should avoid foods to which they have had previous reactions.

FA can cause severe allergic reactions and even death from food-induced anaphylaxis. Despite the risk, there is no current treatment for FA; the disease can only be managed by allergen avoidance or treatment of symptoms. The diagnosis of FA may be problematic because nonallergic food reactions, such as food intolerance, are frequently confused with FAs.

NIAID guidelines separate diseases defined as FA that include IgE-mediated reactions to food (FAs), non-IgE-mediated reactions to certain foods (e.g., celiac disease), and mixed IgE and non-IgE disorders (Table 20.1).

Latex contains low–molecular-weight soluble proteins that cause IgE-mediated allergic reactions. Latex allergy can give rise to a broad range of symptoms. Glove wearers may experience type IV, or delayed hypersensitivity, contact dermatitis that ranges from nonspecific pruritus to eczematous, red, weepy skin. These symptoms and the irritant contact dermatitis are caused by the accelerators and chemicals used in glove manufacturing, not by the latex itself. Avoidance of latex gloves is often sufficient to prevent these symptoms.

Anaphylactic reactions to latex have been reported in those who had previously experienced only irritant or allergic contact dermatitis. Direct skin contact with latex may cause a type I, or immediate hypersensitivity, IgE-mediated reaction within 30 to 60 minutes of exposure. Urticaria may be local or generalized, and the spectrum of progression is notably unpredictable; some persons have experienced anaphylactic reactions after having minimal or no previous symptoms.

TYPES OF HYPERSENSITIVITY REACTIONS

The four types of hypersensitivity reactions (I–IV) are defined by the principal mechanism responsible for a specific cell or tissue injury that occurs during an immune response (Table 20.1). Type I, II, and III reactions are antibody dependent, and type IV reaction is cell mediated. Some overlapping occurs among the various types of hypersensitivity reactions, but there are major differences in how each type is diagnosed and treated.

> **KEY CONCEPTS: Type I Hypersensitivity Reaction**
> - Type I hypersensitivity reactions can range from life-threatening anaphylactic reactions to milder manifestations associated with FAs. This reaction is usually mediated by IgE antibody.
> - In vitro evaluation of type I hypersensitivity reactions involves various methods. The advantages of in vitro testing include no risk of a systemic hypersensitivity reaction and no dependence on skin reactivity influenced by drugs, disease, or age.

TABLE 20.1 Classification of Hypersensitivity Reactions

Parameter	I	II	III	IV
Reaction	Anaphylactic	Cytotoxic	Immune complex	Cell-mediated
Antibody	IgE[a]	IgG, possibly other immunoglobulins	Antigen-antibody complexes (IgG, IgM)[a]	None
Complement involved	No	Yes[a]	Yes[a]	No
Cells involved	Mast cells, basophils, granules (histamine)[a]	Effector cells (macrophages, polymorphonuclear leukocytes)[a]	Macrophages, mast cells	Antigen-sensitized T lymphocytes or particles that remain phagocytize in a macrophage
Cytokines involved	Yes[a]	No	Yes[a]	Yes[b]
Comparative description	Antibody mediated, immediate	Antibody dependent; complement or cell mediated	Immune complex mediated (immune complex disease)	Delayed-type T-lymphocyte–mediated response to antigen
Mechanism of tissue injury	Allergic and anaphylactic reactions	Target cell lysis	Immune complex deposition, inflammation	Antigen receptor T lymphocytes that causes the release of cytokines that then activates macrophages with the release of inflammatory mediators
Examples	Anaphylaxis Hay fever Asthma Food allergy	Hemolytic transfusion reactions HDFN Thrombocytopenia	Arthus reaction Serum sickness Systemic lupus erythematosus	Mechanism of defense against various intracellular pathogens; responsible for immunologic mechanisms in contact sensitivity rejection of foreign tissue grafts; formation of chronic granulomas

[a]Mediator.
[b]Tumor necrosis factor-α.
HDFN, Hemolytic disease of the fetus and newborn; *IgE*, Immunoglobulin E; *IgG*, Immunoglobulin G; *IgM*, Immunoglobulin M.

Type I Anaphylactic Reactions

Type I hypersensitivity reactions can range from life-threatening anaphylactic reactions to milder manifestations associated with FAs.

Etiology

Atopic allergies are mostly naturally occurring, and the source of antigenic exposure is not always known. Atopic illnesses were among the first antibody-associated diseases demonstrating a strong familial or genetic tendency.

Several groups of agents cause anaphylactic reactions. Common agents involved in type I hypersensitivity reactions are drugs (e.g., systemic penicillin) and insect stings. Insects of the order Hymenoptera (e.g., common hornet, yellow jacket, yellow hornet, and paper wasp) are examples of insects causing the most serious reactions. Immune-mediated IgE adverse food reactions (Box 20.1) can be fatal.

Immunologic Activity

Mast cells (tissue basophils) are the cellular receptors for IgE, which attaches to their outer surface. These cells are common in connective tissues, lungs, the uterus, and around blood vessels. They are also abundant in the liver, kidney, spleen, heart, and other organs. The granules contain a complex of heparin, histamine, and zinc ions, with heparin in a ratio of approximately 6:1 with histamine.

Immediate hypersensitivity is the basis of acute allergic reactions caused by molecules released by mast cells when an allergen interacts with membrane-bound IgE (Fig. 20.1). Acute allergic reactions result from the release of preformed granule-associated mediators, membrane-derived lipids, cytokines, and chemokines when an allergen interacts with IgE that is bound to mast cells or basophils by the alpha chain of the high-affinity IgE receptor (FcεRI-α). This antigen receptor also occurs on antigen-presenting cells, where it can facilitate the IgE-dependent trapping and presentation of allergen to T cells.

Histamine, leukotriene C4, interleukin-4 (IL-4), and interleukin-13 (IL-13) are major mediators of allergy and asthma. All are formed by basophils and released in large quantities after stimulation with interleukin-3 (IL-3); IL-3's effect is restricted to basophil granulocytes. Basophil granulocytes should be considered key effector cells in type 2 helper T (Th2) cell immune responses and allergic inflammation. IL-3 strongly induces messenger RNA (mRNA) for granzyme B, a major effector of granule-mediated cytotoxicity.

Anaphylactic reaction. Anaphylaxis is the clinical response to immunologic formation and fixation between a specific antigen and a tissue-fixing antibody. This reaction is usually mediated by IgE antibody and occurs in the following three stages:

1. The offending antigen attaches to the IgE antibody fixed to the surface membrane of mast cells and basophils. Cross-linking of two IgE molecules is necessary to initiate mediator release from mast cells.
2. Activated mast cells and basophils release various mediators.
3. The effects of mediator release produce vascular changes and activation of platelets, eosinophils, neutrophils, and the coagulation cascade.

It is believed that physical allergies (e.g., to heat, cold, ultraviolet light) cause a physiochemical derangement of proteins or polysaccharides of the skin and transform them into autoantigens responsible for the allergic reaction. Most, if not all, of these reactions are caused by the action of a self-directed IgE.

Anaphylactoid reaction. Anaphylactoid reactions (anaphylaxis-like) are clinically similar to anaphylaxis and can result from immunologically inert materials that activate serum and tissue proteases and the alternative pathway of the complement system. Anaphylactoid reactions are not mediated by antigen-antibody interaction; instead, offending substances act directly on the mast cells, causing release of mediators, or on the tissues, such as anaphylatoxins of the complement cascade (e.g., C3a and C5a). Direct chemical degranulation of mast cells may be the cause of anaphylactoid reactions resulting from the infusion of macromolecules, such as proteins.

Atopic reaction. In a person with atopy, exposure of the skin, nose, or airway to an allergen produces allergen-specific IgG antibodies. In response to the allergen, the T cells (when tested in vitro) exhibit moderate proliferation and production of interferon-gamma (IFN-γ) by type 1 helper T (Th1) cells. In comparison, individuals with atopy have an exaggerated response characterized by the production

---

> **BOX 20.1 Diagnosis of IgE-Mediated Food Allergy**
>
> The National Institute of Allergy and Infectious Diseases (NIAID) Expert Panel recommends the following:
>
> - Considering food allergy (FA) in individuals presenting with anaphylaxis or any combination of symptoms that occur within minutes to hours of ingesting food, especially in young children and/or if symptoms have followed the ingestion of a specific food on more than one occasion. In addition, infants, young children, and selected older children diagnosed with certain disorders, such as moderate-to-severe atopic dermatitis (AD), eosinophilic esophagitis (EoE), enterocolitis, enteropathy, and allergic proctocolitis (AP), should be considered for FA.
> - Using medical history and physical examination to aid in the diagnosis of FA.
> - Confirming parent and patient reports of FA, because multiple studies demonstrate that 50% to 90% of presumed FAs are not allergies.
> - Performing a skin puncture test (SPT) to assist in the identification of foods that may be provoking IgE-mediated food-induced allergic reactions; however the SPT alone cannot be considered diagnostic of FA.
> - Not using intradermal testing or measurement of the total serum IgE to make a diagnosis of FA.
> - Using allergen-specific serum IgE (sIgE) tests for identifying foods that potentially provoke IgE-mediated food-induced allergic reactions, but not using these tests as diagnostic of FA.
> - Not using an atopy patch test (APT) in the routine evaluation of noncontact FA.
> - Not using the combination of SPTs, sIgE tests, and APTs for the routine diagnosis of FA.
> - Eliminating one or a few specific foods from the diet may be useful in the diagnosis of FA, especially in identifying foods responsible for some non-IgE-mediated food-induced allergic disorders, such as food protein–induced enterocolitis syndrome (FPIES), AP, and Heiner syndrome, and some mixed IgE- and non-IgE-mediated food-induced allergic disorders, such as EoE.
> - Using oral food challenges for diagnosing FA. The double-blind, placebo-controlled food challenge is the gold standard. However, a single-blind or open-food challenge may be considered diagnostic under certain circumstances. If either of these challenges elicits no symptoms (i.e., the challenge is negative), then FA can be ruled out. If either challenge elicits objective symptoms (i.e., the challenge is positive) *and* those objective symptoms correlate with the medical history *and* are supported by laboratory tests, then a diagnosis of FA is supported.
> - Not using any of the following nonstandardized tests for the routine evaluation of IgE-mediated FA: basophil histamine release or activation, lymphocyte stimulation, facial thermography, gastric juice analysis, endoscopic allergen provocation, hair analysis, applied kinesiology, provocation of neutralization allergen-specific IgG4, cytotoxicity assays, electrodermal test (Vega), mediator release assay (LEAP diet).

Modified from the National Institute of Allergy and Infectious Diseases (NIAID). https://www.niaid.nih.gov.

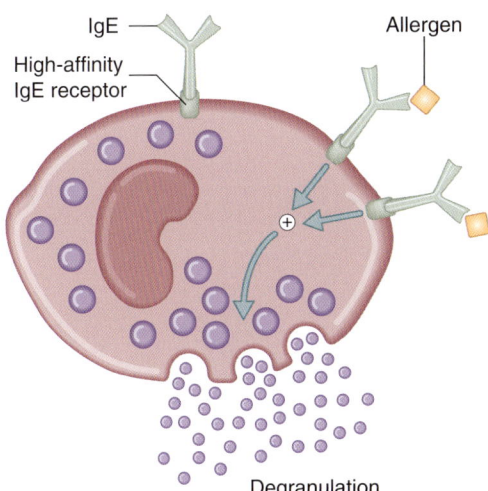

Fig. 20.1 Mast Cell Degranulation. The mast cell carries high-affinity receptors for the Fc portion of IgE. Allergen-specific IgE, occupying these receptors, induces mast cell degranulation immediately. (From Peakman M, Vergani D: *Basic and clinical immunology*, ed 2, London, 2009, Churchill Livingstone.)

of allergen-specific IgE antibodies and positive reactions to extracts of common airborne allergens when tested with a skin prick test. T cells from the blood of atopic patients respond to allergens in vitro by inducing cytokines produced by Th2 cells (e.g., IL-4, IL-5, and IL-13), rather than cytokines produced by Th1 cells (e.g., IFN-γ and IL-2).

There are always exceptions to the rule, but the immunologic hallmark of allergic disease is the infiltration of affected tissue by Th2 cells.

Signs and Symptoms

Although everyone inhales airborne allergens derived from pollen, house dust mites, and animal dander, children and adults without atopy produce an asymptomatic, low-grade immunologic response. In a person with atopy, exposure of the skin, nose, or airway to a single dose of allergen produces symptoms (skin redness, sneezing, and wheezing) within minutes. Depending on the amount of allergen, immediate hypersensitivity reactions are followed by a late-phase reaction that reaches a peak 6 to 9 hours after exposure to the allergen and then slowly subsides.

Localized reaction. A localized reaction occurs as an immediate response to mediators released from mast cell degranulation. Local reactions can consist of urticaria and angioedema at the site of antigen exposure or angioedema of the bowel after ingestion of certain foods. Localized reactions are severe but rarely fatal. Skin reactions are characterized by the appearance of redness and itching at the site of the introduction of the allergen. This phenomenon is the basic principle of the skin test to diagnose an allergy or confirm sensitivity to a specific antigen.

Generalized reaction. A generalized (anaphylactic) reaction is produced by mediators such as cytokines and vasoactive amines (e.g., histamine) from mast cells. Anaphylactic reactions are dramatic and rapid in onset. The physiologic effects of the primary and secondary mediators on the target organs, such as the cardiovascular or respiratory system, gastrointestinal (GI) tract, or the skin, define the signs and symptoms of anaphylaxis. Several important pharmacologically active compounds are discharged from mast cells and basophils during anaphylaxis (see Table 20.2).

Histamine release leads to constriction of bronchial smooth muscle, edema of the trachea and larynx, and stimulation of smooth muscle in the GI tract, which causes vomiting and diarrhea. The resulting breakdown of cutaneous vascular integrity results in urticaria and angioedema; vasodilation causes a reduction of circulating blood volume and a progressive fall in blood pressure, leading to shock. Kinins also alter vascular permeability and blood pressure.

The body's so-called natural moderators of anaphylaxis are the enzymes that decompose the mediators of anaphylaxis. Antihistamines have no effect on histamine release from mast cells or basophils. In human beings, antihistamines are effective antagonists of edema and pruritus, probably related to their blockage of a histamine-induced increase in capillary permeability, but are relatively less effective in preventing bronchoconstriction.

Allergic disease in children. Atopic children characteristically experience a progression of allergic disease called allergy march (see the section ImmunoCAP). The formation of IgE antibodies begins early in life, and sensitization can be detected before clinical symptoms. Sensitization to food allergens such as cow's milk is manifested as colic or chronic otitis. The highest incidence of sensitization is at age 2 years. After 3 years of age, food sensitivities tend to decrease; sensitization to inhalant allergens typically increases during the preschool years. In most children with asthma, symptoms begin before age 5 years. Risk factors for allergic asthma include a family history of allergy, sensitization to food allergens, a total serum IgE higher than 100 kU/L before age 6 years, living in an allergen-rich environment, and smoking.

Testing for Type I Hypersensitivity Reactions

In addition to a patient history and physical examination, laboratory testing, including an in vivo testing protocol, can be used to assist in the identification of foods that may provoke allergic reactions. Laboratory testing can include:

1. Skin (pin prick) testing
2. Patch testing, if non-IgE-mediated FA (e.g., eosinophilic esophagitis) is suspected
3. Food-specific serum IgE testing
4. Serum tryptase, an enzyme released with histamine and other chemicals from mast cells, if they have been activated in an anaphylactic reaction

Skin Testing Protocols

Skin testing can be performed by a skin puncture test (SPT) to assist in the identification of foods that may provoke IgE-mediated, food-induced allergic reactions or by a patch test.

TABLE 20.2 Mediators of Anaphylaxis

Mediator	Primary Action
Histamine	Increases vascular permeability; promotes contraction of smooth muscle
Leukotrienes	Alter bronchial smooth muscle and enhance effects of histamine on target organs
Basophil kallikrein	Generates kinins
Serotonin	Contracts smooth muscle
Platelet-activating factor	Enhances the release of histamine and serotonin from platelets that affect smooth muscle tone and vascular permeability
Eosinophil chemotactic factor of anaphylaxis	Attracts eosinophils to areas of activity; these cells release secondary mediators that may limit the effects of primary mediators
Prostaglandins	Affect smooth muscle tone and vascular permeability

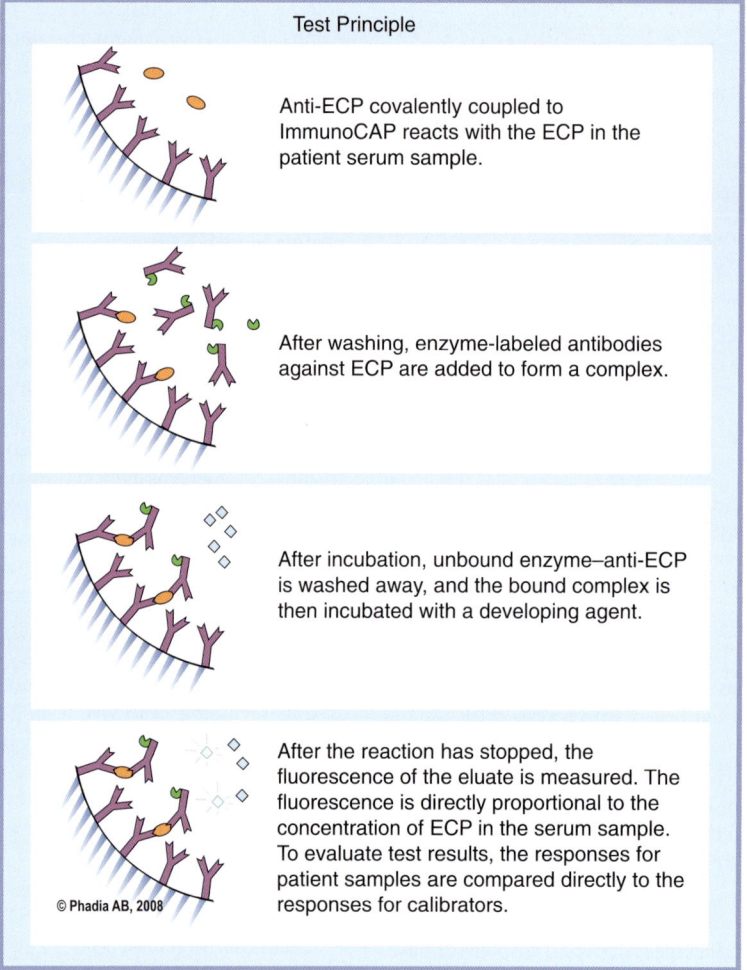

Fig. 20.2 ImmunoCAP Test—Principle, Steps, and Evaluation. *ECP,* Eosinophilic cationic protein. (Courtesy Phadia AB, Uppsala, Sweden.)

The SPT alone cannot be considered diagnostic of FA. Placing a drop of a solution containing a possible allergen on the skin is the basis of skin testing. A series of scratches or needle pricks allows the solution to enter the skin. If the skin develops a red, raised, itchy area, this is a positive reaction, which usually means that the person is allergic to that particular allergen. Skin testing is a simple outpatient technique to screen for many potential allergens but may not be suitable for pediatric patients, pregnant women, or other groups. The procedure carries the risk of triggering a systemic reaction (e.g., anaphylactic reaction) or initiating a new sensitivity.

A patch test may be used for the evaluation of contact FAs. Skin patch testing involves taping a patch that has been soaked in the allergen solution to the skin for 24 to 72 hours. This type of testing is used to detect contact dermatitis.

Laboratory Evaluation of Allergic Reactions

Advantages of in vitro testing include the lack of risk of a systemic hypersensitivity reaction and the lack of dependence on skin reactivity, which can be influenced by drugs, disease, or the patient's age. Detection of an increased amount of total IgE or allergen-specific IgE in serum indicates an increased probability of an allergic disorder, parasitic infection, or aspergillosis. In vitro laboratory testing can be performed by a variety of methods.

The clinical significance of serum allergen-specific IgE (sIgE) in allergic disorders has long been recognized. The quantitative determination of serum IgE antibodies is an essential component for differential diagnosis and for identifying the causative allergens for proper medical treatment. The quality and availability of allergens, reagent stability, and degree of automation all influence the method of testing. Based on thousands of test results, a generic curve indicates what an allergen-specific IgE antibody value can mean in relation to symptoms. Although a final diagnosis should always be based on the physician's overall impression of the patient, a general rule of thumb is that the higher the IgE antibody value, the greater the likelihood of symptoms appearing.

ImmunoCAP. The US Food and Drug Administration (FDA) has approved ImmunoCAP to provide an in vitro quantitative measurement of IgE in human serum (Fig. 20.2). It is considered the gold standard for the analysis of allergen-specific IgE. It is intended for in vitro use as an aid in the clinical diagnosis of IgE-mediated allergic disorders in conjunction with other clinical findings (Table 20.3).

ImmunoCAP assays can be performed for hundreds of allergens, such as weeds, trees, pollens, mold, food, and animal dander. It offers testing for over 650 different allergens and 70 allergen components for sensitive and specific quantitative detection of allergen-specific IgE antibodies.

TABLE 20.3 Comparison of Tests for Specific IgE

Parameter	Skin Prick Testing	Intradermal Testing	Blood Testing (ImmunoCAP)
Sensitivity (%)	93.6	60	87.2
Specificity (%)	80.1	32.3	90.5

Adapted from Choo-Kang LR: Specific IgE testing: objective laboratory evidence supports allergy diagnosis and treatment, *Med Lab Observer MLO* 38:10–14, 2006.

The substances to which a patient is exposed will generally dictate the allergens to test. Some allergens are more common as causes of allergy than others. Factors to consider are the following:
- Patient's age
- Symptoms
- Home environment (e.g., pets, hobbies)
- Geographic location of patient's residence

An example of a pediatric allergy, the march (progression) profile, includes testing for allergens to *Alternaria alternata* (*Alternaria tenuis*; mold), cat dander, cockroach (German), *Dermatophagoides pteronyssinus* (*Dermatophagoides farinae*; mites), dog dander, egg white, codfish, whitefish, cow's milk, peanut, soybean, wheat, and total serum IgE. Food profile allergens might include corn, egg white, cow's milk, orange, peanut, shrimp, soybean, and wheat.

Respiratory allergen inhalants can include *A. alternata* (*A. tenuis*), cat epithelium and dander, dog dander, elm tree, *Hormodendrum hordei* (*Cladosporium herbarum*; fungi), house dust, June grass, Kentucky bluegrass, mountain cedar (juniper) tree, and Russian thistle. Respiratory subtropical Florida allergens include *A. alternata* (*A. tenuis*), *Aspergillus fumigatus*, pine, Australian pine, Bahia grass, Bermuda grass, cat dander, cockroach (German), common short ragweed, *D. farinae* (*D. pteronyssinus*; mites), dog dander, *H. hordei* (*C. herbarum*; fungi), oak tree, pecan (white hickory) tree, *Penicillium notatum*, pigweed, and total serum IgE.

The clinical use of inhaled steroids is becoming increasingly popular owing to their anti-inflammatory effects, although overtreatment may have serious side effects. To ensure the lowest effective dosage throughout treatment, the laboratory can periodically monitor the occurrence in serum of eosinophil cationic protein-2 (ECP-2) released from inflammatory cells. ECP released by eosinophils can be detected in body fluids.

Chemiluminescent enzyme immunoassay. A third-generation sIgE method (Immulite 2000, Siemens Healthcare Diagnostics, Tarrytown, NY) is a solid-phase (bead), two-step chemiluminescent enzyme immunoassay (EIA). Allergens are covalently lined to a soluble polymer-ligand matrix, allowing immunochemical reactions to occur in liquid phases for random access automation.

Treatment

Treatment of patients with allergies involves identifying and eliminating or avoiding possible allergens. Drug therapy and desensitization are two treatment strategies.

Drug therapy. Drug treatments include the following:
- Epinephrine (adrenaline) can be lifesaving in anaphylaxis. Epinephrine stimulates both α-adrenergic and β-adrenergic receptors, decreases vascular permeability, increases blood pressure, and reverses airway obstruction.
- Antihistamines block specific histamine receptors and play an important role in allergies affecting the skin, nose, and mucous membranes. Antihistamines act much slower than epinephrine in treating anaphylaxis and are not very useful in asthma because histamine is not an important allergic mediator released by mast cells in the lung.
- Specific receptor antagonists block the effects of leukotrienes. One drug, montelukast, reduces the amount of airway inflammation in asthma.
- Corticosteroids, often given topically, are widely used in the prevention of symptoms in patients with allergy.
- Other drugs in development aim to block the Th2 cytokine pathway or prevent IgE binding to FcεRI-α.

Desensitization. Desensitization, or immunotherapy, is a well-established technique to improve allergy symptoms caused by specific allergens (e.g., hay fever). If a patient has a history of life-threatening conditions, and if other treatment alternatives are unsatisfactory, desensitization is used to prevent anaphylaxis resulting from insect stings (e.g., yellow jackets). It is best if only one allergen is incriminated.

Specific immunotherapy is associated with downregulation of the cytokines produced by Th2 cells, upregulation of cytokines produced by Th1 cells, and induction of regulatory T (T_{reg}) cells. These changes produce inhibition of allergic inflammation, increases in cytokines that control the production of IgE (IFN-γ and interleukin-12), production of blocking antibodies (IgG), and release of cytokines involved in allergen-specific hyporesponsiveness (interleukin-10 and transforming growth factor-β).

Different routes of desensitization induce different T-cell populations—Th1 and T_{reg} cells in the case of subcutaneous administration and Th2 cells in the case of a sting on the skin.

For desensitization to insect venom, venom is injected subcutaneously in increasing doses at fixed intervals. Treatment starts with very small doses of venom because there is a risk of inducing anaphylactic shock. Over time, the patient is injected with increasing quantities of venom, eventually corresponding to the amount of venom in the insect sting. Once desensitization has been carried out, high levels of allergen-specific IgG will bind venom and prevent it from cross-linking IgE on mast cells. After following the prescribed treatment protocol, more than 90% of patients will not develop anaphylaxis if they are stung again.

KEY CONCEPTS: Type II Hypersensitivity Reaction
- Type II cytotoxic reactions are characterized by the interaction of IgG or IgM antibody to cell-bound antigen.
- The binding of an antigen and antibody can result in activation of complement and destruction of the cell (cytolysis) to which the antigen is bound. Erythrocytes, leukocytes, and platelets can be lysed by this process.

Type II Cytotoxic Reactions

Hypersensitivity reaction types II and III are initiated by the interaction between antibody, except IgE, and antigen. The distinction between types II and III is based on where the complex of antibody and antigen forms—in type II, the target is fixed in the tissues or on the cell surface; in type III the target is soluble, and circulating immune complexes are formed. Three different mechanisms of antibody-mediated injury exist in type II hypersensitivity, as follows:

1. Antibody-dependent, complement-mediated cytotoxic reactions. These are characterized by the interaction of IgG or IgM antibody with cell-bound antigen. This binding of an antigen and antibody can result in the activation of complement and destruction of the cell (cytolysis) to which the antigen is bound. Erythrocytes, leukocytes, and platelets can be lysed by this process. Examples of antibody-dependent, complement-mediated cytotoxic reactions include immediate (acute) transfusion reactions and immune hemolytic anemias (e.g., hemolytic disease of the newborn).

2. **Antibody-dependent, cell-mediated cytotoxicity** (Fig. 20.3). This depends on the initial binding of specific antibodies to target cell surface antigens. The antibody-coated cells are lysed by effector cells, such as natural killer (NK) cells and macrophages, expressing Fc receptors. The Fc receptors of these effector cells attach to the Fc portion of the antibody that is coating the target cell. Target cell destruction occurs when cytotoxic substances are released by the effector cells. This is the mechanism of injury in antibody-mediated glomerulonephritis and many other diseases (Fig. 20.4). Antibody binding damages solid tissues, in which the antigen may be cellular or part of the extracellular matrix (e.g., basement membrane).
3. **Antireceptor antibodies.** These disturb the normal function of receptors. Less often, antibodies may modify the function of cells by binding to receptors for hormones (autoimmune hypersensitivity against solid tissue), as illustrated by autoimmune thyroid disease (see Chapter 22). Hyperacute graft rejection is also an example of type II hypersensitivity (see Chapter 25).

Examples of Antibody-Dependent, Complement-Mediated Cytotoxic Reactions

Transfusion reactions. Transfusion reactions are examples of antibody-dependent, complement-mediated cytotoxic reactions. The term *transfusion reaction* generally refers to the adverse consequences of incompatibility between patient and donor erythrocytes. Transfusion reactions can include hemolytic (red blood cell [RBC]–lysing) reactions that occur during or shortly after a transfusion, shortened posttransfusion survival of RBCs, an allergic response, or disease transmission.

Transfusion reactions can be divided into hemolytic and nonhemolytic types. **Hemolytic reactions** are associated with the infusion of incompatible erythrocytes. These reactions can be further classified into acute (immediate) or delayed in their manifestations (Box 20.2). Several factors influence whether a transfusion reaction will be acute or delayed, including the following:
- Number of incompatible erythrocytes infused
- Antibody class or subclass
- Achievement of the optimal temperature for antibody binding

Immediate hemolytic reactions. The most common cause of an acute hemolytic transfusion reaction is the transfusion of ABO group–incompatible blood. In patients with preexisting antibodies resulting from prior transfusion or pregnancy, other blood groups may be responsible.

Epidemiology. Acute hemolytic reactions are the most serious and potentially lethal transfusion reactions. Most fatalities resulting from acute hemolytic transfusion reactions occur in anesthetized or unconscious patients, with the immediate cause of death being uncontrollable hypotension.

Signs and symptoms. Reactions can occur with the infusion of as little as 10 to 15 mL of incompatible blood. The most common initial symptoms are fever and chills, which mimic a febrile nonhemolytic reaction caused by leukocyte incompatibility. Back pain, shortness of breath, pain at the infusion site, and hypotension are additional symptoms. In addition to shock, the release of thromboplastic substances into the circulation can induce disseminated intravascular coagulation and acute renal failure.

Immunologic manifestations. Acute hemolytic reactions occur during infusion or immediately after blood has been infused. Infusion of incompatible erythrocytes in the presence of preexisting antibodies initiates an antigen-antibody reaction, with activation of the complement, plasminogen, kinin, and coagulation systems. Other initiators of acute hemolytic reactions include bacterial contamination of blood or infusion of hemolyzed erythrocytes. Many reactions

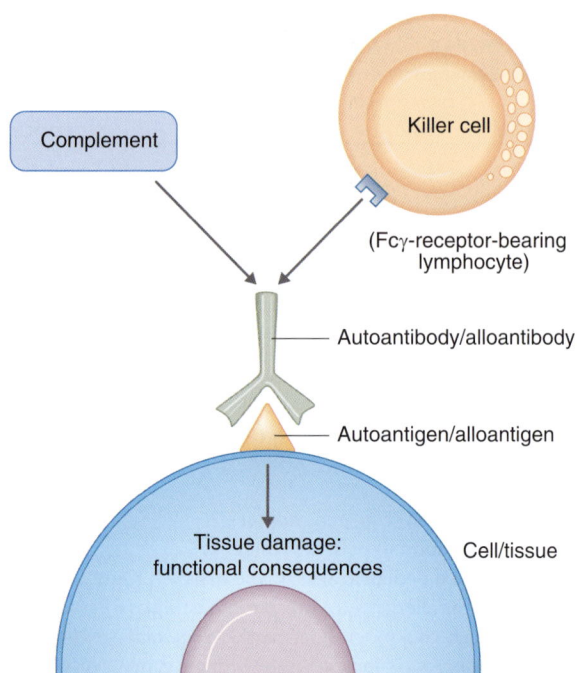

Fig. 20.3 Mechanism of a type II hypersensitivity reaction. (From Peakman M, Vergani D: *Basic and clinical immunology*, ed 2, London, 2009, Churchill Livingstone.)

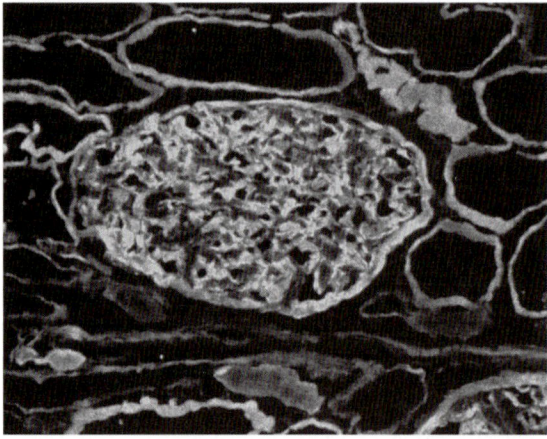

Fig. 20.4 Indirect immunofluorescence was used to detect autoantibodies in a patient with Goodpasture syndrome. Kidney tissue is used as the target antigen for this test. Linear staining along the glomerular basement membrane appears to be lit up compared with the renal tubules in the background. (From Nairn R, Helbert M: *Immunology for medical students*, ed 2, St. Louis, 2007, Mosby.)

demonstrate extravascular and intravascular hemolysis. If an antibody is capable of activating complement and is sufficiently active in vivo, intravascular hemolysis occurs, producing a rapid increase of free hemoglobin in the circulation. Although uncertain, the cause of the immediate clinical symptoms may be products released by the action of complement on the erythrocytes, which triggers multiple shock mechanisms.

Delayed hemolytic reaction. A delayed reaction may not manifest until 7 to 10 days after transfusion. In contrast to an immediate reaction, a delayed reaction occurs in the extravascular spaces. These reactions are associated with decreased RBC survival because of the coating of the RBCs (positive direct antiglobulin test [DAT]), which promotes phagocytosis and premature removal of RBCs by

> **BOX 20.2 Types of Transfusion Reactions**
>
> **Immediate Hemolytic**
> Intravascular hemolysis of erythrocytes
>
> **Delayed Hemolytic**
> Extravascular hemolysis of erythrocytes
>
> **Immediate Nonhemolytic**
> Febrile reactions
> Anaphylaxis
> Urticaria
> Noncardiac pulmonary edema
> Fever and shock
> Congestive heart failure
> Myocardial failure
>
> **Delayed Nonhemolytic**
> Graft-versus-host disease
> Posttransfusion purpura
> Iron overload
> Alloimmunization to erythrocytes, leukocytes, and platelet antigens or plasma proteins
> Infectious disease

the mononuclear phagocyte system. If an antibody does not activate complement or activates it very slowly, extravascular hemolysis occurs. Most IgG antibody–coated erythrocytes are destroyed extravascularly, mainly in the spleen.

A delayed hemolytic transfusion reaction may be of two types. It may represent an anamnestic antibody response in a previously immunized recipient on secondary exposure to transfused erythrocyte antigens, or it may result from primary *alloimmunization*. In an anamnestic response, the antibodies are directed against antigens to which the recipient has been previously immunized by transfusion or pregnancy.

Hemolytic disease of the fetus and newborn. Hemolytic disease of the fetus and newborn (HDFN) results from excessive destruction of fetal RBCs by maternal antibodies. HDFN in the fetus or neonate is clinically characterized by anemia and jaundice. If the hemoglobin breakdown product that visibly produces jaundice (bilirubin) reaches excessive levels in the newborn's circulation, it will accumulate in lipid-rich nervous system tissue and can result in intellectual disability or death.

Etiology. HDFN is caused by the interaction of maternal antibody with antigens on fetal erythrocytes.

For antibody formation to take place, the mother must lack the antigen and the fetus must express the antigen (gene product). The fetus would inherit the gene for antigen expression from the father. HDFN results from the production of maternal antibodies that have been stimulated by the presence of these foreign fetal antigens. The actual production of antibodies depends on a variety of factors: the genetic makeup of the mother, the antigenicity of a specific antigen, and the actual amount of antigen introduced into the maternal circulation.

Epidemiology. The incidence of HDFN resulting from ABO incompatibility ranges from 1 in 70 to 180 births, with an estimated average of 1 in 150 births. The most frequent form of ABO incompatibility occurs when the mother is type O and the baby is type A or type B, usually type A.

Until the early 1970s, the Rh antibody, anti-D, caused many more cases of moderate or severe forms of HDFN than are seen today. Anti-D occurred alone or in combination with another Rh antibody such as anti-C. Anti-D accounted for approximately 93% of cases of non-ABO HDFN. Since the development of modern treatment to prevent primary immunization to the D antigen, the frequency of HDFN caused by anti-D has significantly decreased.

Signs and symptoms. Manifestations of HDFN can range from mild to severe. In addition to possible death in utero, newborns may demonstrate severe anemia and an increase in RBC breakdown products, such as bilirubin. Accumulation of bilirubin causes jaundice and may result in intellectual disablity if the bilirubin is not cleared from the infant's body.

Immunologic mechanisms. HDFN resulting from ABO incompatibility is usually mild because of fewer A and B antigen sites on the fetal or newborn erythrocytes, weaker antigen strength of fetal or newborn A and B antigens, and competition for anti-A and anti-B between tissues and erythrocytes. The number and strength of A and B antigen sites on fetal erythrocytes are less than on adult RBC membranes because they are not fully expressed on the erythrocytes of the fetus and newborn.

Although anti-A and anti-B are present in the absence of their corresponding antigens as environmentally stimulated (IgM) antibodies, infrequent IgG forms may be responsible for HDFN because of ABO incompatibility. Only a small fraction of IgG anti-A and anti-B that crosses the placenta combines with the infant's erythrocytes. High titers of anti-A and anti-B of the IgG type in group O mothers often cause mild HDFN. Anti-A and anti-B antibodies are usually IgM in character and, as such, are unable to pass through the placental barrier. In a survey of antibodies that have caused HDFN, more than 70 different antibodies were identified.

Transplacental hemorrhage (TPH) can occur at any stage of pregnancy. Immunization resulting from TPH can result from negligible doses during the first 6 months in utero; however significant immunizing hemorrhage usually occurs during the third trimester or at delivery. Fetal erythrocytes can also enter the maternal circulation as the result of physical trauma from an injury, abortion, ectopic pregnancy, amniocentesis, or normal delivery. Abruptio placentae, cesarean section, and manual removal of the placenta are often associated with a considerable increase in TPH.

An example of the normal pattern of immunization is demonstrated by the case of an Rh(D)-negative mother whose primary immunization (sensitization) was caused by a previously incompatible Rh(D)-positive pregnancy or a blood transfusion, which stimulates the production of low-titered anti-D, predominantly of the IgM class. Subsequent antigenic stimulation, such as fetal-maternal hemorrhage during pregnancy with an Rh(D)-positive fetus, can elicit a secondary (anamnestic) response, characterized by the predominance of increasing titers of anti-D of the IgG class.

Immune antibodies subsequently react with fetal antigens. Erythrocytic antigens, in addition to leukocyte and platelet antigens, can induce maternal immunization by the formation of IgG antibodies. In HDFN, the erythrocytes of the fetus become coated with maternal antibodies that correspond to specific fetal antigens. Antibodies to IgG, the only immunoglobulin selectively transported to the fetus, are transferred from the maternal circulation to the fetal circulation through the placenta. In the third trimester, IgG is efficiently transported across the placenta from the mother and fetus. It is now generally accepted that a cellular receptor, neonatal Fc receptor (FcRn), is pivotal for maternofetal IgG transport. When the antigen and its corresponding antibody combine in vivo, increased lysis of RBCs results. Because of this hemolytic process, the normal 45- to 70-day life span of the fetal erythrocytes is reduced. To compensate for RBC loss, the fetal liver, spleen, and bone marrow respond by increasing production of erythrocytes. Increased RBC production outside the bone marrow, extramedullary hematopoiesis, can result in enlargement of the liver and spleen and premature release of nucleated erythrocytes from the bone marrow into the fetal circulation. If increased RBC production cannot compensate for the cell being destroyed, a progressively severe anemia develops that can cause the fetus to develop cardiac failure, with generalized edema and death in utero. Less severely affected infants continue to experience erythrocyte destruction after birth, which generates large quantities of unconjugated bilirubin. Bilirubin resulting from excessive hemolysis could result in the accumulation of free bilirubin in lipid-rich tissue of the central nervous system.

Diagnostic evaluation

The following procedures are generally used for the prenatal or postnatal diagnostic evaluation of HDFN:

- ABO blood grouping
- Rh testing
- Screening for irregular antibodies; identification and titering of any antibodies
- Amniocentesis (prenatal)
- Serum bilirubin of cord or infant blood
- DAT of cord or infant blood
- Peripheral blood smear
- Flow cytometry or Kleihauer-Betke test (in emergency situations)

The **direct antiglobulin test (DAT)** (see online Procedure) is performed to detect HDFN, transfusion reactions, and autoimmune hemolytic anemia. Polyspecific antihuman globulin (AHG), a mixture of antibodies to IgG and complement components (e.g., C3d), is used for preliminary screening. If positive, the DAT can be repeated using monospecific anti-IgG and anti-C3d reagents for a more exact determination. If there is an autoimmune hemolytic anemia caused by IgM, only the C3d assay would be positive.

Prevention. Independent researchers have shown that a passive antibody, Rh IgG, could protect most Rh-negative mothers from becoming immunized after the delivery of Rh(D)-positive infants or similar obstetric conditions. In 1968 Rh IgG was licensed for administration in the United States. Since that time, the incidence of HDFN caused by anti-D has decreased dramatically, although complete elimination may never occur because of the cases in which anti-D is formed before delivery. All pregnant Rh-negative women should receive Rh IgG, even if the Rh status of the fetus is unknown, because fetal D antigen is present on fetal erythrocytes as early as 38 days from conception.

Autoimmune hemolytic anemia. Autoimmune hemolytic anemia is an example of a type II hypersensitivity reaction directed against self-antigens on RBCs. It can take two forms, cold autoagglutinins and warm autoagglutinins.

Cold autoimmune hemolytic anemia. Cold autoagglutinins, usually IgM, represent about one-third of cases of autoimmune hemolytic anemia. Cold agglutinins react best at room temperature or lower.

Warm autoimmune hemolytic anemia. In contrast to the cold form, warm autoagglutinins, usually IgG, represent most cases of autoimmune hemolytic anemia. Although the source of antigen exposure may be unknown, antibodies can be formed to microorganisms or drugs. Warm autoagglutinins react best at 37°C (98.6°F).

KEY CONCEPTS: Type III Hypersensitivity Reactions

- Type III hypersensitivity reactions are characterized by deposit of immune complexes in blood vessel walls and tissues.
- Examples of type III reactions include farmer lung, the Arthus reaction, serum sickness, and certain aspects of autoimmune disease.
- Type III reactions are caused by IgG, IgM, and possibly other antibody types.
- Autoimmune disorder (e.g., systemic lupus erythematosus [SLE]) is characterized by autoantibodies that form immune complexes with autoantigens and are deposited in the renal glomeruli.

Type III Immune Complex Reactions

Type III hypersensitivity reactions are caused by the deposition of immune complexes in blood vessel walls and tissues. Repeated antigen exposure leads to sensitization with the production of an insoluble antigen-antibody complex. As these complexes are deposited in tissues, the complement system is activated, macrophages and leukocytes are attracted, and immune-mediated damage occurs. Common skin conditions in this category include allergic vasculitis and erythema nodosum. Pulmonary reactions include hypersensitivity pneumonitis, characterized best by farmer lung, which is a reaction to thermophilic actinomycetes found in moldy hay. Chemicals such as toluene diisocyanate, phthalic anhydride, and trimetallic anhydride can cause bathtub refinisher lung, epoxy resin lung, and plastic worker lung, respectively.

Farmer lung and the **Arthus reaction** are examples of local immune complex diseases. Immune complexes are lattices of antigen and antibody that may be localized to the site of antigen production or may circulate in the blood. Immune complexes are produced as part of the normal immune response and are usually cleared by mechanisms involving complement. However, they cause disease in various situations. Failure to clear immune complexes can result from the saturation of mechanisms involving excessive ongoing production of immune complexes, as well as antigenemia caused by chronic infection.

The formation of immune complexes under normal conditions protects the host because they facilitate the clearance of various antigens and invading microorganisms by the mononuclear phagocyte system. In immune complex reactions (disease), antigen-antibody complexes form in the soluble or fluid phase of tissues or in the blood and assume unique biological functions, such as interaction with complement and with cellular receptors.

Other type III (immune complex) reactions include serum sickness and certain aspects of autoimmune diseases (e.g., glomerulonephritis in SLE). Circulating soluble immune complexes are responsible for or associated with various human diseases in which exogenous and endogenous antigens can trigger a pathogenic immune response and result in immune complex disease (Table 20.4).

Mechanism of Tissue Injury

Type III reactions are caused by IgG, IgM, and possibly other antibody types. Immune complexes can exhibit a spectrum of biological activities, including suppression or augmentation of the immune response by interaction with B and T cells; inhibition of tumor cell destruction; and deposition in blood vessel walls, glomerular membranes, and other sites. These deposits interrupt normal physiologic processes because of tissue damage secondary to the activation of complement and resulting activities such as mediating immune adherence and attracting leukocytes and macrophages to the sites of immune complex deposition. The release of enzymes and possibly other agents damages the tissues. There are three general anatomic sites of antigen-antibody interactions:

1. Antibody can react with soluble antigens in the circulation and form immune complexes that may disseminate and lodge in any tissue with a large filtration area and cause lesions of immune complex disease.
2. Antibody can react with antigen secreted or injected locally into the interstitial fluid. The classic example is the experimental Arthus reaction, the basic model of local immune complex disease (Fig. 20.5).
3. Antibody can also react with structural antigens that form part of the cell surface membranes or with fixed intercellular structures such as the basement membranes. Systemic immune complex disease serum sickness is an example of soluble and tissue-fixed antigen involvement.

Clinical Manifestations

The persistence of immune complexes in the blood circulation is not inherently harmful. Immune complex disease develops when these circulating complexes are not cleared from the circulation by phagocytosis and are subsequently deposited in certain tissues.

Serum sickness. Acute serum sickness develops within 1 to 2 weeks after initial exposure or repeated exposure by injection of heterologous serum protein. There is no preexisting antibody, and the disease appears as antibody formation begins. The hallmark of serum sickness is the protracted interaction between antigen and antibody in the circulation, with the formation of antigen-antibody complexes in an environment of antigen excess. Chronic serum sickness can be experimentally induced if small amounts of antigen are given daily and represent just enough antigen to balance antibody production.

Autoimmune disorders. SLE is an autoimmune disorder characterized by autoantibodies that form immune complexes with autoantigens, which are deposited in the renal glomeruli. As a consequence of this type III hypersensitivity reaction, glomerulonephritis (inflammation of capillary vessels in the glomeruli) develops.

Testing for Type III Hypersensitivity Reactions

Specific autoimmune disorders, such as rheumatoid arthritis (see Chapter 24), have specific assays for detecting and monitoring the autoimmune disorder. Common assays use latex agglutination, nephelometry, and chemiluminescence techniques.

TABLE 20.4 Diseases Associated With Immune Complexes

Disease Type	Examples
Autoimmune	Rheumatoid arthritis, systemic lupus erythematosus, Sjögren syndrome, mixed connective tissue disease, systemic sclerosis, glomerulonephritis
Neoplastic	Solid and lymphoid tumors
Infectious	Bacterial infective endocarditis, streptococcal infection, viral hepatitis, infectious mononucleosis

Fluorescent staining of tissue biopsy specimens can be used to observe the deposition of immune complexes in tissues. Staining patterns and affected tissues can assist in disease diagnosis and prognosis. Another laboratory assay used in assessment is the quantitation of complement (C3 and C4 components).

Treatment

The most direct treatment is avoidance of the offending antigen. Corticosteroids block some of the damage caused by effector cells. Cyclophosphamide is an alkylating agent that impairs DNA synthesis and prevents rapid proliferation of cells (e.g., lymphocytes reduce B-cell proliferation).

> **KEY CONCEPTS: Type IV Hypersensitivity Reactions**
> - Type IV cell-mediated immunity consists of immune activities that differ from antibody-mediated immunity.
> - Cell-mediated immunity is moderated by the link between T lymphocytes and phagocytic cells.
> - Delayed hypersensitivity is a major mechanism of defense against various intracellular pathogens, including mycobacteria, fungi, and certain parasites.
> - In addition cell-mediated immunity is responsible for the immunologic mechanisms of contact sensitivity, rejection of foreign tissue grafts, elimination of tumor cells bearing neoantigens, and formation of chronic granulomas.

Type IV Cell-Mediated Reactions

Type IV cell-mediated immunity consists of immune activities that differ from antibody-mediated immunity. Cell-mediated immunity is moderated by the link between T lymphocytes and phagocytic cells (i.e., monocyte-macrophages). Lymphocytes (T cells) do not recognize the antigens of microorganisms or other living cells but are immunologically active through various types of direct cell-to-cell contact and by the production of soluble factors.

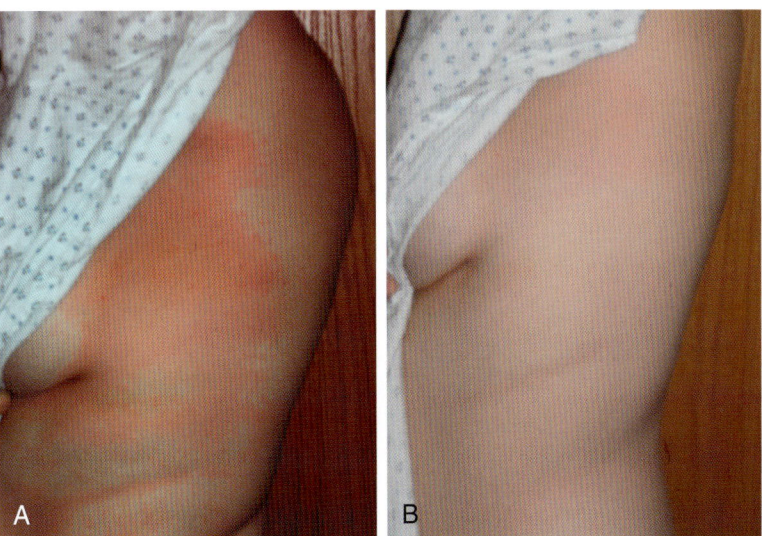

Fig. 20.5 (A) Erythematous morbilliform eruption affecting the torso 2 days after initial exposure to rabbit bones (rATB) and 1 day after rabbit antithymocyte globulin (rATG) was discontinued due to urticaria and an Arthus reaction present at the intravenous infusion site. (B) Complete resolution of the rash a few hours after 50 mg of prednisone was administered orally. (From Soleimanpour SA, Sekiguchi DR, LaRose DF, et al. In Transplantation proceedings: hypersensitivity to rabbit antithymocyte globulin in an islet transplant recipient: a case report, 23[9]:3302–3306, 2011.)

Characteristics

There are three defining characteristics of type IV hypersensitivity reactions. These are:

1. Type IV delayed-type hypersensitivity (DTH) involves antigen-sensitized T cells or particles that remain phagocytized in a macrophage and are encountered by previously activated T cells for a second or subsequent time. T cells respond directly, or by the release of lymphokines, to exhibit contact dermatitis and allergies of infection (Fig. 20.6). One of the mechanisms of cell-mediated immunity is delayed hypersensitivity. Delayed hypersensitivity is a major mechanism of defense against various intracellular pathogens, including mycobacteria, fungi, and certain parasites. In addition, cell-mediated immunity is responsible for immunologic mechanisms in contact sensitivity.
2. Rejection of foreign tissue grafts, elimination of tumor cells bearing neoantigens.
3. Formation of chronic granulomas. Under some of these conditions, the activities of cell-mediated immunity may not be beneficial. Suppression of the normal adaptive immune response (immunosuppression) by drugs or other means is necessary to overcome an unwanted immunologic response in conditions such as organ transplantation, hypersensitivity, and autoimmune disorders.

DTH can be a physiologic reaction to pathogens that are difficult to clear, such as hepatitis B virus and *Mycobacterium tuberculosis*. This triggers the most extreme DTH reactions, characterized by granuloma formation, extensive cell death, and appearance of caseous necrosis. DTH can also occur in response to innocuous environmental antigens (e.g., nickel). Antigens must have a low molecular weight to enter the body. DTH reactions also take place against autoantigens. In insulin-dependent (type 1) diabetes, T cells respond to pancreatic islet cell antigens, damaging the islets and eventually preventing insulin secretion.

DTH reactions are initiated when tissue macrophages recognize the presence of danger signals and initiate the inflammatory response. Dendritic cells loaded with antigen migrate to local lymph nodes, where they present antigen to T cells. Specific T-cell clones proliferate in response to antigens and migrate to the site of inflammation. T cells and macrophages stimulate one another through the cytokine network. Tumor necrosis factor-α (TNF-α) is secreted by macrophages and T cells, and stimulates much of the damage in DTH reactions. Because of the need for antigen presentation by T cells, DTH reactions are often associated with specific human leukocyte antigen (HLA) alleles.

The hallmark of occupational type IV hypersensitivity is allergic contact dermatitis caused by metals (e.g., nickel, mercury, and copper), sunscreen agents, disinfectants, perfumes and fragrances, and pesticides. Pulmonary hypersensitivity can be caused by inorganic dust particles, hard metal, and beryllium. Hard metal exposure involves cobalt from the grinding of steel.

Latex Sensitivity

In the healthcare setting, natural latex can be an allergen in those who have significant cumulative exposure. Since 1985, policies of Standard Precautions have resulted in an exponential increase in the use of latex gloves. The use of latex condoms has also increased. The increase in total exposure to latex and variations in manufacturing apparently have led to an increase in the number of persons with latex sensitivity.

Once sensitized, an individual may experience allergic symptoms when exposed to any product containing latex. At-risk groups sensitized to natural rubber latex include 8% to 17% of healthcare workers, in addition to children who have repeated surgeries. Today, most healthcare facilities use nonlatex gloves and products to avoid latex exposure.

Cell-mediated contact dermatitis (type IV) is a type of allergy to latex. It is not a life-threatening allergy. This type of reaction is usually caused by sensitivity to any of the many chemicals used to make latex products, rather than to rubber.

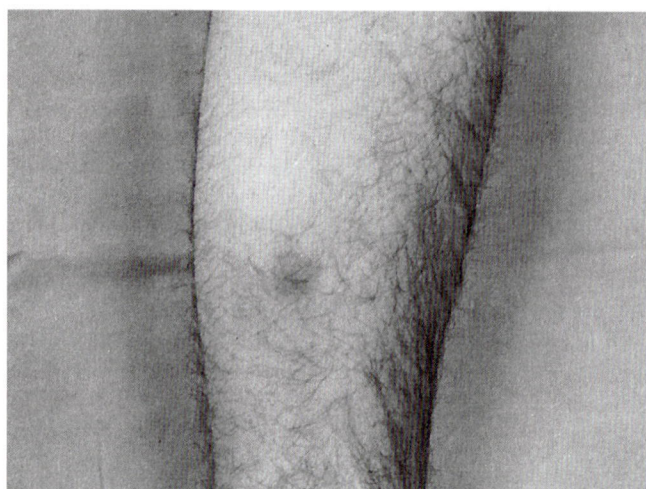

Fig. 20.6 Delayed Skin Reaction. This reaction exhibited an erythematous but nonedematous zone 15 mm in diameter at 48 hours. A control site, inoculated higher on the forearm, showed no reaction at this time. (From Barrett JT: *Textbook of immunology*, ed 5, St. Louis, 1988, Mosby.)

Testing for Delayed Hypersensitivity

The skin test for testing of exposure to tuberculosis (TB) is a classic example of a delayed hypersensitivity reaction. The test is based on the principle that soluble antigens from *M. tuberculosis* induce a reaction in individuals who have acquired or been exposed to the TB microorganism or a related organism at some time. It does not mean that the person has TB.

A small amount of antigen is injected under the skin (intradermally) with a fine-needle syringe. The site is observed at 48 and 72 hours for the presence of induration (a lesion ≥10 mm in diameter).

Other antigens that can be skin tested include diphtheria toxoid, tetanus toxoid, fungal antigens (e.g., *Trichophyton* and histoplasmin), and *Candida albicans*.

In cases of persistent dermatitis, a patch test may be performed. An adhesive patch containing the suspected allergen is applied to the skin. The skin is checked for redness with papules or tiny blisters, indicating a positive test result, over 48 hours.

Diagnosis of latex allergy is determined by the patient history and immunologic testing. FDA-approved in vitro tests to measure latex-specific IgE are available (Pharmacia CAP, Pharmacia-UpJohn Diagnostics, Kalamazoo, MI; AlaSTAT, Diagnostic Products, Los Angeles, CA). The low specificity of these tests, which have a false-negative rate of at least 20% and thus unclear positive predictive value, limits their clinical usefulness. Negative serologic testing with a strongly positive history would suggest the value of skin prick testing to confirm the diagnosis.

Treatment

Strategies to avoid a DTH reaction include avoiding antigen exposure. Anti-inflammatory drugs or corticosteroids may be useful. In some patients, TNF-α monoclonal antibodies and recombinant interferon-β may be administered.

COMPARISON OF TYPES OF HYPERSENSITIVITY

Each type of hypersensitivity reaction has a different type of pathologic immune destruction. In addition, the mechanisms of tissue injury and disease are different (Fig. 20.7).

Type of hypersensitivity	Pathologic immune mechanisms	Mechanisms of tissue injury and disease
Immediate hypersensitivity (Type I)	Th2 cells, IgE antibody, mast cells, eosinophils 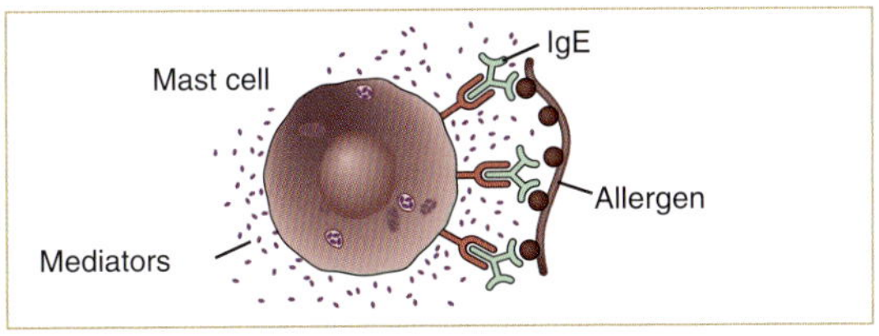	Mast cell–derived mediators (vasoactive amines, lipid mediators, cytokines) Cytokine-mediated inflammation (eosinophils, neutrophils, lymphocytes)
Antibody mediated (Type II)	IgM, IgG antibodies against cell surface or extracellular matrix antigens 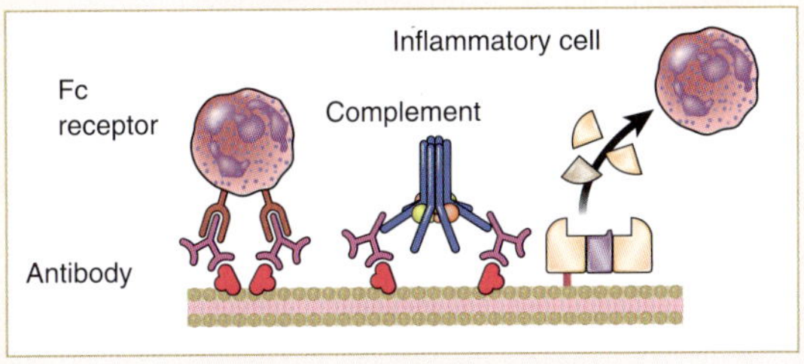	Complement- and Fc receptor–mediated recruitment and activation of leukocytes (neutrophils, macrophages) Opsonization and phagocytosis of cells Abnormalities in cellular function (e.g., hormone or neurotransmitter receptor signaling)
Immune complex mediated (Type III)	Immune complexes of circulating antigens and IgM or IgG antibodies deposited in vascular basement membrane 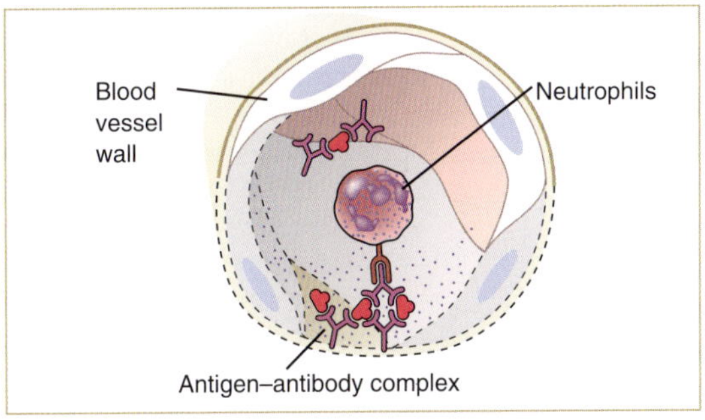	Complement- and Fc receptor–mediated recruitment and activation of leukocytes and tissue damage secondary to impaired blood flow
T-cell mediated (Type IV)	1. CD4+ T cells (cytokine-mediated inflammation) 2. CD8+ CTLs (T cell–mediated cytolysis) 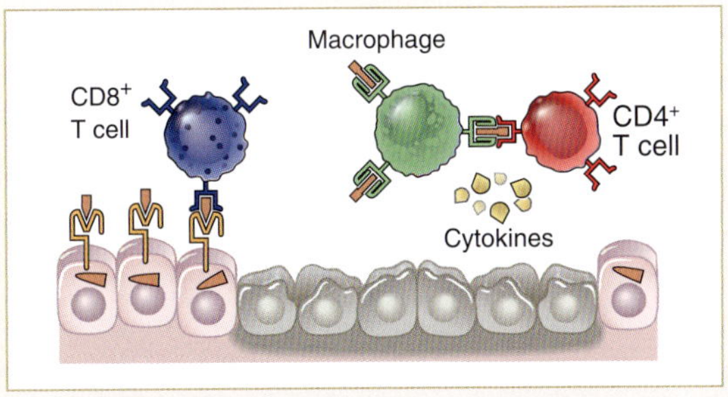	1. Macrophage activation, cytokine-mediated inflammation 2. Direct target cell lysis, cytokine-mediated inflammation

Fig. 20.7 Types of Hypersensitivity Reactions. In the four major types of hypersensitivity reactions, different immune effector mechanisms cause tissue injury and disease. *CTL*, Cytotoxic T lymphocyte; *Ig*, immunoglobulin; *Th2*, type 2 helper T cell. (From Abbas AK, Lichtman AH, Pillai S: *Basic immunology functions and disorders of the immune system,* ed 5, St. Louis, 2016, Elsevier.)

CASE STUDY 20.1

A 60-year-old man was stung by a bee while gardening. He had been stung once before earlier in the summer. Within a few seconds, his hand began to itch and he began to experience abdominal cramping. He subsequently had difficulty breathing. Fortunately, he was able to reach a first-aid kit in his garage. Inside the kit was an EpiPen (injectable epinephrine) for his wife because she was allergic to bee venom. He used the pen and began to feel somewhat better. He immediately had his wife drive him to the hospital.

He was asymptomatic on arrival at the hospital. He had no history of adverse reactions to bee venom or antibiotics. Because of the nature of the incident, a diagnosis of anaphylactic shock caused by bee venom sensitivity was made. A follow-up IgE panel and skin test were performed. The patient was extremely positive for bee venom.

Question
1. Agents that can produce type I hypersensitivity reactions in susceptible individuals include:
   a. Peanuts
   b. Penicillin
   c. Latex
   d. All of the above
   Answers to this multiple-choice question can be found in Appendix A.

Critical Thinking Group Discussion Questions
1. What is the mechanism involved in anaphylaxis?
2. What types of agents can induce anaphylactic shock?

CASE STUDY 20.2

A 35-year-old gravida 4 para 1 + 2 woman was seen by her gynecologist when she was 8 weeks pregnant. Her first pregnancy 4 years ago was unremarkable. The patient reported that her second and third pregnancies had resulted in a stillbirth at 36 weeks and a spontaneous abortion at 10 weeks of gestation, respectively. Her medical history revealed no history of blood transfusions. She remembered being vaccinated for rubella. Her medical records had been destroyed in a fire at the clinic. Repeat blood grouping and Rh testing and an irregular antibody screen were ordered. The test results were:
- Mother: Group A; Rh(D)-negative; irregular antibody screen, positive anti-D (1:8)
- Father: Group A; Rh(D)-positive; CDe/Cde

The patient returned in 2 weeks for a repeat anti-D titer. The titer had risen to 1:16. At 17 weeks' gestation, an amniocentesis was performed. Severe hemolysis was demonstrated, and an intrauterine transfusion of the fetus was carried out using fresh, washed, cytomegalovirus screening test–negative, group O, Rh(D)-negative blood. Because of the continuing risk to the fetus, a cesarean section was performed at 36 weeks' gestation. On delivery, the baby was noted to be jaundiced and pale. The first of three exchange transfusions was performed. Phototherapy was also used to degrade the bilirubin deposited in the skin. The baby made an uneventful recovery with no signs of kernicterus and was discharged from the hospital 5 days after birth.

Question
1. Type II hypersensitivity reactions are related to:
   a. Bee venom
   b. Antibodies (IgM, IgG)
   c. IgE antibodies
   d. Nickel allergy
   Answers to this multiple-choice question can be found in Appendix A.

Critical Thinking Group Discussion Questions
1. What is the mechanism of HDFN?
2. What prophylactic measures are used to prevent HDFN caused by the D antigen?

CASE STUDY 20.3

A patient had a medical history that included frequent sore throats as a child. He had been treated with antibiotics, particularly penicillin. Eventually, he developed a rash. He was told that he had developed an allergy to penicillin and that he should not have it again.

A decade later, he developed a urinary tract infection. He was treated with an antibiotic, trimethoprim, for 8 days. A few days after completing the regimen, he developed a headache and some itchy bumps on his skin. The next day he had sore and swollen joints. His physician confirmed that the rash was urticaria. The patient also had an elevated temperature and swollen glands in his neck. The diagnosis of a drug allergy was made. The patient was given antihistamines. If this medication failed to alleviate the symptoms, more aggressive steroid therapy would be pursued.

The patient's symptoms did not improve, and he was started on an oral corticosteroid, prednisone. When the patient returned to his physician 3 weeks later, he was asymptomatic.

Question
1. Type III diseases associated with immune complexes include:
   a. Autoimmune
   b. Neoplastic
   c. Infection
   d. All of the above
   Answers to this multiple-choice question can be found in Appendix A.

Critical Thinking Group Discussion Questions
1. What is the likely mechanism of this reaction?
2. What types of agents can lead to drug reactions?

CASE STUDY 20.4

A 19-year-old college student went to Student Health Services because she had a slowly developing rash on both earlobes, her hands and her wrists, and around her neck.

Her medical history revealed that she had eczema in childhood. During her early teens, she had facial acne, for which she was given tetracycline. Physical examination revealed a rash of erythema and small blisters, with marked excoriation because of the itching. Her hands were red, scaly, and dry. The rash on her hands was different from the eruptions on her neck and ears. A contact hypersensitivity was suspected.

Follow-up patch tests included a standard battery of agents—rubber, cosmetics, plant extracts, perfumes, nickel, and makeup. Strongly positive reactions for rubber and nickel were observed.

The student was advised to eliminate contact with rubber (e.g., rubber gloves) used at home or on the job. Her jewelry probably contained nickel and was believed to be the source of the irritation to her earlobes, neck, and wrists. She was advised to wear only nickel-free jewelry. A mild corticosteroid cream was prescribed for use until her symptoms disappeared.

Question

1. An example of a type IV reaction can be caused by:
   a. Nickel
   b. Incompatible blood transfusion
   c. Bacterial contamination of water
   d. An autoimmune disorder
   Answers to this multiple-choice question can be found in Appendix A.

Critical Thinking Group Discussion Questions

1. Why did the jewelry cause a rash?
2. What is the mechanism of type IV hypersensitivity involvement in contact eczema?

See instructor site for the discussion of these questions.

CASE STUDY 20.5

A 35-year-old woman reported that she had experienced three bouts of urticaria of unknown origin about 10 years ago. The urticaria affected her mucous membranes and skin. She had experienced similar symptoms after repair of a fractured femur caused by a skiing accident. These symptoms were attributed to an antibiotic reaction.

As an emergency department nurse, she observed occasional localized hives after the use of latex gloves. Even when she used hypoallergenic latex gloves, she continued to have hives every few months. Increased urticaria, at times generalized, continued to occur.

Within 30 minutes of having a routine vaginal examination performed by a healthcare provider wearing latex gloves, she had an anaphylactic reaction that required resuscitation and hospitalization. A vaginal biopsy 1 week later required a latex-free environment for her safety.

A short time later, she was forced to retire from nursing because of symptoms of asthma. She had also developed food allergies to shellfish.

Question

1. If a person is allergic to latex, a reaction rarely takes place more than _____ after exposure to latex.
   a. 30 minutes
   b. 2 hours
   c. 48 hours
   d. 1 week
   Answers to this multiple-choice question can be found in Appendix A.

Critical Thinking Group Discussion Questions

1. What are the most likely type and mechanism of the urticarial hypersensitivity reaction?
2. What are the most likely type and cause of the anaphylactic reaction?

REVIEW QUESTIONS

1. A type I hypersensitivity reaction is a:
   a. Cytotoxic reaction
   b. Cell-mediated reaction
   c. Immune complex reaction
   d. Anaphylactic reaction
2. A type II hypersensitivity reaction is a:
   a. Cytotoxic reaction
   b. Cell-mediated reaction
   c. Immune complex reaction
   d. Anaphylactic reaction
3. A type III hypersensitivity reaction is a:
   a. Cytotoxic reaction
   b. Cell-mediated reaction
   c. Immune complex reaction
   d. Anaphylactic reaction
4. A type IV hypersensitivity reaction is a:
   a. Cytotoxic reaction
   b. Cell-mediated reaction
   c. Immune complex reaction
   d. Anaphylactic reaction
5. What cell type is anaphylactic reactions associated with?
   a. T lymphocyte
   b. B lymphocyte
   c. Monocyte
   d. Mast cells
6. Type III reactions are exemplified by all of the following *except*:
   a. Arthus reaction
   b. Serum sickness
   c. Glomerulonephritis
   d. Shingles
7. Type IV reactions are responsible for all of the following *except*:
   a. Contact sensitivity
   b. Delayed hypersensitivity
   c. Elimination of tumor cells bearing neoantigens
   d. Hemolysis of red blood cells
8. Type I sensitivity reactions can be associated with all of the following *except*:
   a. Food allergies
   b. Hay fever
   c. Asthma
   d. Hemolytic disease of the newborn
9. The most common agents that cause anaphylactic reactions are:
   a. Drugs and food
   b. Drugs and insect stings
   c. Poison ivy and insect stings
   d. Food and insect stings

Questions 10 to 12. Arrange the sequence of events in anaphylaxis in the proper order.
10. _____
11. _____
12. _____
    a. The effects of mediator release produce vascular changes, activation of platelets, eosinophils and neutrophils, and activation of the coagulation cascade.
    b. The offending antigen attaches to the IgE antibody fixed to the surface membrane of mast cells and basophils.
    c. Activated mast cells and basophils release various mediators.
13. Histamine as a mediator of anaphylaxis:
    a. Enhances the effects of histamine on target organs
    b. Increases vascular permeability and promotes contraction of smooth muscle
    c. Generates kinins
    d. Contracts smooth muscle
14. Leukotrienes as a mediator of anaphylaxis:
    a. Enhance the effects of histamine on target organs
    b. Increase vascular permeability and promote contraction of smooth muscle
    c. Generate kinins
    d. Contract smooth muscle
15. Serotonin as a mediator of anaphylaxis:
    a. Enhances the effects of histamine on target organs
    b. Increases vascular permeability and promotes contraction of smooth muscle
    c. Generates kinins
    d. Contracts smooth muscle
16. Platelet-activating factor as a mediator of anaphylaxis:
    a. Affects smooth muscle tone and vascular permeability
    b. Enhances the release of histamine and serotonin
    c. Attracts cells to areas of activity; these cells release secondary mediators that may limit the effects of primary mediators
    d. Alters bronchial smooth muscle
17. Eosinophil chemotactic factor of anaphylaxis as a mediator of anaphylaxis:
    a. Affects smooth muscle tone and vascular permeability
    b. Enhances the release of histamine and serotonin
    c. Attracts cells to areas of activity; these cells release secondary mediators that may limit the effects of primary mediators
    d. Alters bronchial smooth muscle
18. Prostaglandins as a mediator of anaphylaxis:
    a. Affect smooth muscle tone and vascular permeability
    b. Enhance the release of histamine and serotonin
    c. Attract cells to areas of activity; these cells release secondary mediators that may limit the effects of primary mediators
    d. Alter bronchial smooth muscle
19. An important cellular mediator associated with an immune complex tissue injury is a:
    a. neutrophil
    b. lymphocyte
    c. basophil
    d. monocyte
20. Cytotoxic reactions are characterized by the interaction of:
    a. IgG to soluble antigen
    b. IgG to cell-bound antigen
    c. IgM to soluble antigen
    d. IgM or IgG to cell-bound antigen
21. An example of a delayed nonhemolytic (type II hypersensitivity) reaction is:
    a. Febrile reaction
    b. Graft-versus-host disease
    c. Urticaria
    d. Congestive heart failure
22. Under normal conditions, immune complexes protect the host because they:
    a. Facilitate the clearance of various antigens
    b. Facilitate the clearance of invading microorganisms
    c. Interact with complement
    d. Both a and b
23. If a young child is suspected of having an allergy to peanuts, what are the best diagnostic procedures?
    a. Serum IgM and allergen-specific IgM
    b. Serum IgG and allergen-specific IgG
    c. Serum IgA and allergen-specific IgA
    d. Serum IgE and allergen-specific IgE
24. A patient with a known penicillin allergy will suffer from a hypersensitivity reaction related to:
    a. IgM
    b. IgG
    c. IgD
    d. IgE
25. Type IV hypersensitivity reactions are responsible for all of the following *except*:
    a. Contact sensitivity
    b. Elimination of tumor cells
    c. Rejection of foreign tissue grafts
    d. Serum sickness
26. IL-4 can stimulate B lymphocytes to secrete IgE, which is a major factor in _____ hypersensitivity reaction.
    a. Type I
    b. Type II
    c. Type III
    d. Type IV
27. An "in vivo" procedure to assess a patient's cellular immune system is:
    a. Performance of a skin test
    b. Lymphocyte multiplication after antigen exposure
    c. Assessing serum antibodies by electrophoresis
    d. Observe for signs of an anaphylactic reaction
28. A peripheral blood leukocyte that is an important mediator of immune complex tissue injury is a:
    a. neutrophil
    b. lymphocyte
    c. basophil
    d. eosinophil
29. The type of hypersensitivity associated with macrophage activation and cytokine-mediated inflammation is:
    a. Type I anaphylactic (immediate hypersensitivity)
    b. Type II cytotoxic (antibody-mediated and antibody-dependent, complement-mediated hypersensitivity)
    c. Type III complex–mediated hypersensitivity
    d. Type IV (T-cell dependent)

21

Plasma Cell Neoplasms and Other Diseases With Paraproteins

LEARNING OUTCOMES

- Compare the general characteristics of monoclonal and polyclonal gammopathies.
- Name disorders based on proliferation of plasma cells and abnormal production of immunoglobulins.
- Describe the general characteristics and laboratory data in multiple myeloma.
- Identify recent changes to the diagnostic criteria for multiple myeloma with specific biomarkers.
- Describe and compare the etiology, epidemiology, signs and symptoms, immunologic manifestations, diagnostic evaluation, and treatment of multiple myeloma and Waldenström primary macroglobulinemia.
- Compare and contrast the characteristics of other monoclonal disorders, such as monoclonal gammopathy of unknown significance (MGUS), plasma cell leukemia (PCL), and heavy-chain disease.
- Analyze a case study related to immunoproliferation and answer related multiple-choice questions.
- Participate in a discussion of case study–related critical thinking questions.
- Describe the principle and application of the Bence Jones protein screening procedure.
- Correctly answer 80% of end-of-chapter review questions.

OUTLINE

General Characteristics of Gammopathies, 354
    Monoclonal Gammopathies, 354
    Polyclonal Gammopathies, 355
Multiple Myeloma, 355
    Etiology, 355
    Epidemiology, 355
    Pathophysiology, 356
    Signs and Symptoms, 356
        Skeletal Abnormalities, 356
        Hematologic Features, 356
        Renal Disorders, 357
        Neurologic Features, 358
        Infectious Diseases, 358
    Immunologic Manifestations, 358
    Diagnostic Evaluation, 358
    New Diagnostic Criteria, 358
        Hematologic Assessment, 358
        Molecular Testing, 358
        Bence Jones Proteins, 359
        Free Light Chains, 360
        Immunologic Testing, 360
    Prognosis, 361
    Treatment, 362
        Chemotherapy, 362
Plasma Cell Neoplasms With Associated Paraneoplastic Syndrome, 363
    POEMS Syndrome, 363
    TEMPI Syndrome, 363
    AESOP Syndrome, 363
Waldenström Primary Macroglobulinemia, 363
    Etiology, 363
    Epidemiology, 363
    Signs and Symptoms, 363
        Skeletal Features, 363
        Hematologic Abnormalities, 363
        Renal Dysfunction, 364
        Ocular Manifestations, 364
        Neuropsychiatric Problems, 364
        Cardiopulmonary Abnormalities, 364
        Cutaneous Manifestations, 364
    Immunologic Manifestations, 364
    Diagnostic Evaluation, 364
        Hematologic Assessment, 364
        Immunologic Assessment, 364
    Treatment, 365
Other Monoclonal Disorders, 365
    Monoclonal Gammopathy of Undetermined Significance, 365
    Light-Chain Disease, 365
    Heavy-Chain Disease, 365
    Light-Chain Deposition Disease, 365
Case Study 21.1, 365
Procedure: Bence Jones Protein Screening Procedure, 368.e1

KEY TERMS

amyloidosis
Bence Jones (BJ) protein
hypercalcemia
hypergammaglobulinemias
hyperviscosity
light-chain disease (LCD)

M protein
monoclonal gammopathy
multiple myeloma
osteoclasts
paraprotein
plasma cell dyscrasias

polyclonal gammopathy
rouleaux
smoldering multiple myeloma
Waldenström primary macroglobulinemia (WM)

Various plasma cell neoplasms such as plasma cell myeloma (multiple myeloma [MM]) and monoclonal gammopathy have been reorganized by the World Health Organization (WHO) into various diseases with paraproteins in the *WHO Classification of Haematolymphoid Tumours*, 5th edition (2022) (Box 21.1). Representative examples of these diseases are presented here.

> **KEY CONCEPTS: Features of Gammopathies**
> - Hypergammaglobulinemias are monoclonal or polyclonal.
> - A monoclonal gammopathy can be benign or malignant, and results from a single clone of lymphoid plasma cells producing elevated levels of a single class and type of immunoglobulin, referred to as a *monoclonal protein*, *M protein*, or *paraprotein*. These disorders include MM and Waldenström primary macroglobulinemia (WM). MM is the most common form of dysproteinemia.
> - A polyclonal gammopathy is classified as a secondary disease and is characterized by the elevation of two or more immunoglobulins produced by several clones of plasma cells. Polyclonal protein consists of one or more heavy-chain classes; both light-chain types increase as secondary manifestations of infection or inflammation.

BOX 21.1 Plasma Cell Neoplasms and Other Diseases With Paraproteins

Monoclonal Gammopathies
Cold agglutinin disease
IgM monoclonal gammopathy of undetermined significance
Non-IgM monoclonal gammopathy of undetermined significance
Monoclonal gammopathy of renal significance

Diseases With Monoclonal Immunoglobulin Deposition
Immunoglobulin-related (AL) amyloidosis
Monoclonal immunoglobulin deposition disease

Heavy-Chain Diseases
Mu heavy-chain disease
Gamma heavy-chain disease
Alpha heavy-chain disease

Plasma Cell Neoplasms
Plasmacytoma
Plasma cell myeloma
Plasma cell neoplasms with associated paraneoplastic syndrome
- POEMS syndrome
- TEMPI syndrome
- AESOP syndrome

From World Health Organization (WHO) Classification of Haematolymphoid Tumours, B-cell lymphoid proliferations and lymphomas, ed.5, Table 1 Plasma cell neoplasms and other diseases with paraproteins 2022.
AESOP, Adenopathy and extensive skin patch overlying a plasmacytoma; *AL*, amyloid light chain or primary amyloidosis; *POEMS*, Peripheral neuropathy, organ enlargement, endocrine gland dysfunction, monoclonal plasma cell tumors and monoclonal immunoglobulin, skin changes; *TEMPI*, telangiectasias, elevated erythropoietin level and erythrocytosis, monoclonal gammopathy, perinephric fluid collections, and intrapulmonary shunting.

A small number of long-lived plasma cells in the bone marrow (<1% of mononuclear cells) produce most of the immunoglobulins G and A (IgG and IgA) in normal adult serum. These well-differentiated cells do not divide and have a characteristic phenotype: $CD38^{bright}$, $syndecan-1^{bright}$, CD19+, and $CD56^{weak/-}$. Their precursors are slowly proliferating plasmablasts, which migrate to the marrow from lymph nodes after stimulation by antigens and cytokines from helper T (Th) cells in the germinal centers.

Events in the germinal centers initiate somatic mutations of the immunoglobulin genes of B cells and a switch from the production of immunoglobulin M (IgM) to the production of IgG or IgA. After the activated B cells enter the bone marrow, they stop proliferating and differentiate into plasma cells under the influence of adhesion molecules and factors such as interleukin-6 (IL-6). Normal plasma cells die by apoptosis after several weeks or months.

Hypergammaglobulinemias are monoclonal or polyclonal in nature. A monoclonal gammopathy, which can be a benign or malignant condition, results from a single clone of lymphoid plasma cells producing elevated levels of a single class and type of immunoglobulin, referred to as a *monoclonal protein*, M protein, or paraprotein. Disorders in this category of plasma cell dyscrasias include MM and WM. In comparison, a polyclonal gammopathy is classified as a secondary disease and characterized by the elevation of two or more immunoglobulins by several clones of plasma cells.

GENERAL CHARACTERISTICS OF GAMMOPATHIES

Monoclonal Gammopathies

Monoclonal gammopathies are characterized by the production of monoclonal immunoglobulin and are associated with suppressed uninvolved immunoglobulins and dysfunctional T-cell responses. MM is the prototypical monoclonal gammopathy.

Serum and urine electrophoresis and other immunoglobulin assays can demonstrate strikingly abnormal results in disorders such as MM and WM. The gamma region of the electrophoretic pattern can show a dense, highly restricted band from uncontrolled proliferation of one-cell clone, whereas the other normal immunoglobulins are deficient. The clinical interpretation of some patterns can be difficult.

In contrast, some symptomatic patients do not exhibit the characteristic monoclonal band or spike in their serum protein patterns. This is often the case with light-chain disease (LCD), in which only kappa (κ) or lambda (λ) monoclonal light chains are synthesized by the clone. These low-molecular-weight immunoglobulin fragments are filtered through the glomerulus and into the urine, producing a serum electrophoretic pattern that suggests hypogammaglobulinemia, with a very faint monoclonal band or no band at all. These light chains also suggest the presence of a nonsecretory clone, which produces no monoclonal immunoglobulins and frequently demonstrates hypogammaglobulinemia because of the inhibition of normal clones.

Monoclonal gammopathy of renal significance (MGRS) and cold agglutinin disease (CAD) are two new entities that fall under the umbrella of plasma cell neoplasms/other diseases with paraproteins. CAD, IgM, and non-IgM monoclonal gammopathies of unknown significance (MGUS) and MGRS are and were previously grouped as monoclonal gammopathies.

CAD is grouped with other monoclonal gammopathies. This is an autoimmune hemolytic anemia mediated by monoclonal cold agglutinins produced by B-cell lymphoid clonal proliferation.

MGRS is grouped with diseases associated with abnormal monoclonal immunoglobulin deposition. This nonmalignant disorder is classified as a B-cell lymphocyte disorder.

In addition to the previously cited monoclonal gammopathies, there is another related category, monoclonal immunoglobulin deposition. This category includes:
- Immunoglobulin-related (AL) amyloidosis (previously named primary amyloidosis), and
- Monoclonal immunoglobulin deposition disease (previously named light-chain and heavy-chain deposition disease).

Polyclonal Gammopathies

A polyclonal gammopathy is a common protein abnormality. It is defined as an increase in more than one immunoglobulin and involves several clones of plasma cells. In contrast to a monoclonal protein, a polyclonal protein consists of one or more heavy-chain classes and both light-chain types. Polyclonal increases are exhibited as secondary manifestations of infection or inflammation. They are often seen in chronic infections, chronic liver disease (especially chronic active hepatitis), rheumatoid connective tissue (autoimmune) diseases, and lymphoproliferative disorders.

A polyclonal protein is characterized by a broad peak or band, usually of gamma mobility, on electrophoresis, by a thickening and elongation of all heavy-chain and light-chain arcs on immunoelectrophoresis, and by the absence of a localized band on immunofixation. A polyclonal gammopathy resembles a normal pattern, with the serum staining more intensely. In a selective polyclonal increase, only the level of one class of immunoglobulin is significantly elevated. The increase is polyclonal because immunoglobulin is produced by several clones of plasma cells, and both κ and λ types are produced. Immunoglobulin quantitation by specific assay procedures demonstrates which immunoglobulin is increased. Immunofixation is not recommended in cases of polyclonal gammopathy because it presents no additional information.

> **KEY CONCEPTS: Clinical Features of Multiple Myeloma**
> - The cause of MM is unknown, but radiation may be a factor; a viral cause has also been suggested. Other causes may include environmental stimuli or genetic factors.
> - Signs and symptoms of MM include bone pain (back or chest), weakness, fatigue, and pallor associated with anemia or abnormal bleeding.

MULTIPLE MYELOMA

Multiple myeloma is classified as a clonal plasma cell neoplasm associated with abnormal protein production. Plasma cells related to MM include:
- Smoldering MM (SMM)
- IgM monoclonal gammopathy of undetermined significance (IgM-MGUS)
- Non-IgM monoclonal gammopathy of undetermined significance (non–IgM-MGUS)
- Light-chain MGUS
- Solitary plasmacytoma (subtypes solitary plasmacytoma of bone and extramedullary plasmacytoma)
- Solitary plasmacytoma with minimal marrow involvement

MM evolves from a clinically silent premalignant stage, MGUS. However, an intermediate condition between the malignant MM and premalignant MGUS is SMM with a much higher risk of progression to MM compared with MGUS SMM M protein levels of 3g/dL or more and >10% clonal plasma cells in bone marrow. The evidence of end-organ damage exists. MM is a plasma cell neoplasm characterized by the accumulation of malignant plasma cells within the bone marrow microenvironment, monoclonal protein in the blood or urine, and associated organ dysfunction. Normal bone marrow has approximately 1% plasma cells, but in MM the plasma cell concentration can rise to 90%. Bone marrow identification of monoclonal plasma cells by histology is an essential part of MM diagnosis and is frequently based on identifying intracellular κ and λ chains.

Plasma cells produce one of five heavy-chain types together with κ and λ molecules. There is approximately 40% excess production of free light-chain over heavy-chain synthesis to allow proper conformation of the intact immunoglobulin molecules.

Etiology

The precise etiology of MM has not yet been established. Roles have been suggested for a variety of factors, including genetic causes, environmental or occupational causes, MGUS, radiation, chronic inflammation, and infection.

Chromosomal abnormalities are found in at least half of patients with MM. Numerous changes and structural abnormalities, including giant chromosomes, translocations, and deletions, have been associated with plasma cells. MM cells uniformly overexpress CD38. The presence of del(17p), t(4;14), t(14;16), t(14;20), gain 1q, or p53 mutation is considered high risk for MM.

Abnormalities of certain oncogenes, such as *c-myc*, are associated with development early in the course of plasma cell tumors. In addition, abnormalities of oncogenes such as *N-ras* and *K-ras* are associated with development after bone marrow relapse. Abnormalities of tumor suppressor genes, such as *TP53*, have been shown to be associated with spread to other organs. Ongoing research is investigating whether human leukocyte antigen (HLA)-Cw5 or HLA-Cw2 may play a role in the pathogenesis of MM.

New data have emerged concerning the progression from precursor states to plasma cell (multiple) myeloma (PCM). A 1q21 gain is often an early event, and translocations and additional amplifications of 1q21 emerge later during pathogenesis.

Epidemiology

MM is the most common form of dysproteinemia. It accounts for 1% of all types of malignant diseases and 10% of hematologic malignancies. The age-adjusted incidence is estimated to be 5.6 cases per 100,000 population per year in Western countries, and the frequency of myeloma is likely to increase in these countries in the near future as the population ages.

The onset of MM is from 40 to 70 years, with a peak incidence in the seventh decade. It is uncommon (<2% of cases) in patients younger than 40 years. In general, patients with LCD and IgD myeloma are younger than those with IgG or IgA myeloma and have a poorer prognosis due to their high incidence of nephropathy. Males are affected in approximately 62% of cases; the male-to-female ratio is 1.6:1. In addition, Black people are affected twice as often as White people. MM has been reported in two or more first-degree relatives and in identical twins, although no evidence suggests a hereditary basis for the disease.

IgG myeloma is the most common form of MM (Table 21.1). Four subtypes of IgG heavy chains are known to exist among patients with IgG myeloma. The subclasses of cases of IgG myeloma are distributed as follows:

- 65% gamma G1
- 23% gamma G2
- 8% gamma G3
- 4% gamma G4

The only subclass-dependent difference is the greater propensity for patients with IgG3 myeloma to experience hyperviscosity syndrome, similar to the manifestation in WM.

MM runs a progressive course. Most patients die within 1 to 3 years, although newer treatments, including stem cell transplantation, are increasing longevity. The β_2-microglobulin level at initial evaluation has been adopted as a predictor of outcome. If the serum β_2-microglobulin level is elevated at the start of therapy, the prognosis is less favorable. The major causes of death are overwhelming infection (sepsis) and renal insufficiency. In patients with sepsis, mortality exceeds 50%, despite antibiotic therapy.

Pathophysiology

Increasing research evidence suggests that the bone marrow microenvironment of tumor cells plays a pivotal role in the pathogenesis of myelomas. The role of cytokines in the pathogenesis of MM is an important area of research. IL-6 is also an important factor promoting the in vitro growth of myeloma cells. Other cytokines are tumor necrosis factor and IL-1b.

Myelomas arise from an asymptomatic premalignant proliferation of monoclonal plasma cells derived from postgerminal-center B cells. In contrast to normal plasma cells, myeloma cells are often immature and may have the appearance of plasmablasts. These cells usually are CD19–CD56^{bright}, CD38, and syndecan-1, and produce very low amounts of immunoglobulins.

Most patients demonstrate complex karyotype abnormalities with chromosomal gains, deletions, and translocations, some of which are identical to those observed in certain B-cell lymphomas.

Primary early chromosomal translocations occur at the immunoglobulin switch region on chromosome 14 (q32.33). This process results in the deregulation of two adjacent genes. Secondary late-onset translocations and gene mutation are implicated in disease progression and include complex karyotypic abnormalities. These genetic abnormalities may prevent the differentiation and apoptosis of myeloma cells, which continue to proliferate and accumulate in the bone marrow. Chromosomal aberrations are of sufficient number to be detected on flow analysis of DNA content, which is aneuploid in about 80% of patients.

Most patients exhibit a slight nuclear DNA excess of 5% to 10%; hypoploidy is observed in only 5% to 10% of patients and is strongly associated with resistance to standard chemotherapy. Deletions of chromosomes 13 and 17 have been observed. The morphologic immaturity, hypodiploidy, and 13q- and 14q+ abnormalities correlate with the resistance to treatment and short survival that are characteristic of aggressive disease.

The somatic mutations of the immunoglobulin genes of myeloma cells indicate that the putative myeloma cell precursors are stimulated by antigens and are memory B cells or migrating plasmablasts.

Myeloma cells proliferate slowly in the marrow. Less than 1% divide at any one time, and myeloma cells do not differentiate. The absolute number of these cells correlates with disease activity and predicts the progression of disease in smoldering multiple myeloma. Circulating myeloma cells may disseminate the tumor within the bone marrow and elsewhere.

IL-6 is essential for the survival and growth of myeloma cells, which express specific receptors for this cytokine. Initially identified as a growth factor for myeloma cells, IL-6 has been shown to promote the survival of myeloma cells by preventing spontaneous or dexamethasone-induced apoptosis. An increased level of IL-6 in the serum of patients with MM can be explained by the overproduction of IL-6 in the marrow. The IL-6 system also has a role in the pathogenesis of bone lesions in MM. IL-6, soluble IL-6 receptor alpha (sIL-6Rα), and interleukin-1 beta (IL-1β) activate osteoclasts in the vicinity of myeloma cells and thus initiate bone resorption. IL-6 may account for MM-associated anemia and for the lack of thrombocytopenia due to its stimulation of megakaryopoiesis.

Signs and Symptoms

MM is historically defined by the presence of end-organ damage, specifically hypercalcemia, renal failure, anemia, and bone lesions. These are called the CRAB features that can be attributed to the neoplastic process.

The signs and symptoms of MM include bone pain, typically in the back or chest, and weakness, fatigue, and pallor associated with anemia or abnormal bleeding. In all, 20% of patients exhibit hepatomegaly and 5% demonstrate splenomegaly. In some cases, the major manifestations of disease result from acute infection, renal insufficiency, hypercalcemia, or amyloidosis. Weight loss and night sweats are not prominent until the disease is advanced. Bone pain, anemia, and renal insufficiency constitute a triad of signs and symptoms strongly suggestive of MM.

Skeletal Abnormalities

Approximately 90% of patients with MM have broadly disseminated destruction of the skeleton, which is responsible for the predominance of bone pain. These abnormalities consist of punched-out lytic areas (Fig. 21.1), osteoporosis, and fractures in about 80% of patients. The vertebrae, skull, thoracic cage, pelvis, proximal humeri, and femurs are the most frequent sites of involvement.

Hematologic Features

The diagnosis of MM depends on the demonstration of an increased number of plasma cells in bone marrow aspirate and/or biopsy and supporting laboratory results (see the section Diagnostic Evaluation). Although the bone marrow is typically involved, the disorder may

TABLE 21.1 Distribution of Immunoglobulin Types in Patients With Multiple Myeloma.

Type of Protein	Multiple Myeloma (%)
IgM	12
IgG	52
IgA	22
IgD	2
IgE	Rare
Light chains (kappa [κ] or lambda [λ])	11
Heavy chains	Rare
Monoclonal proteins	<1
Nonsecretory myeloma	1

IgA, Immunoglobulin A; *IgD*, immunoglobulin D; *IgE*, immunoglobulin E; *IgG*, immunoglobulin G; *IgM*, immunoglobulin M.

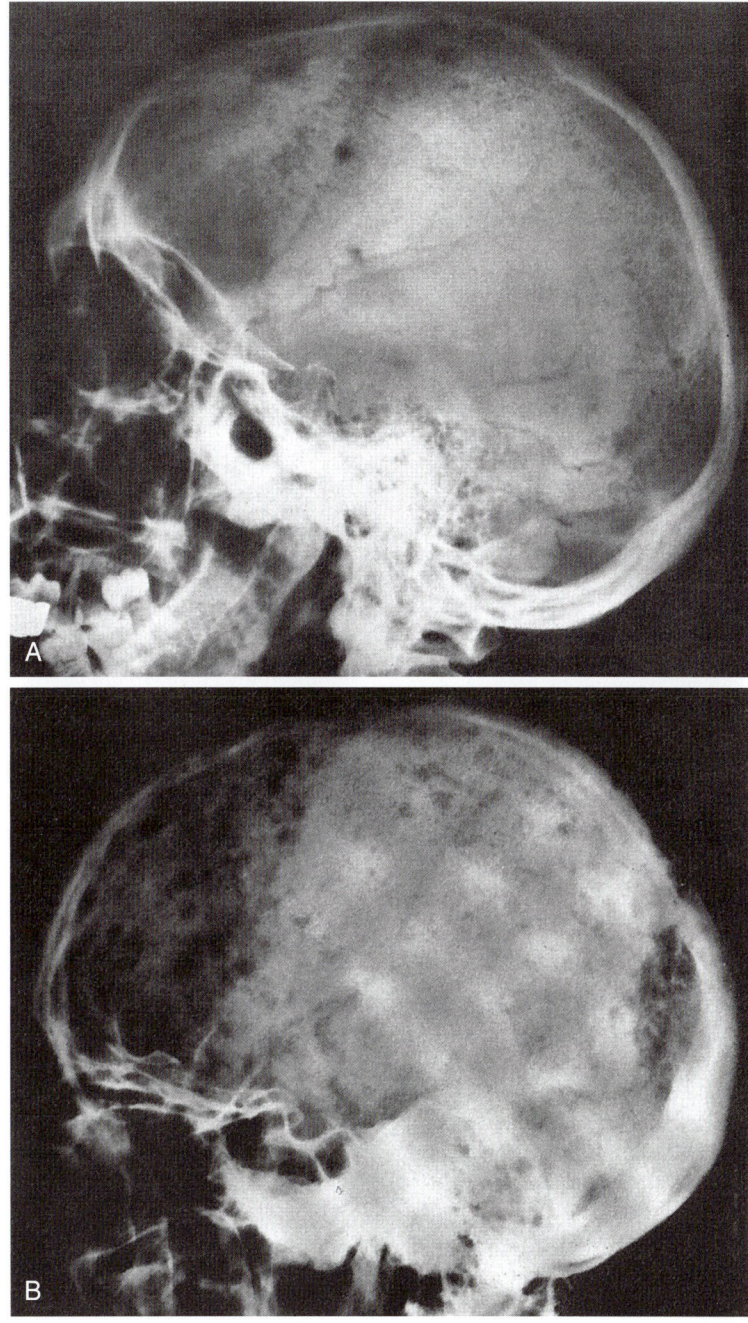

Fig. 21.1 **Multiple Myeloma.** (A) Several scattered, small, well-marginated lytic lesions appear in the calvarium, located in normally mineralized bone. Multiple lytic lesions can also be seen in the mandible. (B) Multiple circumscribed lytic lesions crowd bones throughout the skull. The lesions are still discrete and the margins of most are fairly sharp. (From Newton TH, Potts DG: *Radiology of the skull and brain*, St. Louis, 1971, Mosby.)

involve other tissues. For example, a positive correlation exists between the production of osteoclast-activating factor by bone marrow cells and the extent of skeletal destruction. Other hematologic factors contributing to the signs and symptoms of pallor and anemia include bleeding, qualitative platelet abnormalities, inhibition of coagulation factors by M protein, and thrombocytopenia. Intravascular coagulation may occur.

Renal Disorders

Acute renal failure (ARF) occurs in approximately 5% to 10% of patients. Although ARF may occur at any time in the course of myeloma, it can be the initial manifestation of disease. ARF has been observed after infection, hypercalcemia, dehydration, and IV urography. Serum creatinine levels are elevated in about half of these patients, and approximately one-third have hypercalcemia.

Chronic renal failure is a common development in MM patients. As many as two-thirds of patients display serum creatinine levels higher than 1.5 mg/dL, and 10% to 20% may develop end-stage renal disease (ESRD). Patients with IgD or light-chain myeloma are much more likely to develop renal failure than those with IgG or IgA myeloma. Proteinuria is a common finding, with over half of all MM patients excreting abnormal amounts of Bence Jones (BJ) protein (light chains). Patients with BJ proteinuria are much more likely to have renal tubular defects than those without BJ proteinuria.

Studies have suggested that BJ proteins have a deleterious effect on renal function via at least two mechanisms. First, renal failure may result from intratubular precipitation of BJ protein and subsequent intrarenal obstruction. When the distal collecting tubules become obstructed by large casts consisting mainly of BJ protein, the disorder may be referred to as *myeloma kidney*. The second mechanism of renal failure may be a function of direct tubular cell injury. As a result of these tubular defects, abnormalities in urine-concentrating ability and renal acidification are observed. Although the presence of a large concentration of BJ proteinuria is usually associated with some degree of renal dysfunction, some patients excrete large amounts of BJ protein for years and maintain renal function.

Lambda (λ) light chains have been implicated in nephrotoxicity, but their role has not been firmly established.

Neurologic Features

Pain is a common characteristic of MM, often caused by compression of the spinal cord or nerves. Compression produces back pain, with weakness or paralysis of the lower extremities and bowel or bladder incontinence.

Infectious Diseases

The most frequent cause of death is infection. Patients with MM have increased susceptibility to infectious microorganisms because of an inability to cope with bacterial infections and certain viral diseases. Increased susceptibility principally results from defective antibody synthesis caused by the crowding out and suppression of normal plasma cell precursors.

Repeated bouts of sepsis, often resulting from recurrent infection by microorganisms such as pneumococci or gram-negative bacteria, are common. Pneumonia, pyelonephritis, meningitis, and arthritis are the leading forms of sepsis; when bacteremia ensues, mortality is high.

Immunologic Manifestations

In approximately 20% of patients, MM is diagnosed by chance in the absence of symptoms, usually after screening laboratory studies have revealed an increased serum protein concentration. MM cells express not only cytoplasmic immunoglobulins, the hallmark of plasma cells, but also early B, T, natural killer (NK), myeloid, erythroid, and megakaryocytic cell markers. These phenotypic features are consistent with the hypothesis that MM may originate from a transformed early hematopoietic progenitor cell, which explains the occasional coexistence of MM and acute myelogenous leukemia (AML).

Patients with MM have defects in humoral but not cellular immunity. Humoral immunity is disrupted because plasma cell tumors induce the suppression of antibody synthesis by normal immunoglobulin-secreting cells and the production of antiidiotype antibodies declines proportionately. In addition, selective impairment occurs in the formation of normal antibodies because of increased immunoglobulin catabolism and the release of a protein that incites macrophages to suppress synthesis of normal immunoglobulins by myeloma cells. Depression of normal humoral immunity accounts for the high susceptibility of MM patients to bacterial infection. The normal functioning of cellular immunity is demonstrated by normal resistance to fungal and most viral infections, and by normal delayed-type hypersensitivity to skin-testing antigens.

The most consistent immunologic feature of MM is the incessant synthesis of a dysfunctional single monoclonal protein or of immunoglobulin chains of fragments, with concurrent suppression of the synthesis of normal functional antibody. In 99% of myeloma patients, an M component is usually found in serum, urine, or both.

Diagnostic Evaluation

> **KEY CONCEPTS:** Laboratory Findings in Multiple Myeloma
> - Proteinuria is a common finding in more than 50% of patients excreting abnormal amounts of BJ protein (light chains). Patients have defects in humoral but not cellular immunity.
> - Laboratory diagnosis of MM includes electrophoresis of the serum or urine. A monoclonal protein is seen in the serum and urine in 90% of patients.

New Diagnostic Criteria

Any one or more of the following biomarkers of malignancy or myeloma-defining events (MDEs) are:

1. 60% or greater clonal plasma cells on bone marrow examination;
2. Serum involved/uninvolved free light-chain ratio of 100 or greater, provided the absolute level of the involved light chain is at least 100mg/L (a patient's involved free light chain [FLC], either κ or λ, is the one that is above the normal reference range; the uninvolved FLC is the one that is typically in, or below, the normal range);
3. More than one focal lesion on magnetic resonance imaging (MRI) that is at least 5 mm or greater in size.

Hematologic Assessment

Normochromic normocytic anemia is present in about two-thirds of patients at diagnosis. In part, anemia is related to the hypervolemia caused by the increase in plasma volume from monoclonal protein production. Rouleaux formation is a common finding in peripheral blood smears. The leukocyte count can be normal, although about one-third of patients have leukopenia. Relative lymphocytosis is usually present. If lymphocyte subsets are examined, a reduction in CD4+ (helper) and an increase in CD8+ (suppressor-cytotoxic) blood lymphocytes can be noted. Defects in the proliferative responses of lymphocytes to mitogens or antigens are explained by the large portion of B cells in MM that originate from the malignant stem cell clone. Few mature plasma cells are seen in the circulation except at the terminal phase of the disease, but the covert presence of the malignant B-cell clone can be unmasked by the laboratory use of monoclonal antibodies (MAbs) or by transforming agents such as phorbol esters. In rare cases, in the terminal stages plasmablasts and proplasmacytes may amount to 50% of the leukocytes in the peripheral blood.

Bleeding is common. Platelet abnormalities, impaired aggregation of platelets, and interference with platelet function by the abnormal monoclonal protein contribute to bleeding. Inhibitors of coagulation factors and thrombocytopenia from marrow infiltration of plasma cells or chemotherapy may also contribute to bleeding. Some patients have a tendency toward thrombosis, which may manifest as a shortened coagulation time and increased levels of fibrinogen and factor VIII.

Diagnosis of MM, however, depends on the demonstration of an increased number (>10%) of plasma cells in a bone marrow aspirate (Fig. 21.2) and/or biopsy and supporting laboratory results.

Molecular Testing

Baseline cytogenetic analysis or fluorescent in situ hybridization (FISH) of bone marrow aspirate is essential. Testing must be done with either cytoplasmic immunoglobulin-enhanced FISH or FISH carried out on the nuclei from purified plasma cells. A minimum FISH panel should include t(4;14)(p16;q32), t(14;16)(q32;q23), and 17p13 deletions. A more comprehensive panel should include testing for t(11;14)(q13;q32), chromosome 13 deletion, and chromosome 1 abnormalities.

Newer clinical investigations are stratifying patients with MM into so-called good-risk, intermediate-risk, and high-risk groups based on genetic aberrations detected by interphase fluorescence in situ hybridization (iFISH) (Table 21.2). Genetic abnormalities that reflect disease progression include deletion of 17p13 and chromosome 1 abnormalities (1p deletion and 1q amplification).

Bence Jones Proteins

BJ proteins have been important diagnostic markers for MM since the mid-19th century (see online, Procedure, Bence Jones Protein Screening). In about 10% of MM patients, only BJ proteins are produced, with no complete IgM, IgG, or IgA. BJ proteins are single-peptide chains with a molecular weight of 20 to 22 kDa, but dimerization occurs spontaneously to form molecules of 40 to 44 kDa.

BJ proteins are monoclonal κ or λ immunoglobulin FLCs not attached to the heavy-chain portion of the immunoglobulin molecule. BJ proteins are seen in two types of syndromes:
- With a typical monoclonal gammopathy
- In free LCD

Serum concentrations of FLCs depend on the balance between production by plasma cells and their precursors, and on renal clearance. If there is increased polyclonal immunoglobulin production and/or renal impairment, both κ and λ FLC concentrations can increase by 30% to 40%. Serum FLC tests have been assuming an increasing role in the detection and monitoring of monoclonal gammopathies. Serum FLCs have a short half-life in the blood (κ, 2–4 hours; λ, 3–6 hours) compared with 21 days for IgG molecules. FLC concentrations allow more rapid assessment of the effects of chemotherapy than monoclonal IgG levels.

Very small amounts of BJ proteins in serum can be associated with significant clinical problems, especially pathologic renal changes. FLCs filter through the glomeruli almost without obstruction due to their small molecular size and accumulate in the tubules. Renal impairment can result from the toxicity of FLCs. Pathologic changes can range from relatively benign tubular proteinuria to ARF or amyloidosis.

BJ proteins can be detected in serum, urine, or both. The level of monoclonal light chains in serum or urine is related to filtration, resorption, or catabolism of the protein by the kidneys. During the early stages of renal disease, when the kidneys are only mildly affected, excretion and reabsorption continue normally, but only partial catabolism occurs. At this point, BJ proteins may be detected in the serum but not in the urine. Progressive renal involvement impairs reabsorption, and diminished reabsorption with decreased catabolism results in FLCs in serum and urine. Later, as resorption is totally blocked, FLCs are present in urine only. In terminal stages of renal disease, uremia occurs, renal clearance is affected, and BJ proteins again appear in the serum.

BJ proteins are unusual in their response to heating. They are soluble at room temperature, become insoluble (form a precipitate around 60°C–70°C [140°F–158°F]), and then dissolve at 100°C (212°F). This pattern reverses when the temperature is lowered, which is unique to BJ protein.

Serologically, all BJ proteins are not identical, although there are κ and λ types. BJ proteins will react with antisera to the λ chains of IgG, and λ chains react with antisera to BJ protein.

Approximately 80% of patients with MM produce intact immunoglobulin monoclonal proteins, of which 46% have excess monoclonal FLCs in the urine by immunofixation electrophoresis (IFE). Serum protein electrophoresis is positive less often because of the low serum concentrations of FLCs. Between 3% and 4% of MM patients have nonsecretory disease, and these patients have no detectable monoclonal proteins with serum and urine electrophoretic testing because their tumor cells produce small amounts of monoclonal protein. Their FLC

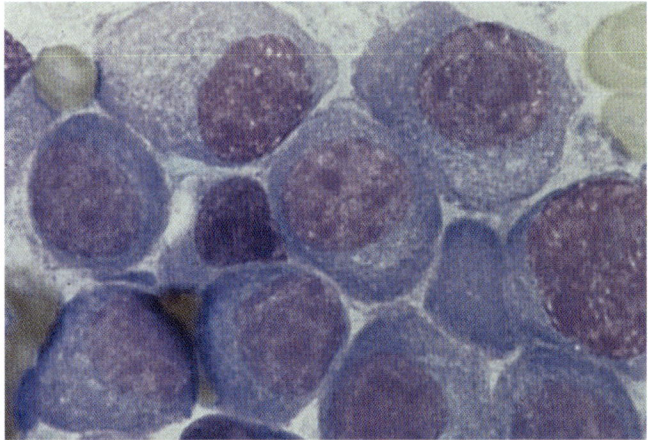

Fig. 21.2 Myeloma cells in a bone marrow aspirate. (From Nairn R, Helvert M: *Immunology for medical students*, ed 2, St. Louis, 2007, Elsevier.)

TABLE 21.2 Correlation of Cytogenetic Findings With Level of Risk, Disease Characteristics, and Median Years of Survival.

Risk Group	Cytogenetic Findings	Disease Characteristics	Median Survival (Years)
Good risk	Has any of the following cytogenetic findings: (1) no adverse FISH or cytogenetics, (2) hyperdiploidy, (3) t(11;14) by FISH, or (4) t(6;14) by FISH	These patients most often have: (1) disease that expresses IgG kappa monoclonal gammopathies, and (2) lytic bone lesions	8–10
Intermediate risk	t(4;14) by FISH	These patients often have IgA lambda monoclonal gammopathies and less bone disease	5
High risk	Has any of the following cytogenetic findings: (1) del 17p by FISH, (2) t(14;16) by FISH, (3) t(4;14), (4) t(14;20), (5) cytogenetic del 13, (6) nonhyperdiploidy without adverse cytogenetic findings, (7) 1q gain, or (8) plasma cell leukemia	These patients have: (1) disease that expresses IgA lambda monoclonal gammopathies (often), and (2) skeletal-related complications (less often)	<2

FISH, Fluorescence in situ hybridization; *IgA*, Immunoglobulin A; *IgG*, immunoglobulin G.
From the National Cancer Institute. https://www.cancer.gov. Updated July, 2019.

concentrations are below the sensitivity of serum electrophoretic tests and below the threshold for clearance into the urine. These patients can be monitored by serum FLC tests rather than by repeated bone marrow biopsies or whole-body scans.

Free Light Chains

FLCs are incorporated into immunoglobulin molecules during B-lymphocyte development and expressed initially on the surface of immature B cells. Production of FLCs occurs throughout the rest of B-cell development and in plasma cells, in which secretion is highest. Tumors associated with the different stages of B-cell maturation will secrete monoclonal FLCs into the serum, where they may be detected by FLC immunoassays (Box 21.2 and Table 21.3).

Production of FLCs in normal individuals is approximately 500 mg/day from bone marrow and lymph node cells. The molecules enter the blood and are readily partitioned between the intravascular and extravascular compartments. In normal individuals, serum FLCs are rapidly cleared and metabolized by the kidneys, depending on their molecular size.

Immunologic Testing

Traditionally, laboratories have detected monoclonal immunoglobulins by protein electrophoresis, which was introduced in the 1930s, and have characterized the proteins by IFE, which was developed in the 1980s.

The identification of κ and λ molecules has been accomplished with the use of antibodies specific to each type of protein. Immunodiffusion was initially used, followed by immunoelectrophoresis (in 1953),

---

BOX 21.2 Benefits of Serum-Free Light-Chain Immunoassays

- Better sensitivity and precision than current electrophoretic assays
- Numeric results for disease monitoring
- Convenience of serum as a test medium
- Identification of amyloidosis and nonsecretory multiple myeloma (NSMM) patients who have detectable monoclonal proteins by conventional tests
- More accurate marker of complete disease remission than existing assays
- Short half-life marker for rapid assessment of treatment responses
- Identification of progression risk in individuals with monoclonal gammopathy of undetermined significance (MGUS)
- Better screening of symptomatic patients

Modified from Bradwell AR: *Serum free light chain analysis*, Birmingham, UK, 2006, Binding Site Group.

TABLE 21.3 Assays for Free Light Chains.

Assay	Advantages	Disadvantages
Total urine protein	Simple, inexpensive, widely used	Inadequate sensitivity for FLC detection
Urine dipstick	Simple, inexpensive, widely used	Most dipsticks will pick up albumin but may not detect low concentrations of FLCs
Serum protein electrophoresis	Simple, manual, or semiautomated method Well established, inexpensive Monoclonal bands detected Quantitative results with scanning	Insensitive (<500–2000 mg/L) Cannot detect FLCs at low concentration Subjective interpretation of results
Urine protein electrophoresis	Simple, manual, or semiautomated method Well established, inexpensive Monoclonal bands detected Sensitive in concentrated urine (10 mg/L) Quantitative results with scanning	Subjective interpretation of results Urine may require concentration, with possible protein loss False bands from concentrating urine Heavy proteinuria obscures results Cumbersome 24-hour urine collection
IFE on serum and urine	Well established Good sensitivity for serum, very sensitive for concentrated urine (5–30 mg/L)	Nonquantitative Serum sensitivity (150 mg/L) inadequate for normal serum FLC levels Rather laborious to perform Visual interpretation may be difficult Expensive use of antisera Cannot be used to quantify monoclonal immunoglobulins because of precipitating antibody
Capillary zone electrophoresis	Automated technology Quantitative	Less sensitive (400 mg/L) than IFE for serum FLCs Can fail to detect 5% of positive samples (false negatives)
Total serum κ and λ assays	Automated immunoassay	Not sensitive enough for routine testing Specificity inadequate for detecting many patients with LCMM
Freelite serum FLC assays	Automated immunoassay Quantitative Sensitive (<1 mg/L) Widely used 100% diagnostic sensitivity for LCMM	Use in combination with SPE/CZE to screen for monoclonal proteins Modified reference range required for patients with renal impairment

CZE, Capillary zone electrophoresis; *FLC*, free light chains; *IFE*, immunofixation electrophoresis; *LCMM*, light-chain multiple myeloma; *SPE*, serum protein electrophoresis.
Adapted from Bradwell AR: *Serum free light chain analysis*, Birmingham, UK, 2006, Binding Site Group Limited.

> **BOX 21.3 Monoclonal Gammopathies**
>
> 1. Malignant monoclonal gammopathies
>   a. Multiple myeloma (IgG, IgA, IgD, IgE, and free light chains)
>   b. Plasmacytoma
>   c. Malignant lymphoproliferative diseases
>   d. Heavy-chain diseases
>   e. Amyloidosis
> 2. Monoclonal gammopathies of undetermined significance
>   a. Benign (IgG, IgA, IgD, IgM, and, rarely, free light chains)
>   b. Associated with neoplasms of cell types not known to produce monoclonal proteins
>   c. Biclonal gammopathies

radial immunodiffusion, and ultimately nephelometry and turbidimetry. An automated nephelometric assay, described in 2001, represented a major breakthrough. This methodology allows for the quantitation of both κ and λ FLCs and can be performed using automated chemistry analyzers.

Each monoclonal protein (M protein or paraprotein) consists of two heavy-chain polypeptides of the same class and subclass and two light-chain polypeptides of the same type. A monoclonal protein is characterized by a narrow peak or localized band on electrophoresis, by a thickened, bowed arc on immunoelectrophoresis, and by a localized band on immunofixation. Many different entities are associated with M proteins (Box 21.3).

Electrophoresis of the serum or urine reveals a tall, sharp peak on the densitometer tracing or a dense localized band in most cases of MM (Fig. 21.3). A monoclonal protein is demonstrable in the serum and urine of 90% of patients. In all, 60% of patients exhibit IgG, 20% IgA, 10% light chain only (BJ proteinemia), and 1% IgD. Electrophoresis of urine shows a globulin peak in 75% of cases, mainly albumin in 10% of patients, and a normal pattern in 15%. When an M spike is observed on serum protein electrophoresis, the suggested sequence of testing includes testing by immunoelectrophoresis and immunofixation (Table 21.4). Screening for cryoglobulins and viscosity may also be warranted.

Immunoelectrophoresis, also called *gamma globulin electrophoresis* or *immunoglobulin electrophoresis*, is a method of determining the blood levels of three major immunoglobulins—IgM, IgG, and IgA—based on their combined electrophoresis and immunologic properties (see Chapter 9). Immunoelectrophoresis is also used frequently to diagnose MM, which affects the bone marrow. Some drugs may cause increased immunoglobulin levels. Immunizations within the prior 6 months can lead to increased immunoglobulin levels that result in false-positive results.

Note: Matrix-assisted laser desorption ionization time of flight mass spectrophotometry coupled to immune enrichment (MASS-FIX) as an alternative to serum IFE has demonstrated increased sensitivity in monoclonal protein detection. Urine IFE can be replaced with u-MASS-FIX as a reliable alternative. This replacement results in detosylation and detection of light-chain glycosylation and monoclonal tracking between serum and urine. In addition, another benefit of u-MAS-FIX is the elimination of the need to concentrate urine for u-IFE, which increases testing productivity.

Prognosis

A new staging system has been developed by the International Myeloma Foundation. Potential prognostic factors were evaluated using various statistical techniques. Serum β2 microglobulin (Sβ2M), serum albumin, platelet count, serum creatinine, and age emerged as

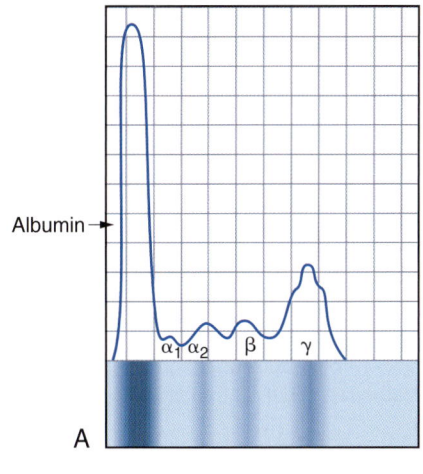

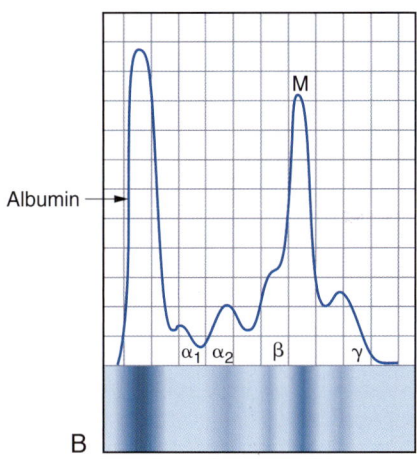

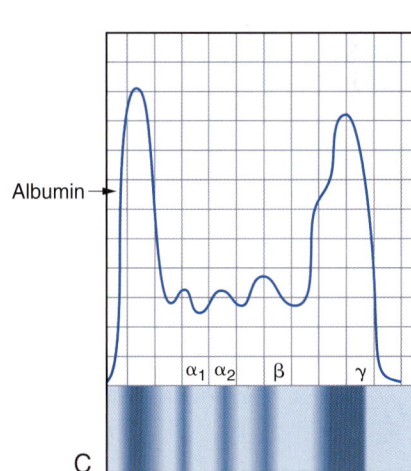

Fig. 21.3 Serum Electrophoretic Patterns. (A) Normal patient. (B) Patient with multiple myeloma. (C) Patient with Waldenström macroglobulinemia.

powerful predictors of survival and were then further analyzed. A combination of serum β2 microglobulin and serum albumin provided the most powerful, simple, and reproducible three-stage classification.

Accurate prognostic determination of the disease course allows for a more rational selection and sequencing of therapy approaches. In August 2015, the Revised International Staging System (R-ISS) (Table 21.5) for MM was published to incorporate two further prognostic factors: genetic risk as assessed by FISH, and level of lactate dehydrogenase (LDH) level.

Stage I indicates a less aggressive disease, and stage III indicates an aggressive disease that may affect bone, kidneys, and other organs.

Treatment

MM treatments can include interventional and/or supportive treatments. Interventional treatments include:

Chemotherapy

- Autologous or allogeneic stem cell transplantation
- Immunomodulatory agents, for example, lenalidomide (Revlimid), pomalidomide (Pomalyst)
- Proteasome inhibitors (PIs), for example, bortezomib (Velcade), carfilzomib (Kyprolis), ixazomib (Ninlaro)
- Histone deacetylase (HDAC) inhibitors, for example, panobinostat (Farydak)
- MAbs, for example, daratumumab (DARZALEX), elotuzumab (Empliciti)
- Corticosteroids, for example, dexamethasone, prednisone
- Radiation

TABLE 21.4 Suggested Sequence of Immunologic Testing for Monoclonal Proteins.

M Spike on Serum Protein Electrophoresis
Serum
Immunoelectrophoresis
Immunofixation
Quantitation of immunoglobulins by radial immunodiffusion or nephelometry
Screening for cryoglobulins
Determination of serum viscosity if IgM, IgA, or IgG or signs and symptoms suggestive of hyperviscosity

IgA, Immunoglobulin A; *IgG*, immunoglobulin G; *IgM*, immunoglobulin M.

The microenvironment of MM is important. Mature B-cell malignancies, including MM, rely heavily on their microenvironment for growth and survival (Fig. 21.4). Healthy bone marrow supports long-lived plasma cells. MM plasma cells establish tight interactions with most of the bone marrow components. The severance of these ties to the bone marrow environment is essential to the impact of therapeutic drugs. The main mechanism of action of thalidomide, lenalidomide, and bortezomib is their impact on the interactions between MM cells and their bone marrow microenvironment, including the extracellular matrix and the cellular component.

Supportive treatments include bisphosphonates to strengthen and reduce the risk of fractures in weakened bones, plasmapheresis to remove abnormal proteins from the blood circulation, and surgery

TABLE 21.5 Revised International Staging System (R-ISS) for Multiple Myeloma.

Stage	Criteria
I	Sβ2M <3.5 mg/l
	Serum albumin ≥3.5 g/dl
	Standard-risk CAs by iFISH
	Normal LDH
II	Not R-ISS stage I or III
III	Sβ2M ≥5.5 mg/L and either:
	High-risk CA by FISH
	OR
	High LDH

CA, chromosomal abnormality; *iFISH*, interphase fluorescence in situ hybridization; *LDH*, lactate dehydrogenase; *Sβ2M*, serum β2 microglobulin.

© 2024, International Myeloma Foundation. All rights reserved.

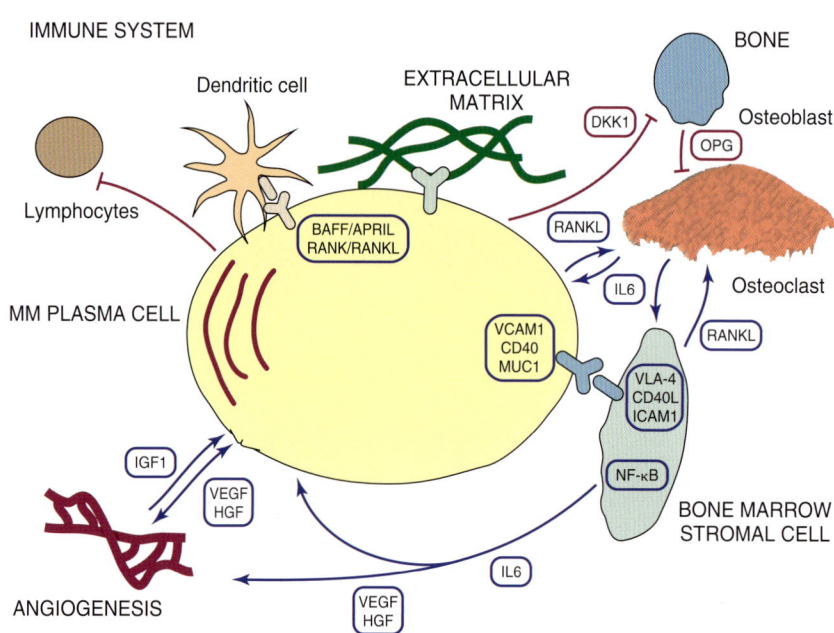

Fig. 21.4 A simplified view of the interaction between the multiple myeloma plasma cell and the surrounding environment. *BAFF*, B-cell–activating factor; *DKK1*, Dickkopf-related protein 1; *HGF*, human growth factor; *IGF1*, insulin-like growth factor; *IL-6*, interleukin-6; *MM*, multiple myeloma; *OPG*, osteoprotegerin; *RANKL*, receptor activator of nuclear factor kappa-B ligand; *VEGF*, vascular endothelial growth factor. (Mendelsohn J, Gray J, Howley P, et al: *The molecular basis of cancer*, St. Louis, 2015, Elsevier.)

may be used to remove individual bone tumors. Surgery may also be needed to prevent or treat fractures.

PLASMA CELL NEOPLASMS WITH ASSOCIATED PARANEOPLASTIC SYNDROME

POEMS Syndrome

POEMS syndrome is a paraneoplastic syndrome caused by an underlying plasma cell neoplasm. The acronym is derived from:
- **P**eripheral neuropathy
- **O**rgan enlargement
- **E**ndocrine gland dysfunction
- **M**onoclonal plasma cell tumors and monoclonal immunoglobulin production
- **S**kin changes

The major criteria for the syndrome are polyradiculoneuropathy, clonal plasma cell disorder (PCD), sclerotic bone lesions, elevated vascular endothelial growth factor, and the presence of Castleman disease. Minor features include organomegaly, endocrinopathy, characteristic skin changes, papilledema, extravascular volume overload, and thrombocytosis.

The diagnosis of POEMS syndrome is made with three of the major criteria, two of which must include polyradiculoneuropathy and clonal PCD, and at least one of the minor criteria.

TEMPI Syndrome

TEMPI (**t**elangiectasias, **e**levated erythropoietin level and erythrocytosis, **m**onoclonal gammopathy, **p**erinephric fluid collections, and **i**ntrapulmonary shunting) syndrome is a rare and newly defined multisystemic disease that belongs to "monoclonal gammopathy of clinical significance". Due to its rarity, the etiology, pathogenesis, and clinical features of this disease remain largely unknown. Most patients have normal bone marrow activity; however, some exhibit erythroid hyperplasia and low levels of light-chain–restricted plasma cells.

AESOP Syndrome

AESOP syndrome (**a**denopathy and **e**xtensive **s**kin patch **o**verlying a **p**lasmacytoma). Is characterized by diffuse hyperplasia of dermal vessels in skin biopsies with associated dermal mucin in the surrounding tissue.

WALDENSTRÖM PRIMARY MACROGLOBULINEMIA

> **KEY CONCEPTS: Waldenström Macroglobulinemia**
> - WM has an indolent progression over many years. The basic abnormality is uncontrolled proliferation of B lymphocytes and plasma cells.
> - Laboratory diagnosis of WM involves serum electrophoresis showing a homogeneous M component composed of monoclonal IgM. Blood samples characteristically display hyperviscosity. In addition, cryoglobulins can be detected.
> - WM is a malignant cell disorder that exhibits abnormally large amounts of 19S IgM. The cause is unknown, but a genetic predisposition may exist.

Etiology

Waldenström primary macroglobulinemia (WM), or simply macroglobulinemia, is a B-cell disorder characterized by the infiltration of lymphoplasmacytic cells into bone marrow and the presence of an IgM monoclonal gammopathy. WM is considered a lymphoplasmacytic lymphoma, as defined by the Revised European American Lymphoma (REAL) and WHO classification systems. WM is a malignant lymphocyte–plasma cell proliferative disorder that exhibits abnormally large amounts of immunoglobulin of the 19S IgM type.

The cause of WM is unknown, but a possible genetic predisposition may exist. Approximately 20% of WM patients have a familial predisposition to the disease and related B-cell malignancies. Greater frequencies of IgM monoclonal proteins and quantitative abnormalities have been observed in some relatives of patients with WM. In addition, research has suggested a significantly increased risk of WM after infections, for example, hepatitis B virus, HIV, and some members of the genus *Rickettsia*. Rocky Mountain spotted fever (RMSF).

Because WM is a malignant offshoot of B-cell development before the myelomas, the sole gene product is IgM. Patients with WM have chromosomal rearrangements that are characteristic of B-cell neoplasia, including t(8:14) and trisomy 12.

Epidemiology

WM occurs about 10% as frequently as MM. WM has an age-specific incidence; it is most often found in older individuals, with a mean age of onset of 60 to 64 years. No significant gender differences exist in the incidence of WM. Disease onset is usually insidious; median survival is approximately 3 years after diagnosis.

Signs and Symptoms

The signs and symptoms of WM have an indolent progression over many years. Initially disease onset is slow and insidious, with the pace of manifestations determined by the rate of proliferation of the IgM-secreting clone. Most clinical signs and symptoms of disease stem from intravascular accumulation of high levels of IgM macroglobulin. When IgM is precipitable at cold temperatures, as it is in 37% of cases, clinical manifestations of cold sensitivity such as Raynaud phenomenon, arthralgias, purpura of the extremities, renal insufficiency, and peripheral vascular occlusions may develop. Cold hypersensitivity can occur when serum IgM levels exceed 2 to 3 g/dL and the protein precipitates at temperatures exceeding 20°C (68°F).

Although the patient experiences weakness and fatigue, it is usually the onset of bleeding from the gums or nose that arouses concern. Patients undergo weight loss, and the incidence of infection is twice the normal rate. As the disease progresses, about 40% of patients develop hepatomegaly, splenomegaly, and lymphadenopathy. Occasionally, the clinical manifestations may simulate those of diffuse lymphoma. Specific dysfunctions and abnormalities occur in a variety of body systems.

Skeletal Features

In contrast to MM, bone pain is almost nonexistent in WM. Diffuse osteoporosis may be seen, but bone lesions are extremely rare.

Hematologic Abnormalities

Patients with WM usually have chronic anemia and bleeding episodes. Bleeding problems in the form of bruising; purpura; and bleeding from the mouth, gums, nose, and gastrointestinal tract are common. The quantities of circulating platelets may be normal or decreased, but the most notable alteration is a disturbance in platelet function. Therefore thrombocytopenia or hyperviscosity may contribute to the bleeding disorder.

In addition to anemia caused by chronic or recurrent bleeding, the decrease in red blood cells (RBCs) becomes more severe as the disease progresses because of a dilutional effect caused by increased immunoglobulin production. In addition, the presence of macroglobulin produces an increased erythrocyte sedimentation rate (ESR). Microscopic examination of a peripheral blood smear usually reveals normocytic and frequently hypochromic RBCs with a striking rouleaux (rolled coin) formation. The total blood leukocyte count is normal or slightly decreased because of moderate neutropenia. In a terminal patient, the blood may be inundated with malignant lymphoplasmacytic cells.

Renal Dysfunction
Renal function becomes mildly or moderately impaired in approximately 15% of WM patients. Nephrosis is uncommon. BJ proteinuria, however, is present in approximately 70% of WM patients, although the quantity of light chains excreted is much less than in MM.

Glomerular lesions are the predominant form of renal injury. IgM collects on the endothelial side of the basement membrane of the kidney; sometimes these macroglobulin accumulations obstruct glomerular capillaries.

Ocular Manifestations
Blurred vision is a frequent abnormality of WM. Rouleaux induced by elevations of IgM causes distention of veins and capillaries; retinal oxygenation diminishes as rouleaux-inducing IgM rises. As a result of increased IgM levels, retinal hemorrhage, exudate formation, and varicosities develop, which can lead to more permanent retinal damage unless IgM levels are lowered by therapy.

Neuropsychiatric Problems
The most common serious neurologic consequence of the slowed cerebral perfusion caused by macroglobulinemia is acute cerebral malfunction, beginning with headache, fluctuating confusion, forgetfulness, and slowed mentation. This can progress to somnolence, stupor, and coma-diffuse brain syndrome, sometimes termed *coma paraproteinemia*. Neurologic abnormalities can be improved by a reduction in plasma viscosity.

Polyneuropathy affects 5% to 10% of patients with WM. This condition is associated with an increase in spinal fluid protein and deposits of monoclonal IgM on myelin sheaths. Monoclonal IgM found in the plasma and attached to damaged nerves has been shown in some cases to share idiotypic determinants. This suggests that the polyneuropathy of WM may be an autoimmune process caused by monoclonal IgM possessing antibody activity for a component of nerve tissue.

Cardiopulmonary Abnormalities
Congestive heart failure becomes a serious problem in patients with chronic uncontrolled WM. Approximately 90% of IgM remains trapped in the circulating plasma and exerts an unbalanced transendothelial osmotic effect sufficient to cause marked expansion of the plasma volume. This in turn creates a dilutional anemia and augments cardiac filling and cardiac output. As a result, increased cardiac output and blood viscosity overwork the myocardium.

About 10% of patients develop pulmonary lesions. Pulmonary tumors, diffuse infiltrates, and pleural involvement are all roughly equally represented. The signs and symptoms of pulmonary dysfunction include coughing and dyspnea.

Cutaneous Manifestations
Cold sensitivity is a frequent manifestation of WM; however, skin lesions are uncommon. A small number of patients develop flat, violaceous, macular skin lesions resulting from dense infiltration by lymphoplasmacytoid cells. Pink, pearly-looking papules caused by dense deposits of IgM may be seen.

Immunologic Manifestations
The basic abnormality in this macroglobulinemia is uncontrolled proliferation of B lymphocytes and plasma cells. As a result, there is a heavy accumulation of monoclonal IgM in the circulating plasma and plasmacytoid lymphocytes in the bone marrow.

In many cases, WM is associated with mixed cryoglobulinemia, which reflects the binding of IgG or IgA antiidiotypic antibody to the mutant IgM. In a small number of patients, dysplastic tumor cells secrete 7S IgM monomers, mu (μ) chains, or other monoclonal immunoglobulins or fragments. Therefore the major IgM production indicates that the immunoglobulin (gene) lesion sometimes degenerates and codes for more than one M component.

Diagnostic Evaluation
Hematologic Assessment
Microscopic examination of a bone marrow aspirate reveals that the lymphoplasmacytic cells vary morphologically from small lymphocytes to obvious plasma cells. Frequently the cellular cytoplasm is ragged and may contain material staining positive with periodic acid-Schiff (PAS) stain, probably identical to the circulating macroglobulin.

The total peripheral blood leukocyte count is usually normal, with an absolute lymphocytosis. Moderate-to-severe degrees of anemia are frequently observed on peripheral blood smears, as is rouleaux formation. The patient's plasma volume may be greatly increased, and the ESR is also increased.

Platelet counts are usually normal. Faulty platelet aggregation and release of platelet factor 3 are caused by the nonspecific coating of platelets by IgM. The most common coagulation defect is a prolonged thrombin time, resulting from the binding of M component to fibrin monomers and consequent gel clotting of IgM-coated fibrin. Bleeding abnormalities can be demonstrated by the following:
- Faulty platelet adhesiveness
- Defective platelet aggregation
- Abnormal release of platelet factor 3
- Impaired clot retraction
- Prolonged bleeding time
- Positive tourniquet test
- Prolonged thrombin-prothrombin time test
- Decreased levels of factor VIII

Immunologic Assessment
Serum electrophoresis usually demonstrates the overproduction of IgM (19S) antibodies. Diagnosis is made by the demonstration of a homogeneous M component composed of monoclonal IgM. Quantitation of immunoglobulins reveals IgM levels ranging from 1 to 12 g/dL (usually >3 g/dL), accounting for 20% to 70% of total protein. Characteristically, blood samples are described as having hyperviscosity.

In addition, cryoglobulins can be detected in the patient's serum. Cryoglobulins are proteins that precipitate or gel when cooled to 0°C (32°F) and dissolve when heated. In most cases, monoclonal cryoglobulins are IgM or IgG. Occasionally, the macroglobulin cryoprecipitable may precipitate at cold temperatures and be capable of cold-induced, anti–I-mediated agglutination of RBCs. IgM may also occasionally be pyroglobulin, which precipitates on heating to 50°C to 60°C (122°F–140°F) but does not redissolve on cooling or intensified heating, as do typical BJ pyroglobulins. Many cryoglobulins have the ability to fix complement and initiate an inflammatory reaction similar to that of antigen-antibody complexes. Cryoglobulins have been classified into the following three types:
- Type I is composed of a single class. IgM and IgG classes are most common; IgA or light-chain, single cryoglobulins are seen less frequently. Type I constitutes about 25% of cryoglobulins and is generally associated with MM, macroglobulinemia, and other, rarer neoplastic proliferations of plasma cells and lymphocytes.

- Type II cryoglobulins consist of two forms. The monoclonal form always has rheumatoid factor activity and usually is an IgM with κ light chains. The second form is polyclonal IgG, which reacts with the monoclonal IgM rheumatoid factor.
- Type III is a mixed cryoglobulin in which both constituent immunoglobulins are polyclonal. More than 90% of type III cryoglobulins contain IgM rheumatoid factor and IgG. Type III cryoglobulins are seen in a variety of autoimmune, systemic rheumatic diseases and persistent infections with immune complexes (e.g., bacterial endocarditis).

Treatment
Some patients undergo plasmapheresis to reverse or prevent symptoms.

Many drugs can be used to treat WM; these include single agents, such as rituximab, chlorambucil, cladribine, fludarabine, bortezomib, or bendamustine. These drugs can be administered alone and in various combinations.

Various therapies can be used or reused, depending on length of remission, patient age, stem cell transplant eligibility, or previous toxicities. Several new drugs and drug combinations are being studied in clinical trials. Today's scientific research is continuously evolving and may change treatment options.

OTHER MONOCLONAL DISORDERS

Monoclonal Gammopathy of Undetermined Significance
MGUS represents the presence of a monoclonal protein in patients with no features of MM or related malignant disorders (e.g., WM, B-cell lymphoma, chronic lymphocytic leukemia). MGUS was originally considered a benign monoclonal gammopathy, but it is now known that this disorder can evolve into a malignant monoclonal gammopathy.

The International Myeloma Working Group has established the differences between MGUS and plasma cell neoplasms (Table 21.6). Characteristics of MGUS include the following:
- Serum monoclonal protein concentration less than 3 g/dL
- Fewer than 10% plasma cells in the bone marrow
- Absence of lytic bone lesions
- Anemia
- Hypercalcemia
- Renal insufficiency
- No clinical signs or symptoms related to the monoclonal gammopathy

The incidence of MGUS increases with age and the median age at diagnosis is approximately 70 years. MGUS occurs more frequently in men than women, and more often in Black individuals than in White individuals. IgG is the most common immunoglobulin affected, followed by IgM. The cause is unknown.

> **KEY CONCEPTS: Other Monoclonal Disorders**
> - Other monoclonal disorders include LCD, which represents about 10% to 15% of monoclonal gammopathies. In LCD, only κ or λ monoclonal light chains or BJ proteins are produced.
> - Heavy-chain disease is characterized by monoclonal proteins composed of the heavy-chain portion of the immunoglobulin molecule.

Light-Chain Disease
LCD represents about 10% to 15% of monoclonal gammopathies, ranking behind IgG and IgA myelomas, which represent about 60% and 15%, respectively. LCD occurs about as frequently as WM. In LCD, only κ or λ monoclonal light chains or BJ proteins are produced.

Diagnostic evaluation of suspected LCD is similar to the protocol for any lymphoproliferative disorder, but certain changes in approach are necessary because of the low levels of paraprotein that can be involved.

Heavy-Chain Disease
As the name implies, heavy-chain disease is characterized by the presence of monoclonal proteins composed of the heavy-chain portion of the immunoglobulin molecule. These are a family of rare, systemic syndromes involving B lymphocytes. A heavy-chain disease is similar to myeloma in that it is a malignancy of B lymphocytes that secrete a characteristic immunoglobulin, but its clinical features are very different. For example, there is no evidence of bone disease in heavy-chain disease.

Alpha heavy-chain disease is the most common of the heavy-chain gammopathies and is frequently seen in men of Mediterranean descent. Mu heavy-chain disease is rare.

Light-Chain Deposition Disease
Light-chain deposition disease (LCDD) is a systemic disorder that involves the immune system and is caused by an excess build-up of immunoglobulin light chains in tissues and organs. Light chains are an important part of the body's immune system, but if these chains become trapped in the tissues of the kidneys, lungs, skin, joints, or blood vessels, the light chains can trigger reactions that lead to tissue or organ inflammation and damage.

Early signs and symptoms of LCDD may include proteinuria, high blood pressure, decreased kidney function, and nephrotic syndrome. About 50% to 60% of patients with LCDD have myeloma, and about 17% have MGUS.

CASE STUDY 21.1

History and Physical Examination
A 58-year-old nuclear power plant worker saw his family physician because of increasing fatigue and weakness. He also reported pain in his lower back and arms when he walked. Physical examination revealed that the man had pale mucous membranes and hepatosplenomegaly. The physician ordered a complete blood count (CBC) and urinalysis (UA). A follow-up appointment was scheduled for the following week.

Laboratory Data
The CBC revealed that the patient had anemia. His leukocyte count and differential count were normal, except for a rouleaux (rolled coin) appearance of the red blood cells (RBCs). The UA was normal. The patient was called and requested to return to the laboratory for additional tests. The physician ordered an erythrocyte sedimentation rate (ESR), kidney screening profile, liver blood profile, and radiographic skeletal survey, with the following results:
- ESR—50 mm/hour
- Kidney profile—Normal
- Liver profile—Normal, except for increased globular protein
- Skeletal survey—Bone lesions in various sites

Questions
1. To follow-up with the diagnosis of this patient, a _____ would be of value.
   a. Hemoglobin electrophoresis
   b. Serum electrophoresis
   c. Immunoelectrophoresis
   d. Both b and c

Continued

CASE STUDY 21.1—cont"d

2. A risk factor for an immunologic disease is significant in this patient because of:
   a. Age
   b. Occupation
   c. Gender
   d. Recreational lifestyle

Answers to these multiple-choice questions can be found in Appendix A.

Critical Thinking Group Discussion Questions
1. What follow-up laboratory tests might be ordered to assist in establishing a definitive diagnosis?
2. What is the nature of the protein found in the urine?
3. What is the most significant laboratory finding in this disorder?
4. What type of immunologic defect exists in this disease process?
5. Does this patient have a risk of occupational exposure?

TABLE 21.6 International Working Group for the Diagnosis of Multiple Myeloma and Related Plasma Cell Disorders Diagnostic Criteria[a].

Disorder	Laboratory Diagnostic Criteria
Active multiple myeloma	Clonal bone marrow plasma cells ≥10% or biopsy-proven bony or extramedullary plasmacytoma and any one or more of the following (CRAB)[a] features and myeloma-defining events: 1. Evidence of end-organ damage that can be attributed to the underlying plasma cell proliferative disorder, specifically: 　• Hypercalcemia: serum calcium >0.25 mmol/L (>1 mg/dL) higher than the upper limit of normal or >2.75 mmol/L (>11 mg/dL) 　• Renal insufficiency: creatinine clearance 177 μmol/L (>2 mg/dL) 　• Anemia: hemoglobin value of >20 g/L below the lower limit of normal, hemoglobin value 　• Bone lesions: one or more osteolytic lesions on skeletal radiography, CT, or PET-CT. If bone marrow has <10% clonal plasma cells, more than one bone lesion is required to distinguish from solitary plasmacytoma with minimal marrow involvement 2. Any one or more of the following biomarkers of malignancy (MDEs): 　• ≥60% clonal bone marrow plasma cell percentage on bone marrow examination 　• Serum involved/uninvolved free light–chain ratio of 100 or greater, provided the absolute level of the involved light chain is at least 100 mg/L (a patient's involved FLC either kappa or lambda is the one that is above the normal reference range; the uninvolved FLC is the one that is typically in, or below, the normal range) 　• More than one focal lesion on MRI that is at least 5 mm or greater in size 　• Bence Jones protein
Smoldering multiple myeloma	1. Serum monoclonal protein (IgG or IgA) ≥30 g/L or urinary monoclonal protein ≥500 mg/24 hours and/or clonal bone marrow plasma cells 10%–60% 2. Absence of myeloma-defining events or amyloidosis
Non–IgM-MGUS	1. Serum monoclonal protein <3 0g/dL 2. Clonal bone marrow plasma cells <10% 3. Absence of end-organ damage such as hypercalcemia, renal insufficiency, anemia, and bone lesions (CRAB) or amyloidosis that can be attributed to plasma cell proliferative disorder
IgM-MGUS	1. Serum monoclonal protein <30 g/L 2. No evidence of anemia, constitutional symptoms, hyperviscosity, lymphadenopathy, hepatosplenomegaly, or other end-organ damage that can be attributed to plasma cell proliferative disorder
Light-chain MGUS	1. Abnormal FLC ratio (<0.26 or >1.65) 2. Increased level of the appropriate free light chain (increased κ FLC in patients with ratio >1.65 and increased λ FLC in patients with ratio <0.26) 3. No immunoglobulin heavy-chain expression on immunofixation 4. Absence of end-organ damage such as hypercalcemia, renal insufficiency, anemia, and bone lesions (CRAB) or amyloidosis that can be attributed to plasma cell proliferative disorder 5. Clonal bone marrow plasma cells <10% 6. Urinary monoclonal protein <500 mg/24 h
Solitary plasmacytoma	1. Biopsy-proven solitary lesion of bone or soft tissue with evidence of clonal plasma cells 2. Normal bone marrow with no evidence of clonal plasma cells 3. Normal skeletal survey and MRI (or CT) of the spine and pelvis (except for the primary solitary lesion) 4. Absence of end-organ damage such as hypercalcemia, renal insufficiency, anemia, and bone lesions (CRAB) or amyloidosis that can be attributed to the plasma cell proliferative disorder
Solitary plasmacytoma with minimal marrow involvement	1. Biopsy-proven solitary lesion of bone or soft tissue with evidence of clonal plasma cells 2. Clonal bone marrow plasma cells <10% 3. Normal skeletal survey and MRI (or CT) of the spine and pelvis (except for the primary solitary lesion) 4. Absence of end-organ damage, e.g., CRAB, attributable to a lymphoplasma cell disorder

TABLE 21.6 International Working Group for the Diagnosis of Multiple Myeloma and Related Plasma Cell Disorders Diagnostic Criteria[a].—cont'd

Disorder	Laboratory Diagnostic Criteria
POEMS syndrome	1. Polyneuropathy 2. Monoclonal plasma cell proliferative disorder Any one of the three other major criteria: 1. Sclerotic bone lesions 2. Castleman's disease 3. Elevated levels of VEGFA Any one of the following six minor criteria: 1. Organomegaly (splenomegaly, hepatomegaly, or lymphadenopathy) 2. Extravascular volume overload (edema, pleural effusion, or ascites) 3. Endocrinopathy (adrenal, thyroid, pituitary, gonadal, parathyroid, pancreatic) 4. Skin changes (hyperpigmentation, hypertrichosis, glomeruloid hemangiomata, plethora, acrocyanosis, flushing, white nails) 5. Papilloedema 6. Thrombocytosis/polycythemia
Systemic AL amyloidosis	1. Presence of an amyloid-related systemic syndrome (e.g., renal, liver, heart, gastrointestinal tract, or peripheral nerve involvement) 2. Positive amyloid staining by Congo red in any tissue (e.g., fat aspirate, bone marrow, or organ biopsy) 3. Evidence that amyloid is light-chain related established by direct examination of the amyloid using mass spectrometry-based proteomic analysis or immunoelectron microscopy 4. Evidence of a monoclonal plasma cell proliferative disorder (serum monoclonal protein, abnormal free light-chain ratio, or clonal plasma cells in the bone marrow)

[a]CRAB = hypercalcemia = serum calcium >0.25 mmol/L (>1 mg/dL) higher than the upper limit of normal or >2.75 mmol/L (>11 mg/dL); renal insufficiency = creatinine clearance <40 mL/min or serum creatinine >177 μmol/L (>2 mg/dL); anemia = hemoglobin of >2 g/dL below the lower limit of normal, or a hemoglobin value <10 g/dL; bone lesions—one or more osteolytic lesions on skeletal x-ray, CT, or PET-CT.
AL, amyloid light chain or primary amyloidosis; *CT*, computed tomography; *FLC*, free light chain; *IgA*, Immunoglobulin A; *IgG*, immunoglobulin G; *MDE*, myeloma-defining event; *MGUS*, monoclonal gammopathy of unknown significance; *MRI*, magnetic resonance image; VEGFA, *VEGF*, vascular endothelial growth factor A.
© 2024, International Myeloma Foundation. All rights reserved.

REVIEW QUESTIONS

1. Polyclonal gammopathies can be exhibited as a secondary manifestation of all of the following *except*:
   a. Chronic infection
   b. Chronic liver disease
   c. Multiple myeloma
   d. Rheumatoid connective disease
2. What is the most frequent cause of death in a patient with multiple myeloma?
   a. Skeletal destruction
   b. Chronic renal failure
   c. Neurologic disorders
   d. Infectious disease
3. Patients with multiple myeloma have defects in:
   a. Cellular immunity
   b. Humoral immunity
   c. Phagocytosis
   d. Both a and c
4. What is the single most consistent immunologic feature of multiple myeloma (MM)?
   a. Most common form of dysproteinemia
   b. Onset at between 20 and 40 years of age
   c. IgM is the most common abnormality of MM
   d. Predominantly composed of the heavy chain of the Ig molecule
5. Bence Jones proteins are soluble at room temperature and form a precipitate near ___ and resolubilize at a higher temperature.
   a. 37°C (98.6°F)
   b. 50°C (122°F)
   c. 60°C (140°F)
   d. 100° (212°F)
6. M proteins are associated with all of the following malignant conditions *except*:
   a. Multiple myeloma
   b. Plasmacytoma
   c. Malignant lymphoproliferative diseases
   d. Lymphoma
7. Cryoglobulins are proteins that precipitate or gel at:
   a. −18°C
   b. −4°C
   c. 0°C
   d. 4°C
8. The most common form of MM is:
   a. IgM
   b. IgG
   c. IgE
   d. IgA

9. In light-chain disease, only monoclonal light chains are synthesized by a one-cell clone.
   a. Lambda
   b. Gamma
   c. Kappa
   d. Alpha
10. Bence Jones proteins can be detected in:
    a. Serum
    b. Urine
    c. Cerebrospinal fluid (CSF)
    d. Both a and b
11. Most patients with multiple myeloma manifest:
    a. Bone pain
    b. Acute renal failure
    c. No symptoms
    d. Hepatomegaly and splenomegaly
12. The figure represents the serum electrophoresis of a patient with:

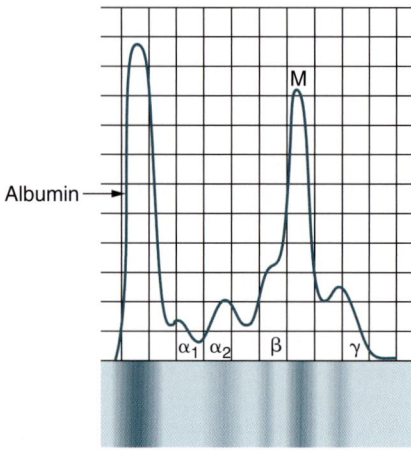

   a. Waldenström macroglobulinemia
   b. Multiple myeloma
   c. No protein abnormality
   d. Polyclonal gammopathy

13. How does Waldenström primary macroglobulinemia differ from other monoclonal gammopathies?
    a. Frequently an increase in IgG with an M spike
    b. Overproduction of IgM
    c. Only κ and λ monoclonal light chains seen on serum protein electrophoresis
    d. Characterized by the presence of monoclonal proteins composed of the heavy-chain portion of the Ig molecule
14. Monoclonal gammopathy of undetermined significance (MGUS) is characterized by all of the following except:
    a. Monoclonal protein in patients with no features of multiple myeloma or related malignant disorders
    b. Disorder that can evolve into a malignant monoclonal gammopathy
    c. Serum monoclonal protein concentration less than 3 g/dL
    d. More than 10% of plasma cells in the bone marrow
15. MGUS is characterized by all of the following *except*:
    a. Renal insufficiency
    b. Presence of lytic bone lesions
    c. Anemia
    d. Hypercalcemia
16. Light-chain disease represents about _____ of monoclonal gammopathies.
    a. 5% to 10%
    b. 10% to 15%
    c. 15% to 25%
    d. 25% to 50%

22
Tolerance, Autoimmunity, and Autoimmune Disorders

LEARNING OUTCOMES

- Define the term immunologic tolerance.
- Compare various layers of self-tolerance.
- Describe positive selection, negative selection, and peripheral tolerance.
- Discuss factors influencing the development of autoimmunity.
- Coordinate the presence of major autoantibodies with at least five different autoimmune disorders.
- Describe the characteristics of autoimmune disorders.
- Compare organ-specific and organ-nonspecific characteristics.
- Describe organ-specific and midspectrum disorders.
- Analyze representative case studies and answer case study–related multiple-choice questions.
- Participate in a discussion of case study–related critical thinking questions.
- Describe the principle, sources of error, limitations, and application of the antinucleoprotein slide test.
- Correctly answer 80% of end-of-chapter review questions.

OUTLINE

Immunologic Tolerance, 370
   Maintenance of Self-Tolerance, 370
      T-Cell Tolerance, 371
      B-Cell Tolerance, 371
Factors Influencing the Development of Autoimmunity, 371
   Progression to Autoimmune Disease, 371
   Genetic Factors, 371
   Patient Age and Sex, 372
   Exogenous Factors, 372
      Immunopathogenic Mechanisms, 372
Major Autoantibodies, 372
Autoimmune Disease, 373
Innate Immune System, 373
Adaptive Immune Response, 374
Comparison of Organ-Specific and Organ-Nonspecific Autoimmune Disorders, 374
Organ-Specific and Midspectrum Disorders, 374
   Cardiovascular Disorders, 374
      Vasculitis, 375
      Carditis, 375
   Collagen Vascular Disorders, 376
      Progressive Systemic Sclerosis (Scleroderma), 376
      Eosinophilia-Myalgia Syndrome, 376
   Endocrine Gland Disorders: Thyroid Disease, 376
      Lymphoid (Hashimoto) Chronic Thyroiditis, 376
      Immunologic Manifestations, 376
      Diagnostic Evaluation, 377
      Graves Disease, 377
   Pancreatic Disorders, 377
      Insulin-Dependent Diabetes Mellitus, 378
      Latent Autoimmune Diabetes in Adults, 379
      Autoimmune Pancreatitis, 379
      Adrenal Glands, 380
      Pituitary Gland, 380
      Parathyroid Gland, 380
      Polyglandular Syndromes, 380
   Reproductive Disorders, 380
   Exocrine Gland Disease, 380
      Sjögren Syndrome, 380
   Gastrointestinal Disorders, 381
      Atrophic Gastritis and Pernicious Anemia, 381
      Autoimmune Liver Disease, 382
      Idiopathic Biliary Cirrhosis, 382
      Inflammatory Bowel Disease, 382
   Immune Markers, 383
      Celiac Disease, 383
      Other Gastrointestinal Tract Immunologic Disorders, 383
   Autoimmune Hematologic Disorders, 384
      Autoimmune Lymphoproliferative Syndrome, 384
      Autoimmune Hemolytic Anemia, 384
      Idiopathic Thrombocytopenic Purpura, 386
   Neuromuscular Disorders, 386
      Amyotrophic Lateral Sclerosis, 386
      Inflammatory Polyneuropathies, 386
      Myasthenia Gravis, 386
      Multiple Sclerosis, 387
   Neuropathies, 389
   Renal Disorders, 390
      Renal Disease Associated with Circulating Immune Complexes, 390
      Membranoproliferative Glomerulonephritis, 390
      Renal Disease Associated With Anti–Glomerular Basement Membrane Antibody, 390
      Tubulointerstitial Nephritis, 391
   Skeletal Muscle Disorders, 391
      Inflammatory Myopathy, 391
   Skin Disorders: Bullous Disease and Other Conditions, 391
Case Study 22.1, 391
Case Study 22.2, 392
Procedure: Rapid Slide Test for Antinucleoprotein, 395.e1

KEY TERMS

antinuclear antibodies (ANAs)
autoantibodies
autoantigens
autoimmune disease
central tolerance
exogenous factors
IF-blocking antibodies
immune complex
immunocompetent cells
immunologic tolerance
immunoregulation
intrinsic factor (IF)
negative selection
peripheral tolerance
positive selection
prealbumin band
vasculitic syndromes

IMMUNOLOGIC TOLERANCE

The importance of tolerance to self antigens was recognized early in the study of immunology. Immunologic tolerance is the acquisition of nonreactivity toward particular self antigens. Self-recognition, or tolerance, is a critical process, and the failure to recognize "immunologic" self antigens can result in autoimmune disease.

> **KEY CONCEPTS: The Importance of Self-Tolerance**
> - Self-recognition (tolerance) is induced by at least two mechanisms.
>   - One mechanism is the elimination of a small clone of immunocompetent cells programmed to react with antigen (Burnet clonal selection theory).
>   - Another mechanism is the induction of unresponsiveness in immunocompetent cells through excessive antigen binding to them and through triggering of a suppressor mechanism.

An immune response requires presentation of a foreign antigen by an antigen-presenting cell (APC) and another signal from the appropriate major histocompatibility complex (MHC) molecule on the host's cells. Both are needed for an immune response. Tolerance is the lack of immune response to self antigens.

There are layers of tolerance in the human immune system influenced by cellular activity and soluble mediators (Table 22.1). Tolerance is initiated during fetal development (central tolerance) by the elimination of cells with the potential to react strongly with self antigens. Peripheral tolerance is a process involving mature lymphocytes and occurs in the circulation.

Central tolerance develops in the thymus during fetal life. Self antigens are presented by dendritic cells to self-reactive T cells that are responsible for positive and negative selection of specific lymphocytes. The ultimate goal is to remove T lymphocytes that respond strongly to self antigens. As genes rearrange and code for antigen receptors, the T-cell receptors (TCRs) produced may or may not be specific for the MHC expressed in that individual's cells. Positive-selection cells that have TCRs capable of responding with self antigens (low-level MHC affinity) are selected for continued growth.

A major mechanism of self-tolerance, autoreactivity, is the elimination of self-reactive immature lymphocytes. Autoreactivity is an aspect of a normal immune system. Our repertoire of immunocompetent lymphocytes provides protective immunity. Regulation of autoreactivity maintains immune homeostasis. The immune system maintains a precarious balance between being overly reactive and minimally reactive. For autoimmunity to develop there must be a failure in the elimination of autoreactive cells. If there is too little deletion at any stage of development, autoreactivity ensues; too much deletion and the protective repertoire of the immune system may be compromised. Failures of tolerance can result in an autoimmune reaction to self antigen, hypersensitivity reactions to non–self antigen, and autoinflammatory disorders in the presence of no antigen.

Maintenance of Self-Tolerance

To eliminate autoreactive cells and sustain the maintenance of self-tolerance, T and B lymphocytes routinely undergo a selection process during their maturation in primary lymphoid tissues, the thymus, and bone marrow. B cells undergo a second process of selection during their maturation.

Signals for survival are called positive selection; T cells in the thymus that lack any affinity for self-peptide–self-MHC complexes are eliminated in a process called negative selection. B cells undergo negative selection before achieving immunocompetence. This process occurs in the bone marrow and continues in the spleen, where B cells migrate as transitional cells after exiting the bone marrow. Highly autoreactive B cells are negatively selected on self antigens encountered during early maturation, but the threshold for deletion differs for each individual. Negative selection of T and B cells occurs in the peripheral lymphoid tissues and in primary lymphoid tissues, permitting the removal of autoreactive cells that do not encounter autoantigens in the thymus or bone marrow. This process of negative selection is called peripheral tolerance. Traditionally there has been a debate as to whether autoimmunity results from a defect of central tolerance in the thymus and bone marrow or in peripheral tolerance in secondary lymphoid tissues. The distinction may be artificial.

Various pathways to immunologic tolerance have been recognized. It has been suggested that T and B cells are affected independently and differently, and may be tolerated under certain circumstances. Several mechanisms may operate simultaneously in a single host. During fetal development of the immune system and during the first few weeks of neonatal life, none of the cells of the immune system have reached maturity. For this reason, the entire immune system is particularly susceptible to tolerance induction at this stage of development.

TABLE 22.1 Layers of Tolerance

Types of Tolerance	Site of Action	Mechanism
Central tolerance	Bone marrow	Deletion
	Thymus	Editing
Peripheral tolerance	Secondary lymphoid tissue	Cellular inactivation by weak signaling without costimulus
Regulatory cells	Secondary lymphoid tissue and sites of inflammation	Suppression by cytokines, intercellular signals
Clonal deletion	Secondary lymphoid tissue and sites of inflammation	Apoptosis postactivation
Cytokine deviation	Secondary lymphoid tissue and sites of inflammation	Differentiation to cells, limiting inflammatory cytokine secretion
Antigen segregation	Peripheral organs such as thyroid, pancreas	Physical barrier to self antigen access to lymphoid system
Clearance of apoptotic bodies	Secondary lymphoid tissue and sites of inflammation	Removal of self antigen and induction of negative signal

T-Cell Tolerance

T cells do not show a marked difference in tolerance at different stages of maturation. The antigen required to produce tolerance and the circumstance of its presentation are specific for each individual T-cell subset. At least three pathways have been recognized for T-cell tolerance:

1. Clonal abortion. Immature T-cell clones may be aborted in a manner similar to that of B cells.
2. Functional deletion. The subsets of a mature T cell may be individually deleted, leading to the loss of only one of the functions of the T-cell group.
3. T-cell suppression. T-cell suppressors actively suppress the actions of other T-cell subsets or B cells.

Regulatory T (T_{reg}) cells are immunoregulatory CD4+ lymphocytes that control autoimmunity in the peripheral blood. The primary function of these cells was originally defined as the prevention of autoimmune diseases by maintaining self-tolerance. T_{reg} cells that express the transcription factor Foxp3 and produce IL-10 are required for systemic immunologic tolerance. T_{reg} cells are characterized by constitutive expression of CD25 and are developed primarily in the thymus from positively selected thymocytes with high avidity for self antigens.

The thymus is responsible for deleting autoreactive T cells that have the potential to cause autoimmune disease. The epithelial cells or dendritic cells in the thymus present antigen in association with a cell surface molecule, MHC class II. The antigen is recognized by the TCR. If there is strong recognition, the autoreactive T cell is killed by apoptosis. Failure to delete autoreactive cells potentially results in autoimmunity.

B-Cell Tolerance

As a B cell matures, it becomes less susceptible to tolerization. In addition, during B-cell maturation the forms of antigen presentation that will produce tolerance vary. Four pathways have been established for the induction of B-cell tolerance; thus the mode of tolerance depends on the maturity of the cell, the antigen, and manner of antigen presentation to the immune system.

The pathways of B-cell tolerance are as follows:

1. Clonal abortion. A low concentration of multivalent antigen may cause the immature clone to abort. Tolerance of immature B cells by this mechanism is high.
2. Clonal exhaustion. Repeated antigen challenge with a T-independent antigen may remove all mature functional B-cell clones. Tolerance of mature B cells is moderate.
3. Functional deletion. The combined absence of the helper T subset and presence of T-dependent antigen (or with T suppressor cells) or an excess of T-independent antigen prevents mature B cells from functioning normally. The ability to tolerize B cells by this mechanism is moderate.
4. Antibody-forming cell blockade. An excess of T-independent antigen interferes with the secretion of antibody by antibody-forming cells. B-cell tolerance by this mechanism is low.

> **KEY CONCEPTS: What Goes Wrong in Autoimmune Disorders**
> - Autoimmunity represents a breakdown of the immune system in its ability to discriminate between self and nonself.
>   - The potential for autoimmunity is always present in every immunocompetent individual because lymphocytes that are potentially reactive with self antigens exist in the body.
>   - Factors that influence the development of antibodies to self antigens include genetic factors, age, exogenous factors, and normally functioning immunopathogenic mechanisms.
>   - The term *autoimmune disorder* is used when demonstrable immunoglobulins, autoantibodies, or cytotoxic T cells display a specificity for self antigens and contribute to disorder pathogenesis.

FACTORS INFLUENCING THE DEVELOPMENT OF AUTOIMMUNITY

Autoimmune disorders affect up to approximately 10% of the population. Although rare genetic autoimmunity syndromes can result from monogenic mutations, disrupting essential mechanisms and peripheral tolerance are more commonly expressed human autoimmune disorders. These complex disorders arise from the interaction between polygenic risk factors and environmental factors. Genome-wide associated studies have identified loci underlying human disorders, but the causal nucleotide changes and mechanisms are still largely unknown.

The immune response involves interaction of cellular elements such as lymphocytes and macrophages, antigens, antibody, immune complexes, and complement. The immune system walks a tightrope to avoid an attack against self. The body must distinguish "immunologic" self from nonself. Autoimmune disorders represent a breakdown of the immune system's ability to discriminate between "immunologic" self and nonself.

The potential for autoimmunity, if given appropriate circumstances, is constantly present in every immunocompetent individual because lymphocytes that are potentially reactive with self antigens exist in the body. Antibody expression appears to be regulated by a complex set of interacting factors; these influences include genetic factors, patient age, and *exogenous factors.*

Progression to Autoimmune Disease

Autoimmune diseases are believed to occur in stages as the result of a multistep process. These stages are:

1. First Phase. A genetic predisposition and other factors, such as female hormones.
2. Second Phase. An incident such as an infection or exposure to ultraviolet radiation leads to loss of self-tolerance and induces autoantibody formation.
3. Intermediate Step. An autoimmune attack subsequently leads to tissue damage caused by the release of self antigens that are not removed as would be normal.
4. Propagation Phase. An autoimmune response to an increasing number of autoantigens and also to more epitopes within each antigen (epitope spread).

Genetic Factors

A strong genetic component is associated with organ-specific or systemic systems involving human leukocyte antigens (HLAs). The presence of certain HLAs is associated with an increased risk of certain autoimmune states. Any genetic change that reduces deletion or enhances activation of autoreactivity may be a risk factor for autoimmunity (Fig. 22.1). The association of genetics and autoimmune disease focuses on common allelic variants, not mutation. Each has a small effect on disease risk. Although the effect on disease risk is small, the biological effects of allelic variants is striking. Genetic findings emphasize that the identification of environmental components that interact with host genetic factors is important to developing a deeper understanding of autoimmunity.

In autoimmune disease, there is a tendency for familial aggregates to occur. In addition, there is a tendency for more than one autoimmune disease to occur in the same individual. For example, patients with Hashimoto disease have a higher incidence of pernicious anemia (PA) than would be expected in a random population matched for age and sex.

Another factor related to genetic inheritance is that autoimmune disorders and *autoantibodies* are found more frequently in women than in men.

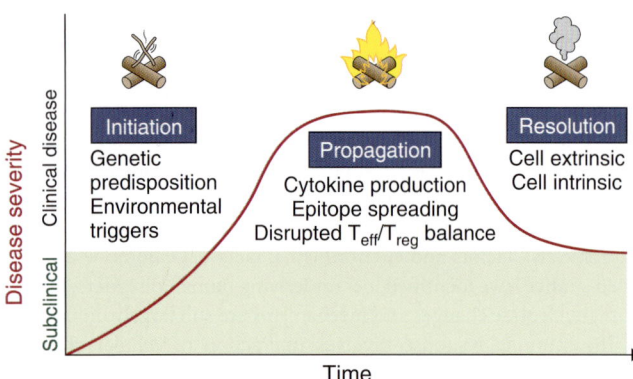

Fig. 22.1 Three major phases of autoimmune disease. Autoimmunity is initiated by a combination of genetic predisposition and environmental triggers. Patients in the initiation phase of disease are typically unaware of clinical symptoms (subclinical). Patients present with clinical disease during the propagation phase, which is characterized by self-perpetuating inflammation and tissue damage due to cytokine production, epitope spreading, and a disrupted effector T-cell/regulatory T-cell (T_{eff}/T_{reg}) balance. Autoimmune reactions resolve with the activation of cell-intrinsic (inhibitory pathways) and cell-extrinsic (T_{reg}) mechanisms to limit effector responses and restore the T_{eff}/T_{reg} balance. Patients in this phase often suffer from relapsing and remitting disease as a result of a persistent struggle between pathogenic effector responses and regulation. (From Rosenblum MD, Remedios KA, Abbas AK. Mechanisms of human autoimmunity, *J Clin Invest* 2015;125[6]:2228–2233.)

Patient Age and Sex

Healthy individuals may have autoantibodies without clinical disease. For example, healthy individuals may exhibit antinuclear antibodies (ANAs), with a prevalence in the general population over 60 years old of 20% to 30%. The incidence of autoantibodies, however, increases steadily with age, reaching a peak at around 60 to 70 years.

Sex can be a factor in autoimmune disorders. Generally, they are most prevalent in women of reproductive age.

Exogenous Factors

Ultraviolet radiation, drugs, viruses, and infectious diseases may all play a role in the development of autoimmune disorders. These factors may alter antigens, which the body then perceives as non–self antigens.

Direct stimulation of autoreactive cells with resulting damage can be elicited by foreign antigens.

Immunopathogenic Mechanisms

Autoimmune disorders are usually prevented by the normal functioning of immunologic regulatory mechanisms. When these controls dysfunction (Fig. 22.2), antibodies to self antigens may be produced and bind to antigens in the circulation to form circulating immune complexes or to antigens deposited in specific tissue sites.

The mechanisms governing the deposition in one organ or another are unknown, but several mechanisms may be operative in a single disease. Wherever antigen-antibody complexes accumulate, complement can be activated, with the subsequent release of mediators of inflammation. These mediators increase vascular permeability, attract phagocytic cells to the reaction site, and cause local tissue damage. Alternatively, cytotoxic T cells can directly attack body cells bearing the target antigen, which releases mediators that amplify the inflammatory reaction. Autoantibody and complement fragments coat cells bearing the target antigen, which leads to destruction by phagocytes or antibody-seeking K-type lymphocytes.

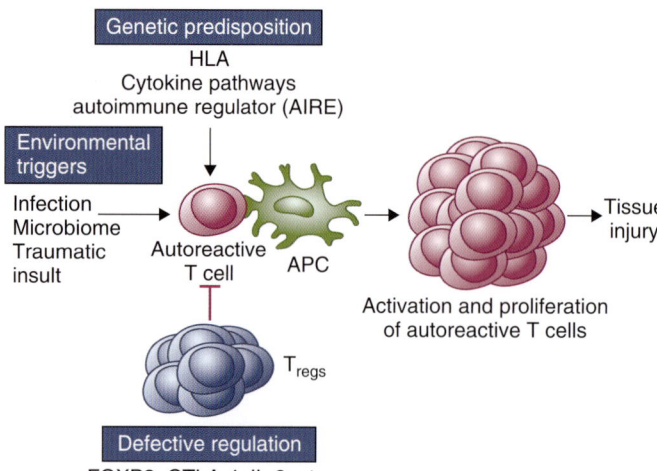

Fig. 22.2 Genetic susceptibility, environmental stimuli, and defective regulation are responsible for initiating autoimmunity. Genetic polymorphisms in immune-related genes (including the human leukocyte antigen [HLA], cytokines/receptors, and those involved in central tolerance) may lower the threshold for the activation of autoreactive T cells. Environmental triggers such as infection, the microbiome, and tissue injury generate a proinflammatory environment that supports the activation of autoreactive lymphocytes. T_{regs} normally function to suppress autoreactive T cells, but defects in development, stability, or function may render these cells dysfunctional and unable to control autoreactive T-cell responses. Alone or in combination, these factors can contribute to the escape, activation, and proliferation of autoreactive lymphocytes that result in tissue injury and clinical disease. *AIRE*, Autoimmune regulator; *APC*, antigen-presenting cell; *HLA*, human leukocyte antigen; *IL-2*, interleukin-2. (From Rosenblum MD, Remedios KA, Abbas AK. Mechanisms of human autoimmunity, *J Clin Invest* 2015;125[6]:2228–2233.)

The hidden antigen (sequestered antigen) theory is one of the earliest views of organ-specific antibodies. Antigens are sequestered within the organ and, because of the lack of contact with the mononuclear phagocyte system, they fail to establish immunologic tolerance.

Any conditions producing a release of antigen would then provide an opportunity for autoantibody formation. This situation occurs when sperm cells or lens and heart tissues are released directly into the circulation and autoantibodies are formed. Unmodified extracts of tissues involved in organ-specific autoimmune disorders, however, do not readily elicit antibody formation.

- An individual may develop an autoimmune response to a variety of immunogenic stimuli (Table 22.2). These responses may be caused by the following:
- Antigens that do not normally circulate in the blood
- Altered antigens that arise because of chemical, physical, or biological processes (e.g., hapten complexing, physical denaturation, and mutation)
- A foreign antigen that is shared or crossreactive with self antigens or tissue components
- Mutation of immunocompetent cells to acquire a response to self antigens
- Loss of the immunoregulatory function by T lymphocyte subsets

MAJOR AUTOANTIBODIES

Major autoantibodies can be detected in different disorders. Many diagnostic laboratory tests (Table 22.3) are based on detecting these autoimmune responses. Common autoantibodies include thyroid, gastric, adrenocortical, striated muscle, acetylcholine receptor, smooth

TABLE 22.2 Autoimmune Disorders and Associated Abnormalities

Clinical Diagnosis	Autoantigen
Addison disease	P-450 enzymes
Crohn disease	p-ANCA, pancreatic acinar cells
Ovarian failure/infertility	P-450 enzymes
Pernicious anemia	Parietal cells
Ulcerative colitis	p-ANCA

TABLE 22.3 Major Autoantibodies

Acetylcholine receptor (AChR)–binding antibody	Antireticulin antibody
Acetylcholine receptor (AChR)–blocking antibody	Anti–rheumatoid arthritis nuclear antigen (anti-RANA; RA precipitin)
Antiadrenal antibody	Antiribosome antibody
Anticardiolipin antibody	Anti–nuclear ribonucleoprotein (anti-nRNP) antibody
Anticentriole antibody	Anti-Scl antibody or anti–Scl-70 antibody
Anticentromere antibody	Antiskin (dermal-epidermal) antibody
	Antiskin (interepithelial) antibody
Anti–DNA antibody	Anti-Sm antibody
Anti–glomerular basement membrane antibody	Anti–smooth muscle antibody
Anti–intrinsic factor antibody	Antisperm antibody
Anti–islet cell antibody	Anti–SS-A (SS-A precipitin; anti-Ro) antibody
Anti–liver-kidney microsomal (anti-LKM) antibody	Anti–SS-B (SS-B precipitin, anti-La) antibody
Antimitochondrial antibody	Antistriational antibody
Antimyelin antibody	Antithyroglobulin and antithyroid microsome antibody
Antimyocardial antibody	Histone-reactive antinuclear antibody (HR-ANA)
Antineutrophil antibody	Jo-1 antibody
Antinuclear antibody (ANA)	Ku antibody
Anti–parietal cell antibody	Mi-1 antibody
Antiplatelet antibody	PM-1 antibody

BOX 22.1 Examples of Autoimmune Disorders

- Active chronic hepatitis
- Addison disease
- Autoimmune atrophic gastritis
- Autoimmune hemolytic anemia
- Dermatomyositis
- Discoid lupus erythematosus
- Goodpasture syndrome
- Hashimoto thyroiditis
- Idiopathic thrombocytopenic purpura
- Insulin-dependent (juvenile, type 1) diabetes mellitus
- Multiple sclerosis
- Myasthenia gravis
- Pemphigus vulgaris
- Pernicious anemia
- Primary biliary cirrhosis
- Primary myxedema
- Rheumatoid arthritis
- Scleroderma
- Sjögren syndrome
- Systemic lupus erythematosus
- Thyrotoxicosis

muscle, salivary gland, mitochondrial, reticulin, myelin, islet cell, and skin. Antibodies to antinuclear antibodies (ANAs) include DNA, histone, and nonhistone protein antibodies.

AUTOIMMUNE DISEASE

The term *autoimmune disease* is used when demonstrable immunoglobulins (autoantibodies) or cytotoxic T cells display specificity for self antigens, or autoantigens, and contribute to the pathogenesis of the disease.

The hallmark of autoimmune disease is tissue injury caused by T lymphocytes or antibody reactivity to "immunologic" self. Immune activation may be initiated by infection that goes on to persist as ischemic injury. Some autoimmune disorders are characterized by activation of the immune system in the absence of an external threat to the organism. In these disorders, inflammation and tissue damage occur in the absence of infection, toxin exposure, or tumor growth.

Autoimmune disorders are characterized by the persistent activation of immunologic effector mechanisms that alter the function and integrity of individual cells and organs. The sites of organ or tissue damage depend on the location of the immune reaction. The variety of signs and symptoms seen in patients with autoimmune disorders reflects the various forms of the immune response.

In the initial stage of some disorders, infiltration by T lymphocytes may induce inflammation and tissue damage, leading to alterations in self antigens and production of autoantibodies. In other disorders, only the production of autoantibodies is noted with tissue damage. These autoantibodies attack cell surface antigens or membrane receptors or combine with antigen to form immune complexes that are deposited in tissue, subsequently causing complement activation and inflammation.

It is also important to note that autoantibodies may be formed in patients secondary to tissue damage or when no evidence of clinical disease exists. Unlike autoimmune disorders, autoantibodies can occur as immune correlates of conditions such as blood transfusion reactions. In addition, autoantibodies can be demonstrated in hemolytic disease of the newborn and graft rejection, and can result from disorders such as serum sickness, anaphylaxis, and hay fever when the immune response is clearly the cause of the disease. Additional disorders are continually being identified (Box 22.1).

Chronic and other intermittent inflammation contributes over time to the destruction of target organs that contain inciting antigens or are the sites of immune complex deposition. Although the adaptive immune system has long been the focus of attention, innate immune mechanisms are now viewed as central to the pathogenesis of these disorders.

INNATE IMMUNE SYSTEM

Some autoimmune disorders display activation of the innate immune system and an excess of inflammation. One example is activation of the innate immune system in systemic lupus erythematosus (SLE) due to complement deficiencies that permit excess accumulation of proinflammatory apoptotic debris.

The role of the innate system in tissue injury, particularly neutrophils and macrophages, is that these types of cells are recruited to sites of ischemic injury. Macrophages have a complex program in which they first release proinflammatory mediators to fight pathogens but may then initiate programs to help in the clearance of dead tissue and tissue repair. Although the latter response is beneficial if short-lived, continued activation of the repair program may be detrimental if it becomes chronic.

ADAPTIVE IMMUNE RESPONSE

Alternatively, there are disorders characterized by an activation of the adaptive immune response with T and B lymphocytes responding to self antigen in the absence of any detectable microbial invasion or tumor invasion.

Disruption of the delicate balance between activating and inhibitory signals that regulate normal B-cell activation and longevity can predispose to pathogenic autoantibody production and autoimmunity. It has become more obvious that B cells contribute substantially to multiple human autoimmune disorders. B cells may contribute to autoimmune pathogenesis by presentation of autoantigen to T cells or through production of proinflammatory cytokines. In most cases of human autoimmune disease, the combination of environmental factors and polygenic effects collectively dysregulate normal B-cell function and confer disease susceptibility. These disorders constitute the vast majority of disorders that are considered to be autoimmune in origin.

> **KEY CONCEPTS: Overview of Organ-Specific Versus Organ-Nonspecific Disorders**
> - At one extreme are organ-specific disorders; at the other end of the spectrum are disorders that manifest as organ-nonspecific disorders.
> - Organ-specific and midspectrum disorders include cardiovascular disorders (e.g., vasculitis and carditis), collagen vascular disorders, endocrine gland disorders, exocrine gland disorders, gastrointestinal disorders, autoimmune hematologic disorders, neuropathies, renal disorders, skeletal muscle disorders, and skin disorders.
> - Midspectrum disorders are characterized by localized lesions in a single organ and organ-nonspecific autoantibodies.
> - Major autoantibodies can be detected in different disorders. Many diagnostic laboratory tests are based on detecting autoimmune antibodies.
> - Antinuclear antibodies (ANAs) include DNA, histone, and nonhistone protein antibodies.

COMPARISON OF ORGAN-SPECIFIC AND ORGAN-NONSPECIFIC AUTOIMMUNE DISORDERS

Organ-specific autoimmune disorders are produced by T cells or antibodies against antigens restricted to a single organ. Examples include type 1 diabetes (T1D) and multiple sclerosis. Systemic autoimmune disease is produced by circulating antibodies or immune complexes and affects multiple end organs. Examples are SLE and myasthenia gravis.

Autoimmune disorders exhibit a full spectrum of tissue reactivity (Fig. 22.3 and Table 22.4). At one extreme are organ-specific disorders, such as Hashimoto disease of the thyroid; at the other extreme are disorders that manifest as organ-nonspecific disorders, such as systemic lupus erythematosus (SLE) (see Chapter 23) and rheumatoid arthritis (RA) (see Table 22.4 and Chapter 24).

In organ-specific disorders, both the lesions produced by tissue damage and the autoantibodies are directed at a single target organ

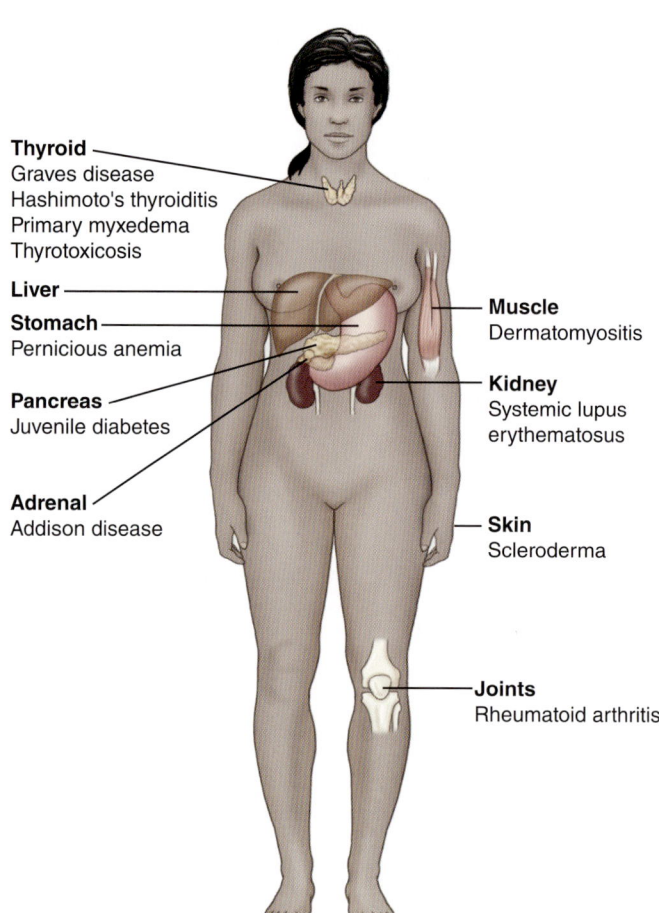

Fig. 22.3 Organ-specific autoimmune disorders.

(e.g., the thyroid). Midspectrum disorders are characterized by localized lesions in a single organ and by organ-nonspecific autoantibodies. For example in primary biliary cirrhosis, the small bile duct is the main target of inflammatory cell infiltration, but the serum autoantibodies are mainly mitochondrial antibodies and are not liver specific.

In comparison, organ-nonspecific disorders are characterized by the presence of lesions caused by the deposition of antigen-antibody immune complexes formed from the binding of an antibody to an antigen and not confined to any one organ.

At one extreme are organ-specific disorders; at the other end of the spectrum are disorders that manifest as organ-nonspecific disorders.

Organ-specific and midspectrum disorders include cardiovascular disorders (e.g., vasculitis and carditis), collagen vascular disorders, endocrine gland disorders, exocrine gland disorders, gastrointestinal disorders, autoimmune hematologic disorders, neuropathies, renal disorders, skeletal muscle disorders, and skin disorders.

Midspectrum disorders are characterized by localized lesions in a single organ and organ-nonspecific autoantibodies.

Major autoantibodies can be detected in different disorders. Many diagnostic laboratory tests are based on detecting autoimmune antibodies.

ANAs include DNA, histone, and nonhistone protein antibodies.

ORGAN-SPECIFIC AND MIDSPECTRUM DISORDERS

Cardiovascular Disorders

The primary immunologic disorders of the blood vessels are termed *vasculitis*; those of the heart are termed *carditis*.

TABLE 22.4 Summary of Organ-Specific and Organ-Nonspecific Disorders

Similarities
1. Circulating autoantibodies react with normal body constituents
2. Increased immunoglobulin concentration in serum often found
3. Antibodies may appear in each of the main immunoglobulin classes
4. Disease process not always progressive; exacerbations and remissions occur
5. Autoantibody tests of diagnostic value

Differences

Organ Specific	Organ Nonspecific
Antibodies and lesions are organ specific	Antibodies and lesions are organ nonspecific
Clinical and serologic overlap (e.g., thyroid, stomach, adrenal glands, and kidney)	Overlap of systemic lupus erythematosus (SLE), rheumatoid arthritis (RA), and other connective tissue disorders
Antigens only available to lymphoid system in low concentrations	Antigens accessible at higher concentrations
Antigens evoke organ-specific antibodies in normal animals with complete Freund adjuvant	No antibodies produced in animals with comparable stimulation
Familial tendency to develop organ-specific autoimmunity	Familial tendency to develop connective tissue disease; questionable abnormalities in immunoglobulin synthesis in relatives
Lymphoid invasion, parenchymal destruction by questionable cell-mediated hypersensitivity or antibodies	Lesions caused by deposition of antigen-antibody (immune) complexes
Tendency to develop cancer in the organ	Tendency to develop lymphoreticular neoplasia

BOX 22.2 Classification of Vasculitic Syndromes

- Systemic necrotizing arteritis
  - Polyarteritis nodosa
  - Allergic angiitis and granulomatosis
  - Overlap syndrome
- Hypersensitivity vasculitis
  - Henoch-Schönlein purpura
  - McDuffie syndrome
- Granulomatosis with polyangitis
- Lymphomatoid granulomatosis
- Giant-cell arteritis
  - Takayasu arteritis
- Mucocutaneous lymph node syndrome (Kawasaki's disease)
- Behçet's disease
- Thromboangiitis obliterans
- Central nervous system vasculitis
- Miscellaneous
  - Cogan syndrome
  - Eales disease
- Hypereosinophilic syndrome with vasculitis

Vasculitis

Deposition of circulating immune complexes is considered directly or indirectly responsible for many forms of vasculitis. The inflammatory lesions of blood vessels produce variable injury or necrosis of the blood vessel wall. This may result in narrowing, occlusion, or thrombosis of the lumen, or aneurysm formation or rupture. Vasculitis occurs as a primary disease process or as a secondary manifestation of another disease (e.g., RA).

Vasculitis is characterized by inflammation within blood vessels, which often results in a compromise of the vessel lumen with ischemia. Ischemia causes the major manifestations of the vasculitic syndromes and determines the prognosis. Any size and type of blood vessel may be involved; therefore the vasculitic syndromes are a heterogeneous group of disorders (Box 22.2).

Antibodies specific to endothelial cells also contribute to immune vasculopathy. Antiendothelial antibodies are autoantibodies directed against antigens in the cytoplasmic membrane of endothelial cells.

Carditis

The heart shares a susceptibility to immune-mediated injury with other organs. Numerous cardiac disorders are characterized by the presence of inflammatory cells within the myocardium resulting from immune sensitization to endogenous or exogenous cardiac antigens. The consequent reaction of cardiac myocytes to immune injury can range from reversible modulation of their electrical and mechanical capabilities to cell death. Carditis can be caused by a variety of conditions, including acute rheumatic fever, Lyme disease, and cardiac transplant rejection.

Myocardial contractility can be impaired by cell-mediated injury or the local release of cytokines. The study of immune cardiac disease has entered a period of rapid expansion. Primary idiopathic myocarditis is an autoimmune disease characterized by infiltration of the heart by macrophages and lymphocytes. Studies involving the mechanisms whereby immune cells and factors localize in the myocardium, modulate myocyte function, and remodel myocardial architecture are underway.

A diagnosis of acute rheumatic fever requires differentiation from other immunologic and infectious disorders. The immunologic basis for rheumatic heart disease has long been suspected. Patients with rheumatic heart disease exhibit antimyocardial antibodies that bind in vitro to foci in the myocardium and heart valves. These antibodies may be responsible for the deposition of immunoglobulin and complement components found in the same area of rheumatic heart disease tissues at autopsy.

Antimyocardial antibodies appear to be strongly crossreactive with streptococcal antigens, but they are not toxic to heart tissue unless the latter is damaged previously by some other cause. Because antimyocardial antibodies are often found in patients with a recent myocardial infarction or streptococcal infection without cardiac sequelae, detection of these antibodies has not been a particularly useful differential diagnostic test for cardiac injury. The presence of myocardial antibodies is diagnostic of Dressler syndrome (cardiac injury) or rheumatic fever.

Collagen Vascular Disorders
Progressive Systemic Sclerosis (Scleroderma)

Scleroderma is a collagen vascular disease of unknown cause that assumes various forms. Eosinophilic fasciitis may be a variant of scleroderma.

The development of scleroderma has been associated with a number of occupations and with drugs such as bleomycin sulfate, tryptophan, and carbidopa. Occupational exposure to vinyl chloride, vibratory stimuli, and silicosis have been associated with the subsequent development of scleroderma.

Epidemiology. Scleroderma occurs in all races and is three times more frequent in women than men.

Signs and symptoms. Systemic sclerosis is a chronic multisystem disease that causes thickening of the skin (scleroderma). Scleroderma is characterized by fibrosis in the skin and internal organs, and by arterial occlusions with a distinct proliferative pattern.

Initial symptoms usually appear in the third decade of life. Raynaud phenomenon is the most frequent manifestation. In more than 50% of patients, Raynaud phenomenon occurs before the onset of other manifestations. Articular complaints are common. Hypomotility of the gastrointestinal (GI) tract is the second most common clinical feature. The disease is slowly progressive and chronically disabling but can be rapidly progressive and fatal.

Immunologic manifestations. Idiopathic scleroderma is considered an autoimmune disease because of the associated autoantibodies and the overlapping syndromes of scleroderma-polymyositis and scleroderma-SLE.

In 40% to 90% of patients, ANAs are formed to: (1) extractable nuclear antigens, (2) the nucleolus, (3) the centromere, and (4) Scl-70. The anticentromere antibody is sensitive and specific for patients with a subset of scleroderma with CREST syndrome (*c*alcinosis, *R*aynaud phenomenon, *e*sophageal dysmotility, *s*clerodactyly, and *t*elangiectasia).

In addition, cell hyperactivity correlates with disease activity. Activated T cells can result in both vascular changes and increased collagen production seen in scleroderma. It is now thought that both vascular disease and fibrosis result from this cellular immune activation. Vascular injury could be mediated by cytokines or direct cell-cell interaction by activated lymphocytes and endothelial cells.

Eosinophilia-Myalgia Syndrome

Many people exposed to the agent causing eosinophilia-myalgia syndrome (EMS) may develop illness. Patients develop severe myalgia, and more than 50% of patients with EMS develop scleroderma-like manifestations.

The most important predictor of EMS is the ingestion of contaminated L-tryptophan. The association of ingestion of L-tryptophan with a systemic disease now called EMS was first observed in 1989. Some patients have died from L-tryptophan.

Endocrine Gland Disorders: Thyroid Disease

Numerous endocrine gland disorders are attributable to an autoimmune process. Several of the classic and more common disorders are discussed in this section.

The clinical spectrum of autoimmune thyroid disease is very broad. There are two major forms of autoimmune thyroid disease: chronic autoimmune thyroiditis and Graves disease.

Lymphoid (Hashimoto) chronic thyroiditis is a classic example of an organ-specific autoimmune disease. Other autoimmune disorders affecting the thyroid gland include transient thyroiditis syndrome and idiopathic hypothyroidism.

Lymphoid (Hashimoto) Chronic Thyroiditis

Etiology. The exact causative mechanism is unknown but is believed to be related to an autoimmune process in which the development of circulating cytotoxic antibodies eventually destroys the thyroid gland, producing hypothyroidism. This disease is associated with the presence of HLA-DR4 and HLA-DR5. However, these associations are not consistent in different races and ethnic groups.

Epidemiology. Lymphoid thyroiditis can occur at any age but is first diagnosed most often in the third to fifth decades of life; it is much more common in women than in men. The fibrous variant of the disease is more often present in middle-aged and older patients.

The mode of inheritance is unknown. However, a genetic tendency to inherit the trait for the development of antibodies against the thyroid gland is highly possible. It is common to have multiple members of a family develop the same disease (e.g., Graves disease and lymphoid thyroiditis).

Signs and symptoms. Lymphoid thyroiditis is believed to be the most common cause of sporadic goiter. Characteristically there is a firm, diffusely enlarged, nontender thyroid gland that may be lobulated. Hypothyroidism, however, is a common late sequela of lymphoid thyroiditis and patients are usually euthyroid when first seen by a physician. Some individuals have clinical and pathologic evidence of the coexistence of Graves disease and lymphoid (Hashimoto) thyroiditis. Histologically, Hashimoto thyroiditis is characterized by diffuse lymphocytic infiltration.

Immunologic Manifestations

Patients with lymphoid thyroiditis, in addition to other autoimmune thyroid disorders, can demonstrate histologic (Fig. 22.4) and immunologic manifestations of the disease. Antibodies to thyroid constituents may be observed in these patients. Antibodies to the following constituents may be demonstrated serologically:

- Thyroglobulin
- Thyroid microsome
- Second colloid antigen (CA2 antigen)
- Thyroid membrane receptors
- Thyronine (T_4) and triiodothyronine (T_3)

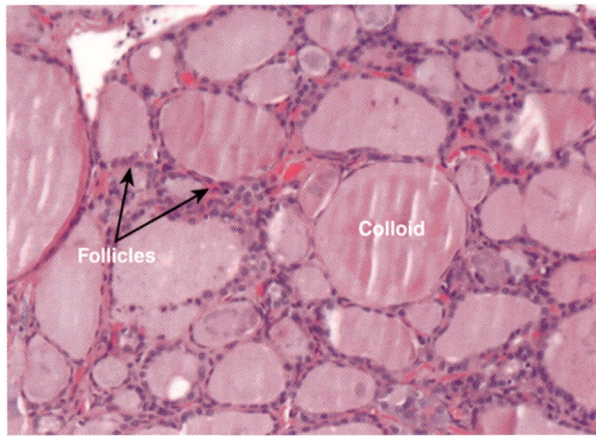

Fig. 22.4 Histologic cross-section of a normal thyroid gland (100×, hematoxylin and eosin). Single-layer, epithelial-lined follicles of variable sizes are filled with pink colloid where thyroglobulin, triiodothyronine (T_3), and thyronine (T_4) are stored. (From Strauss JF, Barbieri RL: *Yen and Jaffe's reproductive endocrinology*, ed 6, St. Louis, 2009, Elsevier.)

Thyroglobulin. Antithyroglobulin (TgAb) was the first antibody discovered against a thyroid protein, thyroglobulin. Immunofluorescent laboratory methods using fluorescein-labeled anti–human globulin can demonstrate the binding of antithyroglobulin antibody to thin sections of thyroid tissue in abnormal conditions or in approximately 4% of the normal population. The frequency of positive titers gradually increases in the female population with aging. The absence of antithyroglobulin antibodies, however, does not exclude the diagnosis of Hashimoto thyroiditis; conversely the presence of antibodies does not establish the diagnosis because it can be positive in Graves disease and is occasionally positive in thyroid cancer and subacute thyroiditis. Testing for antibody may also be used to monitor patients with thyroid cancers.

Thyroid microsomes. Antibodies directed against thyroid microsomes, antithyroid microsomal antibodies, or antithyroperoxidase antibodies (TPO Abs) can be detected in about 7% of the population, with titers ranging from 1:100 to 1:1600. Even a low titer of antithyroid antibodies correlates with a degree of thyroid involvement by an autoimmune process. The absence of antibodies has been documented in diagnosed cases of autoimmune thyroiditis, which may be explained by special characteristics of the antibody or because it forms complexes with thyroglobulins in the circulation and escapes detection. The presence of these circulating complexes has been documented in patients with thyroid autoimmune disorders.

Second colloid antigen. CA2 antigen is directed against a colloid protein and can be detected by immunofluorescent examination. Antibody to CA2 is present in about 50% of patients who have subacute thyroiditis, and it is detectable in some patients with Hashimoto thyroiditis whose sera show no other evidence of abnormal antibodies.

Thyroid membrane receptors. The thyroid membrane receptors are a group of immunoglobulin G (IgG) antibodies that interact with receptors on thyroid membranes. They often produce hyperthyroidism that manifests itself clinically, chemically, and histologically. At present classification of these IgG antibodies is operational, based on their method of detection. Long-acting thyroid stimulator (LATS) and long-acting thyroid stimulator protector (LATS-P) assays are of importance.

Thyronine and triiodothyronine. Antibodies to T_4 and T_3 have been found in several patients, most of whom had evidence of a thyroid autoimmune process such as goiter or hypothyroidism. In these cases, the underlying autoimmune process is most likely responsible for the hypothyroidism rather than hormone binding by the circulating antithyronine antibodies.

Diagnostic Evaluation

Fine-needle aspiration biopsy of the thyroid, in conjunction with clinical evaluation and serologic studies, is useful for the diagnosis of lymphocytic thyroiditis.

Histologic examination of thyroid tissue demonstrates variable infiltration of the entire gland with lymphocytes. Germinal lymphoid centers are characteristic, and destruction and distortion of normal thyroid follicles are apparent. The thyroid cells remain intact but are hypertrophied, although the usual heterogeneity of small, enlarged thyroid follicles, some containing flat epithelium, can also be seen. In advanced cases, there is almost complete destruction of normal thyroid tissue, with replacement by lymphocytes or fibrous tissue. A biopsy is important in ruling out malignancy. Today, endocrinologists rely on sonography as a diagnostic method. It allows for measurement and monitoring of the size of the thyroid over time noninvasively and enables the investigator to look for nodules or anything suspicious.

When the disease produces hypothyroidism, a slight increase in the plasma thyroid-stimulating hormone (TSH) concentration can usually be demonstrated in the early phase, followed by a decrease in serum T_4 and eventually by a decrease in serum T_3 levels. Antithyroglobulin and/or antithyroid microsomal antibodies are found in moderate-to-high titers in more than 50% of patients, but the presence of antimicrosomal antibodies is considered more diagnostic.

Antibodies directed against thyroid microsomal antigen (thyroid peroxidase antibody [anti-TPO]) can be detected by various techniques (Table 22.5). Chemiluminescent immunoassay is typically performed to detect anti-TPO autoantibodies. TPO plays a significant role in the biosynthesis of thyroid hormones by catalyzing the iodination of tyrosyl residues in thyroglobulin and the coupling of iodotyrosyl residues to form T_4 and T_3. Autoantibodies produced against TPO are capable of inhibiting enzyme activity. They are also complement-fixing antibodies that can induce cytotoxic changes in cells and consequently cause thyroid dysfunction (Table 22.6). More than 90% of patients with autoimmune thyroiditis (Hashimoto thyroiditis) have anti-TPO. Antibodies to TPO have also been found in most patients with idiopathic hypothyroidism (85%) and Graves disease (50%).

Graves Disease

Graves disease (Fig. 22.5) is a form of hyperthyroidism. This disease is most likely if a patient has signs and symptoms of hyperthyroidism. Laboratory chemistry assays usually demonstrate low TSH and elevated free T_4 levels. Of patients with Graves disease, 50% exhibit thyroid peroxidase antibody (anti-TPO). TSH receptor antibody (TRAb) can discriminate between Graves disease and toxic nodular goiter. In addition, thyroid-stimulating immunoglobulin can detect thyroid antibodies for diagnosing Graves disease.

Pancreatic Disorders

The autoimmune forms of diabetes (Fig. 22.6) include T1D, estimated at 5% to 10% of those with diabetes, and latent autoimmune diabetes in adults (LADA), estimated to be 5% to 10% of those diagnosed with type 2 diabetes (T2D). It is now believed that some overlap exists

TABLE 22.5 Antigens Implicated in Autoimmune Endocrine Disorders

Disease	Antigen
Hashimoto disease	Thyroglobulin
	Thyroid peroxidase
	Thyrotropin receptor
Graves disease	Thyrotropin receptor
	Thyroid peroxidase
	Thyroglobulin
	64-kDa antigen
	70-kDa heat shock protein
Type 1 diabetes	Insulin/proinsulin
	Insulin receptor
	Glutamic acid decarboxylase
	B-cell release granule
	Pancreatic cytokeratin
	64-kDa antigen
	Glucagon
	65-kDa heat shock protein
Addison disease	Adrenal cortical cells
	55-kDa microsomal antigen
Idiopathic hypoparathyroidism	130- and 200-kDa antigens
	Endothelial antigen
	Mitochondrial antigen

between T1D and T2D. A subset of adult patients diagnosed with T2D actually has LADA.

Insulin-Dependent Diabetes Mellitus

Etiology. Insulin-dependent diabetes mellitus (IDDM), or T1D, is a disease of deficient insulin production caused by immune destruction of the B cells of the pancreatic islets. The only definitively identified environmental factor causing T1D is congenital rubella infection. Reports of an association between diabetes and infection with coxsackievirus B and several other viruses have suggested other triggers for the disease.

Genetic susceptibility factors have been identified. T1D is associated with HLA-DR3, DR4, DQ2, and DQ8 antigens. About 90% of White patients with T1D have one or both DR antigens. The presence of both DR3 and DR4 antigens yields an even higher risk of disease development than the additive susceptibility from either antigen, suggesting that other MHC-related genes may be involved in its pathogenesis. Another HLA antigen, DR2, is found less frequently in people with diabetes than in the general population, indicating that this antigen is associated with some type of protective effect. HLA-DQw8 is associated with a twofold to sixfold increased risk for diabetes. Several lines of investigation have implicated the CD4+ T lymphocyte as central in the immune process that leads to the development of diabetes.

Epidemiology. T1D was previously called *juvenile-onset diabetes* because of when it often presents; 10% of people with diabetes have T1D, and approximately 10,000 new cases are diagnosed each year. Most patients develop T1D in childhood or early adolescence but it may occur at any age. Approximately 95% of patients who develop clinical diabetes before age 30 years have T1D.

Signs and symptoms. The central clinical feature is the requirement for exogenous insulin to maintain euglycemia.

Immunologic manifestations. T cells of the CD4+ type are responsible for initiating the immune response to the islets that results in islet cell autoantibodies and B-cell destruction. Patients with T1D have the following types of autoantibodies (Table 22.7):

- Insulin autoantibodies (IAAs)
- Glutamic acid decarboxylase (GAD) autoantibodies
- Islet cell antigen-2 (IA-2)

Antibodies reacting with the cells of the pancreatic islets have been found in patients with diabetes accompanying autoimmune endocrine disorders. Autoantibodies to islet-related antigens precede the development of clinical T1D by a prolonged period, often several years. A higher incidence of these anti–islet cell antibodies, however, has been demonstrated in T1D patients.

An immunoglobulin in the sera of patients with insulin-resistant diabetes appears to bind to a tissue receptor for insulin, which prevents some of the biological effects of insulin. In addition, antibodies that bind to and possibly kill pancreatic islet cells have been found in most young patients with T1D.

A small subgroup of patients with T1D has demonstrated antireceptor antibody (InR), an IgG class of antibodies directed against the insulin receptor. Antibodies to InR may be directed to the binding site or to determinants away from the binding site for insulin. This condition is predominant in non-White females of all ages.

TABLE 22.6	Antithyroid Antibody Tests
Antigen	**Test to Identify Antibody**
Thyroglobulin	Indirect immunofluorescence on fixed thyroid tissues
	Tanned red blood cell (RBC) hemagglutination
	Immunometric assays (IMAs) or sandwich methods
	Radioimmunoassay (RIA)
Microsomal antigen	Enzyme-linked immunosorbent assay (ELISA)
Second colloid antigen (CA2)	Indirect immunofluorescence
Thyroid membrane receptors	LATS
	LATS-P
	In vitro assays for thyroid-stimulating immunoglobulin (TSI) or TSH–binding inhibition (TBI)
Triiodothyronine (total T_3)	RIA using different separation methods
	Electrophoresis with radioactive-labeled thyronines

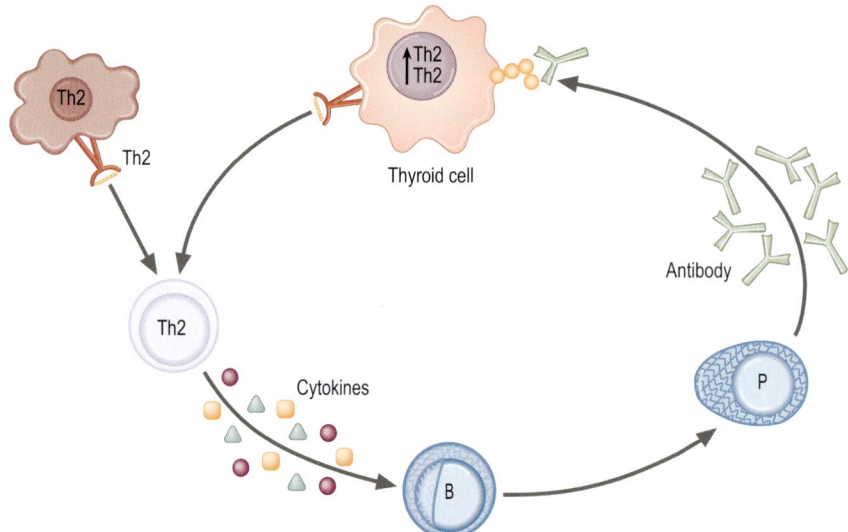

Fig. 22.5 The mechanism of thyroid dysfunction in Graves disease. A type 2 helper T-cell response is initiated and induces production of a stimulatory autoantibody against the thyroid-stimulating hormone receptor. (From Peakman M, Vergani D: *Basic and clinical immunology*, ed 2, London, 2009, Churchill Livingstone.)

CHAPTER 22 Tolerance, Autoimmunity, and Autoimmune Disorders

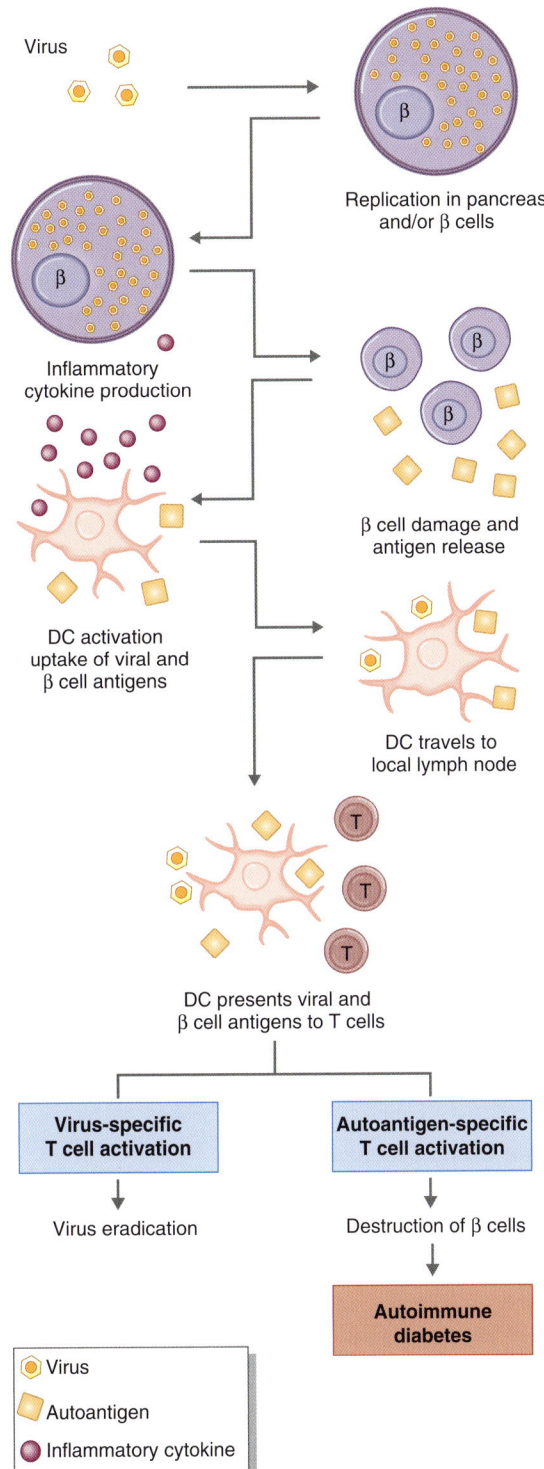

Fig. 22.6 Disease model for the development of type 1 diabetes. A virus infection in the pancreas has two effects: (1) cells are damaged, releasing β-cell antigens; and (2) local dendritic cells are activated by the damaged cells and by viral RNA/DNA. The dendritic cells take samples from the inflamed tissue to the local lymph node. There, they process and present antigens that will include viral and β-cell proteins. T cells are activated to eradicate the virus. Inadvertently, T cells are activated against β cells, and the slow process of β-cell damage starts. The virus is eradicated and all evidence of the initiating virus is long gone by the time the patient presents with clinical diabetes. *DC*, Dendritic cell. (From Peakman M, Vergani D: *Basic and clinical immunology*, ed 2, London, 2009, Churchill Livingstone.)

TABLE 22.7 Autoantibody Assays to Differentiate Type 1 Diabetes[a,b]

Assay	Characteristic
Insulin autoantibodies (IAAs)	Autoantibodies specific for beta cells of the pancreas; may aid in proband diagnosis or predict development of type 2 diabetes
Glutamic acid decarboxylase autoantibodies	Aid in the diagnosis and confirmation of type 1 diabetes; may be found in patients who eventually develop type 1 diabetes
Islet antigen-2 autoantibodies	Associated with type 1 diabetes; may be present in patients years before the onset of clinical symptoms

[a]American Diabetic Association (2008): Note: Type 1 diabetes results typically have antibodies and low C-peptide levels. Absence of antibodies or normal C-peptide levels does not rule out type 1, but likelihood of type 1 diabetes is low.
[b]United States Preventive Services Task Force (USPSTF; 2008): Note: C-peptide testing – use to confirm lack of insulin production, suggesting type 1 diabetes. Use of C-peptide levels or insulin levels to diagnose type 1 diabetes is not recommended.

IA-2 is directed against a phosphatase-type transmembrane 37-kDa islet B-cell antigen (ICA512).

Latent Autoimmune Diabetes in Adults

LADA is now recognized as a slowly developing form of autoimmune diabetes found in patients who are older than 35 years of age. LADA is frequently misdiagnosed as T2D. LADA patients progress more rapidly to insulin dependence (T1D) than the typical T2D patient.

Autoimmune Pancreatitis

Autoimmune pancreatitis is a heterogeneous disease. This type of chronic pancreatitis is characterized by an autoimmune inflammatory process in which prominent lymphocyte infiltration with associated fibrosis of the pancreas causes organ dysfunction.

Etiology. Although the cause of the disease is unknown, it is thought to be a systemic autoimmune disease. It is frequently associated with other autoimmune disorders (e.g., RA).

Epidemiology. Autoimmune pancreatitis is rare but an increasing number of cases have been reported since 2000. Although this condition can occur in both sexes, it is at least twice as common in men as women. Most patients are older than 50 years at diagnosis.

Signs and symptoms. Symptoms are variable. Many patients have jaundice; some have abdominal pain. Histologic examination of pancreatic tissue reveals a collar-like periductal infiltrate composed of lymphocytes and plasma cells. Computed tomography (CT) typically reveals a diffuse enlargement of the pancreas, with a halo around its peripheral rim. Various findings on imaging radiography are correlated with serologic and histologic analyses. It is important to diagnose autoimmune pancreatitis correctly on the basis of imaging, histology, and serology because it can mimic pancreatic cancer.

Immunologic manifestations. In the Japanese population, an association between HLA haplotype DRB1*0405-DQB1*0401 has been observed with immunologic abnormalities including the following:
- Hypergammaglobulinemia (elevated serum IgG or gamma globulin level) in patients with enhanced peripheral rim halo of the pancreas on CT;

- Elevated serum IgG4 concentrations in patients with a diffusely enlarged pancreas;
- Autoantibodies against carbonic anhydrase II (ACA II), lactoferrin (antilactoferrin antibody [ALA]), anti–smooth muscle antibody (ASMA), or ANA;
- Increased number of CD4+ T lymphocytes (T_{regs}) that control autoimmunity in the peripheral blood.

Adrenal Glands

Idiopathic adrenal atrophy is the primary cause of Addison disease. It is believed that many of these cases have an autoimmune cause. Women are afflicted twice as often as men and the disease usually presents in the third or fourth decade of life. Although great potential exists for morbidity, it has a relatively low incidence. The adult form of Addison disease is associated with HLA class II antigens DR3 and DR4.

Idiopathic Addison disease is usually diagnosed in patients because of low serum cortisol levels in the presence of elevated levels of corticotropin. Approximately 80% of patients manifest serum antibodies against cortical elements, probably microsomal. Some patients demonstrate antibodies against adrenal cell surfaces. These antibodies generally bind to components in the adrenal cortex but affect only individual zones. Antibodies are generally low in titer and are not a direct reflection of adrenal cell damage. Autoimmune destruction of the ovarian stroma has been observed in women with premature ovarian failure.

Pituitary Gland

Sheehan syndrome—lymphocytic adenohypophysitis—is a disease that causes a rapid decline in pituitary function. This disease is most frequently seen in postpartum women and antibodies against pituitary cells are observed in some patients. The disease is distinguished by a mononuclear infiltrate of the pituitary gland and hypophysis.

Parathyroid Gland

Idiopathic hypoparathyroidism occurs as a childhood disease in type I polyglandular syndrome and, less often, as an isolated disease in adults. It is associated with complement-mediated cytotoxicity of parathyroid cells, indicating a specific immune response to the parathyroid. Several antigens have been associated with this disease, including endothelial cell proteins and mitochondria.

Polyglandular Syndromes

Three syndromes of associated endocrinopathies have been defined as the polyglandular syndromes. Type I polyglandular syndrome involves mucocutaneous candidiasis and associated endocrinopathies that begin in early childhood. Patients initially develop candidiasis and hypoparathyroidism, but more than 50% also develop Addison disease. Gonadal failure, alopecia, and chronic hepatitis are also seen. Patients have organ-specific autoantibodies and poorly defined defects in cell-mediated immunity.

Type II polyglandular syndrome involves the combined occurrence of IDDM or autoimmune thyroid disease with Addison disease. It is also called *Schmidt syndrome*. This type of disease is seen primarily in women in the second or third decade of life. Most cases are familial, but the mode of inheritance is unknown. There is a strong association with HLA-DR3.

Type III polyglandular syndrome is defined as autoimmune thyroid disease occurring with two other autoimmune disorders, including IDDM, PA, and a nonendocrine, organ-specific autoimmune disease, such as myasthenia gravis. These patients do not have Addison disease.

The HLA-DR3 allele is present in more than 50% of cases. Patients in this category are overwhelmingly female.

Reproductive Disorders

Antibodies against cytoplasmic components of different cells of the ovary have been demonstrated in Addison disease and in premature ovarian failure, which may be an immune disease causing reproductive failure and eventually early menopause. A prevalence of smooth muscle antibody, ANA, and antiphospholipid antibodies has been found in women with unexplained infertility. In addition, autoantibodies to the ovary and gonadotropin receptors exist in many women with polyendocrinopathies.

Patients with endometriosis have a defect in natural killer (NK) cell activity. This results in decreased cytotoxicity for autologous endometrial cells. Reduced T-lymphocyte–mediated cytotoxicity to endometrial cells has also been found.

A sizable proportion of pregnancy losses may be caused by immunologic factors. The fetus is an immunogenic allograft that evokes a protective immune response from the mother, which is necessary for implantation and growth. The mechanism of pregnancy loss is hypothesized to involve two antiphospholipid antibodies. Lupus anticoagulant and anticardiolipin antibodies are directed against platelets and vascular endothelium. This causes vascular destruction and thrombosis, leading to fetal death and abortion. There is no evidence of a direct immunologic attack on the embryo. A human fetus is capable of survival in utero if it does not share a significant number of maternal MHC antigens, especially HLA-B and HLA-DR and DQ loci.

Antisperm antibodies have been detected in the serum of men and women, in the cervical mucus of women, in the seminal fluid of men, and attached to sperm cells. In seminal fluid, the immobilizing antibodies to sperm are usually of the IgG class and the agglutinating antibodies are immunoglobulin A. Elevated levels of antibodies to sperm have been found in more than 40% of men after vasectomy but only occasionally in men with primary testicular agenesis. Allergy-like reactions to seminal fluid have also been observed. These reactions range from local reactions to systemic reactions, including life-threatening anaphylaxis. The allergen is usually one or more prostatic proteins, but it can include immunoglobulin E to spermatozoa.

Exocrine Gland Disease

Sjögren Syndrome

Etiology. Sjögren syndrome is a chronic inflammatory disease of unknown cause that affects lacrimal, salivary, and other excretory glands. It results in keratoconjunctivitis sicca and xerostomia.

As with RA and SLE, causative factors include infection, abnormalities of immune regulation, and genetic factors. Development of Sjögren syndrome is strongly associated with HLA-B8 and HLA-DR3, and an infectious origin has been suggested. Clear evidence for excessive B-cell activity has been demonstrated, but it is not known whether this is caused by B- or T-cell abnormalities.

Epidemiology. A primary form is not associated with other disorders; a secondary form is associated with RA and other connective tissue disorders. About 90% of patients are women and a 44-fold increased incidence of lymphoma has been noted in patients with Sjögren syndrome.

Signs and symptoms. The main clinical manifestations of Sjögren syndrome are dry eyes, dry mouth, and recurrent salivary gland pain and swelling (Table 22.8). Hoarseness, chronic cough, and an increased incidence of infection have been observed. Dryness of the vagina leads to dyspareunia and itching. Dysphagia and atrophic gastritis can also be present. Extraglandular involvement results in interstitial pneumonitis

TABLE 22.8 Criteria for Diagnosis of Sjögren Syndrome[a]

Ocular symptoms	Dry eyes daily for 3 months, sand or gravel feeling in eyes
Oral symptoms	Dry mouth daily for 3 months or recurrent or persistent swollen glands
Ocular signs	Post-Schirmer test or rose Bengal score >4
Histopathology	Aggregates of ≥50 mononuclear cells/4 mm^2 of glandular tissue
Autoantibodies	Presence of anti-Ro (SS-A), anti-La (SS-B), antinuclear antibodies (ANAs), or rheumatoid factor

[a]Four or more of these criteria must be met.
(From Vitali C, Bombardieri S, Moutsopoulos HM, et al: Preliminary criteria for the classification of Sjögren's syndrome: results of a prospective concerted action supported by the European community, *Arthritis Rheum* 1993;36:340–347.)

and fibrosis. Renal tubular acidosis and vasculitis involving the peripheral nerves and central nervous system (CNS) can also result from Sjögren syndrome.

Immunologic manifestations. The immunologic characteristics of Sjögren syndrome include hypergammaglobulinemia, rheumatoid factor, autoantibodies to salivary duct and other antigens, and lymphocyte and plasma cell infiltration of involved tissue. Antibodies are usually polyclonal and may result in hyperviscosity syndrome and hypergammaglobulinemic purpura. Speckled or homogeneous ANA patterns are present in 65% of patients and occur more frequently in primary Sjögren syndrome. Antibodies to Sjögren syndrome A antigen have been associated with vasculitis in primary Sjögren syndrome. Antibodies to Sjögren syndrome B antigen are almost always found in association with Sjögren syndrome A antigen and only occur in SLE and Sjögren syndrome. Rheumatoid factor is found in 90% of cases. A rather new autoantibody, anti–α-fodrin, has been found in the sera of most patients with primary Sjögren syndrome. This antibody may be pathophysiologically associated with some extraglandular manifestations characteristically seen in patients with Sjögren syndrome.

Autoantibodies to salivary duct antigens are frequently detected in patients with secondary Sjögren syndrome, and they are also common in 25% of patients with RA without Sjögren syndrome. Mitochondrial antibodies are detected in 10% of patients with primary Sjögren syndrome and rarely in patients with secondary Sjögren syndrome and RA. Patients with primary Sjögren syndrome also have higher levels of antibodies to the thyroid gland, gastric parietal cells, pancreatic epithelial cells, and smooth muscle. Lymphocytic infiltration of the exocrine glands of the eyes, mouth, nose, lower respiratory tract, GI tract, and vagina occurs. The infiltrate is composed of B and T cells. In tissue culture, these cells produce large amounts of immunoglobulin M (IgM) and IgG. T cells are predominantly helper cells.

Gastrointestinal Disorders
Atrophic Gastritis and Pernicious Anemia

A malfunctioning immune system can target the stomach lining resulting in autoimmune gastritis, characterized by chronic inflammation of the gastric mucosa. Individuals with autoimmune gastritis may progress to PA.

Atrophic gastritis. Autoimmune gastritis is characterized by the presence of serum autoantibodies against gastric parietal cells, H$^+$/K$^+$–ATPase (proton pump), and the cobalamin-absorbing protein, intrinsic factor.

Immunologic findings. Antibodies against a lipoprotein cytoplasmic component of gastric parietal cells can be detected by immunofluorescence in up to 90% of PA patients and in about 60% of patients with atrophic gastritis without hematologic abnormalities. These antibodies may also be demonstrated in patients with other autoimmune disorders, such as thyroiditis. In addition, antibodies can be found in asymptomatic patients and in those older than 60 years.

Histologic findings. Atrophic gastritis, which almost always accompanies PA, is characterized by destruction of the gastric mucosa, with lymphocytic infiltration and the absence of parietal and chief cells. The lesions are associated with decreased synthesis of gastric acid and intrinsic factor. Intrinsic factor normally binds ingested vitamin B$_{12}$ at one site and binds to receptors in the distal ileum at another site. Therefore vitamin B$_{12}$ transport across the ileum is affected.

Vitamin B$_{12}$ (cobalamin) transport. Cobalamin transport is mediated by three different binding proteins capable of binding the vitamin at its required physiologic concentrations: intrinsic factor, transcobalamin II, and the R proteins (Table 22.9).

Intrinsic factor (IF), a glycoprotein, is synthesized and secreted by the parietal cells of the mucosa in the fundus region of the stomach in several mammalian species, including human beings. In a healthy state, the amounts of IF secreted by the stomach greatly exceed the quantities required to bind ingested cobalamin in its coenzyme forms. At a very acidic pH, cobalamin splits from dietary protein and combines with IF to form a vitamin-IF complex. Binding by IF is extraordinarily specific and is lost with even slight changes in the cobalamin molecule. This complex is stable and remains unabsorbed until it reaches the ileum. In the ileum, the vitamin-IF complex attaches to specific receptor sites present only on the outer surface of microvillous membranes of ileal enterocytes.

The release of this complex from the mucosal cells, with subsequent transport to the tissues, depends on transcobalamin II (TCII). TCII is a plasma polypeptide synthesized by the liver and probably by several other tissues. TCII, which turns over very rapidly in plasma, acts as the acceptor and principal carrier of the vitamin to the liver and other tissues, as with IF. Receptors for TCII are observed on the plasma membranes of a wide variety of cells. TCII is also capable of binding a few unusual cobalamin analogs. TCII also stimulates cobalamin uptake by reticulocytes.

The R proteins comprise an antigenically crossreactive group of cobalamin-binding glycoproteins that bind cobalamin and various cobalamin analogs. Their function is unknown, but they appear to serve as storage sites and as a means of eliminating excess cobalamin and unwanted analogs from the blood circulation through receptor sites on liver cells. R proteins are produced by leukocytes and perhaps other tissues. They are present in plasma as transcobalamin I and transcobalamin III, and are also found in saliva, milk, and other body fluids. Transcobalamin I probably serves only as a backup transport system for endogenous cobalamin. Endogenous vitamin is synthesized in the human GI tract by bacterial action, but none is adsorbed.

Pernicious anemia. PA is a megaloblastic anemia characterized by a variety of hematologic and chemical manifestations (Table 22.10). PA is caused by a deficiency of vitamin B$_{12}$ that results from the patient's inability to secrete IF. In autoimmune cases of PA, anti-IF or antiparietal antibodies have been reported. Demonstration of these antibodies supports the theory that PA is an autoimmune disease. Nutritional disorders (e.g., vegan diet, gastric bypass surgery, AIDS, small-bowel disorders, and competition for vitamin B$_{12}$) can be nonimmunologic causes of PA.

TABLE 22.9 Vitamin B$_{12}$ (Cobalamin)–Binding Proteins

Parameter	Intrinsic Factor	Transcobalamin (TC II)	R Proteins
Source	Stomach	Liver, other tissues	Leukocytes, ? other tissues
Function	Intestinal absorption	Delivery to cells	Excretion storage
		Is the principal transport carrier protein system of cobalamin	
Membrane receptors	Ileal enterocytes	Many cells	Liver cells

TABLE 22.10 Hematologic and Chemical Findings in Pernicious Anemia

Assay	Finding
Hematologic Indices	
Hemoglobin (Hb)	Severely decreased
Hematocrit (Hct)	Severely decreased
Erythrocyte (RBC) count	Decreased
Leukocyte (WBC) count	Slightly decreased
Platelet count	Slightly decreased or normal
Mean corpuscular volume (MCV)	Increased
Chemical Indices	
Serum iron	Increased
Total iron-binding capacity (TIBC)	Normal or decreased
Percentage of iron (Fe) saturation	Increased
Serum ferritin	Increased

WBC, White blood cell.

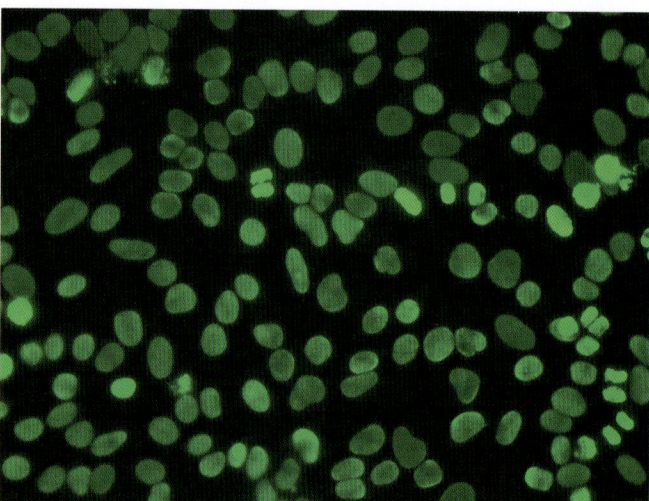

Fig. 22.7 Antinuclear antibody (ANA). Homogeneous or diffused—a solid staining of the nucleus with or without apparent masking of the nucleoli. (Courtesy INOVA Diagnostics, Inc., San Diego, CA.)

Assays for anti-IF measure antibodies to IF. The presence of **IF-blocking antibodies** is diagnostic of PA and antibodies can be demonstrated in about 60% of cases. Antiparietal cell assays measure antibodies to parietal cells (large cells on the margins of the peptic glands of the stomach). Most patients with PA (80%) have parietal cell antibodies. In the presence of these antibodies, gastric biopsy almost always demonstrates gastritis. Low antibody titers to parietal cells are often found with no clinical evidence of PA or atrophic gastritis and are sometimes seen in older patients.

Autoimmune Liver Disease

Autoimmune processes are believed to be the possible cause of chronic liver disease. Hypergammaglobulinemia, prominent lymphocyte and plasma cell inflammation of the liver, and the presence of one or more circulating tissue antibodies are typically manifested. These manifestations suggest an organ-localized autoimmune pathogenesis.

Autoimmune hepatitis (AIH), formerly known as *chronic active hepatitis*, is an inflammatory condition most common in young women. It is characterized by prominent lymphocyte and plasma cell inflammatory changes, which start in the portal tracts. In some patients, this condition results from a chronic viral infection or inflammation, but in others, a number of immunologic abnormalities are present to varying degrees in addition to hypergammaglobulinemia and an elevated erythrocyte sedimentation rate (ESR). A defect in **immunoregulation** is often demonstrated, which may lead to unrestrained immunoglobulin production.

ANA using HEp-2 cells will have differing levels of reactivity, depending on factors such as the disease activity or multiple ANA specificities. A homogeneous staining pattern is the most frequent pattern, particularly in active AIH. The frequency of positive ANA tests is about 70% in AIH. In remission, the frequency of ANA positivity decreases and the ANA pattern is replaced by a speckled pattern in almost 40% of cases. Other significant antibodies can include an atypical perinuclear antineutrophil cytoplasmic autoantibody (p-ANCA) in one type of AIH, with a frequency of 65% positivity. In addition, AIH is characterized by autoantibodies to cytoskeletal proteins. These proteins support cellular structure, contractility, and locomotion. Autoantibodies to cytoskeleton can be studied by immunofluorescent light (IFL) methodology (Fig. 22.7).

These patients display ANAs and ASMAs. A high and persistent titer of antismooth antibodies is suggestive of the autoimmune form of chronic active hepatitis or viral disorders, such as infectious mononucleosis.

In some cases, this disease is referred to as *lupoid hepatitis*. Patients with aggressive chronic active hepatitis have a poor prognosis and a significant rate of mortality is reported 5 years after diagnosis.

Idiopathic Biliary Cirrhosis

Idiopathic biliary cirrhosis is a slowly progressive disease that starts as an apparently noninfectious inflammation in the bile ducts of young to middle-aged women. An increased familial incidence has been noted.

Patients exhibit increased serum IgM and depression of cellular immunity, with prominent decreases in suppressor T cells common, as well as associated autoimmune disorders. It is believed that tissue damage results from an unmodulated attack against host tissue antigens. Antimitochondrial antibodies directed against the cellular ultrastructures—mitochondria—can be displayed. A high titer of antimicrobial antibody strongly suggests primary biliary cirrhosis (PBC); an absence of mitochondrial antibodies is strong evidence against PBC. Other forms of liver disease, however, frequently exhibit low mitochondrial antibody titers.

Inflammatory Bowel Disease

Inflammatory bowel disease (IBD) is the collective name given to Crohn disease and ulcerative colitis (UC). A major gene has been identified in these disorders. The Centers for Disease Control and Prevention (CDC) estimates that IBD, which is more common among Ashkenazi Jewish people than other groups, affects more than 1 million Americans. When researchers examined more than 300,000 single-nucleotide polymorphisms (SNPs) and the variations that occur when a nucleotide (molecular subunit of DNA) is altered, it was discovered that the frequency of variations in the receptor gene for interleukin-23 (IL-23) is significantly different for those with IBD. A coding variant that apparently protects against IBD is found less frequently in patients with IBD than in healthy patients.

Many factors (e.g., genetic susceptibility and diet) affect the onset and development of IBD. The crux of the disease is an abnormal immune response to harmless bacteria in the gut that benefits the host by providing energy and nutrients. In IBD patients, these microorganisms become a target for attack by the immune system. The inflammation seen in IBD patients has been linked to the following:
- Presence of increased levels of inflammation-promoting cytokines
- Protein molecules used by cells of the immune system to communicate with each other

Studies have suggested that one cytokine, IL-12, is a crucial mediator of this disease. IL-12 causes inflammation by activating a class of different immune cells, type 1 helper T (Th1) cells, which in turn secrete proinflammatory molecules such as interferon-γ (IFN-γ) and tumor necrosis factor-α (TNF-α). These pathways have been suggested as therapeutic targets for human IBD.

The discovery of IL-23 has led some to question the central role of IL-12 and Th1 cells in IBD. Newer studies have indicated that IL-12 and IL-23 are closely related molecules that share a common subunit known as *p40*. IL-23 has been associated with the activation of a new class of proinflammatory T cells called *Th17*. These cells secrete the proinflammatory cytokine IL-17, which mediates the inflammatory response in organs such as the brain and joints. Intestinal inflammation is still associated with large increases in IL-17 production in the intestines. Innate immune cells present in inflamed intestines (e.g., granulocytes and monocytes) have been found to contribute to the increased production of IL-17.

ILC3, a subset of innate lymphocytes in the lamina propria of the intestine or in the mesenteric lymph node, performs a similar function, except that the T cells that are deleted are those that recognize bacterial antigens and could thus cause IBD. As in the thymus, the ILC3 cells use MHC class II to present antigen to T cells. If a bacterial antigen is presented and strongly recognized by the T cell, the T cell undergoes apoptosis. Failure to delete these cells results in inflammation that can be labeled autoinflammatory.

Crohn disease and UC are characterized by a dysbiosis, a change in the microbiome, the bacteria that colonize the gut. In Crohn disease lymphocytes, which ignore bacteria in the intestine in healthy persons, have an exuberant immune response that correlates with bowel inflammation and disease. It is more appropriate to label this disease autoinflammatory than autoimmune.

Immune Markers

The following serologic markers have been found to be useful in the diagnosis and differentiation of Crohn disease and UC:
- Deoxyribonuclease (DNase I)-sensitive p-ANCA. IBD-associated p-ANCA defines an antibody to a nuclear antigen that is sensitive to DNase I.
- Anti–*Saccharomyces cerevisiae* antibody (ASCA). This is present in the sera of up to 70% of Crohn disease patients.
- Pancreatic antibody. This is observed in approximately 30% of Crohn disease patients.

> **BOX 22.3 Clinical Immune Disorders Associated with Celiac Disease**
> - Selective IgA deficiency
> - Autoimmune thyroid disease
> - Chronic autoimmune hepatitis
> - Lupus erythematosus
> - Sjögren syndrome
> - Type 1 diabetes

- Anti–outer membrane porin from *Escherichia coli* (anti-OmpC). An IgA response to OmpC is observed in 55% of Crohn disease patients.

Celiac Disease

Celiac disease is a lifelong autoimmune intestinal disease found in individuals who are genetically susceptible. There are also associated clinical disorders of an immune basis (Box 22.3). Damage to the mucosal surface of the small intestine is caused by an immunologically toxic reaction to the ingestion of gluten and interferes with the absorption of nutrients. Celiac disease is unique in that a specific food component, gluten, has been identified as the trigger. *Gluten* is the common name for the offending proteins in specific cereal grains that are harmful to those with celiac disease. These proteins are found in all forms of wheat (e.g., durum, semolina, spelt, kamut, einkorn, and farro) and related grains (rye, barley, and triticale) and must be eliminated.

In recent years, key laboratory diagnostic assays comprise testing for autoantibodies against tissue transglutaminase (antitTG) or endomysium (EmA) antibodies against deamidated gliadin peptides and the celiac disease–associated HLA DQ2 and DQ8.

New European guidelines have resulted in two algorithms of testing: symptomatic patients versus asymptomatic patients (Fig. 22.8). For symptomatic patients, the algorithm begins with determination of specific anti-TG antibodies of class IgA in parallel with total IgA or specific IgG measured in parallel testing. If the anti-TG antibody titer is more than 10 above the upper normal limit, the endomysium (EmA) is positive, and compatible HLA results are found, it is not necessary to perform a small-bowel biopsy, as was done in the past. Diagnostic tests should be done on individuals on a gluten-containing diet. A biopsy is needed only if serologic and genetic findings are inconclusive.

The most common autoimmune disorders associated with celiac disease are T1D, autoimmune hepatitis, Sjögren's syndrome, multiple sclerosis (MS), RA, Addison disease, idiopathic dilated cardiomyopathy, Hashimoto's thyroiditis, and IgA nephropathy (Berger's disease).

Other Gastrointestinal Tract Immunologic Disorders

Examples of other immunologic disorders related to the GI and hepatobiliary tracts include GI allergy, Whipple disease, immunoproliferative intestinal disease (alpha heavy-chain disease), and infectious hepatitis. Allergy of the GI tract is an IgE-mediated hypersensitivity to food substances that involves the GI tract and, in some cases, the skin and lungs. Examples of systemic autoimmune disease caused by mucosal immune abnormalities are IgA nephropathy (Berger disease), Henoch-Schönlein purpura, and disorders associated with circulating IgA complexes in the kidney and vasculature. Immunoproliferative intestinal disease is characterized by monoclonal B cells that produce an aberrant alpha heavy chain.

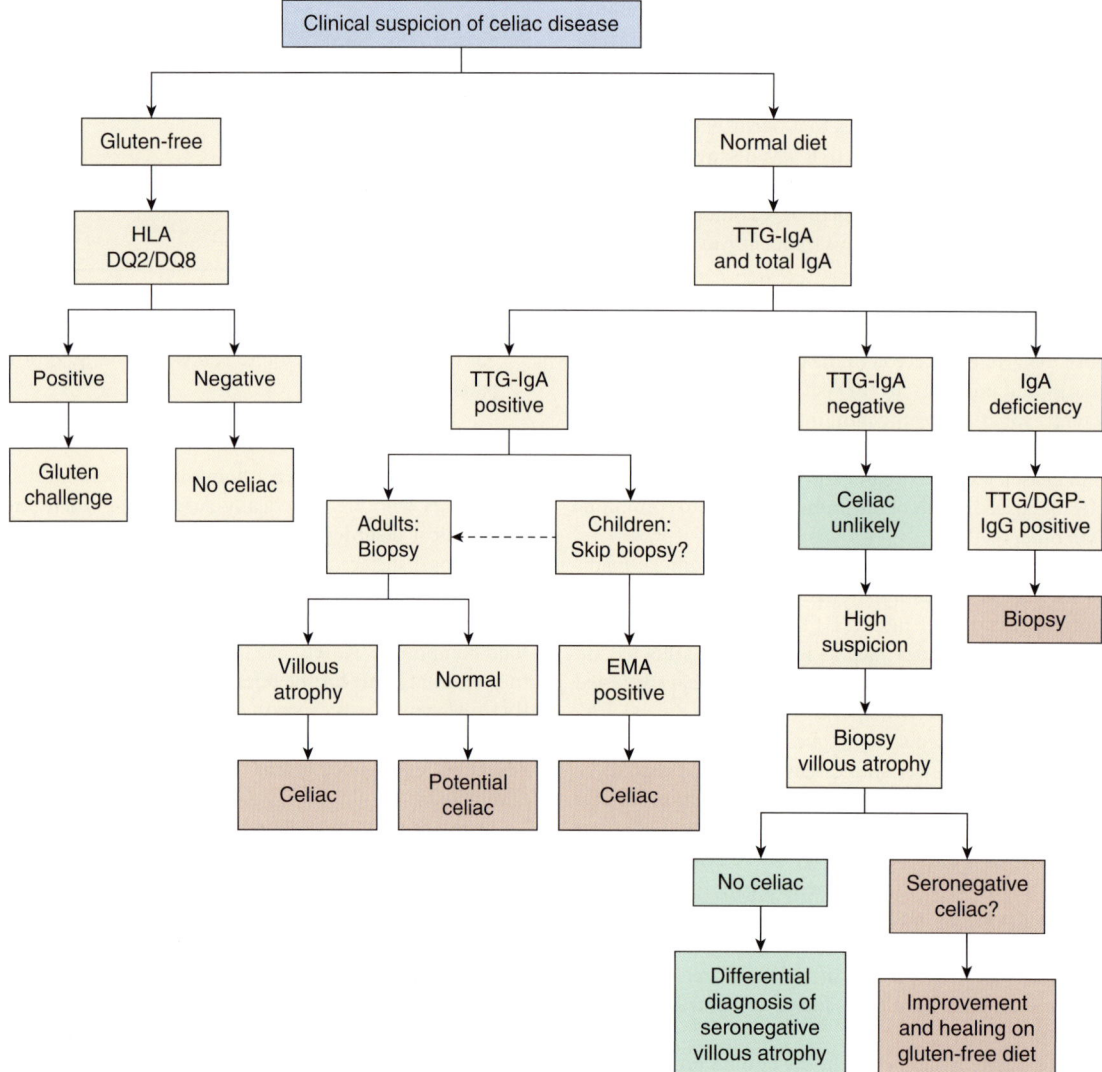

Fig. 22.8 Diagnostic algorithm for celiac disease. (Lebwohl B, Rubio-Tapia A: Epidemiology, presentation, and diagnosis of celiac disease, *Gastroenterology* 160(1):63–75, 2021.)

Autoimmune Hematologic Disorders

Various hematologic conditions can be caused by alloantibodies and autoantibodies (Table 22.11).

Autoimmune Lymphoproliferative Syndrome

Autoimmune lymphoproliferative syndrome (ALPS) is a disease in which a genetic defect in programmed cell death, or apoptosis, leads to breakdown of lymphocyte homeostasis and normal immunologic tolerance. ALPS is the first pediatric syndrome described in which the primary defect is in apoptosis.

Defective apoptosis in lymphocytes (and in ALPS type II dendritic cells) leads to accumulation of these cells in the lymphoid organs after they would normally be eliminated. As a result, cells with autoimmune potential are unchecked and can induce a variety of autoimmune disorders; the risk for malignant transformation to lymphoma is increased.

Patients with ALPS have chronic enlargement of the spleen and lymph nodes, various manifestations of autoimmunity, and elevation of a normally rare population of double-negative T cells (DNTs). When lymphocytes from ALPS patients are cultured in vitro, they are resistant to apoptosis compared with cells from healthy controls.

Most ALPS patients have mutations in a TNF receptor gene that is a member of a superfamily (TNFRSF6). This gene, previously known as *APT1*, encodes the cell surface receptor for the major apoptosis pathway in mature lymphocytes. This receptor has many names, including Fas. The Fas apoptotic pathway is important for eliminating excess T cells after they have been activated and also eliminating antigen-driven and autoreactive T-cell clones. Fas is a functional trimer residing at the cell membrane that, when engaged by trimeric Fas ligand (FasL), initiates a proteolytic cascade leading to chromosomal DNA degradation and cell death.

Autoimmune Hemolytic Anemia

Autoimmune hemolytic anemia can be classified into the following four groups:
- Warm-reactive autoantibodies (most common)
- Cold-reactive autoantibodies (<20% of cases)
- Paroxysmal cold hemoglobinuria (rare)
- Drug-induced hemolysis (<20% of cases)

Warm autoimmune hemolytic anemia. This anemia is associated with antibodies reactive at warm temperatures (i.e., 37°C [98.6°F]). In more than 75% of cases, the erythrocytes are coated with both IgG and complement, although some may demonstrate coating with IgG alone or, less often, with complement coating. In warm autoimmune hemolytic anemia, negligible serum autoantibody exists because the antibody reacts optimally at 37°C (98.6°F) and is being continuously adsorbed by red blood cells (RBCs) in vivo. Elution of the antibody from the RBCs (mechanical removal of antibodies) can demonstrate an autoantibody, but testing for specificity is not routinely necessary.

Cold autoimmune hemolytic anemia. Cold hemagglutinin disease (CHAD), acute or chronic, is the most common type of hemolytic anemia associated with cold-reactive autoantibodies. The acute form is often secondary to *Mycoplasma pneumoniae* infection or lymphoproliferative disorders such as lymphoma. The chronic form is seen in older patients and produces mild-to-moderate hemolysis. In addition, Raynaud phenomenon and hemoglobinuria occur in cold weather.

In CHAD, a cold-reactive IgM autoantibody reacts with RBCs in the peripheral circulation when the body temperature falls to 32°C (89.6°F) or lower and binds complement to the cells. Therefore complement is the only globulin detected on the erythrocytes. Elutions prepared from RBCs collected at 37°C (98.6°F) will not demonstrate antibody reactivity in the eluate.

Paroxysmal cold hemoglobinuria. Previously associated with syphilis, paroxysmal cold hemoglobinuria is now seen more often as an acute transient condition secondary to viral infections, particularly in young children. It may also occur as an idiopathic chronic disease in older people.

The autoantibody is an IgG protein that reacts with RBCs in colder parts of the body; this produces complement components C3 and C4 to bind irreversibly to the erythrocytes. At warmer temperatures, RBCs are hemolyzed and the antibody elutes from the cells. Eluates are also nonreactive. This IgG autoantibody, a biphasic hemolysin, can be demonstrated by performing the classic Donath–Landsteiner test. The autoantibody has anti-P specificity and reacts with all except the rare p or p^k phenotypes. Exceptions that include examples with anti-IH specificity have been described.

Drug-induced hemolysis. Coating of RBCs demonstrated by a positive direct anti–human globulin test (DAT) result may be drug induced and accompanied by hemolysis (Table 22.12). The reactivity has been described as being caused by four basic mechanisms: (1) drug adsorption, (2) immune complexing, (3) membrane modification, and (4) autoantibody formation.

Drug adsorption. Penicillin is a representative example of an agent that displays drug adsorption. In this type of mechanism, the drug strongly binds to any protein, including RBC membrane proteins. This binding produces a drug-RBC-hapten complex that can stimulate antibody formation. The antibody is specific for this complex, and no reactions will take place unless the drug is adsorbed on erythrocytes. Massive doses of IV penicillin are needed to coat the erythrocytes sufficiently for antibody attachment to occur.

Approximately 3% of affected patients will demonstrate a positive DAT result and less than 5% will develop hemolytic anemia because of the drug. The hemolysis of RBCs is usually extravascular and occurs slowly. It is not life-threatening and will abate when penicillin is discontinued. There appears to be no connection between this type of antibody production and allergic penicillin sensitivity caused by IgE production.

Other drugs that display drug adsorption are cephalothin derivatives (e.g., cephalothin [Keflin] and quinidine).

Immune complexing. Immune complexing is associated with a variety of drugs, including phenacetin, quinine, rifampin, and stibophen. In this interaction, the drug and antibody form a complex in the serum and attach nonspecifically to the RBCs. Once attached this complex initiates the complement cascade, which culminates in intravascular hemolysis. The immune complex may dissociate from the RBC membrane after complement activation and attach to another

TABLE 22.11	Immunohematologic Disorders
Category	**Examples**
Immune hemolysis	Warm autoimmune hemolytic anemia
	Cold agglutinin disease
	Paroxysmal cold hemoglobinuria
	Drug-induced hemolytic anemias
	Hemolytic disease of the newborn
Immune thrombocytopenia	Idiopathic (autoimmune) thrombocytopenic purpura
	Neonatal alloimmune thrombocytopenia
Immune neutropenia	Autoimmune neutropenia
Immune-mediated transfusion reactions	Acute hemolytic transfusion reaction
	Febrile reactions
	Pulmonary hypersensitivity reaction
	Allergic reactions
	IgA-deficient recipient
	Delayed hemolytic reactions
	Posttransfusion purpura
	Transfusion-associated graft-versus-host disease
Anemias	Pernicious anemia
Deficiency of hemostasis and coagulation	Autoimmune protein S deficiency

TABLE 22.12	Drug-Induced Positive Direct Antiglobulin Test			
Parameter	**Drug Adsorption**	**Immune Complex**	**Membrane Modification**	**Autoantibody Formation**
Common cause	IgG	Complement	Nonserologic	IgG
Antibody screening	Negative[a]	Positive[b]	Negative	Variable[c]
Eluate reactivity with reagent RBCs	Nonreactive	Nonreactive	Nonreactive	Reactive[d]
Penicillin-treated RBCs	Reactive with patient's serum and eluate	Nonreactive	Nonreactive	Nonreactive

[a]Unless irregular antibodies are present in the sample.
[b]If the drug and complement are present in the test system.
[c]If the autoantibody is high enough in titer, screening tests may be positive with all cells tested.
[d]Will react with all normal cells tested, occasionally showing Rh-like specificity.
RBCs, Red blood cells.

erythrocyte. This allows a small amount of drug to produce severe anemia. When the offending drug is discontinued, the hemolytic process disappears quickly.

Membrane modification. Drugs of the cephalosporin type (e.g., cephalothin) occasionally cause a positive DAT result with polyspecific and monospecific anti–human globulin antisera by membrane modification. In this type of mechanism, the drug alters the membrane so that there is nonspecific absorption of globulins, including IgG, IgM, IgA, and complement. Hemolysis is not a common complication in this type of membrane augmentation.

Autoantibody formation. Drugs such as methyldopa (Aldomet), levodopa, and mefenamic acid (Ponstel) have been implicated in positive DAT results caused by autoantibody formation. The autoantibody formed recognizes a part of the RBC and therefore reacts with most normal RBCs. Some drug-induced autoantibodies have been shown to have specificities that appear to be of the Rh type, but most have no apparent specificity. Antibody production ceases with withdrawal of the drug.

Idiopathic Thrombocytopenic Purpura

Idiopathic thrombocytopenic purpura is now also known as *immunologic thrombocytopenic purpura (ITP)*. Patients with ITP usually demonstrate petechiae, bruising, menorrhagia, and bleeding after minor trauma. ITP may be acute or chronic. Children are most often affected with the acute type, whereas adults predominantly experience the chronic type. This common disease may complicate other antibody-associated disorders such as SLE.

Thrombocytopenia, a condition of absent or severely decreased platelets ($<10–20 \times 10^9$/L), may result from a wide variety of conditions, such as after extracorporeal circulation in cardiac bypass surgery or from alcoholic liver disease. However, most thrombocytopenic conditions can be classified into the following three major categories:

- Decreased production of platelets
- Disorders of platelet distribution
- Increased destruction or use of platelets

Decreased platelet production may result from invasion of the bone marrow by neoplastic cells and is usually not associated with an immunologic cause. Disorders of platelet distribution are associated with a sequestering of platelets in the spleen for various nonimmunologic reasons. Increased destruction or use of platelets, however, is associated with immunologic mechanisms. These mechanisms of destruction are caused by antigens, antibodies, or complement.

Drugs or foreign substances that can cause platelet destruction include quinidine, sulfonamide derivatives, heroin, morphine, and snake venom. Sulfonamide derivative reactions involve the interaction of platelet antigens with drug antibodies. Morphine reactions involve the activation of complement.

Bacterial sepsis causes increased destruction of platelets resulting from the attachment of platelets to bacterial antigen-antibody immune complexes. Certain microbial antigens may initially attach to platelets, followed by specific antibodies to the microorganism. This mechanism has been reported to cause the thrombocytopenia that frequently complicates *Plasmodium falciparum* malaria.

Antibodies of autoimmune or isoimmune origin may cause increased destruction of platelets. Examples of thrombocytopenias of isoimmune origin include posttransfusion purpura and isoimmune neonatal thrombocytopenia. Neonatal autoimmune thrombocytopenia is a condition caused by immunization of a pregnant female by a fetal platelet antigen and by transplacental passage of maternal IgG platelet antibodies. The antigen is inherited by the fetus from the father and is absent on maternal platelets. Posttransfusion purpura is a rare form of isoimmune thrombocytopenia.

Neuromuscular Disorders

Several important neurologic disorders are related to the immune system. The immune system may play an important role in the pathogenesis and cause of myasthenia gravis and MS. In addition, amyotrophic lateral sclerosis (ALS) has become one of the prime subjects of modern neurologic research.

Amyotrophic Lateral Sclerosis

Along with Alzheimer disease and Parkinson disease, ALS is one of the so-called *degenerative disorders of the aging nervous system*. The immune system has been implicated in ALS. Monoclonal paraproteinemia seems to be disproportionately frequent in patients with ALS. It has also been suggested that ALS patients have a higher incidence of lymphoproliferative disease—lymphoma, Waldenström macroglobulinemia, and myeloma. There also seems to be an increased frequency of antibodies to a neuronal ganglioside, GM-1.

Inflammatory Polyneuropathies

The inflammatory polyneuropathies are a group of idiopathic disorders that includes the acute disease Guillain-Barré syndrome (GBS). It is characterized clinically by the subacute onset of generally symmetric weakness, ranging from modest lower extremity weakness to total, life-threatening involvement of motor and even cranial nerves. Sensory symptoms are less prominent. Unstable blood pressure and potentially fatal arrhythmias have also been observed. Progression of GBS can be rapid; however, most patients do recover.

The cause of GBS is unknown, but it is likely that an abnormal immune response against the peripheral nervous system (PNS) is involved. This may be triggered by an antecedent viral infection. There is infiltration of the PNS with lymphocytes and macrophages and patchy myelin destruction. Some patients display deposition of IgG, IgM, and IgA in PNS tissues. Greatly elevated immunoglobulin levels in the cerebrospinal fluid (CSF), sometimes with oligoclonal bands, suggest locally altered immunoregulation. The antigenic targets of these immunoglobulins remain unknown.

Myasthenia Gravis

Myasthenia gravis is a disease of the neuromuscular junction characterized by neurophysiologic and immunologic abnormalities (Box 22.4). A postsynaptic defect is caused by a decrease in receptors for acetylcholine and frequently an anatomic defect in the neuromuscular junction plate. Acetylcholine receptor (AChR)–binding antibody is directed against acetylcholine receptors at neuromuscular junctions of skeletal muscle and AChR-blocking antibodies. The ligand bungarotoxin or acetylcholine is important in producing a neuromuscular block. About one-third of patients with myasthenia gravis demonstrate AChR-blocking antibodies.

The role of these antibodies in producing disease is unclear. Complement-mediated, antibody-determined damage may be an important mechanism in myasthenia gravis because IgG, C3, and C9

BOX 22.4　Abnormalities Associated with Myasthenia Gravis

- Thymic hyperplasia with germinal follicles
- Increase in thymic B cells
- Thymoma
- Expression of acetylcholine receptor (AChR)-binding antibody and AChR-blocking antibody
- Associated with other autoimmune disorders

can be demonstrated at the neuromuscular junction, and the motor endplate is often abnormal. This suggests that antibody to AChR is capable of increasing the normal rate of degradation, resulting in fewer available receptors.

Multiple Sclerosis

MS is the most common demyelinating disease of the CNS related to abnormalities of the immune system. It is characterized by regions of demyelinization of varying size and age scattered throughout the white matter of the CNS. Demyelinization plaques have a tendency to form in the cerebrum, optic nerves, brainstem, spinal cord, and cerebellum.

Etiology. Although research studies support genetic and environmental components of susceptibility, epidemiologic findings are most consistent with an environmental influence against a background of genetic susceptibility as the cause.

Environmental risk factors linked to increased disease prevalence include viral infections, limited sunlight exposure, a geographical latitude further from the Equator, and low serum vitamin D. Epstein-Barr virus (EBV) may increase the risk of MS but it is uncertain as to how EBV infection causes a prevalence of MS. The idea that EBV mediates molecular activation of antigen-presenting and autoreactive T cells is considered to be a possibility.

Over 200 genetic variations have been associated with MS, with the strongest association being associated with class I and class II alleles of the MHC, HLA-DRB1 locus, and other susceptibility genes linked to cytokine expression (IL7R, CD6, and IL2RA).

Epidemiology. The incidence, prevalence, and mortality rates of MS vary with latitude. MS is rare in tropical and subtropical areas. The higher risk for MS in Europeans and in relatives of patients with MS and the existence of MS-resistant ethnic groups (e.g., Eskimos, Norwegian Lapps, and Australian aborigines) support a genetic predisposition. A low prevalence of MS occurs in Africa, India, China, Japan, and Southeast Asia.

MS is the major acquired neurologic disease in young adults and most patients develop symptoms between the ages of 18 and 50 years. Women are more often affected than men, and the prevalence of MS in women has almost doubled between 1950 and 2000. Approximately 1 in 1000 individuals of northern European origin residing in temperate climates will develop prototypical MS in their lifetime. In the United States the incidence is 1 per 1000 individuals and up to 400,000 people in the United States currently have MS.

Pathophysiology. MS results from T-cell–dependent inflammatory demyelination of the CNS. Inflammatory demyelination caused by T lymphocytes induces B lymphocytes to produce antimyelin antibodies.

The ongoing pathologic process involves the formation of CNS lesions, called *plaques,* characterized by inflammation and demyelination. Plaques result from a localized inflammatory immune response initiated by the entry of activated blood T cells into the CNS. These T cells cross the blood-brain barrier by binding to endothelial cells in blood vessels via reciprocal adhesion molecules. The release of enzymes called *matrix metalloproteinases (MMPs)* allows them to penetrate the basement membrane and extracellular matrix. At the same time, other blood immune system cells penetrate the CNS, causing additional local synthesis and release of damaging inflammatory mediators. The net result is the destruction of myelin sheaths, injury to axons and glial cells, and formation of permanent scar tissue.

Research investigations have demonstrated that osteopontin, which is known to play a role in enhancing inflammation, may play a critical role in the immune attack in MS and its progression. Osteopontin has been found to be very active in areas of myelin damage during relapse and remission and in myelin-synthesizing cells and nerve cells. More research is required to determine the exact role of this protein, in addition to the therapeutic possibilities it presents.

Signs and symptoms. The original version of the most widely used tool to diagnose MS is the McDonald Multiple Sclerosis criteria originally published in 2001 and updated most recently in 2017. To diagnose MS based on these guidelines, an individual must demonstrate evidence of:

- Dissemination of neurological damage occurring in multiple parts of the CNS or *space.* Specifically, this means presentation of lesions in at least two of four regions in the nervous system.

These regions include three areas of the brain (periventricular, juxtacortical or cortical, and infratentorial) and the spinal cord. Lesions in the optic nerves are common in MS but the criteria for dissemination cannot be fulfilled with optic nerve lesions in a person with symptoms of optic neuritis, or inflammation in the optic nerves.

Dissemination at different points in time means that neurological damage is happening at more than one point in time. This can be seen by a second disease exacerbation, the appearance of new lesions on magnetic resonance imaging (MRI) scans, or by clear-cut evidence of brain damage that happened at different times or new inflammatory lesions alongside older lesions that are no longer actively inflamed.

Note: Detection of oligoclonal bands is an alternative to dissemination in time by a new clinical attack or MRI. According to the 2017 McDonald criteria, testing positive for oligoclonal bands can be sufficient to fulfill the criteria for dissemination in time, even if a patient only has evident damage from one time point.

If a patient does not meet the two space and time criteria, a clinical case will not be diagnosed as MS but will be considered to be a mimic MS.

Initial signs and symptoms of MS are difficulty walking and abnormal sensations (e.g., numbness, possible pain, and ineffective vision). Primary symptoms caused by demyelination include fatigue, bladder and bowel dysfunction, loss of balance, loss of memory, slurred speech, difficulty swallowing, and seizures. Depression is a common symptom.

Categorization of Multiple Sclerosis. MS can be divided into different categories based on clinical signs and symptoms ranging from asymptomatic to progressive disease. There are at least five categories in the spectrum of MS:

1. *Radiologically isolated MS.* This form of MS demonstrates MRI findings without clinical signs and symptoms.
2. *Clinically isolated MS.* This form of MS represents the first attack of MS.
3. *Primary relapsing-remitting MS.* This form of MS begins as a relapsing illness with episodes of neurologic dysfunction lasting several weeks, followed by substantial or complete improvement. According to the McDonald Criteria, a patient who has experienced at least two clinical attacks and has clear-cut evidence of damage in at least two distinct brain areas can be definitively diagnosed with MS. Relapsing MS is the most common form; 85% of patients are symptomatic at onset.
4. *Primary progressive MS.* Primary progressive MS advances insidiously from onset, with or without occasional plateaus and minor improvements.
    Unlike the more common relapsing forms, primary progressive MS (PPMS) is not characterized by disease relapses. Instead, this disease type is defined by disability that gradually gets worse over time, starting from the onset of the disorder.
    According to the 2017 McDonald criteria, PPMS may be formally diagnosed in patients who experience worsening disability for at

least 1 year (based on previous symptoms or ongoing observation) and who exhibit at least two of the following:
- At least one MS-like lesion in the brain
- At least two lesions in the spinal cord
- A positive test for oligoclonal bands in the CSF

5. *Secondary progressive MS.* Secondary progressive MS develops in about 50% of relapsing MS patients about 10 years into the disease. Progressive relapsing is the rarest form of the disease. Patients begin with primary progression but subsequently experience one or more relapses.

Overview of Diagnostic Methods. The McDonald criteria guidelines incorporate radiological and clinical laboratory evaluations.

Radiological Examination. MRI is a key imaging modality for establishing a diagnosis of MS. A contrast agent called gadolinium can be used during an MRI to better distinguish active and inactive lesions. Gadolinium-enhancing lesions represent areas of active inflammation.

Clinical Laboratory Evaluations. Traditionally laboratory testing is used to *rule out* or *rule in* MS by analysis of cerebrospinal fluid (CSF) and serum specimens. No single laboratory test confirms a diagnosis, but appropriate laboratory test results must be evaluated carefully. Conditions that need to be excluded include collagen vascular disease, vitamin B_{12} deficiency, and endocrine disorders (e.g., thyroid and adrenal gland disease). It is also important to rule out infectious disorders (e.g., Lyme disease, syphilis, and human T lymphotropic virus type 1 [HTLV-1] infection).

Ruling Out MS. Laboratory testing using paired CSF and serum are performed to assess the integrity of the blood-brain barrier (BBB).

Total Protein in CSF. The total CSF protein concentration (>100 mg/dL) may indicate a challenged integrity of the BBB. Elevated levels are more suggestive of infectious or inflammatory CNS conditions than MS. Disruption of the BBB and infiltration of immune cells are key steps in inflammatory CNS conditions.

Albumin Quotient. Although this parameter is not sensitive or specific for MS, a high albumin quotient is indicative of a systemic inflammation.

$$\text{Albumin Quotient} = \frac{\text{CSF Albumin(mg/dL)}}{\text{Serum albumin}(g/L)}$$

Leukocyte Cell Counts. Increased white blood cells counts in CSF (>50 cells/μL) is suggestive of infectious or inflammatory CNS conditions rather than MS. The total CSF leukocyte count is within the reference range in about 66% of patients.

Glucose in CSF and Serum. Decreased CSF glucose in serum glucose (ratio <0.5) is not a typical finding for MS but suggests either an infectious or neoplastic disease source.

Ruling In MS. Oligoclonal banding and CSF IgG index assays (CSF) are considered to be the most sensitive and specific assays for diagnosing MS. Both assays require paired serum and CSF specimens.

Detection of Oligoclonal Banding. Oligoclonal bands or antibodies are characteristically detected in the CSF of patients with MS. Protein testing for bands includes protein electrophoresis (used by one-third of labs) or isoelectric focusing (used by two-thirds of labs) (see Chapter 9).

An oligoclonal immunoglobulin pattern consists of multiple homogeneous, narrow, and probably faint bands in the gamma zone on electrophoresis. Electrophoresis on cellulose acetate will rarely resolve an oligoclonal pattern. Therefore, electrophoretic media with greater resolution, such as agar or agarose gel, are required, and both require the use of concentrated CSF. It is important to perform electrophoresis on a serum specimen concurrently with the CSF specimen to ensure that the demonstrated homogeneous bands are present only in the CSF, which implies endogenous synthesis rather than a serum band that might appear secondarily in the CSF. Infrequently, if a prominent CSF band is present it may appear in the serum as a homogeneous band. This is most often encountered in subacute sclerosing panencephalitis.

> **BOX 22.5 Immunologic Manifestations of Multiple Sclerosis**
>
> - Antimyelin antibodies
> - Myelinotoxicity and glial toxicity of serum and cerebrospinal fluid in vitro
> - In vitro cell-mediated immunity by blood and cerebrospinal fluid cells to myelin components
> - Oligoclonal increase in cerebrospinal fluid immunoglobulin
> - Increase in certain human leukocyte antigens (HLAs) and islet antigens (Ias) (HL-A A3, B7, DW2, and DRW2)

High-resolution electrophoresis attempts to achieve better resolution of proteins beyond the classic five-band pattern. The primary reason for performing high-resolution protein electrophoresis is to detect oligoclonal bands in CSF to increase the diagnostic usefulness of protein patterns. About 80% of CSF proteins originate in the plasma. The electrophoretic pattern of normal CSF is similar to a normal serum protein pattern; however, several differences are detectable, including a prominent prealbumin band and two transferrin bands.

Immunofixation has been used in some research studies to show that the oligoclonal bands seen in CSF protein patterns are made up primarily of IgG. Although this may be of academic interest, characterization of the immunoglobulin bands does not significantly improve the diagnostic usefulness of the procedure. Isoelectric focusing, however, is becoming the method of choice for oligoclonal band detection.

Significance of oligoclonal bands. If oligoclonal bands are present in CSF but not in the serum, they are the result of increased production of IgG by the CNS. CNS production of IgG occurs in the subarachnoid space of the brain in conjunction with local accumulation of immunocytes. Each has its own specificity that gives rise to oligoclonal bands. Although the immunoglobulin is IgG it is polyclonal in nature, with several groups of cells producing it. Oligoclonal bands are therefore defined as discrete populations of IgG, with restricted heterogeneity demonstrated by electrophoresis.

One procedure for confirming local CNS production of oligoclonal IgG is to test a matched serum specimen diluted 1:100 concurrently with a nonconcentrated CSF sample. Oligoclonal bands present in CSF but not in the serum indicate CNS production. This matched sample procedure is especially useful if damage to the BBB is suspected because of acute or chronic inflammation, such as meningitis, intracranial tumor, or cerebrovascular disease.

The presence of these antibodies is evidence of CNS inflammation that is an independent predictor of relapse in individuals with clinically isolated syndrome or a single episode of MS-like symptoms. Box 22.5 presents immunologic manifestations of MS suggestive of its autoimmune nature. Antimyelin antibodies directed against components of the myelin sheath of nerves or myelin basic protein can be demonstrated in patients with MS or other neurologic disorders. Myelin antibodies are not detectable in the CSF of MS patients.

Serum oligoclonal bands may represent immune complexes and are associated with disorders such as Hodgkin disease or a nonspecific early immune response to other disorders (Box 22.6).

Oligoclonal bands in serum are not absolutely indicative of MS; their presence should be used in conjunction with the clinical evaluation and other diagnostic procedures. Although oligoclonal bands can occur in more than 90% of MS patients at some time during the

BOX 22.6 Conditions Associated with Oligoclonal Cerebrospinal Fluid Gamma Globulins

- Multiple sclerosis
- Neurosyphilis-paresthesia
- Paraneoplastic syndrome—subacute sclerosing panencephalitis
- Chronic mycobacterial and fungal meningitis
- Chronic viral meningitis and meningoencephalitis (uncommon)
- Acute viral meningitis (uncommon)
- Primary optic neuritis
- Acute disseminated encephalomyelitis
- Peripheral neuropathy
- Guillain-Barré syndrome
- Burkitt lymphoma
- Psychoneurosis
- Cerebral infarction

TABLE 22.13 Neuropathy Syndromes Associated with Antibodies Directed Against Peripheral Nerve Components

Clinical Syndrome	Antibodies
Chronic sensorimotor demyelinating neuropathy	Antimyelin-associated glycoprotein
Chronic axonal sensory neuropathy	Antisulfatide or anti–chondroitin sulfate
Multifocal motor neuropathy	Anti-GM1 (IgM)
Acute axonal motor neuropathy	Anti-GM1 (IgG)
Fisher syndrome	Anti-GQ1b
Guillain-Barré syndrome	Anti-LM1, GD1b, GD1A, GT1b, sulfatide, B tubulin
Large-fiber sensory neuropathy with ataxia	Anti-GQ1b, GD3, GD1b, GT1b
Subacute sensory neuropathy/encephalomyelitis	Antineuronal nuclear antibody type 1 (anti-Hu)

(From Cohen B, Mitsumoto H. Neuropathy syndromes associated with antibodies against the peripheral nerve, *Lab Med* 1995;26(7):459–463.)

course of their disease, the presence of bands does not correlate with the activity of the disease. The exact number of bands present in MS varies; some studies have demonstrated 7 to 15 bands.

IGG Index Assays (CSF). Normally, most IgG in CSF comes from peripheral blood crossing the BBB. However, the presence of protein does not necessarily indicate inflammation. Albumin is a smaller protein molecule synthesized in the liver and its presence in CSF suggests a disrupted BBB.

The IgG index assay (CSF) is a quantitative measurement of intrathecal IgG. When a CSF specimen tests positive, it indicates an inflammatory CNS condition. According to ARUP Laboratories, IgG in the CSF reference range is 0.0 to 0.6 mg/dL. The CSF IgG synthesis range is less than or equal to 8.0 mg/dL with an IgG index of 0.28 to 0.66.

In general, patients with no neurologic disease have an IgG concentration of less than 10% of total CSF proteins. Almost 70% of MS patients typically have IgG concentrations of 11% to 35% of total CSF proteins.

Note: In contrast, the presence of IgM antibody in CSF is associated with more aggressive progression to MS in patients with clinically isolated syndrome (CIS). It is further correlated with MRI lesion loads and the severity of the course of the disease.

Note: Biomarkers such as kappa immunoglobulin free light chain concentration in CSF and kappa CSF index measurement are potential alternative replacements for oligoclonal band analysis. Other potential biomarkers include neurofilament light chain, glial fibrillary acidic protein, and myelin basic protein.

Treatment. US Food and Drug Administration (FDA)-approved drugs for treatment of MS include:

- Alemtuzumab (Lemtrada)
- Cladribine (Mavenclad)
- Dimethyl fumarate (Tecfidera)
- Diroximel fumarate (Vumerity)
- Fingolimod (Gilenya); this was the first oral drug available for the long-term treatment of MS
- Glatiramer acetate (Copaxone, Glatopa)
- Interferon beta-1a (Avonex, Rebif)
- Interferon beta-1b (Betaseron)
- Ocrelizumab (Ocrevus).

Ocrevus and Tysabri account for over 85% of the patient share of MS medications and are therefore the commonly prescribed drugs for MS.

Oral medications include Tecfidera (dimethyl fumarate), Vumerity (diroximel fumarate), Bafiertam (monomethyl fumarate), Gilyena (fingolimod), Mayzent (siponimod), and Zeposia (ozanimod).

Ocrelizumab (Ocrevus) is a humanized anti-CD20 monoclonal antibody that is a newer drug that is. It targets the CD20 marker on B lymphocytes and is immunosuppressive.

On August 24, 2023, the FDA approved Tyruko (natalizumab-sztn), the first biosimilar to Tysabri (natalizumab) injection, for the treatment of adults with relapsing forms of MS.

Corticosteroid therapy (e.g., methylprednisolone and prednisone) is a common symptomatic treatment for disease relapses. The relapsing form of MS can be treated with immunomodulators such as interferon beta-1b (Betaseron), interferon beta-1a (Avonex), and glatiramer acetate (Copaxone).

Possible future therapeutic strategies may include combination treatments using existing therapies, standard immunosuppressive drugs, and new immunomodulating agents. Autologous bone marrow transplantation, plasma exchange, TCR peptide vaccine, and gene therapy are other possibilities.

Neuropathies

A neuropathy is a derangement in the function and structure of peripheral motor, sensory, or autonomic neurons. Autoimmune disorders are one of the disease categories that cause neuropathy. In many cases, evidence supports autoimmune pathogenesis. Demonstration of the relationships between specific neuropathic syndromes and antibodies directed against glycolipid and neural antigens are important scientific advances.

In autoimmune neuropathies, antibodies directed against peripheral nerve components are associated with specific clinical syndromes (Table 22.13). Knowledge of these syndromes and antibody tests can be used to identify a treatable neuropathy. In addition, many autoimmune neuropathic syndromes are associated with malignancies, which they often precede. Recognition of these syndromes can lead to early identification and treatment.

Most antibodies implicated in the development of autoimmune-mediated neuropathies are directed against carbohydrate epitopes of glycoproteins or glycolipids. Glycolipids are concentrated in neural membranes in which the lipid portion is immersed in the membrane

TABLE 22.14 Clinical Types of Systemic Sclerosis (SSc) and Associated Antibody Markers

Clinical Type	Antibodies
SSc with diffuse cutaneous involvement (dcSSc)	Anti–RNA polymerase I, anti–topoisomerase I
SSc with limited cutaneous involvement (lcSSc)	Anti–Th ribonucleoprotein anticentromere antibody
SSc-polymyositis overlap syndrome	Anti–PM-Scl

BOX 22.7 Categories of Immunologic Renal Disorders

Associated with Circulating Immune Complexes
- Systemic lupus erythematosus
- Certain vasculitis
- Infections
- Tumors (possibly)
- Immunoglobulins and antiimmunoglobulins

Membranoproliferative Glomerulonephritis
- Activation of alternate complement pathway
- Possible genetic factors

Associated With Anti–Glomerular Basement Membrane Antibody
- Most cases of Goodpasture syndrome
- Some rapidly progressive glomerulonephritides
- Membrane altered by virus or drugs (possibly)

Tubulointerstitial Nephritis
Associated with Immune Complex–Mediated Disease
- Drugs and possibly infection
- Involvement of transplanted kidneys

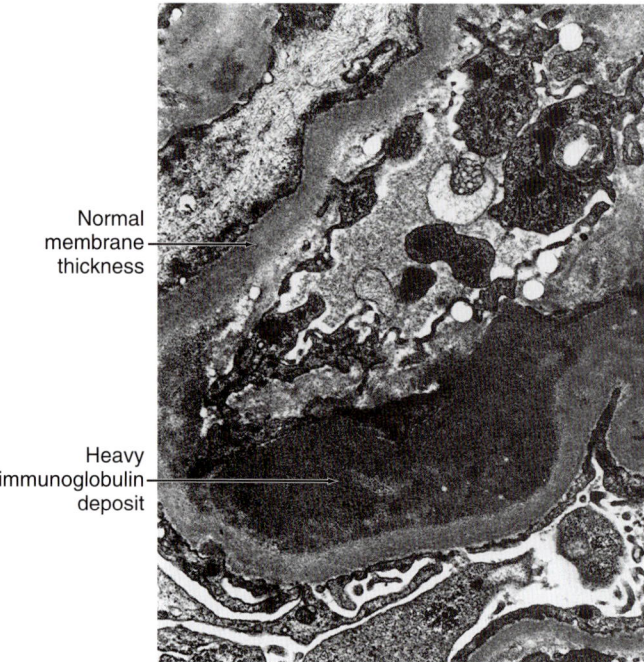

Fig. 22.9 Electron photomicrograph demonstrating an immunoglobulin deposit in the basement membrane of a patient with systemic lupus erythematosus (SLE). (From Barrett JT: *Textbook of immunology*, ed 5, St. Louis, 1988, Mosby.)

bilayer and the carbohydrate portion is exposed extracellularly. The extracellular domain of the carbohydrate epitopes makes them vulnerable to antibody binding.

Systemic sclerosis (scleroderma) is an autoimmune disease characterized by a wide spectrum of clinical, pathologic, and serologic abnormalities. More than 90% of patients with systemic sclerosis spontaneously produce ANAs. The structure and function of the intracellular antigens to which these ANAs are directed have been characterized. These serum autoantibodies are helpful markers because they correlate with certain clinical features of systemic sclerosis (Table 22.14). A more recently developed marker autoantibody, anti–RNA polymerase III antibody, has been identified in many patients who have systemic sclerosis with diffuse or extensive cutaneous involvement.

Renal Disorders

It is generally accepted that most immunologically mediated renal disorders fall into several categories (Box 22.7).

Renal Disease Associated with Circulating Immune Complexes

Renal disorders associated with circulating immune complexes are caused by nonrenal antigens and their corresponding antibodies. These complexes are deposited in one or more of several loci in the glomerulus. Deposition may depend on the size and other characteristics of the complex. Studies have suggested that potentially damaging immune complexes may be formed in situ and involve antigens already present or fixed in the glomerulus. In addition, immune complex activation of complement in the glomerular basement membrane may be augmented by the presence of cells with receptors for C3 located in that area. Activation probably releases biologically active products such as chemotactic substances and causes an inflammatory type of tissue injury. A renal complication of this type can be manifested in SLE.

Membranoproliferative Glomerulonephritis

Another type of glomerular disease, membranoproliferative glomerulonephritis, is believed to be caused by nonimmunologically activated complement. Activation is thought to be analogous to the alternative pathway activation of C3 by certain bacterial products and polysaccharides.

Renal Disease Associated With Anti–Glomerular Basement Membrane Antibody

Anti–glomerular basement membrane (GBM) antibodies are directed against the GBM of the glomerulus of the kidney (Fig. 22.9). These antibodies are induced in vivo against the basement membrane of the glomerulus and possibly that of the renal tubule or lung. The factors that stimulate antibody production are not well defined, but it appears likely that binding of drugs (e.g., methicillin), certain infectious agents, or renal damage caused by other immune mechanisms may lead to an immune antibody response. The end result may be direct damage to the bone marrow, with or without complement activation. Production of anti–bone marrow antibodies, however, appears to be self-limited and lasts for several weeks to months after removal of the inciting agent (i.e., by the kidney).

High antibody titers of anti-GBM are suggestive of Goodpasture disease, early SLE, or anti-GBM nephritis. The absence of antibodies, however, does not rule out Goodpasture disease. This type of renal disease represents less than 5% of glomerular disorders.

Tubulointerstitial Nephritis

Tubulointerstitial nephritis involving the renal tubules has been associated with a variety of causes, including immune complex–mediated disease. Precipitating factors can include drugs and possibly infection, in addition to the involvement of transplanted kidneys.

Skeletal Muscle Disorders
Inflammatory Myopathy

Polymyositis and dermatomyositis are the most common expressions of a group of chronic inflammatory disorders and can be subclassified into the following six categories:
- Primary idiopathic polymyositis
- Primary idiopathic dermatomyositis
- Polymyositis or dermatomyositis associated with neoplasia
- Childhood polymyositis or dermatomyositis
- Dermatomyositis or polymyositis associated with collagen vascular disease
- Polymyositis or dermatomyositis associated with infections.

All these disorders have skeletal muscle damage by a lymphocyte inflammatory process, resulting in symmetric weakness, predominantly of proximal muscles.

Polymyositis may be accompanied by inflammation at other sites, especially in the joints, lungs, and heart. The term *dermatomyositis* is used for the disease when the clinical features of disease are accompanied by characteristic inflammatory manifestations in the skin.

The causes of these disorders remain unknown, but they may develop in genetically susceptible persons after exposure to environmental agents that induce immune activation and inflammation. Infection is the most likely initiating event. As part of the inflammatory response to the infection, susceptible individuals develop a persistent cell-mediated immune attack that continues to destroy muscle after the acute infection is eradicated.

Polymyositis and dermatomyositis are more common in females, with peaks of occurrence in childhood and the fifth decade. Clinically, these disorders present with proximal muscle weakness sometimes associated with pain, fatigue, and low-grade fever, and lead to atrophy in progressive disease.

Evidence has suggested the polymyositis and dermatomyositis result from immune destruction. Muscle biopsies in patients with dermatomyositis have shown vasculitis, with IgG and complement deposition in the vessel walls in children and infrequently in adults. There is a preponderance of B lymphocytes and an increased CD4+ to CD8+ T-cell ratio. An increased frequency of activated T cells has been noted in polymyositis and dermatomyositis.

Patients with myositis have many immunologic abnormalities. One unique immunologic feature is the targeting by autoantibodies of certain cytoplasmic proteins and RNAs involved in the process of protein synthesis. These autoantibodies are found only in patients with myositis and are known as *myositis-specific autoantibodies* (MSAs) (Box 22.8). MSAs are antigen-driven, arise months before the onset of myositis, correlate in titer with disease activity, disappear after prolonged complete remission, and bind to and inhibit the function of targeted human autoantigenic enzymes on in vitro assays.

Skin Disorders: Bullous Disease and Other Conditions

A wide variety of autoimmune disorders are associated with skin manifestations (Box 22.9).

Two immunologic assays that can be used in conjunction with other clinical information include measurement of antibodies to the basement membrane area of the skin and of antibodies to the intercellular substance of the skin.

> **BOX 22.8 Myositis-Specific Autoantibodies**
>
> **Antisynthetases**
> - Anti–Jo-1
> - Anti–PL-7
> - Anti–PL-12 (1)
> - Anti–PL-12 (II)
> - Anti-OJ
> - Anti-EJ
> - Anti-SRP
> - Anti–MI-2
>
> **Others**
> - Anti-FER
> - Anti-KJ
> - Anti-MAS

> **BOX 22.9 Autoimmune Disorders Associated with Skin Manifestations**
> - Discoid lupus
> - Bullous pemphigoid
> - Pemphigus group
> - Dermatitis herpetiformis

Antiskin (dermal-epidermal) antibodies are present in more than 80% of patients with bullous pemphigoid, but the absence of antibodies does not rule out the disease. Antiskin (interepithelial) antibodies can be detected in 90% of patients with pemphigus. A rising antibody titer may indicate an impending relapse of pemphigus and a decreasing titer suggests effective control of the disease. The absence of demonstrable antibody usually excludes the diagnosis.

> **CASE STUDY 22.1 HISTORY AND PHYSICAL EXAMINATION**
>
> A 50-year-old White woman visited her primary care provider because of extreme fatigue. She reported experiencing mild pain in her abdominal region.
> Physical examination revealed slight hepatomegaly. Her physician ordered a complete blood count and urinalysis.
>
> **Laboratory Results**
> See Table 22.15 for the results of these tests.
>
> **Question**
> 1. An immunologic assay of importance in the diagnosis of pernicious anemia is:
>   a. Antiintrinsic factor
>   b. Antiparietal cell antibody
>   c. Antiislet cell antibody
>   d. Both a and b
>
> See Appendix A for the answer to the multiple-choice question.
>
> **Critical Thinking Group Discussion Questions**
> 1. Which chemical and immunologic assays would be helpful in establishing a diagnosis for this patient?
> 2. What is the prevalence of anti–intrinsic factor in patients with pernicious anemia?
> 3. What is the prevalence of parietal cell antibodies in patients with pernicious anemia?

TABLE 22.15 Laboratory Data[a]

	Patient Results	Reference Range
Complete Blood Count		
Hemoglobin (Hb)	6.2 g/dL	11.5–16.0 g/dL
Hematocrit (Hct)	0.22 L/L	0.37–0.47 L/L
Red blood cell (RBC) count	1.7×10^{12}/L	$4.2–5.4 \times 10^{12}$/L
White blood cell (WBC) count	3.8×10^{9}/L	$4.5–11.0 \times 10^{9}$/L
Red Blood Cell Indices		
Mean corpuscular volume (MCV)	129.4 fL	80–96 fL
Mean corpuscular hemoglobin (MCH)	36.5 pg	27–32 pg
Mean corpuscular hemoglobin concentration (MCHC)	28%	32%–36%

[a]Blood smear comments: three macrocytic RBCs, polychromatophilia, a few nucleated RBCs.

CASE STUDY 22.2 HISTORY AND PHYSICAL EXAMINATION

A right-handed 25-year-old woman had no significant medical history. She came to the emergency department because of a sudden onset of slurred speech.

She reported being in excellent health until a month ago, when she began to notice weakness and numbness in her right hand and leg. She felt unsteady when walking and experienced urinary urgency.

Physical examination revealed an overweight young female with a right facial droop. In addition, she staggered on turning around and had difficulty walking in a straight line. A spinal tap and MRI were ordered.

Laboratory Results
See Table 22.16 for the laboratory findings.

Additional Notes
- Cerebrospinal fluid (CSF) agarose electrophoresis: Positive for oligoclonal bands (reference range negative)
- CSF isoelectric focusing: Positive for oligoclonal bands (reference range negative)
- Serum protein electrophoresis interpretation: No apparent monoclonal peak (reference range, no apparent monoclonal peak)
- Serum immunofixation: No paraprotein detected (reference range, no paraprotein detected)

Imaging Studies
MRI revealed a masslike lesion in the region of the corpus callosum, with extensions into the right and left hemispheres of the brain. The location of the lesion was consistent with the patient's presenting symptoms.

A follow-up biopsy of the brain was ordered. Histologically, a biopsy of white matter demonstrated sheets of macrophages, clumps of lymphocytes and plasma cells, and myelin debris.

Question
1. In the diagnosis of multiple sclerosis, the most significant body fluid to analyze is:
   a. Blood
   b. Cerebrospinal fluid
   c. Urine
   d. Joint fluid

Answers to this question can be found in Appendix A.

Critical Thinking Group Discussion Questions
1. What is the cause of the patient's symptoms?
2. Does the patient's age provide a clue to the diagnosis?
3. What is the significance of the laboratory analysis of the CSF?

TABLE 22.16 Cerebrospinal Fluid Examination

Assay	Patient Results	Reference Range
Color, clarity	Clear, colorless	Clear, colorless
Total cells	6	0–8
Nucleated cells	2	0–2
Differential, lymphocytes (%)	75	40–60
CSF protein (mg/dL)	125	20–40
CSF glucose (mg/dL)	70	40–80
CSF IgG (mg/dL)	8.5	0–33
Serum albumin (g/dL)	4.2	3.5–5.0
Serum IgG (mg/dL)	941	700–1450
Cerebrospinal Fluid Profile		
CSF serum IgG index	1.2	0–0.7
CSF IgG-to-albumin ratio	0.28	0–0.23
Albumin index	7.38	0–7.0
CNS IgG synthesis rate (mg/dL)	22.65	0–2.8

CNS, Central nervous system; *CSF*, cerebrospinal fluid.

REVIEW QUESTIONS

1. All of the following characteristics are common to organ-specific and organ-nonspecific disorders *except*:
   a. Autoantibody tests are of diagnostic value
   b. Antibodies may appear in each of the main immunoglobulin classes
   c. Antigens are available to the lymphoid system in low concentrations
   d. Circulatory autoantibodies react with normal body constituents

2. Antibody expression in the development of autoimmunity is regulated by all of the following factors *except*:
   a. Genetic predisposition
   b. Increasing age
   c. Environmental factors (e.g., ultraviolet [UV] radiation)
   d. Active infectious disease

3. The mechanism responsible for autoimmune disease is:
   a. Circulating immune complexes
   b. Antigen excess
   c. Antibody excess
   d. Antigen deficiency

4. In an autoimmune condition influencing the development of a disorder include the following factors except:
   a. Genetic factors
   b. Exogenous factors
   c. Increased discrimination of self- from non–self antigen
   d. Immunopathogenic mechanisms

5. A characteristic associated with acetylcholine receptor–blocking antibodies is:
   a. Helpful in monitoring Addison disease
   b. Found in one-third of patients with myasthenia gravis
   c. Useful in monitoring the activity and exacerbations of SLE
   d. Suggestive of Goodpasture disease

6. A characteristic associated with anticardiolipin antibody is:
   a. Helpful in monitoring Addison disease
   b. Found in one-third of patients with myasthenia gravis
   c. Useful in monitoring the activity and exacerbations of SLE
   d. Present in SLE and associated with arterial and venous thrombosis

7. A characteristic associated with anti-DNA antibodies is:
   a. Helpful in monitoring Addison disease
   b. Found in one-third of patients with myasthenia gravis
   c. Useful in monitoring the activity and exacerbations of SLE
   d. Present in SLE and associated with arterial and venous thrombosis

8. A characteristic associated with anti–glomerular basement membrane antibodies is:
   a. Helpful in monitoring Addison disease
   b. Found in one-third of patients with myasthenia gravis
   c. Useful in monitoring the activity and exacerbations of SLE
   d. Suggestive of Goodpasture disease

9. A characteristic associated with antinuclear ribonucleoprotein is:
   a. Antibody to basic nonhistone nuclear protein, diagnostic of systemic sclerosis
   b. Present in bullous pemphigoid
   c. Presence of antibody confirms diagnosis of SLE
   d. Characteristic of mixed connective tissue disease

10. A characteristic associated with anti-Scl is:
    a. Antibody to basic nonhistone nuclear protein, diagnostic of systemic sclerosis
    b. Present in bullous pemphigoid
    c. Presence of antibody confirms diagnosis of SLE
    d. Seen in viral disease

11. A characteristic associated with anti-Sm is:
    a. Antibody to basic nonhistone nuclear protein, diagnostic of systemic sclerosis
    b. Present in bullous pemphigoid
    c. Presence of antibody confirms diagnosis of SLE
    d. Characteristic of mixed connective tissue disease

12. A characteristic associated with anti–smooth muscle is:
    a. Antibody to basic nonhistone nuclear protein, diagnostic of systemic sclerosis
    b. Present in bullous pemphigoid
    c. Presence of antibody confirms diagnosis of SLE
    d. Seen in viral disease

13. A characteristic associated with SS-A is:
    a. Detectable in patients with myasthenia gravis
    b. Demonstrable in Sjögren syndrome–sicca complex
    c. Highly suggestive of drug-induced lupus erythematosus
    d. Found in one-third of patients with uncomplicated polymyositis and some patients with dermatomyositis

14. A characteristic associated with histone-reactive antinuclear antibody is:
    a. Detectable in patients with myasthenia gravis
    b. Demonstrable in Sjögren syndrome–sicca complex
    c. Highly suggestive of drug-induced lupus erythematosus
    d. Found in most patients with polymyositis

15. A characteristic associated with PM-I antibody is:
    a. Detectable in patients with myasthenia gravis
    b. Demonstrable in Sjögren syndrome–sicca complex
    c. Highly suggestive of drug-induced lupus erythematosus
    d. Found in most patients with polymyositis

16. The term *autoimmune disease* is used when:
    a. Demonstrable immunoglobulins display specificity for self antigens
    b. Cytotoxic T cells display specificity for self antigens
    c. B cells contribute to the pathogenesis of the disease
    d. Both a and b

17. Self-recognition tolerance is characterized by:
    a. Acquisition of nonreactively directed action toward a specific self antigen
    b. Failure to recognize self antigens
    c. Lack of immune response to self antigens
    d. Reactions initiated during adolescence

18. A description of acetylcholine receptor–binding antibody (AChR) is:
    a. Strongly suggestive, in a high titer, of primary biliary binding antibody cirrhosis
    b. Useful in the diagnosis of myasthenia gravis
    c. Demonstrated in most patients with CREST syndrome
    d. Found in 60% of patients with pernicious anemia

19. A description of anticentromere antibody is:
    a. Strongly suggestive, in a high titer, of primary biliary binding antibody cirrhosis
    b. Useful in the diagnosis of myasthenia gravis
    c. Demonstrated in most patients with CREST syndrome
    d. Found in 60% of patients with pernicious anemia

20. Antiintrinsic factor antibody is:
    a. Strongly suggestive, in a high titer, of primary biliary binding antibody cirrhosis
    b. Useful in the diagnosis of myasthenia gravis
    c. Demonstrated in most patients with CREST syndrome
    d. Found in 60% of patients with pernicious anemia
21. Antimitochondrial antibody is:
    a. Strongly suggestive, in a high titer, of primary biliary binding antibody cirrhosis
    b. Useful in the diagnosis of myasthenia gravis
    c. Demonstrated in most patients with CREST syndrome
    d. Found in 60% of patients with pernicious anemia
22. A description of antimyelin antibody is:
    a. Associated with multiple sclerosis
    b. A marker for granulomatosis with polyangiitis
    c. A characteristic of untreated systemic lupus erythematosus
    d. Diagnostic of Dressler syndrome or rheumatic fever
23. A description of antimyocardial antibody is:
    a. Associated with multiple myeloma
    b. A marker for granulomatosis with polyangiitis A characteristic of untreated systemic lupus erythematosus
    c. Diagnostic of Dressler syndrome or rheumatic fever
24. A description of cytoplasmic antineutrophil cytoplasmic antibody (c-ANCA) is:
    a. Associated with multiple myeloma
    b. A marker for granulomatosis with polyangiitis A characteristic of untreated systemic lupus erythematosus
    c. Diagnostic of Dressler syndrome or rheumatic fever
25. A description of antinuclear antibody (ANA) is:
    a. Associated with multiple myeloma
    b. A marker for granulomatosis with polyangiitis
    c. A characteristic of untreated systemic lupus erythematosus
    d. Diagnostic of Dressler syndrome or rheumatic fever

Questions 26–29: Match each organ in the illustration with the appropriate autoimmune disorder from the following table.

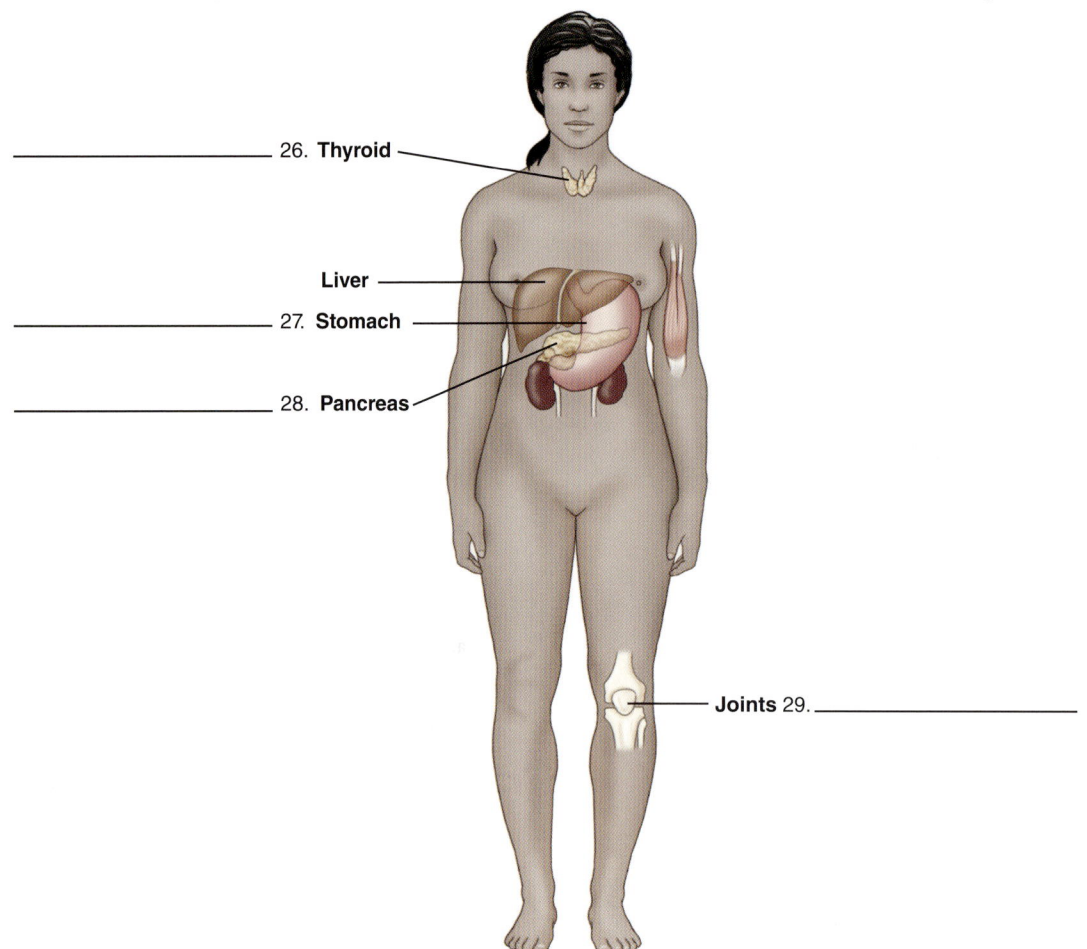

26. Thyroid
27. Stomach
28. Pancreas
29. Joints

Possible answers to question 26

a. Takayasu arteritis

b. Behçet disease

c. Graves disease

d. Scleroderma

Possible answers to question 27

a. Eosinophilia-myalgia

b. Hashimoto thyroiditis

c. Raynaud phenomenon

d. Pernicious anemia

Possible answers to question 28

a. Addison disease

b. Sheehan syndrome

c. Insulin-dependent diabetes

d. Sjögren syndrome

Possible answers to question 29

a. Idiopathic biliary cirrhosis

b. Crohn disease

c. Rheumatoid arthritis

d. Multiple sclerosis

30. A characteristic of Hashimoto thyroiditis (chronic lymphocytic thyroiditis):
    a. More common in men
    b. Hypothyroidism commonly develops later in life
    c. Anti–thyroid-stimulating hormone (TRab) is usually present
    d. Usually diagnosed between the ages of 20 and 30 years old
31. In Graves disease:
    a. Only a few exhibit anti-TPO
    b. A high level of TSH is demonstrated
    c. Decreased T_4 levels are present
    d. It is a form of hyperthyroidism
32. Which thyroid antibody produces hyperthyroidism by binding to the TSH receptor?
    a. Antithyroid globulin (Tg)
    b. Anti–thyroid-stimulating hormone receptor antibody (TRab)
    c. Antithyroperoxidase (TPO)
    d. Anti–thyroid-stimulating hormone (TSH)
33. The immunologic manifestations of multiple sclerosis include all of the following *except*:
    a. Antimyelin antibodies
    b. An oligoclonal increase in CSF immunoglobulin
    c. In vitro antibody-mediated immunity
    d. An increase in certain HLA and Ia antigens
34. Most immunologically mediated renal disorders fall into one of the following categories, *except for*:
    a. Association with circulating immune complexes
    b. Association with circulating antigen
    c. Association with anti–glomerular basement membrane antibody
    d. Membranoproliferative glomerulonephritis
35. Polymyositis and dermatomyositis are the most common expressions of:
    a. Rheumatoid heart disease
    b. Skeletal muscle disorders
    c. Rheumatoid arthritis
    d. Either a or b
36. In terms of the epidemiology of autoimmune pancreatitis:
    a. It is twice as common in men than in women
    b. It is more common in women than in men
    c. Most patients are younger than 50 years of age
    d. The number of reported cases has been decreasing over the past decade
37. The immunologic abnormality associated with autoimmune pancreatitis in the Japanese population is:
    a. Autoantibodies against carbonic anhydrase
    b. HLA haplotype
    c. Hypogammaglobulinemia
    d. Elevated serum IgE levels

23

Systemic Lupus Erythematosus

LEARNING OUTCOMES

- Compare the different forms of lupus, citing manifestations, incidence, and other features.
- Name the two most common drugs that can cause drug-induced lupus.
- Explain the epidemiology and signs and symptoms of systemic lupus erythematosus (SLE).
- Describe the immunologic manifestations of SLE, including diagnostic evaluation.
- Discuss the laboratory evaluation of antinuclear antibodies.
- Analyze selected SLE case studies. Correctly answer related multiple-choice questions.
- Participate in a discussion of critical thinking questions.
- Describe the principle, sources of error, limitations, and clinical applications of the antinuclear antibody visible method.
- Describe the principle and clinical applications of the rapid slide test for antinucleoprotein and the autoimmune enzyme immunoassay ANA screening test.
- Correctly answer 80% of the end-of-chapter review questions.

OUTLINE

Different Forms of Lupus, 397
    Discoid Lupus, 397
    Systemic Lupus Erythematosus (SLE), 397
    Drug-Induced Lupus, 397
    Neonatal Lupus, 397
Etiology, 397
    Genetic Predisposition, 397
    Environmental Factors, 397
    Hormonal Influences, 399
    Antibiotics, 399
    Vitamins, 399
Epidemiology, 399
Signs and Symptoms, 399
    Infection, 400
    Cutaneous Features, 400
    Renal Characteristics, 402
    Lymphadenopathy, 402
    Serositis, 402
    Cardiopulmonary Characteristics, 402
    Gastrointestinal Manifestations, 402
    Musculoskeletal Features, 402
    Neuropsychiatric Features, 402
    Late-Onset Lupus, 402
    Immunologic Manifestations, 403
    Cellular Aspects, 403
    Humoral Aspects, 403
    Immunologic Consequences, 404
Diagnostic Evaluation, 404
    Histologic Changes, 404
    Hematologic and Hemostatic Findings, 404
        Hemostatic Testing, 404
    Serologic Findings, 404
        Complement, 404
        Antibodies, 405
        Antinuclear Antibodies, 405
    Laboratory Evaluation, 406
        Indirect Immunofluorescent Tests for Antinuclear Antibody, 406
        Indirect Immunofluorescent Technique, 406
    Rapid Slide Test for Antinucleoprotein, 408
    Autoimmune Enzyme Immunoassay, 410
    Automated Testing: Multiplex Immunoassay, 410
Treatment, 411
    Rituximab, 411
    Equalise for Lupus Nephritis, 411
Case Study 23.1, 411
Case Study 23.2, 412
Procedure: Antinuclear Antibody Visible Method, 413.e1
Procedure: Rapid Slide Test for Antinucleoprotein, 413.e3
Procedure: Autoimmune Enzyme Immunoassay ANA Screening Test, 413.e3

KEY TERMS

antineutrophil cytoplasmic antibodies (ANCAs)
antinuclear antibody (ANA)
antiphospholipid antibodies
antiphospholipid syndrome
discoid lupus
hygiene hypothesis
idiopathic SLE
lupus anticoagulants
lupus erythematosus microbiota
nonhistone proteins
Raynaud phenomenon
systemic lupus erythematosus (SLE)

Systemic autoimmune diseases, autoimmune rheumatic diseases, and systemic rheumatic diseases (SRDs) basically refer to the same category of diseases, and these terms are used interchangeably. Systemic lupus erythematosus (SLE), scleroderma (SSc), polymyositis/dermatomyositis (PM/DM), and rheumatoid arthritis (RA) are representative disorders in this category. These diseases involve multiple systems (e.g., joints, connective tissue, and collagen vascular system) in the disease process. Whether Sjögren syndrome (SjS) should be classified as organ-specific (salivary glands, lacrimal glands) or systemic is arguable.

Table 23.1 lists the American College of Rheumatology criteria for the classification of SLE.

> **KEY CONCEPTS: Important Facts about Systemic Lupus Erythematosus**
> - SLE is the classic model of autoimmune disease.
> - No single cause of SLE has been identified, but a primary defect in immune system regulation is considered important in its pathogenesis. Other influences include the effect of estrogens, genetic predisposition, and extraneous factors.
> - SLE is a disease of acute and chronic inflammation.

DIFFERENT FORMS OF LUPUS

Although this chapter focuses on SLE, there are several forms of lupus, including discoid, systemic, drug-induced, and neonatal lupus.

Discoid Lupus

Discoid (cutaneous) lupus is always limited to the skin and is identified by biopsy of the rash that may appear on the face, neck, and scalp. Discoid lupus does not generally involve the body's internal organs but can evolve into the systemic form of the disease, even if treated. Evolution to systemic lupus cannot be predicted or prevented. The antinuclear antibody (ANA) test result may be negative or positive at a low titer. Discoid lupus accounts for approximately 10% of all cases of lupus.

Systemic Lupus Erythematosus (SLE)

SLE is usually more severe than discoid lupus. It is a multisystem autoimmune disorder that can affect the skin, joints, and almost any organ or body system, including the lungs, kidneys, heart, and brain. SLE may include periods in which few, if any, symptoms are evident (remission) and other times when the disease becomes more active (flare). Most often, when people mention "lupus," they are referring to the systemic form of the disease. Approximately 70% of lupus cases are systemic. In about 50% of these cases, a major organ will be affected.

Drug-Induced Lupus

Drug-induced lupus occurs after the use of certain prescribed drugs (Box 23.1). The most frequently used drugs associated with drug-induced lupus are hydralazine hydrochloride and procainamide hydrochloride. Factors such as the rate of drug metabolism, the drug's influence on immune regulation, and the host's genetic composition are all believed to influence pathogenesis. Some drugs (e.g., oral contraceptives, and isoniazid) induce serum ANAs without symptoms. High antibody titers may exist for months without the development of clinical symptoms.

Procainamide-induced disease does not induce antibodies to double-strand DNA (dsDNA). The ANAs in the drug-induced syndromes are histone dependent and are never the only ANAs present in the blood. Even with discontinuation of the drug, antibody titers usually remain elevated for months or years.

Only about 4% of patients who take these drugs will develop the antibodies suggestive of lupus. Of those 4%, only an extremely small number will develop overt drug-induced lupus. The symptoms of drug-induced lupus are similar to those of systemic lupus, but milder. Patients with drug-related lupus have a predominance of pulmonary and polyserositic signs and symptoms. Patients with drug-induced lupus have no associated renal or central nervous system (CNS) disease. In addition, lupus-inducing drugs do not appear to exacerbate idiopathic SLE. The symptoms usually fade when the medications are discontinued.

Neonatal Lupus

Neonatal lupus is a rare condition acquired from the passage of maternal autoantibodies, specifically anti-Ro/SS-A or anti-La/SS-B, that can affect the skin, heart, and blood of the fetus and newborn. Neonatal lupus is associated with a rash that appears within the first several weeks of life and may persist for about 6 months before disappearing. Congenital heart block can occur but is much less common than a rash. Neonatal lupus is not systemic lupus.

ETIOLOGY

The cause of SLE is unclear. No single causative agent has been identified. However, a primary defect in the regulation of the immune system is considered important in the pathogenesis of the disorder. Development of autoantibodies by patients diagnosed with SLE is due to defective B-cell tolerance for self-antigens. It is believed that breakdown of B-cell tolerance occurs very early in the disease and may precede or trigger other immune abnormalities.

Both genetic and environmental factors have been implicated in the disease mechanism. In the past decade, a growing body of evidence has indicated an important role of gut microbes in the development of autoimmune diseases. Although it is already known that environmental factors can trigger the development of SLE, alterations of the gut microbial composition may be correlated with SLE disease.

Genetic predisposition can be a factor. Environmental factors, hormones, antibiotics, and diet can have an impact on lupus. Antibodies directed against T lymphocytes, including the membrane molecules that mediate their responses, are regularly detected in patients with SLE. Their role in the pathogenesis of autoimmunity is still unclear.

Genetic Predisposition

SLE is known to occur within families, but there is no identified gene or genes associated with lupus. Previously, genes on chromosome 6 called *immune response genes* were associated with the disease. The discovery of a gene on chromosome 1 has been associated with SLE in certain families. Only 10% of SLE patients will have a parent or sibling who already has or may develop lupus. Statistics show that only about 5% of the children born to those with SLE will develop the illness.

Environmental Factors

Microbes and a number of environmental triggering factors have been associated with SLE, including ultraviolet (UV) light and smoking. These factors may act in different ways. For example, UV light may cause DNA to form thymine dimers, which significantly alter the antigenicity of DNA and could result in the formation of anti-DNA.

Gut microbiota have a potentially important impact on lupus, especially the potential role of the phylum Bacteroidetes because the relative abundance of these bacteria is increased in human SLE. In human SLE, recent findings have shown that the relationship of the phylum Firmicutes, a gram-positive organism, some of which can form

TABLE 23.1 1997 Update of the 1982 American College of Rheumatology Revised Criteria for Classification of Systemic Lupus Erythematosus.

Criterion	Definition
Malar rash	• Fixed erythema, flat or raised, over the malar eminences, tending to spare the nasolabial folds
Discoid rash	• Erythematous raised patches with adherent keratotic scaling and follicular plugging; atrophic scarring may occur in older lesions
Photosensitivity	• Skin rash as a result of unusual reaction to sunlight by patient history or physician observation
Oral ulcers	• Oral or nasopharyngeal ulceration, usually painless, observed by physician
Nonerosive arthritis	• Involving two or more peripheral joints, characterized by tenderness, swelling, or effusion
Pleuritis or pericarditis	• Pleuritis—convincing history of pleuritic pain or rubbing heard by a physician, or evidence of pleural effusion OR • Pericarditis—documented by electrocardiogram (ECG) or rub or evidence of pericardial effusion
Renal disorder	• Persistent proteinuria >0.5 g/day, or >3+ if quantitation is not performed OR • Cellular casts—may be red cell, hemoglobin, granular, tubular, or mixed
Neurologic disorder	• Seizures—in the absence of offending drugs or known metabolic derangements (e.g., uremia, ketoacidosis, and electrolyte imbalance) OR • Psychosis—in the absence of offending drugs or known metabolic derangements (e.g., uremia, ketoacidosis, and electrolyte imbalance)
Hematologic disorder	• Hemolytic anemia—with reticulocytosis OR • Leukopenia—<4000/mm^3 total on two or more occasions OR • Lymphopenia—<1500/mm^3 on two or more occasions OR • Thrombocytopenia—<100,000/mm^3 in the absence of offending drugs

Immunologic disorder	• Anti-DNA—antibody to native DNA in abnormal titer OR
	 • Anti-Sm—presence of antibody to Sm nuclear antigen OR
	 • Positive finding of antiphospholipid antibodies on:
	   • An abnormal serum level of IgG or IgM anticardiolipin antibodies
	   • A positive test result for lupus anticoagulant using a standard method
	   • A false-positive test result for at least 6 months and confirmed by *Treponema pallidum* immobilization or fluorescent treponemal antibody absorption test
	 • Standard methods should be used in testing for the presence of antiphospholipids

Positive antinuclear antibody	• An abnormal titer of antinuclear antibody by immunofluorescence or an equivalent assay at any point in time and in the absence of drugs known to be associated with drug-induced lupus syndrome

From Hochberg MC: Updating the American College of Rheumatology revised criteria for the classification of systemic lupus erythematosus (letter), *Arthritis Rheum* 40:1725, 1997; and the American College of Rheumatology. https://www.rheumatology.org.

BOX 23.1 Drugs That Can Produce Clinical and Serologic Features of Systemic Lupus Erythematosus

- Antiarrhythmics (e.g., procainamide hydrochloride)
- Anticonvulsants (e.g., phenytoin)
- Antihypertensives (e.g., hydralazine hydrochloride)
- Miscellaneous (e.g., chlorpromazine, isoniazid, penicillin, and sulfonamides)

---

endospores, compared with the phylum Bacteroidetes, a gram-negative microbe, is important.

The role of microbial environmental factors in the etiology of SLE is evidenced by the dramatic difference in disease incidence between West African and African American individuals, both derived from the same ethnic group but exposed to different environments. With an obviously higher burden of infections, the frequency of SLE is much lower in West African than African individuals living in Europe or the United States.

In addition, an increase in the occurrence of SLE in the developed world has been reported. Infections from pathogenic microbes, or their absence, are known to be associated with SLE occurrence. Higher hygiene standards, with the elimination of many pathogenic and nonpathogenic microbes from the environment in industrialized countries, may be contributing to this increase in SLE. There is speculation that the lower exposure to infectious organisms leads to the rise of allergies and some autoimmune diseases. The hygiene hypothesis supports the assumption that a child's environment can be "too clean," and that the absence of exposure to a variety of microorganisms deprives a person's immune system of the chance to develop resistance to diseases. Therefore improvement in hygiene and the absence or reduction of certain microbes may contribute to the higher incidence and faster progression of lupus disease.

Bacteria constitute a large part of the symbiotic microbiota living in our body. Diverse components of gram-positive and gram-negative bacteria have been reported to contribute to the initiation and maintenance of lupus disease through stimulating toll-like receptors (TLRs), especially TLR2 and TLR4. TLRs are pattern-recognition receptors that can recognize invading microorganisms bearing pathogen-associated molecular patterns.

Lipopolysaccharide (LPS), a gram-negative cell wall component, can be recognized by TLR4. In SLE patients, soluble CD14 (sCD14), which is released by monocytes in response to LPS, is increased in the blood. The level of sCD14 is highly correlated with disease activity and suggests the involvement of LPS in lupus development. LPS might be involved in lupus by inducing neutrophil activation and migration, the key processes that promote the development of SLE.

Another possible role for LPS-TLR4 in lupus is to induce autoantibody production or isotype switching toward more pathogenic immunoglobulins, such as immunoglobulin G (IgG). In addition, increased TLR2 leads to enhanced interleukin-17A (IL-17A) and IL-17F production and is associated with inflammatory response of CD4+ T cells.

In developed countries, where hepatitis B virus (HBV) and *Helicobacter pylori* infections are decreasing, the risk of developing SLE can become greater. T-cell exhaustion during chronic infection may explain the ability of these pathogens to downregulate inflammation and ameliorate SLE.

Hormonal Influences

Hormonal factors may explain why lupus occurs more frequently in women than in men. Lupus is often called a woman's disease because a disproportionate number of women between puberty and menopause suffer from it. The increase in disease symptoms may be caused by hormones, particularly estrogen. There is a risk that the disease will worsen during pregnancy and the immediate postpartum period. In addition, postmenopausal therapy is associated with an increased risk for developing SLE. The exact reason for the greater prevalence of lupus in women, and the cyclic increase in symptoms, is unknown.

A condition called **antiphospholipid syndrome** can be secondary to lupus and may complicate pregnancy. Antibodies against specific autoantigens often present on coagulation factors can cause blood to clot faster than normal or, in some cases, not at all. **Antiphospholipid antibodies** (Fig. 23.1) can be found in many patients with lupus and pose a particular risk to pregnant lupus patients because their presence is often associated with miscarriages.

Both the developing fetus and the pregnant mother with lupus are at increased risk of various complications during and after pregnancy. Passive placental transfer of maternal antibodies can produce transient abnormalities such as hepatosplenomegaly, cytopenia, and a photosensitive rash in the newborn. These conditions do resolve in the newborn after the antibody titer declines (see earlier discussion of neonatal lupus).

Antibiotics

Antibiotics, which can remove gut bacteria, are known to trigger lupus flares. These include sulfa drugs such as trimethoprim–sulfamethoxazole, tetracycline-related antibiotics, and penicillin-related antibiotics. Antibiotics can cause diarrhea and remove beneficial microbes from the intestinal tract. Metabolites produced by gut bacteria, especially butyrate produced by *Clostridia*, can promote the differentiation of regulatory T cells (T_{regs}) in the colon, spleen, and lymph nodes to suppress inflammation. African American individuals have used antibiotics much more frequently than people in West African countries, which may have an impact on the differences in lupus prevalence and severity between the two populations.

Vitamins

Diet is one of the main factors with known effects on gut microbiota. Vitamin D (VD), vitamin A (VA), and omega-3 polyunsaturated fatty acids (PUFAs) have been found to modulate lupus onset or flares. VD deficiency is increasingly common, resulting in increased risks for multiple disorders. VD plays an important role in the homeostasis of the immune system through a nuclear receptor existing in all immune cells, VD receptor (VDR). Inhibition of neutrophil extracellular traps (NETs) prevents endothelial damage that promotes the progression of lupus disease.

VA has long been recognized as an immune regulator. VA exerts its effects mainly via all-transretinoic acid (tRA), an active metabolite of VA. For SLE, the role of VA may be important to the healthy balance between the host and symbiotic microbiota in the gut of SLE patients.

EPIDEMIOLOGY

SLE can occur at any age and in either gender, although it occurs 10 to 15 times more frequently in women than in men after puberty. The Lupus Foundation of America estimates that approximately 1.4 million Americans have a form of lupus. The prevalence ranges from 20 to 200 cases per 100,000 persons, with a higher prevalence for people of African, Hispanic, or Asian (particularly Chinese) ancestry. SLE is two to three times more prevalent among people of color. The incidence of SLE in African American women between 20 and 64 years old is 1 in 245. The reasons for ethnic differences are not clear.

Although the disease affects both males and females, women of childbearing age are diagnosed nine times more often than men. Women between 20 and 64 years of age are most commonly diagnosed, with 80% of those having SLE develop between ages 15 and 45 years.

Survival is estimated to be higher than 90% at 10 years after diagnosis. The highest mortality rate is in patients with progressive renal involvement or CNS disease. The two most frequent causes of death are renal failure and infectious complications.

SIGNS AND SYMPTOMS

SLE is a disease of acute and chronic inflammation. Symptoms often mimic other, less serious illnesses. Fever is one of the most common clinical manifestations of SLE. Disease activity accounts for more than 66% of febrile episodes in patients with SLE. Antibodies with elevated titers that are characteristic of lupus disease activity rather than infection include anti-dsDNA and anti–ribosomal P antibodies, in addition to reduced levels of complement and leukopenia.

Many of the clinical manifestations of SLE are a consequence of tissue damage from vasculopathy mediated by immune complexes. Other conditions (e.g., thrombocytopenia and antiphospholipid syndrome) are the direct effects of antibodies to cell surface molecules or serum components.

Manifestations of the disease range from a typical mild illness limited to a photosensitive facial rash and transient diffuse arthritis to life-threatening involvement of the CNS or renal, cardiac, or respiratory system (Fig. 23.2). In the early phases, it is often difficult to distinguish SLE from other systemic rheumatic disorders, such as progressive systemic sclerosis (PSS), PM, primary SjS, primary Raynaud phenomenon, and RA. Polyarthritis and dermatitis are the most common clinical manifestations.

The course of the disease is highly variable. It usually follows a chronic and irregular course, with periods of exacerbations and

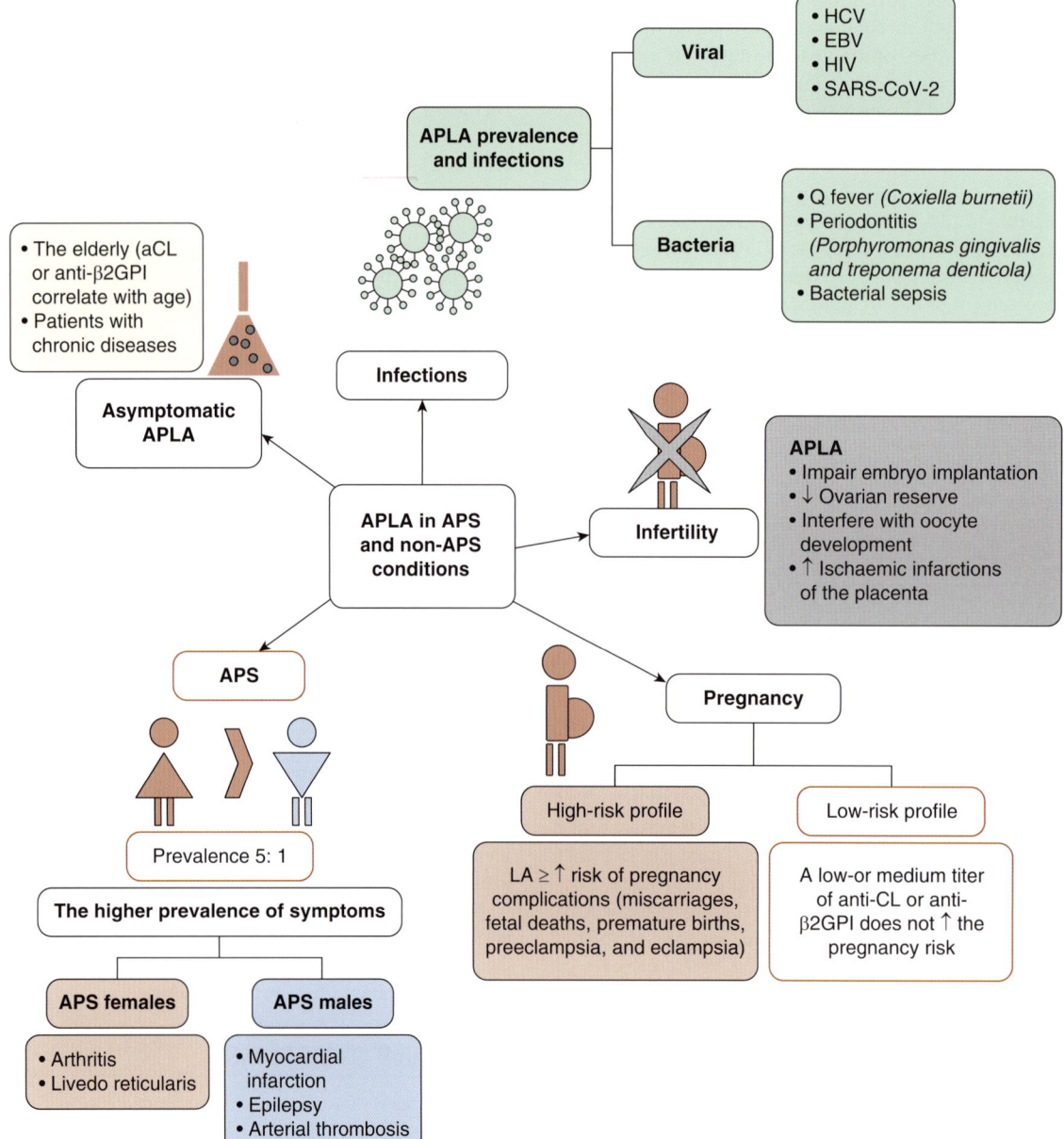

Fig. 23.1 The Prevalence and Gender-Related Characteristics of APS. (Used with permission from Grygiel-Górniak B, Mazurkiewicz Ł: Positive antiphospholipid antibodies: observation or treatment? *J Thromb Thrombolysis* 56(2):301–314, 2023.)

remissions. Clinical signs and symptoms can include fever, weight loss, malaise, arthralgia (joint pain) and arthritis (inflammation of the joints), and the characteristic erythematous, maculopapular ("butterfly") rash over the bridge of the nose (Table 23.2). In addition, there is a tendency toward increased susceptibility to common and opportunistic infections. Multiple organ systems may be affected simultaneously.

The onset of lupus can be caused by sun exposure, resulting in sudden development of a rash and then possibly other symptoms. In some patients, an infection, even a cold, does not improve, and complications then arise. These complications may be the first signs of lupus. In some women, the first symptoms develop during pregnancy or soon after delivery.

Infection

About 20% of episodes of fever are caused by infections in patients with SLE. Infections are the leading cause of death in hospitalized patients. Infections can be caused by bacterial, viral, fungal, or parasitic pathogens. Immunosuppression produced by treatment (e.g., steroids) can interfere with host defense against opportunistic infections (e.g., *Mycobacterium tuberculosis*, *Histoplasma capsulatum*, and *Listeria monocytogenes*).

Cutaneous Features

Approximately 20% to 25% of patients with SLE develop dermal disorders as the initial manifestation of the disease. As many as 65% of patients will develop a cutaneous abnormality during the course of the disease. The characteristic erythematous, maculopapular butterfly rash across the nose and upper cheeks is the cutaneous feature for which the disease is named: **lupus erythematosus**, the "red wolf" (Fig. 23.3). This rash may also be observed on the arms and trunk. Exposure to UV light will worsen erythematous and other types of cutaneous lesions.

The spectrum of cutaneous abnormalities includes urticaria, angioedema, nonthrombocytopenic purpura associated with the presence of cryoglobulins, scale formation, and ulcerations of oral and

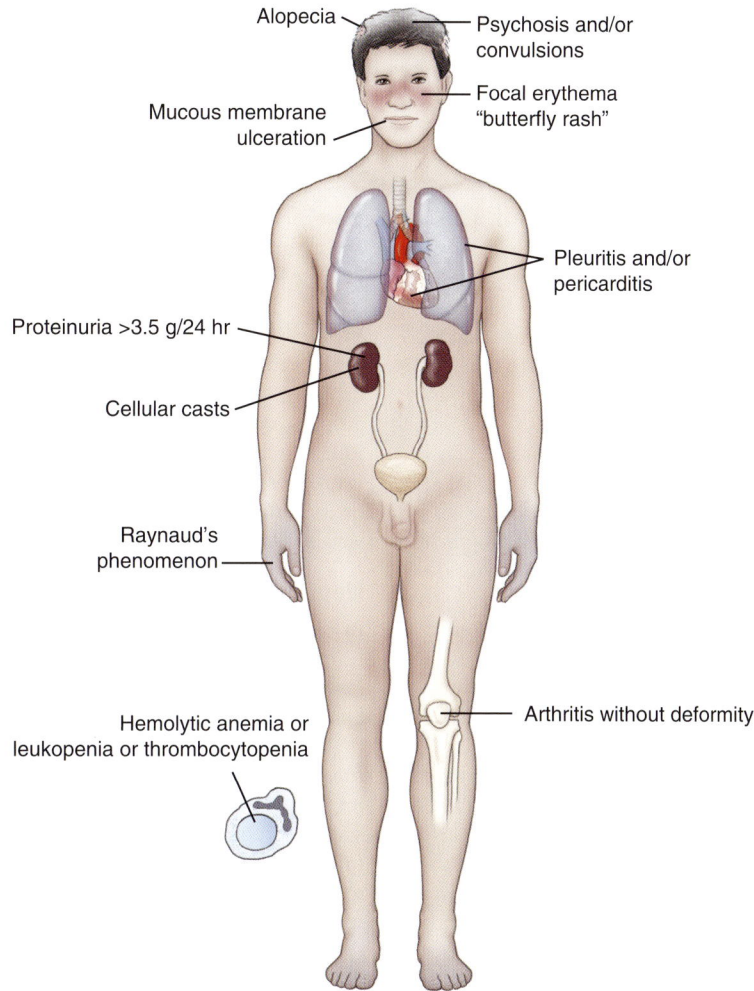

Fig. 23.2 Signs and symptoms of systemic lupus erythematosus (SLE).

TABLE 23.2 Systemic Lupus Erythematosus Symptoms.	
Symptom	Percentage of Cases
Achy joints (arthralgia)	95
Frequent fevers >37.8°C (100°F)	90
Arthritis (swollen joints)	90
Prolonged or extreme fatigue	81
Skin rashes	74
Anemia	71
Kidney involvement	50
Pain in the chest on deep breathing (pleurisy)	45
Butterfly-shaped rash across the cheeks and nose	42
Sun or light sensitivity (photosensitivity)	30
Hair loss	27
Abnormal blood-clotting problems	20
Raynaud phenomenon (fingers turning white and/or blue in the cold)	17
Seizures	15
Mouth or nose ulcers	12

Adapted from Lupus Foundation of America: General Lupus Fact Sheet, 2012. (https://www.lupus.org/webmodules/webarticlesnet/?z = 8&a = 351org).

genital mucous membranes. Although neither the collection of immunoglobulins and complement at the dermal-epidermal junction nor the presence of specific antibody nuclear ribonucleoprotein (RNP), Sm, native DNA, and single-strand DNA (ssDNA) appears to play a direct role in the pathogenesis of cutaneous lupus lesions, Ro (SS-A) and perhaps La (SS-B) antibodies may be prominent factors.

Diffuse or patchy alopecia is also a common cutaneous manifestation. Hair loss is caused by pustular lesions of the scalp and is usually related to the stress of the disease process. Although the cause of pustular lesions is unknown, these inflammatory infiltrates are characterized by the presence of predominantly Ia-positive (activated) T lymphocytes with both CD4+ and CD8+ phenotypes.

Approximately 2% to 3% of SLE patients demonstrate lupus panniculitis. This condition is characterized by tender or nontender subcutaneous nodules that sometimes ulcerate and discharge a yellowish lipid material. In addition, various nonspecific skin changes are observable secondary to vascular insults. **Raynaud phenomenon** is demonstrated by approximately one-third of patients with SLE and appears to be increased in those who have antibodies to nuclear RNP in their serum.

The presence of lesions does not distinguish between the limited cutaneous (discoid lupus erythematosus) and cutaneous manifestations of SLE. The term **discoid lupus** is used to differentiate the benign dermatitis of cutaneous lupus from the cutaneous involvement of SLE. In discoid

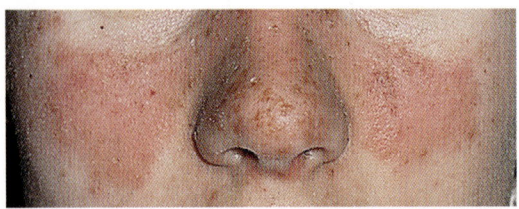

Fig. 23.3 Facial rash over the bridge of the nose in a patient with active SLE. (From Behrman R, Kliegman R, Jenson HB: *Nelson's textbook of pediatrics*, ed 17, Philadelphia, 2004, Saunders.)

lupus, the round lesion is an erythematous inflammatory dermatosis. These lesions are primarily located in light-exposed areas of the skin.

Renal Characteristics

Complement-mediated injury to the renal system is a usual consequence of the high levels of immune complexes in the blood that are deposited in tissues such as the kidneys. Renal disease progression is highly unpredictable. It may be acute, but more typically it progresses slowly. As the kidneys degenerate, the urinary sediment is typical of acute glomerulonephritis and later of chronic glomerulonephritis. Acute glomerulonephritis is characterized by the presence of erythrocytes, leukocytes, and granular and red blood cell (RBC) casts in urinary sediment. The presence of proteinuria may lead to nephrotic syndrome. If end-stage renal disease (renal failure) occurs, it can be managed by dialysis or allograft transplantation.

The systemic necrotizing vasculitis of SLE involves small blood vessels and leads to renal involvement. The most common method of classification of the renal involvement of SLE is the World Health Organization (WHO) system, which is based on histopathologic criteria. The stages of renal disease range from the earliest and least severe form, class II, characterized by mesangial deposits of immunoglobulin and C3, to class V, the most severe form of involvement.

Lymphadenopathy

Enlargement of peripheral and axial lymph nodes and splenomegaly both occur in patients with SLE, but these conditions are usually transient. Patients with SLE may be at greater risk of developing lymphoma than the general population, especially those with secondary SjS.

Serositis

Serositis is an inflammation of the membrane consisting of mesothelium, a thin layer of connective tissue that lines enclosed body cavities. Mesothelium, a type of epithelium, is originally derived from the mesoderm lining the primitive embryonic body cavity. It becomes the covering of the serous membranes of the body surfaces such as the peritoneum, pleura, and pericardium. Inflammation of these serosal surfaces leads to sterile peritonitis, pleuritis, or pericarditis and is frequently accompanied by severe pain. Serositis is associated with an increased frequency of thrombophlebitis, which may lead to pulmonary embolization.

Cardiopulmonary Characteristics

Inflammation of the myocardium in patients with SLE can produce persistent tachycardia and, occasionally, intractable congestive heart failure. Ischemic disease or, more often, atherosclerotic coronary disease may occur. Patients with severe nephrosis or those treated with corticosteroids for a prolonged period are at an increased risk of developing atherosclerosis.

Pulmonary function studies reveal occult diffusion and obstructive abnormalities in a high proportion of SLE patients, but clinical problems secondary to pulmonary involvement are unusual. Massive hemoptysis may result from acute alveolar hemorrhage. This particular complication occurs in the absence of any detectable bleeding diathesis and is associated with a high rate of mortality.

Gastrointestinal Manifestations

Nonspecific gastrointestinal symptoms are relatively common in patients with SLE, but acute abdominal crises caused by visceral and peritoneal vasculitis are less common. Infarction and perforation of the bowel and viscera are associated with a high rate of mortality. Acute and chronic pancreatitis may also develop as a secondary complication of acute lupus or as a complication during therapy.

Musculoskeletal Features

A characteristic arthritis of SLE is a transient and peripheral polyarthritis with symmetric involvement of small and large joints. Chronic arthritis can result in disability and deformity in SLE patients. Rheumatoid-like hand deformities develop in about 10% of patients. Osteonecrosis develops in 25% of all SLE patients. Arthropathy of osteonecrosis, or avascular necrosis, is often initially detected in weight-bearing joints such as the hips and knees.

Neuropsychiatric Features

In SLE, various neuropsychiatric manifestations develop secondary to involvement of the central and peripheral nervous systems. CNS involvement in SLE includes inflammation of the brain or intracranial blood vessels (vasculitis) and ischemic complications of vasculitis.

The most common abnormalities are disturbances of mental function, ranging from mild confusion, with memory deficiency and impairment of orientation and perception, to psychiatric disturbances such as hypomania, delirium, and schizophrenia. The most common manifestations are cognitive dysfunction, headache, seizures, and psychiatric conditions. Aseptic meningitis, stroke, encephalopathy, movement disorders, and myelopathy can be observed.

Seizures of the grand mal type may be the initial manifestation of SLE and may be present long before the multisystem disease develops. In addition, some patients may have epilepsy and severe headaches.

Antiribosomal P antibodies have been detected in patients with lupus suffering from psychosis or depression.

Late-Onset Lupus

Late-onset lupus can occur at any age, in either gender, and in any race. The average age of onset is 59 years; the average age at diagnosis is 62 years. Late-onset lupus affects women eight times more often than men and is found primarily in White individuals, but it occurs in all races.

Symptoms in most cases are relatively mild, but symptoms of lupus in older people can mimic those of other diseases (e.g., RA, SjS, and polymyalgia rheumatica). Distinguishing among these disorders can be difficult and may result in a delayed or missed diagnosis. Drug-induced lupus occurs more often in older people because they are more likely to have conditions (e.g., high blood pressure and heart disease) that require treatment that may cause the symptoms of lupus. Symptoms generally fade when the medication is discontinued. Patients with late-onset lupus have a good survival rate and rarely die of the disease or complications of therapy when treated conservatively.

> **KEY CONCEPTS: Immunologic Characteristics of SLE**
> - Lymphocyte subset abnormalities are a major immunologic feature of SLE.
> - The regulation of antibody production of B lymphocytes, ordinarily a function of the subpopulation of T-suppressor cells, appears defective in SLE.
> - Circulating immune complexes are the hallmark of SLE.
> - Antibodies also combine with their corresponding antigens to form immune complexes.

Immunologic Manifestations

B lymphocytes, T lymphocytes, and dendritic cells are involved in the pathogenesis of SLE. The pathogenesis of this systemic autoimmune disorder is characterized by the loss of tolerance to nuclear antigens, deposition of immune complexes in tissues, and multiorgan involvement.

Patients with SLE are known to produce multiple autoantibodies that react with native or altered self-antigens. Demonstrable antibodies include antibodies to nuclear components; cell surface and cytoplasmic antigens of polymorphonuclear and lymphocytic leukocytes, erythrocytes, platelets, and neuronal cells; and IgG.

There are two leading hypotheses, not mutually exclusive, as to why so many different antibodies develop. One hypothesis supports the belief that antibody-forming B lymphocytes are stimulated in a relatively nonspecific manner, so-called *polyclonal B-cell activation*. The second hypothesis is that the immune response in SLE is specifically stimulated by antigens. The most compelling evidence in its favor is that the antibody molecules formed over time show evidence of the gene rearrangement and somatic mutation characteristic of an antigen-driven response. Recent studies have suggested that the neutrophilic leukocyte activity is implicated in linked biochemical and cellular events. Findings suggest that in SLE, anti–self-antibodies activate neutrophils that consequently release NETs containing complexes of DNA and antimicrobial peptide. These complexes activate plasmacytoid dendritic cells, which leads to interferon-α release and perpetuation of inflammation and disease. In the future, NETs may serve as a biomarker or predictor of tissue damage in SLE.

Antibodies also combine with their corresponding antigens to form immune complexes. When the mononuclear phagocyte system is unable to eliminate them entirely, these immune complexes accumulate in the blood circulation. These circulating immune complexes are deposited in the subendothelial layers of the vascular basement membranes of multiple target organs, where they mediate inflammation. Laboratory features of SLE are the presence of ANAs, immune complexes, decreased complement level, tissue deposition of immunoglobulins and complement, circulating anticoagulants, and other autoantibodies. The human antineutrophil cytoplasmic antibodies (ANCAs), described for the first time in 1982, are directed against antigenic components mainly present in primary granules of neutrophils. ANCAs are serologic markers of primary necrotizing systemic vasculitis, particularly in Wegener granulomatosis. In addition, these antibodies have a prognostic interest because, in most cases, their titer is correlated with clinical activity during the disease.

Cellular Aspects

SLE is a disease that results from defects in the regulatory mechanism of the immune system. Studies of the immunopathogenesis of lupus nephritis have demonstrated a variety of aberrations in T-cell and B-cell function. It is uncertain whether the disease represents a primary dysfunction of T cells or B cells, but alterations in function do occur. Lymphocyte subset abnormalities are a major immunologic feature of SLE. Among the T-cell subsets, a lack of or reduced generalized suppressor T-cell function and hyperproduction of helper T cells occurs. The formation of lymphocytotoxic antibodies with a predominant specificity for T lymphocytes by patients with SLE at least partially explains the interference with certain functional activities of T lymphocytes associated with SLE. Lymphocytotoxic antibodies are capable of destroying T lymphocytes in the presence of complement and coating peripheral blood T cells.

The regulation of antibody production by B lymphocytes, ordinarily a function of the subpopulation of suppressor T cells, appears to be defective in patients with SLE. Although no single cause can be implicated in the pathogenesis of SLE, patients exhibit a state of spontaneous B-lymphocyte hyperactivity, with ensuing uncontrolled production of a wide variety of antibodies to host and exogenous antigens. Host response to some antigens, such as vaccination with influenza, is normal in many cases and the patient manifests a specific, well-controlled humoral immune response.

Humoral Aspects

Circulating immune complexes are the hallmark of SLE. Patients with SLE exhibit multiple serum antibodies that react with native or altered self-antigens. Demonstrable antibodies include antibodies to the following:

- Nuclear components
- Cell surface and cytoplasmic antigens of polymorphonuclear and lymphocytic leukocytes, erythrocytes, platelets, and neuronal cells
- Immunoglobulin G (IgG)

SLE is characterized by autoantibodies to almost any organ or tissue in the body. These antibodies may not be specifically diagnostic for SLE. In addition, some may have pathologic significance.

Antibodies to host antigens, particularly nuclear antigens such as DNA, are the principal type of antibody produced in SLE. ANAs are a heterogeneous group of antibodies produced against a variety of antigens within the cell nucleus. ANAs may be found in diseases other than SLE (e.g., other rheumatic or nonrheumatic diseases), in some patients undergoing specific drug therapy, and in healthy older individuals. The absence of ANAs almost excludes the diagnosis of SLE unless the patient is being chemically immunosuppressed. ANA titers and specific anti-DNA antibodies fluctuate during the course of the disease. In some cases, a rise in titer may forewarn of an impending disease flare-up.

Antigens to which antibodies are formed are present on nucleic acid molecules (DNA and RNA) or proteins (histones and nonhistones), and on determinants consisting of nucleic acid and protein molecules. Drug-induced cases of lupus have a high incidence of antibodies to histones. Some of these antibodies are directed against the double-strand helical DNA (native DNA or dsDNA). The presence of anti–native DNA (anti-nDNA) antibodies was reported in 1957. High titers of dsDNA are seen primarily in SLE and closely parallel disease activity. Most SLE patients simultaneously demonstrate antibodies to nucleoprotein and native DNA.

Other nuclear antibodies are directed at the determinants of ssDNA. Antibody titers of 1:32 or higher indicate a substantial concentration of antibody in an autoimmune response. Antibody to the Smith (Sm) antigen, a nuclear acidic protein extractable by aqueous solution, is considered a marker for SLE because anti-Sm has been found almost exclusively in patients with SLE. The presence of anti-Sm is seen in 25% to 30% of patients with SLE, but it rarely occurs in those with other systemic rheumatic (collagen) diseases.

The ANA antideoxyribonucleoprotein (anti-DNP) gives rise to the lupus erythematosus (LE) cell, which is found in more than 90% of untreated patients with active SLE. SLE patients with serositis may form LE cells in vivo. The LE cell testing procedure is now an obsolete test. In SLE patients with serositis, LE cells formed in vivo may be observed in aspirate fluid (e.g., pleural fluid). LE cells have been shown to be an expression of the interaction between IgG antibodies and DNP. Anti-DNP is referred to as the *LE serum factor*.

Antibodies to the Robert (Ro) soluble substance–A (SS-A) nuclear antigens are associated with SLE skin disease and neonatal SLE syndrome. Antibodies to the Lane soluble substance–B (SS-B) antigens are associated with SLE and with the primary and secondary forms of SjS. Their presence with SS-A antigen in SLE indicates mild disease. When present as the only antibody, SS-B is associated with primary SjS.

Autoantibodies to RBCs result in hemolytic anemia and can be detected by the anti–human globulin (AHG) test. Membrane-specific autoantibodies to neutrophils and platelets and autoantibodies to lymphocytes (cold-reactive type) are specific for SLE. Antibody titers correlate with disease activity.

Immunologic Consequences

Antibodies combine with their corresponding antigens to form immune complexes. When the mononuclear phagocyte system is unable to eliminate these immune complexes completely, immune complexes accumulate in the blood circulation. These circulating immune complexes are deposited in the subendothelial layers of the vascular basement membranes of multiple target organs, where they mediate inflammation. The sites of deposition are determined in part by the following physiochemical properties of the particular antigens or antibodies involved:

- Size
- Molecular configuration
- Immunoglobulin class
- Complement-fixing ability

After deposition, the immune complexes appear to initiate a localized inflammatory response that stimulates neutrophils to the site of inflammation, activates complement, and results in the release of kinins and prostaglandins. These activities become the basis of antibody-dependent, cell-mediated tissue injury.

DIAGNOSTIC EVALUATION

The manifestations of SLE expressed in laboratory findings are numerous. Histologic, hematologic, and serologic abnormalities reflect the multisystem nature of this disease.

Histologic Changes

The earliest pathologic abnormalities are those of acute vasculitis. Supportive tissue becomes edematous, initially infiltrated with neutrophils and later with plasma cells and lymphocytes. Persistent inflammation results in local deposition of a cellular homogeneous material histologically similar to fibrin. Nuclear debris from resulting cellular necrosis reacts with ANAs (discussed later in this section) to form hematoxylin bodies. The presence of immunoglobulins in vascular lesions, predominantly immunoglobulin M (IgM) and IgG, can be demonstrated by indirect immunofluorescence (IIF).

Renal pathology can also be observed in SLE. The two basic renal abnormalities that manifest are (1) proliferative glomerulonephritis, which resembles the renal changes in immune complex nephritis; and (2) membranous nephritis.

Hematologic and Hemostatic Findings

In SLE, a moderate anemia (normocytic normochromic anemia) representing chronic disease is a consistent factor. Some patients display coating of erythrocytes, which can be demonstrated by a positive AHG test, but actual hemolysis is infrequent. Lymphocytopenia is common and often reflects disease activity. Thrombocytopenia (50–100×10^9/L) may also be seen.

Hemostatic Testing

Lupus anticoagulants, antiphospholipid antibodies, are often seen in association with SLE. Antiphospholipid antibodies develop in up to 20% of patients with SLE. These form a group of antibodies detected by tests for lupus anticoagulant and anticardiolipin antibodies.

Circulating anticoagulants are believed to be associated with the presence of false-positive serologic test results for syphilis. Because of the presence of lupus anticoagulant, patients with SLE frequently demonstrate prolonged prothrombin time (PT) and partial thromboplastin time (PTT) results, but lupus anticoagulant rarely causes hemostatic problems. Inhibitors are not necessarily associated with bleeding unless some other defect is present. Because lupus anticoagulant is an inhibitor or prothrombin activator, it is often associated with excessive thrombosis rather than with bleeding. Patients with SLE have a high incidence of thrombotic episodes. Although less common, specific coagulation factor antibodies directed against coagulation factors VIII, IX, XI, and XII have been described. Thrombocytopenia can also occur because of the removal of antiphospholipid antibody–coated platelets.

> **KEY CONCEPTS: Laboratory Testing**
> - The ANA procedure is a valuable screening tool for SLE and can indicate various systemic autoimmune connective tissue disorders.
> - ANAs can be found in SLE and other disorders such as SSc, SjS, PM/DM, and RA.
> - ANAs are classified into antibodies to DNA, antibodies to histones, antibodies to nonhistone proteins, and antibodies to nuclear antigens.
> - Detection of autoantibodies by immunofluorescence is extremely sensitive and may show positive results when ANA procedures (e.g., complement fixation or precipitation) yield negative results. At present, immunofluorescence is the most widely used technique for ANA screening.

Serologic Findings

Serologic testing frequently reveals high levels of anti-DNA antibodies, reduced complement levels, and the presence of complement breakdown products of C3 (C3d and C3c). In addition, cryoglobulins, which in some cases represent immune complexes, are frequently present in the serum of patients with SLE. Because monoclonal gammopathies have occasionally been described, a marked increase in gamma globulins may result in a hyperviscosity syndrome or renal tubular acidosis. Serum cryoglobulins of a mixed IgG-IgM type are found in patients with hypocomplementemia. The level of cryoglobulin correlates well with the severity of SLE. The following procedural results are helpful in assessing renal disease:

- Antibody to dsDNA
- Levels of C3 and C4 (with C4 probably being the most sensitive result)
- Cryoglobulin levels

A general correlation exists between abnormal results in each of these procedures and disease activity in many patients, but considerable disagreement surrounds the usefulness of these measurements in predicting renal disease activity. The best laboratory procedures for monitoring the activity of renal disease are the serum creatinine level, urinary protein excretion, and careful examination of urine sediment.

Complement

Inherited deficiencies of several complement components are associated with lupus-like illnesses. Some, but not all, deficiencies are coded for by autosomal-recessive genes of the sixth chromosome, which are in linkage disequilibrium with human leukocyte antigen (HLA)-DRw2. The association of complement deficiencies with SLE may represent the fortuitous association of linked HLA-D region genes, rather than some unusual susceptibility induced by the complement deficiency.

Serum levels of complement typically are reduced, particularly during states of active disease. Deficiencies involving classic and alternative pathway complement components in SLE patients have resulted from consumption of components at the tissue sites of immune complex deposition, impaired synthesis, or both. A depressed level of complement is not specific for the diagnosis of SLE but is a helpful guide in treating patients. Levels of complement (C3, C4) are generally reduced in relationship to disease activity, and fluctuation in these levels is often used to monitor disease activity. Patients with decreased levels are at risk for renal and CNS involvement. Deficiencies of C1, C3, and C4 are associated with SLE and other rheumatic diseases.

Antibodies

Nonspecific elevation in immunoglobulin levels, particularly IgM and IgG, frequently occurs in SLE. An actual deficiency of immunoglobulin A (IgA) appears to be more common in SLE than in normal individuals.

The ANA procedure (discussed in detail in the next section) is commonly used to detect autoimmune disorders, and 97% of people with lupus test positive for ANA. Although ANAs are a hallmark of the disease, more research is needed to understand the relationship between ANA positivity and lupus risk and disease development.

Antinuclear Antibodies

Although it is usually called the ANA test, the same procedure also exhibits reactivity against all types of subcellular structures and cell organelles, including cell surfaces, cytoplasm, nuclei, or nucleoli. The antigens recognized are mainly proteins, protein macromolecular complexes, protein-nucleic acid complexes, and nucleic acids. In fact, most autoantibodies that are clinically useful target RNA-protein or DNA-protein complexes. The staining may be purely nucleolar or purely cytoplasmic. Therefore the ANA test is not just for "nuclear" staining.

In addition, it has been reported that 31.7% of normal individuals were ANA positive at 1:40 dilution, which was decreased to 13.3% at 1:80 and 5% at 1:160 dilution. Since about 95% were still positive at 1:160 dilution, raising the negative cutoff titer from 1:40 to 1:160 may improve the distinction between a clinically significant ANA result and a positive ANA result occurring in a normal individual.

Anti-dsDNA antibodies are the only autoantibodies that may be used to monitor the disease activity of SLE. High levels of anti-dsDNA antibodies, often with hypocomplementemia, correlate with clinical activity in a subset of SLE, such as patients with proliferative nephritis. ANAs are a heterogeneous group of circulating immunoglobulins that include IgM, IgG, and IgA. These immunoglobulins react with the whole nucleus or nuclear components (e.g., proteins, DNA, and histones) in host tissues; therefore they are true autoantibodies. Generally ANAs have no organ or species specificity and are capable of crossreacting with nuclear material from human beings (e.g., human leukocytes) or various animal tissues (e.g., rat liver, and mouse kidney). ANAs are found in other diseases (e.g., RA), are associated with certain drugs, and are found in older adults without disease (Table 23.3). Thus assays for ANAs are not specific for SLE. ANAs are present in more than 95% of SLE patients. Because the detection of ANAs is not diagnostic of only SLE, their presence cannot confirm the disease, but the absence of ANAs can be used to help rule out SLE. The significance of the presence of ANAs in a patient's serum must be considered in relation to the patient's age, gender, clinical signs and symptoms, and other laboratory findings.

Systematic classification. ANAs can be divided into five groups to provide a systematic classification: antibodies to DNA, antibodies to centromere, antibodies to histone, antibodies to nonhistone proteins, and antibodies to nucleolar antigens.

Antibodies to DNA. Antibodies to DNA can be divided into two major groups: antibodies that react with native (double-strand) DNA, and antibodies that recognize denatured (single-strand) DNA only.

Antibodies that react with native DNA appear to interact with antigenic determinants present on the deoxyribose phosphate backbone of the beta helix of DNA. These autoantibodies characteristically stain the kinetoplast of the hemoflagellate *Crithidia luciliae*, a substrate used to detect anti–native DNA antibodies by IIF. This procedure continues to be the gold standard for testing. Antibodies reactive with denatured DNA probably react with the purine and pyrimidine bases. These bases are readily accessible on ssDNA; they are buried within the beta helix of dsDNA and are therefore inaccessible. Anti–denatured DNA antibodies are unable to cross-react with native DNA. Conformational changes in the deoxyribose phosphate backbone of denatured DNA appear to be important for antigenicity.

Antibodies to centromere. Centromere antibodies are found to react with several centromere proteins of 18 kDa, 80 kDa, and 140 kDa named CENP-A, CENP-B, and CENP-C, respectively. The CENP-B antigen is believed to be the primary autoantigen and is detected in all patient sera that contain centromere antibodies.

Antibodies to histones. Antibodies to histones have been shown to react with all major classes of histones—H1, H2A, H2B, H3, and H4. Antihistone antibodies can be induced by drugs such as procainamide and hydralazine. Procainamide-induced LE is characterized by IgG antibodies against the histone complex H2A-H2B in symptomatic patients with SLE. In asymptomatic patients, the antibody may be restricted to the IgM class. Antibodies specific to other nuclear antigens are usually absent in drug-induced lupus in contrast to patients with SLE, who have ANAs of multiple specificity.

Patients with SLE are characterized by the presence of antibodies to multiple antigens, including Sm, RNP, dsDNA, chromatin, and SS-A/Ro (Table 23.4). There are 11 criteria for the diagnosis of SLE, and for a definitive diagnosis, patients must meet at least four of these criteria (see Table 23.1). Two of the criteria are a positive ANA test result and the detection of antibodies to Sm, dsDNA, or cardiolipin. Antibodies to Sm are detected in 20% to 30% of SLE patients, and antibodies to dsDNA may occur in up to 60% of patients. Antibodies to Sm and RNP typically occur together because they react with different proteins that are associated in an RNP particle called a *spliceosome*. A positive Sm indicates a high probability of SLE.

The presence of antibodies to dsDNA is one of the criteria for the diagnosis of SLE, and these antibodies are associated with active disease. The presence of dsDNA is a major concern in patients with SLE. The formation and deposition of immune complexes can affect various organ systems. Antibodies to dsDNA have also been reported in RA patients being treated with tumor necrosis factor-α (TNF-α) inhibitors. Patients with SLE have antibodies to chromatin more often than

TABLE 23.3 Antibodies in Systemic Rheumatic Diseases.			
Systemic Lupus Erythematosus	**Progressive Systemic Sclerosis**	**Polymyositis**	**Rheumatoid Arthritis**
Antinuclear antibodies	Antinuclear antibodies	Antinuclear antibodies	Antinuclear antibodies
Anti–native DNA	Anti–Scl-1	Anti–Jo-1	Rheumatoid factors
Anti-Sm	—	—	—

TABLE 23.4 Immunologic Assays for Detection and Monitoring of Systemic Lupus Erythematosus.

Assay	Reference Range
Antibodies	
Anti–dsDNA antibody	Negative (1:10)
Anti-La (SS-B) antibody	Negative
Anti–liver cytosol antibody	<15 U/mL
Anti-LKM antibody	<1:40
Antimitochondrial antibody	Negative
Antinuclear antibody	Negative (1:40)
Anti–ribosomal P protein antibody	<20 U/mL
anti-RNP antibody	Negative
Anti-Ro (SS-A) antibody	Negative
Anti-Smith IgG	Negative
Anti–soluble liver antigen-antibody	<5 U/mL
Complement	
Total complement	63–145 U/mL
C3	86–145 mg/dL
C4	20–58 mg/dL

anti-LKM, Anti–liver-kidney microsomal; *anti-RNP*, antinuclear ribonucleoprotein; *dsDNA*, double-strand DNA; *IgG*, immunoglobulin G.

antibodies to dsDNA. These chromatin antibodies are also associated with glomerulonephritis and have been identified, along with dsDNA antibodies, in immune complexes eluted from patients' kidneys. Patients with drug-induced lupus develop antibodies to chromatin and, in some cases, to the histone component of chromatin, but not to dsDNA.

The demonstration of only antihistone antibodies may be useful in distinguishing drug-induced lupus from SLE.

Antibodies to nonhistone proteins. Another primary class of ANAs in systemic autoimmune disorders are characterized by reactivity with soluble nonhistone nuclear protein and RNA-protein complexes. Clinically important antibodies that react with nuclear **nonhistone proteins** are listed in Table 23.5.

Antibodies to nucleolar antigens. The antibodies to nucleolar antigens are as follows:
- U3-RNA-protein complex (enzyme-transcribing ribosomal genes in the nucleolus)
- 7-2-RNP
- RNA polymerase I
- PM-Scl

These antinucleolar antibodies are primarily associated with PM-SSc overlap, in which they have the highest incidence and titers. However, they are rarely demonstrated in PSS, DM, or SSc.

Laboratory Evaluation

Both microscopy-based and immunoassay-based methods have significant importance in laboratory medicine. The traditional methods for detecting ANA are IIF and enzyme-linked immunosorbent assay (ELISA). Demonstrable antibodies include antibodies to nuclear components; cell surface and cytoplasmic antigens of polymorphonuclear and lymphocytic leukocytes, erythrocytes, platelets, and neuronal cells; and IgG. The detection of ANAs is a valuable screening tool for SLE.

Immunofluorescence is extremely sensitive and may show positive results in patients in whom procedures for ANAs (e.g., complement fixation or precipitation) give negative results. At present, immunofluorescence is the most widely used technique for ANA screening. Serologic testing frequently reveals high levels of anti-DNA antibodies, reduced complement levels, and the presence of complement breakdown products of C3 (C3d, C3c).

In addition, cryoglobulins, which may represent immune complexes, are frequently present in the serum of patients with SLE. The level of cryoglobulins correlates well with the severity of SLE. Assays helpful in assessing renal disease associated with SLE are antibodies to dsDNA, levels of C3 and C4, and cryoglobulins.

Indirect Immunofluorescent Tests for Antinuclear Antibody

IIF tests for ANA are based on the use of fluorescein-conjugated antiglobulin. These methods are extremely sensitive. In one assay, the serum specimen is delivered into a well on a microscope slide that contains a mouse liver substrate. Substrates of rat or mouse liver or kidney, or cell-cultured fibroblasts, can also be used as the antigen and are fixed to the slides. If antibody is present in the serum of the patient, the unlabeled antibody will attach to the nuclei of the cells in the substrate. After the substrate is washed in buffer, the slide is incubated with fluorescein-labeled goat AHG. If the patient's antibodies have attached themselves to the nuclear antigens in the substrate, the fluorescein-tagged goat AHG will attach to these antibodies. Fluorescence will be seen microscopically using UV light. The slides should be examined as soon as possible. If immediate examination is not possible, the slides can be stored in the dark at 4°C (39°F) for up to 48 hours before being read.

Several different patterns of fluorescence reactivity are seen (Figs. 23.4–23.8), depending on whether the ANAs have reacted with the whole nucleus or with nuclear components, such as the nuclear proteins, DNA, or histone (a simple protein). This difference in nuclear fluorescence pattern reflects specificity for various diseases. Patterns are described as being diffused or homogeneous, peripheral, speckled, or nucleolar fluorescence. Nuclear rim (peripheral) patterns correlate with antibody to native DNA and DNP and bear a correlation with SLE, SLE activity, and lupus nephritis. Homogeneous (diffused) patterns suggest SLE or another connective tissue disorder. Speckled patterns are found in many diseases, including SLE. Nucleolar patterns are seen in patients with PSS and SjS.

After ensuring that the results for positive and negative control specimens are providing the expected reactions, the results for the patient are reported. Results from the screening tests are reported as positive or negative. The normal person is expected to have a negative reaction; no green or gold fluorescence is observed. The degree of positive fluorescence may be semiquantitated on a scale of 1+ to 4+. Positive samples give a green-gold fluorescence of a characteristic pattern (homogeneous, peripheral, speckled, or nucleolar).

Indirect Immunofluorescent Technique

The detection of autoantibodies by immunofluorescence has become an extremely valuable tool. This method is extremely sensitive and may be positive in cases in which procedures for ANAs, such as complement fixation or precipitation, are negative. At present, the IIF method on a Hep-2 cell substrate is the primary screening test for the diagnosis of SRDs. A negative IIF result almost rules out a diagnosis of SLE, but the patterns observed on Hep-2 slides can provide a key to the diagnosis of other SRDs.

Principles. The antigen in the substrate tissue is fixed to a slide for testing. ANA is not specific to a particular organ; therefore any tissue containing nuclei may be used as substrate. The tissues most often used are rat or mouse liver or kidney or cell-cultured fibroblasts grown on slides. If antibody is present in a patient's serum, the unlabeled antibody will attach to the nuclei in the substrate. After the substrate is washed in buffer, it is incubated with fluorescein-tagged goat AHG. If the patient's antibodies have affixed themselves to the nuclear antigens

TABLE 23.5 Antibodies to Nonhistone Proteins (NhPs) and NhP-RNA Complexes in Systemic Rheumatic Diseases.

Antibody	Disease	Incidence (%)
Centromere-kinetochore	CREST variant of PSS	70–90
	Diffuse scleroderma	10–20
Jo-1	Polymyositis	31
Ki antigen	SLE	20
Ku	Polymyositis/scleroderma overlap	55
Ma antigen	SLE	20
Mi-I	Dermatomyositis	11
NuMa antigen	RA	
	Sjögren syndrome	
	Carpal tunnel syndrome	
	SLE	3
PCNA	RA	90
RANA	PSS	20
Scl-70	SLE	30
Sm	Sjögren syndrome	70
SS-A/Ro	SLE	50
	Other connective tissue diseases	
	Sjögren syndrome	40–50
SS-B/La	SLE	15
	Mixed connective tissue disease	>95
UI-RNP	SLE	35

CREST, Calcinosis, Raynaud phenomenon, esophageal dysmotility, sclerodactyly, and telangiectasia; *NuMa*, nuclear mitotic apparatus; *PCNA*, proliferating cell nuclear antigen; *PSS*, progressive systemic sclerosis; *RA*, rheumatoid arthritis; *RANA*, RA-associated nuclear antigen; *SLE*, systemic lupus erythematosus; *Sm*, Smith; *UI-RNP*, ribonucleoprotein.
Adapted from Reimer G, Tan E: Antinuclear antibodies. In Stein J, editor: *Internal medicine,* Boston, 1987, Little, Brown.

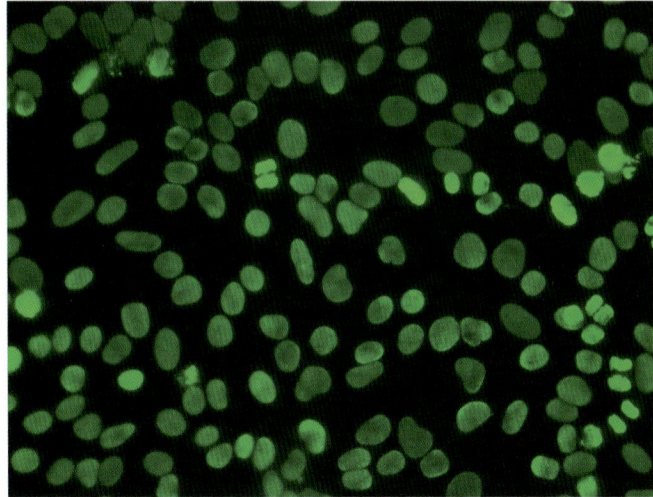

Fig. 23.4 Antinuclear Antibody (ANA). Homogeneous or diffused: A solid staining of the nucleus with or without apparent masking of the nucleoli. Nuclear antigens present: double-strand DNA (dsDNA), native DNA (nDNA), and deoxyribonucleoprotein (DNP) histone. Disease association: High titers are suggestive of systemic lupus erythematosus (SLE); lower titers are suggestive of SLE or other connective tissue diseases. (Courtesy INOVA Diagnostics, Inc., San Diego, CA.)

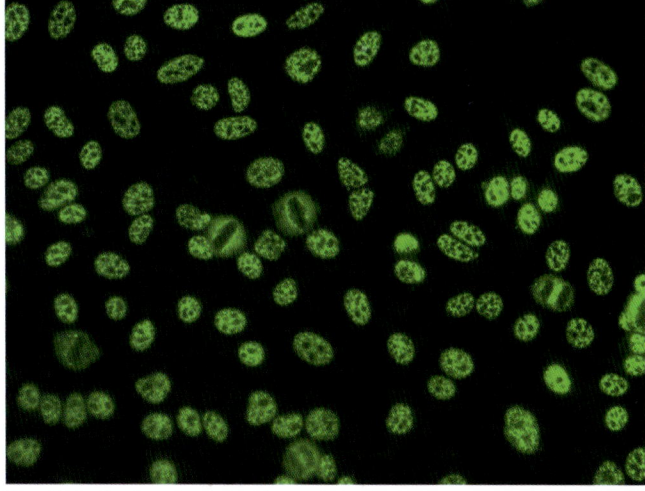

Fig. 23.5 Antinuclear Antibody (ANA). Coarse speckled. (Courtesy INOVA Diagnostics, Inc., San Diego, CA.)

- RNP, SS-A/Ro
- SS-B/La
- Scl-70
- Centromere
- Jo-1, cyclic citrullinated peptide (CCP)

of the substrate, the fluorescein-tagged goat AHG will attach to these antibodies. When the slide is examined microscopically, fluorescence will be visible on UV light.

Interpretation of staining patterns of major rheumatic autoantibodies

- dsDNA
- Chromatin, Sm

Because ANAs react with the whole nucleus or with nuclear components (e.g., proteins, DNA, and histone), reaction patterns reflect the distribution of the various antigens in the nuclei. Major ANAs are detected on all Hep-2 slides, but detection of antibodies to SS-A/Ro varies according to the fixation method. Alcohol diminishes or destroys the SS-A/Ro speckled ANA pattern, leading to a negative ANA result. It is always important to include a control for antibodies to SS-A/Ro.

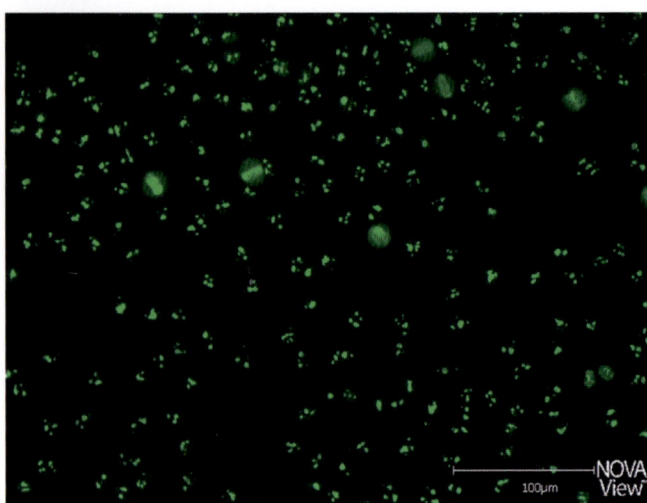

Fig. 23.6 Antinuclear Antibody (ANA). Nucleolar. (Courtesy INOVA Diagnostics, Inc., San Diego, CA.)

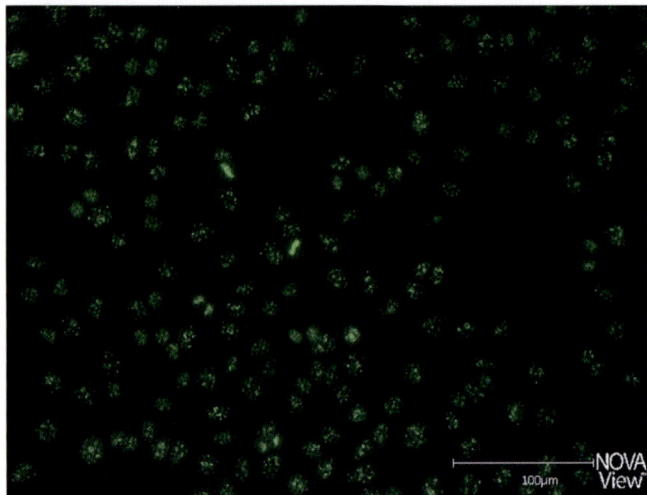

Fig. 23.7 Antinuclear Antibody (ANA). Centromere. (Courtesy INOVA Diagnostics, Inc., San Diego, CA.)

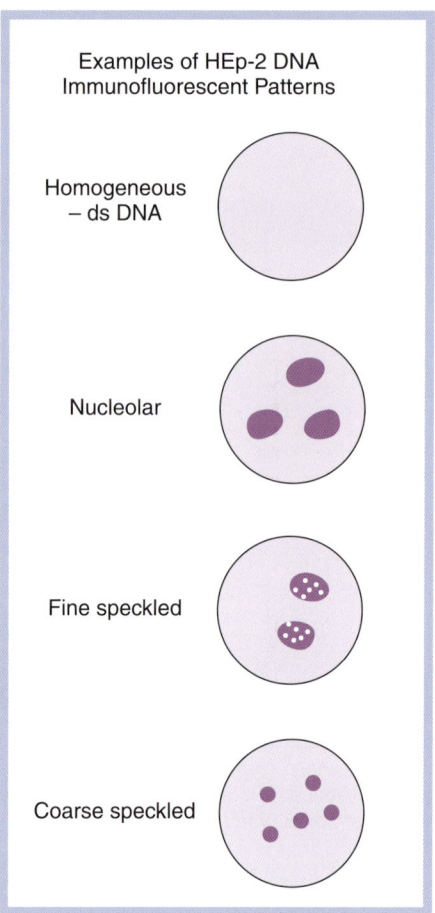

Fig. 23.8 Illustration of antinucleoprotein antibody patterns. *dsDNA*, Double-strand deoxyribonucleic acid.

Several patterns of reactivity can be observed when a slide is examined in the ANA procedure (Fig. 23.9).

Diffused or homogeneous pattern. The diffused or homogeneous pattern characterizes anti–DNA nucleoprotein antibodies (i.e., antibodies to nDNA, dsDNA, ssDNA, DNP, or histones). Antibodies to DNP have been shown to have the same specificity as the LE factor. Although vacuoles may be seen, the whole nucleus fluoresces evenly. This pattern is typically seen in rheumatoid disorders. High titers of homogeneous ANA suggest SLE, whereas low titers may be found in SLE, RA, SjS, and mixed connective tissue disease (MCTD).

Peripheral pattern. The peripheral (marginal or rim) pattern results from antibodies to DNA, nDNA, dsDNA, or DNP. The central protein of the nucleus is only lightly stained or not stained at all, but the nuclear margins fluoresce strongly and appear to extend into the cytoplasm. This pattern is associated with SLE in the active stage of the disease and with SjS.

Speckled pattern. The speckled pattern occurs in the presence of antibody to any extractable nuclear antigen devoid of DNA or histone. The antibody is detected against the saline extractable nuclear antigens, anti-RNP, and anti-Sm. A grainy pattern with numerous round dots of nuclear fluorescence, without staining of the nucleoli, is seen in this pattern type.

Antibodies to Sm antigen have been shown to be highly specific for patients with SLE and appear to be marker antibodies. Anti-RNP has been found in patients with a wide variety of rheumatic diseases, including SLE, RA, SjS, PSS, MCTD, and DM.

Nucleolar pattern. The nucleolar pattern reflects an antibody to nucleolar RNA (4-6S RNP). A few round, smooth nucleoli that vary in size will fluoresce when examined under UV light. The nucleolar pattern is present in about 50% of patients with SSc (PSS), SjS, and SLE. This pattern can also be observed in undiagnosed illnesses manifesting Raynaud phenomenon.

Centromere. The anticentromere antibody reacts with centromeric chromatin of metaphase and interphase cells. The particular pattern on tissue culture cells is discrete and speckled. This antibody appears to be highly selective for the CREST variant of PSS. The CREST syndrome is a variant of systemic sclerosis characterized by the presence of *c*alcinosis, *R*aynaud phenomenon, *e*sophageal motility abnormalities, *s*clerodactyly, and *t*elangiectasia. This antibody is found infrequently in the serum of patients with SLE, MCTD, and PSS.

Rapid Slide Test for Antinucleoprotein

The SLE latex test provides a suspension of polystyrene latex particles coated with DNP (see Procedure). When the latex reagent is mixed with serum containing the ANAs, binding to the DNP-coated latex particles produces macroscopic agglutination. The procedure is positive in SLE and SRDs (e.g., RA, SSc, and SjS).

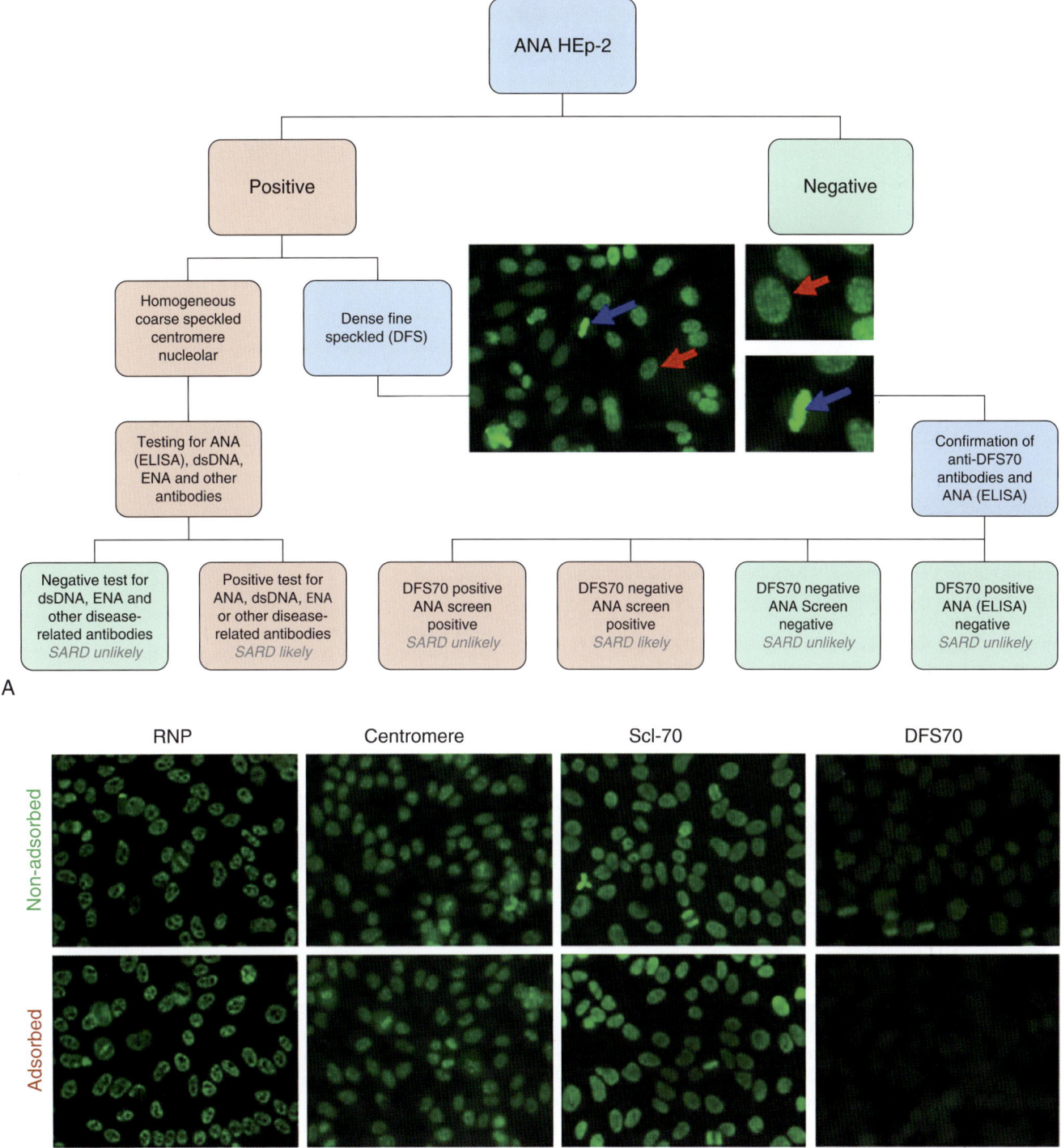

Fig. 23.9 Characteristic staining pattern, suggested testing algorithm and immunoadsorption of anti-DFS70 antibodies. a.) The characteristic dense fine speckled staining pattern of interphase cells is indicated by the red arrow and the strong chromatin staining of mitotic cells by the blue arrow (the density of speckles in interphase cells can vary between different HEp-2 substrates). Samples with a dense fine speckled pattern should be tested for anti-DFS70 antibodies by a confirmatory test and by ANA Screen ELISA containing various autoantigens. Patients with a negative ANA Screen ELISA and negative DFS70 result as well as patients with negative ANA Screen ELISA and positive DFS70 result have a low likelihood for having SARD. Patients with a positive ANA Screen ELISA either in combination with a positive or a negative DFS70 test result have an increase likelihood of having SARD. b.) A sample diluted in Sample Diluent without recombinant DFS70 showed a characteristic dense fine speckled (DFS) staining pattern. After immunoadsorption of anti-DFS70 antibodies, the IIF shows no specific pattern. Samples with SARD associated autoantibodies such as anti-RNP, anti-Centromere or anti-Scl-70 antibodies showed no inhibition of the pattern. (Mahler M, Hanly JG, Fritzler MJ: Importance of the dense fine speckled pattern on HEp-2 cells and anti-DFS70 antibodies for the diagnosis of systemic autoimmune diseases, *Autoimmun Rev* 11(9):642–645, 2012.)

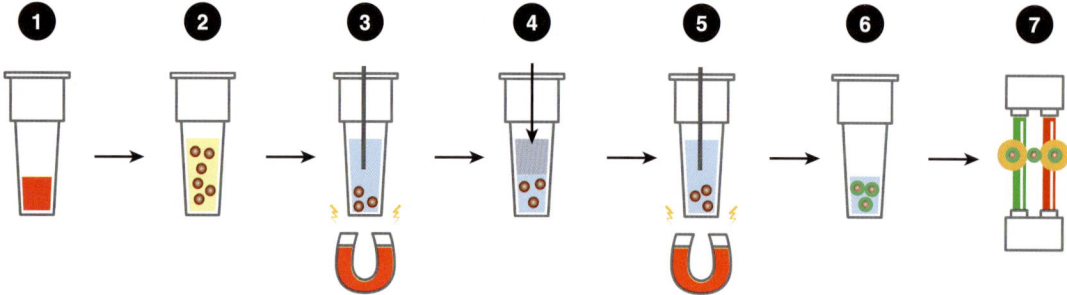

1. Patient sample (5 µL) automatically added to reaction vessel
2. Sample diluent & beads added, mixed, and incubated at 37°C
3. Wash step (3x)
4. Conjugate added, mixed, and incubated at 37°C
5. Wash step
6. Bead resuspended in wash buffer
7. Flow-based, dual-laser detection

Fig. 23.10 BioPlex 2200 Antinuclear Antibody Screen with Medical Decision Support Software. An indirect assay format is used for the BioPlex 2200 ANA Screen. (© 2012 Bio-Rad Laboratories, Inc.; reviewed August 17, 2024.)

Autoimmune Enzyme Immunoassay

The autoimmune enzyme immunoassay (EIA) provides a qualitative screening test for the presence of ANAs. In one well, the assay collectively detects total ANAs against dsDNA (nDNA) histones, SS-A/Ro, SS-B/La, Sm, Sm/RNP, Scl-70, Jo-1, and centromeric antigens, along with sera positive for immunofluorescent assay (IFA) Hep-2 ANAs. This assay serves as an alternative to the IFA for screening a patient's serum for ANAs.

Automated Testing: Multiplex Immunoassay

Multiplex technology represents an advanced technology assay method for simultaneously screening a patient to confirm or to exclude the presence of a large number of ANAs associated with various autoimmune diseases. ANA testing by multiplexing has good agreement with the traditional methods. The automated multiplex system represents a rapid, sensitive, and specific method with the absence of subjective error in interpretation of results.

Two basic assay formats have been developed to facilitate simultaneous quantification of multiple antigens: planar array assays and microbead assays. Planar array assays spot different capture ligands at defined positions on a two-dimensional array. Microbead assays like those based on Luminex MAP technology involve multiple microbeads, each coated with different capture ligands. Flow cytometry (see Chapter 11) then detects an assay-specific fluorescent signal, which allows simultaneous detection of multiple analytes in a single reaction.

Currently available commercial systems based on fluorescent microbead technology include two US manufacturers: BioPlex 2200 (Bio-Rad Laboratories, Hercules, CA) and AtheNA Multi-Lite (Zeus Diagnostics, Raritan, NJ). As an example, BioPlex 2200, a fully automated Luminex-based system, performs simultaneous analysis of 13 autoimmune analytes in a single tube:

- dsDNA
- SSA (52 kDa)
- SSA (60 kDa)
- SSB
- Sm
- Sm/RNP
- RNP-A
- RNP-68 kDa
- Scl70
- Centromere B
- Chromatin
- Jo-1
- Ribosomal P proteins

The BioPlex 2200 system couples microspheres with different laser-reactive colors to antigens of interest and combines them in a single microtiter well. The specimen and a fluorochrome-coupled secondary antibody are then added. The analysis uses flow dual-laser cytometry in which the first laser identifies the color of the bead, which addresses the identity of the coated antigen, and the second laser identifies the presence and quantity of autoantibody bound to the antigen (Fig. 23.10).

In this system, anti-dsDNA antibody is calibrated with the WHO Wo/80 standard. The results are quantitative and expressed in terms of IU/mL. Results of ≥10 IU/mL are considered to be positive. All of the other antibody results are semiquantitative measurements expressed as the antibody index (AI), with results of ≥1 AI being a positive result. An ANA screening assay is reported as negative if the results for all of the 13 autoantibodies are negative. If any of the 13 autoantibodies is positive, it is considered to be a positive ANA screen, and the AIs of individual antibodies should be reported.

The medical decision support software (MDSS) included in the system suggests a disease association based on how individuals with similar autoantibody profiles have been diagnosed. The MDSS uses a database of 1200-plus real-world individuals and contains the specific ANA screen results for all 13 autoantibodies. In addition, patterns of autoantibodies detected by this system, when analyzed by an interpretative algorithm, are useful in the evaluation of patients with autoimmune disorders.

A limitation of this technology is that only a limited number of antigens is tested, which can lead to false-negative results compared with other methods. This is particularly serious when searching for some specific disease profiles, such as autoimmune liver diseases. In addition, recombinant proteins used in the assay may be poorly recognized by human autoantibodies, leading to false-negative results. For some, the absence of the reporting of an ANA pattern and an antibody titer may be disconcerting.

TREATMENT

For most patients with lupus, effective treatment and prevention methods can minimize symptoms, reduce inflammation, and maintain normal body functions. For photosensitive patients, avoidance of (excessive) sun exposure and the regular application of sunscreens will usually prevent rashes. Regular exercise helps prevent muscle weakness and fatigue. Immunization protects against specific infections. Support groups and counseling can help alleviate the effects of stress. Lupus patients should avoid smoking, excessive consumption of alcohol, overuse or underuse of prescribed medication, and postponing regular medical checkups.

Medications are often prescribed for patients with lupus, depending on the organ(s) involved and the severity of involvement. Common medications include the following:

- Nonsteroidal antiinflammatory drugs (NSAIDs). NSAIDs are prescribed for a variety of rheumatic diseases, including lupus. Examples include acetylsalicylic acid (aspirin), ibuprofen (Advil, Motrin), and naproxen sodium (Aleve). These drugs are usually recommended for muscle and joint pain and arthritis. Newer NSAIDs contain a prostaglandin in the same capsule (Arthrotec). The other NSAIDs work in the same way as aspirin but may be more potent.
- Acetaminophen. Acetaminophen (Tylenol) is a mild analgesic that can often be used for pain. It has the advantage of causing less stomach irritation than aspirin but is not nearly as effective at suppressing inflammation as aspirin.
- Steroids (e.g., prednisone) are used to reduce inflammation and suppress activity of the immune system. Side effects occur more frequently when steroids are taken over long periods at high doses. These side effects include weight gain, a round face, acne, easy bruising, thinning of the bones (osteoporosis), high blood pressure, cataracts, onset of diabetes, increased risk of infection, stomach ulcers, hyperactivity, and increased appetite.
- Antimalarials. Chloroquine (Aralen) or hydroxychloroquine (Plaquenil), typically used to treat malaria, may also be useful for some individuals with lupus. Antimalarials are most often prescribed for the skin and joint symptoms of lupus.
- Immunosuppressants. Drugs that suppress the immune system may be helpful in serious cases of lupus. Examples include azathioprine (Imuran, Azasan), mycophenolate (CellCept), leflunomide (Arava), and methotrexate (Trexall). A newer medication, belimumab (Benlysta), also reduces lupus symptoms in some patients.
- Studies have suggested that immunosuppressive therapy targeted against the calcineurin pathway of helper T cells, such as tacrolimus, may be effective in the treatment of primary membranous nephropathy.
- Anticoagulants. Anticoagulants range from aspirin at a very low dose to heparin or Coumadin. Generally such therapy is lifelong in those with lupus and follows an episode of embolus or thrombosis.
- Biological disease-modifying antirheumatic drug (DMARD) therapy.
  - Belimumab (Benlysta) is a human monoclonal antibody that specifically recognizes and inhibits the biological activity of B-lymphocyte stimulator (BLyS). BLyS is a naturally occurring protein discovered by human genome scientists that is required for B lymphocytes to develop into mature plasma B cells, which produce antibodies, the body's first line of defense against infection.
  - In March 2011 the US Food and Drug Administration (FDA) approved the use of belimumab in combination with standard therapies (including steroids and nonbiological DMARDs [e.g., hydroxychloroquine, azathioprine, and methotrexate]) to treat active autoantibody-positive SLE.
- Other monoclonal antibody therapy.

Rituximab

B-cell depletion with rituximab (Rituxan) has shown mixed results for the treatment of SLE. An open study using rituximab showed excellent results as rescue therapy for patients with active SLE who were unresponsive to standard immunosuppressant therapy. There have also been case reports of patients with severe refractory SLE in which off-label use of rituximab showed benefits with tolerable safety profiles.

Pharmacologic agents targeting specific pathways such as cytokines and complement, in addition to combinations of rituximab with costimulatory inhibition with anti-CD4OL or CTLA-41g, may prove to be more effective in treating SLE.

On April 29, 2019, the US FDA approved Benlysta, belimumab, intravenous (IV) infusion for the treatment of children with SLE.

Equalise for Lupus Nephritis

The Lupus Research Alliance is investigating an experimental compound, itolizumab, at various doses in a small group of patients with SLE and lupus nephritis, a common complication of lupus. This drug, Equalise (Equillium, La Jolla, CA), is in a Phase 1b trial to evaluate its safety and tolerability as a potentially effective treatment in addition to its pharmacokinetics and pharmacodynamics. This clinical trial will also evaluate how well biomarkers in the urine can provide patient information. The biomarker ALCAM is a small molecule on the outside of T cells of the immune system that helps the T cells move through these tissues of the body, including the kidney. Equalise blocks this ALCAM pathway.

CASE STUDY 23.1

History and Physical
A 39-year-old Black woman with SLE was diagnosed with the illness 20 years ago. Her initial manifestations of illness developed during the postpartum period of her second pregnancy. The pregnancy was complicated by proteinuria, which was believed to be caused by toxemia of pregnancy.

The patient had polyarthralgia, alopecia, and erythematous rashes of the face, arms, and legs. A renal biopsy was performed because her urinalysis revealed proteinuria and RBC casts. The renal biopsy revealed diffuse, proliferative glomerulonephritis. In addition to abnormal laboratory results related to renal function, she manifested ANA (titer 1:1280) and antibodies to DNA and the C3 component of complement.

Questions
1. The antibody found in common in systemic rheumatic diseases is:
   a. Antinuclear antibody (ANA)
   b. Antinative DNA
   c. Anti–SCl-1
   d. Anti–Jo-1
2. Patients with systemic lupus erythematosus (SLE) are characterized by the presence of antibodies to _____ antigens.
   a. dsDNA
   b. RNA polymerase I
   c. PM-Scl
   d. Anticentromere

See Appendix A for the answers to these multiple-choice questions.

Critical Thinking Group Discussion Questions
1. Are the antibodies manifested by the patient typical of SLE?
2. Do patients with SLE have significant morbidity?

CASE STUDY 23.2

History and Physical
A 27-year-old White woman sought medical attention because of persisting pain in her wrists and ankles and an unexplained skin irritation on her face. On physical examination, swelling of the joints of the hands and ankles was evident, along with erythema of the skin over the bridge of the nose and the upper cheeks. The patient had a slightly elevated temperature.

Laboratory Data
A complete blood count (CBC), urinalysis (UA), and rheumatoid arthritis (RA) screening test were ordered, with the following results:
- Hemoglobin and hematocrit—Normal
- Total leukocyte count—70×10^9/L
- Differential leukocyte count—Normal
- Gross and microscopic UA—Normal
- RA screening test—Positive

Follow-Up
An ANA screening test was ordered. The results were positive.

Questions
1. Serologic testing frequently reveals _____ in patients with systemic lupus erythematosus (SLE).
   a. Increased titer of anti-DNA
   b. Increased complement C3 levels in the serum
   c. Absence of C3d and C3c
   d. Absence of rheumatoid factor
2. A homogeneous antinuclear antibody (ANA) (Hep-2) pattern characterizes antibodies to:
   a. SSB/La
   b. dsDNA
   c. RNA polymerase III
   d. SCL-70

See Appendix A for the answers to these multiple-choice questions.

Critical Thinking Group Discussion Questions
1. What is the most probable diagnosis in this case?
2. Does this patient fit into the general characteristics of patients with this disease?
3. What is the principle of the ANA test?

REVIEW QUESTIONS

1. SLE is more common in:
   a. Female infants
   b. Male infants
   c. Adolescent through middle-aged women
   d. Adolescent through middle-aged men
2. One of the most potent inducers of abnormalities and clinical manifestations of SLE is:
   a. Chloramphenicol
   b. Procainamide hydrochloride
   c. Isoniazid
   d. Penicillin
3. The cellular aberrations in SLE include:
   a. B-cell depletion
   b. Deficiency of suppressor T-cell function
   c. Hyperproduction of helper T cells
   d. Both b and c
4. The principal demonstrable antibody in SLE is antibody to:
   a. Nuclear antigen
   b. Cell surface antigens of hematopoietic cells
   c. Cell surface antigens to neuronal cells
   d. Lymphocytic leukocytes
5. The sites of immune complex deposition in SLE are influenced by all of the following factors *except*:
   a. Molecular size
   b. Molecular configuration
   c. Immune complex specificity
   d. Immunoglobulin class
6. Renal disease secondary to SLE injury is caused by:
   a. Antibody to native dsDNA
   b. Presence of erythrocytes and leukocytes
   c. Increased levels of ANA
   d. Increased levels of immune complexes
7. SLE is a classic model of autoimmune disease and is a(n):
   a. Abnormality of hematopoiesis
   b. Abnormality of lymphatic system
   c. Connective tissue disorder
   d. Systemic rheumatoid disorder
8. The overall incidence of SLE has an increased frequency among:
   a. Blacks
   b. Indigenous South Americans
   c. First Nation Canadians
   d. White Americans
9. Patients with SLE characteristically manifest:
   a. Butterfly rash over the bridge of the nose
   b. Skin lesions on the arms and legs
   c. Ulcerations on the trunk
   d. Photophobia
10. Laboratory features of SLE include:
    a. High titers of ANAs
    b. High titers of rheumatoid factor
    c. Increased levels of complement factors
    d. Decreased immunoglobulin levels
11. Laboratory procedures that are helpful in assessing renal disease include:
    a. Antibody to double-strand DNA
    b. Concentrations of C3 and C4
    c. Crystals in urinary sediment
    d. Both a and b
12. Jo-1 is associated with:
    a. Systemic lupus erythematosus
    b. Dermatomyositis
    c. Progressive systemic sclerosis
    d. Polymyositis
13. Mi-I is associated with:
    a. Systemic lupus erythematosus
    b. Dermatomyositis
    c. Progressive systemic sclerosis
    d. Polymyositis

14. SS-B/La is associated with:
    a. Systemic lupus erythematosus
    b. Dermatomyositis
    c. Progressive systemic sclerosis
    d. Polymyositis
15. RANA is associated with:
    a. Systemic lupus erythematosus
    b. Dermatomyositis
    c. Progressive systemic sclerosis
    d. Polymyositis
16. The ANA staining of a diffused or homogeneous pattern is associated with:
    a. Anti–DNA-nucleoprotein antibody
    b. Antibody to nucleolar RNA
    c. Antibody to any extractable nuclear antigen devoid of DNA or histone
    d. Anticentromere antibody
17. The ANA staining of a nucleolar pattern is associated with:
    a. Anti–DNA-nucleoprotein antibody
    b. Antibody to nucleolar RNA
    c. Antibody to any extractable nuclear antigen devoid of DNA or histone
    d. Anticentromere antibody
18. The classic substrate used in the anti–double-strand DNA procedure is:
    a. Hamster kidney tissue
    b. *Bacillus subtilis*
    c. *Crithidia luciliae*
    d. Fluorescent monoclonal antibodies
19. The name of the ANA pattern in the microscopic image is:

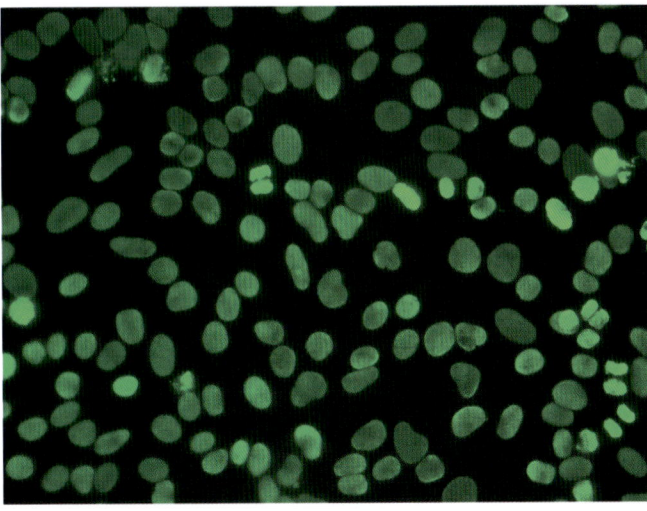

   a. Homogeneous
   b. Centromere
   c. Coarse speckled
   d. Nucleolar

20. The name of ANA pattern in the microscopic image is:

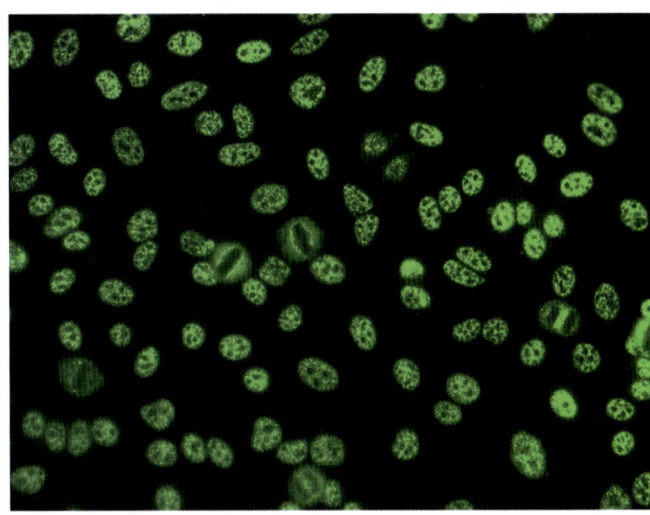

   a. Homogeneous
   b. Diffused
   c. Coarse speckled
   d. Nucleolar
21. A positive ANA with a centromere pattern is associated with:
    a. Systemic lupus erythematosus
    b. CREST syndrome
    c. Antisynthetase syndrome
    d. Mixed connective tissue disease
22. Patients with active SLE are known to exhibit widespread complement activation that results in deficiencies of complement components such as:
    a. C3
    b. C4
    c. C8
    d. Both a and b
23. Autoantibodies against the alternative complement pathway C3 convertase in patients with membranoproliferative glomerulonephritis that can also be found in patients with SLE are called:
    a. C3 nephritic factors (C3NeF)
    b. C4 nephritic factors C4NeF)
    c. C_1Q complement deficiency
    d. None of the above
24. If a patient is suffering from active SLE, a CH_{50} assay would be expected to be:
    a. Within the normal reference range
    b. Above the normal reference range
    c. Below the normal reference range
    d. Variable depending on the age of a patient
25. What specific diagnostic test does not meet the criteria for a definitive diagnosis of a patient with a differential diagnosis of SLE?
    a. Positive antinuclear antibody (ANA)
    b. Ribonucleic protein (RNP) antibodies
    c. Smith (Sm) antibodies
    d. Double-stranded DNA (dsDNA) antibodies

24

Rheumatoid Arthritis

LEARNING OUTCOMES

- Name significant factors related to the development of arthritis.
- Describe the etiology, epidemiology, and signs and symptoms of rheumatoid arthritis.
- Discuss the immunologic manifestations and diagnostic evaluation of rheumatoid arthritis.
- Briefly describe juvenile rheumatoid arthritis.
- Explain diagnostic procedures used in the identification and evaluation of rheumatoid arthritis.
- Analyze representative rheumatoid arthritis case studies.
- Correctly answer case study–related multiple-choice questions.
- Be prepared to participate in a discussion of critical thinking questions.
- Describe the principle, sources of error, clinical applications, and limitations of a rapid rheumatoid factor procedure.
- Correctly answer 80% of the end-of-chapter review questions.

OUTLINE

Etiology, 415
Epidemiology, 415
Signs and Symptoms, 416
Anatomy and Physiology of Joints, 417
Immunologic Manifestations, 418
Diagnostic Evaluation, 419
Rheumatoid Factor, 419
Cyclic Citrullinated Peptide Antibodies, 419
    Other Markers, 419
    Immune Complexes, 419
    Complement Levels, 420
    Antinuclear Antibodies, 420
Juvenile Idiopathic Arthritis, 420
    Etiology, 420
    Epidemiology, 420

Signs and Symptoms, 420
Immunologic Manifestations, 420
    Rheumatoid Factors, 420
    Immune Complexes, 420
    Antinuclear Antibodies, 421
Treatment, 421
    Traditional Treatment, 421
    Corticosteroids and Glucocorticoids, 421
    Nonbiological Disease-Modifying Antirheumatic Drugs, 421
    Biological Disease-Modifying Antirheumatic Drugs, 421
Diagnostic Procedures, 424
Case Study 24.1, 424
Case Study 24.2, 424
Procedure: Rapid Agglutination, 425.e1

KEY TERMS

ankylosing spondylitis
arthrocentesis
articular
biologics
cryoglobulins

extraarticular
juvenile idiopathic arthritis (JIA)
leukotrienes
pathogenesis
polyarthritis

rheumatoid factor
scleroderma
synovitis
synovium

The word *arthritis* literally means joint inflammation: *arth-* (joint) and *-itis* (inflammation). Arthritis is a large and growing public health problem in the United States. There are more than 100 forms of arthritis and related diseases. With the aging of the US population, even assuming that the prevalence of obesity and other risk factors remain unchanged, the prevalence of physician-diagnosed arthritis and arthritis-attributable activity limitation is expected to increase significantly by 2030.

Based on the data from the Centers for Disease Control and Prevention (CDC) combined with data from the National Health Interview Survey (NHIS) years 2013–2015 Sample Adult Core components to estimate the average annual arthritis prevalence in the civilian, noninstitutionalized US adult population aged 18 years or older, an estimated 54.4 million citizens had physician-diagnosed arthritis. There is a significantly higher age-adjusted prevalence in women than in men. The prevalence of arthritis increases significantly with age. Initial onset of symptoms can begin between 30 and 50 years of age. Females are more likely than males to suffer from arthritis. Non-Hispanic White, African American, Indigenous Alaska Natives, and Alaska Native individuals are more likely to have arthritis than Hispanic, Asian, and Pacific Islander individuals. Obese and overweight people are diagnosed with arthritis more frequently than underweight or normal-weight individuals. Physically inactive people develop arthritis more often than do physically active people.

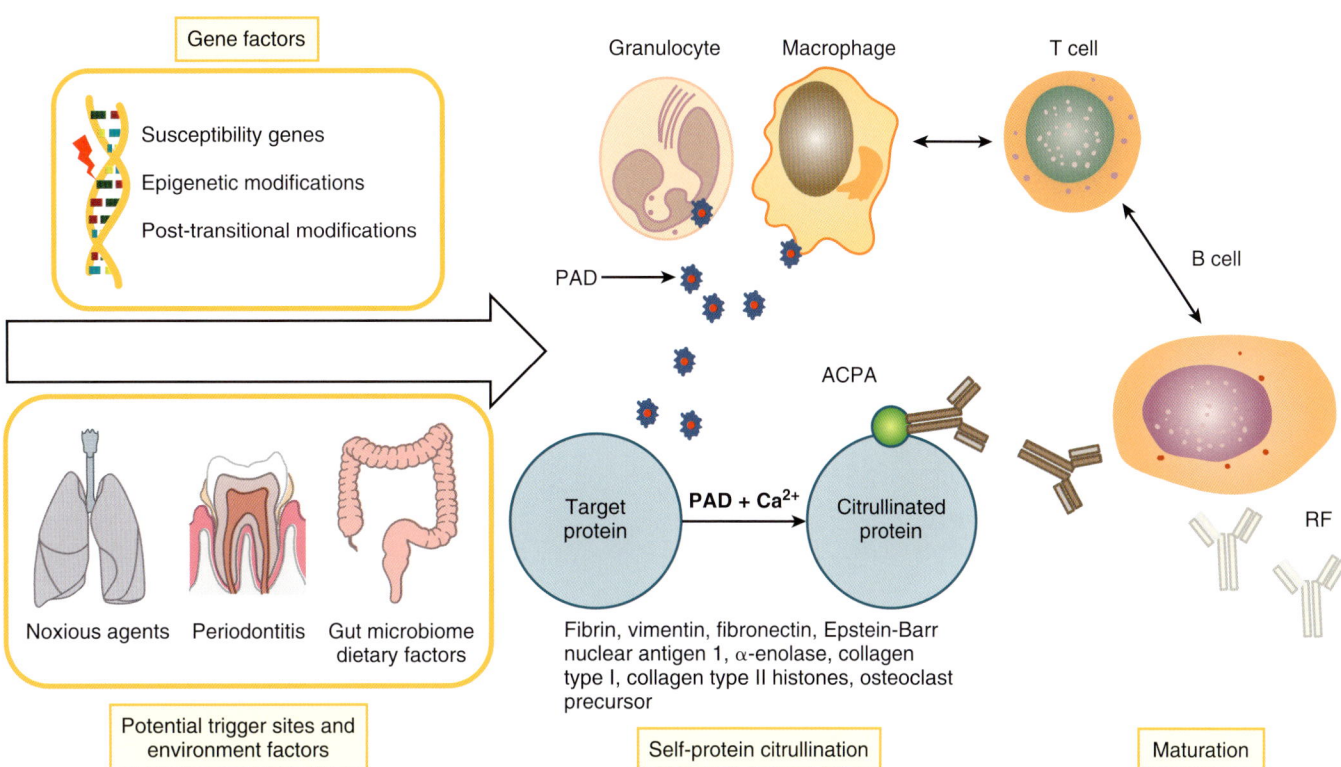

Fig. 24.1 Rheumatoid arthritis (RA) can be triggered in the potential trigger sites (e.g., lung, oral, and gut) by the interaction between genes and environmental factors; this is characterized by the onset of self-protein citrullination, which results in the production of autoantibodies against citrullinated peptides. Lung exposure to noxious agents, infectious agents (*Porphyromonas gingivalis*, *Aggregatibacter actinomycetemcomitans*, and Epstein-Barr virus), gut microbiome, and dietary factors may induce the self-protein citrullination and maturation of anticitrullinated protein antibodies (ACPAs). Citrullination is catalyzed by the calcium-dependent enzyme peptidyl-arginine-deiminase (PAD), changing a positively charged arginine to a polar but neutral citrulline as the result of a posttranslational modification. In RA, PAD can be secreted by the granulocyte and macrophage. ACPA occurs as a result of an abnormal antibody response to a range of citrullinated proteins, including fibrin, vimentin, fibronectin, Epstein-Barr nuclear antigen 1, α-enolase, type II collagen, and histones, all of which are distributed throughout the whole body. Many citrullination neoantigens would activate major histocompatibility complex (MHC) class II–dependent T cells, which in turn would help B cells produce more ACPA. The stage is also called *loss of tolerance*. (From Guo Q, Wang Y, Xu D, et al: Rheumatoid arthritis: pathological mechanisms and modern pharmacologic therapies, *Bone Research* 6[15]: 2018.)

> **KEY CONCEPTS: Characteristics of Rheumatoid Arthritis**
> - Rheumatoid arthritis (RA) is a chronic, usually progressive, inflammatory disorder of the joints, ranging from mild illness to a progressive, destructive polyarthritis associated with systemic vasculitis.
> - Two pathogenic mechanisms for RA have been hypothesized:
>   - The extravascular immune complex hypothesis proposes an interaction of antigens and antibodies in synovial tissues and fluid.
>   - An alternative hypothesis is that cell-mediated damage occurs because of accumulation of lymphocytes, primarily T cells, in the rheumatoid synovium, resembling a delayed-type hypersensitivity reaction. The presence of cytokines, which affect articular inflammation and destruction, supports this hypothesis.

ETIOLOGY

Rheumatic diseases are among the oldest diseases recognized, but the cause of RA remains unknown. Genetic factors are important, as are hormonal and psychosomatic factors (Fig. 24.1). Evidence indicates that immunologic factors are involved in the articular and extraarticular manifestations of the disease. RA may represent an unusual host response to one or perhaps many causative agents. An infectious cause is possible, although this has not been established.

EPIDEMIOLOGY

RA occurs worldwide, but no definite geographic or climatic variation in incidence has been established. RA affects all races, but the incidence varies across racial and ethnic groups.

Although no specific genetic relationship has been established, a small increase in incidence has been noted in first-degree relatives of patients with RA. Persons with the human leukocyte antigen (HLA)-DR4 haplotype have a significantly higher incidence of RA.

Patients with RA have a shortened life span. The most frequent cause of death is cardiovascular disease. The increased prevalence of atherosclerosis in RA patients is suspected to be related to atherogenic side effects of some antirheumatic medications, the effects of chronic systemic inflammation on the vascular endothelium, or shared mechanisms of action between RA and atherosclerosis.

Complications resulting from an increased frequency of local or extraarticular infections in RA patients have been demonstrated. Mortality may result from conditions such as septicemia,

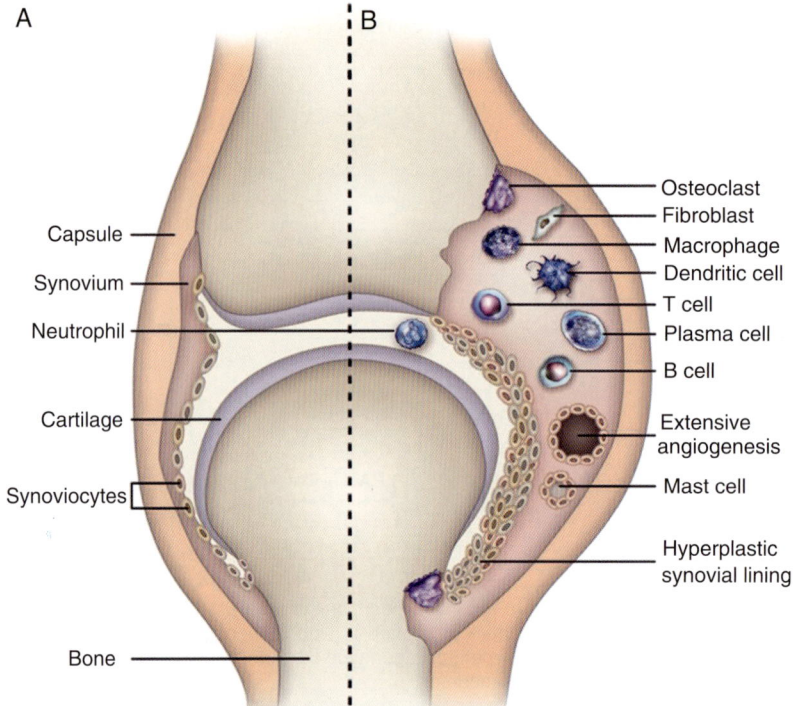

Fig. 24.2 Schematic view of a normal joint (A) and a joint affected by rheumatoid arthritis (RA) (B). The joint affected by RA (B) shows increased inflammation and cellular activity. (From Smolen JS, Steiner G: Therapeutic strategies for rheumatoid arthritis, *Nat Rev Drug Discov* 2:473–488, 2003.)

pneumonia, lung abscess, or pyelonephritis. In the past 15 years, the pharmacotherapy of RA has been improved by the development of more effective medications.

SIGNS AND SYMPTOMS

The term *rheumatic disease* does not have a clear boundary; more than 100 different conditions are labeled as rheumatic diseases, including RA, osteoarthritis, autoimmune disorders (e.g., systemic lupus erythematosus [SLE] and scleroderma), osteoporosis, back pain, gout, fibromyalgia, and tendinitis.

RA is a chronic, multisystemic, autoimmune disorder and a progressive inflammatory disorder of the joints (Fig. 24.2). It is, however, a highly variable disease that ranges from a mild illness of brief duration to a progressive destructive polyarthritis associated with systemic vasculitis (Fig. 24.3). The pathogenesis of RA has the following three distinct stages:

1. Initiation of synovitis by the primary causative factor;
2. Subsequent immunologic events that perpetuate the initial inflammatory reaction;
3. Transition of an inflammatory reaction in the synovium to a proliferative, destructive tissue process.

RA often begins with prodromal symptoms such as fatigue, anorexia, weakness, and generalized aching and stiffness not localized to articular structures. Joint symptoms usually appear gradually over weeks to months. The patient may display a wide variety of extraarticular manifestations (Box 24.1).

The revised criteria of the American Rheumatism Association for diagnosis of RA are presented in Table 24.1. If these conditions are present for at least 6 weeks, the patient is designated as having classic RA. Prognostic markers, such as a persistently high number of swollen joints, high serum levels of acute-phase reactants of immunoglobulin M (IgM) rheumatoid factor (RF), early radiographic and functional abnormalities, in addition to the presence of certain HLA class II

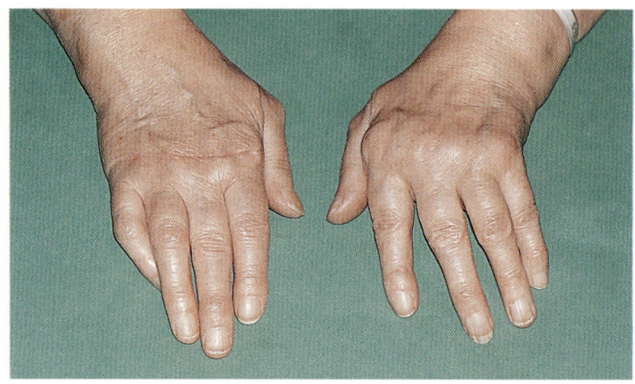

Fig. 24.3 Symmetrical Involvement of Joints in Rheumatoid Arthritis. Advanced symmetrical involvement of joints of the hands (proximal interphalangeal and metacarpophalangeal joints) is typical of rheumatoid arthritis. Note the ulnar deviation. (From Forbes CD & Jackson WF: *Color atlas and text of clinical medicine*, ed 3, St. Louis, 2002, Mosby.)

BOX 24.1 Extraarticular Manifestations of Rheumatoid Arthritis

- Constitutional manifestations (e.g., weight loss and fatigue)
- Subcutaneous rheumatoid nodules
- Ocular abnormalities (e.g., inflammatory lesions of episclera and sclera)
- Vasculitis
- Neuropathy (e.g., mononeuritis multiplex)
- Myopathy
- Cardiac manifestations (e.g., pericarditis)
- Pulmonary manifestations (e.g., pleural effusion)
- Osteoporosis
- Felty syndrome (a complex of chronic rheumatoid arthritis, splenomegaly, anemia, thrombocytopenia, and neutropenia)

TABLE 24.1   2010 ACR/EULAR Classification Criteria for Rheumatoid Arthritis[a].

Parameter	Score (Points)
A. Joint Involvement[b,c]	
• 1 large joint[d]	0
• 2 to 10 large joints	1
• 1 to 3 small joints (with or without involvement of large joints)[c]	2
• 4 to 10 small joints (with or without involvement of large joints)	3
• 10 joints (at least one small joint)[e]	5
B. Serology (at Least One Test Result Is Needed for Classification)[f]	
• Negative RF and negative ACPA	0
• Low-positive RF or low-positive ACPA	2
• High-positive RF or high-positive ACPA	3
C. Acute-Phase Reactants (At Least One Test Result Is Needed for Classification)[g]	
• Normal CRP and normal ESR	0
• Abnormal CRP or abnormal ESR	1
D. Duration of Symptoms[h]	
• <6 weeks	0
• ≈6 weeks	1

[a]The criteria are aimed at the classification of newly presenting patients. In addition, patients with erosive disease typical of RA with a history compatible with prior fulfillment of the 2010 criteria should be classified as having RA. Patients with long-standing disease, including those whose disease is inactive (with or without treatment), who, based on retrospectively available data, have previously fulfilled the 2010 criteria, should be classified as having RA.
[b]"Joint involvement" refers to any swollen or tender joint on examination, which may be confirmed by imaging evidence of synovitis. Distal interphalangeal joints, first carpometacarpal joints, and first metatarsophalangeal joints are excluded from assessment. Categories of joint distribution are classified according to the location and number of involved joints, with placement into the highest category possible based on the pattern of joint involvement.
[c]"Small joints" refers to the metacarpophalangeal joints, proximal interphalangeal joints, second through fifth metatarsophalangeal joints, thumb interphalangeal joints, and wrists.
[d]"Large joints" refers to shoulders, elbows, hips, knees, and ankles.
[e]In this category, at least one of the involved joints must be a small joint; the others can include any combination of large and additional small joints, in addition to other joints not specifically listed elsewhere (e.g., temporomandibular, acromioclavicular, and sternoclavicular).
[f]Negative refers to IU values that are equal to the upper limit of normal (ULN) for the laboratory and assay; low-positive refers to IU values that are higher than the ULN but equal to three times the ULN for the laboratory and assay; high-positive refers to IU values that are greater than three times the ULN for the laboratory and assay. If rheumatoid factor (RF) information is only available as positive or negative, a positive result should be scored as low-positive for RF.
[g]Normal/abnormal is determined by local laboratory standards.
[h]"Duration of symptoms" refers to the patient's self-report of the duration of signs or symptoms of synovitis (e.g., pain, swelling, and tenderness) of joints that are clinically involved at the time of assessment, regardless of treatment status.
Note: These are classification criteria for rheumatoid arthritis (RA) (score-based algorithm). The scores of categories A to D are added together. A score of 6 to 10 points is needed to classify a patient as having definite RA. Although patients with a score of 6 to 10 points are not classifiable as having RA, their status can be reassessed and the criteria might be fulfilled cumulatively over time. Differential diagnoses vary among patients with different presentations but may include conditions such as systemic lupus erythematosus (SLE), psoriatic arthritis, and gout. If it is unclear which relevant differential diagnoses to consider, an expert rheumatologist should be consulted.
ACPA, Anti–citrullinated protein antibody; *ACR-EULAR*, American Academy of Rheumatology/European League Against Rheumatism; *CRP*, C-reactive protein; *ESR*, erythrocyte sedimentation rate; *RF*, rheumatoid factor.
Adapted from American College of Rheumatology: The 2010 American College of Rheumatology/European League Against Rheumatism classification criteria for rheumatoid arthritis, 2011. https://www.rheumatology.org/practice/clinical/classification/ra/ra_2010.asp.

alleles, may help identify patients with more severe RA who are still in the early stages of the disease.

ANATOMY AND PHYSIOLOGY OF JOINTS

Diarthrodial joints are lined at their margins by a synovial membrane (synovium), with synovial cells lining this space. The lining cells synthesize protein and are phagocytic. Synovial (joint) fluid is a transparent viscous fluid. Its function is to lubricate the joint space and transport nutrients to the articular cartilage. Mechanical, chemical, immunologic, or bacteriologic damage may alter the permeability of the membrane and capillaries and may produce varying degrees of an inflammatory response. In addition, inflammatory joint fluids contain lytic enzymes that produce depolymerization of hyaluronic acid, which greatly impairs the lubricating ability of the fluid.

A variety of disorders produce changes in the number and types of cells and chemical composition of the fluid. Analysis of synovial fluid plays a major role in the diagnosis of joint diseases. Arthrocentesis constitutes a liquid biopsy of the joint. It is a fundamental part of the clinical database, together with the medical history, physical examination, and plain radiographic films. Analysis of aspirated synovial fluid is essential in the evaluation of any patient with joint disease because it is a better reflection of the events in the articular cavity than abnormal blood test results. Abnormal test results—for example, antinuclear antibody (ANA), an increased erythrocyte sedimentation rate (ESR), an elevated uric acid level, an increased C-reactive protein concentration, and rheumatoid factor (RF)—can be seen in normal individuals or in unrelated joint diseases.

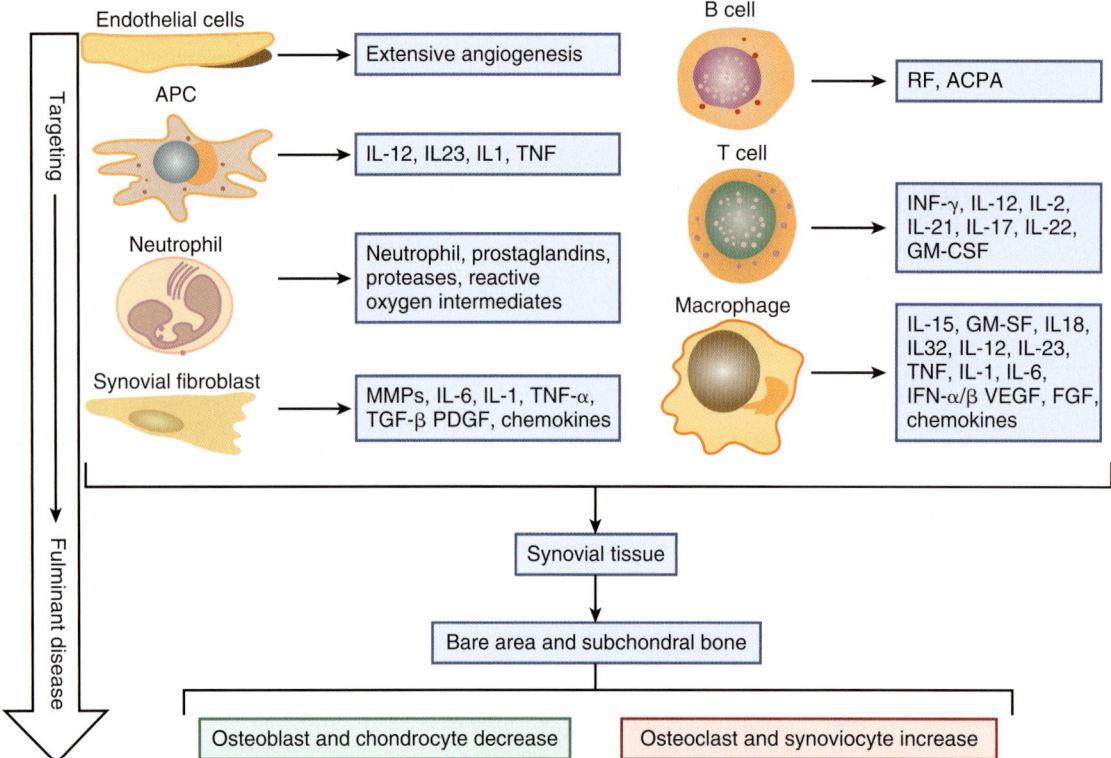

Fig. 24.4 Immune Mechanisms. Many cells and their cytokines play critical roles in the development of rheumatoid arthritis. The synovial compartment is infiltrated by leukocytes, and the synovial fluid is inundated with proinflammatory mediators that are produced to induce an inflammatory cascade, which is characterized by interactions of fibroblast-like synoviocytes with the cells of the innate immune system, including monocytes, macrophages, mast cells, dendritic cells, and so on, in addition to cells of the adaptive immune system, such as T cells and B cells. Endothelial cells contribute to the extensive angiogenesis. The fulminant stage contains hyperplastic synovium, cartilage damage, bone erosion, and systemic consequence. Bone resorption virtually creates bone erosions, which are usually found at spots where the synovial membrane inserts into the periosteum; this is known as a bare area, according to certain anatomic features. The destruction of the subchondral bone can eventually result in the degeneration of the articular cartilage as the result of a decrease in osteoblasts and an increase in osteoclasts and synoviocytes. *ACPA,* Anti–citrullinated protein antibodies; *APC,* antigen-presenting cell; *FGF,* fibroblast growth factor; *GM-CSF,* granulocyte–macrophage colony-stimulating factor; *IFN,* interferon; *IL,* interleukin; *MMPs,* matrix metalloproteinases; *PDGF,* platelet-derived growth factor; *RF,* rheumatoid factor; *TGF,* transforming growth factor; *TNF,* tumor necrosis factor; *VEGF,* vascular endothelial growth factor. (From Guo Q, Wang Y, Xu D, et al: Rheumatoid arthritis: pathological mechanisms and modern pharmacologic therapies, *Bone Research* 6[15]: 2018.)

Disorders such as gout, calcium pyrophosphate dihydrate deposition disease, and septic arthritis can be definitively diagnosed by synovial fluid analysis and may allow for consideration or exclusion of RA and SLE. Synovial fluid analysis can also support a diagnosis of diseases as disparate as amyloidosis, hypothyroidism, ochronosis, hemochromatosis, or even simple edema. In addition arthrocentesis may alleviate elevated intraarticular pressure. Removal of fluid will relieve symptoms and potentially reduce joint damage. Removal of the products of inflammation is an important component of the treatment of infectious arthritis and may be beneficial for other forms of arthritis.

Routine analysis of synovial fluid should include wet preparation examination for cell count and differential, crystals, Gram stain, and microbiologic culture. Very turbid fluids or, if septic arthritis is considered for other reasons, synovial fluid should be sent for Gram staining and culture. Gram staining is needed if a high likelihood of infection exists. Other observations and procedures can include volume and appearance, viscosity, mucin test, chemical analysis for protein, and glucose.

When examined by the immunofluorescent technique, the rheumatoid synovium can be seen to contain large amounts of immunoglobulin G (IgG) and IgM, alone or together. Immunoglobulins can also be seen in synovial lining cells, blood vessels, and interstitial connective tissues. B cells make immunoglobulin in the synovium of patients with RA. As many as 50% of the plasma cells that can be located in the synovium secrete an IgG RF that combines with similar IgG molecules (self-associating IgG) in the cytoplasm.

IMMUNOLOGIC MANIFESTATIONS

A current model of the pathogenesis of RA (Fig. 24.4) proposes that an infective agent or other stimulus binds to receptors on dendritic cells (DCs), which activates the innate immune system. DCs migrate into lymph nodes and present antigen to T lymphocytes, which are activated by two signals: the presentation of antigen and costimulation through CD28. Activated T lymphocytes proliferate and migrate into the joint. Subsequently, T lymphocytes produce interferon-γ (IFN-γ) and other proinflammatory cytokines. This in turn stimulates macrophages and other cells, including B lymphocytes. B cells appear to be pivotal in the pathogenesis of RA because they can be 10,000 times as potent as DCs in presenting antigens.

Stimulated macrophages and fibroblasts release cytokines, including tumor necrosis factor-α (TNF-α), a central component of the cascade of cytokines. This results in the production of additional inflammatory mediators and further recruitment of immune and inflammatory cells into a joint. Anti–TNF-α treatment strategies (e.g., monoclonal) prevent interaction with receptors on cell surfaces.

The leukotrienes play a major role in the inflammatory response to injury. This class of biologically active molecules has been implicated in the pathogenesis of RA and in other inflammatory diseases (e.g., asthma, psoriasis, inflammatory bowel disease). Leukotrienes are major constituents of a group of oxygenated fatty acids that are synthesized de novo from membrane phospholipid through a cascade of enzymes. Research studies have focused on these molecules because leukotriene inhibitors and antagonists will probably become important agents in the group of antiinflammatory drugs (see the section Treatment).

> **KEY CONCEPTS: Serology of Rheumatoid Arthritis**
> - Immunoglobulins can also be observed in synovial lining cells, blood vessels, and interstitial connective tissues. As many as 50% of the plasma cells that can be located in the synovium secrete IgG. The serum of most RA patients has detectable soluble immune complexes. RFs have been associated with IgM, IgG, and immunoglobulin A (IgA).
> - Anti–cyclic citrullinated peptide antibodies are a highly specific and early RA indicator.

DIAGNOSTIC EVALUATION

Low serum iron levels and a normal or low iron-binding capacity are common features in RA. The ESR is elevated to a variable degree in most RA patients and roughly parallels the level of disease activity. Serum protein electrophoresis may demonstrate elevations in the alpha-2 and gamma globulin fractions, with a mild-to-moderate decrease in serum albumin. The gamma globulin increase is polyclonal.

Immunologic features of RA include RF, anti–cyclic citrullinated peptide (anti-CCP), immune complexes, characteristic complement levels, and ANAs. For example, patients with Felty syndrome (the association of RA with splenomegaly and leukopenia) almost always develop a high-titer RF assay, a positive ANA assay, and rheumatoid nodules. In addition, these patients have a high titer of immune complex and low total serum complement levels.

RHEUMATOID FACTOR

RFs are immunoglobulins of any isotype with antibody activity directed against antigenic sites on the Fc region of human or animal IgG. RFs have been associated with three major immunoglobulin classes: IgM, IgG, and IgA. IgM and IgG RFs are the most common.

IgM RF is manifested in approximately 70% of adults but is not specific for RA. Being RF positive correlates with the following:
- Severity of the disease (in general)
- Nodules
- Other organ system involvement (e.g., vasculitis, Felty syndrome, and Sjögren syndrome)

Agglutination tests for RF, such as the sensitized sheep cell test and latex agglutination, generally detect IgM RFs. Latex agglutination is sensitive but can produce a fairly high number of false-positive results. Because conventional procedures are semiquantitative, they may be insensitive to changes in titer and may detect only those RFs that agglutinate. Immunoturbidimetric assays and enzyme-linked immunosorbent assays (ELISAs) are automated methods of analysis. The presence of abnormal levels of all three RF isotypes—IgM, IgG, and IgA—has a specificity of 99% for RA.

RF has been associated with some bacterial and viral infections, including hepatitis and infectious mononucleosis, and some chronic infections, such as tuberculosis, parasitic disease, subacute bacterial endocarditis, and cancer. Elevated values may also be observed in the normal older population. The concentration of RF tends to be highest when the disease peaks and tends to decrease during prolonged remission.

CYCLIC CITRULLINATED PEPTIDE ANTIBODIES

RA occurs when, during inflammation, some proteins become altered via a process known as *citrullination*. These modified proteins can induce an autoimmune reaction.

CCP antibodies are a highly specific indicator for RA. Antibodies to CCPs (anti-CCP1) were first described in 1998. Since the introduction of commercial ELISA products using the so-called second-generation peptides (CCP2), there has been increased interest in using this marker in the diagnosis of RA. Anti-CCP IgG antibodies are present in about 69% to 83% of patients with RA and have specificities ranging from 93% to 95%. These autoantibodies may be present in the preclinical phase of disease, are associated with future RA development, and may predict radiographic joint destruction. Antibodies can be detected in sera from individuals up to 16 years before the first clinical symptoms of RA appear.

Compared with other assays for RF, CCP is considered to be more sensitive. This antibody is reported to have high specificity (>95%) and sensitivity (80%) for RA. Early diagnosis and effective treatment provide a window of opportunity for controlling this autoimmune disease. Anti-CCP and RF assays constitute an RA panel.

Autoantibodies against mutated and citrullinated vimentin (MCV), a member of the citrullinated protein family, are highly specific markers for RA. A lateral flow immunoassay (LFIA) for the qualitative detection of anti-MCV antibodies, anti-MCV ELISA (Orgentec Diagnostics, Mainz, Germany), has been developed as a point-of-care test.

Recent research has discovered that testing for antibodies targeting citrullinated tenascin-C (cTNC) can diagnose RA in about half of cases, comprising those that get past CCP. Tenascin-C is a large, multimodular, extracellular matrix glycoprotein that is specifically upregulated during inflammation but is absent in most healthy tissues. Tenascin-C stimulates inflammation, inducing de novo cytokine synthesis via activation of toll-like receptor 4 (TLR4), controlling cytokine synthesis posttranscriptionally via induction of microRNAs, and regulating adaptive immunity by driving type 17 helper T (Th17)–cell polarization. Tenascin-C can be found in immune complexes in the RA joint. Testing for antibodies that target cTNC could diagnose RA in around 50% of cases, including some cases not identified by current best tests. It also has a very low rate of false positives—98% accurate at ruling out RA.

Other Markers

Antibodies to anti–perinuclear factor (APF) and keratin (anti–keratin antibody [AKA]) are highly specific for RA. Antibodies to APF are reported to be present in the sera of 49% to 91% of RA patients, with specificity greater than 70%.

Immune Complexes

Soluble circulating immune complexes and cryoprecipitable proteins consisting of immunoglobulins, complement components, and RFs

TABLE 24.2 Subgroups of Juvenile Idiopathic Arthritis.

New Classification	Old Classification	Comments
Systemic arthritis	Systemic-onset JIA	Comprises only ≈10% of JIA cases
Oligoarthritis	Pauciarticular JIA	Accounts for 40% of new JIA patients
Polyarthritis (RF negative) or polyarthritis (RF positive)	Polyarticular JIA	
Enthesitis-related arthritis	Excluded in JIA classification, but at onset some patients in this group may be similar to late-onset pauciarticular JIA	
Psoriatic arthritis	Excluded in JIA classification	
Other	Does not fulfill criteria for any categories or fulfills criteria for more than one category	JIA is the most common type of JA but is not the only type. Other forms include juvenile lupus, juvenile scleroderma, and juvenile dermatomyositis. Children can also experience noninflammatory disorders characterized by chronic pain associated with heredity, injury, or unknown causes.

JA, Juvenile arthritis; *JIA*, juvenile idiopathic arthritis; *RF*, rheumatoid factor.

are demonstrable in the sera of some patients with RA. Anti–gamma globulin isotypes, IgM, IgG, and IgA classes, are important complexes.

The IgA, IgM, and IgG isotypes of RF are detected years before any symptoms of RA become apparent. The various vascular and parenchymal lesions of RA suggest that the lesions result from injury induced by immune complexes, especially those containing antibodies to IgG. Vasculitis is associated with complexes made up of IgG and 7S IgM RFs. A positive laboratory assay for mixed cryoglobulins indicates the presence of a large number of immune complexes and is associated with an increased incidence of extraarticular manifestations, particularly vasculitis.

Complement Levels

Serum complement levels are usually normal in patients with RA, except in those with vasculitis. Hemolytic complement levels are reduced in the serum of less than one-third of patients, especially in patients with very high levels of RF and immune complexes. Levels of C4 and C2 are most profoundly depressed in these patients.

Antinuclear Antibodies

ANAs have been found in 14% to 28% of RA patients, who usually have advanced disease. However, disease manifestation is the same in ANA-positive and ANA-negative patients.

> **KEY CONCEPTS: Associated Disorders**
> - Felty syndrome is RA with associated splenomegaly and leukopenia. High-titer RF, a positive ANA assay result, and rheumatoid nodules are frequently found in patients with Felty syndrome.
> - Juvenile idiopathic arthritis (JIA) is a condition of chronic synovitis that begins during childhood.

JUVENILE IDIOPATHIC ARTHRITIS

Etiology

The term *juvenile rheumatoid arthritis* (JRA) has fallen out of favor worldwide for a number of reasons. JRA is not, as the language implies, simply a pediatric replica of the condition that affects adults. Only about 10% of children have an arthritic disease that closely mirrors RA in adults. Researchers have concluded that the JRA category is drawn too narrowly and should include some related diagnoses, such as ankylosing spondylitis. JIA and JRA cannot be used interchangeably because there are differences between the diagnoses they include (Table 24.2).

Juvenile idiopathic arthritis (JIA) is a condition of chronic synovitis beginning during childhood. It is believed that there are a number of causes, including factors such as infection, autoimmunity, and trauma. Research at Tulane University Medical Center in Louisiana has suggested that JIA may be associated with a retroviral particle called *human intracisternal A-type particle (HIAP)*. Antibodies to this particle have been found in a very high percentage of patients with JIA. These antibodies have also been found in many patients with three other autoimmune disorders: SLE, Sjögren syndrome, and Graves disease. Researchers believe that these four disorders may result from the presence of HIAP, together with genetic factors and some internal or external stimulus, which all combine to dictate the specific symptomatology.

Epidemiology

The incidence of JIA in the US pediatric population is 0.1 to 1.1 per 1000.

Signs and Symptoms

Diagnostic criteria include onset before 16 years of age, presence of arthritis (i.e., joint swelling for 6 consecutive weeks or longer), and exclusion of other conditions known to cause or mimic childhood arthritis. Several distinct subgroups of JIA have been recognized.

Immunologic Manifestations

Immunologic features of JIA can include the presence of RF, immune complexes, and ANAs.

Rheumatoid Factors

Approximately 20% of children are positive for RF. Most patients who are positive for RF probably represent adult RA occurring in childhood. So-called *hidden RF* can be detected in 65% of children with negative latex fixation test results. Children in this category do not develop the clinical manifestations of adults with RA.

Immune Complexes

Soluble immune complexes may be detected in patients with active synovitis. Analysis of these complexes is not useful for the diagnosis, prognosis, or monitoring of patients.

Antinuclear Antibodies

ANAs are detectable in few patients with JIA, except that most girls with pauciarthritis and chronic iritis demonstrate a positive ANA test result.

> **KEY CONCEPTS: Treatment**
> - The major goals of treatment of arthritis are (1) to reduce pain and discomfort; (2) to prevent deformities and loss of joint function; and (3) to help the patient maintain a productive and active life.
> - Treatment options include reduction of joint stress, physical and occupational therapy, drug therapy, and surgical intervention.
> - Some treatment classes are traditional. Newer therapy consists of drugs that are biological response modifiers, and some of these drugs can be used in conjunction with traditional medication.
> - Traditional treatment of RA consists of nonsteroidal antiinflammatory drugs (NSAIDs) (e.g., salicylates and ibuprofen). The major effect of these agents is to reduce acute inflammation. Prostaglandins are a group of related compounds that are important mediators of a wide variety of physiologic processes, including immunomodulation. NSAIDs inhibit prostaglandin synthesis by blocking two isoforms of cyclooxygenase (COX): COX-1 and COX-2. Newer NSAID agents (e.g., Vioxx and Celebrex) selectively block the COX-2 enzyme, which is primarily upregulated in response to tissue damage during inflammation, but preserve COX-1 activity and enhance the safety profile.
> - Cortisone and prednisolone have antiinflammatory and immunoregulatory activity. Glucocorticosteroids pass through the cell membrane into the cytoplasm and activate the cytoplasmic glucocorticosteroid receptor, which represses gene expression through the transcriptional interference of activator protein 1 (AP-1) and nuclear factor kappa B (NF-κB). The proteins inhibited by glucocorticosteroids include interleukin-1 (IL-1), IL-2, IL-6, IL-8, TNFα, and IFN-γ. Glucocorticosteroids were the original selective COX-2 inhibitors. Oral corticosteroids can produce a variety of complications, including high blood pressure, increased susceptibility to infection, and osteoporosis.
> - Methotrexate is a popular nonbiological disease-modifying antirheumatic drug (DMARD) because of its early onset of action (4 to 6 weeks), good efficacy, ease of administration, and high patient tolerability.
> - Tofacitinib is the first in a new class of nonbiological DMARDs, a targeted, synthetic drug approved for the treatment of RA.
> - Biological DMARDs are genetically engineered proteins derived from human genes. They are designed to inhibit specific components of the immune system that play pivotal roles in fueling inflammation, which is a central feature of RA.

TREATMENT

The major goals of treatment of arthritis are to (1) reduce pain and discomfort; (2) prevent deformities and loss of joint function; and (3) help the patient maintain a productive and active life. Inflammation must be suppressed and mechanical and structural abnormalities corrected or compensated for with assistive devices. Treatment options include reduction of joint stress, physical and occupational therapy, drug therapy, and surgical intervention.

There are several general classes of drugs (Table 24.3). Some treatment classes are traditional. Newer therapy consists of drugs that are biological response modifiers, and some of these drugs can be used in conjunction with traditional medication. A Janus kinase (JAK) drug has recently been approved by the US Food and Drug Administration (FDA).

Traditional Treatment

Traditional treatment of RA consists of NSAIDs (e.g., salicylates and ibuprofen). The major effect of these agents is to reduce acute inflammation. Aspirin is the oldest drug of the nonsteroidal class, but the use of aspirin as the initial choice of drug therapy has largely been replaced by the newer NSAIDs.

Prostaglandins are a group of related compounds that are important mediators of a wide variety of physiologic processes, including immunomodulation. Prostaglandins are derived primarily from arachidonic acid via the COX enzymes pathway. NSAIDs inhibit prostaglandin synthesis by blocking two isoforms of COX: COX-1 and COX-2. Newer NSAID agents (e.g., Vioxx and Celebrex) selectively block the COX-2 enzyme, which is primarily upregulated in response to tissue damage during inflammation, but preserve COX-1 activity and enhance the safety profile.

Corticosteroids and Glucocorticoids

Corticosteroids (e.g., cortisone and prednisolone [prednisone]) have anti-inflammatory and immunoregulatory activity. Glucocorticosteroids pass through the cell membrane into the cytoplasm and activate the cytoplasmic glucocorticosteroid receptor, which represses gene expression through the transcriptional interference of AP-1 and NF-κB. The proteins inhibited by glucocorticosteroids include IL-1, IL-2, IL-6, IL-8, TNF-α, and IFN-γ. Glucocorticosteroids were the original selective COX-2 inhibitors. Oral corticosteroids can produce a variety of complications, including high blood pressure, increased susceptibility to infection, and osteoporosis.

Nonbiological Disease-Modifying Antirheumatic Drugs

Methotrexate is a popular disease-modifying antirheumatic drug (DMARD) because of its early onset of action (4–6 weeks), good efficacy, ease of administration, and high patient tolerability. Methotrexate is a folic acid antagonist. The immunosuppressive and cytotoxic effects of methotrexate are caused by the inhibition of dihydrofolate reductase.

Tofacitinib (Xeljanz) is the first in a new class of nonbiological DMARDs, a targeted, synthetic drug approved for the treatment of RA. It is a JAK inhibitor and reduces T-cell activation, proinflammatory cytokine production, and cytokine signaling by inhibiting binding of the type I cytokine receptor family and γ-chain cytokines to paired JAK1/JAK3 receptors. The net effect of tofacitinib's mechanism of action is decreased synovial inflammation and structural joint damage in RA patients.

Biological Disease-Modifying Antirheumatic Drugs

Biologics are genetically engineered proteins derived from human genes. They are designed to inhibit specific components of the immune system that play pivotal roles in fueling inflammation, which is a central feature of RA. Biological DMARDs are usually most effective when paired with a nonbiological DMARD (e.g., methotrexate). DMARDs can slow the progression of RA and save the joints and other tissues from permanent damage. Common side effects vary but may include liver damage, bone marrow suppression, and severe lung infections.

Drugs in this class of biological DMARDs have various mechanisms of action. The following are examples of this type of drug.

- Abatacept (Orencia), a selective costimulation modulator, inhibits T-cell (T-lymphocyte) activation, competes with CD28 for CD80 and CD86 binding, and can be used to modulate T-cell activity selectively by binding to CD80 and CD86, thereby blocking interaction with CD28. This interaction provides a costimulatory signal necessary for full activation of T lymphocytes. Activated T lymphocytes are implicated in the pathogenesis of RA. In vitro studies demonstrate that abatacept reduces T-cell proliferation and inhibits the production of the cytokines TNF-α, IFN-γ, and IL-2.
- Adalimumab (Humira) binds specifically to TNF-α and blocks its interaction with the p55 and p75 cell surface TNF receptors. This

TABLE 24.3 Drugs for Treatment of Rheumatoid Arthritis.

Drug Type	Generic Name (Trade Name)	Clinical Pharmacology
NSAIDs	Over-the-counter NSAIDs include ibuprofen (e.g., Advil and Motrin) and naproxen sodium (Aleve)	The effect of NSAIDs is mainly due to their common property of inhibiting cyclooxygenases involved in the formation of prostaglandins, which leads to the normalization of an increased pain threshold.
	Stronger NSAIDs are available by prescription	NSAIDs can relieve pain and reduce inflammation. Side effects may include stomach irritation, heart problems, and kidney damage.
Steroids	Prednisone	Steroids depress natural immune system activity. Corticosteroid medications (e.g., prednisone) reduce inflammation and pain and slow joint damage. Side effects may include thinning of bones, weight gain, and diabetes. Doctors often prescribe a corticosteroid to relieve acute symptoms, with the goal of gradually tapering off the medication.
DMARDs— nonbiological	Methotrexate (Trexall)	Methotrexate is a folic acid derivative and a folic acid antagonist. In the cell it is a competitive inhibitor of the dihydrofolate reductase. The inhibition of the reduction of dihydrofolate to tetrahydrofolate causes blocking of DNA synthesis and cell replication. If a high concentration of methotrexate is in a cell over a long period, methotrexate-polyglutamates develop that cause a lengthy folic acid antagonism.
	Leflunomide (Arava)	Leflunomide inhibits pyrimidine synthesis and growth factor signal transduction nucleotide synthesis.
	Hydroxychloroquine (Plaquenil)	Hydroxychloroquine is one of the two antimalarial agents. Chloroquine and hydroxychloroquine increase the pH within intracellular vacuoles and alter processes such as protein degradation by acidic hydrolases in the lysosome, assembly of macromolecules in the endosomes, and posttranslational modification of proteins in the Golgi apparatus. It is proposed that the antirheumatic properties of these compounds results from their interference with "antigen processing" in macrophages and other antigen-presenting cells.
		Acidic cytoplasmic compartments are required for the antigenic protein to be digested and for the peptides to assemble with the alpha and beta chains of MHC class II proteins. As a result, antimalarials diminish the formation of peptide-MHC protein complexes required to stimulate CD4+ T cells and result in downregulation of the immune response against autoantigenic peptides.
	Sulfasalazine (Azulfidine)	The mode of action of SSZ and its metabolites, 5-ASA and SP, remains under investigation but may be related to the antiinflammatory and/or immunomodulatory properties that have been observed in animal and in vitro models, to its affinity for connective tissue, and/or to the relatively high concentration it reaches in serous fluids, the liver, and intestinal walls.
	Minocycline (Dynacin, Minocin)	Minocycline hydrochloride is a semisynthetic derivative of tetracycline. It inhibits protein synthesis and subsequent bacterial growth by binding to 30S and possibly 50S ribosomal subunits of susceptible bacteria.
Biological agents or biological response modifiers	Abatacept (Orencia)	Abatacept is a selective costimulation modulator. It inhibits T-cell (T-lymphocyte) activation by binding to CD80 and CD86, thereby blocking interaction with CD28.
		This interaction provides a costimulatory signal necessary for full activation of T lymphocytes. Activated T lymphocytes are implicated in the pathogenesis of RA.
		In vitro studies demonstrate that abatacept decreases T-cell proliferation and inhibits the production of the cytokines TNF-α, interferon-γ, and interleukin-2.
Antirheumatic drugs	Adalimumab (Humira)	HUMIRA stands for human monoclonal antibody in rheumatoid arthritis. In rheumatoid diseases, TNF-α appears to be a major contributor to inflammation. It triggers inflammation and pain. Humira binds to TNF-α and blocks its inflammatory effect, thereby reducing pain and inflammation.
	Anakinra (Kineret)	Anakinra is a recombinant, nonglycosylated form of the human IL-1Ra It is produced by recombinant DNA technology using an *Escherichia coli* bacterial expression system.
		Anakinra blocks the biological activity of IL-1 by competitively inhibiting IL-1 binding to the IL-1RI, which is expressed in a wide variety of tissues and organs. IL-1 produced in response to inflammation has a broad range of activities including cartilage degradation by its induction of the rapid loss of proteoglycans, in addition to stimulation of bone resorption. The levels of the naturally occurring IL-1Ra in synovium and synovial fluid from RA patients are not sufficient to compete with the elevated amount of locally produced IL-1.
	Baricitinib (Olumiant)	Baricitinib is a JAK inhibitor. The mode of action is within the intracellular signaling pathway. JAKs phosphorylate and activate STATs, which modulate gene expression within the cell. Baricitinib modulates the signaling pathway at the point of JAKs, preventing the phosphorylation and activation of STATs. Within in vitro assays, it has greater inhibitory potency at JAK1, JAK2, and TYK2, relative to JAK3.
	Certolizumab (Cimzia)	Certolizumab pegol is an Fc-free, PEGylated anti-TNF with a high affinity for human TNF-α, which is a proinflammatory cytokine. The drug binds to human TNF-α and neutralizes the pathologic inflammation caused by the cytokine.

TABLE 24.3 Drugs for Treatment of Rheumatoid Arthritis.—cont'd

Drug Type	Generic Name (Trade Name)	Clinical Pharmacology
	Etanercept (Enbrel)	Etanercept is a soluble TNF receptor. It is a dimeric fusion protein consisting of the extracellular ligand–binding portion of the human 75 kilodalton (p75) TNFR linked to the Fc portion of human IgG1. Etanercept was designed to bind specifically to TNF and block its interaction with cell surface TNF receptors, thereby modulating the biological responses induced or regulated by TNF.
	Golimumab (Simponi)	Golimumab is a TNF blocker.
	Infliximab (Remicade)	Infliximab is a chimeric monoclonal antibody biological. It works by binding to TNF-α.
	Rituximab (Rituxan)	Rituximab binds specifically to the antigen CD20 (human B lymphocyte–restricted differentiation antigen, Bp35), a hydrophobic transmembrane protein located on pre-B and mature B lymphocytes. CD20 regulates one or more early steps in the activation process for cell cycle initiation and differentiation and possibly functions as a calcium ion channel. CD20 is not shed from the cell surface and does not internalize upon antibody binding. Free CD20 antigen is not found in the circulation. B cells are believed to play a role in the pathogenesis of rheumatoid arthritis and associated chronic synovitis. The Fab domain of rituximab binds to the CD20 antigen on B lymphocytes, and the Fc domain recruits immune effector functions to mediate B-cell lysis in vitro. Possible mechanisms of cell lysis include CDC and ADCC.
	Sarilumab (Kevzara)	Sarilumab is a fully human IL-6R inhibitor. It targets and binds with high affinity to soluble and membrane-bound IL-6 receptors (sIL-6R and mIL-6R), thereby inhibiting IL-6 signaling.
	Tocilizumab (Actemra)	Tocilizumab is a novel monoclonal antibody that competitively inhibits the binding of IL-6 to its receptor IL-6R. This inhibits the entire receptor complex and prevents IL-6 signal transduction to inflammatory mediators that summon T and B lymphocytes. It may be used as monotherapy or in combination with methotrexate or other nonbiological DMARDs. Use of tocilizumab in combination with biological DMARDs or with potent immunosuppressants (e.g., azathioprine and cyclosporine) is not recommended.
	Tofacitinib (Xeljanz)	Tofacitinib is a United States FDA–approved synthetic DMARD. It works by blocking JAK pathways involved in the body's immune response. Tofacitinib fights inflammation from inside the cell, attacking a different part of the pathway than biological agents, which block proinflammatory cytokines (e.g., TNF-α and IL-6) from outside the cell. Tofacitinib is a JAK3 inhibitor. JAKs are intracellular enzymes that transmit signals arising from cytokine or growth factor receptor interactions on the cellular membrane to influence hematopoiesis and immune cell function. It is believed that tofacitinib suppresses STAT-1–dependent genes and inhibits the production of inflammatory mediators in joint tissue.

5-ASA, 5-aminosalicylic acid; *ADCC*, Antibody-dependent cell-mediated cytotoxicity; *CDC*, complement-dependent cytotoxicity; *DMARD*, disease-modifying antirheumatic drug; *FDA*, Food and Drug Administration; *IL-1Ra*, interleukin-1 receptor antagonist; *IL-1RI*, interleukin-1 type I receptor; *JAK*, Janus kinase; *MHC*, major histocompatibility complex; *NSAID*, Nonsteroidal antiinflammatory drug; *RA*, rheumatoid arthritis; *SP*, sulfapyridine; *SSZ*, sulfasalazine; *STATs*; *TNF-α*, tumor necrosis factor alpha; *TNFR*, tumor necrosis factor receptor.
Adapted from the Mayo Clinic: Rheumatoid arthritis: Treatments and drugs. https://www.mayoclinic.org/diseases-conditions/rheumatoid-arthritis/diagnosis-treatment; and Arthritis Foundation: Rheumatoid arthritis treatment. https://www.arthritis.org. Specific mode of action information is from each pharmaceutical manufacturer's website.

drug also lyses surface TNF-expressing cells in vitro in the presence of complement.
- Anakinra (Kineret) blocks the biological activity of IL-1 alpha and beta by competitively inhibiting IL-1 from binding to the IL-1 type I receptor (IL-1RI), which is expressed in a wide variety of tissues and organs.
  Anakinra is a recombinant, nonglycosylated form of the human IL-1 receptor antagonist (IL-1Ra). It is produced by recombinant DNA technology using an *Escherichia coli* bacterial expression system.
  IL-1 produced in response to inflammation has a broad range of activities, including cartilage degradation by its induction of the rapid loss of proteoglycans, in addition to stimulation of bone resorption. The levels of the naturally occurring IL-1Ra in synovium and synovial fluid from RA patients are not sufficient to compete with the elevated amount of locally produced IL-1.
- Certolizumab pegol (Cimzia) binds to human TNF-α with a kD of 90 pM. TNF-α is a key proinflammatory cytokine with a central role in inflammatory processes.
- Etanercept (Enbrel) is a soluble TNF receptor. It is a dimeric fusion protein consisting of the extracellular ligand–binding portion of the human 75 kD (p75) TNF receptor (TNFR) linked to the Fc portion of human IgG1. The biological activity of etanercept is that it inhibits binding of TNF-α and TNF-β (lymphotoxin alpha [LT-α]) to *cell surface* TNFRs, rendering TNF biologically inactive.
- Golimumab (Simponi) is a human monoclonal antibody that binds to both the soluble and transmembrane bioactive forms of human TNF-α. This interaction prevents the binding of TNF-α to its receptors, thereby inhibiting the biological activity of TNF-α (a cytokine protein).
- Infliximab (Remicade) neutralizes the biological activity of TNF-α by binding with high affinity to the soluble and transmembrane forms of TNF-α and inhibits binding of TNF-α with its receptors. Infliximab does not neutralize TNF-β (lymphotoxin-α), a related cytokine that uses the same receptors as TNF-α.
- Rituximab (Rituxan) acts by having the Fab domain of rituximab bind to the CD20 antigen on B lymphocytes, and the Fc domain recruits immune effector functions to mediate B-cell lysis in vitro.

Possible mechanisms of cell lysis include complement-dependent cytotoxicity (CDC) and antibody-dependent cell-mediated cytotoxicity (ADCC).
- Rituximab binds specifically to the antigen CD20 (human B lymphocyte–restricted differentiation antigen, Bp35), a hydrophobic transmembrane protein located on pre-B and mature B lymphocytes. CD20 regulates one or more early steps in the activation process for cell cycle initiation and differentiation and possibly functions as a calcium ion channel. CD20 is not shed from the cell surface and does not internalize upon antibody binding. Free CD20 antigen is not found in the circulation.
- B cells are believed to play a role in the pathogenesis of RA and associated chronic synovitis.
- Sarilumab (Kevzara) is a fully human IL-6R inhibitor. It targets and binds with high affinity to soluble and membrane-bound IL-6 receptors (sIL-6R and mIL-6R), thereby inhibiting IL-6 signaling.
- Tocilizumab (Actemra) directly blocks the action of IL-6. Tocilizumab is a novel monoclonal antibody that competitively inhibits the binding of IL-6 to its receptor, IL-6R. This inhibits the entire receptor complex and prevents IL-6 signal transduction to inflammatory mediators that summon T and B lymphocytes.

DIAGNOSTIC PROCEDURES

Diagnostic testing for RA primarily involves RF assays (see Procedure: Rapid Agglutination).

CASE STUDY 24.1

History and Physical Examination
A 62-year-old woman experienced pain in her left knee unrelated to trauma. The pain occurred primarily with weight bearing. She is being treated for hypertension but is otherwise healthy.
 An examination of her knee showed tenderness over the medial epicondyle superior to the joint margin. There was a small effusion in her left knee.

Laboratory Data
Her laboratory data was normal, including the rheumatoid factor assay, except for an elevated uric acid level. An x-ray film of her knee was read as normal.

Questions
1. Rheumatoid arthritis (RA) has a genetic association with:
    a. HLA-A
    b. HLA-B
    c. HLA-C
    d. HLA-DR4
2. IgM rheumatoid factor (RF) is manifested in approximately _____% of adults but is not specific for rheumatoid arthritis.
    a. 30
    b. 50
    c. 70
    d. 90
 Answers to these questions can be found in Appendix A.

Critical Thinking Group Discussion Questions
1. What is the cause of the patient's painful knee?
2. What might the effusion in her left knee demonstrate microscopically?
3. Would a restricted diet be of value?

CASE STUDY 24.2

History and Physical Examination
A 31-year-old patient was referred to a rheumatologist because of pain and stiffness in her fingers and wrists. Before her last pregnancy, 3 years earlier, she had experienced similar symptoms, but those had gone away. Since the birth of her last child, she had found it progressively more awkward to carry out a variety of work tasks and hobbies, such as needlepoint. The symptoms were worse in the morning. She had no trouble with her other joints.
 Her family history revealed that her mother had RA. On physical examination, the patient was pale. She had bilateral and symmetric tender swelling of her wrists and proximal to the joints of her hands. She had normal range of movement. Her other body systems appeared to be within normal limits.

Laboratory Data
Laboratory assays were ordered (Table 24.4). A diagnosis of early rheumatoid arthritis (RA) was made. The patient was advised to take one aspirin daily. This initially provided some relief of her symptoms.
 She returned to her physician 4 months later with worsening symptoms in her hands and pain in both knees. Synovial fluid was removed from her knees. A diagnosis of progressive RA was made.

Questions
1. A highly specific indicator for rheumatoid arthritis is:
    a. Rheumatoid factor
    b. C-reactive protein
    c. Cyclic citrullinated peptide (CCP) antibodies
    d. Depletion of complement
2. An immunoglobulin (Ig) class associated with rheumatoid arthritis is:
    a. IgM
    b. IgG
    c. IgA
    d. All of the above
 See Appendix A for the answers to these multiple-choice questions.

Critical Thinking Group Discussion Questions
1. Do genetic associations exist with RA?
2. Is RA more common in women?
3. What is the immunopathogenesis of RA?
4. What is rheumatoid factor?

TABLE 24.4 Laboratory Data for Case Study 24.2.

Assay	Result (Reference Range)
Erythrocyte sedimentation rate (ESR)	53 mm/hour
C-reactive protein (CRP)	4+
IgM rheumatoid factor (RF)	Positive
Citrullinated peptide (CCP), immunoglobulin G (IgG)	Increased (43 units)
Antinuclear antibody (ANA)	Negative
Antibodies to extractable nuclear antigens	Negative
Double-strand DNA (dsDNA)–binding activity	15%
Serum Complement	
C3	1.1 (0.75–1.65)
C4	0.4 (0.20–0.65)

REVIEW QUESTIONS

1. Rheumatoid arthritis most frequently develops in:
   a. Adolescent females
   b. Adolescent males
   c. Middle-aged women
   d. Middle-aged men
2. The incidence of rheumatoid arthritis in the United States is currently approximately:
   a. 10 million
   b. 25 million
   c. 55 million
   d. More than 100 million
3. Women are _____ likely than men to develop rheumatoid arthritis.
   a. Extremely less
   b. Less
   c. Equally
   d. More
4. Rheumatoid factor is defined as:
   a. Antigens with specificity for antibody determinants on the Fc fragment of human or certain animal IgG
   b. Autoantibodies with specificity for antigen determinants on the Fc fragment of human or certain animal IgG
   c. Antigens with specificity for antibody determinants on the Fc fragment of human or certain animal IgD
   d. Autoantibodies with specificity for antigen determinants on the Fc fragment of human or certain animal IgD

Questions 5–7. Arrange the steps in the pathogenesis of rheumatoid arthritis in the proper order.

5. _____
6. _____
7. _____
   a. Immunologic events perpetuate the initial inflammatory reaction
   b. The primary etiologic factor initiates synovitis
   c. An inflammatory reaction in the synovium develops into a proliferative destructive process of tissue
8. Criteria for the diagnosis of rheumatoid arthritis include all of the following *except*:
   a. Morning stiffness
   b. Rheumatoid nodules
   c. Radiographic changes
   d. Urinary tract infection
9. RF correlates with all of the following *except*:
   a. The severity of the disease in general
   b. The presence of nodules
   c. Other organ system involvement (e.g., vasculitis)
   d. The age of the patient
10. In RA, vascular and parenchymal lesions suggest that lesions result from injury induced by immune complexes, especially those containing antibodies to:
    a. IgM
    b. IgG
    c. IgE
    d. IgD
11. Serum complement levels are usually _____ in patients with rheumatoid arthritis except for patients with vasculitis.
    a. Normal
    b. Decreased
    c. Increased
    d. Either a or b
12. The most common form of juvenile idiopathic arthritis is:
    a. Systemic
    b. Oligoarthritis
    c. Psoriatic
    d. Enthesitis related
13. In the RF agglutination procedure, a false-positive result may be observed in a serum specimen because of:
    a. Complement interference
    b. High levels of C-reactive protein (CRP)
    c. Antigen excess
    d. Antibody excess
14. Rheumatoid factor binds to the:
    a. Fc portion of IgG
    b. Fc portion of IgM
    c. Fab portion of IgG
    d. Fab portion of IgM
15. Rheumatoid factor usually belongs to the _____ class of immunoglobulins.
    a. IgM
    b. IgG
    c. IgD
    d. IgE
16. What is the newest, highly specific laboratory assay for rheumatoid arthritis?
    a. Latex agglutination
    b. Cyclic citrullinated peptide (CCP)
    c. Flow cytometry
    d. Massive parallel sequencing

PART V

Transplantation and Tumor Immunology

Chapter 25: Transplantation: Human Leukocyte Antigens, Solid Organ, Tissues, and Hematopoietic Stem Cells, 428

Chapter 26: Tumor Immunology and Applications of Massive Parallel Sequencing/ Next-Generation Sequencing, 454

25

Transplantation: Human Leukocyte Antigens, Solid Organ, Tissues, and Hematopoietic Stem Cells

Mary Lou Turgeon

LEARNING OUTCOMES

- Identify and describe the histocompatibility antigens.
- Explain the clinical applications of histocompatibility antigens and human leukocyte antigens.
- Identify and describe several laboratory methods for evaluating potential transplant recipients and donors.
- List frequently used terms in transplantation.
- Describe the microorganism screening that should take place predonation.
- Identify various types of transplants.
- Name three types of stem cell transplants.
- Discuss the laboratory evaluation of patients and donors for transplantation.
- Describe the types of graft rejections.
- Briefly explain the mechanism of organ or tissue rejection.
- Define graft-versus-host disease.
- Explain the etiology, epidemiology, signs and symptoms, manifestations, diagnosis, and prevention of graft-versus-host disease.
- Identify and explain some methods of immunosuppression.
- Analyze a representative organ transplantation case study.
- Correctly answer case study–related multiple choice questions.
- Participate in a discussion of critical thinking questions.
- Explain the principle and application of the Longitudinal Assessment of Posttransplant Protocol.
- Correctly answer 80% of the end-of-chapter review questions.

OUTLINE

Histocompatibility Antigens, 429
   Nomenclature of Human Leukocyte Antigen Alleles, 430
   Major Histocompatibility Complex Regions, 431
   Classes of Human Leukocyte Antigen Molecules, 431
   Role of Major Histocompatibility Complex and Human Leukocyte Antigens, 431
   Impact of Human Leukocyte Antigens, 432
   Evaluation of Potential Transplant Recipients and Donors, 432
      Human Leukocyte Antigen Techniques, 433
      Complement-Mediated Cytotoxicity, 433
      Solid-Phase Enzyme-Linked Immunosorbent Assay, 434
      Flow Cytometry, 434
      Molecular Techniques, 435
      Bead Technology, 435
      Donor-Specific Antibody Tests, 435
Transplantation Terminology, 435
General Facts About Transplantation, 435
   Tissue and Organ Transplantation, 435
   Hematopoietic Stem Cells, 436
Pretransplantation Screening, 436
Types of Transplants, 437
   Bone, 437
   Cornea, 437
   Heart, 438
   Heart Valves, 438
   Intestine, 438
   Kidney, 438

   Liver, 438
   Lung, 438
   Pancreas, 439
   Skin, 439
   Hematopoietic or Peripheral Blood Stem Cells, 439
Sources of Stem Cells for Transplantation, 439
   Bone Marrow, 439
   Peripheral Blood Stem Cells, 439
   Umbilical Cord Blood, 440
      Issues Related to Cord Blood Transplantation, 440
   Engraftment, 440
   Impact of HLA Matching, 441
Graft Rejection, 441
   First-Set and Second-Set Rejections, 441
   Hyperacute Rejection, 441
   Accelerated Rejection, 442
   Acute Rejection, 443
   Chronic Rejection, 443
Mechanisms of Rejection, 443
   General Characteristics, 443
   Role of T Cells, 444
   Antibody Effects, 444
   Immunosuppression, 444
   Pharmacologic Activity of Representative Immunosuppressant Drugs, 445
      Azathioprine, 446
      Corticosteroids, 446

Cyclosporine (Cyclosporin A), 446
Tacrolimus, 446
Sirolimus, 446
Mycophenolate Mofetil, 446
Antilymphocyte (Antithymocyte) Globulin, 446
Nulojix, 447
Monoclonal Antibodies, 447
Immunosuppressive Protocols, 447
New Approaches in Immunosuppression, 447
Transplantation Complications, 447
Post–Organ Transplantation, 447
Infectious Diseases, 447
Cancer, 447
Osteoporosis, 447
Diabetes, 447
Hypertension, 447
Hypercholesterolemia, 447
Post–Stem Cell Transplantation, 448

Xenotransplantation, 448
Biomarkers for Rejection, 448
***FOXP3* Messenger Ribonucleic Acid (mRNA), 448**
Graft-Versus-Host Disease, 449
Etiology, 449
Epidemiology, 449
Signs and Symptoms, 449
Immunologic Manifestation, 450
Diagnostic Evaluation, 450
Prevention, 450
High-Risk Patients, 450
Intermediate-Risk Patients, 450
Low-Risk Patients, 451
Effects of Radiation on Specific Cellular Components, 451
Current Directions, 451
Case Study 25.1, 451
Procedure: Longitudinal Assessment of Posttransplant Immune Status, 453.e1

KEY TERMS

accelerated rejection
acute GVHD
acute rejection
alloepitopes
allotype
antibody-dependent, cell-mediated cytotoxicity (ADCC)
autografts
avascularity
CD34+ cells
chronic rejection
cytotoxicity
engraftment
exons
graft-versus-host disease (GVHD)
haplotypes
HLA allele
human leukocyte antigens (HLAs)
hyperacute rejection
immunosuppressive agents
major histocompatibility complex (MHC)
null alleles
peripheral blood stem cells (PBSCs)
proteomics
T-cell receptor (TCR)
xenotransplantation

The first organ transplantation, using a kidney from an identical twin, was performed in 1954 by Dr. Joseph Murray at Peter Bent Brigham Hospital in Boston, Massachusetts. The recipient survived for 9 years. Dr. Murray was ultimately recognized for his work by receiving the Nobel Prize in Physiology or Medicine in 1990.

At present a variety of tissues and organs are transplanted in human beings, including bone marrow, peripheral stem cells, bone matrix, skin, kidneys, liver, cardiac valves, heart, pancreas, corneas, and lungs. Transplantation is one of the areas, in addition to hypersensitivity (see Chapter 20) and autoimmunity (see Chapter 22), in which the immune system functions in a detrimental way.

Early in the history of transplantation, tissue antigens were recognized as important to successful grafting. If significantly different foreign antigens were introduced into an immunocompetent host, the transplanted tissue or organ would undoubtedly fail. Currently tissue (histocompatibility) matching, with concomitant immunosuppression of the host in many cases, is used to enhance the probability of success in organ and tissue transplantation.

Transplantation presents the following two basic problems:

> **KEY CONCEPTS: Major Histocompatibility Antigens in Transplant Rejection**
> - All vertebrates capable of acute rejection of foreign skin grafts have a localized complex involving many genes that exert major control over the organism's immune reactions.
> - Some antigens are much more potent than others in provoking an immune response and therefore are called the *major histocompatibility complex (MHC)*. In human beings, the MHC is referred to as *human leukocyte antigens (HLAs)*.

> - The MHC is divided into four major regions: D, B, C, and A. The A, B, and C regions code for class I molecules, whereas the D region codes for class II molecules.
> - Class I and class II antigens can be found on surface membrane proteins of body cells and in body fluids.
> - The MHC gene products have an important role in clinical immunology. For example, transplants are rejected if performed against MHC barriers; thus immunosuppressive therapy is required. These antigens are of primary importance in influencing the genetic basis of survival or rejection of transplanted organs.
> - Although HLA was originally identified by its role in transplant rejection, it is now recognized that the products of HLA genes play a crucial role in our immune system. T cells do not recognize antigens directly but do so when the antigen is presented on the surface of an antigen-presenting cell (APC), the macrophage. In addition to presenting the antigen, the macrophage must present another molecule for this response to occur. This molecule is a cell surface glycoprotein coded in each species by the MHC.

- Genetic variation between donor and recipient
- Recognition of genetic differences by a transplant recipient's immune system that causes rejection of a transplanted organ

HISTOCOMPATIBILITY ANTIGENS

The major histocompatibility complex (MHC) is a cluster of genes found on the short arm of chromosome 6 at band 21 6p21 (Fig. 25.1). These genes code for proteins that have a role in immune recognition.

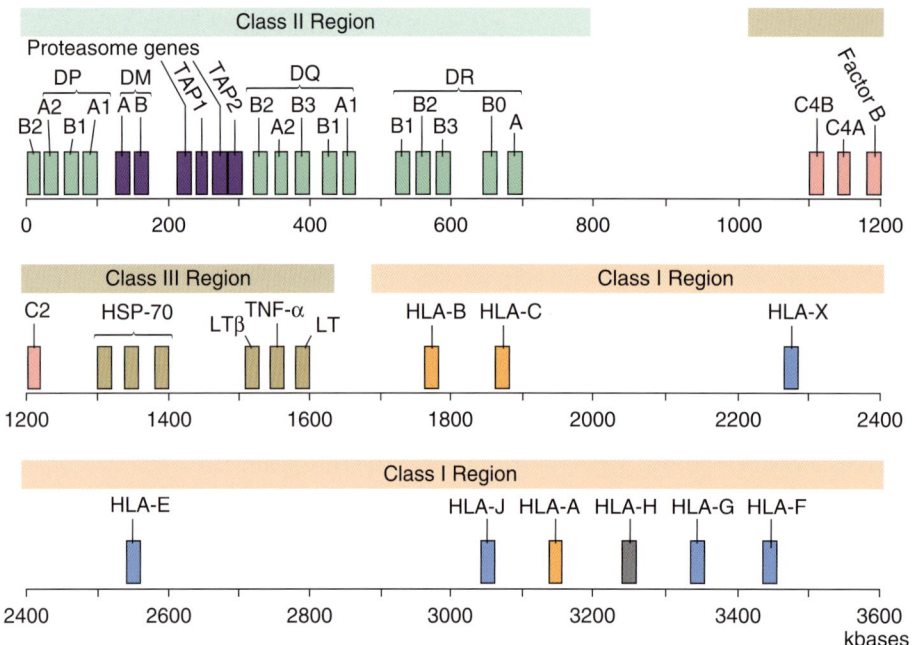

Fig. 25.1 Human Major Histocompatibility Complex. (From Abbas AK, Lichtman AHH, Pillai S: *Cellular and molecular immunology*, ed 7, Philadelphia, 2012, Saunders.)

The MHC encodes the **human leukocyte antigens (HLAs)**, which are the molecular basis for T-cell discrimination of self from nonself. The HLA complex contains over 200 genes, more than 40 of which encode leukocyte antigens, with the rest an assortment of genes not directly related to the HLA genes nor having a role in immunity.

The functional role of HLA molecules is to present peptides to T cells (both CD4 and CD8 T cells), enabling them to recognize and eliminate "foreign" particles and to prevent the recognition of "self" as foreign. Transplanted tissue may trigger a destructive mechanism (i.e., rejection) if the recipient's cells recognize the MHC protein products on the surface of the transplanted tissue as foreign or if immunocompetent cells transplanted on the donor tissue target the foreign cells of the recipient for elimination.

Nomenclature of Human Leukocyte Antigen Alleles

Each **HLA allele** has a unique four-, six-, or eight-letter or digit name (Table 25.1). The length of the allele designation depends on the sequence of the allele and that of its nearest relative. All alleles receive a four-letter or -digit name; six- and eight-digit names are only assigned when necessary.

The first two digits describe the type, which often corresponds to the serologic antigen carried by an **allotype**. The third and fourth digits are used to list the subtypes, with numbers assigned in the order in which DNA sequences have been determined.

Alleles whose numbers differ in the first four digits must differ in one or more nucleotide substitutions that change the amino acid sequence of the encoded protein. Alleles that differ only by synonymous nucleotide substitutions (also called *silent* or *noncoding substitutions*) within the coding sequence are distinguished by the use of fifth and sixth digits. Alleles that only differ by sequence polymorphisms in the introns or in the 5′ or 3′ untranslated regions that flank the **exons** and introns are distinguished by the use of seventh and eighth digits.

In addition to the unique allele designation, optional suffixes may be added to an allele to indicate its expression status. Alleles shown not to be expressed, termed **null alleles**, have been given the suffix N. Alleles shown to be alternatively expressed may have the suffix L, S, C, A, or Q.

The suffix L is used to indicate an allele shown to have *l*ow cell surface expression compared with normal levels. The S suffix is used

TABLE 25.1	Human Leukocyte Antigen Naming System[a].
Nomenclature	Indicates
HLA	Human leukocyte antigen (HLA) region and prefix for an HLA gene
HLA-DRB1	Particular HLA locus (e.g., DRB1)
HLA-DRB1*13	Group of alleles that encode the DR13 antigen
HLA-DRB1*1301	Specific HLA allele
HLA-DRB1*1301N	Null allele
HLA-DRB1*130102	Allele that differs by a synonymous mutation
HLA-DRB1*13010102	Allele that contains a mutation outside the coding region
HLA-A*2409N	Null allele
HLA-A*3014L	Allele encoding a protein with significantly reduced or low cell surface expression
HLA-A*24020102L	Allele encoding a protein with significantly reduced or low cell surface expression, where the mutation is found outside the coding region
HLA-B*44020102S	Allele encoding a protein expressed as a secreted molecule only
HLA-A*3211Q	Allele that has a mutation previously shown to have a significant effect on cell surface expression, but where this has not been confirmed and its expression remains questionable

[a]As of June 2007, no alleles have been named with the C or A suffixes.

TABLE 25.2	Comparison of Major Histocompatibility Complex Class I and Class II.	
Parameter	Class I	Class II
Loci	HLA-A, -B, and -C	HLA-DN, -DO, -DP, -DQ, and -DR
Distribution	Most nucleated cells	B lymphocytes, macrophages, other antigen-presenting cells, activated T lymphocytes
Function	To present endogenous antigen to cytotoxic T lymphocytes	To present endogenous antigen to helper T lymphocytes

TABLE 25.3	Examples of Nomenclature of Human Leukocyte Antigen (HLA) Alleles.
Allele (New Nomenclature)	Frequently Used Shorthand
Class I	
HLA-A*0101	HLA-A1
HLA-B*0801	HLA-B8
Class II	
HLA-DRB1*0101	HLA-DR1
HLA-DRB1*0301	HLA-DR3

Adapted from Peakman M, Vergani D: *Basic and clinical immunology*, ed 2, New York, 2009, Churchill Livingstone.

to denote an allele specifying a protein that is expressed as a soluble *s*ecreted molecule but that is not present on the cell surface. A C suffix indicates an allele product that is present in the *c*ytoplasm but not on the cell surface. An A suffix indicates *a*berrant expression, when there is some doubt as to whether a protein is expressed. A Q suffix is used when the expression of an allele is *q*uestionable, given that the mutation seen in the allele has previously been shown to affect normal expression levels.

Major Histocompatibility Complex Regions

The MHC is divided into four major regions (Table 25.2): D, B, C, and A. The A, B, and C regions are the classic, or class Ia, genes that code for class I molecules. The D region codes for class II molecules. Class I includes HLA-A, HLA-B, and HLA-C. The three principal loci (A, B, and C) and their respective antigens are numbered 1, 2, 3, and so on. The class II gene region antigens are encoded in the HLA-D region and can be subdivided into three families: HLA-DR, HLA-DC (DQ), and HLA-SB (DP).

Classes of Human Leukocyte Antigen Molecules

Structurally there are two classes of HLA molecules: class I and class II (Table 25.3). Both classes are cell surface heterodimeric structures. Class I HLA molecules consist of an alpha chain, a highly polymorphic glycoprotein encoded within the MHC on chromosome 6. This alpha chain noncovalently associates with beta-2 microglobulin, a nonpolymorphic glycoprotein encoded by a non-HLA gene on chromosome 15. Class II HLA molecules are composed of alpha chains and beta chains encoded within the MHC. The conformation of class I and class II HLA molecules provides each with a groove in which linear peptides, consisting of 8 to 25 peptides, are displayed for recognition by the cell surface expression on lymphocytes of a transmembrane heterodimeric receptor. All nucleated cells of the body display transmembrane class I HLA molecules in association with the non–transmembrane beta-2 microglobulin molecule.

Class I and class II antigens can be found on body cells and in body fluids. Class I and class II molecules are surface membrane proteins. Class I molecules are transmembrane glycoproteins, but the class II dimer molecule differs from class I in that both dimers span the cell membrane. Class I and class II gene products are biochemically distinct, although they appear to be distantly related through evolution. Class III gene products such as C2, C4A, C4B, and Bf complement components are incomplete, but these structures are defined by genes lying between or very near the HLA-B and HLA-DR loci.

Multiple alleles occur at each locus. Genes of class I, II, and III antigens at each locus are inherited as codominant alleles. Inheritance within families closely follows simple mendelian dominant characteristics. Conservation of entire haplotypes through generation after generation is the general rule. Very strong linkage disequilibrium is displayed between several HLA loci, creating super or extended haplotypes that may differ from race to race. For example, the most frequent Caucasoid superextended haplotype, AL, Xw7, BB, BfS, C2-1, C4AQOB1, DR3, is almost absent in Asian populations.

Role of Major Histocompatibility Complex and Human Leukocyte Antigens

The histocompatibility complex that encodes cell surface antigens was first discovered in graft rejection experiments with mice. When the antigens were matched between donor and recipient, the ability of a graft to survive was remarkably improved. A comparable genetic system of alloantigens was subsequently identified in human beings.

The presence of HLA was first recognized when multiply transfused patients experienced transfusion reactions despite proper crossmatching. It was discovered that these reactions were caused by leukocyte antibodies rather than by antibodies directed against erythrocyte antigens. These same antibodies were subsequently discovered in the sera of multiparous women.

The MHC gene products have an important role in clinical immunology. For example, transplants are rejected if performed against MHC barriers; thus immunosuppressive therapy is required. These antigens are of primary importance and are second only to the ABO antigens in influencing the genetic basis of survival or rejection of transplanted organs.

Although HLA was originally identified by its role in transplant rejection, it is now recognized that the products of HLA genes play a crucial role in our immune system. T cells do not recognize antigens directly but do so when the antigen is presented on the surface of an APC, the macrophage. In addition to presentation of the antigen, the macrophage must present another molecule for this response to occur. This molecule is a cell surface glycoprotein coded in each species by the MHC. T cells are able to interact with the histocompatibility molecules only if they are genetically identical (MHC restriction).

Both class I and class II antigens function as targets of T lymphocytes that regulate the immune response. Class I molecules regulate interactions between cytolytic T cells and target cells, and class II molecules restrict the activity of regulatory T cells (helper, suppressor, and amplifier subsets). Thus class II molecules regulate the interaction between helper T (Th) cells and APCs. Cytotoxic T (Tc) cells directed against class I antigens are inhibited by CD8 cells;

Tc cells directed against class II antigens are inhibited by CD4 cells. Many genes in both class I and class II gene families have no known function.

The class I and class II molecules can also bind to self-antigens produced in the normal process of cellular protein degradation. Usually, these are not recognized by the T-cell receptor (TCR). In transplant patients, most immune responses are generated not from bacterial antigens, viral antigens, or self-antigens, but from the presentation of alloepitopes derived from the transplanted tissue to circulating T lymphocytes. T-cell activation leads to the production of cytokines and chemokines, which may recruit components of innate immunity such as natural killer (NK) cells or macrophages and complement. In addition, defensins and cathelicidins have chemoattractant properties on T lymphocytes.

Class III molecules bear no clear relationship to class I and class II molecules aside from their genetic linkage (presence of the gene in or near the MHC complex). Class III molecules are involved in immunologic phenomena because they represent components of the complement pathways.

Impact of Human Leukocyte Antigens

Matching of the donor and the recipient for MHC antigens exerts a significantly positive effect on graft acceptance. HLA matching is essential in organ transplantation and hematopoietic stem cell (HSC) transplantation. Important HLA antigens are HLA-A, HLA-B, HLA-C, and HLA-DRB1. The HLA-DQ is used for evaluation by some transplant centers but not by others. The impact of DQ is minimal.

Everyone has two types of each of these major HLA antigens; there are many different subtypes of HLA-A and of the others. The best possible match is 6/6; the worst possible match is 0/6. Minimum matching levels must be met before a donor or unit of cord blood cells can be transplanted. For adult donors, a match of at least 6 of these 8 HLA markers is required. For cord blood units, which require less strict matching criteria, a match of at least 4 of 6 markers is required at HLA-A, HLA-B, and HLA-DRB1. Some transplant centers set more stringent requirements for a 7 out of 8 match between patient and donor (Fig. 25.2).

In transplantation immunology, the major impact on graft loss comes from the effects of HLA-B and -DR antigens. The effects of HLA-DR mismatches are most important in the first 6 months after transplantation. The HLA-B effect emerges in the first 2 years, and HLA-A mismatches have a deleterious effect on long-term graft survival.

In kidney transplants, HLA compatibility exerts the strongest influence on long-term kidney survival. The 1-year survival for kidneys transplanted from an HLA-identical sibling approaches 95%. Approximately 50% to 65% of cadaveric kidneys mismatched for all four HLA-A and HLA-B antigens function for 6 months but deteriorate thereafter with time. Only 15% to 25% of these mismatched cadaveric kidneys remain functioning 4 years after transplantation.

Evaluation of Potential Transplant Recipients and Donors

HLA matching is the primary consideration in assessing whether a donor is acceptable for a given patient and overshadows any other non-HLA factors, including ABO incompatibility.

HLA matching is important because a close HLA match does the following:
- Improves the chances for a successful transplantation
- Promotes engraftment, the process of donated cells beginning to grow and produce new blood cells in the host
- Reduces the risk of posttransplantation graft-versus-host disease (GVHD)

According to the Organ Procurement and Transplantation Network (OPTN) proposed Best Practice Guidelines for Histocompatibility Laboratories published on March 16, 2023, Policy 4, the responsibility of the histocompatibility laboratory is to provide an evaluation of histocompatibility data and pertinent patient immunologic risk factors that will allow the clinician and patient to decide which approaches to transplantation are in the patient's best interest, such as standard criteria donor, expanded criteria donor, or donation after cardiac death donor wait lists, desensitization, or potential paired donation exchanges. In addition to accurate HLA typing and evaluation, this information may include the following from patient history and histocompatibility test results: Although the entire patient history is not always available, the laboratory should make every effort to work with clinicians and healthcare providers to secure as accurate a sensitization record as possible.

The patient's level of immunologic risk for transplantation is defined by:

a. Sensitization history
b. Detection and characterization of HLA-specific antibodies
c. The titers of the various HLA-specific antibodies, as appropriate
d. Repeat mismatches
e. Aggressiveness of response to previous transplant
f. Numbers of pregnancies and age of youngest child
g. Antibody trend—decreasing or increasing
h. Donor relationship—husband to wife or child to mother

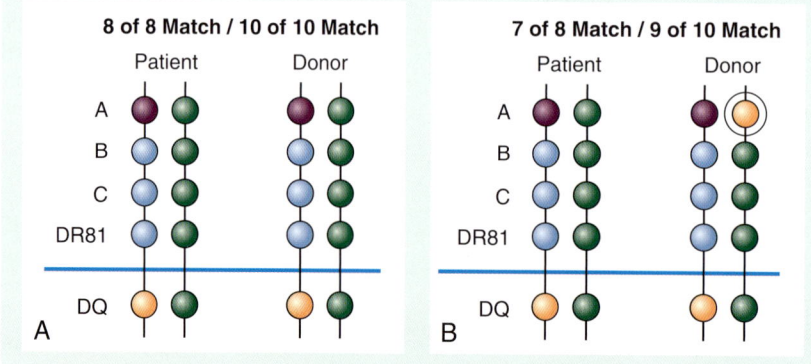

Fig. 25.2 Human Leukocyte Antigen (HLA) Matching of Patient and Donor. (A) All the patient's markers match the donor's markers. The 8 of 8 match means that there is a match at A, B, C, and DRB1. A 10 of 10 match means that there is a match at A, B, DRB1, C, and DQ. (B) One of the patient's A markers does not match one of the donor's A markers. Therefore this is a 7 of 8 match or a 9 of 10 match. (Copyright National Marrow Donor Program. Copyright © 2012. www.marrow.org/patient. Reprinted with permission.)

An assessment of the above factors should provide a list of HLA antigens that would be unacceptable in a donor. The only new practice for some laboratories will be the listing of unacceptable HLA antigens defined by the historic or current presence of HLA-specific antibodies. Such definition is now routinely performed in many laboratories but unacceptable antigens are not always listed for allocation purposes.

Human Leukocyte Antigen Techniques

A potential recipient needs to have HLA typing (Fig. 25.3A), and a family search may be conducted for a suitable donor. If a suitable match is not found, the patient is placed on a waiting list (Fig. 25.3B). When an organ becomes available, the donor is HLA typed and a computerized search is made for a suitable recipient (Fig. 25.3C).

Because different individuals in a species carry different HLA antigens on their cell surfaces, introduction of foreign antigens can stimulate T cells. These T cells are prominently implicated in graft rejection, and they can also stimulate antibody formation under certain circumstances. Histocompatibility crossmatching is performed to rule out preexisting antibodies (see Fig. 25.3D) capable of causing **hyperacute rejection**.

Regarding antibody screening to avoid hyperacute rejection, it is important to identify recipient anti-HLA antibodies to antigens expressed on donor cells. The pioneer method to detect antibodies was complement-dependent **cytotoxicity**. Since the mid-1990s, it has been gradually replaced by more sensitive solid-phase immunoassays (SPIs), such as enzyme-linked immunosorbent assay (ELISA) and the bead-based technology, flow cytometry (Flow PRA and Flow Analyzer; Luminex Technology, Austin, Texas). These assays use microparticles coated with purified HLA molecules. The era of solid-phase microparticle technology for HLA antibody detection permits sensitive and specific detection of HLA antibody.

Complement-Mediated Cytotoxicity

Class I antigens are determined by several techniques; the classic method is the lymphocyte microcytotoxicity method (complement-mediated cytotoxicity). With this technique, a battery of reagent antisera and isolated target cells is incubated with a source of complement

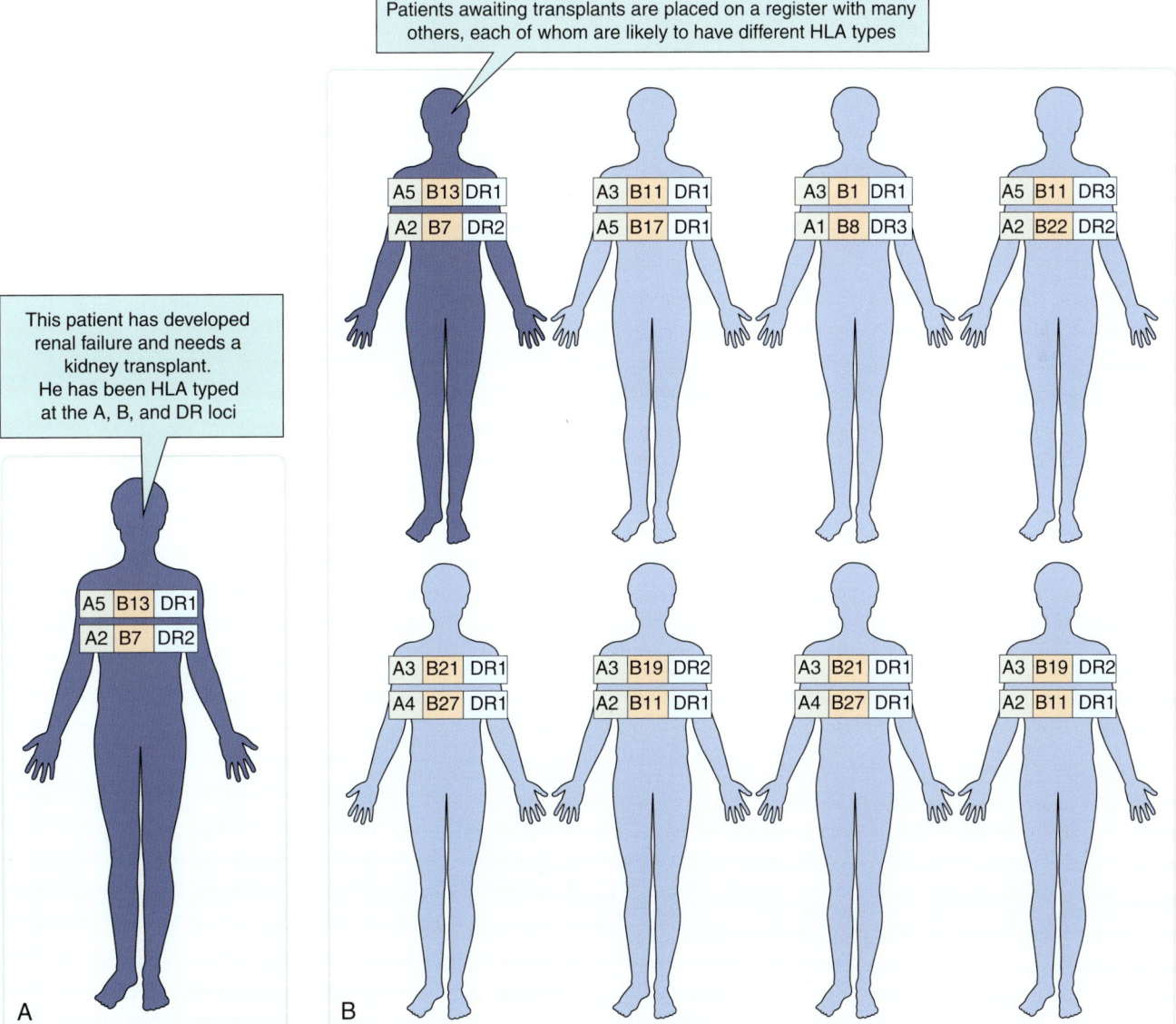

Fig. 25.3 Patients (recipients) requiring a solid organ transplant, such as a kidney, are human leukocyte antigen (HLA) typed (A) and then placed on a transplant registry waiting list (B).

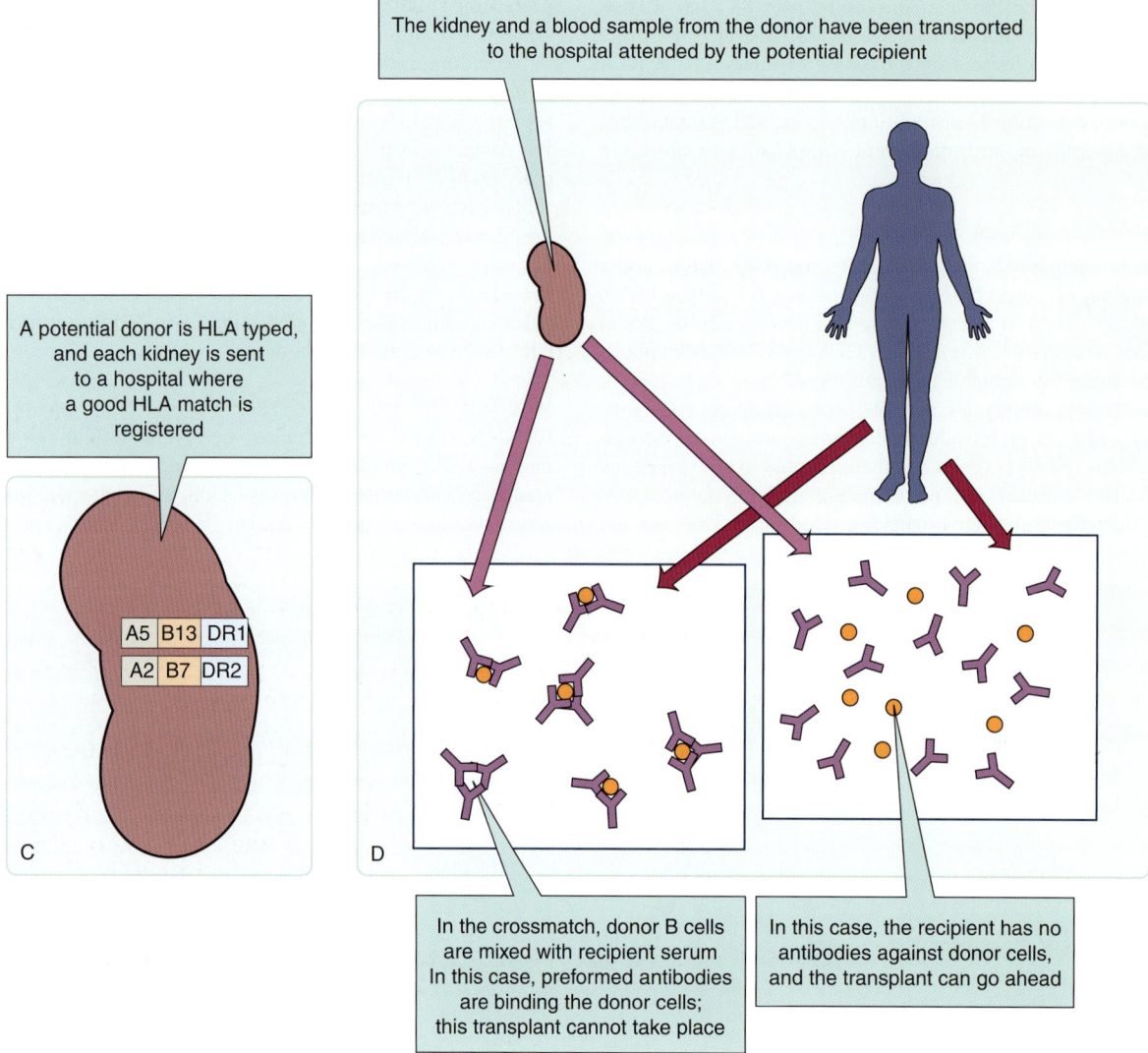

Fig. 25.3 cont'd (C) When a potential organ becomes available, the donor is HLA typed. If the donor and recipient demonstrate a suitable match by computer, a blood sample is procured from the donor and cross-matched with the recipient's blood to determine compatibility. (D) If no HLA antibodies are detected against the donor cells, the organ is harvested and transplanted to the recipient. (From Nairn R, Helbert M: *Immunology for medical students*, ed 2, St. Louis, 2007, Mosby.)

under oil to prevent evaporation. If a specific alloantibody and cell membrane antigen combine, complement-mediated damage to the cell wall allows for penetration of a vital dye and the cells are killed. Cell death is determined by staining. A stain such as trypan blue will penetrate dead cells but not living cells. Unaffected cells remain brilliantly refractile when observed microscopically.

This assay can be insensitive, and scoring is subjective. Test sensitivity can be enhanced by the addition of anti–human globulin (AHG) antibody. This assay is used for pretransplantation crossmatching and for antibody specificity analysis. For HLA class I typing or anti–class I antibody identification, a purified T-cell population is preferred because human T lymphocytes express class I but not class II molecules. Conversely, B lymphocytes are required for class II typing or antibody identification because human B cells express class I and class II HLA molecules.

Class II HLA-DR and HLA-DQ specificities can be recognized by similar serologic methods, except that isolated B cells are the usual target cells because their surface is rich in these molecules and also in class I determinants. At present HLA-Dw and HLA-DP cannot be serologically defined, and their detection relies on the ability of these molecules to stimulate newly synthesized DNA when added to primary mixed lymphocyte (HLA-Dw) or when readded to secondary primary lymphocyte (HLA-DP) in vitro cultures.

Class III complement specificities are recognized by the availability of diagnostic reagents, but reagents remain scarce.

Solid-Phase Enzyme-Linked Immunosorbent Assay

The ELISA is available for panel-reactive antibody (PRA) determination and antibody specificity analysis. ELISA-based HLA tests are considered reproducible, sensitive, and objective. Newer assays use pure HLA antigens produced by recombinant technology to improve specificity analysis.

Flow Cytometry

Single-cell analysis by flow cytometry is a sensitive method for crossmatching and antibody identification (see Chapter 11). Tagged T or B lymphocytes are incubated with the patient's serum to allow the formation of antigen–antibody complexes on the cell surface. Unbound proteins are washed away, and the bound antibodies are detected with a second antibody: anti–human immunoglobulin G (IgG) labeled with a chromophore. An alternative flow cytometry format uses microparticles coated with HLA antigens of known specificity (obtained through recombinant techniques) instead of lymphocytes.

Molecular Techniques

The first molecular method for HLA typing was polymerase chain reaction (PCR) amplification of DNA. Tissue typing using the sequence-specific oligonucleotide (SSO) and sequence-specific primer (SSP) technologies has been in routine use in many tissue typing laboratories worldwide for more than 20 years since the development of PCR. The DNA-based methods have more sensitivity, accuracy, and resolving power than serologic typing methods.

Today, more precise DNA-based HLA typing methods using molecular techniques include:
- Sequence-specific oligonucleotide probe hybridization (SSO)
- Sequence-specific primer amplification (SSP)
- Sequencing-based typing (SBT)
- Reference strand–based conformation analysis (RSCA)

In 2013, a new project demonstrated the potential benefits of massively parallel sequencing (MPS)/next-generation sequencing (NGS) in the HLA laboratory. MPS/NGS may resolve the issue through the combination of clonal amplification, which provides phase information, and the ability to sequence larger regions of genes, including introns, without the additional effort or cost associated with current methods.

Methodologies approved by the US Food and Drug Administration (FDA) exist, and there are several advantages, including typing additional loci with no additional time testing. Another advantage of MPS/NGS is high throughput because one instrument with little hands-on time can type 96 loci in 3 days compared with the standard typing methods that can take up to 2 weeks for a few specimens. MPS/NGS costs continue to decrease, and as MPS/NGS instruments are introduced into more laboratories for molecular oncology and diagnosis of inherited diseases, it is expected that there will be an increase in the use of MPS/NGS in HLA typing laboratories.

Another simplified method using short tandem repeat (STR) genotyping provides additional information, allowing determination of the extent of HLA identity in families. The HLA STR assay is a reliable and rapid test that is used to inexpensively screen potential sibling donors for HLA identity.

Bead Technology

HLA antibodies in solid organ transplant recipients and, in particular, the use of the single-antigen bead assay to detect antibodies to HLA loci such as Cw, DQA, DPA, and DPB, are not readily detected by other methods. The use of SPI for antibody detection should be supplemented with cell-based assays to examine the correlations between the two types of assays and to establish the likelihood of a positive crossmatch (XM). The technical factors that can influence the results and clinical interpretation when using Luminex bead technology include variation in antigen density and the presence of denatured antigen on the beads.

Donor-Specific Antibody Tests

Donor-specific antibodies (DSAs) are anti-HLA antibodies specifically generated against donor cells. Although a donor's HLA type and crossmatching status are known before transplantation, physicians are becoming interested in knowing when an organ recipient is starting to make DSA antibodies. The presence of DSA in 30% of renal transplant recipients is associated with significantly lower graft survival.

Due to the larger availability of single HLA antigens, this technique is more sensitive and specific, but this high sensitivity can cause false-positive results. Luminex beads can denature intact HLA molecules, which unmasks hidden epitopes, and are able to react with "natural" HLA antibodies present in nonimmunized patients. The extreme sensitivity of the Luminex assay can make it difficult to determine positive and negative results determined by mean fluorescence intensity (MFI). The MFI could vary between centers, depending on different company reagents and operator ability.

TABLE 25.4 Transplantation Terms.

Term	Definition
Autograft	Graft transferred from one position to another in the same individual (e.g., skin, hair, bone)
Syngraft	Graft transplanted between different but identical recipient and donor (e.g., kidney transplant between monozygous twins)
Allograft (homograft)	Graft between genetically different recipient and donor of the same species; grafted donor tissue or organ contains antigens not present in recipient
Xenograft (heterograft)	Graft between individuals of different species (e.g., pig heart valve to a human heart)

TRANSPLANTATION TERMINOLOGY

The transplanting or grafting of an organ or tissue ranges from self-transplantation, such as skin grafts from one part of the body to another to correct burn injuries, or hair transplants from one area of the scalp to another to correct pattern baldness, to the grafting of a body component from one species to another, such as transplanting a pig's heart valve to a human. Table 25.4 defines the most recent terms used in transplantation.

GENERAL FACTS ABOUT TRANSPLANTATION

Tissue and Organ Transplantation

In the United States the most commonly transplanted tissues are bones, tendons, ligaments, skin, heart valves, blood vessels, and corneas. Around 3.3 million tissue grafts are distributed each year and approximately 2.5 million grafts are transplanted. Organ transplantation is widely viewed as the preferred treatment for end-stage organ failure because of the quality of life that the treatment offers for patients. The increased demand for organ transplantation is fueled by the transplantation success rate.

According to Health and Human Service's OPTN data, on December 17, 2021 the United States officially passed a historic milestone for the nation with 40,000 transplants in one year. The three organ types most commonly transplanted all set annual volume records. There were totals of 24,669 kidney transplants, 9236 liver transplants, and 3817 heart transplants. Liver transplant totals have set annual records for the past 9 years, and heart transplants have set a new record each of the past 10 years.

Living donor transplants, which decreased significantly in 2020 due to the COVID-19 pandemic, increased in 2021, but still at lower totals than prior years. However, increases in organ donations occurred in many areas throughout the United States. A total of 13,861 people became deceased organ donors nationwide in 2021, representing the 11th consecutive record year for deceased donation and an increase of 10.1% over 2020. Donors representing less traditional medical criteria continue to fuel the overall increase. Donations from individuals who died of cardiorespiratory failure, as opposed to brain death, continued a substantial increase. Also for the third straight year, the most common age range of deceased donors was 50 to 64 years.

> **BOX 25.1 Examples of Diseases Treatable by Stem Cell Transplantation**
>
> **Acute Leukemias**
> - Acute lymphoblastic leukemia
> - Acute myelogenous leukemia
>
> **Chronic Leukemias**
> - Chronic myelogenous leukemia
> - Chronic lymphocytic leukemia
>
> **Stem Cell Disorders**
> - Aplastic anemia
> - Fanconi anemia
> - Paroxysmal nocturnal hemoglobinuria
>
> **Myeloproliferative Disorders**
> - Primary myelofibrosis
> - Polycythemia vera
>
> **Lymphoproliferative Disorders**
> - Non-Hodgkin lymphoma
> - Hodgkin disease
>
> **Phagocyte Disorders**
> - Chédiak-Higashi syndrome
> - Chronic granulomatous disease
> - Immunodeficiencies
> - Severe combined immunodeficiency
>
> **Inherited Platelet Abnormalities**
> - Congenital thrombocytopenia
> - Plasma cell disorders
> - Multiple myeloma
> - Plasma cell leukemia
> - Waldenström macroglobulinemia
>
> **Other Malignancies**
> - Breast cancer
> - Ewing sarcoma
> - Neuroblastoma
> - Renal cell carcinoma
>
> **Inherited Erythrocyte Abnormalities**
> - Beta-thalassemia major
> - Pure red cell aplasia
> - Sickle cell disease
>
> **Liposomal Storage Diseases**
> - Mucopolysaccharidoses
> - Hurler syndrome
> - Gaucher disease
> - Niemann-Pick disease

The waiting time for allogeneic organ transplantation varies widely for many reasons. Each patient's situation is different. Some patients are more ill than others when they are put on the transplant waiting list. Some patients become sick more quickly than others or respond differently to treatments. Patients may have medical conditions that make finding a good match more difficult. How long a patient waits for a transplant depends on factors such as blood or tissue types, existing medical condition, medical urgency, size of donated organ, time on the waiting list, distance between donor's site and potential donor organ site, number of donors in a local area over time, and the transplantation center's criteria for accepting organ offers.

Depending on the type of organ needed, some factors are more important than others.

In 1984 the US Congress passed the National Organ Transplant Act. The goal of this legislation was to match a low supply of organs with the most critically ill patients, regardless of where they resided.

As of early 2023, 106,962 men, women, and children were on the waiting list for a transplant, which is the lowest number of waiting patients since 2009. The list topped 124,000 at its height in 2014.

Most of these registrants are waiting for a kidney transplant, followed by those waiting for a liver transplant and those for a heart transplant. Other transplant registrants are waiting for lung, kidney, and pancreas; pancreatic islet cells heart and lung; and intestine transplants.

The most common reasons for needing a solid organ transplant vary by the type of organ. Kidney recipients usually have diabetes, glomerulonephritis, hypertensive nephrosclerosis, or polycystic kidneys. Liver recipient patients typically have noncholestatic cirrhosis, cholestatic liver disease, biliary atresia, acute hepatic necrosis, or hepatitis C infection. Patients with cardiomyopathy, congenital heart disease, valvular heart disease, or coronary artery disease are the most frequent heart transplant recipients. The number of patients living with a function graft has generally increased over the past decade. According to the OPTN, the percentage of graft survivals between 2008 and 2015 has improved for four types of organs:

- Kidney—95% 1-year survival, 88% 3-year survival, 80% 5-year survival
- Heart—90% 1-year survival, 84% 3-year survival, 76% 5-year survival
- Liver—89% 1-year survival, 81% 3-year survival, 74% 5-year survival
- Lung—87% 1-year survival, 68% 3-year survival, 53% 5-year survival

Graft survival time depends on many factors, including the source of the organ and the type of organ transplanted. For example, a living donor kidney functions, on average, 12 to 20 years, and a deceased donor kidney from 8 to 12 years.

Hematopoietic Stem Cells

Stem cell transplantation is currently being used to treat patients with many types of hematologic disorders and malignant diseases (Box 25.1).

PRETRANSPLANTATION SCREENING

According to the OPTN policies (for organ procurement organizations [OPOs]) and FDA regulations and guidance (for tissue and eye banks), a medical and social history interview needs to be conducted with the deceased donor's next of kin or another knowledgeable person. These interviews gather information about:

1. Risk behaviors that may have exposed the donor to certain diseases
2. The donor's past medical history
3. Relevant travel history, which can be important for exposure to certain pathogens

This interview is one of several ways to assess the donor's risk for having an infectious disease; its usefulness depends on (1) how well the person being interviewed knew the donor; and (2) the interviewee's comprehension of the meaning of the questions.

CHAPTER 25 Transplantation: Human Leukocyte Antigens, Solid Organ, Tissues, and Hematopoietic Stem Cells

TABLE 25.5 Infectious Disease Screening Recommendations Prior to Tissue, Eye or Solid Organ Transplantation.

Type of Organism	Infectious Disease	Pretransplantation Recommendations
Bacteria		
	Treponema pallidum (syphilis)	All transplant candidates should be screened with a nontreponemal test and, if reactive, confirmed by TP-PA
	Mycobacterium tuberculosis (tuberculosis)	All transplant candidates should be evaluated for latent TB infection by TST and IGRA
Parasite		
	Toxoplasmosis	Heart transplant candidates should be screened for prior evidence of *Toxoplasma* by IgG
	Chagas	If the transplant patient was born in or has a history of residing in an endemic area of Latin America, or if the person's mother was born in Latin America, US FDA-approved assays for blood donor screening are recommended
Virus		
	Human Immunodeficiency Virus (HIV)	4th Generation Antigen/Antibody Test with Reflex to Confirmation or Rapid Antibody Test (see Chapter 19)
	Cytomegalovirus (CMV)	Serologic testing for CMV IgG
	Epstein-Barr virus (EBV)	Serologic testing for EBNA IgG, EBV VCA IgM and IgG, and EA IgG
	Hepatitis B Virus (HBV)	Hepatitis panel, acute with reflex HBV surface antigen confirmation
	Hepatitis C Virus (HCV)	Hepatitis panel, acute with reflex to HCV quantitative nucleic acid amplification test (NAAT)

FDA, Food and Drug Administration; *IgG*, immunoglobulin G; *IGRA*, interferon-gamma release assay; *TB*, tuberculosis; *TP-PA*, treponema pallidum particle agglutination; *TST*, tuberculin skin test.
From Centers for Disease Control and Prevention, National Center for Emerging and Zoonotic Infectious Diseases (NCEZID), Division of Healthcare Quality Promotion (DHQP). https://www.cdc.gov/transplantsafety/protecting-patient/screening-testing.html.

Laboratory testing for infectious diseases

Tissue and eye bank requirements. FDA regulations require tissue and eye banks to adequately and appropriately test donor specimens for risk associated with HIV, HBV, HCV, and syphilis. Living tissue donors must also be tested for West Nile virus (WNV). Donors of tissues that may contain live white blood cells, such as semen and hematopoietic stem/progenitor cells (e.g., umbilical cord blood), are also tested for human T-lymphotropic virus (HTLV) and cytomegalovirus (CMV). A donor with positive test results for any of these infectious pathogens, but not necessarily CMV, is not eligible.

Solid organ transplantation requirements. The goal of organ transplantation is to be a life-saving endeavor; however, serious illness, graft loss, and death can occur from undetected infectious agents in donor organs and tissues. Infectious pathogens, such as viruses, bacteria, fungi, or an amoebic parasites, have been unknowingly transmitted through transplants. Examples, such as HIV, hepatitis C, rabies virus, (*Mycobacterium tuberculosis* [tuberculosis]) and *Balamuthia mandrillaris*, have been detected.

In late 2022 the Centers for Disease Control and Prevention Division of Healthcare Quality Promotion (DHQP) endorsed laboratory testing requirements for certain infectious pathogens in deceased organ and tissue donors and living donors (Table 25.5).

OPTN policy requires OPOs and hospitals that recover living donor organs to perform the tests to see if the donor may have certain infections: HIV, hepatitis B virus (HBV), hepatitis C virus (HCV), syphilis, CMV, Epstein-Barr virus (EBV), Chagas disease (for heart donors), and toxoplasmosis (for deceased donors only). Living potential kidney donors at increased risk for tuberculosis are also tested for this infection.

TYPES OF TRANSPLANTS

Eleven different organs or human body parts can be transplanted: blood vessels, bone, bone marrow or stem cells, cornea, heart, kidneys, liver, lung, middle ear, pancreas, and skin. Successful organ transplants have increased since the advent of the immunosuppressive drug cyclosporine (cyclosporin A).

Living donor transplants have attracted significant media attention. According to United Network for Organ Sharing (UNOS) and the Health Resources and Services Administration of the US Department of Health and Human Services, a living donor may donate a single kidney, segment of the liver, portion of the pancreas, or the lobe of a lung.

Bone

Bone matrix autografts or allografts are common. Transplantation of bone matrix is used after certain limb-sparing tumor resections and to correct congenital bone abnormalities. The major criteria for bone donation are a lack of infection, no history of intravenous (IV) drug use, and no history of prolonged steroid therapy or human growth hormone treatment. Bone can be easily harvested and frozen. Freezing not only preserves the bone but offers the additional benefit of concomitant diminution of histocompatibility antigens.

The major technical requirement for allograft transplantation is maintaining the periosteal sheath of the recipient bone to strip the donor bone completely of all periosteal elements. Transplantation of bone is an easy procedure. Processed bone lacks significant quantities of immunogenic substances; therefore the need for immunosuppression is almost completely eliminated.

Cornea

Corneal transplants have been a common form of therapy for many years. The first human corneal eye bank was established in New York City in 1944. This type of transplantation has an extremely high success rate because of the ease in obtaining and storing viable corneas.

Corneal grafts are generally performed to replace nonhealing corneal ulcerations. Graft rejection is minimal because of (1) the avascularity (lack of blood vessels) of this tissue; (2) a reasonably low concentration of class I transplantation antigens; and (3) an essential absence of class II antigens. To prevent rejection, grafts are made as small as possible and are placed centrally to avoid contact with the highly vascularized limbic region. Eccentrically placed grafts are subject to a high rate of immunologic failure because vascularity will allow for lymphocyte contact. **Immunosuppressive agents** are not routinely administered.

Heart

The first successful allograft cardiac transplantation was performed in 1967 by Dr. Christiaan Barnard in Cape Town, South Africa. The criteria for selecting the donor and recipient combination for cardiac transplantation are essentially the same as those used for cadaveric renal transplantation. The most significant exclusion for cardiac transplantation, however, is the presence of an active infection. Cardiac transplant donors must have sustained irreversible brain death, but near-normal cardiac function must be maintained. Prophylactic antibiotics and cytotoxic drugs are given to the donor just before harvesting of the heart. Because of the urgency of most situations, most grafts are performed despite multiple HLA incompatibilities. Transplant recipients are maintained on immunosuppressive therapy, anticoagulants, and antithrombotic agents and also on a low-lipid diet.

Due to advances in immunosuppression after heart transplantation, there has been an increase in the rate of 1-year survival among recipients to almost 90%, but acute cellular rejection is still observed during the first year after transplantation and at lower rates after the first year. Endomyocardial biopsy remains the primary method for monitoring organ rejection for heart transplants. An alternative method for detecting the rejection of a heart transplant, aside from endomyocardial biopsy, is quantitative assessment of mononuclear cell gene expression in peripheral blood specimens.

Heart Valves

Xenogenic valve replacement is a standard modality for the treatment of aortic and mitral valve defects. Sources of these xenogenic valves are bovine (cow) or porcine (pig); the valves are chemically or physically modified to reduce antigenicity.

Patients receiving xenoallografts of heart valves are not immunosuppressed after surgery because only minimal or nonexistent graft rejection reactions take place in these modified valves.

Intestine

The first successful intestine transplantation was performed at the University of Toronto in 1986, although the patient only survived for 10 days. The first intestinal transplant recipient to survive for an extended time was a 3½-year-old girl, who lived for 192 days in 1987. Intestinal transplantation has improved over the past decade, along with the number of intestinal transplantations performed in North America. Due to recent surgical advances, control of acute cellular rejection, and decrease in lethal infections, the rate of patient survival for the first year now exceeds 90%.

When the small intestine is transplanted alone, it is referred to as an *isolated intestinal transplant*, but intestinal transplantations are usually performed with other organs, with a composite allograft or with organs implanted separately from the same donor. Suitable intestinal organ donors have stable cardiopulmonary status and liver function. Potential organ transplant recipients with systemic infection and malignancy are excluded. Generally the recipient of the transplant is a person suffering from short gut syndrome, in which the intestine had been resected for a variety of reasons.

Kidney

The first successful human kidney transplantation was performed in 1954 between monozygotic twins. Induction of tolerance was attempted through the use of sublethal total-body irradiation and allogeneic bone marrow transplantation, followed by renal transplantation. By 1960 renal transplantation was firmly established as a viable treatment for end-stage renal disease. Because of the continuing problems associated with total-body irradiation, chemical immunosuppression became the mode of treatment. The criteria for recipients of renal allografts generally exclude older patients and patients with a history of malignancy. In addition, patients with active sepsis or patients in whom chronic infection may be reactivated by treatment with steroids or immunosuppressive therapy are also not considered transplantation candidates.

Traditionally kidney donations are not accepted from individuals older than 65 years because of a decreased likelihood of recipient survival. Donors are excluded if chronic renal disease or sepsis is present. Transplant donations are usually not accepted from those with generalized or systemic diseases such as diabetes mellitus, hypertension, and tuberculosis. Because of the severe shortage of donor kidneys, organs from donors older than 55 years or from donors with a history of hypertension or diabetes mellitus have been used with increasing frequency. Young trauma victims are the most desirable source of cadaveric organ transplants, including the kidneys. Cadaveric organs are not accepted from donors with a history of any malignancy other than that involving the central nervous system.

In addition to tissue compatibility, newer methods of harvesting kidneys have reduced the sensitizing effect related to passenger leukocytes against transplantation antigens borne on these cells. HLA-A and HLA-B loci matches have the best chance for long-term survival of the graft and recipient. The increased survival rate with HLA-A and HLA-B matches is determined not as much by class I compatibility as by the HLA-D region–related antigens associated with these regions. The strongest association between transplantation survival and tissue antigens is with the D region–related antigens (DR, MB, and MT). Lewis antigens on the erythrocytes and H-Y antigens associated with X and Y chromosomes are among the other antigen systems that demonstrate a reasonably significant association with graft survival.

BK virus (BKV) infection is an important clinical problem in kidney transplant recipients and is most likely due to the enhanced immunosuppressive state and BKV-specific immune deficiency with alloimmune activation. Diagnostic tools such as detection of BKV DNA in urine and/or plasma and careful renal histologic evaluation are critical to making the diagnosis of infection. A reduction in immunosuppression therapy and/or antiviral therapy and careful monitoring of patients is of paramount importance to prevent progressive renal graft failure. Screening for viremia or viruria can be used to identify early infection.

Liver

Potential liver transplant recipients must have no extrahepatic disease or infection present. The largest group of transplant recipients has been those with congenital biliary atresia. Patients with cirrhosis may also be good candidates. HLA crossmatching appears to increase the rate of graft survival, but the influence of tissue typing is somewhat unclear. Immunosuppressive regimens such as azathioprine and corticosteroids or cyclosporin A increase survival. Major complications of this procedure have been biliary tract fistulae or leaks, which have occurred in 30% to 50% of patients.

Lung

Successful lung transplantation has been difficult to achieve because of technical, logistic, and immunologic problems. Technically the lung donor and recipient must have essentially identical bronchial circumferences to obtain a good match. An additional technical problem is that the lungs are extremely sensitive to ischemic damage, and preservation after harvesting has been unsuccessful. Occasionally lung–heart combination transplantation has been attempted. The combined procedure is less difficult than single-organ transplantation.

The lungs are susceptible to infection; sepsis is very common among potential donors. Severe rejection is common because of the high density of Ia-positive cells in the vasculature and the high concentration of passenger leukocytes trapped in the alveoli and blood vessels. Intensive immunosuppressive therapy is needed to maintain the graft. Many lung recipients have died from massive infections and sepsis.

Pancreas

Whole-pancreas or isolated islet cell transplantation is possible. Whole pancreas after islet (PAI) transplantation is a treatment option for patients seeking insulin independence after a failed cellular transplant. A report from the International Pancreas Transplant Registry (IPTR) and UNOS of PAI transplant outcomes over a 10-year period, regardless of the reason for transplantation, demonstrated overall 1-year and 5-year PAI patient survival rates of 97% and 83%, respectively, and graft survival rates of 84% and 65%, respectively. According to IPTR/UNOS analysis, a PAI transplant is a safe procedure with low recipient mortality and high graft-function rates in both the short and long term. Patients with a failed islet transplant should know about this alternative in their quest for insulin independence through transplantation.

Three types of pancreatic transplantations can be carried out: pancreas–kidney transplantation (SPK; the most common; 73%), pancreas transplantation after kidney transplantation (PAK; 18%), and pancreas transplantation alone (PTA; 9%).

Skin

The development of nonimmunogenic skin-replacement materials has lowered the demand for skin allografts. Skin allografts elicit the rejection phenomenon because skin has an extremely high density of MHC class I antigens. Therefore sensitization and recognition of antigenic differences are likely, with resultant rejection of the grafted skin. If done, skin allografts are performed and supported with immunosuppressive therapy.

> **KEY CONCEPTS: Transplantation of Hematopoietic or Peripheral/Stem Cells**
> - The goal of transplanting bone marrow or peripheral blood progenitor cells is to achieve a potential cure or help patients recover from high-dose chemotherapy that has destroyed healthy stem cells or marrow cells.
> - Bone marrow and peripheral blood progenitor cells are capable of reconstituting a patient's immune system because they contain the precursor to the cells that make up the blood. Stem cells that circulate in the bloodstream are called *peripheral blood stem cells* (*PBSCs*).
> - There are three major types of transplants: allogeneic, syngeneic, and autologous.
> - Without healthy bone marrow, a patient cannot make the blood cells that are needed to fight off infections, carry oxygen, and prevent bleeding.
> - Factors that influence the eligibility for stem cell transplantation include age, disease status, performance status for the recipient, organ function, infectious disease status, compatibility of the donor and recipient, and psychosocial status.
> - The procedure for obtaining or harvesting bone marrow is the same for all types of transplants. The goal of the harvest procedure is to collect 10 to 15 mL of bone marrow per kilogram of the recipient's weight.

Hematopoietic or Peripheral Blood Stem Cells

Depending on the source of stem cells, HSC transplants may be called a *bone marrow transplant*, a *peripheral blood stem cell transplant*, or a *cord blood transplant*. Embryonic tissue transplantation is not currently performed in humans.

The goal of transplanting stem cells is to achieve a potential cure in many hematologic disorders or malignancies or to help patients recover from high-dose chemotherapy that has destroyed stem or marrow cells, a condition known as *myeloablation*. Stem cell transplants are expensive. The total cost for the procedure varies, but it can easily reach $100,000 or more for an autologous transplant. Allogeneic transplants tend to cost even more, up to $200,000 or higher.

Stem cells have the ability to evolve into different types of cells. Bone marrow and peripheral blood progenitor cells are capable of reconstituting a person's immune system because they contain the precursor to the cells that make up the blood: lymphocytes, granulocytes, macrophages, and platelets. Progenitor cells that circulate in the bloodstream are called **peripheral blood stem cells (PBSCs)**. PBSCs are found in much smaller quantities in the circulating blood than in the bone marrow. HSCs are found in very small numbers in the peripheral blood and greater numbers in the marrow. Peripheral blood progenitor cells have been increasingly used in place of bone marrow as a source of stem cells for allogeneic transplants. The reasons for this trend are the large amount of HSCs that can be collected, more rapid hematologic recovery, elimination of the surgical procedure and anesthesia risk for the donor, and reduced transplantation costs.

There are three types of stem cell transplants:
- Allogeneic
- Syngeneic
- Autologous

In an allogeneic transplantation a patient receives bone marrow or PBSCs from a related or an unrelated donor, depending on the availability of a good HLA match (Fig. 25.4). Because HLA tissue types are inherited, patients are more likely to find a matched donor from within their own family, racial, or ethnic group. In syngeneic transplantation, patients receive stem cells from their identical twin. Patients who undergo an autologous transplantation have donated their own cells after PBSC mobilization with granulocyte colony-stimulating factor (G-CSF) or granulocyte–macrophage colony-stimulating factor (GM-CSF).

In the HSC population, the cell marker CD34+ antigen identifies stem cells that can repopulate the bone marrow after chemotherapy. The required minimal dose of **CD34+ cells** is difficult to define, but most transplantation centers will infuse a minimal dose of 2×10^6 CD34+ cells per kilogram of the patient's weight in the autologous and allogeneic PBSC setting.

SOURCES OF STEM CELLS FOR TRANSPLANTATION

Bone Marrow

In the procedure for harvesting bone marrow, the donor is given general or regional anesthesia and marrow is usually aspirated with large needles from the posterior iliac crest; the anterior crest can also be used in certain cases. The goal of the procedure is to collect about 10% of the donor's marrow, or about 2 pints. This takes about 1 to 2 hours. The body will replace these cells within 4 to 6 weeks. If blood was taken from the donor before the marrow donation, it may be retransfused back to the donor at this time. The aspirated marrow is collected in bags containing a buffered isotonic solution and heparin to prevent coagulation.

After the marrow has been collected, it is filtered to remove any bone chips, fat, and clots that may have been collected or formed during the procedure. The bone marrow is frequently processed to remove undesired volume and cells for an allogeneic or syngeneic transplant; if the marrow is matched and no further manipulation is needed, it is transfused within 12 to 24 hours after collection, depending on the location of the recipient. If it is not transfused within 24 hours, it is cryopreserved.

Peripheral Blood Stem Cells

PBSCs are obtained for transplant by a procedure called *apheresis* or *leukapheresis*. For 4 or 5 days before apheresis, normal donors are given G-CSF, filgrastim (Neupogen), which increases the amount of

Influence of Graft, Donor, and Host Factors on Allogeneic HSC Engraftment

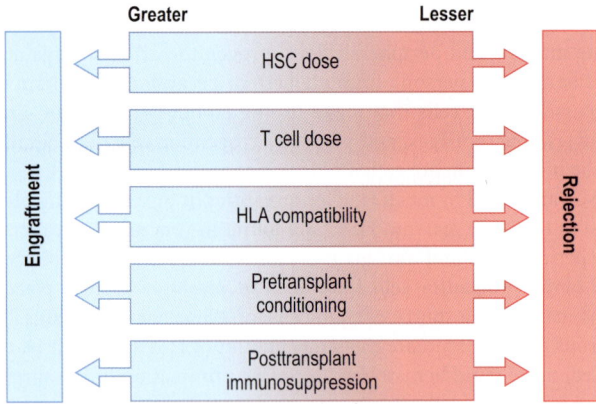

Fig. 25.4 Effect of Donor and Graft characteristics on Allogeneic Hematopoietic Stem Cell Transplantation (Allo-HSCT). Hematologic engraftment requires that the host-versus-graft reaction be overwhelmed, either by administration of a more intensive conditioning regimen before transplantation, use of more immunosuppressive medications after transplantation, closer matching of donor with host, or infusion of donor lymphocytes that can affect development of graft-versus-host disease. *HLA*, Human leukocyte antigen; *HSC*, hematopoietic stem cell. (From Rich RR, Fleisher TA, Shearer, et al., editors: *Clinical immunology*, ed 5, Philadelphia, 2019, Elsevier.)

stem cells released into the bloodstream. Typically in the autologous setting, the patient is mobilized, with G-CSF given for 7 to 10 days after myelosuppressive chemotherapy. Disease status and prior treatment influence the ability to mobilize autologous PBSCs. The levels of HSCs rise up to 50-fold in the recovery phase after myelosuppressive chemotherapy and the administration of G-CSF. Sometimes a second drug, plerixafor (Mozobil), is used along with filgrastim in patients with non-Hodgkin lymphoma or multiple myeloma.

Umbilical Cord Blood

At birth, cord blood is collected and put into a sterile container, mixed with a preservative, and frozen. Umbilical cord blood transplantation has become a successful alternative therapeutic option for transplant patients who have no suitable related allogeneic donors. Benefits include greater availability of stem cells and possible antileukemic effects in patients with hematologic malignancies when a noninherited maternal antigen of the cord blood donor matches the patient's mismatched antigen.

The disadvantages of storing umbilical blood are:
- A single cord blood unit might not have enough stem cells for most adults, so personal cord blood use could be limited to childhood or early adolescence.
- Most medical specialists feel that the chance that the average child or close relative will be helped by storing their own cord blood is very low. Estimates have ranged from 1 out of 1000 to 1 out of 200,000. This means that most privately collected cord blood will likely be wasted.
- Some diseases that are treatable by transplant require allogeneic stem cells. Infusing autologous cord blood stem cells that contain the same defect would not cure the disease.
- The "shelf life" of cord blood is not known. Because cord blood storage is a recent development, scientists do not know whether blood taken at birth will be useful if a family member develops a disease treatable by stem cell transplant many decades later.
- Some scientists suspect that advances in immunology and genetics will reveal substitutes for stored cord blood.

Issues Related to Cord Blood Transplantation

The two critical concerns in the transplantation of umbilical cord blood are the initial time to engraftment and restoration of immune function.

Two factors have been found to be of extreme importance to patient and graft survival:
1. The total dose of progenitor (CD34+) cells in a cord blood unit has been associated with patient survival.
2. The total dose of clonogenic progenitors with the graft correlates with engraftment of the transplant.

A significant delay in recovery of all hematopoietic blood cell lines is a major complication. The initial engraftment of cells that develop into the myeloid cell line (red blood cells [RBCs], platelets, and granulocyte/monocyte) is 1 month. Development of T and B lymphocytes commonly takes 6 months or more after transplantation.

Immune reconstitution after stem cell transplantation is a complex process involving various components of the innate and adaptive immune systems. Two main pathways of T-cell regeneration contribute to post–T-lymphocyte recovery: thymopoiesis and peripheral blood expansion of mature T cells. Thymopoiesis provides a new pool of naïve T cells that is essential for sustained long-term immunity. Challenges to thymopoiesis can lead to a higher risk of opportunistic infections and an adverse outcome. Secondary cytopenia is a common complication of stem cell transplantation, which accounts for much of the morbidity and mortality associated with the procedure. Causes of secondary cytopenia include viral infection, septicemia, graft-versus-host disease (GVHD), and myelotoxic drugs. Older patients appear to be more prone to cumulative toxicities of posttransplantation drug regimens, but nonmyeloablative conditions, optimized HLA matching, and higher doses of CD34+ cell infusion may reduce the risk of cytopenia after day 28.

Engraftment

After the bone marrow or PBSCs are transplanted into the recipient via a central catheter, the cells migrate to the bone marrow where they begin to produce new blood cells in a process known as *engraftment*. The primary measure of hematopoietic recovery, or engraftment, is reached when the neutrophil count reaches at least 0.5×10^9/L for 3 consecutive days and a platelet count of 20×10^9/L is maintained without platelet transfusion. An STR analysis is performed in allogeneic transplants as a standard of care to monitor engraftment and detect any return of a recipient's malignancy.

Engraftment usually occurs within 2 to 4 weeks after the infusion of stem cells. The type of transplant, source, and dose of stem cells are factors influencing engraftment times. Complete recovery of immune function takes much longer, up to several months for autologous transplant recipients and 1 to 2 years for allogeneic transplant recipients. Studies have shown that patients receiving allogeneic PBSCs are less likely to have infections after transplantation than bone marrow recipients.

> **KEY CONCEPTS: Mechanisms of Transplantation Rejection**
> - T cells are able to interact with the histocompatibility molecules only if they are genetically identical (MHC restriction). Both class I and class II antigens function as targets of T lymphocytes that regulate the immune response.
> - Class I molecules regulate interaction between cytolytic T cells and target cells; class II molecules restrict the activity of regulatory T cells (helper, suppressor, and amplifier subsets).
> - Class II molecules regulate the interaction between Th cells and APCs.
> - HLA matching is of value in organ transplantation and in the transplantation of bone marrow, PBSCs, and umbilical cord blood cells.

Impact of HLA Matching

The donor-recipient HLA mismatch level affects the outcome of unrelated cord blood transplantation. Possible permissive mismatches involve the relationship between direction HLA mismatch vector or direction and transplantation outcomes. In most cord blood transplants, a mismatched HLA antigen is present in recipient and donor. This type of mismatch is bidirectional between the graft and the host. The preferred type of mismatch is a donor who is homozygous at an HLA locus but the patient has two antigens identified (one matching the donor) at that locus; only donor cells have an HLA target; and the mismatch is in the graft-versus-host (GVH) direction with a rejection mismatch. If all mismatched loci have this type of mismatch, these are GVH-only mismatches. Engraftment of myeloid cells is significantly faster, with grafts having GVH-only mismatches.

A major advantage of cord blood has been the ability to transplant grafts that are partially HLA-mismatched because of a relatively low incidence and severity of GVHD for the level of mismatch, a probable consequence of immunologic tolerance of this neonatal HSC source. Most cord blood transplantations to date (estimated at >30,000 globally) have been performed with grafts having one or two HLA-A, HLA-B, and HLA-DRB1 mismatches.

A new idea is to transplant stem cells into a fetus early in gestation. The benefit is that in utero transplantation would occur when the immune system of the fetus is immature, which would provide the theoretical opportunity to induce fetal tolerance of foreign cells. This would avoid rejection and the need for immunosuppressive therapy. To date, a major problem has been achieving adequate levels of engraftment.

GRAFT REJECTION

Organs vary with respect to their susceptibility to rejection based on inherent immunogenicity (Box 25.2), which is influenced by factors such as vascularity.

The role of sensitized lymphocytes and antibodies in graft rejection differs and is influenced by the type of organ transplanted. Lymphocytes, particularly recirculating small lymphocytes, are effective in shortening graft survival. Cell-mediated immunity is responsible for the rejection of skin and solid tumors. However, humoral antibodies can also be involved in the rejection process. The complexity of the action and interaction of cellular and humoral factors in grafts is considerable. Possible categories of graft rejection (Table 25.6 and Fig. 25.5) have been demonstrated in human kidney transplant rejection:

- Hyperacute
- Accelerated
- Acute
- Chronic
- Immunopathologic

First-Set and Second-Set Rejections

Skin transplantation is the most common experimental model for transplantation research (Fig. 25.6). Rejection of skin and solid tumors can be divided into first-set and second-set rejections. Activation of cellular immunity by T cells is the predominant cause of first-set allograft rejection. Lymphocytes can directly attack cellular antigens to which they are sensitized by previous exposure or by cytotoxic lymphokines. The primary role of lymphocytes in first-set rejection is consistent with the histology of early reaction and shows infiltration by mononuclear cells, with very few polymorphonuclear leukocytes or plasma cells. Sensitization occurs within the first few days of transplantation, and the tissue is lost in 10 to 20 days.

When sensitized lymphocytes are already present because of prior graft rejection, an accelerated rejection of tissue results from regrafting, called *second-set rejection*. Lymphocytes from a sensitized animal transferred to a first-graft recipient will accelerate rejection of the graft. Graft rejection is primarily a T-cell function, with some assistance from antibodies.

Hyperacute Rejection

Hyperacute rejection of an organ or tissue occurs within minutes after transplantation. The predominant mechanism of rejection is the presence of preformed humoral antibodies in the host, which react with donor tissue cellular antigens. These antibodies are usually anti-A–related or anti-B–related antibodies to the ABO blood group systems or antibodies to class I MHC antigens (hypersensitivity type II). Potential recipients harboring antibodies to HLA-A, HLA-B, and HLA-C (class I) but not HLA-DR (class II) antigens are at high risk for this process.

The interaction of cellular antigens with antibodies activates the complement system and leads to grafted cell lysis and clotting in the grafted tissue. Kidney allografts can be rejected by the hyperacute

---

BOX 25.2 One-Year United States National Organ Transplant Patient/Graft Survival[a] Rates

- Kidney patient rate (95.9%); graft rate (93.8%)
- Liver patient rate (93.7%); graft rate (91.9%)
- Heart patient rate (91.3%); graft rate (90.9%)
- Lung patient rate (88.4%); graft rate (87.7%)

[a] Graft survival refers to the survival of the transplanted organ. https://health.ucsd.edu/care/transplant-programs/quality/
Modified from the January 2023 Scientific Registry of Transplant Recipients (SRTR) Report.

TABLE 25.6 Categories and Characteristics of Graft Rejection Based on Immune Destruction of Kidney Grafts.

Type	Time of Tissue Damage	Predominant Mechanism	Cause
Hyperacute	Within minutes	Humoral	Preformed cytotoxic antibodies to donor antigens
Accelerated	2–5 days	Cell mediated	Previous sensitization to donor antigens
Acute	Several days or a few weeks	Cell mediated (possibly antibody cell–mediated cytotoxicity)	Development of allogeneic reaction to donor antigens
Chronic	Later than 3 months	Cell mediated	Disturbance of host-graft tolerance
Immunopathologic damage to the new organ	Later than 3 months	Immune complex disorder Complex formation with soluble antigens	Immunopathologic mechanisms related to circumstances necessitating transplantation

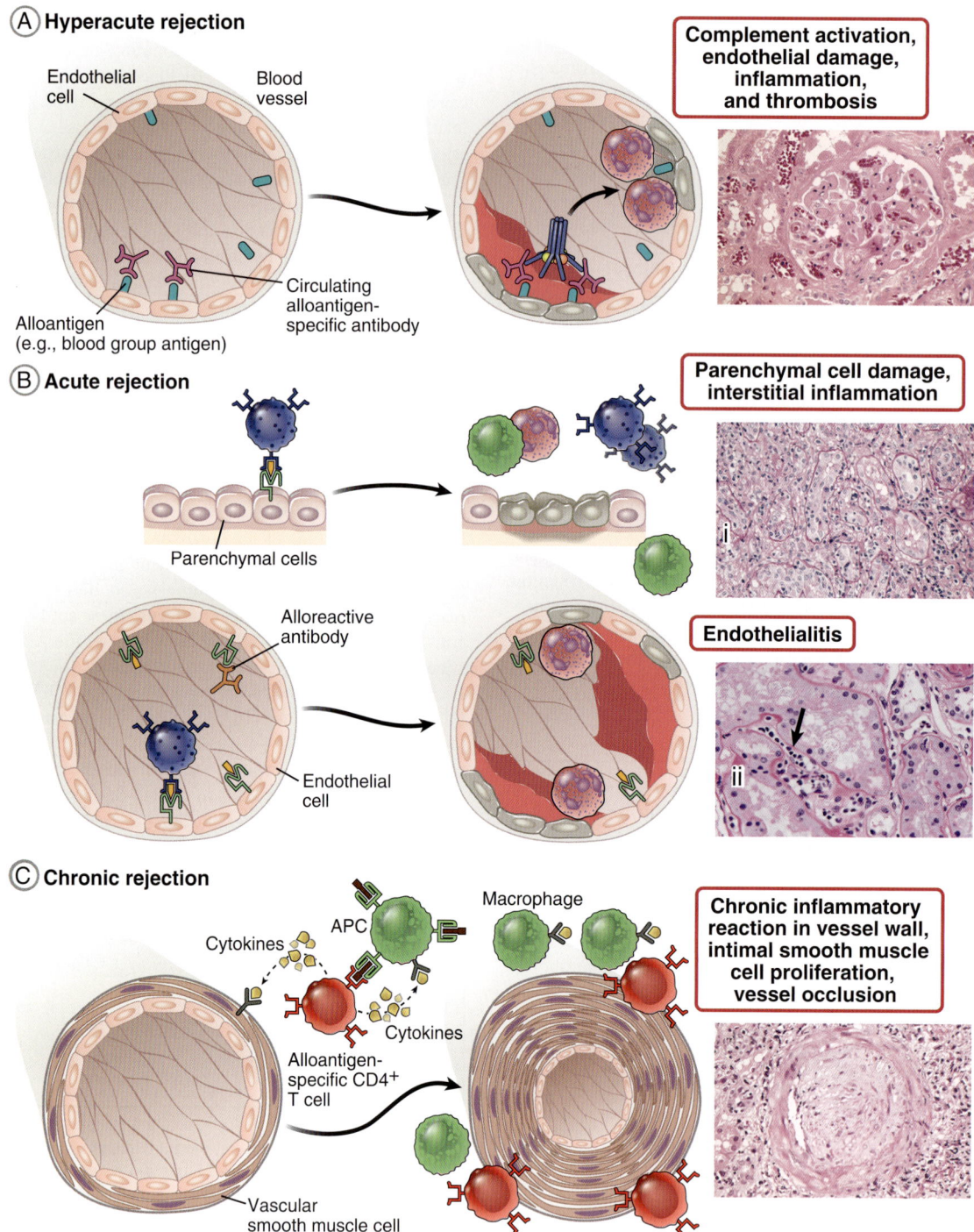

Fig. 25.5 Immune Mechanism of Graft Rejection. (From Abbas AK, Lichtman AHH, Pillai S: *Cellular and molecular immunology*, ed 7, Philadelphia, 2012, Saunders.)

rejection process within minutes of transplantation. The irreversible kidney damage of hyperacute rejection is characterized by sludging of erythrocytes, development of microthrombi in the small arterioles and glomerular capillaries, and infiltration of phagocytic cells.

Genetically altered pig organs could be available for transplantation into human beings within 2 years, but it is likely to be at least 5 years before full-scale studies can begin. Future xenotransplantation will depend on overcoming problems of hyperacute rejection. In hyperacute rejection, the recipient of the organ produces xenoreactive antibodies, which lodge on the cells lining the blood vessels of the new organ and trigger the release of complement. This release triggers inflammation, swelling, and ultimately blockage of the blood vessels, leading to death of the organ.

Accelerated Rejection

Accelerated rejection, which occurs 2 to 5 days after organ or tissue transplantation, is comparable to the second-set rejection phenomenon observed in animal models. In these cases, retransplantation is less severe than hyperacute rejection and is considered to be accelerated rejection. Accelerated rejection is caused by activation of the T-cell–mediated response.

Acute Rejection

Acute rejection can result after the first exposure to alloantigens. In this reaction, donor antigens select reactive T-cell clones and initiate visible manifestation of rejection in 7 to 21 days after transplantation. The early processes in acute rejection appear to be T-cell mediated; however, later aspects may involve antibodies and complement.

Acute rejection is equivalent to a first-set allograft rejection in experimental animals and is primarily mediated by cells, as in accelerated rejection. Immunopathologic changes include the presence of immune complex deposition and other hypersensitivity reactions already present in the recipient.

Acute rejection takes place when there is HLA incompatibility. Recipient T cells can respond to donor peptides presented by a recipient MHC or to donor MHC molecules themselves. The better the HLA match, the more successful the prospects for nonrejection. Because of the shortage of organs and the huge demand for organs, partially mismatched organs (e.g., kidneys) may be used. The survival of the kidney is related to the degree of mismatching, especially at the HLA-DR loci. Despite mismatching, 1-year survival with five mismatches was almost 80% because of the effect of potent immunosuppressive drugs.

A recipient may respond to minor histocompatibility antigens; minor antigens are encoded by genes outside the HLA. These minor histocompatibility antigen mismatches are not detected by standard tissue typing techniques but may cause rejection despite a good HLA match. Up to one-third of transplants can be rejected because of minor antigens.

Acute early rejection after transplantation is histologically characterized by dense cellular infiltration and rupture of peritubular capillaries. It appears to be a cell-mediated hypersensitivity reaction involving T cells. In comparison, acute late rejection occurs 11 days or more after transplantation in patients suppressed with prednisone and azathioprine. In kidney allografts, acute late rejection is probably caused by the binding of immunoglobulin, presumably antibody and complement, to the arterioles and glomerular capillaries, where they can be visualized by immunofluorescent techniques. These immunoglobulin deposits on the vessel walls include platelet aggregates in glomerular capillaries, which cause acute renal shutdown. Damage to antibody-coated cells through **antibody-dependent, cell-mediated cytotoxicity (ADCC)** is also possible.

Chronic Rejection

Chronic rejection of an organ or tissue occurs later than 3 months after transplantation. It occurs in most graft recipients as a result of a disturbance of host-graft tolerance. The process is a slow but continual loss of organ function over months or years. However, chronic rejection is often responsive to various immunosuppressive therapies.

In kidney allografts this insidious rejection is associated with subendothelial deposits of immunoglobulin and the C3 component of complement on the glomerular basement membranes. This may occasionally be an expression of an underlying immune complex disorder that may have originally necessitated the transplantation, or it may result from complex formation with soluble antigens derived from the grafted kidney.

MECHANISMS OF REJECTION

General Characteristics

Variations in the expression of class II histocompatibility antigens by different tissues and the presence of APCs in some tissues greatly influence the success of a transplant. APCs that enter the graft through the donor's circulation are likely to elicit graft rejection. If these so-called *passenger*

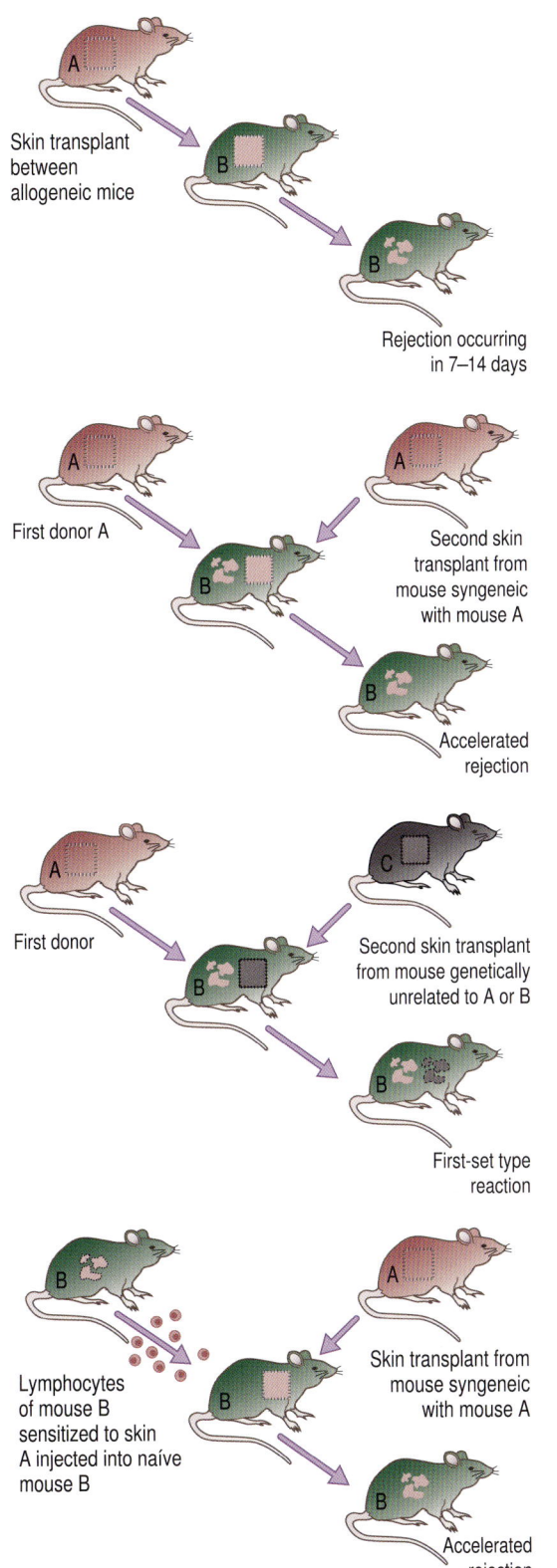

Fig. 25.6 Hyperacute rejection results from placement of tissue in an animal that already has antibodies to antigens of grafted tissue. Second-set rejection is an accelerated first-set reaction and is seen in animals that have already rejected tissue at least once. (Adapted from Barrett JT: *Textbook of immunology*, ed 5, St. Louis, 1988, Mosby.)

lymphocytes leave the graft after transplantation and enter the draining lymphatic system, they are particularly effective at sensitizing the host.

Rejection of a graft displays the following two key features of adaptive immunity:
- Memory
- Specificity

Only sites accessible to the immune system in the recipient are susceptible to graft rejection. Certain privileged sites in the body allow allogeneic grafts to survive indefinitely.

Role of T Cells

Graft rejection is primarily regulated by the interaction of the host's T cells with the antigens of the graft. Unmodified rejection, however, results from the destructive effects Tc cells, activated macrophages, and antibody.

In tissue transplants, the graft consists of tissue cells that carry class I antigens (HLA-A, HLA-B, and HLA-C) and of lymphocytes that carry class I and class II antigens (HLA-D and related antigens of an associated Ir gene). Activated T cells specific for class I antigens have the potential to express cytotoxic activity, which damages the endothelium and parenchymal cells of the graft. Binding of these cells to the class I antigens on target cells of the donor organ triggers the release of lymphokines and subsequently activates a nonspecific inflammatory response in the allograft.

T cells specific for class II antigens of the donor tissue cannot react directly with the parenchymal cells of the graft not expressing class II antigens. However, these cells can activate lymphocytes in the transplant through lymphocyte release. Therefore damage to the graft can result from a cytotoxic reaction directed against cells of the transplanted organ, a severe nonspecific inflammatory response, or both.

Activation of Th cells by class II antigens such as HLA-DR probably stimulates the release of interleukin-1 (IL-1). IL-1 subsequently stimulates the release of various lymphokines from Th cells, which in turn activate macrophages, Tc cells, and antibody-releasing B cells, and also increase the immunogenicity of the graft. In addition, macrophages and other accessory cells are subsequently stimulated by T-cell products and release IL-1, which in turn stimulates the formation of IL-2 receptors and the release of IL-2 by Th cells. IL-2 interacts with specific IL-2 receptors expressed on activated Th and Tc cells. This interaction stimulates the initiation of DNA synthesis and the eventual clonal proliferation of IL-2 receptor–bearing cells. IL-2 also causes the release of interferon-gamma (IFN-γ), which activates macrophages and stimulates the release of B-cell differentiation factors required for the proliferation of antigen-activated B cells. The release of IL-2–dependent IFN-γ by activated T cells may initiate a vicious cycle, because IFN-γ induces the expression of class II molecules on endothelial cells, in addition to the expression of certain class II–negative macrophages.

Histologic examination of an allogeneic skin graft during the process of rejection demonstrates that the dermis becomes infiltrated by mononuclear cells, many of which are small lymphocytes. This accumulation of lymphocytes precedes the destruction of the graft by several days. Although this graft rejection process is caused by Tc cells, in some cases Th cells are also elicited by MHC gene differences. Graft rejection may be a special form of response related to delayed hypersensitivity reactions, in which case the ultimate effectors of graft destruction are the monocyte-macrophages recruited to the site. It is debatable whether the macrophages seen in grafts are effectors of graft destruction or arrive only as a consequence of the inflammatory process and cell damage.

Antibody Effects

Cell-mediated immunity is the major effector mechanism in graft rejection. Antibodies, however, can also be involved in graft rejection. Antibodies can cause rapid (hyperacute) graft rejection, but they are usually less significant than cell-mediated immunity. Exceptions include cases in which the recipient has been previously sensitized to a particular antigen, when reactions occur to hematopoietic cells, or when the graft is directly connected to the host's blood circulation (e.g., kidney allograft).

In dispersed cellular grafts, such as infusion of erythrocytes, leukocytes, and platelets, antibodies (humoral immunity) may dominate the rejection process because antigens are fully exposed to a preexisting or developing antibody response. Cells are highly susceptible to complement-activated membrane damage. If cytolysis does not occur immediately, antibodies may function as opsonins to encourage phagocytic destruction of transfused cells.

Humoral immunity is suspected of playing a major role in the rejection of xenografts. Xenografts have a large number of antigens shared between donor and recipient. One species can have agglutinins for cells of distantly related species, which can attack the xenogenic tissue as soon as it is transplanted.

Immunosuppression

Forms of immunosuppression include chemical, biological, and irradiation of the lymphoid system or the donated organ. The immunosuppressive activities of therapeutic agents used in transplantation directly interfere with the allograft rejection response. Solid organ transplant patients take immunosuppressant drugs for their entire life, but HSC transplant patients receive immunosuppression for only about 1 year. The difference in the length of reliance on these drugs—lifelong versus about 1 year—is that in solid organ transplantation, medication keeps the recipient's immune system from recognizing the organ as foreign "nonself," but in HSC transplantation the recipient's immune system must elude recognition of foreign antigens only until the newly transplanted HSCs are recognized by the recipient's immune system as "self."

Since the discovery of cyclosporine there have been great advances in graft survival for patients receiving organ transplants (Box 25.3). Immunosuppressive measures may be antigen specific or antigen nonspecific (Table 25.7). Antigen-nonspecific immunosuppression includes drugs and other methods of specifically altering T-cell function. Many cytotoxic drugs are primarily active against dividing cells and therefore have some functional specificity for any cells activated to

BOX 25.3 Immunosuppression in Human Solid Organ Transplantation

1945–1960s	Research on antimetabolites, including 6-mercaptopurine, azathioprine, and corticosteroids, used to improve kidney graft survival
Late 1960s	Antilymphocyte globulin proved successful
1976	Cyclosporine developed
1983	Cyclosporine approved by the US Food and Drug Administration (FDA)
1984	OKT3 (muromonab-CD3) approved by the FDA
1994	Tacrolimus (FK-506) approved by the FDA
1995	Mycophenolic acid approved by the FDA (almost 30 years after development)
1996	Cyclosporine microemulsion (Neoral) approved by the FDA
1997	Antithymocyte globulin approved by the FDA
	Daclizumab (Zenapax) approved by the FDA
1999	Sirolimus (Rapamune) approved by the FDA
2004	Enteric-coated mycophenolic acid approved by the FDA
2008–2010	Generic formulations of both tacrolimus and mycophenolate mofetil approved by the FDA
2011	Nulojix (belatacept) approved by the FDA

TABLE 25.7	Types of Immunosuppressive Treatments.
Drug	Mechanism of Action
Corticosteroids	Reduce inflammation by inhibiting macrophage cytokine secretion
Cyclosporine and tacrolimus (FK506)	Blocks T-cell cytokine production by inhibiting the phosphatase calcineurin and then blocking activation of the NFAT transcription factor
Mycophenolate mofetil	Blocks lymphocyte proliferation by inhibiting guanine nucleotide synthesis in lymphocytes
Rapamycin	Blocks lymphocyte proliferation by inhibiting IL-2 signaling
Anti–IL-2 receptor (CD25) antibody	Inhibits T-cell proliferation by blocking IL-2 binding; may also opsonize and help eliminate activated IL-2R–expressing T cells
CTLA4-Ig (belatacept)	Inhibits T-cell activation by blocking B7 costimulator binding to T-cell CD28 (clinical trials), a selective T-cell costimulation blocker
Antithymocyte globulin	Binds to and depletes T cells by promoting phagocytosis or complement-mediated lysis (used to treat acute rejection)
Anti-CD52 (alemtuzumab)	Depletes lymphocytes by complement-mediated lysis

CTLA4-Ig, Cytotoxic T-lymphocyte–associated protein-4-immunoglobulin (fusion protein); *IL*, interleukin; *NFAT*, nuclear factor of activated T cells.
From US Food and Drug Administration: FDA approves Nulojix for kidney transplant patients. www.fda.org.

divide by donor antigens. The use of these drugs is limited by the toxic effects that they may have on other dividing cells or on the physiologic functioning of organs such as the liver.

Antigen-specific immunosuppression is an ideal form of immunosuppression. Antigen-specific tolerance is that induced by the infusion of donor cells. This is generally impractical in transplantation, but it may be useful in the phenomenon of immunologic enhancement. Enhancement of tolerance has been attempted in renal allograft patients. In a donor-specific blood transfusion program, the patient is transfused several times before elective transplantation with blood from the prospective kidney donor. The overall effect of these transfusions appears to be a tolerance of the recipient to donor transplantation antigens other than those in the HLA-linked regions, such as minor histocompatibility loci, RBC loci, and leukocyte surface antigens. This treatment has greatly prolonged graft survival in these patients.

Laboratory methods for measuring immunosuppressant drug concentrations in blood include immunoassay, high-performance liquid chromatography (HPLC), and liquid chromatography with mass spectrometry (LC-MS). Clinical laboratories are increasingly using LC-MS for routine measurement of immunosuppressants.

Immunosuppression is used for the following phases:
- Induction
- Maintenance of transplant
- Antirejection

Immunosuppressive treatment of the transplantation patient begins with the induction phase, before the procedure, and immediately after transplantation. Induction and maintenance strategies use different medicines at specific doses or at doses adjusted to achieve target therapeutic levels.

Induction immunosuppressive agents consist of depleting and nondepleting protein drugs (polyclonal and monoclonal antibodies) such as humanized monoclonal anti–CD-52 antibody (alemtuzumab) or B-cell–depleting monoclonal anti–CD-20 antibody (rituximab).

Maintenance therapy then continues for the life of the allograft. Maintenance immunosuppression is the key to prevention of acute and chronic rejections throughout the life of the graft. Maintenance immunosuppressive therapies include glucocorticoids and small-molecule drugs that bind immunophilin, such as cyclosporine, or that inhibit purine synthesis, such as mycophenolate mofetil, or pyrimidine synthesis, such as the antimetabolite azathioprine. There are also special agents, including IV immunoglobulin drugs such as rituximab, leflunomide, eculizumab (a C5 inhibitor), and bortezomib (a protease inhibitor).

Antirejection therapy is used in acute and chronic rejection therapy. Three agents used to treat acute rejection are steroids, antithymocyte globulin, and muromonab-CD3.
- Steroids: These agents are the mainstay of therapy for acute rejection episodes, preventing release of IL-1 by macrophages and blocking synthesis of IL-2 by Th cells. Steroids reverse 60% to 75% of rejection episodes.
- Antithymocyte globulin: This agent binds all circulating T and B lymphocytes, which are then lysed or removed by the mononuclear phagocytic system. Antithymocyte globulin is reserved for steroid-resistant acute rejection.
- Muromonab-CD3: This agent displaces the T3 molecule from antigen receptors, captures all mature T cells, and prevents alloantigen recognition. The reversal rate of first acute rejection episodes is 94%. Development of human antimurine antibodies allows for the reappearance of CD3 T cells, which may reduce the efficacy of the drug, which necessitates higher doses and increases the risk of infection. The success rate in recurrent episodes is approximately 40% to 50%.

Chronic rejection is a concern for the life span of a transplant. Long-term data on transplanted patients treated with sirolimus demonstrated a chronic rejection rate of 14%, which is much lower than rates traditionally reported in cyclosporine-based regimens. In a recent study of kidney transplant patients, patient and graft survival, and the mean glomerular filtration rate, patients receiving belatacept medication had significantly better outcomes than those receiving a cyclosporine regimen.

Pharmacologic Activity of Representative Immunosuppressant Drugs

Cytotoxic drugs are the most common form of therapy and usually include alkylating agents, purine and pyrimidine analogs, folic acid analogs, or the alkaloids. The drugs of choice, excluding alkylating drugs, include azathioprine.

Most immunosuppressive drugs administered alone cannot produce antigen-specific tolerance because they act equally on all susceptible clones. Except for certain drugs (e.g., cyclosporine), most immunosuppressive agents can be rendered antigen specific only by including an antigen-specific element in the tolerizing regimen. In these cases, the drugs act as cofactors in tolerogenesis. Experimental evidence has suggested that these regimens may act as follows:
- Lowering the threshold for tolerance induction
- Blocking the differentiation sequence in cells triggered by antigen

Azathioprine

Since its introduction in 1961, azathioprine, an oral purine analog that is an antimetabolite with multiple activities, has been the mainstay of antirejection therapy. Azathioprine requires activation to 6-mercaptopurine, which is further metabolized to active 6-thioguanine nucleotides. Metabolites of azathioprine, such as the in vivo metabolite 6-mercaptopurine, are incorporated into cellular DNA. This inhibits purine nucleotide synthesis and metabolism and alters the synthesis and function of RNA. Therefore azathioprine acts at an early stage in T-cell or B-cell activation during the proliferative cycle of effector lymphocyte clones. Azathioprine is useful in preventing acute rejection because it inhibits the primary immune response; however, it has little or no effect on secondary responses. Adverse effects include bone marrow suppression, myopathy, alopecia, pancreatitis, and hepatitis. A drug interaction can occur with allopurinol.

Corticosteroids

Corticosteroids can be used in conjunction with azathioprine or other immunosuppressants such as cyclosporine. Corticosteroids directly inhibit antigen-driven T-cell proliferation, but steroids do not act directly on the IL-2–producing T cell. They do, however, inhibit production of lymphokines by preventing monocytes from releasing IL-1, thereby blocking IL-1–dependent release of IL-2 from antigen-activated T cells. Other activities of monocytes, such as inhibition of chemotaxis, are also likely to be important in the immunosuppressive process.

High doses of corticosteroids are used to treat acute rejection. In addition, steroids probably reverse in vivo rejection episodes by preventing the production of IL-2, which would inhibit activated T cells as an essential trophic factor.

Cyclosporine (Cyclosporin A)

Cyclosporine, isolated in 1971 from the fungus *Tolypocladium inflatum*, has become the mainstay of immunosuppressive therapy in transplantation. Cyclosporine affects T cells preferentially by inhibiting the induction of Tc cells. Unlike corticosteroids, cyclosporine does not inhibit the capacity of all accessory cells to release IL-1. Cyclosporine blocks calcineurin to the IL-2 gene transcription pathway and the release of certain other lymphokines (e.g., IFN-γ). Cyclosporine binds to cyclophilin, and the complex binds to and inhibits calcineurin (a protein phosphatase). This prevents activation of the IL-2 transcription factor.

The secretion of B-cell growth and differentiation factors by activated T cells is also inhibited by cyclosporine. Therefore under the influence of cyclosporine, Th-cell–dependent B cells are not fully activated because of a lack of necessary Th-cell stimulation. In pharmacologic doses, however, cyclosporine does not grossly interfere with the activation and proliferation of suppressor T cells. Studies have shown prolonged renal allograft survival with cyclosporine, despite potential mismatches of the HLA system. Adverse effects of corticosteroids include fluid retention, electrolyte abnormalities, hyperglycemia, hypertension, peptic ulcer disease, osteoporosis, and adrenal insufficiency. Hepatotoxicity has been observed in 4% to 7% of patients. Drug interactions can occur with grapefruit juice, erythromycin, oral contraceptives, and a variety of other drugs. Drug monitoring is critical because of the narrow therapeutic range.

A newer cyclosporine microemulsion offers the advantage of improved trough measurement correlation with the actual patient circulating concentration.

Tacrolimus

Tacrolimus (FK-506), a macrolide with mechanisms similar to that of cyclosporine, is derived from a fungus, *Streptomyces tsukubaensis*, found in soil samples in Japan. FK-506 is 50- to 100-times more powerful than cyclosporine. Its primary target appears to be the Th lymphocytes, with little effect on other aspects of the immune response. FK-506 acts early in the process of T-cell activation and inhibits the production of IL-2. As a result, T lymphocytes do not proliferate, secretion of IFN-γ is inhibited, MHC class II antigens are not induced, and further activation of macrophages does not occur.

Because FK-506 is a more potent immunosuppressant than cyclosporine, patient recovery time is faster. FK-506 has higher toxicity compared with cyclosporine. Nephrotoxicity, hyperkalemia, hypokalemia, hypomagnesemia, hypertension, and other side effects may occur, but FK-506 causes no serious side effects (e.g., kidney damage, elevated blood pressure, and mood swings). Patients receiving FK-506 have increased susceptibility to infections (e.g., CMV) and an increased risk of developing lymphoma or posttransplantation lymphoproliferative diseases. Inhibitors and inducers of P-450 3A4 may demonstrate an altered rate of metabolism that requires an adjustment in drug dose. In July, 2015 Envarsus XR, an extended-release formulation of tacrolimus, a calcineurin-inhibitor immunosuppressant, was approved by the FDA.

Sirolimus

Sirolimus (Rapamune), previously referred to as *rapamycin*, was under development for more than 20 years before gaining approval by the FDA. Sirolimus is derived from the fungus *Streptomyces hygroscopicus* from the soil of Easter Island. Structurally sirolimus resembles tacrolimus and has the same intracellular binding protein or immunophilin, known as FKBP-12, but sirolimus has a novel mechanism of action. Sirolimus is a substrate for P-450 3A4 and inhibits the activation and proliferation of T lymphocytes and subsequent production of IL-2, IL-4, and IL-15. Sirolimus also inhibits antibody production. Sirolimus has been approved as an adjunctive agent (in combination with steroids) for the prevention of acute renal allograft rejection. The main side effects include increased risk of infections and lymphoma, hypercholesterolemia, hypertriglyceridemia, interstitial pneumonitis, insomnia and tremor, and thrombocytopenia.

Mycophenolate Mofetil

Mycophenolate mofetil (MMF; RS-61443) inhibits de novo guanosine synthesis by inhibiting inosine monophosphate dehydrogenase. This drug inhibits T- and B-lymphocyte proliferation and antibody formation by B lymphocytes, and has been efficacious as prophylactic and rescue therapy in refractory renal allograft rejection in clinical trials.

MMF (CellCept) is a drug that is now being used more frequently in treatment plans as a substitute for azathioprine. MMF prevents the production of cells but is believed to be more effective for preventing rejection in patients. Studies have suggested that MMF is effective in preventing acute rejection and may slow the progression to chronic rejection. Adverse side effects include a lowering of blood cell development, which can cause abdominal pain, vomiting, and diarrhea, but generally it is a well-tolerated drug.

Antilymphocyte (Antithymocyte) Globulin

Other immunosuppressive measures directed at T cells include the use of antilymphocyte (antithymocyte) globulin (ATG), an IgG polyclonal antibody, at the time of transplantation and the use of lymphoid irradiation before transplantation. The usefulness of ATG for preventing or reversing rejection in renal allograft recipients has been well established. Adverse side effects can include complement-mediated lysis of lymphocytes, serum sickness, leukopenia, and thrombocytopenia.

Among patients at high risk for acute rejection or delayed graft function who have received a kidney transplant from a cadaveric donor, induction therapy consisting of a 5-day course of antithymocyte globulin, compared with basiliximab, reduces the incidence and severity of acute rejection but not the incidence of delayed graft function.

A regimen of total lymphoid irradiation plus antithymocyte globulin reduces the incidence of acute GVHD and allows graft antitumor activity in patients with lymphoid malignant diseases or acute leukemia treated with hematopoietic cell transplantation.

Nulojix

One of the newer drugs is belatacept (Nulojix). This drug was approved by the FDA in 2011 to prevent acute rejection in adult patients who have had a kidney transplant. This drug is approved for use with other immunosuppressants (e.g., basiliximab, MMF, and corticosteroids). This type of drug is called a *selective T-cell costimulation blocker*.

Monoclonal Antibodies

A monoclonal antibody (muromonab-CD3) is used because the CD3 surface membrane marker is found on all mature postthymic T cells. Interaction between OKT3 and the surface of mature T lymphocytes causes T-cell depletion. The use of OKT3 reverses almost all acute renal transplant rejection and is indicated for the treatment of steroid-resistant rejection. A side effect of this drug is cytokine-release syndrome, a condition of flulike symptoms, dyspnea, aseptic meningitis, and pulmonary edema.

Immunosuppressive Protocols

Protocols for immunosuppression of transplant recipients vary widely, depending on the transplantation center, type of organ transplanted, underlying cause of organ failure, and preexisting conditions. Protocols are becoming more complex because of more immunosuppressive drug choices. In general, protocols include the following:
- Lymphokine synthesis inhibitors (e.g., cyclosporine and tacrolimus)
- Nucleoside synthetase inhibitors (e.g., azathioprine and MMF)
- Steroids (e.g., prednisone)
- Induction or pretransplantation therapy, which may include antithymocyte globulin, CD3 or CD25, or daclizumab

New Approaches in Immunosuppression

Survival after solid organ transplantation has increased in the era of tacrolimus and mycophenolate. These drugs have enhanced specificity and potency for T and B lymphocytes compared with their predecessors, cyclosporine and azathioprine. Between 2008 and 2010 the FDA approved several generic formulations of both tacrolimus and MMF. Deciding whether generic products can be safely substituted for the innovator product is a clinical dilemma similar to that which occurred when generic formulations of cyclosporine became available.

Suggested new strategies include the following:
- Cellular transplants
- Transgenic organs
- Development of chimerism
- Localized immunosuppression
- Prevention of chronic rejection

TRANSPLANTATION COMPLICATIONS

Post–Organ Transplantation

Because complications are associated with transplantation, their early diagnosis and treatment are essential. The primary risks of transplantation are rejection and infection. Five other major complications of organ transplantation are cancer, osteoporosis, diabetes, hypertension, and hypercholesterolemia.

Infectious Diseases

Infections can be viral, such as CMV (80%), EBV (20% to 30%), hepatitis B, or hepatitis C. Even rabies has been associated with organ transplantation. Other pathogens include *Pneumocystis jirovecii* (formerly known as *P. carinii*). Organisms associated with central nervous system infection in renal transplant recipients, in decreasing order of frequency, are *Listeria*, *Cryptococcus*, *Mycobacterium*, *Nocardia*, *Aspergillus*, *Mucor*, *Toxoplasma*, and *Strongyloides* spp. Published guidelines advise transplant teams to do the following to minimize transplant risk:
1. Screen for infectious disease agents in the donor and recipient before transplantation.
2. Culture and identify known and novel pathogens in recipients after transplantation.
3. Archive serologic samples before transplantation for identification of new infections later.

Cancer

Organ transplant recipients have a 20% greater risk of the development of cancer. The incidence of non-Hodgkin lymphoma is increased by 40%. The greatest risk for lymphoma is within the first 6 to 12 months after transplantation. Transplant recipients also have a greater risk of skin cancer and a slightly increased risk of cervical cancer. An increased risk of the development of cancer may be the result of chemotherapy and radiation therapy.

Osteoporosis

In the general population, osteoporosis affects one in four women and one in eight men. The general risk factors are age, postmenopausal state, sedentary lifestyle, and inadequate calcium intake. Transplant recipients are at an increased risk of developing osteoporosis because of pretransplantation immobility and the long-term effects of steroid therapy. Regular bone density scanning should be a routine component of posttransplantation care.

Diabetes

Diabetes mellitus is a concern in two risk groups: patients with preexisting diabetes (25%) and those who develop diabetes after transplantation (20%). Patients with preexisting diabetes may require increased doses of insulin until stabilized on medications. Posttransplantation steroid-induced hyperglycemia can produce physiologic conditions that negatively affect a graft. Steroid medication might aggravate a familial tendency toward diabetes. The use of steroids results in decreased use of insulin by peripheral tissues, eventual insulin resistance with decreasing receptor sites, reduction in insulin production, and accelerated glycogenolysis by the liver to assist in glucose availability. These metabolic activities perpetuate hyperglycemia. In addition to threatening graft survival, diabetes can have other negative health consequences, such as adult blindness, vasculopathy, neuropathy, retinopathy, bladder infections, and a shortened life span.

Hypertension

An abnormal increase in blood pressure is usually a preexisting medical condition in transplant recipients. This condition is often associated with renal failure. Hypertension can negatively affect the patient's general health and graft survival.

Hypercholesterolemia

Increased blood cholesterol is a serious posttransplantation concern because of long-term vascular effects to the patient and engrafted organ. Hypercholesterolemia can result from the return of the patient's appetite and the lifting of dietary restrictions.

Post–Stem Cell Transplantation

Complications after stem cell transplantation can range from infection, GVHD, rejection, and organ damage to infertility and death. Early complications usually occur within the first 100 days after transplantation. After a patient receives an allogeneic transplant, rejection rates can range between 1% and 2% in HLA-matched recipients and 5% to 10% in mismatched recipients. Minor ABO mismatches are present in 15% to 20% of HLA-matched donor-recipient pairs. Patients who receive hematopoietic progenitor cells from a minor ABO-incompatible donor are at risk of developing immediate immune hemolysis caused by isohemagglutinins infused with the marrow or PBSCs, or delayed hemolysis caused by isohemagglutinins produced by the donor lymphocytes (i.e., B cells). Immediate hemolysis can be avoided by simple removal of plasma from the graft before infusion. Delayed hemolysis caused by antibody production from donor-derived B lymphocytes requires the ex vivo removal of lymphocytes or suppression of T-lymphocyte function by cyclosporine.

Xenotransplantation

Xenotransplantation is any procedure that involves the transplantation, implantation, or infusion into a human recipient of either (1) live cells, tissues, or organs from a nonhuman animal source; or (2) human body fluids, cells, tissues, or organs that have had ex vivo (outside the body) contact with live nonhuman animal cells, tissues, or organs. The development of xenotransplantation is, in part, driven by the fact that the demand for human organs for clinical transplantation far exceeds the supply (Box 25.4). There is a global shortage of organs for transplantation. Pig heart valves are already used to repair human hearts, and porcine pancreatic islet cells are used to treat diabetes, so it is not a big leap to envision transspecies whole-organ transplantation. Pigs are considered the most likely organ transplant donors for human beings because their organs are similar in size to human organs, they are easy to breed, and the extensive biological differences between pigs and human beings make it unlikely for porcine diseases to infect human beings.

Another application of cross-species organ use was successfully demonstrated in a Phase I clinical trial that used transgenic pig livers as an ex vivo support system for patients with acute liver failure. The pig liver was used to bridge the gap between organ failure and obtaining an appropriate human liver for transplantation in these patients. Protocols are being developed for a phase I in vivo (inside the body) clinical trial.

Other procedures, some in clinical trials, use cells or tissues from other species to treat life-threatening illnesses such as cancer, AIDS, diabetes, liver failure, and Parkinson disease. Even if whole organs are not transplanted, animal cells or tissues will likely be used to treat many diseases. In 1995 physicians in California transplanted bone marrow from a baboon into an AIDS patient in a highly controversial procedure that prompted the creation of strict guidelines for transplantation by the FDA, National Institutes of Health (NIH), and Centers for Disease Control and Prevention.

Ethical and medical concerns surround xenotransplantation. Ethical concerns relate to selling organs. Donors may be paid as little as $1000 for a donated kidney in countries such as Brazil, India, or Moldova. A serious medical concern is the risk that transplanted tissue may carry unknown latent infections that, once introduced into the recipient, could be activated and give rise to infection.

BIOMARKERS FOR REJECTION

From the early era of solid organ transplantation, the main question has been whether grafts were rejected by antibodies or by cells. The

BOX 25.4 Milestones in Xenotransplantation

1963–1964	Chimpanzee to human renal transplants
1964	Pig heart valve transplant
1968	Sheep heart transplant
1984	"Baby Fae" transplanted with a baboon heart
1992	Baboon to human liver transplant
1994	Pig pancreatic islets transplanted to insulin-dependent patients
1995	Neuronal cells from fetal pig transplanted to patients with Parkinson disease
1996	Baboon bone marrow transplanted to patient with AIDS

association between hyperacute rejection after transplantation and the presence of preformed cytotoxic antibodies to donor HLA antigens has been well known for more than 30 years. Very recently a new definition of acute rejection has introduced the concept that appearance of DSA is critical in renal transplantation to establish the diagnosis of acute antibody-mediated rejection (AAMR).

Emerging technologies, such as gene expression profiling, proteomics, metabolomics, and genomics, are rapidly advancing the pace of discovery of new biomarkers for rejection. These approaches are expected to generate improved diagnostic tests and knowledge that will lead to more effective therapies.

One of the most promising areas of transplant research, especially kidney transplantation, has been the discovery of biomarkers for rejection that are detectable in blood and urine. Biopsy-confirmed rejection, the current gold standard for diagnosis of allograft rejection, is invasive and subject to sampling errors. Development of noninvasive assays that detect molecular biomarkers for rejection could revolutionize the management of transplant recipients by the following:

- Detecting a prerejection profile that will allow therapeutic interventions before rejection causes graft dysfunction
- Improving the sensitivity and specificity of rejection diagnosis
- Developing new classification systems for rejection that will improve the prognosis
- Providing information for designing individualized immunosuppressive regimens that could prevent rejection while minimizing drug toxicity
- Performing a Longitudinal Assessment of Posttransplant Immune Status

FOXP3 MESSENGER RIBONUCLEIC ACID (mRNA)

By studying concentrations of particular messenger RNAs (mRNAs) or proteins associated with immune activation or tissue stress, several gene products with altered expression in blood, urine, and biopsy tissue during rejection episodes have been identified. Urine concentrations of *FOXP3* mRNA, a member of the forkhead family of cell differentiation genes and a lineage-specific transcript for graft-protecting regulatory T cells, can predict reversal of acute renal allograft rejection with high sensitivity and specificity.

Measurement of the products of individual genes such as *FOXP3* probably will not supplant conventional biopsies for the diagnosis of rejection, but the development of panels of informative gene products in blood and urine, coupled with renal function and immune response markers, ultimately should achieve the sensitivities and specificities required for diagnosis and clinical management of kidney rejection.

Analyses of more than 1300 genes that were differentially expressed in kidney allografts have revealed three distinct molecular signatures of acute rejection that were more predictive of allograft survival than traditional histologic analysis. These data have also generated new hypotheses for the molecular mechanisms of rejection. For example, B-cell infiltration is characteristic of aggressive acute rejection.

A new gene expression test, AlloMap (XDx, San Francisco, California), is a panel of 20 gene assays, 11 informative and 9 used for normalization and quality control, which produces gene expression data used in the calculation of an AlloMap Score. The AlloMap test is based on quantitative real-time polymerase chain reaction (qRT-PCR) methodology using RNA purified from peripheral blood mononuclear cells (PBMCs).

The test is designed to detect the absence of moderate-to-severe cellular rejection, which might reduce the need for frequent biopsies.

GRAFT-VERSUS-HOST DISEASE

GVHD can be an unintentional consequence of blood transfusion or transplantation in severely immunocompromised or immunosuppressed patients. The degree of immunodeficiency in the host, rather than the number of transfused immunocompetent lymphocytes, determines whether GVHD will occur (Table 25.8).

> **KEY CONCEPTS: Graft-Versus-Host Disease**
> - Complications that develop from transplantation of bone marrow or PBSCs range from infection, GVHD, rejection, and organ damage to infertility and death.
> - Immunosuppressive measures may be antigen specific or antigen nonspecific. Antigen-nonspecific immunosuppression includes drugs and other methods of specifically altering T-cell function.
> - Immunosuppressive measures directed at T cells include the use of ATG at the time of transplantation and of lymphoid irradiation before transplantation.
> - Host immunity to the donor can cause GVHD, believed to result from the patient being sensitized to unshared HLA antigens before transplantation or transfusion.
> - When allogeneic T lymphocytes are transfused from donor to recipient with a graft or blood transfusion, the patient can develop acute or chronic GVHD.
> - Patients at risk for GVHD include those who are immunodeficient or immunosuppressed with severe lymphocytopenia and bone marrow suppression.

In allogeneic HSC transplantations performed due to a malignancy, a mild GVHD is welcome. GVHD can markedly improve a recipient's survival because the donor T cells can eliminate residual tumor cells caused by minor histocompatibility antigens.

Etiology

When immunocompetent T lymphocytes are transfused from a donor to an immunodeficient or immunosuppressed recipient, the transfused or grafted lymphocytes recognize that the antigens of the host are foreign and react immunologically against them (see Table 25.6). Instead of the usual transplantation reaction of host against graft, the reverse GVH reaction occurs and produces an inflammatory response.

In a normal lymphocyte transfer reaction, the results of a GVHD are usually not serious because the recipient is capable of destroying the foreign lymphocytes. However, engraftment and multiplication of donor lymphocytes in an immunosuppressed recipient are a real possibility because lymphocytes capable of mitosis can be found in stored blood products. If the recipient cannot reject the transfused lymphocytes, the grafted lymphocytes may cause uncontrolled destruction of the host's tissues and eventually death. A patient can develop acute or chronic GVHD. The stronger the antigen difference, the more severe the reaction.

TABLE 25.8 Requirements for Potential Graft-Versus-Host Disease.

Factor	Comment
Source of immunocompetent lymphocytes	Blood products, bone marrow transplant, organ transplant
Human leukocyte antigen differences between patient and recipient	The stronger the antigen difference, the more severe the reaction
Inability to reject donor cells	Patients are severely immunocompromised or immunosuppressed

Epidemiology

It is now accepted that GVHD can occur whenever immunologically competent allogeneic lymphocytes are transfused into a severely immunocompromised host. Patients at risk include those who are immunodeficient or immunosuppressed with severe lymphocytopenia and bone marrow suppression. Despite chemotherapy at the time of bone marrow transplantation, patients are highly likely to develop acute GVHD, and some of these immunocompromised patients will die of GVHD or associated infections.

Chronic GVHD affects 20% to 40% of patients within 6 months after transplantation. Two factors closely associated with the development of chronic GVHD are increasing age and a preceding episode of acute GVHD.

Cases of transfusion-related GVHD have increased significantly in the past 2 decades. This reaction has been reported subsequent to blood transfusion in bone marrow transplant recipients after total-body irradiation and in adults receiving intensive chemotherapy for hematologic malignancies. GVHD has also occurred in infants with severe congenital immunodeficiency and in those who received intrauterine transfusions followed by exchange transfusion. Almost 90% of patients with posttransfusion GVHD will die of acute complications of the disease. The usual cause of death is generalized infection.

Signs and Symptoms

GVHD causes an inflammatory response. Posttransfusion symptoms begin within 3 to 30 days after transfusion. Because of lymphocytic infiltration of the intestine, skin, and liver, mucosal destruction results, including ulcerative skin and mouth lesions, diarrhea, and liver destruction. Other clinical symptoms include jaundice, fever, anemia, weight loss, skin rash, and splenomegaly.

A patient who receives allogeneic peripheral blood progenitor cells may be at a greater risk for chronic GVHD, possibly because of the high amount of lymphocytes in the product. Many more lymphocytes are collected in a PBSC collection compared with a bone marrow collection. Conversely, this increase in lymphocytes could aid in the patient's immune reconstitution and also impart a graft-versus-leukemia effect.

GVHD can be attributed to many factors, including HLA mismatch between donor and recipient, conditioning regimen, viral exposure of donor and recipient, and dose of T cells infused into the patient.

Acute GVHD affects at least 40% to 60% of allogeneic HSC transplant patients after conditioning with myeloablative regimens, and it is a major cause of early morbidity and nonrelapse mortality in these patients. Acute GVHD occurs within the first weeks after transplantation, is the result of complex interactions among the donor T cells, and involves the recognition of MHC antigens on the recipient's organs (liver, gastrointestinal tract, skin, mucosal membranes). Glucocorticoids such as methylprednisolone or prednisone combined with cyclosporine are used to treat acute GVHD. New drugs and strategies available now or in clinical trials can supplement standard treatment.

In bone marrow transplant patients, acute GVHD develops within the first 3 months of transplantation. The initial manifestations are lesions of the skin, liver, and gastrointestinal tract. An erythematous maculopapular skin rash, particularly on the palms and soles, is usually the first sign of GVHD. Disease progression is characterized by diarrhea, often with abdominal pain, and liver disease. Other signs and symptoms of complications related to therapy include fever, granulocytopenia, and bacteremia. Interstitial pneumonia, frequently associated with CMV, can also occur.

Chronic GVHD occurs later and is defined as the presence or persistence of GVHD beyond 100 days since transplantation. Chronic GVHD can be prevented or controlled by medications. Corticosteroids are the primary therapy used for chronic GVHD. Cyclosporine may be combined with prednisone. Clinical trials are investigating GVHD that does not respond to steroid treatment (Box 25.5).

Chronic GVHD resembles a collagen vascular disease, with skin changes such as erythema and cutaneous ulcers, and a liver dysfunction characterized by bile duct degeneration and cholestasis. Patients with chronic GVHD are susceptible to bacterial infections. For example, increasing age and preexisting lung disease increase the incidence of interstitial pneumonia.

Immunologic Manifestation

In immunocompromised patients the transfused or grafted lymphocytes recognize the antigens of the host as foreign and react immunologically against them. Instead of the usual transplantation reaction of host against graft, the reverse GVHD occurs.

Diagnostic Evaluation

Laboratory evidence of immunosuppression or immunodeficiency, such as a decreased total lymphocyte concentration, suggests that a patient may develop GVHD. Evidence of inflammation, such as an increased C-reactive protein (CRP) level, elevated leukocyte count with granulocytosis, and increased erythrocyte sedimentation rate (ESR), may suggest that the disease has developed in GVHD candidates. Complications of anemia and liver disease, characterized by increased levels of bilirubin and blood enzymes (e.g., transaminases, alkaline phosphatase) and the presence of opportunistic pathogens (e.g., CMV) can further support the diagnosis.

Pathologic features include lymphocytic and monocytic infiltration into perivascular spaces in the dermis and dermoepidermal junction of the skin and into the epithelium of the oropharynx, tongue, and esophagus. Infiltration can also be observed into the base of the intestinal crypts of the small and large bowels and into the periportal area of the liver, with secondary necrosis of cells in infiltrated tissues. GVHD testing done in an HLA laboratory is conducted by performing STR analysis on affected skin regions where the donor's lymphocytes are in the recipient's skin.

Prevention

The incidence of GVHD can be minimized by depleting mature lymphocytes from the marrow through the use of monoclonal antibodies or physical methods. The risk of GVHD can be minimized, if not eliminated, by irradiation of the marrow transplant or blood products. Blood product irradiation is believed to be the most efficient and probably the most economic method available for the prevention of posttransfusion GVHD.

No cases of posttransfusion GVHD have been reported after the administration of blood products irradiated with an effective and appropriate radiation dose. Several categories of patients have the clinical indications for the use of irradiated products.

High-Risk Patients

Patients at the highest risk with an absolute need for irradiated blood products include the following:
- Recipients of autologous or allogeneic bone marrow grafts. Recipients of autologous bone marrow may be expected to have the same risk of posttransfusion GVHD as patients receiving allogeneic bone marrow.
- Children with severe congenital immunodeficiency syndromes involving T lymphocytes. The degree of immunodeficiency in the host, rather than the number of transfused immunocompetent cells, determines whether GVHD will occur.

Intermediate-Risk Patients

Patients considered to be at a lower risk of developing GVHD include the following:
- Infants receiving intrauterine transfusions, followed by exchange transfusions, and possibly infants receiving only exchange transfusions. The immune mechanism of the fetus and newborn may not be sufficiently mature to reject foreign lymphocytes, and

---

BOX 25.5 Drugs Used in Graft-Versus-Host Disease (GVHD)

Acute GVHD
- Antithymocyte globulin (rabbit ATG; thymoglobulin)
- Denileukin diftitox (Ontak)
- Monoclonal antibodies, such as daclizumab (Zenapax), infliximab (Remicade), or, more rarely, alemtuzumab (Campath)
- Mycophenolate mofetil (CellCept)
- Sirolimus (Rapamune)
- Tacrolimus (Prograf)
- Oral nonabsorbable corticosteroids such as budesonide or beclomethasone dipropionate
- Intraarterial corticosteroids
- Pentostatin (Nipent)
- Extracorporeal photopheresis (a procedure under study that removes, treats, and reinfuses the patient's blood)
- Infusions of mesenchymal stem cells (experimental only)

Chronic GVHD
- Daclizumab (Zenapax)
- Etanercept (Enbrel)
- Extracorporeal photopheresis
- Infliximab (Remicade)
- Mycophenolate mofetil (CellCept)
- Pentostatin (Nipent)
- Rituximab (Rituxan; experimental only)
- Tacrolimus (Prograf)
- Thalidomide (Thalomid)
- Imatinib mesylate (Gleevec) for some skin changes

prior transfusions may induce a state of immune tolerance in the newborn. Transfused lymphocytes may continue to circulate for a prolonged period in some immunologically tolerant hosts without the development of GVHD. There is insufficient evidence to recommend irradiation of blood given to all premature infants.
- Patients receiving total-body radiation or immunosuppressive therapy for disorders such as lymphoma and acute leukemia. Although routine irradiation of blood products given to these patients can be justified, it cannot be regarded as absolutely indicated because the risk of developing GVHD is so low. Blood product irradiation, however, is advised for selected patients with hematologic malignancies, especially when transfusions are given during or near the time of sustained and severe therapy-induced immunosuppression.

Low-Risk Patients

Patients also at risk but considered the least susceptible include the following:
- Patients with solid tumors. The incidence of the development of GVHD in these patients is difficult to determine. However, it has developed in nonhematologic malignancies such as neuroblastoma. In one case GVHD developed after infusion of a single unit of packed RBCs.
- Patients with aplastic anemia receiving antithymocyte globulin theoretically may be at increased risk of posttransfusion GVHD during therapy-induced periods of lymphocytopenia.
- Although a theoretical risk of posttransfusion GVHD may exist in patients with AIDS, the disease has not actually been observed in this disorder. The routine use of irradiated blood is not recommended.

Effects of Radiation on Specific Cellular Components

Lymphocytes. Ionizing radiation is known to inhibit lymphocyte mitotic activity and blast transformation. Irradiation of normal donor lymphocytes with 1500 rad from a cesium-137 source results in a 90% reduction in mitogen-stimulated ^{14}C-thymidine incorporation. An 85% reduction in mitogen-induced blast transformation after exposure to 1500 rad and a 97% to 98.5% reduction in mitogenic response have been noted after an appropriate exposure to radiation.

Granulocytes. Ionizing radiation may impair granulocyte function in a dose-dependent manner. The degree of actual damage to granulocytes is controversial. Chemotactic activity decreases linearly with increasing doses of irradiation from 500 to 120,000 rad, but the reduction only reaches statistical significance at 10,000 rad. A linear dose-response curve demonstrates that granulocyte locomotion is affected by very small doses of irradiation. An appropriate dose of radiation is likely to eliminate lymphocytic mitotic activity and prevent GVHD without causing significant damage to granulocytes or altering their chemotactic or bactericidal ability. Irradiation before transfusion has been demonstrated to contribute to defective oxidative metabolism, but this effect is highly variable.

Mature red blood cells. Mature RBCs appear to be highly resistant to radiation damage. In the general opinions of hematologists, after RBCs were exposed to 10,000 rad, ^{52}Cr-labeled in vivo RBC survival was the same as that of untreated controls. Stored erythrocytes can be treated with up to 20,000 rad without changing their viability or in vitro properties, including adenosine triphosphate (ATP) and 2,3-diphosphoglycerate (2,3-DPG) levels, plasma hemoglobin (Hb), and potassium ions (K^+).

Platelets. Ionizing radiation may impair platelet function. Although this impairment is dose dependent, the effects of irradiation on platelets have been difficult to characterize. Several studies have demonstrated unchanged in vivo platelet survival after exposure to 5000 to 75,000 rad. A 33% decrease in the expected platelet count increase was noted after transfusion of platelets exposed to 5000 rad, and similarly irradiated autologous platelets had a diminished ability to correct the bleeding times in a small number of volunteers who had consumed aspirin.

CURRENT DIRECTIONS

Genetic engineering of HSCs holds the promise of potentially treating many hereditary and acquired diseases. The promise of this form of therapy is exciting, but it does have limitations. The technologies used to date have occasionally resulted in clonal expansion, myelodysplasia, or leukemogenesis.

At present, technology is challenged by the inability to expand or clone genetically modified HSCs from adult or cord blood specimens. New genetic material must be permanently introduced to correct the underlying disease mutation in the treatment of genetic disorders. Safer and more effective methods will rely on the therapeutic use of pluripotent stem cells.

A recent approach consists of direct reprogramming of skin cells to a multipotent progenitor stage by the introduction of a single transcription factor. Reprogrammed progenitor cells may have desirable traits. Reprogrammed human adult stem cells could be stimulated to an expandable condition without reducing the long-term self-renewal properties and their safety.

CASE STUDY 25.1

A 40-year-old, CG, was seen by her family physician after several episodes of painless hematuria. On direct questioning, she complained of worsening malaise and swelling of her legs and hands over the previous 2 weeks. She also reported that despite a high fluid intake, she was urinating much less frequently than normal. She had no significant medical history.

On examination, the patient was pale and had generalized swelling of her extremities. Her temperature was 38.5°C (101°F) and her blood pressure was 160/110 mm Hg. She had no palpable masses or hepatosplenomegaly.

A diagnosis of idiopathic and rapidly progressive glomerulonephritis was made. She was given antihypertensive agents, corticosteroids, and azathioprine for 2 weeks, but her renal function deteriorated and end-stage renal failure was diagnosed. Hemodialysis was initiated.

In preparation for a possible renal transplant, she was tissue typed for major histocompatibility complex (MHC) antigens using anti–human leukocyte antigen (HLA) antibodies. She was found to be HLA-A10, A28, B7, Bw52, Cw2, Cw6, DR2, DRw10, and blood group B positive. A suitable cadaveric kidney was found

Continued

CASE STUDY 25.1—cont'd

from a donor of HLA-A9, A28, B7, B17, Cw2, Cw6, DR2, DR4, and blood group B positive. A crossmatch of the patient's serum with donor lymphocytes was satisfactory.

She underwent successful kidney transplantation. Her posttransplantation treatment was a combined triple-immunosuppressive regimen of prednisolone, cyclosporine, and azathioprine. She progressed well immediately after transplantation.

Twelve days after engraftment, the patient developed a fever and was noted to be lethargic. Physical examination revealed generalized edema. Her blood pressure was 165/110 mm Hg. Her urine output had dropped significantly and a renal biopsy was performed. Histologic examination demonstrated significant interstitial mononuclear cell infiltration. This finding was consistent with the diagnosis of acute graft rejection. She was immediately treated with parenteral methylprednisolone. This treatment failed to improve her renal function, and an antilymphocyte monoclonal antibody was administered. Her renal function improved, and she was eventually discharged receiving cyclosporine therapy.

Questions

1. Class II major histocompatibility complex (MHC) antigens are encoded for in the _____ region.
   a. A
   b. B
   c. C
   d. D
2. In a kidney transplant, antibody to ABO antigens of donor tissue will produce _____ rejection.
   a. Hyperacute
   b. Acute
   c. Delayed
   d. Chronic

Answers to these questions can be found in Appendix A.

Critical Thinking Group Discussion Questions

1. What factors are important in matching donor to recipient in renal transplantation?
2. How does this patient's graft rejection compare with other types of graft rejection?

REVIEW QUESTIONS

1. MHC class I includes:
   a. HLA-A, -B, -C
   b. HLA-DP, -DQ, -DR
   c. Complement
   d. Cytokines
2. The preferential matching of bone marrow donor and recipient is the _____ system.
   a. ABO
   b. Rh
   c. HLA
   d. Kell
3. An HLA-DR mismatch is the most important the first_____ after transplantation.
   a. Month
   b. 2 months
   c. 6 months
   d. 2 years
4. The definition of an allograft is:
   a. Graft transplanted between different but identical recipient and donor
   b. Graft transferred from one position to another in the same individual
   c. Graft between genetically different recipient and donor of the same species
   d. Graft between individuals of different species
5. Graft-versus-host disease is most frequently associated with which transplant?
   a. Cornea
   b. Bone marrow
   c. Bone matrix
   d. Lung
6. The definition of a hyperacute graft rejection is:
   a. Caused by preformed cytotoxic antibodies
   b. An immunopathologic mechanism
   c. Caused by previous sensitization to donor antigens
   d. Disturbance of host-graft tolerance
7. The definition of an accelerated graft rejection is:
   a. Caused by preformed cytotoxic antibodies
   b. An immunopathologic mechanism
   c. Caused by previous sensitization to donor antigens
   d. Disturbance of host-graft tolerance
8. The definition of an acute graft rejection is:
   a. Caused by preformed cytotoxic antibodies
   b. An immunopathologic mechanism
   c. Donor antigens select reactive T-cell clones and initiate visible rejection
   d. Disturbance of host-graft tolerance
9. The definition of a chronic graft rejection is:
   a. Caused by preformed cytotoxic antibodies
   b. An immunopathologic mechanism
   c. Caused by previous sensitization to donor antigens
   d. Disturbance of host-graft tolerance
10. The immune system functions in a detrimental way in:
    a. Hypersensitivity reactions
    b. Autoimmunity
    c. Transplantation
    d. All of the above
11. The probability of success in organ and tissue transplantation increases as a result of:
    a. Histocompatibility testing
    b. Immunosuppression
    c. Surgical technique
    d. Both a and b

12. The D region of the major histocompatibility complex (MHC) codes for class _____ molecules.
    a. I
    b. II
    c. III
    d. IV
13. Class I includes HLA-_____ antigens.
    a. A, B, and C
    b. B, C, and D
    c. DR, DC (DQ), and A
    d. DR, DC (DQ), and SB
14. Class I molecules:
    a. Regulate interaction between cytolytic T cells and target cells
    b. Restrict activity of regulatory T cells and target cells
    c. Regulate interaction between helper T cells and antigen-presenting cells
    d. Represent components of the complement pathways
15. The 1-year survival for kidney transplantation from HLA-identical siblings approaches:
    a. 50%
    b. 75%
    c. 95%
    d. 100%
16. The most common form of bone marrow transplant is:
    a. Allogeneic
    b. Autologous
    c. Xenograft
    d. Syngraft
17. Potential GVHD has all of the following characteristics except:
    a. Source of immunocompetent T lymphocytes
    b. Source of immunocompetent B lymphocytes
    c. HLA differences between patient and recipient
    d. Inability to reject donor cells
18. In GVHD posttransfusion, symptoms begin within _____ day(s) after transfusion.
    a. 1
    b. 2 to 4
    c. 3 to 5
    d. 3 to 30
19. GVHD can be prevented by:
    a. Irradiating the patient pretransfusion
    b. Irradiating the blood component pretransfusion
    c. Administering antibiotics pretransfusion
    d. Administering steroids posttransfusion
20. The first successful immunosuppression therapy in renal transplantation was:
    a. Azathioprine
    b. Corticosteroids
    c. Cyclosporine
    d. Antilymphocyte globulin
21. The following diseases are treatable by stem cell transplantation:
    a. Acute lymphoblastic leukemia and acute myelogenous leukemia
    b. Aplastic anemia and non-Hodgkin lymphoma
    c. Severe combined immunodeficiency disease and chronic myeloid leukemia
    d. All of the above
22. Progenitor blood cells are:
    a. Pluripotent
    b. Found only in bone marrow
    c. Not useful in reconstituting a person's immune system
    d. Determined by the exact number of CD34+ and stem cells
23. Pretransplantation evaluation includes:
    a. HLA tissue typing and hepatitis screening
    b. Electrocardiography and CBC
    c. Bone marrow biopsy and complete history, including physical examination
    d. All of the above
24. In adults, bone marrow is usually aspirated from:
    a. Sternum
    b. Anterior iliac crest
    c. Posterior iliac crest
    d. Vertebrae
25. Peripheral blood stem cells (PBSCs) are obtained by:
    a. Phlebotomy
    b. Apheresis
    c. Leukapheresis
    d. Both b and c
26. Engraftment of bone marrow or PBSCs is:
    a. Cell production in the bone marrow
    b. Matching the donor and patient
    c. Measured by the number of lymphocytes in circulation
    d. Antibody production
27. Complications of bone marrow or PBSC transplantation include:
    a. Infection and graft-versus-host disease (GVHD)
    b. Acute rejection and organ damage
    c. Chronic rejection and death
    d. All of the above
28. Differences between donor's and recipient's ABO or Rh blood groups have _____ effect on marrow engraftment.
    a. No
    b. Some
    c. A major
    d. A total
29. Stem cell selection can be improved using the CD_____ cell surface marker.
    a. 4+
    b. 8+
    c. 34+
    d. 56+
30. Increased cell selection and purging of grafts using cell surface membrane markers has resulted in:
    a. Decreased risk of tumor reinfusion
    b. Lesser GVHD
    c. Transfusing fewer erythrocytes as contaminants
    d. All of the above

26

Tumor Immunology and Applications of Massive Parallel Sequencing/Next-Generation Sequencing

LEARNING OUTCOMES

- Compare the characteristics of benign and malignant tumors.
- Describe the epidemiology of cancer in adults and children.
- Explain the characteristics of the three major causative factors in human cancer.
- Compare the stages of carcinogenesis.
- Describe the aspects of cancer-related genes.
- Define and give examples of proto-oncogenes.
- Describe the role of oncogenes.
- Describe the characteristics of the major body defenses against cancer.
- Identify and discuss the characteristics of tumor markers.
- Discuss what's new in cancer diagnostic testing.
- Compare various modalities for treating cancer.
- Analyze representative case studies.
- Correctly answer case study–related multiple-choice questions.
- Participate in a discussion of critical thinking questions.
- Describe the principle and clinical applications of the prostate-specific antigen procedure.
- Correctly answer end-of-chapter review questions.

OUTLINE

Cancer Stem Cells, 455
Types of Tumors, 455
    Benign Tumors, 455
    Malignant Tumors, 455
Epidemiology, 457
    Cancer in Adults, 457
    Cancer in Children, 457
    Risk Factors, 457
Causative Factors in Human Cancer, 457
    Environmental Factors, 457
    Microbial Carcinogens, 457
    Host Factors and Disease Associations, 457
Impact of Somatic Mutations, 458
    Driver, Actionable, and Passenger Mutations, 459
Stages of Carcinogenesis, 459
Cancer-Predisposing Genes, 459
Proto-Oncogenes, 460
    p53 or *tp53* Gene, 460
Role of Oncogenes, 460
    Mechanisms of Activation, 460
    Viral Oncogenes, 461
    Tumor-Suppressing Genes, 461
Body Defenses Against Cancer, 461
    T Lymphocytes, 461
    Natural Killer Cells, 462
    Macrophages, 462
    Antibodies, 462
Tumor Markers, 462
Variety of Tumor Markers, 462
    Categories of Tumor Antigens, 465
        Tumor-Specific Antigens, 467
        Tumor-Associated Antigens, 467
        Carcinofetal Antigens, 467
        Spontaneous Tumor Antigens, 467
    Classic Tumor Markers, 467
        Alpha-Fetoprotein, 467
        CA 125, 467
        Human Epididymis Protein 4, 467
        Thyroglobulin, 467
        Prostate-Specific Antigen and Prostatic Acid Phosphatase, 468
        Carcinoembryonic Antigen, 468
        CA 19-9, 468
        CA 15-3, 468
        CA 27.29: Breast Carcinoma–Associated Antigen, 468
        HER2 (HER2/neu), 468
    Other Cancer Biomarkers, 469
        Human Chorionic Gonadotropin (hCG), 469
        Miscellaneous Enzyme Markers, 469
        Miscellaneous Hormone Markers, 469
    Breast, Ovarian, and Cervical Cancer Markers, 469
        Epidermal Growth Factor Receptor, 469
        Molecular Diagnosis of Breast Cancer, 470
    Bladder Cancer, 470
DNA Microarray Technology, 470
What's New in Cancer Diagnostic Testing?, 470
    Massive Parallel Sequencing/Next-Generation Sequencing, 470
    Identification of Somatic Mutations, 470
    Detection of Low Levels of Genomic Alterations, 471
    Improved Management of Cancer Treatment, 471
    Continuous Field Flow–Assisted Dielectrophoresis, 471
Modalities for Treating Cancer, 471
    Chemotherapeutic Agents, 471
        Cell Cycle Active, Phase Specific, 471
        Cell Cycle Active, Phase Nonspecific, 471

CHAPTER 26 Tumor Immunology and Applications

Non–Cell Cycle Active, 471
Cytokines, 472
Effects of Drug-Induced Immunosuppression, 472
Monoclonal Antibody Therapy, 472

Case Study 26.1, 474
Case Study 26.2, 474
Procedure: Prostate-Specific Antigen Rapid Test of Seminal Fluid (Seratec), 476.e1

KEY TERMS

actionable mutations
adenomas
alpha-fetoprotein (AFP)
antioncogenes
benign
carcinoembryonic antigen (CEA)
carcinoma
carcinoma in situ
cytochrome P-450
DNA microarray technology
driver mutation
immunosurveillance
malignant
neoplasms
oncofetal proteins
oncogenes
p53 or *tp53* gene
passenger mutations
proto-oncogenes
purine analogs
spontaneous tumor antigens
tumor necrosis factor
tumor-specific antigens (TSAs)

Oncology is that branch of medicine devoted to the study and treatment of tumors. The term *tumor* is commonly used to describe a proliferation of cells that produces a mass rather than a reaction or inflammatory condition. Tumors are neoplasms and are described as benign or malignant. Most tumors are of epithelial origin (ectoderm, endoderm, or mesoderm); the remaining tumors are of connective tissue origin (Fig. 26.1). The key distinction between benign and malignant tumors is the ability of malignant tumors to invade normal tissue and metastasize to other secondary sites.

> **KEY CONCEPTS: Types of Tumors**
> - Tumors are neoplasms described as benign or malignant.
> - A benign neoplasm is a nonspreading tumor; a malignant neoplasm is a growth that infiltrates tissues, metastasizes, and often recurs after attempts to remove it surgically.
> - A malignant neoplasm can be referred to as *carcinoma* or *cancer*.

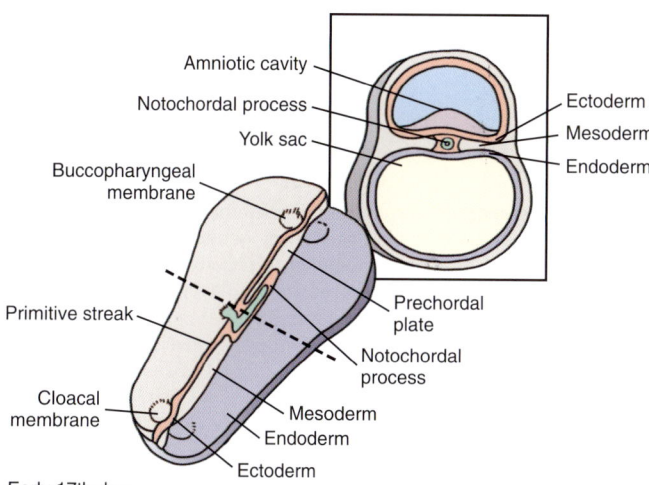

Fig. 26.1 Embryonic Primary Germ Layers. (Adapted from Larsen WJ: *Human embryology*, ed 3, Philadelphia, 2001, Churchill Livingstone.)

CANCER STEM CELLS

Biology research studies have discovered that stem cells are critical for the generation of complex multicellular organisms and the development of tumors. To cure a cancer through stable long-term remission, the stem cell compartment of a tumor needs to be eradicated. Stem cells have three distinctive properties:
1. Self-renewal when daughter cells retain the same biological properties as the parent cell
2. Capability to develop into multiple lineages
3. Potential to proliferate extensively

If normal self-renewal is subverted, it becomes abnormal self-renewal. If increased self-renewal occurs, combined with the intrinsic growth potential of stem cells, it may yield a malignant phenotype. It is possible that cancer stem cells can arise by mutation from normal stem cells or mutated progenitor cells (Fig. 26.2).

TYPES OF TUMORS

Benign Tumors

Benign tumors are often named by adding the suffix *-oma* to the cell type (e.g., lipoma), but there are exceptions (e.g., lymphomas, melanomas, and hepatomas). Benign tumors arising from glands are called adenomas; those from epithelial surfaces are termed *polyps* or papillomas.

Benign tumors are characterized by the following:
- Usually are encapsulated
- Grow slowly
- Usually are nonspreading
- Have minimal mitotic activity
- Resemble the parent tissue

Other types of tumors include nonneoplastic lesions associated with an overgrowth of tissue that is normally present in the organ (e.g., hyperplastic tissue) and choristomas, normal tissue in a foreign location (e.g., pancreatic tissue in the stomach).

Malignant Tumors

A malignant neoplasm of epithelial origin is referred to as carcinoma, or cancer. Those arising from squamous epithelium (e.g., esophagus and lung) are called *squamous cell carcinomas*, those arising from glandular epithelium (e.g., stomach, colon, and pancreas) are called *adenocarcinomas*, and those arising from transitional epithelium in the urinary system are called *transitional cell carcinomas*.

Other types of malignant tumors include amine precursor uptake and decarboxylational tumors. These are neuroendocrine tumors that commonly develop from neural crest and neural ectoderm (e.g., small cell carcinoma of the lung). Sarcomas, malignant tumors of connective tissue origin (e.g., fibrosarcoma), and teratomas are derived from all three germ cell layers (e.g., teratoma of the ovary or testis).

Malignant tumors are characterized by the following:
- Increase in the number of cells that accumulate
- Usually, invasion of tissues
- Dissemination by lymphatic spread or by seeding within a body cavity
- Metastasis
- Characteristic nuclear cellular features
- Receptors for integrin molecules (e.g., fibronectin), which help malignant cells adhere to extracellular matrix; type IV collagenases, which dissolve basement membranes; and proteases
- Secretion of transforming growth factor-α (TGF-α) and transforming growth factor-β (TGF-β) to promote angiogenesis and collagen deposition
- Often, recurrence after attempts to eradicate the tumor by surgery, radiation, or chemotherapy

Biologically distinct and relatively rare populations of tumor-initiating cells have been identified in cancers of the hematopoietic system, brain, and breast. Cells of this type have the capacity for self-renewal, the potential to develop into any cell in the overall tumor population, and the proliferative ability to drive continued expansion of the population of malignant cells. The properties of these tumor-initiating cells closely parallel the three features that define normal stem cells. Malignant cells with these functional properties are termed *cancer stem cells* (Fig. 26.3). Cancer stem cells can be the source of all the malignant cells in a primary tumor.

Despite decreases in the incidence of some cancers and associated mortality, cancer remains highly lethal and very common. About 41% of Americans will develop some form of cancer, including nonmelanoma skin cancer, in their lifetime; 20% of Americans will die of cancer. Cancer is the second leading cause of death in the United States.

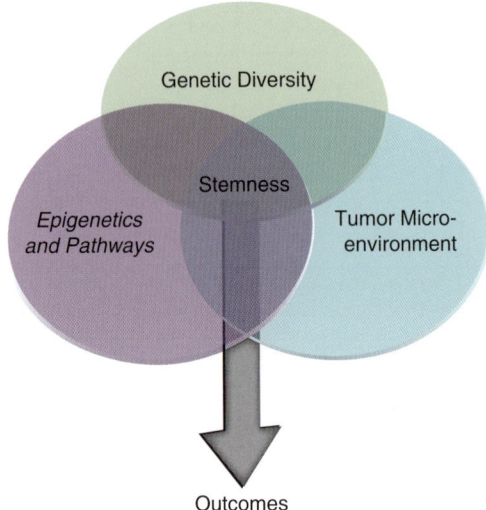

Fig. 26.2 Stemness as a guiding principle that governs therapeutic response. Three fields of biology—cancer genetics, epigenetics, and microenvironment—are coming together to provide increasing clarity to the processes that determine stemness and in turn influence clinical outcome. These three factors can influence stemness simultaneously, but they can also act independently over time. Through evolutionary time, different forces can affect a cell's stemness properties and thereby shape tumor progression and therapeutic response. (From Kreso A, Dick JE: Evolution of the cancer stem cell model, *Cell Stem Cell* 14[3]:75–291, 2014.)

> **KEY CONCEPTS: A Profile of Cancer Incidence**
> - The incidence of cancer has been correlated with certain environmental factors (e.g., occupational exposure to known carcinogenic agents) and host susceptibility.
> - Cancer often begins when a carcinogenic agent damages the DNA of a critical gene in a cell.
> - A mutant cell multiplies, and the succeeding generations of cells aggregate to form a malignant tumor.

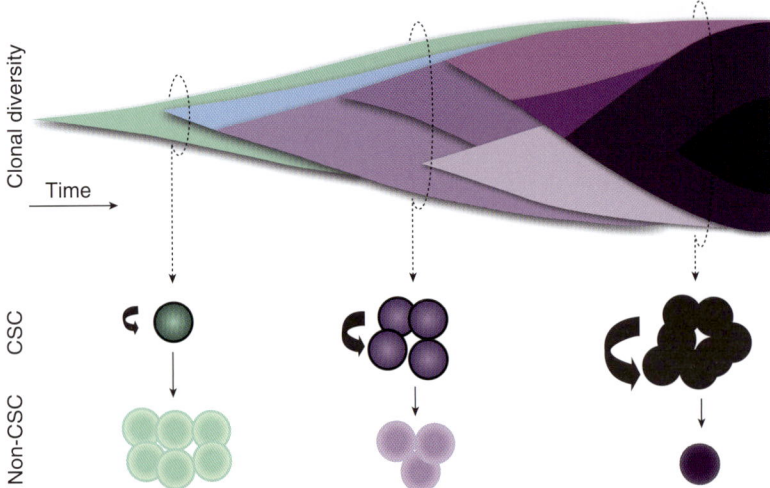

Fig. 26.3 Unified Model of Clonal Evolution and Cancer Stem Cells (CSCs). *Top of figure,* Clonal diversity acquisition of favorable mutations can result in clonal expansion of the founder cell. In parallel, another cell may gain a different mutation that allows it to form a new subclone. Over time, genetic mutations accumulate and subclones evolve in parallel. *Middle of figure,* CSC. Other subclones may contain an intermediate hierarchy, in which the number of CSCs is relatively high but a hierarchy still exists. Some subclones may have the genetic alterations that confer high self-renewal potential, in which most cells are tumorigenic. In this scenario, applying the CSC concept to such homogeneous subclones is not warranted because most cells can self-renew and few non-CSC progeny are generated. *Bottom of figure,* Non-CSC. It may be that CSCs are not static entities but can evolve over the lifetime of a cancer as genetic changes influence CSC frequency. Some subclones may contain a steep developmental hierarchy *(left)*, where only a few self-renewing CSCs exist among a large number of non-CSCs. (From Kreso A, Dick JE: Evolution of the cancer stem cell model, *Cell Stem Cell* 14[3]:275–291, 2014.)

EPIDEMIOLOGY

Lung, colorectal, and breast cancers are the leading causes of cancer deaths in the United States. The types of cancer that have been increasing in incidence are cancer of the lung, breast, prostate, and pancreas, in addition to multiple myeloma, malignant melanoma, and Hodgkin lymphoma. The types of cancer that are decreasing in incidence are cancer of the stomach, cervix, and endometrium.

Cancer in Adults

The lifetime probability of developing cancer is higher in men than in women. The three most common cancers in men are prostate, lung and bronchus, and colorectal, accounting for about 54% of all newly diagnosed cancers. The three most common cancers in women are breast, lung and bronchus, and colorectal, accounting for about 52% of cancer cases in women. Breast cancer alone is expected to account for 26% of all new cancer cases among women. Cancer accounts for more deaths than heart disease in persons younger than 85 years.

Second cancer risk is higher for survivors of some types of cancer. For example, survivors of Hodgkin lymphoma are at an increased risk for subsequent treatment-related malignant neoplasms. Although less toxic treatment protocols have been developed since being introduced in the 1980s, the incidence of a second cancer in patients treated for Hodgkin lymphoma did not appear to be lower among patients treated between 1989 and 2000.

Cancer in Children

Cancer is the second leading cause of death among children between 1 and 14 years old in the United States. Acute lymphoblastic leukemia continues to be the most common cause of pediatric cancer deaths, followed by tumors of the central and sympathetic nervous system, malignant lymphoma, soft tissue sarcomas, and renal tumors.

During the past three decades, increases in the incidence of some childhood cancers, such as leukemia and brain tumors, have suggested prenatal exposure to environmental carcinogens as a causative factor. More than 300 industrial chemicals have been detected in umbilical cord blood.

Risk Factors

Risk factors are important in inducing somatic mutations and the development of cancer. The sum of exposures to various environmental factors is believed to account for the development of most cancers, including tobacco use, some types of infection, exposure to ultraviolet (UV) light, and lifestyle factors such as obesity, lack of exercise, and an unhealthy diet.

Smoking is responsible for one-third of cancers. Other risk factors include a high-fat, low-fiber diet, obesity, and a sedentary lifestyle. Certain types of cancer are more prevalent in specific populations. For example, Blacks have a 20% greater prevalence of cancer than White individuals. The risk of breast cancer increases with age, and deaths are related to geography. Risk factors for breast cancer include family history, particularly breast cancer in a first-degree relative, first pregnancy after age 30 years, presence of fibrocystic disease, probably the use of oral contraceptives or hormone-replacement therapy, prior breast or chest wall radiation, prior breast cancer, and ethanol consumption.

Survivors of childhood and adolescent cancer constitute one of the higher-risk populations. The curative therapy (e.g., chemotherapy and radiation) administered for cancer also affects growing and developing tissues. These patients are at increased risk for early mortality caused by second cancers and cardiac or pulmonary disease. Two-thirds of survivors have at least one chronic or late-occurring health problem.

TABLE 26.1 Selected Environmental Factors Associated With Cancer

Factor	Type of Cancer
Aerosol and Industrial Pollutants	
Asbestos (silica)	Mesothelioma
Lead, copper, zinc, arsenic, cyclic aromatics, tobacco	Lung cancer
Vinyl chloride	Liver angiosarcoma
Benzene	Leukemia
Aniline dyes, coal	Skin and bladder carcinoma
Drugs	
Androgenic steroids	Hepatocellular carcinoma
Stilbestrol (prenatal)	Vaginal adenocarcinoma
Estrogen (postmenopausal)	Endometrial carcinoma
Hydantoins	Lymphoma
Chloramphenicol, alkylating agents	Leukemias, lymphomas

CAUSATIVE FACTORS IN HUMAN CANCER

Factors that cause most neoplasms can be classified as environmental factors (e.g., chemical and radiation), host factors and disease associations, and viruses.

Environmental Factors

The incidence of cancer has been correlated with certain environmental factors. Table 26.1 lists environmental factors that have been definitively linked with cancer, including aerosol and industrial pollutants and drugs.

Radiation exposure is also known to be associated with specific types of cancer (e.g., acute leukemia, thyroid cancer, sarcomas, and breast cancer). Women concerned about organochlorine substances (e.g., polychlorinated biphenyls [PCBs], dioxins, and pesticides [DDT, banned in 1972]) can be reassured that available evidence does not suggest an association between exposure to these chemicals and breast cancer.

Most chemical carcinogens are inactive in their native state and must be activated by enzymes in the cytochrome P-450 or other enzyme systems (e.g., bacterial enzymes or enzymes induced by alcohol).

In radiation carcinogenesis, ionizing particles (e.g., alpha and beta particles, gamma rays, and x-rays) hydrolyze water into free radicals, which are mutagenic to DNA by activating proto-oncogenes. UV light, especially UVB, induces the formation of thymidine dimers, which distort the DNA molecule, leading to skin cancers (e.g., basal cell carcinoma and malignant melanoma).

Microbial Carcinogens

Many scientists believe that microbes cause or contribute to between 15% and 25% of all cancers diagnosed worldwide each year. The International Agency for Research on Cancer (IARC) has classified several microbes as carcinogenic, including human papillomavirus (HPV) and hepatitis B virus (HBV). Infectious agents—bacteria, viruses, and parasites—associated with specific cancers are listed in Table 26.2. Nonpermissive cells that prevent an oncogenic RNA or DNA virus from completing its replication cycle often produce changes in the genome that result in the activation of proto-oncogenes or inactivation of suppressor genes.

Host Factors and Disease Associations

Various host factors have been linked to a higher-than-expected incidence of cancer. A wealth of research has determined that cancer

TABLE 26.2 Microbial Agents Associated With Cancers

Type of Organism	Infectious Agents	Associated Cancers
Bacterium	Helicobacter pylori	Stomach cancer; mucosa-associated lymphoid tissue (MALT) lymphoma
Parasites	Schistosomes (Schistosoma hematobium)	Bladder cancer
	Liver flukes (Opisthorchis viverrini)	Cholangiocarcinoma (a type of liver cancer)
Virus	Epstein-Barr virus	Burkitt lymphoma, non-Hodgkin lymphoma, Hodgkin lymphoma, nasopharyngeal carcinoma
	Hepatitis B virus (HBV)	Hepatocellular carcinoma
	Hepatitis C virus (HCV)	Hepatocellular carcinoma
	Human papillomavirus (HPV) types 16 and 18, and other HPV types	Cervical cancer, vaginal cancer, vulvar cancer, oropharyngeal cancer, anal cancer, penile cancer, squamous cell carcinoma of the skin
	Human T-cell lymphotropic virus type 1 (HTLV1)	Adult T-cell leukemia/lymphoma
	Kaposi sarcoma–associated herpes virus (KSHV), also known as human herpes virus 8 (HHV8)	Kaposi sarcoma

Modified from the World Health Organization, International Agency for Research on Cancer. Biological agents, volume 100 B. A review of human carcinogens IARC monographs on the evaluation of carcinogenic risks to humans, Lyon, France, 2012, IARC.

TABLE 26.3 Cancer-Related Conditions

Disease	Related Cancer
Paget disease	Osteogenic sarcoma
Cryptorchidism	Testicular cancer
Neurofibromatosis	Brain tumors, sarcoma
Esophageal webbing	Esophageal carcinoma
Achlorhydria and pernicious anemia	Gastric carcinoma
Cirrhosis	Hepatoma
Cholelithiasis	Gallbladder cancer
Chronic inflammatory bowel disease	Colon cancer
Migratory thrombophlebitis	Adenocarcinoma, especially pancreatic
Myasthenia gravis, pure red cell aplasia, T-cell disorder	Thymoma
Nephrotic syndrome	Membranous carcinomas; lymphomas, especially Hodgkin

develops through a complex interplay of genetic and environmental factors. The risk of developing cancer is strongly influenced in some cases by inheritance of a mutation in a single gene (e.g., *BRCA1* or *BRCA2*). Mutations in these genes confer a high risk of familial breast cancer and ovarian cancer. According to the National Cancer Institute, specific inherited mutations in *BRCA1* and *BRCA2* increase the risk of female breast and ovarian cancers. These mutations also have been associated with increased risks of several additional types of cancer. About 12% of women in the general population will develop breast cancer sometime during their lives. In contrast, according to the most recent estimates, 55% to 65% of women who inherit a *BRCA1* mutation and around 45% of women who inherit a *BRCA2* mutation will develop breast cancer by age 70 years. About 1.3% of women in the general population will develop ovarian cancer sometime during their lives. In contrast, according to the most recent estimates, 39% of women who inherit a *BRCA1* mutation and 11% to 17% of women who develop a *BRCA2* mutation will develop ovarian cancer by age 70 years. These estimated percentages of lifetime risk are different from those available previously and may change again with additional research.

The presence of certain genetic disorders (e.g., Down syndrome) is associated with an increased incidence of leukemia. The link between certain genetic abnormalities and leukemia is consistent with a germinal or somatic mutation in a stem cell line.

Familial clustering of germ cell tumors, such as malignant tumors arising in the testis, has been observed, particularly among siblings. Cryptorchidism and Klinefelter syndrome are predisposing factors in the development of germ cell tumors arising from the testis and mediastinum, respectively.

The incidence of cancer is 10,000 times greater than expected in patients with an immunodeficiency syndrome. The increased incidence of lymphomas in congenital, acquired, and drug-induced immunosuppression is consistent with the failure of normal immune mechanisms or antigen overstimulation with a loss of normal feedback control. Table 26.3 lists other cancer-related conditions.

IMPACT OF SOMATIC MUTATIONS

All cancers are caused by somatic mutations. Variation in mutation prevalence is attributable to differences between cancers in the duration of the cellular lineage between the fertilized egg and the sequenced cancer cell, and/or to differences in somatic mutation rates during the whole or parts of that cellular lineage.

Mutations in a cancer genome can be acquired at any stage in the cellular lineage from the fertilized egg to the sequenced cancer cell. The diversity and complexity of somatic mutational processes underlying carcinogenesis in human beings are now being revealed through mutational patterns buried within cancer genomes.

Different mutational processes often generate different combinations of mutation types, termed *signatures*. Most individual cancer genomes exhibit more than one mutational signature. In most classifications of malignancies, at least two mutational signatures can be observed, with a maximum of six in cancer of the liver, uterus, and stomach.

Each mutational signature is the imprint left on the cancer genome by a mutational process that may include one or more DNA damage and/or normal or abnormal DNA maintenance mechanisms. Certain signatures are associated with the age of the patient at cancer diagnosis, known mutagenic exposures, or defects in DNA maintenance. Abnormalities in DNA maintenance may also be responsible for mutational signatures and the roles of defective DNA mismatch repair and defective homologous recombination–based DNA double-strand break repair. Other signatures may result from abnormal activity of enzymes that modify DNA or of error-prone polymerases.

Patient age at the time of diagnosis is consistent with the hypothesis that a substantial proportion of signature mutations in cancer genomes has been acquired over the lifetime of the cancer patient at a relatively constant rate in normal somatic tissues. The absence of consistent correlation of signatures with age suggests that mutations associated with these have been generated at different rates in different people, possibly as a consequence of differing carcinogen exposures or after a neoplastic change has been initiated.

The prevalence of somatic mutations is highly variable and ranges between and within cancer classes from about 0.001 per megabase (Mb) to more than 400 per Mb. Certain childhood cancers carry the fewest mutations, but cancers such as lung cancer related to chronic mutagenic exposures and exposure to UV light associated with malignant melanoma exhibit the highest prevalence.

Driver, Actionable, and Passenger Mutations

A **driver mutation** is causally implicated in oncogenesis. Cancer cells originate from normal cells that have accumulated "driver" mutations, which either activate oncogenes by dominant gain of function or inactivate tumor suppressor genes by recessive loss of function. A typical tumor contains two to eight of these driver mutations.

Driver mutations cluster in the subset of genes that are cancer genes. A minority of cancer mutations are considered drivers. This type of mutation confers functional growth advantage to a cancer cell. A cell that acquires a driver mutation will already have biologically inert somatic mutations within its genome. These will be carried along in the clonal expansion that follows and are present in all cells of the final cancer. The importance of identifying driver mutations is that some drivers should be targeted simultaneously during chemotherapy but others need to be targeted in a staggered fashion.

A subset of these drivers and their component cellular pathways may be "actionable" mutations. These **actionable mutations** have significant diagnostic, prognostic, or therapeutic implications in subsets of cancer patients and for the selection of specific therapies. Most mutations found in tumors are not actionable because the impact of the mutation is unknown, or the mutations are passenger mutations that appear as the result of inherent genetic instability in cancer.

Passenger mutations are found in cancer genomes because somatic mutations without functional consequences often occur during cell division. A passenger mutation has not been selected, does not confer clonal growth advantage, and does not contribute to the development of cancer. Some somatic mutations may actually impair cell survival. Passenger mutations are more or less randomly distributed. Mixtures of passenger and driver mutations together comprise the mutated gene sets (MGSs) of tumors.

STAGES OF CARCINOGENESIS

Some precancerous conditions progress through a series of growth alterations before becoming cancerous. For example, cervical cancer progresses from squamous metaplasia to squamous dysplasia to **carcinoma in situ** and finally to invasive cancer. Endometrial cancer progresses from endometrial hyperplasia to atypical endometrial hyperplasia to carcinoma in situ and finally to invasive cancer.

Cancer (Box 26.1) results from a series of genetic alterations that can include the following:
- Activation of oncogenes that promote cell growth
- Loss of tumor suppressor gene activity, which inhibits cell growth

Mutation or overexpression of oncogenes produces proteins that can stimulate uncontrolled cell growth, whereas mutation or deletion of tumor suppressor genes results in the production of nonfunctional proteins that can no longer control cell proliferation. The mutant cell multiplies and the succeeding generations of cells aggregate to form a malignant tumor.

Interleukin-24 (IL-24), initially called *MOB-5*, is a protein that is usually secreted by immune system cells in response to injury or infection. Research on colon cancer cells has demonstrated that IL-24, in conjunction with its receptors, appears to give a cancer cell the ability to fuel its own growth. The secreted proteins are released from one cell to transmit a signal to grow, migrate, or survive to another cell. These proteins cannot act alone and must act through a receptor or receptors on the receiving cell.

> **BOX 26.1 Process of Cancer**
>
> Cancer is a multistep process involving the following:
> 1. Initiation (irreversible mutations involving proto-oncogenes)
> 2. Promotion (growth enhancement to pass on the mutation to other cells)
> 3. Progression (e.g., development of tumor heterogeneity for metastasis, drug resistance)

> **KEY CONCEPTS: Genetics of Cancer**
> - Proto-oncogenes act as central regulators of growth in normal cells and are antecedents of oncogenes.
> - The genetic targets of carcinogens, oncogenes, have been associated with various tumor types, largely from preexisting genes present in the normal human genome.
> - Oncogenes are considered altered versions of normal genes that promote excessive or inappropriate cell proliferation.
> - Various RNA and DNA viruses have been associated with human malignancies (e.g., Epstein-Barr virus and certain papillomaviruses).
> - Viruses carry viral oncogenes into target cells, where they become firmly established.
> - Clonal descendants of target cells carry the viral genes, which maintain the malignant phenotype of the cell clones.
> - A very different class of cancer genes was discovered rather recently. Tumor-suppressing genes (antioncogenes) in normal cells appear to regulate the proliferation of cell growth.
> - When an antioncogene is inactivated, a block to proliferation is removed and cells begin a program of deregulated growth, or the genetically depleted cell itself may proliferate uncontrollably.

CANCER-PREDISPOSING GENES

Cancer-predisposing genes may act in the following ways:
- Affect the rate at which exogenous precarcinogens are metabolized to actively carcinogenic forms that can damage the cellular genome directly
- Affect a host's ability to repair resulting damage to DNA
- Alter the immune ability of the body to recognize and eradicate incipient tumors
- Affect the function of the apparatus responsible for the regulation of normal cell growth and associated proliferation of tissue

Relatively few cancer-predisposing genes have been described. An absence of functional alleles at specific loci, however, allows the genesis of the malignant process (Table 26.4). For example, individuals with certain mutations in the gene *BRCA2* are at a very high risk (up to 85%) for developing breast cancer and other cancers (e.g., ovarian cancer) because a DNA repair path cannot properly repair ongoing wear and tear to the DNA.

A mutation in a gene thought to be responsible for colon cancer may initially cause it. This gene, *APC*, normally limits the expression of a protein, survivin. When *APC* is altered, survivin works overtime and, instead of dying, stem cells in the colon overpopulate, resulting in cancer. Survivin is overexpressed in colon cancer. It prevents programmed cell death, or apoptosis, the process whereby cells normally die. Rather than dying on schedule, cancer cells instead grow out of control. The *APC* gene controls the amount of survivin by shutting down its production.

TABLE 26.4 Tumors Associated With Homozygous Loss of Specific Chromosomal Loci

Tumor Type	Chromosomal Linkage
Multiple endocrine neoplasia type 2	1
Renal cell carcinoma	3
Lung carcinoma	3
Colon carcinoma, familial polyposis	5
Multiple endocrine neoplasia type 2a	10
Wilms tumor, hepatoblastoma, rhabdomyosarcoma	11
Retinoblastoma	13
Ductal breast carcinoma	13
Colon carcinoma	17
Acoustic neuroma, meningioma	22

TABLE 26.5 Examples Oncogenes Formed by Somatic Mutation of Normal Genetic Loci

Oncogene	Disorder
ab1	Chronic myelogenous leukemia
Myc	Burkitt lymphoma
N-myc	Neuroblastoma
EGFR, HER2	Mammary carcinoma
Ras type	Wide variety of tumors

EGFR, Epidermal growth factor receptor; *HER2*, human EGFR-2.

PROTO-ONCOGENES

Proto-oncogenes act as central regulators of the growth in normal cells that code for proteins involved in growth and repair processes in the body. Proteins such as growth factors or transcription factors are necessary for normal growth.

Genetic mutations in proto-oncogenes produce oncogenes. Oncogene activation causes the overexpression of growth-promoting proteins, resulting in hypercellular proliferation and tumorigenesis. Tumor suppressor genes normally counteract proto-oncogenes by encoding proteins that prevent cellular differentiation. When mutations in tumor suppressor genes cause loss of function, the expressed tumor suppressor proteins are no longer able to suppress cellular growth.

For example, the activation of proto-oncogenes (e.g., *ras*) involved in the growth process or inactivation of suppressor genes (e.g., *tp53*), which keeps growth in check by binding and activating genes that put the brakes on cell division, is responsible for neoplastic transformation of a cell. Defects in the gene *tp53* cause about 50% of all cancers.

p53 or tp53 Gene

The p53 or tp53 gene (tumor suppressor gene) is located on chromosome 17 and produces a protein that downregulates the cell cycle. A mutation of *tp53* is associated with an increased incidence of many types of cancer. The p53 protein is dysfunctional in most human cancers. Even when *tp53* is not itself mutant, its regulators (e.g., p14^{ARF}, a p53-stabilizing protein) are often altered. The p53 protein is a key responder to various stresses, including DNA damage, hypoxia, and cell cycle aberrations. Specific molecular pathways that activate *tp53* depend on the nature of the stress and the cell type. Consequently, these determine the specific downstream effectors and cellular response: apoptosis, growth arrest, or senescence.

It is widely believed that the central role of *tp53* in tumor suppression is to mediate the response to DNA damage. If *tp53* is missing when damage occurs, cells do not undergo arrest or apoptosis. Cells that have sustained mutations in oncogenes or tumor suppressor genes because of the damage obtain a growth advantage that fuels the development of cancer.

Apparently, DNA damage itself is not the critical event that leads to cancer, as long as the oncogenic stress pathways that activate *tp53* are intact. For any given cancer type, *tp53* dysfunction generally correlates with poor treatment response and a poor prognosis; therefore restoration of *tp53* function is a potential avenue for therapeutic development. Drugs currently being developed will enhance the function of kinases that activate *tp53* in response to DNA damage.

ROLE OF ONCOGENES

The genetic targets of carcinogens are oncogenes. Oncogenes have been associated with various tumor types (e.g., HER2/*neu* with breast, kidney, and ovarian cancers). Oncogenes are considered altered versions of normal genes that arise as a result of mutations that increase the expression level or activity of a proto-oncogene. Underlying genetic mechanisms associated with oncogene activation include the following: point mutations, deletions, or insertions that lead to a hyperactive gene product. Over a lifetime, a variety of mutations can convert a normal gene into a malignant oncogene.

Once an oncogene is activated by mutation, it promotes excessive or inappropriate cell proliferation. Oncogenes have been detected in about 15% to 20% of a variety of human tumors and appear to be responsible for specifying many of the malignant traits of these cells. More than 30 distinct oncogenes, some of which are associated with specific tumor types, have been identified (Table 26.5). Each gene has the ability to evoke many of the phenotypes characteristic of cancer cells.

Major classes of oncogene products involved in the normal growth process of cells include the following:
- Growth factors (e.g., *sis* oncogene)
- Epidermal growth factor receptors (EGFRs)
- Membrane-associated protein kinases (e.g., *src* oncogene)
- Membrane-related guanine triphosphate (GTP)–binding proteins (e.g., *ras* oncogene)
- Cytoplasmic protein kinases (e.g., *ras* oncogene)
- Transcription regulators located in the nucleus (e.g., *c-myc* oncogene)

In addition, tumor suppressor genes (antioncogenes) are guardians of unregulated cell growth (e.g., *TP53*, *Rb* oncogenes).

Mechanisms of Activation

Point mutations, translocations (e.g., t8;142 in Burkitt lymphoma), and gene amplification (multiple copies of the gene with overexpression of products) are mechanisms of activation as follows:
- Overexpression of the c-erbB-2 (HER2/*neu*) oncogene is noted in up to 34% of patients with invasive ductal breast carcinoma and predicts poor survival.
- Activation of the *ras* proto-oncogene (point mutation) is associated with about 30% of all human cancers. Approximately 25% of patients with acute myelogenous leukemia display this point mutation. *Ras* is mutated frequently in colon and pancreatic cancers; it appears that *ras* activation leads to unregulated expression of IL-24 and its receptors.
- Translocation of the *abl* proto-oncogene from chromosome 9 to chromosome 22 with formation of a large *bcr-abl* hybrid gene on chromosome 22 (Philadelphia chromosome) results in chronic myelogenous leukemia.
- Inactivation of suppressor genes (point mutations) leads to unrestricted cell division, inactivation of each of the *RB1* suppressor

> **BOX 26.2 Oncogenic Viruses**
>
> - RNA: leukemia, carcinoma viruses, mammary tumor viruses
> - DNA: herpes viruses, adenoviruses, papilloma viruses

genes on chromosome 13 is associated with malignant retinoblastoma in children, and inactivation of the *p53* suppressor gene on chromosome 17 accounts for 25% to 50% of all malignancies involving the colon, breast, lung, and central nervous system.

Viral Oncogenes

Various RNA and DNA viruses have been associated with human malignancies (Box 26.2). Some viral agents have a clear causative role, such as the Epstein-Barr virus and certain papillomaviruses, which are the causative agents in Burkitt lymphoma and cervical carcinoma, respectively.

Viruses carry viral oncogenes into target cells, where they become firmly established. Clonal descendants then carry the viral genes, which maintain the malignant phenotype of the cell clones.

Tumor-Suppressing Genes

A very different class of cancer genes has been discovered. These tumor-suppressing genes in normal cells appear to regulate the proliferation of cell growth. When this type of gene is inactivated, a block to proliferation is removed and cells begin a program of deregulated growth, or the genetically depleted cell itself may proliferate uncontrollably. Thus tumor-suppressing genes are referred to as *antioncogenes*. In time, their discovery will lead to the reformulation of ideas about how the growth of normal cells is regulated.

Much speculation surrounds the operation of tumor-suppressing genes in normal tissue. It is known that normal cells exert a negative growth influence on each other within a tissue. Normal cells also secrete factors that are negative regulators of their own growth and that of adjacent cells. Diffusible factors may also be released by normal cells to induce the end-stage differentiation of other cells in the immediate environment; these factors include the following:

- Interferon-β (IFN-β)
- Transforming (tumor) growth factor (TGF)
- Tumor necrosis factor (TNF)

Normal gene products appear to prevent malignant transformation in some way. It is speculated that normal cells must have receptors that detect the presence of these growth-inhibiting and differentiation-inducing factors, which allow them to process the signals of negative growth and respond with appropriate modulation of growth. Genes may specify proteins necessary to detect and respond to the negative regulators of growth. If this process becomes dysfunctional as a result of inactivation or the absence of a critical component, such as the loss of chromosomal loci, a cell may continue to respond to mitogenic stimulation but lose its ability to respond to negative feedback to cease proliferation. Animal experiments have suggested that human beings carry a repertoire of genes, each of which is involved in the negative regulation of the growth of specific cell types. Somatic inactivation of these genes may be involved in the initiation of tumor cell growth or the transformation of benign tumors into malignant ones. Therefore the somatic inactivation of tumor-suppressing genes may be as important to carcinogenesis as the somatic activation of oncogenes.

BODY DEFENSES AGAINST CANCER

The importance of the immune system in conferring protection against pathogens such as viruses, bacteria, and parasitic worms is

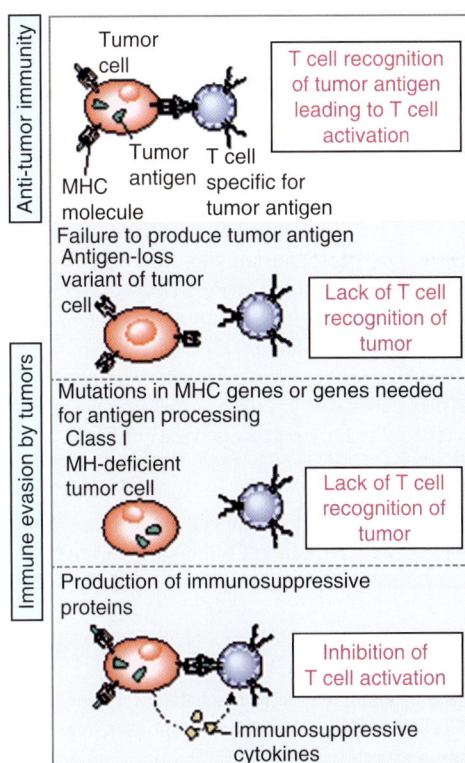

Fig. 26.4 Mechanisms by Which Tumors Escape Immune Defenses. *MHC*, Major histocompatibility complex. (From Abbas AK, Lichtman AHH, Pillai S: *Cellular and molecular immunology,* ed 7, Philadelphia, 2012, Saunders.)

well established. In contrast, there is a long-lasting debate on whether cancer prevention is a primary function of the immune system. The concept of immunologic surveillance of cancer was developed more than 50 years ago. Although there is no single satisfactory explanation for the success of tumors in escaping the immune rejection process, it is believed that early clones of neoplastic cells are eliminated by the immune response. The growth of malignant tumors is primarily determined by the proliferative capacity of the tumor cells and by the ability of these cells to invade host tissues and metastasize to distant sites. It is believed that malignant tumors can evade or overcome the mechanisms of host defenses (Fig. 26.4).

Tumor immunity has the following general features:

1. Tumors express antigens that are recognized as foreign by the immune system of the tumor-bearing host.
2. The normal immune response frequently fails to prevent the growth of tumors.
3. The immune system can be stimulated to kill tumor cells and rid the host of the tumor.

Host defense mechanisms against tumors are both humoral and cellular. Effector mechanisms include the following:

- T lymphocytes
- Natural killer (NK) cells
- Macrophages
- Antibodies

T Lymphocytes

Cytolytic T lymphocytes (CTLs) provide effective antitumor immunity in vivo. CTL-mediated rejection of transplanted tumors is the only established example of completely effective specific antitumor immunity in vivo. Mononuclear cells derived from the inflammatory infiltrate in human solid tumors, called *tumor-infiltrating lymphocytes,* also include CTLs with the capacity to lyse the tumor from which they were derived. CD4+ T cells may play a role in antitumor responses by providing cytokines for effective CTL development.

Natural Killer Cells

NK cells can be activated by direct recognition of tumors or as a consequence of cytokines produced by tumor-specific T lymphocytes. These cells use the same lytic mechanisms as CTLs to kill cells but do not express T-cell antigen receptors, and they have a broad range of specificities. Research has also focused on the role of IL-2–activated NK cells in tumor killing. These cells, referred to as *lymphokine-activated killer cells*, are derived in vitro by culture of peripheral blood cells or tumor-infiltrating lymphocytes from tumor patients with high doses of IL-2.

NK cells may play a role in immunosurveillance against developing tumors, especially those expressing viral antigens.

Macrophages

Activated macrophages produce the cytokine tumor necrosis factor. As the name implies, TNF can kill tumors but not normal cells. TNF kills tumors by direct toxic effects and indirectly by effects on tumor vasculature.

Antibodies

Antibodies are probably less important than T lymphocytes in mediating the effect of antitumor immune responses, but tumor-bearing hosts produce antibodies against various tumor antigens. These serve as tumor markers.

Although malignant tumors may express protein antigens that are recognized as foreign by the tumor host, and despite the fact that immunosurveillance may limit the outgrowth of some tumors, the immune system often does not prevent the occurrence of cancer. The simplest explanation is that the rapid growth and spread of a tumor overwhelm the effector mechanisms of the immune response.

> **KEY CONCEPTS: Tumor Markers**
> - No single satisfactory explanation exists for the success of tumors in escaping the immune rejection process.
> - It is believed that early clones of neoplastic cells are eliminated by the immune response.
> - Cells, rather than immunoglobulins, are believed to dominate tumor immunity.
> - Four types of identified tumor antigens are tumor-specific antigens on chemically induced tumors, tumor-associated antigens on virally induced tumors, carcinofetal antigens, and spontaneous tumor antigens.
> - A tumor marker is a characteristic of a neoplastic cell that can be detected in plasma or serum.
> - Tumor markers may be useful in the diagnosis and selection of different treatment approaches, monitoring therapies, and determining prognosis.

TUMOR MARKERS

Tumor markers have traditionally been proteins or other substances that can be made by both normal and cancer cells but at higher amounts in cancer or certain benign conditions. Markers can be found in blood, urine, stool, tumors, or other tissues or bodily fluids. Although an elevated level of a circulating tumor marker may suggest the presence of cancer and can sometimes help to diagnose cancer, the marker by itself is not enough to diagnose cancer. Measurements of circulating tumor markers are usually combined with the results of other tests, such as biopsies or imaging to diagnose cancer.

A tumor marker provides information that can be used to determine:
- Aggressiveness of the cancer
- Stage of cancer
- Potential for types of treatment
- Responsiveness to treatment
- Prognosis and detection of minimal residual disease

Liquid biopsy tests can detect multiple cancer–associated biomarkers. For example, the Foundation One Liquid CDx test is approved for the detection of genetic mutations in 324 genes and two genomic signatures in any solid tumor type. The test can also identify which patients with non–small cell lung cancer, melanoma, breast cancer, colorectal cancer, or ovarian cancer may benefit from 15 different US Food and Drug Administration (FDA)-approved targeted treatment options.

VARIETY OF TUMOR MARKERS

When a normal cell is transformed into a malignant cell, it develops unique antigens not normally present on the mature normal cell. Tumors frequently produce tumor-specific antigens (TSAs) to which the host may develop antibodies. Virus-induced cancers are the most antigenic; chemical-induced cancers are the least antigenic.

Some tumor markers are associated with only one type of cancer, but other markers are associated with two or more types of cancer. Most tumor markers are proteins and can be detected in blood, body fluids, cells, or tissue (Table 26.6). Nonneoplastic conditions can also exhibit tumor marker activity (Table 26.7). Tumor markers can be measured quantitatively in tissues and body fluids using biochemical, immunochemical, or molecular tests.

Increasingly, however, genomic markers such as tumor gene mutations, patterns of tumor gene expression, and nongenetic changes in tumor DNA are being used as tumor markers. Information gathered from laboratory testing can provide information on a patient's prognosis.

There are some limitations to the use of tumor markers. Under some conditions, noncancerous (benign) conditions can cause the levels of certain tumor markers to increase. In addition, not every patient with a particular type of cancer will have a higher level of a tumor marker associated with that cancer. In addition, tumor markers have not been identified for every type of cancer.

The search for tumor markers goes back more than 150 years. The earliest identified tumor marker was Bence Jones protein, a light-chain immunoglobulin found in patients with multiple myeloma (see Chapter 21). Over the past 15 years, the use of tumor markers in the United States has risen dramatically. Tumor markers play an especially important role in the diagnosis and monitoring of patients with prostate, breast, and bladder cancers.

An ideal tumor marker would be an assay in which a positive result would only occur in patients with a malignancy, would correlate with stage and response to treatment, and would be easily reproducible. No tumor marker to date has met this ideal marker description, nor has any tumor marker been established as a practical screening test in a general healthy population or in most high-risk populations. The rationale for this poor predictive value of tumor markers is the lack of sensitivity and specificity in the low cancer rates that prevail in population groups. Because of the low prevalence of cancer, in general, even assays that are highly sensitive and specific may have a low predictive value.

Older, well-established markers include alkaline phosphatase (ALP) and collagen-type markers in bone cancer, immunoglobulins in myeloma, catecholamines and their derivatives in neuroblastoma and pheochromocytoma, and serotonin metabolites in carcinoid. In addition, there are many breast tissue prognostic markers (e.g., hormone receptors, cathepsin-D, HER2/*neu* oncogenes, and plasminogen

TABLE 26.6 Tumor Markers Currently in Common Use[a]

Tumor Marker	Cancer Type(s)	Tissue Analyzed	Clinical Use
ALK gene rearrangements and overexpression	Non–small cell lung cancer and anaplastic large cell lymphoma	Tumor	Help determine treatment and prognosis
Alpha-fetoprotein (AFP)	Liver cancer and germ cell tumors	Blood	Help diagnose liver cancer and follow response to treatment; assess stage, prognosis, and response to treatment of germ cell tumors
B-cell immunoglobulin gene rearrangement	B-cell lymphoma	Blood, bone marrow, or tumor tissue	Aid in diagnosis, evaluation of treatment, check for tumor recurrence
Beta-2 microglobulin (B2M)	Multiple myeloma, chronic lymphocytic leukemia, and some lymphomas	Blood, urine, or cerebrospinal fluid	Determine prognosis and follow response to treatment
Beta–human chorionic gonadotropin (β-hCG)	Choriocarcinoma and germ cell tumors	Urine or blood	Assess stage, prognosis, and response to treatment
Bladder tumor antigen (BTA)	Bladder cancer and cancer of the kidney or ureter	Urine	As surveillance with cytology and cystoscopy of patients already known to have bladder cancer
BRCA1 and *BRCA2* gene mutations	Ovarian cancer	Blood	Determine whether treatment with a particular type of targeted therapy is appropriate
BCR-ABL fusion gene (Philadelphia chromosome)	Chronic myeloid leukemia, acute lymphoblastic leukemia, and acute myelogenous leukemia	Blood and/or bone marrow	Confirm diagnosis, predict response to targeted therapy, and monitor disease status
BRAF V600 mutations	Cutaneous melanoma and colorectal cancer	Tumor	Select patients who are most likely to benefit from treatment with certain targeted therapies
C-kit/CD117	Gastrointestinal stromal tumor and mucosal melanoma	Tumor	Aid in diagnosis and determining treatment
CA 15-3/CA 27.29	Breast cancer	Blood	Assess whether treatment is working or disease has recurred
CA 19-9	Pancreatic cancer, gallbladder cancer, bile duct cancer, and gastric cancer	Blood	Assess whether treatment is working
CA 125	Ovarian cancer	Blood	Help in diagnosis, assessment of response to treatment, and evaluation of recurrence
CA 27.29	Breast cancer	Blood	Detect metastasis or recurrence
Calcitonin	Medullary thyroid cancer	Blood	Aid in diagnosis, check whether treatment is working, and assess for recurrence
Carcinoembryonic antigen (CEA)	Colorectal cancer and some other cancers	Blood	Keep track of how well cancer treatments are working or check if cancer has come back
CD19	B-cell lymphomas and leukemias	B-cell lymphomas and leukemias	B-cell lymphomas and leukemias
CD20	Non-Hodgkin lymphoma	Blood	Determine whether treatment with a targeted therapy is appropriate
CD22	Hairy cell leukemia and B-cell neoplasms	Blood and bone marrow	Aid in diagnosis
CD25	Non-Hodgkin (T-cell) lymphoma	Blood	Determine whether treatment with a targeted therapy is appropriate
CD30	Mycosis fungoides and peripheral T-cell lymphoma	Tumor	Determine whether treatment with a targeted therapy is appropriate
CD33	Acute myeloid leukemia	Blood	Determine whether treatment with a targeted therapy is appropriate
Chromogranin A (CgA)	Neuroendocrine tumors	Blood	Help in diagnosis, assessment of treatment response, and evaluation of recurrence
Chromosome 17p deletion	Chronic lymphocytic leukemia	Blood	Determine whether treatment with a certain targeted therapy is appropriate
Chromosomes 3, 7, 17, and 9p21	Bladder cancer	Urine	Help in monitoring for tumor recurrence
Circulating tumor cells of epithelial origin (CELLSEARCH)	Metastatic breast, prostate, and colorectal cancers		Inform clinical decision-making and assess prognosis
Cytokeratin fragment 21-1	Lung cancer	Blood	Help in monitoring for recurrence

Continued

TABLE 26.6 Tumor Markers Currently in Common Use[a]—cont'd

Tumor Marker	Cancer Type(s)	Tissue Analyzed	Clinical Use
Des-gamma-carboxy prothrombin (DCP)	Hepatocellular carcinoma	Blood	Monitor the effectiveness of treatment and detect recurrence
DPD gene mutation	Breast, colorectal, gastric, and pancreatic cancers	Blood	Predict the risk of a toxic reaction to 5-fluorouracil therapy
EGFR gene mutation analysis	Non–small cell lung cancer	Tumor	Help determine treatment and prognosis
Estrogen receptor (ER)/progesterone receptor (PR)	Breast cancer	Tumor	Determine whether treatment with hormone therapy and some targeted therapies are appropriate
FGFR2 and FGFR3 gene mutations	Bladder cancer	Tumor	Determine whether treatment with a certain targeted therapy is appropriate
Fibrin/fibrinogen	Bladder cancer	Urine	Monitor progression and response to treatment
FLT3 gene mutations	Acute myeloid leukemia	Blood	Determine whether treatment with certain targeted therapies is appropriate
Gastrin	Gastrin-producing tumor (gastrinoma)	Blood	Help in diagnosis, monitor the effectiveness of treatment, and detect recurrence
HE4	Ovarian cancer	Blood	Plan cancer treatment, assess disease progression, and monitor for recurrence
HER2/neu gene amplification or protein overexpression	Breast cancer, gastric cancer, and gastroesophageal junction adenocarcinoma	Tumor	Determine whether treatment with certain targeted therapies is appropriate
5-HIAA	Carcinoid tumors	Urine	Aid in diagnosis and monitoring of disease
IDH1 and IDH2 gene mutations	Acute myeloid leukemia	Bone marrow and blood	Determine whether treatment with certain targeted therapies is appropriate
Immunoglobulins	Multiple myeloma and Waldenström macroglobulinemia	Blood and urine	Help diagnose disease, assess response to treatment, and look for recurrence
IRF4 gene rearrangement	Lymphoma	Tumor	Help in diagnosis
JAK2 gene mutation	Certain types of leukemia	Blood and bone marrow	Help in diagnosis
KRAS gene mutation	Colorectal cancer and non–small cell lung cancer	Tumor	Determine whether treatment with a particular type of targeted therapy is appropriate
Lactate dehydrogenase (LDH)	Germ cell tumors, lymphoma, leukemia, melanoma, and neuroblastoma	Blood	Assess stage, prognosis, and response to treatment
Microsatellite instability (MSI) and/or mismatch repair deficient (dMMR)	Colorectal cancer and other solid tumors	Tumor	Guide treatment and identify those at high risk of certain cancer-predisposing syndromes
MYC gene expression	Lymphomas, leukemias	Tumor	Help in diagnosis and to help determine treatment
MYD88 gene mutation	Lymphoma, Waldenström macroglobulinemia	Tumor	Help in diagnosis and to help determine treatment
Myeloperoxidase	Leukemia	Blood	Help in diagnosis
Neuron-specific enolase (NSE)	Small cell lung cancer and neuroblastoma	Blood	Help in diagnosis and assess response to treatment
NTRK	Any solid tumor	Tumor	Help determine treatment
Nuclear matrix protein 22	Bladder cancer	Urine	Monitor response to treatment
PCA3 messenger RNA (mRNA)	Prostate cancer	Urine (collected after digital rectal exam)	Determine need for repeat biopsy after negative biopsy
PML/RARα fusion gene	Acute promyelocytic leukemia (APL)	Blood and bone marrow	Diagnose APL, predict response to all-trans-retinoic acid or arsenic trioxide therapy, assess effectiveness of therapy, monitor minimal residual disease, and predict early relapse
Prostatic acid phosphatase (PAP)	Metastatic prostate cancer	Blood	Help in diagnosing poorly differentiated carcinomas
Programmed death ligand 1 (PD-L1)	Non–small cell lung cancer	Tumor	Determine whether treatment with a particular type of targeted therapy is appropriate

TABLE 26.6 Tumor Markers Currently in Common Use[a]—cont'd

Tumor Marker	Cancer Type(s)	Tissue Analyzed	Clinical Use
Prostate-specific antigen (PSA)	Prostate cancer	Blood	Help in diagnosis, assess response to treatment, and look for recurrence
ROS1 gene rearrangement	Non–small cell lung cancer	Tumor	Determine whether treatment with a particular type of targeted therapy is appropriate
Soluble mesothelin-related peptides (SMRPs)	Mesothelioma	Blood	Monitor progression or recurrence
Somatostatin receptor	Neuroendocrine tumors affecting the pancreas or gastrointestinal tract (GEP-NETs)	Tumor (by diagnostic imaging)	Determine whether treatment with a particular type of targeted therapy is appropriate
T-cell receptor gene rearrangement	T-cell lymphoma	Bone marrow, tissue, body fluid, blood	Help in diagnosis; sometimes used to detect and evaluate residual disease
Terminal transferase	Leukemia, lymphoma	Tumor Blood	Help in diagnosis
Thiopurine S-methyltransferase (TPMT) enzyme activity or TPMT genetic test	Acute lymphoblastic leukemia	Blood and buccal (cheek) swab	Predict the risk of severe bone marrow toxicity (myelosuppression) with thiopurine treatment
Thyroglobulin	Thyroid cancer	Blood	Evaluate response to treatment and look for recurrence
UGT1A1*28 variant homozygosity	Colorectal cancer	Blood and buccal (cheek) swab	Predict toxicity from irinotecan therapy
Urine catecholamines: vanillylmandelic acid (VMA) and homovanillic acid (HVA)	Neuroblastoma	Urine	Help in diagnosis
Urokinase plasminogen activator (uPA) and plasminogen activator inhibitor (PAI-1)	Breast cancer	Tumor	Determine aggressiveness of cancer and guide treatment
FoundationOne CDx (F1CDx) genomic test	Any solid tumor	Tumor	Companion diagnostic test to determine whether treatment with a particular type of targeted therapy is appropriate
5-Protein signature (OVA1)	Ovarian cancer	Blood	Preoperatively assess pelvic mass for suspected ovarian cancer
17-Gene signature (Oncotype DX GPS test)	Prostate cancer	Tumor	Predict the aggressiveness of prostate cancer and help manage treatment
21-Gene signature (Oncotype DX test)	Breast cancer	Tumor	Evaluate risk of recurrence
46-Gene signature (Prolaris)	Prostate cancer	Tumor	Predict the aggressiveness of prostate cancer and help manage treatment
70-Gene signature (Mammaprint)	Breast cancer	Tumor	Evaluate risk of recurrence

[a]A tumor marker is anything present in or produced by cancer cells or other cells of the body in response to cancer or certain benign (noncancerous) conditions that provides information about a cancer, such as how aggressive it is, whether it can be treated with a targeted therapy, or whether it is responding to treatment. See the Tumor Markers fact sheet for more information. This table lists tumor markers that are in common use, mainly to determine treatment or to help make a diagnosis of cancer. New tumor markers frequently become available and may not be reflected in this list. In addition, the list does not include the many tumor markers that are tested by immunophenotyping and immunohistochemistry to help diagnose cancer and to distinguish between different types of cancer. Some of the tumor markers listed are targets for targeted therapy in multiple cancers but serve as tumor markers for only a subset of cancers.
Data from the National Cancer Institute, Reviewed May,11 2021 Accessed July 10, 2023. https://www.cancer.gov.

receptors and inhibitors). Enzyme-linked immunosorbent assay (ELISA) for circulating tumor-associated proteins and immunofluorescence for CD markers in diagnosing leukemias and lymphomas are additional methods.

A list of the most currently used tumor markers is presented in Table 26.8. Nine of these biomarkers are protein biomarkers identifiable in blood. Other recently approved protein biomarkers can be detected in urine, such as nuclear matrix protein 22, fibrin and fibrinogen degradation products, and bladder tumor antigen for monitoring bladder cancer, and by immunohistochemical methods using tumor tissues, such as estrogen receptor for breast cancer.

Additional cancer biomarkers approved by the FDA are DNA based, such as human EGFR-2 and HER2/neu for breast cancer, and can be assayed by fluorescent in situ hybridization (FISH). Multiple-marker combinations are useful in the management of some cancers (Table 26.9), but the use of more than two markers is questionable.

Categories of Tumor Antigens

Commonly targeted shared tumor antigens include the following:
- MAGE-1, -2, and -3; BAGE; and RAGE are nonmutated cancer-test antigens expressed in a variety of tumor cells.
- Lineage-specific tumor antigens, such as melanocyte/melanoma lineage antigens. These include MART-1/Melan-A, gp100, gp75, mda-7, tyrosinase and tyrosinase-related protein (TRP-1 and -2), or the prostate antigens prostate-specific membrane antigen (PSMA) and prostate-specific antigen (PSA).

TABLE 26.7 Nonneoplastic Conditions With Elevated Serum and Plasma Concentrations of Tumor Markers

Tumor Marker	Concentration in Normal Serum (ng/mL)	Nonneoplastic Conditions
CEA	<2.5	Inflammatory bowel disease, pancreatitis, gastritis, smoker chronic bronchitis, alcoholic liver disease, hepatitis
AFP	<40	Pregnancy, regenerating liver tissue after viral hepatitis, chemically induced liver necrosis, partial hepatectomy, cystic fibrosis, ataxia-telangiectasia, premature infants, tyrosinemia
β-hCG	Negative	Pregnancy
Serum acid phosphatase	Negative	Pregnancy
Placental alkaline phosphatase	Negative	Pregnancy

AFP, Alpha-fetoprotein; *β-hCG*, beta subunit of chorionic gonadotropin; *CEA*, carcinoembryonic antigen.

TABLE 26.8 Common Serum Tumor Markers and Their Clinical Utility

Tumor Type	Cancer Deaths (United States) (%)	Tumor Markers	Tumor Detection
Lung + bronchus	28	Neuron-specific enolase	Late
Colon + rectum	9	CEA	Late
Breast	7	CA 15-3; CEA	Late
Pancreas	6	CA 19-9; CEA	Late
Prostate	5	PSA	Good
Stomach	2	CEA; CA 19-9	Late
Ovary	2.5	CA 125; PLAP	Intermediate
Liver	3	α-FP	Intermediate
Myeloma	1.9	Monoclonal protein/FLCs	Early
AL amyloidosis	0.3	Monoclonal protein/FLCs	Early
Germ cell	0.1	α-FP; HCG	Early
Choriocarcinoma	<0.1	HCG	Early
Neuroendocrine	<0.1	Chromogranin A, gastrin	Early

α-FP, Alpha-fetoprotein; *CEA*, carcinoembryonic antigen; *FLC*, free light chain; *HCG*, human chorionic gonadotropin; *PLAP*, placental alkaline phosphatase; *PSA*, prostate-specific antigen.
Modified from Bradwell AR: *Serum free light chain analysis (plus Hevylite),* Birmingham, UK, 2010, Binding Site Group Ltd.

TABLE 26.9 Related Multiple Tumor Markers

Markers	Comments
AFP and β-hCG	Valuable combination in therapy and follow-up in patients with germ cell tumors of the testes
CEA, AFP, and LDH	Combination seems to help differentiate primary liver cancer from liver metastases related to another organ
Ratio of free to total PSA	The ratio may distinguish BPH from prostate cancer
CEA and numerous mucin-type markers	May complement each other

AFP, Alpha-fetoprotein; *β-hCG*, beta subunit of chorionic gonadotropin; *BPH*, benign prostatic hypertrophy; *CEA*, carcinoembryonic antigen; *LDH*, lactate dehydrogenase; *PSA*, prostate-specific antigen.

- Protein derived from genes mutated in tumor cells and/or genes transcribed at different levels in tumor compared with normal cells (e.g., mutated *ras*, *bcr/abl* rearrangement, or mutated *p53*).
- Proteins derived from oncoviruses, such as HPV proteins E6 and E7.
- Nonmutated proteins with a tumor-selective, increased expression, including carcinoembryonic antigen (CEA), prostate-specific antigen (PSA), Her2/*neu*, and alpha-fetoprotein.

When tumors arise in a tissue, a number of immune cells can recognize and eliminate them. Cancer immunoediting is divided into three phases (Fig. 26.5):
1. elimination (immunosurveillance),
2. equilibrium (quiescent state), and
3. escape (immune evasion).

Research into each of these phases has clarified the understanding of the complex relationship between the immune system and tumorigenesis.

Variant tumor cells arise that are more resistant to being killed. Over time a variety of different tumor variants develop. Eventually, one variant may escape the killing mechanism or recruit regulatory cells to protect it and be able to spread unchallenged.

Tumor cells manifest tumor antigens and also self-human leukocyte antigen (HLA) antigens. Four types of tumor antigens have been identified:
1. TSAs on chemically induced tumors
2. Tumor-associated antigens (TAAs) on virally induced tumors
3. Carcinofetal antigens
4. Spontaneous tumor antigens

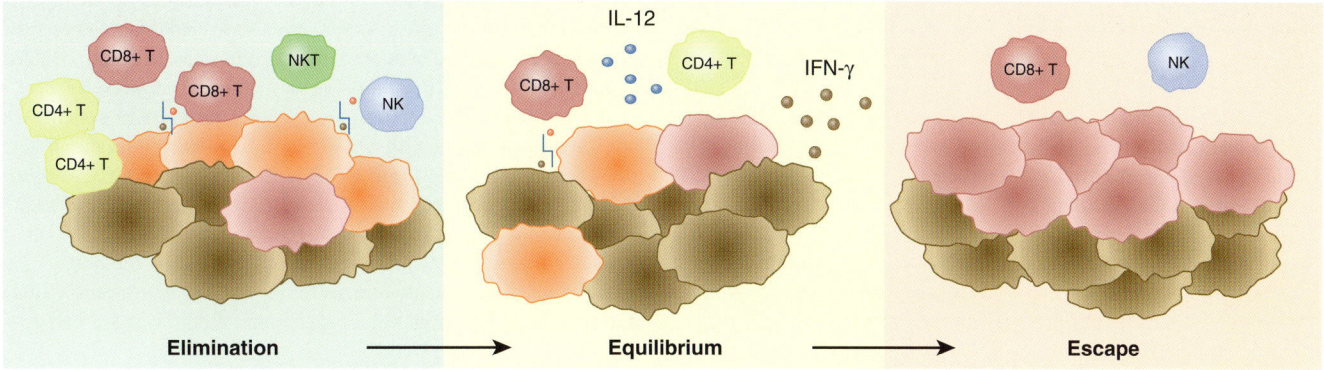

Fig. 26.5 Immunoediting. (Reprinted from Tavakoli F, Sartakhti JS, Manshaei MH, et al.: Immunoediting: a game theoretical approach, *In-Silico-Biology* 14(1–2):1–12, 2020. The publication is available at IOS Press through http://dx.doi.org/10.3233/ISB-200475.)

Tumor-Specific Antigens

Chemically induced tumors are known to develop TSAs, which are uniquely associated with each tumor. These antigens are not found in normal cells. TSAs demonstrate little or no cross-reactivity between different tumors caused by the same carcinogen, perhaps because every tumor caused by chemical agents has unique surface characteristics.

Tumor-Associated Antigens

TAAs are cell surface molecules coded for by tumorigenic viruses. These antigens are not expressed on the virion but are synthesized by the host cell. In contrast to TSAs, TAAs are virus specific. Therefore each specific virus induces the same antigens, regardless of the tissue of origin or the animal species.

Carcinofetal Antigens

Well-differentiated tissue produces and secretes little or no fetal gene products. The abnormal behavior of malignant cells is believed to derepress genes normally expressed only during fetal life. Because the products of these fetally active genes are recognized as self, they do not elicit humoral or cell-mediated responses.

During malignant transformation, however, gene derepression is responsible for the production of increased concentrations of these gene products, which are known as *oncofetal proteins*. CEA is an example of a carcinofetal antigen.

Spontaneous Tumor Antigens

Tumors caused by no known mechanism, known as *spontaneous tumor antigens*, are thought to produce antigens. Disagreement exists regarding whether these tumors are similar to those produced experimentally by chemical, viral, or physical agents. Although substantial evidence supports the contention that these tumors do not produce unique antigens, some evidence has refuted this contention. The importance of these findings remains unclear.

Classic Tumor Markers

Ten protein cancer biomarkers were the initially FDA-approved assays:
1. Alpha-fetoprotein
2. CA 125
3. Human epididymis protein 4
4. Thyroglobulin
5. PSA
6. CEA
7. CA 19-9
8. CA 15-3
9. CA 27.29
10. HER2/*neu*

Other markers include the beta subunit of human chorionic gonadotropin (β-hCG) and miscellaneous enzyme and hormone markers.

Alpha-Fetoprotein

Alpha-fetoprotein (AFP) is normally synthesized by the fetal liver and yolk sac. AFP is secreted in the serum in nanogram-to-milligram quantities in hepatocarcinoma, endodermal sinus tumors, nonseminomatous germ cell (testicular) cancer, teratocarcinoma of the testis or ovary, and malignant tumors of the mediastinum and sacrococcyx. In addition, a small percentage of patients with gastric and pancreatic cancer with liver metastasis may have elevated AFP levels.

The concentration of AFP may be elevated in nonneoplastic conditions such as hepatitis and cystic fibrosis.

AFP is a reliable marker for following a patient's response to chemotherapy and radiation therapy. Levels should be obtained every 2 to 4 weeks (metabolic half-life in vivo, 4 days).

Both AFP and β-hCG should be quantitated initially in all patients with teratocarcinoma because one or both markers may be secreted in 85% of patients.

CA 125

CA 125, a mucinlike glycoprotein, is expressed on the surface of the main body cavity, coelomic, epithelium, and human ovarian carcinoma cells. CA 125 is relatively more sensitive in low-stage ovarian cancer. It reacts against a monoclonal antibody (MAb) developed against a cell line from one patient's ovarian cystadenocarcinoma. It is elevated in carcinomas and benign disease of various organs (e.g., pelvic inflammatory disease, endometriosis) but is most useful in ovarian and endometrial carcinomas.

Human Epididymis Protein 4

Human epididymis protein 4 (HE4) was approved in 2009. It is recommended for monitoring patients for recurring epithelial ovarian cancer. Disease recurrence or progression can be indicated if HE4 levels are 150.1 pM or higher. This marker is not specific for ovarian cancer. Therefore it is not suitable for use in screening or diagnosis of ovarian cancer.

Thyroglobulin

Thyroglobulin (Tg) is produced and used exclusively by the thyroid gland. A Tg assay is frequently ordered before thyroid surgery to determine whether the tumor is producing Tg. This assay can be performed to monitor cancer recurrence because of rising levels over time after thyroid surgery. Tg levels can be elevated not only in thyroid cancer but also in Graves disease and thyroiditis.

Prostate-Specific Antigen and Prostatic Acid Phosphatase

Prostate cancer is a leading cause of cancer death in US men. Although there has been controversy in recent years about the application of prostate assays, there are two tumor markers for cancer of the prostate: PSA and prostatic acid phosphatase.

Prostate-specific antigen. PSA screening has been controversial in recent years. Although the PSA assay has reduced prostate cancer mortality, the limitations of using PSA as a prostate cancer screening tool are now widely acknowledged. The problem with PSA as a screening tool is that it is specific for prostate-related issues, not prostate cancer. Because of this, many false-positive results were reported and many unnecessary prostate biopsies were performed. Today, the value of the PSA assay is as a treatment guide that detects a marked elevation in men who have a known diagnosis of prostate cancer.

PSA is a prostate tissue–specific marker but not a prostate cancer–specific marker. It is a protease enzyme secreted almost exclusively by prostatic epithelial cells. Blood levels of PSA are increased when normal glandular structure is disrupted by benign or malignant tumor inflammation. The serum PSA level is directly proportional to tumor volume, with a greater increase per unit volume of cancer compared with benign hyperplasia. However, elevated PSA levels can be detected in prostate infection, irritation, benign prostatic hypertrophy (BPH), and recent ejaculation.

Free PSA assists in distinguishing cancer of the prostate from BPH. Comparison of free PSA to PSA levels is used to assess the risk of cancer because the ratio of free PSA to PSA in prostate cancer is decreased. PSA levels appear useful for monitoring progression and response to treatment in patients with prostate cancer.

Other techniques that have been used for the detection of prostate cancer include PSA velocity (incremental increase of PSA over time), PSA density (ratio of serum PSA to prostate volume), age-adjusted PSA (PSA increases with age), biostatistically derived algorithms, free and total PSA, complexed PSA, and, most recently, human kallikrein II, a molecule similar but not identical to PSA.

In 2012 the FDA-approved Beckman Coulter's Prostate Health Index (PHI) for prostate cancer testing. The PHI is 2.5 times more specific for detecting prostate cancer than prior methods of testing inpatients with PSA values in the 4 to 10 ng/mL range. The PHI results combine the total PSA, free PSA, and p2PSA isoform in the total assay result. In 2014 the FDA approved the 4K assay to assess a patient's risk for aggressive prostate cancer before a prostate biopsy. Other research is being done on the first exosomal RNA test of prostate cancer, EXO106. Genomic testing is the next frontier in prostate cancer testing.

Other prostate cancer biomarkers. Prostatic acid phosphatase is another older marker for prostate cancer. In the past, it was used as a routine screening test for males. Today it is used for specific diagnosis and monitoring of prostatic carcinoma. The rate of acceleration of PSA values is critical in monitoring the impact of treatment or for surveillance purposes.

Carcinoembryonic Antigen

The cell surface protein carcinoembryonic antigen (CEA) is found predominantly on normal fetal endocrine tissues in the second trimester of gestation. If CEA is detected in mature individuals, it is of limited diagnostic value but is helpful in differentiating between benign and malignant pleural and ascites effusions. CEA was first described in 1965 as a tumor marker specifically elevated in patients with colon cancer; it was later found to be elevated in patients with breast, lung, liver, and pancreatic cancers. Plasma levels higher than 12 ng/mL are strongly correlated with malignancy. Elevated neoplastic states frequently associated with an increased CEA level are endodermally derived gastrointestinal neoplasms and neck and breast carcinomas. In addition, 20% of smokers and 7% of former smokers have elevated CEA levels.

CEA is used clinically to monitor tumor progress in patients who have diagnosed cancer with a high blood CEA level. If treatment leads to a decline to normal levels (<2.5 ng/mL), a rise in CEA level may indicate cancer recurrence to the clinician. A persistent elevation is indicative of residual disease or poor therapeutic response. In patients who have undergone colon cancer resection surgery, the rate of clearance of CEA levels usually returns to normal within 1 month but may take as long as 4 months. Blood specimens should be obtained 2 to 4 weeks apart to detect a trend.

CA 19-9

CA 19-9 is a glycolipid, Lewis blood group carbohydrate. Elevated levels have been found in patients with pancreatic, hepatobiliary, colorectal, gastric, hepatocellular, pancreatic, and breast cancers. Its main use is as a marker for colorectal and pancreatic carcinoma. This marker has greater specificity for pancreatic cancers than CEA. CA 19-9 is also known as *gastrointestinal cancer–associated antigen*.

CA 15-3

CA 15-3 and CA27.29 are the two biomarkers associated with breast cancer. CA 15-3 is a high-molecular-weight (HMW) glycoprotein coded by the *MUC-2* gene and expressed on the ductal cell surface of most glandular epithelial cells.

CA 15-3 is used to monitor patient response to treatment and recurrence of cancer after mastectomy. The sensitivity is much better in higher stage disease, which makes it a good measure of tumor burden. CA 15-3 is positive in other conditions, including liver disease, some inflammatory conditions, and other carcinomas. A change in the CA 15-3 concentration is more predictive than the absolute concentration. Over time, tumor markers exhibit a steady state in the body, a balance between antigen production by the tumor and degradation and excretion. Changes in tumor burden are reflected by changes in the tumor marker concentration.

A high CA 15-3 level (>32 U/mL) usually indicates advanced breast cancer and a large tumor burden. This biomarker lacks sensitivity and specificity, and is approved only for monitoring the patient's response to treatment and recurrence.

CA 27.29: Breast Carcinoma–Associated Antigen

Carcinoma of the breast often produces mucinous antigens that are HMW glycoproteins with O-linked oligosaccharide chains. MAbs directed against breast carcinoma–associated antigen (CA 27.29) can quantitate the levels of this antigen in serum. The antibodies recognize epitopes of a breast cancer–associated antigen encoded by the human *MUC-2* gene. Increased levels of CA 27.29 (>38 U/mL) may indicate recurrent disease in a woman with treated breast carcinoma and may indicate the need for additional testing or procedures. Some clinical investigators do not endorse the routine use of this new marker.

This tumor marker is not recommended for breast cancer screening but this marker may be helpful in conjunction with other clinical methods for predicting early occurrence of breast cancer.

HER2 (HER2/neu)

HER2/neu is encoded by an oncogene and is overexpressed in invasive breast cancers. It is associated with increased tumor aggressiveness and a reduced survival rate. This biomarker is a predictive assay to assess tumor susceptibility to therapy, such as lapatinib and trastuzumab (Herceptin, a humanized MAb, targets *HER2/neu*).

The *HER2* gene is also called the *ERBB2* (Erb-B2 receptor tyrosine kinase 2) gene. The *HER2* gene makes HER2 proteins. *HER2* proteins are receptors on breast cells. Normally, *HER2* receptors participate in the control of normal breast cell growth, division, and repair. But in about 25% of breast cancers, the *HER* gene malfunctions and makes too many copies of itself. This process is called *HER2 gene amplification*, which leads to *HER2* protein overexpression and uncontrolled growth and division.

Breast cancers with *HER* gene amplification or *HER2* protein overexpression are called *HER2 positive*. *HER2*-positive breast cancers are likely to grow faster, metastasize, and recur. Overexpression of *HER2* in human mammary epithelial cells induces proliferative advantage, transformed characteristics, tumorigenic growth, and proliferative and antiapoptotic changes that mimic early stages of epithelial cell transformation. *HER2* amplification is also seen in early in situ ductal carcinomas without any evidence of invasive disease. *HER2* status is maintained during progression to invasive disease, nodal metastasis, and distant metastasis.

There are four tests for *HER2*:
- Immunohistochemistry (IHC) investigation for the detection of *HER2* protein. Results can be 0 (negative), 1+ (also negative), 2+ (borderline), or 3+ (positive—*HER2* protein overexpression).
- Fluorescence in situ hybridization.
- Subtraction probe technology chromogenic in situ hybridization (SPoT-Light *HER2* CISH test): The results of the SPoT-Light test on FISH results can be positive (*HER2* gene amplification) or negative (no *HER2* gene amplification).
- Inform Dual in situ hybridization (Inform *HER2* Dual ISH test): The results of the Inform *HER2* Dual ISH test can be positive (*HER2* gene amplification) or negative (no *HER2* gene amplification).

In general, only cancers that test IHC 3+, FISH positive, SPoT-Light *HER2* CISH positive, or Inform *HER2* Dual ISH positive respond to the drugs that target *HER2*-positive breast cancers. An IHC 2+ test result is considered borderline. In borderline cases, additional retesting with a more precise *HER2* test—the FISH test, SPoT-Light *HER2* CISH test, or the Inform *HER2* Dual ISH test—is warranted.

Research has shown that some breast cancers that are *HER2* positive can become *HER2* negative over time. In comparison, a *HER2*-negative breast cancer can become *HER2* positive over time. If the breast cancer comes back in the future as advanced disease, doctors should consider ordering another biopsy and retesting the tissue's *HER2* status.

Other Cancer Biomarkers

Human Chorionic Gonadotropin (hCG)

Human chorionic gonadotropin (hCG) is a glycoprotein hormone comprised of one α-subunit and one β-subunit. In early pregnancy, hCG is produced by placental trophoblasts, and the α- and β-subunits combine and stimulate corpus luteum synthesis of the steroid hormone, progesterone. Quantitative detection of intact either in a combined or total hCG plus free β-subunits is used to detect and monitor pregnancy. A serum level of β-hCG higher than 1 ng/mL is strongly suggestive of pregnancy.

Ectopic production of several hCG variants is well documented in malignant tumors such as some trophoblastic hydatiform moles and gestational trophoblastic disease and nontrophoblastic (ovarian, breast, or colorectal) disease. Differences in isoform and glycoform vary widely between different instrumentation testing platforms. However, the instrumentation testing platforms of Abbott Architect, Roche Elecsys STAT, Roche Elecsys Total, Siemens Dimension, and Beckman Access are all adequate for use of hCG as a tumor marker in gestational trophoblastic disease and certain germ cell tumors. When monitoring tumors the same instrument platform should be used to ensure continuity.

Miscellaneous Enzyme Markers

Lactic dehydrogenase (LDH) is a frequently measured enzyme of the glycolytic pathway. The level of LDH is elevated in a wide variety of malignancies and other medical disorders. Its level has been shown to correlate with tumor mass in solid tumors, so it can be used to monitor progression of these tumors.

Neuron-specific enolase is an isoenzyme specific for all tumor cells derived from the neural crest. An enzyme increase has been detected in neuroblastoma, pheochromocytoma, oat cell carcinomas, medullary thyroid and C-cell parathyroid carcinomas, and other neural crest–derived cancers. Serum levels are frequently elevated in disseminated disease.

Placental ALP can be detected during pregnancy. ALP is also associated with the neoplastic conditions of seminoma and ovarian cancer.

Miscellaneous Hormone Markers

Elevated or inappropriate serum levels of hormones can function as tumor markers. Adrenocorticotropic hormone (ACTH), calcitonin, and catecholamines may be secreted by differentiated tumors of endocrine organs and squamous cell lung tumors. Oat cell carcinomas may produce β-hCG, antidiuretic hormone (ADH), serotonin, calcitonin, parathyroid hormone (PTH), and ACTH. These hormones can be used to follow a patient's response to therapy.

In addition, some breast cancers demonstrate progesterone and estradiol (estrogen) receptors, which are strongly correlated with a positive response to antihormone therapy. Patients with neuroblastoma and pheochromocytoma secrete catecholamine metabolites that can be detected in the urine. Neuroblastomas also release neuron-specific enolase and ferritin; these markers can be used for diagnosis and prognosis.

Breast, Ovarian, and Cervical Cancer Markers

For more than 15 years, circulating breast cancer antigens have been used to monitor therapy and evaluate recurrence of the cancer. Estrogen and progesterone receptors are universally accepted as prognostic markers and therapeutic choice indicators. A relatively new approach has been the use of the oncogene *HER2/neu* as a prognostic indicator and a marker related to the choice of therapy. This has been particularly useful since the introduction of trastuzumab as a chemotherapeutic agent that targets the *HER2/neu* receptor. Breast cancer patients who express *HER2/neu* in their cancers have a poor prognosis with shorter disease-free and overall survival times than patients who do not express *HER2/neu*. The evaluation of *HER2/neu* has two clinical functions: (1) predictive marker for response to trastuzumab therapy, and (2) prognostic marker.

A newer and more powerful predictor of the outcome of primary breast cancer in young women has been reported. Microarray analysis of a previously established 70-gene profile has demonstrated that a good-prognosis gene expression signature is a strongly independent factor in predicting disease outcome.

Epidermal Growth Factor Receptor

EGFR and *HER2*, *HER2/neu*, and c-erB-2 are transmembrane tyrosine kinase receptors expressed on normal epithelial cells but overexpressed in some cancer cells. A portion of both receptors is released from the cell surface and circulates in normal people and in abnormally high levels in cancer patients. The shed portions can be measured in serum or plasma using antibody-based immunoassays. These assays allow real-time assessment of the patient's *HER2/neu* or EGFR status and repeat testing for patient monitoring; they can be performed in a standardized and quantitative manner.

HER2 and EGFR have been the targets of considerable pharmaceutical activity to develop therapies that will interfere with the oncogenic potential of these growth factor receptors. These therapies include small-molecule inhibitors designed to target and block the function of *HER2* protein overexpression. One drug, trastuzumab, is a humanized antibody that targets cells that overexpress *HER2/neu* and has been successfully used in combination with chemotherapy to increase the efficacy of the antibody-based treatment. An anti-EGFR antibody known as *IMC-225* is directed against cells that overexpress the EGFR oncoprotein.

Molecular Diagnosis of Breast Cancer

In June 2011, the FDA-approved Inform Dual ISH, a genetic test developed by a Roche affiliate (Ventana Medical Systems, Tucson, AZ). This test helps determine whether breast cancer patients are *HER2* positive, which makes them candidates for trastuzumab therapy. The Dual ISH test was designed to detect amplification quantitatively by light microscopy of the *HER2* gene using two-color chromogenic in situ hybridization (CISH) in formalin-fixed, paraffin-embedded human breast and gastric cancer. An advantage of this procedure is that it is possible to view *HER2* and chromosome 17 signals directly under a microscope and for a longer period.

A Ki-67 IHC test for the determination of the proliferative index can be conducted. Because about 60% of women with invasive breast cancer are candidates for selective estrogen modulators, the Ki-67 IHC test is used to detect tumor cells in the cell cycle.

Bladder Cancer

Tumor markers for the management of patients with bladder cancer have been actively investigated. Assays approved for clinical use include the following:
- Matritech nuclear matrix protein (NMP-22)
- Bard bladder tumor antigen (BTA) test

Almost all human tumors contain telomerase, a growth enzyme that promotes the malignant proliferation of cancer. Normal cells usually do not have this enzyme, but telomerase renews the DNA of tumor cells and permits indefinite replication.

Telomerase was first observed in ovarian cancer cells, and its presence was later established in almost all cancers. It is not clear whether other vital cells need telomerase to function. For example, telomerase inhibition could adversely affect stem cells, which help produce blood cells and lymphocytes and may need the enzyme to function. Second, telomerase inhibition has not been proved or tested physiologically in human beings. Finally, a drug based on telomerase would have to reduce the ability of the cancer to spread. Screening for telomerase inhibitors and plans for future studies to discover and develop chemicals that block the action of telomerase may suggest a design of more effective anticancer drugs.

> **KEY CONCEPTS: DNA Microarray Technology**
> - Cancer can arise not only from mutations in oncogenes and tumor suppressor genes, but also from genes involved in cell cycle control, DNA repair, and apoptosis.
> - Microarrays have the potential to uncover signature gene expression patterns for specific cancers and ultimately assist in the staging of tumors, prognosis, and treatment.
> - Microarrays may help disclose global gene expression pattern differences between healthy and diseased cells as more sensitive and specific diagnostic markers are developed.

DNA MICROARRAY TECHNOLOGY

New developments in molecular genetics involve DNA microarray technology (see Chapter 12). Cancer can arise not only from mutations in oncogenes and tumor suppressor genes, but also from genes involved in cell cycle control, DNA repair, and apoptosis. Microarrays have the potential to uncover signature gene expression patterns for specific cancers and ultimately assist in the staging of tumors, prognosis, and treatment. Microarrays may help disclose global gene expression pattern differences between healthy and diseased cells as more sensitive and specific diagnostic markers are developed, such as the CD44+/CD24– gene expression profile in breast cancer versus normal breast tissue. When differentially expressed genes were used to generate a 186-gene invasiveness gene signature (IGS), the IGS was strongly associated with metastasis-free survival and overall survival for four different types of tumors.

Proteomic technology uses two-dimensional polyacrylamide gel electrophoresis (2D-PAGE) and mass spectrometry. Although these techniques are not revolutionary, advances have improved their sensitivity. Expansion of computer-assisted bioinformatics has simplified the process of protein identification from mass spectra. Mass spectra are proving to be comparable to CA 125 for the detection of early-stage ovarian cancer.

In colorectal cancer, fecal DNA screening has been demonstrated to be useful. Oncogene mutations that characterize colorectal neoplasia are detectable in exfoliated epithelial cells in the stool. Neoplastic bleeding is intermittent, but epithelial shedding is continual, potentially making fecal DNA testing more sensitive.

> **KEY CONCEPTS: New Cancer Diagnostic Testing**
> - The use of next-generation sequencing (NGS), or massive parallel sequencing, is not to sequence the entire cancer genomes but to look for the presence of a specific few actionable mutations.
> - Three aspects of importance in NGS are identification of somatic mutations, detection of low levels of genomic alterations, and improved management of cancer treatment.
> - Continuous field flow–assisted dielectrophoresis (DEP) allows for the isolation and characterization of rare circulating tumor cells (CTCs).
> - A newer technology, continuous field flow–assisted dielectrophoresis, is FDA approved for use with only three tumor types: prostate, breast, and colorectal cancers.

WHAT'S NEW IN CANCER DIAGNOSTIC TESTING?

Massive Parallel Sequencing/Next-Generation Sequencing

The use of NGS is not to sequence entire cancer genomes, but rather to look for the presence of a specific few actionable mutations. One small panel of 5 to 50 genes can be used for each tumor type and assayed at once, currently within about 3 days. Also with the small sample size needed, free circulating tumor DNA can be assayed from blood in many cancer types. This eliminates the need for invasive and expensive biopsies.

NGS, as described in Chapter 12, is another step toward personalized cancer treatment. Three aspects of importance in NGS are:
1. Identification of somatic mutations
2. Detection of low levels of genomic alterations
3. Improved management of cancer treatment

Identification of Somatic Mutations

The genetic fingerprint reveals the somatic alteration of cancer genomes. Genetic changes that are associated with cancer include a single nucleotide change or structural chromosomal changes. Only some acquired genetic alterations are clinically significant.

Detection of Low Levels of Genomic Alterations

NGS has higher sensitivity of mutations in cells than traditional Sanger genome sequencing. This allows for better detection of changes occurring in only a small number of cells.

Improved Management of Cancer Treatment

Accurate diagnosis of cancer, including leukemias, is dependent on accurate molecular profiling. This contributes to improved treatment and the ability to predict a prognosis.

The goal of NGS technology is to be able to quickly generate data from a small sample of tissue from a tumor.

Continuous Field Flow–Assisted Dielectrophoresis

The ability to isolate and characterize rare CTCs may provide critical insights into primary tumors and the process of metastasis and monitoring of disease progression. Performing molecular analysis of CTCs offers a unique approach for genotyping patient-specific tumors and mutations, in addition to guiding treatment options.

To date, only one technology has been FDA approved for use with only three tumor types: prostate, breast, and colorectal cancers. The new technology is antibody dependent; that means the detection and capture of CTCs depend on antigen expression of the surface of cancer cells of epithelial origin (e.g., EpCAM). A new next-generation antibody-independent technology has recently been developed. It relies on continuous field flow–assisted DEP to isolate and recover CTCs from the blood of cancer patients. This technology has already proven to be successful in detecting and isolating a wider range of cancers in greater cell quantities, and research prototypes are now being used in phase I, phase II, and phase III clinical studies. The isolation of rare cells from blood using DEP field flow assist is based on the differences in dielectric properties between peripheral white blood cells (e.g., lymphocytes, monocytes, granulocytes, and solid tissue–deprived cancer cells). This technology is revolutionary because:

1. It permits the isolation of cancer cells from all types of cancer (e.g., lung, prostate, melanoma, breast, pancreatic, and liver).
2. The higher CTC isolation and capture capability provides greater opportunities for downstream analysis of cancer cells for treatment options and monitoring of effectiveness.
3. DEP technology captures the cancer cells in a viable state that allows for additional biological testing.

Future applications of this technology are being explored to facilitate implementation of personalized medicine with improved clinical outcomes.

> **KEY CONCEPTS: Treating Cancer**
> - Modalities for treating cancer include surgery, radiation, and chemotherapeutics.
> - In addition to the classic therapies, newer therapies (e.g., monoclonal antibodies [MAbs]) are being used.
> - Chemotherapy can reduce tumor burden by eliminating the highly proliferative cells with subclones but spare relatively dormant cells that can seed a new cancer.
> - Cytokines constitute another group of cancer chemotherapy drugs.
> - The use of MAbs for cancer therapy is one of the great success stories of the past decade.
> - Immunotherapy for tumors can take the form of active or passive therapy.
> - The development of inhibitors to target proteins encoded by mutated cancer genes has now been achieved, with repeated success.

MODALITIES FOR TREATING CANCER

Modalities for treating cancer include surgery, radiation, and chemotherapeutics. Much of the improvement in outcomes is due to new surgical procedures and radiation treatments, particularly in some tumor types such as gliomas. Many different modes of therapy, including angiogenesis inhibitors, which keep tumors from building new blood vessels to supply themselves with food and oxygen, have demonstrated effectiveness in the treatment of cancer.

Chemotherapeutic Agents

Chemotherapy drugs are used in cancer therapy for cure, palliation, and research to develop more effective therapy. Chemotherapy can reduce tumor burden by eliminating the highly proliferative cells with subclones but spare relatively dormant cells that can seed a new cancer (Fig. 26.6).

The mechanisms of drug action are linked to the mitotic cell cycle; thus antitumor drugs may be placed in the following three classes:
- Cell cycle active, phase specific
- Cell cycle active, phase nonspecific
- Non–cell cycle active

Cell Cycle Active, Phase Specific

Drugs in the cell cycle active, phase-specific category act on the S, G2, or M phases of mitosis. S phase active drugs are divided into antimetabolites, antifolates, and synthetic enzyme inhibitors. Antimetabolites act through the incorporation of a nucleotide analog into DNA, resulting in an abnormal nucleic acid (e.g., 5-fluorouracil, 6-mercaptopurine, 6-thioguanine, and fludarabine). The antifolates act as competitive inhibitors of the enzyme dihydrofolate reductase, which is necessary for the generation of CH_3 groups required for thymidine synthesis (e.g., methotrexate). Synthetic enzyme inhibitors include DNA polymerase inhibitor (cytosine arabinoside) and nucleotide reductase inhibitors (hydroxyurea).

G2 phase active drugs include bleomycin, which is thought to cause fragmentation of DNA, and etoposide (Eposin, Etopophos, VePesid, and VP-16), which is thought to cause double-strand breaks in DNA by complexing with topoisomerase.

M phase active drugs include vinca alkaloids (e.g., vincristine and vinblastine), which are thought to inhibit the mitotic spindle apparatus, and paclitaxel (Taxol), which stabilizes microtubules.

Cell Cycle Active, Phase Nonspecific

Drugs in the cell cycle active, phase nonspecific category are intercalating agents, alkylating agents, and 5-fluorouracil. Examples of intercalating agents are anthracyclines (adriamycin, daunomycin, idarubicin, mitoxantrone) and actinomycin D (dactinomycin; Cosmegen, Lyovac). The alkylating agents in this category include cyclophosphamide and ifosfamide. These drugs act by distorting normal DNA through the insertion of flat, aromatic ring systems between the levels of base pairs into the DNA double helix.

Non–Cell Cycle Active

Drugs in the non–cell cycle active category can be divided into five types: alkylating agents, L-asparaginase, corticosteroids, hormone antagonists, and miscellaneous. Alkylating agents (e.g., nitrogen mustard and mustard derivatives—mechlorethamine [Mustargen], cyclophosphamide [Cytoxan], chlorambucil [Leukeran], and melphalan [Alkeran])—act by interstrand crosslinking of DNA, thereby preventing normal DNA replication. This interference is not only cytotoxic but also potentially mutagenic and carcinogenic. L-Asparaginase inhibits protein synthesis.

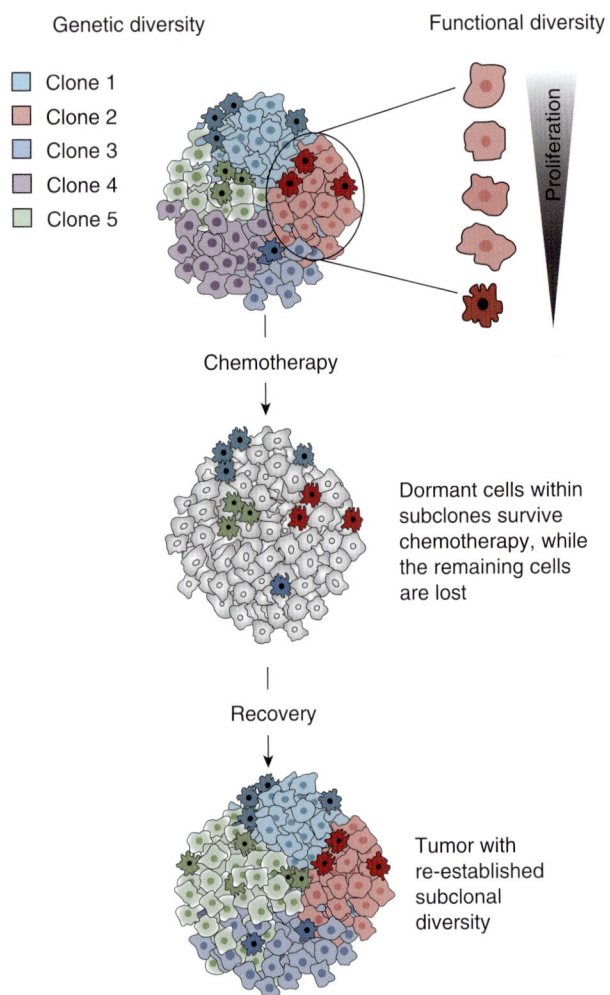

Fig. 26.6 Functional diversity between cells within subclones affects the response to therapy. Each clone (depicted by the different colors) contains a mixture of cells that vary with respect to their stemness and/or proliferative ability, including relatively dormant cells. Together these factors represent the functional diversity present within single genetic subclones. Chemotherapy can reduce tumor burden by eliminating the highly proliferative cells within subclones while sparing the relatively dormant cells; after therapy, these cells can seed a new cancer. Thus subclonal diversity can be altered with chemotherapy and can allow for the selection of cells with additional genetic mutations that confer a survival advantage. Not depicted in the diagram is the concept that chemotherapy-resistant cells can exist before treatment and can be selected after chemotherapy. Thus chemotherapy can introduce new mutations to confer treatment resistance, but it can also select preexisting cells that accumulated mutations, which confer chemotherapy resistance during the long evolution of the tumor before it was diagnosed. (From Kreso A, Dick JE: Evolution of the cancer stem cell model, *Cell Stem Cell* 14[3]:275–291, 2014.)

Glucocorticosteroids are the most frequently used steroids. Steroids control the damaging inflammatory immune response. The target cells are monocytes and T lymphocytes. Monocytes block IL-1 production, block TNF-γ, and reduce chemotaxis. The consequences are inhibition of T-cell activation, activation and recruitment of monocytes and neutrophils, and inhibition of the migration of cells to the site of inflammation. The steroids used in cancer oncology include glucocorticoids (prednisone), estrogens (diethylstilbestrol), androgens (testosterone propionate), and also progestagenic agents (medroxyprogesterone, megestrol acetate).

Hormone estrogen antagonists (e.g., tamoxifen) competitively bind to specific cytoplasmic receptors.

Cytokines

Cytokines constitute another group of cancer chemotherapy drugs (see Chapter 2). Interferon, IL-2, and colony-stimulating factors (CSFs) have been used to treat certain types of cancer in patients. Currently, IFNs are used to treat patients with hairy cell leukemia, chronic myelogenous leukemia, and multiple myeloma. IL-2 is used in the treatment of renal cell carcinoma and melanoma. CSFs reduce the duration of chemotherapy-induced neutropenia and may permit more dose-intensive therapy.

The clinical development of recombinant IFN-α represents the most rapid development of any antineoplastic drug in the United States. IFN was first recognized as a naturally occurring antiviral substance in 1957 and identified for its antineoplastic properties. IFN-α appears to have activity in a wide range of malignancies.

Effects of Drug-Induced Immunosuppression

Drugs used to treat malignancies such as solid tumors or leukemia can have profoundly suppressive effects on the inflammatory response, delayed hypersensitivity, and specific antibody production (Table 26.10). Examples of the immune depression induced by drugs include depletion of T cells by corticosteroids, caused by the blocking of egress from the bone marrow into the circulation, and dysfunction of the antibody response, caused by folate antagonists and purine analogs. Thus infection secondary to immune suppression is a major cause of death in cancer patients beginning therapy and those who are in clinical remission.

Monoclonal Antibody Therapy

The use of MAbs for the therapy of cancer is one of the great success stories of the past decade. The fundamental basis of antibody-based therapy of tumors dates back to the original observations of antigen expression by tumor cells through serologic techniques in the 1960s. The identification of cell surface differentiation antigens, which were initially used to distinguish lymphocyte subsets, set the stage for a revolution in biological and biomedical sciences. Recent studies have shown that, in addition to changes in the surface antigenic structure of cancer cells, tumor stromal and tumor vascular cells express novel antigens that distinguish them from their normal counterparts.

MAb technology began with the winning contribution of Köhler, Milstein, and Jerne, who won the Nobel Prize in Physiology or Medicine in 1984. This led to great expectations that MAbs would provide effective targeted therapy for cancer. After early enthusiasm for MAbs, clinical trials were disappointing in the 1980s and early 1990s with one exception: antiidiotype antibodies in follicular lymphoma. When success was finally observed in hematologic malignancies, the importance of the antigen target specificity and of developing humanized MAbs was recognized. Definition of cell surface antigens that are expressed by human cancers has revealed a broad array of targets that are overexpressed, mutated, or selectively expressed compared with normal tissues.

The major success of MAb therapy has been seen with anti-CD20 MAbs. The anti-CD20 rituximab (Table 26.11) was the first MAb to be approved by the FDA for use in relapsed indolent lymphoma. Today, rituximab is widely accepted to be the single most important factor leading to an improved prognosis in a range of B-cell lymphomas and, more recently, in B-cell chronic lymphocytic leukemia (CLL). However, some patients develop resistance to rituximab, which provides a challenge for research.

TABLE 26.10 Effects of Chemotherapy on the Immune Response

Chemotherapeutic Agent	ANTIBODY		DELAYED HYPERSENSITIVITY	
	Primary Response	Secondary Response	Primary Response (Initial)	Secondary Response (Recall)
Corticosteroid	0	0	++	+
Methotrexate	++	+	+	0
6-Mercaptopurine	0	+	+	0
Azathioprine	0	+	+	0
6-Thioguanine	0	+	+	0
Cytosine arabinoside	+	++	0	0
Cyclophosphamide	++	0	+	0
L-Asparaginase	+	0	0	0
Daunomycin	+	0	+	0

+ = strong reaction; ++ = very strong reaction.

TABLE 26.11 Examples of Monoclonal Antibodies for Cancer Treatment

Antigen Category	Examples of Antigens	Examples of Therapeutic MAbs Raised Against These Targets	Tumor Types Expressing Antigen
Hematopoietic differentiation antigens	CD20	Rituximab	Non-Hodgkin lymphoma
	CD30	Ibritumomab tiuxetan and tositumomab	Lymphoma
	CD33	Brentuximab vedotin	Hodgkin lymphoma
	CD52	Gemtuzumab ozogamicin	Acute myelogenous leukemia
		Alemtuzumab	Chronic lymphocytic leukemia
Glycoproteins expressed by solid tumors	CEA	Labetuzumab	Breast, colon, lung tumors
Glycolipids	Gangliosides	3F8, ch14.18, and KW-2871	Neuroectodermal tumors and some epithelial tumors
Carbohydrates	Ley	Hu3S193 and IgN311	Breast, colon, lung, and prostate tumors
Targets of antiangiogenic MAbs	VEGF	Bevacizumab	Tumor vasculature
Growth and differentiation signaling	EGFR	Cetuximab, panitumumab, nimotuzumab, and 806	Glioma, lung, breast, colon, and hand and neck tumors
	ERBB2	Trastuzumab and pertuzumab	Breast, colon, lung, and head and neck tumors
Stromal and extracellular matrix antigens	Fibroblast activation protein	Sibrotuzumab and F19	Colon, breast, lung, pancreas, and head and neck tumors

CEA, Carcinoembryonic antigen; *EGFR*, epidermal growth factor receptor; *Ley*, Lewis Y antigen; *MAbs*, monoclonal antibodies; *VEGF*, vascular endothelial growth factor.
Adapted from Scott AM, Wolchok JD, Old LJ: Antibody therapy of cancer, *Nat Rev Cancer* 12(4):278–287, 2012.

Antibody-based therapeutics can function by mediating alterations in antigen or receptor function, modulating the immune system or delivering a specific drug that is conjugated to an antibody that targets a specific antigen. The mechanisms of tumor cell killing by antibodies are presented in Fig. 26.6.

Immunotherapy for tumors can take the form of active or passive therapy. Active host immune responses may be achieved by the following:
- Vaccination with killed tumor cells or with tumor antigens or peptides. New research studies have suggested that anti-CD20 MAb may induce an adaptive antitumor immune response or vaccination effect, which may underlie the durable remissions experienced by some patients after anti-CD20 MAb treatment.
- Enhancement of cell-mediated immunity to tumors by expressing costimulators and cytokines and treating with cytokines that stimulate the proliferation and differentiation of T lymphocytes and NK cells.
- Nonspecific stimulation of the immune system by the local administration of inflammatory substances or by systemic treatment with agents that function as polyclonal activators of lymphocytes.
- For the first time in the history of cancer treatment, gene therapy has apparently succeeded in shrinking and even eradicating large metastatic tumors. Inserting genes into a patient's cells enables the body to fight a disease on its own, without medication.

Passive immunotherapy consists of the following:
- Adoptive cellular therapy by transferring cultured immune cells with antitumor reactivity into a tumor-bearing host.
- Administration of tumor-specific MAbs for immunotherapy.

A newer form of therapy, the development of inhibitors to target proteins encoded by mutated cancer genes, has been achieved with repeated success. The first victory was imatinib mesylate (Gleevec), approved by the FDA in 2001, a potent inhibitor of the Abelson (ABL) kinase in chronic myeloid leukemia (CML). This is an important example of therapeutic targeting of the products of genomic alterations in a specific cancer.

After the referencing of the genome sequence, cancer genomes have been identified for several new mutated cancer genes. Unfortunately, many mutated cancer genes do not make tractable targets for new drug development. The International Cancer Genome Consortium and the Cancer Genome Atlas are using NGS technologies for tumors from 50 different cancer types to generate more than 25,000 genomes at genomic, epigenomic, and transcriptomic levels. This should generate a complete catalog of oncogenic mutations, some of which may prove to be new therapeutic targets.

The list of drugs used for cancer therapy continues to grow. The new therapeutic agents target various modes of action and applications (Table 26.12).

TABLE 26.12 Examples of Currently Approved Monoclonal Antibodies and Mechanisms of Action

Antibody	Target	Mechanisms of Action
Trastuzumab (Herceptin; Genentech): humanized IgG1	*ERBB2* gene	Inhibition of *ERBB2* signaling and ADCC
Bevacizumab (Avastin; Genentech/Roche): humanized IgG1	VEGF	Inhibition of *VEGF* signaling
Cetuximab (Erbitux; Bristol-Myers Squibb) chimeric human–murine IgG1	EGFR	Inhibition of *EGFR* signaling and ADCC
Panitumumab (Vectibix™, Amgen, Inc.), human IgG2	*EGFR* gene	Inhibition of *EGFR* signaling
		Inhibition of *CTLA4* signaling
Rituximab (Mabthera; Roche): chimeric human–murine IgG1	CD20	ADCC, direct induction of apoptosis and CDC
Alemtuzumab (Campath; Genzyme): humanized IgG1	CD52	Direct induction of apoptosis and CDC
Ofatumumab (Arzerra; Genmab): human IgG1	CD20	ADCC and CDC
Gemtuzumab ozogamicin (Mylotarg; Wyeth): humanized IgG4	CD33	Delivery of toxic payload, calicheamicin toxin
Brentuximab vedotin (Adcetris; Seattle Genetics): chimeric IgG1	CD30	Delivery of toxic payload, auristatin toxin
^{90}Y-labeled ibritumomab tiuxetan (Zevalin; IDEC Pharmaceuticals): murine IgG1	CD20	Delivery of the radioisotope ^{90}Y
^{131}I-labeled tositumomab (Bexxar; GlaxoSmithKline): murine IgG2–ADCC, CDC	CD20	Delivery of the radioisotope ^{131}I, ADCC, and direct induction of apoptosis

ADCC, Antibody-dependent cell-mediated cytotoxicity; *CDC*, complement-dependent cytotoxicity; *EGFR*, epidermal growth factor receptor; *IgG*, immunoglobulin G; *VEGF*, vascular endothelial growth factor.

CASE STUDY 26.1

A 59-year-old White man visited his primary care provider because of his need to urinate frequently and urgently. Over the past several years, his urine output had been small volumes, with a decreasing flow rate.

On physical examination, the patient had an enlarged prostate with a smooth, uniform surface. A PSA assay was ordered. The results of the current and previous assays were as follows (reference range, 0–3.5 ng/mL):
- Current PSA level—5.5 ng/mL
- PSA level 1 year ago—2.3 ng/mL

Questions
1. Prostate-specific antigen (PSA) is:
   a. A prostate cancer–specific marker
   b. A prostate tissue–specific marker
   c. Indirectly proportional to tumor volume
   d. A marker to distinguish between prostate cancer and benign prostatic hypertrophy (BPH)

2. Tumor markers for prostate cancer can include:
   a. β-human chorionic gonadotropic hormone
   b. Ratio of free to total PSA
   c. Carcinoembryonic antigen (CEA)
   d. α1-fetoprotein

Answers to these questions can be found in Appendix A.

Critical Thinking Group Discussion Questions
1. Is the change in the patient's PSA results in 1 year significant?
2. What is the clinical significance of the patient's results?
3. What is the expected follow-up regimen for a patient with this profile?
4. After a radical prostatectomy, what PSA values would be expected?

CASE STUDY 26.2

A 65-year-old Black woman visited her primary care provider for an annual examination, including a routine pelvic examination. Although she had gained some weight since her last examination, she reported that her general health was good but that she had been experiencing some gastrointestinal problems over the past 6 weeks.

A palpable mass was discovered during her pelvic examination. A CA 125 assay and a transvaginal ultrasound examination were ordered.

The patient's CA 125 was 425 U/mL (reference range, <35 U/mL). The presence of a mass in the right side of the abdomen and abdominal ascites were confirmed.

The patient had a total abdominal hysterectomy with a bilateral salpingo-oophorectomy; 4 weeks after the operation, she began a chemotherapy series. The patient was judged to be in remission for 6 months when recurrence of the tumor was noted with diagnostic imaging. Subsequent chemotherapy was ineffective, and the patient died 8 months later.

Question
1. The tumor marker of significance for ovarian cancer is:
   a. Carcinoembryonic antigen (CEA)
   b. α1-fetoprotein (AFP)
   c. CA 125
   d. β-hCG human chorionic gonadotropic hormone

Answers to this question can be found in Appendix A.

Critical Thinking Group Discussion Questions
1. Is CA 125 an effective diagnostic blood serum tumor marker?
2. Is CA 125 a specific tumor marker for ovarian cancer?
3. What is the major clinical use of CA 125?

REVIEW QUESTIONS

1. Benign tumors are characterized as:
   a. Slowly growing
   b. Resembling the parent tissue
   c. Usually invading tissues (metastasizing)
   d. Both a and b
2. A benign tumor arising from glands is called a(n):
   a. Sarcoma
   b. Adenoma
   c. Adenocarcinoma
   d. Papilloma
3. A benign tumor arising from epithelial surfaces is called a(n):
   a. Sarcoma
   b. Adenoma
   c. Adenocarcinoma
   d. Papilloma
4. A malignant tumor of connective tissue is called a(n):
   a. Sarcoma
   b. Adenoma
   c. Adenocarcinoma
   d. Papilloma
5. A malignant tumor of glandular epithelium is called a(n):
   a. Sarcoma
   b. Adenoma
   c. Adenocarcinoma
   d. Papilloma
6. Which of the following is *not* a risk factor in the development of cancer?
   a. Smoking
   b. Low-fat diet
   c. Obesity
   d. Sedentary lifestyle
7. Risk factors associated with breast cancer include:
   a. First-degree family history of breast cancer
   b. Pregnancy after 30 years of age
   c. Use of estrogen (oral contraceptives or hormone replacement)
   d. All of the above
8. Cells involved in the immune response to tumors are:
   a. T cells, B cells, and macrophages
   b. Cytotoxic T cells, NK cells, and macrophages
   c. Neutrophils, lymphocytes, and monocytes
   d. CD8+ lymphocytes, monocytes, and basophils
9. Which of the following is *not* an environmental factor associated with carcinogenesis?
   a. Ultraviolet light
   b. Organically grown herbs
   c. Benzene
   d. Asbestos
10. The risk factor associated with the development of basal cell carcinoma or malignant melanoma is:
    a. Infrared light
    b. Sunless tanning lotions
    c. Ultraviolet light
    d. Strobe lights
11. Patients with Down syndrome have a higher incidence of:
    a. Leukemia
    b. Breast cancer
    c. Prostate cancer
    d. Teratomas
12. Tumor cells typically carry _____ genetic change(s).
    a. One
    b. Two
    c. Three to six
    d. Multiple
13. Cancer-predisposing genes may:
    a. Affect a host's ability to repair damage to DNA
    b. Increase cell cohesiveness
    c. Decrease cell motility
    d. Enhance the host's immune ability to recognize and eradicate incipient tumors
14. Oncogenes are:
    a. Genetic targets of carcinogens
    b. Altered versions of normal genes
    c. Detectable in 15% to 20% of a variety of human tumors
    d. All of the above
15. A mutation or overexpression of an oncogene:
    a. Results in the production of nonfunctional proteins that can no longer control cell proliferation
    b. Produces proteins that can stimulate uncontrolled cell growth
16. A mutation or overexpression of tumor suppressor genes:
    a. Results in the production of nonfunctional proteins that can no longer control cell proliferation
    b. Produces proteins that can stimulate uncontrolled cell growth
17. Which of the following is used to determine the risk of developing cancer?
    a. *p53* gene
    b. *c-erbB-2* gene
    c. Squamous cell carcinoma antigen
    d. Epidermal growth factor receptor (EGFR)
18. A tumor marker assay is most useful:
    a. To screen patients for malignancies
    b. To monitor a cancer patient for disease recurrence
    c. To determine the degree of tumor burden
    d. All of the above
19. Tumor-specific antigens are:
    a. Cell surface molecules coded for by tumorigenic viruses
    b. Gene products resulting from gene depression
    c. Antigens uniquely related to each tumor
    d. Probably not a producer of unique antigens
20. Tumor-associated antigens are:
    a. Cell surface molecules coded for by tumorigenic viruses
    b. Gene products resulting from gene depression
    c. Antigens uniquely related to each tumor
    d. Probably not a producer of unique antigens
21. Carcinofetal antigens are:
    a. Cell surface molecules coded for by tumorigenic viruses
    b. Gene products resulting from gene depression
    c. Antigens uniquely related to each tumor
    d. Probably not a producer of unique antigens
22. Carcinoembryonic antigen is:
    a. An oncofetal protein elevated in some types of cancer that is found on normal fetal endocrine tissue in the second trimester of gestation
    b. An elevated oncofetal protein strongly correlated with various malignancies that is found on normal fetal endocrine tissue in the second trimester of gestation
    c. Used clinically to monitor tumor progress in some types of patients and is persistently elevated even in residual disease or poor therapeutic response
    d. Both b and c

23. Alpha-fetoprotein (AFP) characteristically includes all of the following *except*:
    a. Is synthesized by the fetal liver and yolk sac
    b. Can be elevated in some nonneoplastic conditions
    c. Is a very reliable marker in liver cancer for monitoring a patient's response to chemotherapy and radiation therapy
    d. Most likely in breast cancer
24. β-hCG is *not*:
    a. Elevated in normal pregnancy
    b. A sensitive tumor marker
    c. Elevated in squamous cell carcinoma of the lung
    d. Elevated in teratocarcinoma and choriocarcinoma
25. Prostate-specific antigen is:
    a. Prostate tissue specific
    b. Prostate cancer specific
    c. Not useful for monitoring response to therapy in patients with prostate cancer
    d. Not directly suggestive of increasing tumor volume in prostate malignancies
26. Carcinoembryonic antigen (CEA):
    a. Is frequently elevated in endometrial-derived gastrointestinal carcinomas
    b. Is most useful in ovarian and endometrial carcinomas
    c. May indicate recurrent breast carcinoma at increased levels
    d. May be elevated in patients with colorectal malignancies
27. Alpha-fetoprotein (AFP):
    a. Is frequently elevated in endometrially derived gastrointestinal carcinomas
    b. Is most useful in ovarian and endometrial carcinomas
    c. May indicate recurrent breast carcinoma at increased levels
28. CA 125:
    a. Is frequently elevated in endometrially derived gastrointestinal carcinomas
    b. Is most useful in ovarian and endometrial carcinomas
    c. May indicate recurrent breast carcinoma at increased levels
    d. May be elevated in patients with gastrointestinal malignancies
29. CA 19-9:
    a. Is frequently elevated in endometrially derived gastrointestinal carcinomas
    b. Is most useful in ovarian and endometrial carcinomas
    c. May indicate recurrent breast carcinoma at increased levels
    d. May be elevated in patients with gastrointestinal malignancies
30. CA 27-29:
    a. Is frequently elevated in endometrially derived gastrointestinal carcinomas
    b. Is most useful in ovarian and endometrial carcinomas
    c. Associated with recurrent breast carcinoma
    d. May be elevated in patients with gastrointestinal malignancies
31. Which tumor marker is used to monitor patients with breast cancer for recurrence of disease?
    a. CA 15-3
    b. Estrogen receptor (ER)
    c. Cathepsin-D
    d. CA 50
32. 6-Mercaptopurine is:
    a. Cell cycle active, phase specific
    b. Cell cycle active, phase nonspecific
    c. Non–cell cycle active
    d. b or c
33. Corticosteroids are:
    a. Cell cycle active, phase specific
    b. Cell cycle active, phase nonspecific
    c. Non–cell cycle active
    d. b or c
34. Alkylating agents are:
    a. Cell cycle active, phase specific
    b. Cell cycle active, phase nonspecific
    c. Non–cell cycle active
    d. b or c
35. Vinca alkaloids are:
    a. Cell cycle active, phase specific
    b. Cell cycle active, phase nonspecific
    c. Non–cell cycle active
    d. b or c
36. Tamoxifen acts as a(n) _____ pharmaceutical agent.
    a. Cell cycle active, phase-specific
    b. Non–cell cycle active
    c. Estrogen receptor–blocking
    d. Both b and c
37. Active host immunotherapy responses may be achieved by:
    a. Transferring immune cells into the host
    b. Vaccination with killed tumor cells
    c. Administration of tumor-specific MAbs
    d. Administration of IFN-α
38. Benzene is associated with:
    a. Endometrial cancer
    b. Hepatocellular carcinoma
    c. Burkitt lymphoma
    d. Leukemia
39. Estrogen is associated with:
    a. Endometrial cancer
    b. Hepatocellular carcinoma
    c. Burkitt lymphoma
    d. Mesothelioma
40. Epstein-Barr virus (EBV) is associated with:
    a. Endometrial cancer
    b. Hepatocellular carcinoma
    c. Burkitt lymphoma
    d. Leukemia
41. Hepatitis B virus (HBV) is associated with:
    a. Endometrial cancer
    b. Hepatocellular carcinoma
    c. Burkitt lymphoma
    d. Mesothelioma
42. Asbestos is associated with:
    a. Endometrial cancer
    b. Hepatocellular carcinoma
    c. Burkitt lymphoma
    d. Mesothelioma

PART VI

Vaccines

Chapter 27: Vaccines: Development and Applications, 478

27

Vaccines: Development and Applications

LEARNING OUTCOMES

- Describe and compare the characteristics of four leading-edge vaccines.
- Identify the federal agency that regulates vaccine products.
- Describe vaccine policy and the role of vaccines in public safety.
- Explain some new targets and technologies for vaccines.
- Briefly describe the history and use of several specific vaccines.
- Identify at least three essential characteristics of a vaccine.
- Based on immunologic principles, describe the host response to vaccination.
- Analyze the problems associated with AIDS vaccine development and use.
- Describe the development and application of human papillomavirus vaccine.
- Compare and contrast preventive and therapeutic cancer vaccines.
- Discuss the novel leukemia vaccine therapy.
- Analyze a case study.
- Correctly answer case study–related multiple-choice questions.
- Be prepared to participate in a discussion of critical thinking questions.
- Describe the principle and clinical application of the tetanus antibodies assay.
- Correctly answer 80% of the end-of-chapter review questions.

OUTLINE

Leading-Edge Vaccines, 479
    Malaria Vaccines, 479
        RTS,S/AS01, 479
        R21/Matrix-M, 479
        RSV Vaccines, 479
    Shigella, 480
    Tuberculosis, 480
Goal of Vaccination, 481
What is a Vaccine?, 481
History of Vaccines, 481
Types of Vaccines, 481
    Inactivated Vaccines, 482
    Live, Attenuated Vaccines, 482
    Nucleic Acid Vaccines, 482
        DNA Vaccines, 482
        RNA Vaccines, 484
    Covid Vaccine Development, 484
    Virus-Like Particle (VLP) Vaccines, 485
    Subunit Vaccines and Carriers, 485
        Recombinant Protein Vaccine, 485
        Polysaccharide and Conjugate Vaccines, 487
    Replicating and Nonreplicating Viral Vector–Based Vaccines, 488
Model of Vaccine Development, 488
    Step 1. Identify and Sequence the Virus, 488
    Step 2: Determine the Target, 488
    Step 3: Conduct Preclinical Trials, 488
    Step 4: Initiate Human Clinical Trials, 488
    Step 5: Obtain Regulatory Approval, 489
    Step 6: Establish Manufacturing and Distribution, 489
Host Response to Vaccination, 489
Rates of Vaccination, 489
Sites of Vaccine Administration, 490
Representative Diseases Associated With Newer Approved or Investigational Vaccines, 490
    Chikungunya Vaccine, 490
Dengue Fever Vaccine, 490
    Herpes Zoster (Shingles) Vaccine, 490
    HIV/AIDS, 491
        Vaccine Development, 491
        Vaccine Problems, 491
        Clinical Trials, 493
        Vaccine Expectations, 493
    Influenza, 493
International Travel Vaccines, 494
    Epidemiology of Vaccine-Preventable Diseases, 494
    Travel-Only Vaccines and Chemoprophylaxis for Adults, 494
Cancer Vaccines, 495
    Prophylactic Vaccines, 495
        Gardasil, 495
        Cervarix, 496
        Therapeutic vaccines, 496
    Cancer Treatment Vaccines, 496
        Clinical Trials, 496
    Leukemia, 496
Vaccines in Biodefense, 497
    Smallpox, 497
        Category A Agents, 497
        Smallpox Vaccine, 497
    Anthrax, 497
Vaccine Safety Issues, 497

Concerns About Vaccines, 497
Vaccine Side Effects and Adverse Events, 497
Monitoring of Adverse Events with Vaccines, 498

Case Study 27.1, 498
Procedure: Tetanus Antibodies (IgG), 499.e1

KEY TERMS

adjuvants
antigenic drift
conjugate vaccine
cytotoxic T-cell responses
dendritic cells (DCs)
herd immunity
humoral and cellular immunity
innate immune response

intranasal spray application
nanoparticles
pathogen
pathogen recognition receptors
pertussis
polysaccharides
polysaccharide vaccine
protein-based subunit vaccine

subunit vaccines
toll-like receptor (TLR)
vaccination
vaccine
variolation
virus-like particles (VLPs)

LEADING-EDGE VACCINES

Vaccine innovations decreased during the global COVID-19 pandemic. However, in 2023, scientists began to play catch-up and report some innovative breakthroughs. Advances in game-changing vaccine developments create the possibility that emerging vaccines may enable vaccine development to leapfrog beyond the status quo. Four vaccines are on the leading edge of development—malaria, **Respiratory Syncytial Virus (RSV)**, *Shigella*, and tuberculosis (TB).

Malaria Vaccines

October 6, 2021, marks a historic day in the development of malaria vaccines. This day marks the release of the World Health Organization (WHO) recommendation for widespread use of the RTS,S/AS01 AS01(Mosquirix; GlaxoSmithKline) malaria vaccine among children living in sub-Saharan Africa and other regions with moderate-to-high levels of *Plasmodium falciparum* malaria transmission. Malaria is common in sub-Saharan African countries in infants, and related deaths are high. *P. falciparum* is the most severe form of malaria and death. On July 5, 2023 it was announced that 12 countries across different regions in Africa are scheduled to receive 18 million doses of the first-ever malaria vaccine over the next 2 years.

RTS,S/AS01

Clinical trials have documented that the RTS,S/AS01 vaccine containing a segment of the malaria parasite initiates antibody formation in patients who receive the vaccine. The antibodies attack and neutralize the malaria parasite entering the body before it infects the liver and causes a severe infection.

Malaria parasites have a complex life cycle, and there is poor understanding of the complex immune response to malaria infection. Malaria parasites are also genetically complex, producing thousands of potential antigens. Unlike vaccines for other diseases with effective vaccines, exposure to malaria parasites does not confer lifelong protection. Acquired immunity only partially protects against future disease. In many cases patients still become infected with the parasite; these malaria infections can persist for months without disease symptoms.

R21/Matrix-M

R21/Matrix-M is only the second vaccine for malaria. Ghana's Food and Drugs Authority (FDA Ghana) assessed clinical trial data and approved the vaccine for use in children aged 5 to 36 months, who are at highest risk of death from malaria. Ghana became the first country in the world to approve this highly anticipated malaria vaccine.

The R21/Matrix-M malaria vaccine was developed using adjuvant technology by the University of Oxford. The R21/Matrix-M vaccine targets the *Plasmodium* sporozoite (Fig. 27.1), the first form of the malaria parasite entering the human body. Only a few (10–100) sporozoites are injected by infected mosquitoes before the parasite multiplies, which makes them the ideal target for a vaccine.

R21/Matrix-M is a subunit vaccine that delivers parts of a protein secreted by the sporozoite that are bundled up with a part of the hepatitis B virus that is known to trigger a strong immune response. This vaccine also contains Novavax's Matrix-M, an adjuvant that boosts the immune system response to make it more powerful and long-lasting. Vaccines work by placing the antigen, which is the piece of the virus or bacteria that our system recognizes and responds to, in front of our immune cells. This technology, which was also used in Novavax's COVID-19 vaccine, induces an influx of antigen-presenting cells (APCs) at the injection site and enhances antigen presentation in local lymph nodes, which means that the immune system is triggered as strongly as possible.

Respiratory Syncytial Virus (RSV). According to the US Food and Drug Administration (FDA), RSV is a highly contagious virus that causes respiratory infections in individuals of all age groups. In most parts of the United States, circulation of RSV is seasonal, typically starting during the fall and peaking in the winter. The virus is especially common in children, and most individuals can be expected to be infected with RSV by the time they reach 2 years of age.

While RSV most often causes cold-like symptoms in infants and young children, it can also lead to serious lung infections such as pneumonia and bronchiolitis. In infants and children the risk of RSV-associated lung infection is highest during the first year of life. According to the Centers for Disease Control and Prevention (CDC), RSV is the most frequent cause of lower respiratory tract illness in infants worldwide. RSV is the leading cause of infant hospitalization in the United States.

The CDC states that RSV infections can be dangerous for certain adults. Each year, it is estimated that between 60,000 and 160,000 older adults in the United States are hospitalized and 6000 to 10,000 die due to RSV infection. Adults at highest risk for severe RSV infection include:
- Older adults
- Adults with chronic heart or lung disease
- Adults with weakened immune systems
- Adults with certain other underlying medical conditions
- Adults living in nursing homes or long-term care facilities

RSV Vaccines

In May, 2023 the RSV vaccines Arexvy and Abrysvo were approved for medical use in the United States. These two vaccines are indicated for active immunization for the prevention of lower respiratory tract

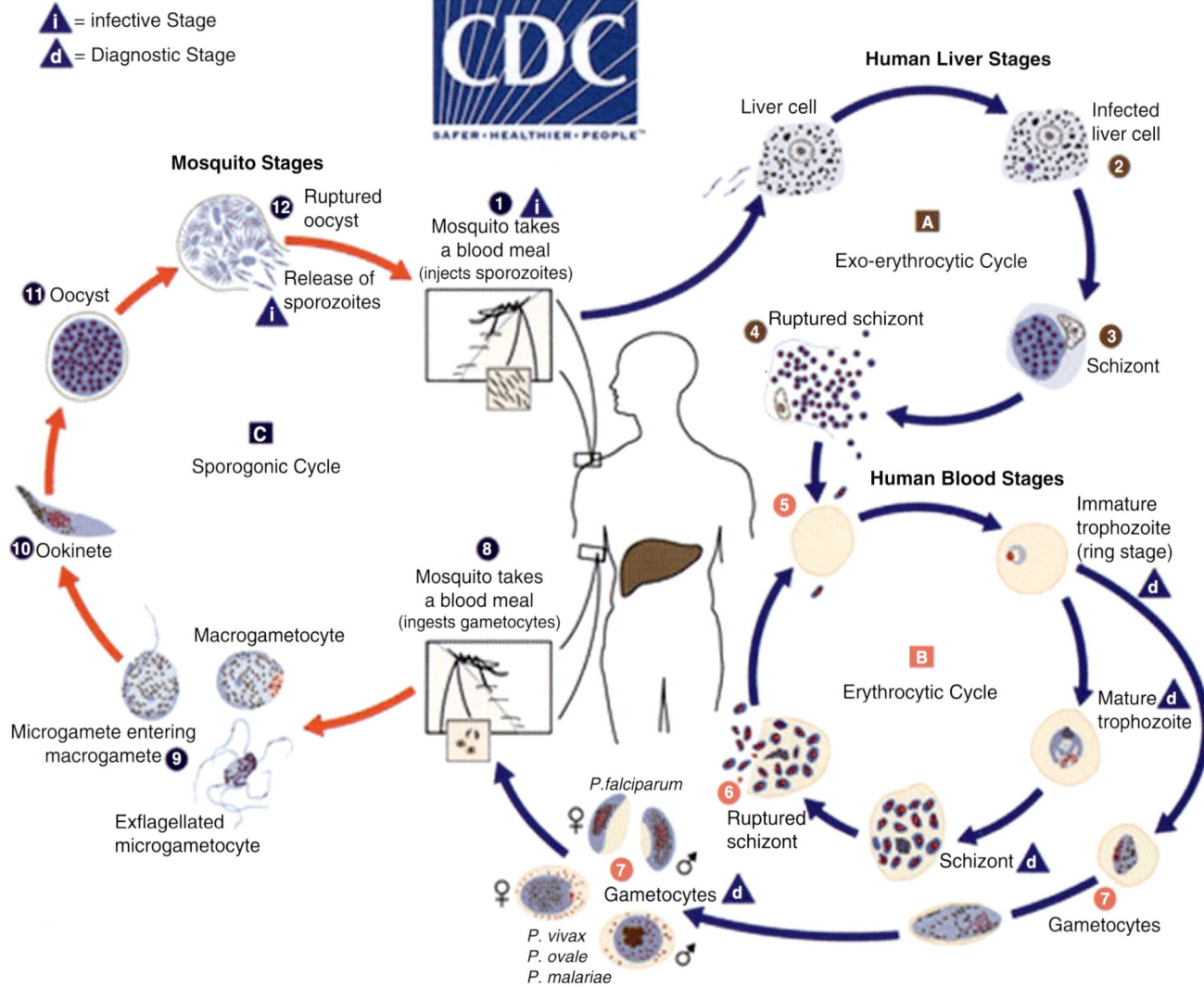

Fig 27.1 Malaria Lifecycle. (From Centers for Disease Control and Prevention, retrieved from www.cdc.gov. Accessed August 26, 2023.)

disease (LRTD) caused by rRSV in individuals 60 years of age and older. Abrysvo is manufactured by Pfizer and Arexvy is manufactured by GlaxoSmithKline. Both vaccines claim 83% to 86% risk reductions in RSV lower respiratory infection. One difference between the vaccines is that Arexvy contains an adjuvant, which is a substance added to vaccines that boosts a person's immune response, but Abrysvo does not.

In July, 2023 the FDA-approved Nirsevimab, a long-acting monoclonal antibody manufactured by Beyfortus, Sanofi, and AstraZeneca, for the prevention of RSV-associated lower respiratory tract infection (LRTI) among infants and children aged <24 months.

Most recently, in August, 2023, the FDA-approved Abrysvo as the first vaccine for use in pregnant individuals to prevent lower LRTD and severe LRTD caused by RSV in infants from birth through 6 months of age. Abrysvo is approved for use at 32 to 36 weeks gestational age of pregnancy.

Shigella

Shigellosis is a global human health problem. The CDC recently estimated the occurrence of over 440,000 annual cases of shigellosis in the United States. Transmission usually occurs by contaminated food and water, or through person-to-person contact.

No vaccines against *Shigella* infection currently exist. Although several candidate *Shigella* vaccines are at different stages of preclinical and clinical trials, currently no licensed vaccines are available. Immunity to *Shigella* is mediated largely by immune responses directed against the serotype-specific polysaccharide.

Shigella infections are typically treated with a course of antibiotics. However, due to the emergence of multidrug-resistant *Shigella* strains, a safe and effective vaccine is highly desirable.

Tuberculosis

Bacillus Calmette-Guérin (BCG) is a TB disease vaccine but it is not widely used in the United States. However, it is often given to infants and small children in other countries where TB is common.

In the United States, BCG is only considered for people who meet specific criteria and in consultation with a TB expert. BCG vaccination should only be considered for children who have a negative TB test (see Chapter 13) and who are continually exposed, and cannot be separated from adults who:

- Are untreated or ineffectively treated for TB disease (where the child cannot be given long-term primary preventive treatment for TB infection); or
- Have isoniazid- and rifampin-resistant strains of TB disease.

The CDC recommends that healthcare workers considered for BCG vaccination should be counseled regarding the risks and benefits associated with both BCG vaccination and treatment of latent TB infection. BCG vaccination of healthcare workers should be considered on an individual basis in settings in which:

- A high percentage of TB patients are infected with TB strains resistant to both isoniazid and rifampin;
- There is ongoing transmission of drug-resistant TB strains to healthcare workers and subsequent infection is likely; or
- Comprehensive TB infection-control precautions have been implemented but have not been successful.

Many people born outside of the United States have been BCG-vaccinated. People who were previously vaccinated with BCG may receive a TB skin test to test for TB infection, as vaccination with BCG may cause a positive reaction to a TB skin test. TB blood tests (interferon-gamma release assays), unlike the TB skin test, are not affected by prior BCG vaccination and are not expected to give a false-positive result in people who have received BCG.

GOAL OF VACCINATION

Human beings become immune to microbial antigens through artificial and natural means. The concept of vaccination, or deliberately introducing a potentially harmful microbe into a patient, was initially met with suspicion and outrage. The goal of vaccination is to produce artificially acquired, active immunity against a specific disease. A complete list of the vaccines approved by the FDA can be found at www.FDA.gov.

Today vaccination against contagious infectious diseases has a positive influence worldwide. Part of the success of vaccination is that it promotes herd immunity. This is an indirect form of protection from infectious diseases at the community level because the majority of that population has immunity to a specific microbe as a consequence of widespread vaccination programs.

> **KEY CONCEPTS**
> **General Vaccine Facts**
> - Vaccines provide artificially acquired active immunity to a specific disease.
> - According to the Centers for Disease Control and Prevention (CDC), vaccines have reduced preventable infectious diseases to an all-time low.
> - Vaccine development is an important focus of research for AIDS, malaria, and other devastating diseases.
> - Jenner discovered a fundamental principle of immunization with the smallpox vaccine and paved the way for the development of rabies (Louis Pasteur) and other vaccines (e.g., diphtheria and typhoid).
> - Children now receive vaccines for many childhood diseases (e.g., rubella). Adults require boosters (e.g., tetanus).

WHAT IS A VACCINE?

The purpose of a vaccine is to stimulate active immunity and create an immune memory so that exposure to an active disease microorganism will stimulate an already primed immune system to fight the disease. A traditional vaccine is a biological suspension of weakened or killed entire pathogens so that they cannot cause disease. The intended goal is to safely boost the immune system's natural ability to protect the body. The pathogen is usually a bacterium or a virus.

HISTORY OF VACCINES

According to WHO, immunization is one of the greatest breakthroughs in medical science. This practice is estimated to save about 3 million lives a year. Vaccines have reduced some preventable infectious diseases to an all-time low; few people now experience the devastating effects of measles, pertussis, and other infectious diseases.

The history of vaccination begins as early as 1000 BCE, when the Chinese used smallpox inoculation, or variolation, a method of scratching the skin and applying pulverized powder from a smallpox scab. By the 18th century, the practice of variolation became known to Europeans and Americans.

In 1721 Cotton Mather, a Boston minister, encouraged smallpox variolation as a preventive step subsequent to the Boston smallpox epidemic. Mather was widely criticized by suspicious citizens for his role in promoting variolation. Edward Jenner, an English physician, used cowpox scabs to create immunity to smallpox beginning in 1796. This was a fundamental principle of immunization, which evolved over 200 years ago and has resulted in the eradication of smallpox globally. The first vaccine for chicken cholera was created in the laboratory of Louis Pasteur in 1879. In 1885 Pasteur developed a rabies vaccine. This launched a period of productive development of many other vaccines (e.g., diphtheria, tetanus, and typhoid fever).

Since the introduction of the first vaccine, there has been opposition to vaccination. In 1910 Sir William Osler expressed his frustration with the antivaccinationist movement. Although fear and mistrust arose every time a new vaccine was introduced in the 18th century, the antivaccine movement receded between the 1940s and the early 1980s. Three trends promoted a positive attitude toward vaccines:

- A boom in scientific discovery and the production of vaccines;
- A desire to protect children from significant outbreaks of infectious diseases, including polio, measles, mumps, rubella, and pertussis (whooping cough);
- An increase in the birth rate among more educated and affluent parents, who accepted the use of vaccines.

An increase in antivaccinationist thinking emerged in the 1970s, when more vaccines were added to the childhood vaccination schedule. When countries dropped pertussis vaccination from the vaccination schedule, the incidence of whooping cough increased 10 to 100 times. Fears grew in the late 1990s, when vaccines were suspected of causing autism. Once again, in 2009 and 2010, the H1N1 influenza pandemic evoked strong public fear of vaccination. Reemergence of a previously controlled disease, such as pertussis, has led to hospitalizations and deaths. The worst pertussis outbreaks in the past 50 years have occurred in California.

Despite public fears and some noncompliance, US children now receive vaccinations against numerous diseases that were once common childhood infectious diseases. In the United States the recommended childhood immunization schedule now includes vaccines to protect against 15 diseases, including seasonal influenza. Immunization schedules vary by age and by country.

> **KEY CONCEPTS**
> **How Vaccines Work**
> - Most vaccines can be divided into two categories: live, attenuated vaccines and nonreplicating vaccines.
> - A vaccine must produce protective immunity with minimal side effects, produce a strong immune response, and be stable during its shelf life.
> - Classic preventive vaccines are designed to mimic the effects of natural exposure to microbes. The earliest host response to vaccination is called the *innate immune response*.

TYPES OF VACCINES

Scientific discoveries have led to development of numerous types of vaccines that produce immune responses to protect us against infectious diseases. Each vaccine production method has its own advantages and disadvantages related to its ability to induce certain immune responses, manufacturing capacity, and safety for human use.

Recent pandemics have raised the awareness of global threats to human health and increased the strategies for the development of new vaccine methods. The need for extremely rapid development and distribution of vaccines against viral pathogens, such as HIV, Zika, Ebola, severe acute respiratory syndrome coronavirus 1 (SARS-CoV-1) and severe acute respiratory syndrome coronavirus 2 (SARS-CoV-2), and the emergence of antibiotic-resistant bacteria, have refocused the need for newer approaches to prevent infections. WHO has identified eight different research platforms used by researchers and scientists in the pursuit of a vaccine to prevent COVID-19 infection caused by the SARS-CoV-2 virus.

Inactivated Vaccines

Traditional vaccines began with the process of using entire killed or weakened pathogens. Scientists first described the ability of inactivated, or killed, whole pathogens to induce immunity in the 19th century. This led to the development of inactivated vaccines, which are produced by killing a pathogen to create a vaccine. One example of such a vaccine, Havrix, is an inactivated vaccine against hepatitis A virus that was licensed in the United States in 1995.

Inactivated vaccines are manufactured by killing an infectious microbe with chemicals, heat, or radiation. This type of vaccine is more stable and safer than live vaccines; the dead microbes cannot mutate back to their disease-causing state. Inactivated vaccines usually do not require refrigeration and can be stored and shipped in a freeze-dried form.

The disadvantage of inactivated vaccines is that they stimulate a weaker immune system response compared with live vaccines. This makes it likely that several additional doses, or booster shots, will be needed to maintain an individual's immunity. Inactivated influenza vaccines are manufactured either as the split-virion or the subunit type. The two types of vaccines are assumed to have similar clinical effectiveness. However, split-virion vaccines contain more internal protein and stimulate a greater cellular immune response, although the clinical significance of this is unknown. The following vaccines are examples of inactivated vaccines:

Whole Virus
- Polio
- Influenza
- Hepatitis A
- Rabies
- Japanese encephalitis

Whole Bacteria
- Pertussis
- Cholera
- Typhoid

Live, Attenuated Vaccines

In the 1950s advances in tissue culture techniques enabled the development of another version of whole-pathogen vaccines—live, attenuated vaccines. These were created by modifying a disease-producing "wild" virus or bacterium that had been weakened in the laboratory to prevent the organism from causing disease. A live, attenuated vaccine is the closest thing to exposure to a natural infection. These vaccines provoke strong cellular and antibody immune responses and often produce lifelong immunity in a patient after only one or two doses of the vaccine.

Live, attenuated vaccines are relatively easy to create for certain viruses. Viruses are simple microbes containing a small number of genes and can be more easily controlled. Viruses are often attenuated through a method of growing generations of them in cells in a hostile environment. As they evolve to adapt to the new environment, they become weaker infectious agents compared with their natural host, human beings.

Modern genetic engineering techniques have created chimeric viruses. These viruses contain genetic information and display biological properties of different parent viruses. An experimental live, attenuated chimeric vaccine has been developed with a dengue virus backbone and Zika virus surface proteins.

The majority of live, attenuated vaccines available in the United States contain live viruses. The following vaccines are examples of live, attenuated vaccines:

Viral
- Measles, mumps, rubella (MMR combined vaccine)
- Rotavirus
- Smallpox
- Varicella (chickenpox)
- Yellow fever
- Zoster
- Polio (oral)
- Influenza (intranasal)

Bacterial
- Bacillus Calmette-Guérin (BCG)
- Oral typhoid

Live, attenuated vaccines are more difficult to create for more complex pathogens, such as bacteria and parasites. Bacteria have thousands of genes and are much harder to control. It may be possible to use recombinant DNA technology to remove several key genes. A risk associated with live, attenuated vaccines is that a microbe in the vaccine could revert to a virulent form and cause disease. In addition, not all patients can safely receive live, attenuated vaccines. For their own protection, patients with damaged or weakened immune systems cannot be given live vaccines. A physical limitation is that live, attenuated vaccines usually need to be refrigerated to stay potent. If the vaccine needs to be shipped and stored in resource-limited countries, a live vaccine may not be suitable.

Two live, attenuated bacterial vaccines are available in the United States. An attenuated, live culture preparation of the BCG strain of *Mycobacterium bovis* is available for percutaneous inoculation to prevent TB in persons not previously infected with *M. tuberculosis* who are at high risk for exposure. An alternate version of BCG is TICE BCG. This vaccine is for the treatment and prophylaxis of carcinoma in situ of the urinary bladder after transurethral resection. This strategy induces a granulomatous reaction at the local site of administration. Intravesical TICE BCG has been used to prevent recurrence of stage TaT1 papillary tumors of the bladder at high risk of recurrence.

Nucleic Acid Vaccines

Gene-based vaccines simply encode a chosen viral protein in DNA or messenger RNA (mRNA). This category is one of the newer vaccine methodologies. DNA and mRNA vaccines are able to induce both specific humoral and cellular immune responses and allow a high degree of adaptability to encode for any antigen. In terms of manufacturing, both platforms allow production of different vaccines using the same established production process and facility.

DNA Vaccines

Once the genes from a microbe have been analyzed, scientists can attempt to create a DNA vaccine against it (Fig. 27.2). DNA vaccines dispense with both the whole organism and its components, and they use the genes that code for antigens. It has been discovered that when the genes for a microbe's antigens are introduced into the human body, some cells will take up that DNA. The DNA then instructs those cells to make the antigen molecules. The cells secrete the antigens and display

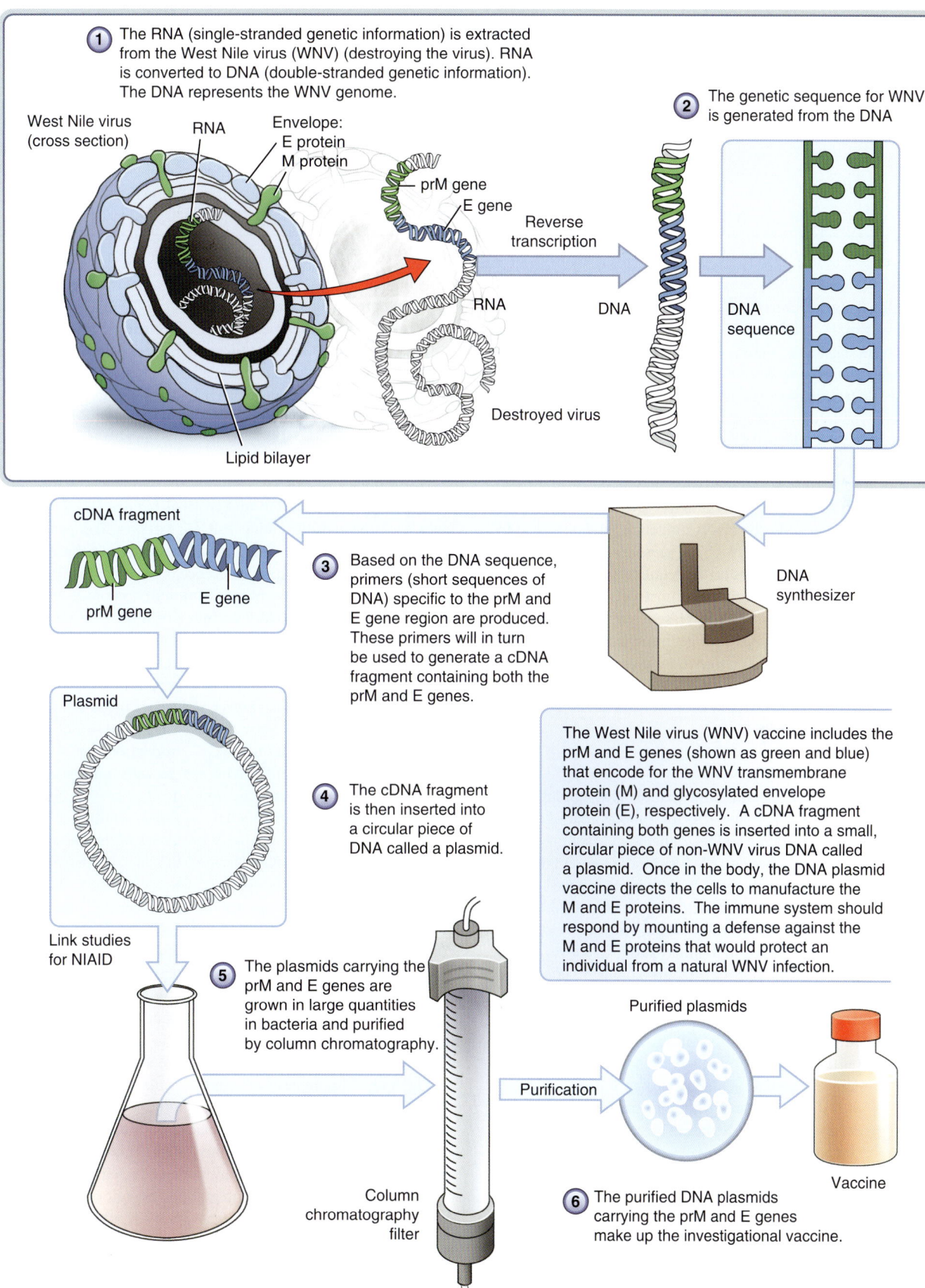

Fig. 27.2 The Making of a DNA Vaccine Against West Nile Virus. *cDNA*, Complementary DNA; *NIAID*, National Institute of Allergy and Infectious Disease. (From the National Institute of Allergy and Infectious Disease, retrieved from https://www.vaccines.gov. Accessed January 15, 2016.)

TABLE 27.1 Two COVID Vaccines FDA Approved and Available in the United States

Company	Description
Moderna Therapeutics	Moderna's vaccine, mRNA-1273, is a synthetic messenger RNA (mRNA) that encodes for a protein found on the surface of the novel coronavirus (LNP-encapsulated mRNA vaccine encoding S protein). By compelling cells to produce that protein, the vaccine should spur an immune response, causing the body to generate antibodies that would protect against infection. The company set a drug industry record with mRNA-1273, identifying a vaccine candidate just 42 days after the novel coronavirus was sequenced.
BioNTech/Pfizer	Pfizer and Germany's BioNTech are working on a multitude of mRNA vaccines for the novel coronavirus, planning to develop them in parallel. The company uses strands of mRNA to generate protective antibodies. Shanghai's Fosun Pharma signed a deal to market BioNTech's vaccine in China if it is eventually approved. Pfizer agreed to codevelop the vaccine in the rest of the world.

them on their surfaces. In this way a patient's own body cells become vaccine-making factories, creating the antigens necessary to stimulate the immune system.

A DNA vaccine against a microbe evokes a strong antibody response to the free-floating antigen secreted by cells, and the vaccine also stimulates a strong cellular response against the microbial antigens displayed on cell surfaces. The DNA vaccine does not cause the disease because it does not contain the microbe—just copies of a few of its genes.

Additionally, DNA vaccines are relatively easy and inexpensive to design and produce. DNA vaccines were developed during previous outbreaks, such as the SARS coronavirus (SARS-CoV-1) in 2003, H5N1 avian influenza in 2005, the H1N1 influenza pandemic in 2009, and the Zika and Ebola viruses in 2016. The presence of nonfunctional sequences in original DNA vectors raised regulatory safety concerns, but newer developments allow minimal constructs that exclusively encode for the target antigen with increased safety. However, the potential for long-term persistence and genomic integration and the dependence on injection devices or electroporation are some important disadvantages of this technology. In the testing of DNA vaccines against Zika virus, this technology was demonstrated to be able to induce promising immune responses.

RNA Vaccines

As with DNA vaccines, RNA-based vaccine technologies support a comparably simple, fully synthetic manufacturing process that allows the production of different vaccines using the same established production process and facility. However, because RNA vaccines represent the most recently developed technology, their use in humans is less well characterized than it is for DNA-based vaccines. Vaccines based on mRNA are an intermediary between DNA and protein. An mRNA molecule is composed of nucleotides linked in a unique order to convey genetic information for the cells to produce the proteins or antigens encoded by mRNA. When mRNA in a vaccine has been internalized by body cells, the cells rely on this genetic template to translate the genetic information and produce the antigens encoded by the mRNA vaccine. These antigens are then located on the cellular surface, where they are recognized by the immune system. This recognition generates an immune response, including antibodies directed against the antigens. The inability for genomic integration and lack of persistence in the cells of an mRNA vaccine offers important advantages in terms of vaccine safety.

Recent technologic advances have largely overcome issues with the instability of mRNA and the difficulty of delivering it into cells. Although to date SARS-CoV-2, the cause of COVID-19, has mutated relatively slowly compared with other RNA viruses (e.g., HIV and the influenza virus), there is always the possibility that an effective vaccine could suddenly be rendered useless if the virus mutates in just the right way.

mRNA has the advantage of using genome sequence information alone rather than relying on slower in vitro cultures of live viruses or bacteria. Nucleic acid–based vaccines that use this next-generation approach were the frontrunners in COVID-19 vaccine research and development (Table 27.1). An example of what may be the first mRNA vaccine approved for use against SARS-CoV-2 is mRNA-1273, developed by Moderna Therapeutics and the National Institutes of Health (NIH). mRNA-1273 encodes for the virus spike protein that is used by viruses to latch onto human host cells.

Two major types of mRNA have been used in prophylactic vaccine development against pathogens that cause infectious diseases:
- Nonreplicating mRNA
- Self-amplifying mRNA

Nonreplicating mRNA contains the sequence of the antigen of choice flanked by 5′ and 3′ untranslated regions (UTRs). The advantages of using nonreplicating mRNA vaccines, compared with self-amplifying mRNA, are rooted in the simplicity of the construct, the small size of the RNA, and the absence of any additional encoded proteins that could induce unintended immune responses.

Self-amplifying mRNA vaccines are most commonly based on the alpha virus genome from which the genes encoding the structural protein have been replaced with an antigen of choice. Despite these gene deletions, the viral RNA is replicated and transcribed by the viral RNA polymerase. Lower yields and increased occurrence of abortive constructs as a consequence of the large size of these vaccine molecules pose challenges to vaccine production that make manufacturing processes more difficult compared with nonreplicating mRNA vaccines. Any genetic information encoded by the self-amplifying mRNA vaccine will be amplified many times, resulting in high levels of antigen expression from relatively low doses of the vaccine compared with nonreplicating mRNA vaccines. Self-amplifying mRNA is most commonly delivered with synthetic delivery vehicles. This technology requires the use of electroporation of the genetic material into cell culture cells during the manufacturing process. There are some safety concerns associated with delivery because of the presence of replicon and helper RNAs that could lead to the generation of infectious viruses.

RNA vaccines represent the most recently developed technology. An mRNA molecule is composed of nucleotides linked in a unique order to convey genetic information for cells to produce the proteins/antigens encoded by mRNA. When mRNA in a vaccine has been internalized by body cells, the cells rely on this genetic template to translate the genetic information and produce the antigens encoded by the mRNA vaccine. These antigens are then located on the cellular surface, where they are recognized by the immune system. This recognition generates an immune response, including antibodies directed against the antigens.

The inability for genomic integration and lack of persistence in the cells of an mRNA vaccine offers important advantages in terms of vaccine safety.

Covid Vaccine Development

Numerous potential COVID-19 vaccines in development mainly focus on an antibody immune response. These proteins are made by B cells that attach onto the SARS-CoV-2 virus to prevent it from entering body cells.

In contrast, T cells fight infections in two different ways. Helper T cells spur B cells and other immune defenders into action, but natural killer (NK) T cells target and destroy infected cells. The severity of disease can be reflected by the strength of these T-cell responses.

To spark production of antibodies, vaccines against the virus need to stimulate helper T cells. In the case of COVID-19, helper T cells target a spike protein seen in the majority of patients hospitalized with COVID-19.

Moderna chose an mRNA vaccine because it potentially offers greater flexibility and quicker development timelines than traditional vaccines. Moderna's vaccine, mRNA-1273, is a synthetic mRNA vaccine that encodes for a protein found on the surface of the novel coronavirus (lipid nanoparticle [LNP]-encapsulated mRNA vaccine encoding S protein). By compelling cells to produce that protein, the vaccine should spur an immune response, causing the body to generate antibodies that would protect against infection.

Pfizer and Germany's BioNTech also chose to develop an mRNA vaccine. Based on initial clinical trial results, two LNP-formulated, nucleoside-modified RNA vaccine candidates against SARS-CoV-2 were evaluated in the United States. One candidate, BNT162b1, encodes the SARS-CoV-2 receptor binding domain, trimerized to increase its immunogenicity through multivalent display. The other candidate, BNT162b2, encodes the SARS-CoV-2 full-length spike protein and more closely mimics the intact virus with which the elicited virus-neutralizing antibodies must interact (Fig. 27.3).

Virus-Like Particle (VLP) Vaccines

In the early 1990s scientists at the NIH discovered that recombinant protein antigens from the outer shell of human papillomavirus (HPV) can form particles that closely resemble the virus. Virus-like particles (VLPs) are multiprotein structures that mimic the organization and conformation of authentic native viruses but lack the viral genome. VLPs prompt an immune response similar to that elicited by the natural virus, but VLPs are noninfectious because they do not contain the genetic material the virus needs to replicate inside cells. This method potentially yields safer and cheaper vaccine candidates than other methods. Several VLP-based vaccines are currently available and other VLP-based vaccine candidates are in research and development (e.g., SARS-CoV-2 and influenza virus).

Subunit Vaccines and Carriers

Subunit vaccines, like inactivated whole-cell vaccines, do not contain live components of the pathogen. They differ from inactivated whole-cell vaccines by containing only the antigenic parts of the pathogen. These parts are necessary to elicit a protective immune response.

This precision comes at a cost, as the antigenic properties of the various potential subunits of a pathogen must be examined in detail to determine which particular combinations will produce an effective immune response within the correct pathway.

Often a response can be elicited, but there is no guarantee that immunological memory will be formed in the correct manner.

With the exception of toxin-based vaccines that are subunits or fractions of their respective microorganisms, most other subunit vaccines include only the components or antigens of a pathogen that best stimulate an immune response instead of the entire microbe. This type of vaccine is either purified biochemically from microorganisms or produced by recombinant DNA technology. Subunit vaccines minimize side effects. In some cases these vaccines use epitopes, the specific parts of the antigen that antibodies or T cells recognize and bind to. Subunit vaccines can contain anywhere from 1 to 20 or more antigens. Most subunit vaccines focus on a particular pathogen. In some cases, a subunit vaccine (e.g., cellular purified *Bordetella pertussis* vaccine) is just as effective as a whole-cell vaccine but much less likely to cause adverse reactions. Another recent advance in subunit technique is the ability to solve the atomic structures of proteins. Scientists have identified a key area of the protein that is highly sensitive to neutralizing antibodies.

Most subunit vaccines focus on a particular pathogen, but subunit vaccines are being developed for protection against more than one disease. In 2017 National Institute for Allergy and Infectious Diseases (NIAID) researchers launched an early-phase clinical trial of a vaccine to prevent mosquito-borne diseases malaria, Zika, chikungunya (CHIK), and dengue fever. This experimental vaccine is designed to elicit an immune response to mosquito saliva and it contains four recombinant proteins from mosquito salivary glands.

Critical to the protective effect of subunit vaccines are additives called adjuvants, which amplify the immune response because the antigens alone are not sufficient to induce adequate long-term immunity. Adjuvants are tested for safety and are continuously monitored by the CDC and FDA. Currently, aluminum and monophosphoryl lipid A are two adjuvants licensed for clinical use in the United States.

Recombinant Protein Vaccine

Protein-based subunit vaccines present an antigen to the immune system without viral particles using a specific, isolated protein of the pathogen. A weakness of this technique is that isolated proteins, if denatured, may bind to different antibodies than the protein of the pathogen.

Recombinant DNA technology, which enables DNA from two or more sources to be combined, was harnessed to develop the first recombinant protein-based subunit vaccine, the hepatitis B vaccine.

Scientists at NIAID and other institutions are developing new strategies to present protein subunit antigens to the immune system. As part of efforts to develop a universal flu vaccine, scientists designed an experimental vaccine featuring the protein ferritin, which can self-assemble into microscopic pieces called nanoparticles that display a protein antigen. Nanoparticle-based technology also is being researched as a platform for the development of vaccines against the Middle East respiratory syndrome coronavirus (MERS-CoV), RSV, and Epstein-Barr virus (EBV).

Examples of recombinant protein subunit vaccines are:
- Hepatitis B virus
- Influenza virus
- Acellular pertussis
- Human papillomavirus

Hepatitis B virus. In the 1980s recombinant DNA technology was used to develop the first recombinant protein vaccine, the hepatitis B vaccine. The first hepatitis B vaccine received FDA approval for use in the United States in 1981, with a recombinant version coming to market in 1986 that replaced the original blood-derived vaccine. The vaccine antigen is a hepatitis B virus protein produced by yeast cells into which the genetic code for the viral protein has been inserted. Several hepatitis B virus VLP-based vaccines are currently available; examples are Engerix, by GlaxoSmithKline, and Recombivax HB, by Merck.

Influenza virus. Research is focused on development of a universal flu vaccine. This kind of experimental vaccine includes the protein, ferritin, which can self-assemble into microscopic pieces, nanoparticles, that display a protein antigen. This type of technology is being assessed as a platform for development of vaccines against MERS-CoV, RSV and EBV.

Acellular pertussis. This is a vaccine that contains cellular material but not complete cells; specifically, antigenic or allergenic parts of cells.

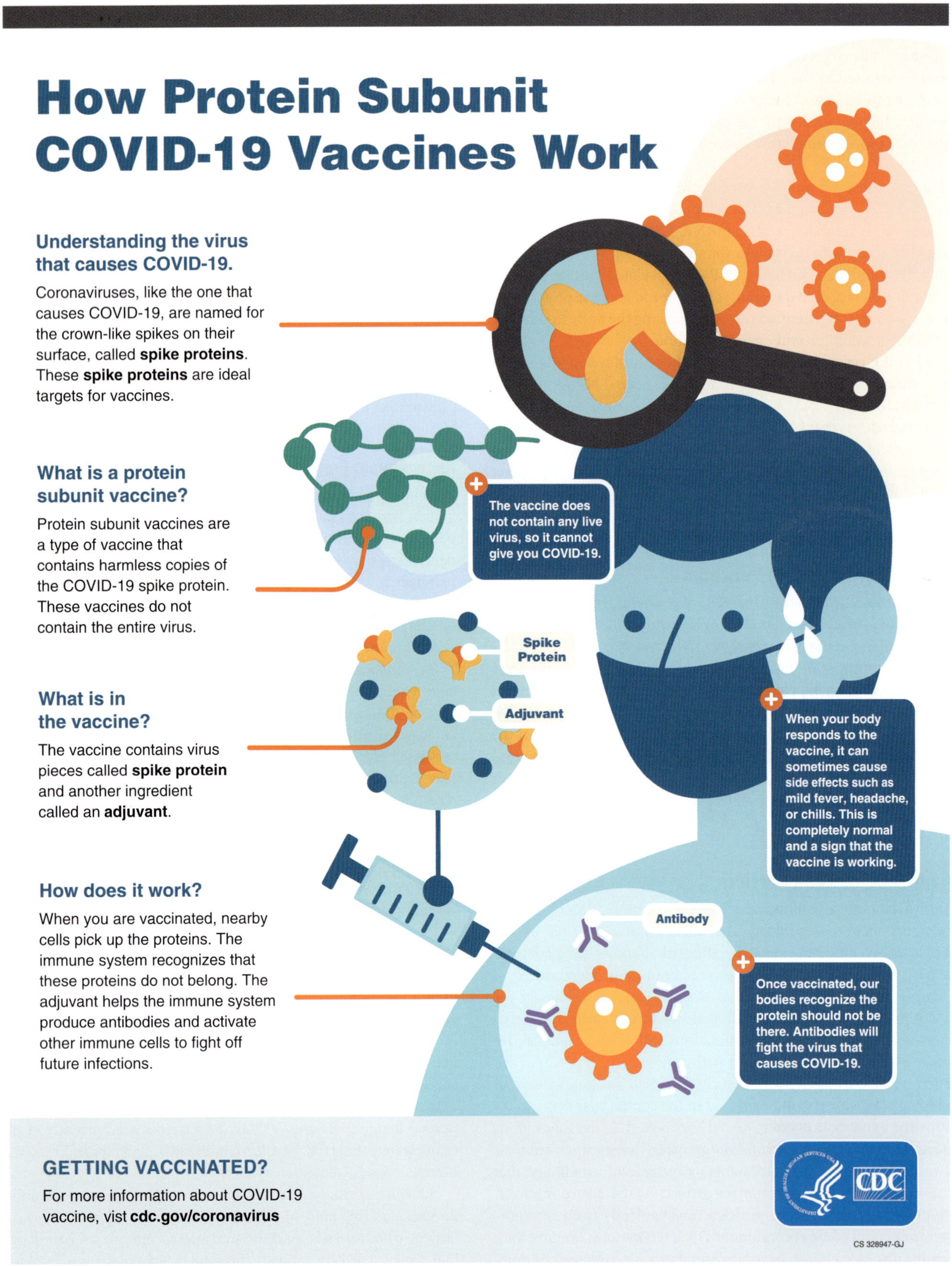

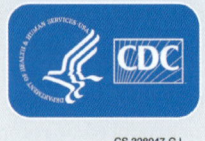

Fig. 27.3 How Protein Subunit COVID-19 Vaccines Work. (From Centers for Disease Control and Prevention, retrieved from www.cdc.gov. Accessed October 14, 2023)

Two forms of vaccine are in use, the whole-cell vaccine (wP) and the acellular vaccine (aP). Most wP vaccines are available in combination with diphtheria and tetanus vaccines and contain aluminum salts as an adjuvant and thiomersal as a preservative. Acellular pertussis vaccines have been mainly products where the acellular pertussis component has been formulated with diphtheria and tetanus antigens. Individual antigens may be derived from different strains of *Bordetella pertussis* and have been purified by different methods. For these reasons, protective efficacy in humans of various manufacturers' products may be based on different mechanisms.

Human papillomavirus. Vaccines to prevent HPV infection also are based on recombinant protein antigens. VLP vaccines directed at prevention of HPV infections are Gardasil (Merck), approved in 2006, and Cervarix (GlaxoSmithKline), approved in 2009. The Gardasil, Gardasil 9, and Cervarix vaccines provide nearly 100% protection against persistent cervical infections with HPV types 16 and 18 and the cervical cell changes these persistent infections can cause. Gardasil is also approved for males aged 9 to 26 years to help prevent genital warts and anal cancer. Cervarix, which targets HPV types 16 and 18, is approved for females aged 10 to 25 years to help prevent cervical cancer.

Polysaccharide and Conjugate Vaccines

The first licensed vaccine against *Haemophilus influenzae* type b (Hib) was a **polysaccharide vaccine**. NIH researchers next developed a so-called **conjugate vaccine**, in which the Hib polysaccharide was attached, or "conjugated," to a protein antigen. Today, conjugate vaccines are available to protect against Hib and pneumococcal and meningococcal infections.

The process of conjugation of a polysaccharide and a protein molecule can improve outcomes. Conjugation changes the immune response from T-cell independent to T-cell dependent, which produces increased immunogenicity in infants and antibody booster response to multiple doses of vaccine.

Several polysaccharide vaccines have been approved by the FDA for use in the United States. These vaccines to prevent bacterial infections are based on the **polysaccharides** that form the outer coating of many bacteria. However, antibodies induced with polysaccharide antigens have less functional activity than those induced by protein antigens. This is because the predominant antibody produced in response to most polysaccharide vaccines is immunoglobulin M (IgM), with only a low concentration of immunoglobulin G (IgG).

Examples of polysaccharide and conjugate vaccines are:
- Meningococcal vaccine
- Pneumococcal vaccine
- *Salmonella typhi* (Vi) vaccine

Meningococcal protein conjugate (Haemophilus influenzae type b conjugate vaccine). PedvaxHIB is an *H. influenzae* type b conjugate vaccine (meningococcal protein conjugate). It is a capsular polysaccharide of *H. influenzae* type b that is covalently bound to an outer membrane protein complex of *Neisseria meningitidis* serogroup B. The covalent bonding is necessary for enhanced immunogenicity. The vaccine product, liquid PedvaxHIB, is indicated for routine vaccination against invasive disease caused by *H. influenzae* type b in infants and children 2 to 71 months of age. It is administered intramuscularly (IM).

Meningococcal vaccines. The vaccine Bexsero is a suspension composed of four distinct antigens, including factor H binding protein (fHbp), neisserial adhesin A (NadA), neisserial heparin-binding antigen (NHBA), and PorA P1.4 immunodominant antigen of OMV NZ (strain NZ98/254). These proteins, found on the surface of meningococci, contribute to the bacterium's ability to cause disease. Protection against invasive meningococcal disease is conferred mainly by complement-mediated antibody-dependent killing of *N. meningitidis*. The effectiveness of Bexsero was assessed by measuring serum bactericidal activity using human complement (hSBA). The susceptibility of serogroup B meningococci to complement-mediated antibody-dependent killing after vaccination is dependent on both the antigenic similarity of the bacterial and vaccine antigens and the amount of antigen expressed on the surface of the invading meningococci. Bexsero is an FDA-approved vaccine to prevent invasive disease caused by *N. meningitidis* serogroup B. It is approved for use in individuals 10 through 25 years of age.

Menactra is a meningococcal polysaccharide diphtheria toxoid conjugate vaccine. It is indicated for active immunization for the prevention of invasive meningococcal disease caused by the four most common types of meningococcal bacteria (serogroups A, C, Y, and W-135). Menactra is approved for use in individuals 9 months through 55 years of age. Menactra does not prevent N meningitidis serogroup B disease.

Pneumococcal vaccines. Vaccines available for the prevention of pneumococcal disease are Prevnar 13 and Pneumovax.

Prevnar 13 (pneumococcal 13-valent conjugate vaccine [diphtheria CRM197 protein]) is a pneumococcal conjugate vaccine (PCV) that protects against 13 types of pneumococcal bacteria. This vaccine is indicated in children aged 6 weeks through 17 years (prior to the 18th birthday) for active immunization against invasive disease caused by *Streptococcus pneumoniae* serotypes 1, 3, 4, 5, 6A, 6B, 7F, 9V, 14, 18C, 19A, 19F, and 23F, and for children aged 6 weeks through 5 years (prior to the 6th birthday) for the prevention of otitis media caused by 7 of the 13 serotypes in the vaccine.

In adults aged 18 years or older, Prevnar 13 is indicated for active immunization to prevent pneumonia and invasive diseases caused by *S. pneumoniae* serotypes in the vaccine. The CDC recommends that all adults aged 65 years or older receive Prevnar 13, then 1 year later, Pneumovax 23.

Pneumovax 23 is a mixture of purified pneumococcal capsular polysaccharides from 23 serotypes of *S. pneumoniae*. This vaccine is approved for use in persons aged 50 years or older and in those aged 2 years or older who are at increased risk for pneumococcal disease.

Salmonella typhi (Vi) vaccine. Two forms of the typhoid vaccine are available in the United States; each one is most effective when given at a particular age. One is an inactivated (killed) vaccine, and the other is a live, attenuated (weakened) vaccine.

Typhoid Vi polysaccharide vaccine is administered to prevent typhoid fever. It contains the cell surface Vi polysaccharide extracted from *Salmonella enterica* serovar Typhi (*S. typhi* Ty2 strain). This polysaccharide vaccine provides active immunization for patients 2 years of age or older to prevent typhoid fever caused by *Salmonella enterica* serovar Typhimurium (*S. typhimurium* or *S. typhi*).

The second form of this vaccine is Ty21a. Ty21a is a weakened form of live bacteria and is given by mouth to patients aged 6 years or older.

Typhoid vaccine should be used only by people traveling to high-risk areas who will be:
- Staying for longer than 6 weeks
- Staying in rural areas or small towns
- Choosing to eat uncooked foods and unpeeled fruits and drink unbottled water

Toxoid vaccines. Toxoid vaccines (e.g., diphtheria, Hib, and tetanus vaccines) are used when a bacterial toxin is the main cause of illness. The antigens in toxoid vaccines are chemically inactivated toxins. Such "detoxified" toxins, called *toxoids*, are safe for use in vaccines.

A toxoid vaccine containing a harmless toxoid stimulates the immune system to produce antibodies that react to and block the toxin. Vaccines against diphtheria and tetanus are examples of toxoid vaccines.

Hiberix is a *Haemophilus* b conjugate vaccine (tetanus toxoid conjugate). It is intended for active immunization against invasive disease caused by *H. influenzae* type b. This product is approved for use in children aged 6 weeks through 4 years (prior to the 5th birthday).

ActHIB is a *Haemophilus* b conjugate vaccine (tetanus toxoid conjugate). It is intended for the prevention of invasive disease caused by *H. influenzae* type b. ActHIB vaccine is indicated for active immunization of infants and children aged 2 months through 5 years.

Replicating and Nonreplicating Viral Vector–Based Vaccines

Viral vector vaccines combine many of the positive qualities of DNA vaccines and live, attenuated vaccines. The term *vector* refers to the virus or bacterium used as a carrier. Viral vector–based vaccine technology uses either live replicating (frequently attenuated) virus or nonreplicating vectors. This versatile platform offers many advantages over more established vaccine technologies. Since the 1980s a variety of viruses have been used as vaccine vectors. Commonly used viral vectors are adenovirus, measles virus, and vesicular stomatitis virus (VSV).

Recombinant vector vaccines are live replicating viruses engineered to carry extra genes derived from a pathogen; these extra genes produce proteins to generate immunity. Recombinant vector vaccines are similar to DNA vaccines, except they use an attenuated virus or bacterium to introduce microbial DNA to cells of the human body. Recombinant vector vaccines closely mimic a natural infection and do an effective job of stimulating the immune system.

Once the microbial DNA is expressed in infected human cells, an immune response should occur, including antibody, T helper cell (CD4+ T cell), and cytotoxic T lymphocyte ([CTL] CD8+ T cell)-mediated immunity. Viral vector vaccines are generally able to produce stronger immune responses than DNA vaccines. However, for some diseases, viral vectors are being used in combination with other vaccine technologies in a strategy called *heterologous prime-boost*. Viral vector vaccines are being investigated as both prime and booster vaccines.

If attenuated bacteria are used as vectors, the inserted genetic material causes the bacteria to display the antigens of other microbes on their surface. The result is that a harmless bacterium mimics a harmful microbe, provoking an immune response.

Nonreplicating viral vector vaccines use a well-established inactivated or killed viral vector (e.g., adenovirus) to express proteins, for example, SARS-CoV-2. This enables proteins to be recognized by the immune system and elicit an immune response.

The use of attenuated viral vectors raises safety concerns due to the risk of adverse events and residual viral replication upon delivery. There are no viral vector vaccines currently on the market for use in humans. Several recombinant vector vaccines have been approved for veterinary use to protect animals from rabies and distemper. Scientists continue to search for and develop recombinant vectored vaccines to protect humans from viruses such as HIV, Zika virus, and Ebola virus.

MODEL OF VACCINE DEVELOPMENT

The FDA's Center for Biologics Evaluation and Research is responsible for regulating vaccines in the United States. Before new vaccines are licensed, they are tested extensively for safety in the laboratory, in animals, and in successive stages of human clinical trials called phases. According to US biopharmaceutical companies, using the novel coronavirus (SARS-CoV-2) as an example, the development of a COVID-19 vaccine can be organized into six steps comprising research, development, and approval/production.

Step 1. Identify and Sequence the Virus

Subsequent to identification and viral isolation, laboratory scientists rapidly sequenced the unique genetic code of this novel coronavirus. On January 10, 2020, Chinese health officials released the full genetic sequence of SARS-CoV-2. Compared with the discovery of severe acute respiratory syndrome (SARS) in 2002, for which it took several months to sequence the full SARS-CoV-1 genetic code, the much faster timeline in the case of SARS-CoV-2 demonstrates how new technologies have dramatically shortened the time required to decode viruses and create a potential vaccine. Genetic sequencing provides the information needed to design diagnostic tests and potential vaccines and treatments.

Step 2: Determine the Target

Vaccines work by imitating an infection without actually causing an infection. The process to determine how to best deliver a vaccine is complex, because different approaches may work better for different pathogens. Historically some vaccines, such as the measles vaccine, used live but weakened versions of a pathogen; others, such as the polio vaccine, used viral material that had been chemically inactivated or killed. Newer vaccines, such as the hepatitis B vaccine, use recombinant vaccine production technology. Because of the urgent need for a safe, effective vaccine against COVID-19, along with the volume of information that remains unknown about the disease, a wide range of approaches to vaccine development are being tested by biopharmaceutical researchers throughout the world to greatly improve the odds that one or more of these approaches will be successful.

Step 3: Conduct Preclinical Trials

Once research scientists identify a vaccine delivery mechanism, cell cultures or animal models are used for phase I to test the vaccine's potential safety and efficacy. It is common for vaccine candidates to fail during this part of the process.

Step 4: Initiate Human Clinical Trials

Researchers design clinical trials to answer specific research questions. Human clinical trials follow a rigorous series, from early, small-scale phase I studies to late-stage, large-scale phase III studies, before approval is granted by the FDA. Three main phases of human clinical trials precede FDA approval.

- **Phase I:** In most cases, 20 to 100 healthy volunteers participate in phase I, which lasts several months. The primary purpose of a phase I study is to evaluate the safety and dosage of a new drug/vaccine candidate before it proceeds to further clinical studies. In addition to safety issues, researchers can answer other questions in a phase I trial related to how the drug works in the body and the side effects associated with increased dosage.
- **Phase II:** In this phase, researchers administer the drug to a larger group of patients (typically up to several hundred) for several months to 2 years to initially assess its effectiveness and to further study its side effects. A key focus of phase II studies is determining the optimal dose or doses of a drug/vaccine candidate, to determine how best to administer the drug to maximize possible benefits while minimizing risks. Unlike with most kinds of phase II clinical trials, volunteers in clinical trials for vaccines are healthy at the beginning of the clinical trial. Accordingly, demonstrating efficacy may require longer and larger clinical trials for vaccines than for other products.
- **Phase III:** The length of study for phase III clinical trials is usually 1 to 4 years. This phase involves 300 to 3000 patients with the disease or condition. Participants are assigned to receive the medication being evaluated or are members of a control group, which receives either the current standard of care treatment or a placebo

(a substance that has no therapeutic effect). Testing is designed to determine the adverse, longer-term effects of a drug or vaccine. The most common reasons for failure in phase III of development are a failure to meet the primary efficacy endpoint and/or unexpected adverse or serious adverse events. Information gained in this phase can serve as the basis for product labeling.
- **Phase IV (optional):** These trials can be done after a drug/vaccine is licensed. They examine the vaccine in hundreds to even a few thousand people to better understand how the immune system responds to a vaccine, whether it is effective and durable at producing immunity, and to further understand the vaccine's safety profile. Depending on the vaccine and disease under study, thousands or even tens of thousands of participants may participate to increase understanding of a vaccine's safety profile. As of August 5, 2020, several coronavirus vaccine candidates had entered phase III clinical trials.

Step 5: Obtain Regulatory Approval

At this point the majority of vaccine candidates will have failed, which highlights the substantial risks and complexities involved. If a vaccine successfully makes it through the clinical trial phases, researchers can apply for approval from the FDA. Applications for approval must meet the FDA's robust standards for safety, purity, and potency, and must include data generated during preclinical testing and clinical trials, in addition to significant information on the manufacturing process.

The FDA and the European Medicines Agency (EMA) concluded that during the novel coronavirus pandemic, companies did not have to prove that their vaccines worked in animals before beginning human clinical studies. If any of the DNA or mRNA vaccines were successful, their makers would face a new challenge: manufacturing massive quantities of vaccines. Manufacturing companies insist that their vaccines are easier to make than traditional vaccines.

Step 6: Establish Manufacturing and Distribution

While the vaccine is going through clinical studies, biopharmaceutical researchers are also developing the manufacturing methods that will be used if the new vaccine is successful. For some types of vaccines used in large populations, these methods then undergo massive scale-up to enable the manufacture of what can be many millions of doses. The transition from laboratory to manufacturing facility is incredibly complex and must ensure consistency in the vaccine composition and in safety and efficacy profiles. Because developing the manufacturing strategy can be a multiyear process, biopharmaceutical companies start early to expand their manufacturing capacity. In the case of a COVID-19 vaccine, Operation Warp Speed, launched by the US federal government, subsidized research and development. Companies received advance orders and the funds to initiate manufacturing pending approval of the vaccine, in order to speed the production process when a vaccine was approved and ready for distribution.

Vaccines are manufactured in batches called *lots*. All vaccine lots are routinely tested and must pass all tests before they can be used, and vaccine manufacturers must comply with strict manufacturing standards. The FDA also analyzes adverse events (possible side effects) associated with individual lots to look for any unusual patterns.

Safely delivering a vaccine to patients around the world is an equally challenging undertaking, especially in less developed regions, because vaccines often require special handling (e.g., temperature control) during distribution. Biopharmaceutical companies must work closely with local governments and nongovernmental organization (NGO) partners to lay the groundwork for potential distribution on a global scale.

HOST RESPONSE TO VACCINATION

It is not entirely clear why the length of acquired protection varies with different vaccines. A single dose of some vaccines provides lifelong immunity, but others require an additional dose (i.e., a booster) to maintain immunity. Boosters can be described as a "reminder" to the immune system. A 5-month pertussis outbreak in a Florida preschool with a high vaccination rate highlighted the need for efforts to reduce transmission and provide booster vaccinations for adults in regular close contact with young children.

Depending on the vaccine, some immunizations must be repeated. The protection provided by the influenza vaccine is short because flu viruses may change from season to season. Therefore all vaccine-eligible individuals, including the more vulnerable older population, must get a vaccination every year.

A patient's immune system responds to a vaccine in various ways. B cells and cytotoxic T cells are responsible for regulation of an immune response. Most preventive vaccines, such as hepatitis B virus (HBV) and HPV, stimulate production of antibodies that bind to specific, targeted microbes and block their ability to cause infection. Helper T cells and dendritic cells (DCs) help activate killer T cells and enable them to recognize specific antigen threats. Cytotoxic T cells kill infected or abnormal cells by releasing toxic chemicals or prompting apoptosis.

Classic preventive vaccines are designed to mimic the effects of natural exposure to microbes. The earliest host response to vaccination is called the innate immune response. This response is an evolutionarily ancient system of host defense that occurs within minutes or hours after vaccination. The DC is critical to this response. DCs can sense components of bacteria, viruses, parasites, and fungi through pathogen recognition receptors. One class of these receptors is the toll-like receptor (TLR); at least 10 have been described. As a group, TLRs can sense a wide variety of microbial stimuli (e.g., lipopolysaccharides and viral or bacterial DNA). Intracellular TLR signaling within DCs is mediated by at least four adapter proteins. Once DCs decode and integrate the signals generated by sensing microbial molecules with TLRs, the cells convey this information to naïve antigen-specific T cells, which launch an immune response.

Over time vaccine-induced immunity wanes; this may result in increased susceptibility later in life (e.g., varicella [shingles]). A second dose of vaccine could improve protection from primary vaccine failure and waning vaccine-induced immunity.

RATES OF VACCINATION

According to the CDC, flu vaccine coverage for all adults is about 47%, which is similar to coverage among adults at the end of last season (2022–2023). The highest overall coverage among adults in the U.S. was during the 2020–2021 flu season, when end-of-season estimates were that 50% of the adult population had gotten a flu vaccine.

As of January 6, 2024, the CDC reports that flu vaccination coverage has decreased in children since the COVID-19 pandemic.

CDC's flu vaccination coverage estimates updated on January 19, 2024, show a drop in flu vaccine uptake among some groups of adults this season, and a continued decline in flu vaccination coverage among pregnant women and children since 2020.

Adults require updates on certain vaccinations (see the CDC website at https://www.cdc.gov), especially serious diseases in adults aged 65 years or older including diphtheria, herpes zoster (shingles), influenza, pneumococcus, and tetanus (lockjaw). Healthcare professionals are now protected against hepatitis B by vaccines. The use of vaccines also has spread to pets and livestock (e.g., rabies, Lyme disease, and feline leukemia).

SITES OF VACCINE ADMINISTRATION

Vaccines can be delivered by injection, orally, or as a nasal spray. mRNA vaccines can be administered by various routes using conventional needle-based injections and, unlike DNA vaccines, they do not require any additional administration device, such as a gene gun or electroporation. The immune system must recognize the pathogen and be able to develop a defense against it. Appropriate vaccine administration is essential to the optimal safety and efficacy of a vaccine.

The routes of administration vary in order to maximize the effectiveness of the vaccine. The site of administration depends on the vaccine(s) that is (are) to be administered and the age and size of the patient to be vaccinated.

Intramuscular (IM) injection of vaccines is the most often practiced route of administration in humans. Only a few vaccines are administered subcutaneously, orally, or intradermally. IM injection involves administration into the muscle mass. Vaccines containing adjuvants should be injected IM to reduce adverse local effects.

Subcutaneous (SC) injection administers the vaccine into the subcutaneous layer above the muscle and below the skin.

Intradermal (ID) injection administers the vaccine in the topmost layer of skin. BCG is the only vaccine that uses this route of administration. ID injection of BCG vaccine reduces the risk of neurovascular injury.

ID injection delivers mRNA vaccines directly into the skin, an organ densely populated with professional APCs such as Langerhans cells in the epidermis and various DC subtypes in the dermis. Immunization can take place via direct injection of **naked mRNA**, especially via routes that lead to effective targeting of APCs, such as ID and intranodal administration. When vaccines are delivered IM, humoral and cellular immune responses induced by naked mRNA remain low compared with LNP-formulated mRNA. The efficacy of mRNA vaccines can benefit significantly from complexing agents such as lipid- and polymer-based nanoparticles, which enhance uptake by cells and improve delivery to the translation machinery in the cytoplasm. Currently LNPs are the most promising and frequently used class of agents for in vivo delivery of mRNA vaccines.

Intranasal spray application of a vaccine offers a needle-free approach through the nasal mucosa.

Intravesical administration is restricted to BCG.

REPRESENTATIVE DISEASES ASSOCIATED WITH NEWER APPROVED OR INVESTIGATIONAL VACCINES

Many different FDA-approved vaccines to protect against infectious diseases are currently available. In 2017 the NIH launched a clinical trial of a vaccine to prevent mosquito-borne diseases, such as malaria, Zika virus infection, CHIK, and dengue fever. The experimental vaccine, designed to trigger an immune response to mosquito saliva rather than a specific virus or parasite, contains four recombinant proteins from mosquito salivary glands. The search for other vaccines (e.g., against HIV and COVID-19) are experimental.

Chikungunya Vaccine

The U.S. Food and Drug Administration (FDA) approved VLA1553, also known as Ixchiq, as the first chikungunya vaccine on November 9, 2023. Ixchiq is a single-dose, live-attenuated vaccine that is approved for people 18 years and older who are at a higher risk of exposure to the chikungunya virus.

According to the U.S. Centers for Disease Control and Prevention (CDC), the U.S. Advisory Committee on Immunization Practices (ACIP) approved recommendations for use of the Chikungunya vaccine in travelers and laboratory workers in February 2024. This live attenuated chikungunya vaccine (manufactured by Valneva as IXCHIQ) is the only Chikungunya vaccine currently licensed in the United States. IXCHIQ is licensed for use in adults aged 18 years and older but pregnant women should avoid the risk for Chikungunya virus infection, if possible.

The CDC reports that all travelers to countries or territories with risk of Chikungunya virus transmission should take steps to avoid mosquito bites. The risk for Chikungunya for most U.S. travelers is low. However, some travelers are at increased risk for infection or more severe disease. Factors to assess when considering use of chikungunya vaccine include the likelihood of exposure to Chikungunya virus, a traveler's risk factors for severe disease outcomes, and traveler preferences.

U.S. Centers for Disease Control and Prevention (CDC). Chikungunya Vaccine, Chikungunya Vaccine Information for Healthcare Providers. https://www.cdc.gov/chikungunya/hcp/vaccine/index.html. Accessed September 25, 2024.

DENGUE FEVER VACCINE

Since early 2020, the majority of the cases of dengue fever have been reported in Brazil, Paraguay, and Colombia. WHO estimates that up to 400 million dengue infections occur annually, resulting in 500,000 hospitalizations. Dengue fever is endemic in the US territories of Puerto Rico, the US Virgin Islands, and American Samoa. Nearly all dengue cases reported in the 48 contiguous US states were in travelers infected elsewhere.

Dengue is caused by any of four related viruses, termed *serotypes*—DEN-1, DEN-2, DEN-3, and DEN-4—which are transmitted to people by *Aedes aegypti* mosquitoes. A person exposed to one dengue virus type gains immunity to that type but not to the other three. In fact, a second infection with a virus type that differs from the first can lead to a more severe course of disease.

Each of the four CYD viruses (CYD-1, CYD-2, CYD-3, and CYD-4) in the vaccine Dengvaxia was constructed using recombinant DNA technology by replacing the sequences encoding the premembrane (prM) and envelope (E) proteins in the yellow fever (YF) 17D204 vaccine virus genome with those encoding for the homologous sequences of dengue virus serotypes 1, 2, 3, and 4, respectively.

Today Dengvaxia is a vaccine indicated for the prevention of dengue disease caused by dengue virus serotypes 1, 2, 3, and 4. Dengvaxia is approved for use in individuals aged 9 through 16 years with laboratory-confirmed previous dengue infection and who live in endemic areas. The vaccine is not approved for use in US travelers who are visiting but not living in an area where dengue is common.

Herpes Zoster (Shingles) Vaccine

Any person who has had chickenpox is at risk of developing shingles. Over 1 million cases occur each year in the United States. Shingles can occur in patients of all ages, with an increasing risk as people age.

When shingles develops, a rash or blisters appear on the skin, generally on one side of the body. This is a sign that the virus, which has been dormant in the nerve cells, has reactivated and traveled from the nerves and followed a path out to the skin. The nerves along the path become inflamed, and shingles can also be painful. For some people this pain can be severe and chronic. Pain that lasts for months after the rash has healed is called *postherpetic neuralgia*.

Previously two shingles vaccines were available. However, Zostavax is no longer available for use in the United States as of November 18, 2020.

The Shingrix vaccine is still available. Shingrix is a recombinant, adjuvanted vaccine, a sterile suspension for IM injection, that was approved in 2017. The vaccine is supplied as a lyophilized recombinant varicella-zoster virus surface glycoprotein E (gE) antigen component, which must be reconstituted with the accompanying vial of AS01B adjuvant suspension component. Healthy adults aged 50 years or older should get two doses of Shingrix, separated by 2 to 6 months. People should get Shingrix even if in the past they:
- had shingles
- received Zostavax
- are not sure if they have had chickenpox.

There is no maximum age for getting the Shingrix vaccine.

HIV/AIDS

The new and unique vaccine design, described in a paper in *Nature Communications* on April 9, 2023, uses tiny protein "nanoparticles" to display multiple copies of HIV's surface protein Env, thus presenting itself to the immune system much as real HIV particles would without causing HIV infection. The results of this early-phase clinical study showed that the experimental HIV nanoparticle vaccine is safe in people. While this vaccine alone will not offer HIV protection and is intended to be part of an eventual broader, multistep vaccination regimen, the researchers also determined that it elicited a robust immune response in nearly all 36 healthy adult volunteers. The results show that the nanoparticle vaccine, known by the lab name "eOD-GT8 60-mer," successfully expanded production of a rare type of antibody-producing immune B cell in nearly all recipients.

Vaccines such as one that could provide immunity to HIV continue to be a problem because of the enormous genetic diversity and other unique features of the HIV-B viral envelope protein.

Currently, no HIV or AIDS vaccines have been approved for use, although many are in clinical trials (https://www.clinicaltrials.gov). However, the results of an early-phase clinical study, published in the journal *Science Translational Medicine*, showed that an experimental HIV nanoparticle vaccine is safe in people. While this vaccine alone will not offer HIV protection and is intended to be part of an eventual broader, multistep vaccination regimen, the researchers also determined that it elicited a robust immune response in nearly all 36 healthy adult volunteers.

The results show that the nanoparticle vaccine, known by the lab name "eOD-GT8 60-mer," successfully expanded production of a rare type of antibody-producing immune B cell in nearly all recipients.

The goal of an effective HIV vaccine is to induce a response in the recipient that is unnatural immunity. The problem with HIV vaccine candidates is that although these vaccines can be modestly protective, they generally do not induce neutralizing antibodies or reactive cytotoxic T-cell responses against HIV.

The status of HIV vaccines to date is as follows:
1. There are no proven effective therapeutic or preventive HIV vaccines.
2. There is a lack of knowledge related to the ability of a vaccine to induce HIV-specific immune responses that are effective in preventing or treating HIV infection.
3. Therapeutic HIV vaccine research is still in its early stages.

Vaccine Development

The goal of producing HIV vaccines is to destroy HIV or keep the virus in check so that it causes no further damage (Box 27.1). An ideal vaccine would stop progressive immunodeficiency and restore the immune system to a healthy state.

The requirements for a preventive HIV vaccine are to generate humoral and cellular immunity against HIV in the host before exposure to the virus. After initial exposure to HIV, the generation of cellular immune responses against the virus may take time to develop, which makes neutralizing antibodies against free virus important to reduce the initial spread of the virus in the body.

In the United States research is based on the use of subunit proteins found in the envelope of HIV. Vaccine research scientists are trying to develop the following three types of HIV vaccines:
1. Preventive or prophylactic vaccines to protect individuals from HIV infection
2. Therapeutic vaccines to prevent HIV-infected patients from progressing to AIDS
3. Perinatal vaccines for administration to HIV-infected pregnant women to prevent transmission of HIV to the fetus

Scientists hope that therapeutic and perinatal administration of a vaccine will reach a high level of success. Challenges associated with HIV vaccine development include the following:
- A high rate of viral mutation and recombination
- No clearly defined natural immunity to HIV
- HIV infects cells that are critical to the immune body defenses; also it is transmitted as a free virus and within infected cells

Vaccine Problems

Problems associated with HIV vaccine development are plagued by the lack of scientific understanding of HIV infection, as well as the complex biology of HIV infection and AIDS. Once inside a host cell, HIV is capable of integrating itself into the genetic material of infected cells. For a vaccine to be effective it needs to produce a constant state of immune protection, not only to block viral entry to most cells but also to continue to block newly produced viruses over the infected person's lifetime.

Researchers have identified the following specific problem areas:
- A lack of knowledge related to the critical components of the body's immune response to HIV infection.
- The high risk of using entire weakened or inactive HIV in a vaccine.
- The extensive rate of viral mutation as HIV replicates. Strains worldwide vary by as much as 35% in terms of the proteins that make up the outer coat of the virus. Even an infected person can experience a change in viral protein by as much as 10% over the years. This genetic diversity may require an effective vaccine to be based on multiple viral strains.
- The protective effect of a vaccine may last only a short time and frequent mandatory booster vaccinations would be impractical and expensive.
- Vaccinated persons could become more susceptible to HIV infection because of vaccine-induced enhancement of infection.
- No vaccine clinical trial to date has demonstrated stimulation of the cellular components of the immune system in the way needed to destroy HIV.
- Animal models have severe limitations, including the possibility of integration of DNA into the human genome from monkeys.
- No research studies have successfully demonstrated which immune responses correlate with protection from HIV infection.

In 2000 vaccine research scientists lowered their expectations and settled for a vaccine that would not completely prevent HIV infection. It is estimated that a vaccine with only 30% effectiveness against HIV (vs. the usual 85%–95% effectiveness of other infectious disease vaccines) can begin to eradicate the virus if it is widely administered and accompanied by disease-prevention education. Based on this premise, the FDA has indicated that it will approve an HIV/AIDS vaccine at this level of efficacy.

BOX 27.1 Timeline for Human Immunodeficiency Virus Vaccine Research

1984
The human Immunodeficiency virus (HIV) was identified as the cause of acquired immunodeficiency syndrome (AIDS).

1987
The first HIV vaccine clinical trial opened at the National Institutes of Health (NIH) Clinical Center in Bethesda, Maryland. This phase I trial enrolled 138 healthy, HIV-negative volunteers. The gp160 subunit vaccine showed no serious adverse effects.

1988
The National Institute of Allergy and Infectious Diseases (NIAID) AIDS Vaccine Evaluation Group (AVEG), the first US cooperative HIV vaccine clinical trials group, began enrolling volunteers in its first trial.

1992
NIAID launched the first phase II HIV vaccine clinical trial. This trial included HIV-negative volunteers with a history of high-risk behavior, such as injection drug use, multiple sex partners, or sexually transmitted infections.

1998
The first large-scale HIV vaccine trial began. VaxGen initiated a phase III trial of AIDSVAX (VAX004) in North America and the Netherlands involving more than 5400 volunteers.

1999
NIAID began the first African preventive HIV vaccine trial in Uganda. The first large-scale HIV vaccine trial in a developing country began. VaxGen initiated a phase III trial of AIDSVAX (VAX003) involving over 2500 volunteers in Thailand.

2000
NIAID formed the HIV Vaccine Trials Network (HVTN), a network of clinical sites in more than 25 sites in the United States, Africa, Asia, South America, and the Caribbean, dedicated to developing a preventive HIV vaccine by testing and evaluating candidate vaccines in all phases of clinical trials.
  The first African HIV vaccine trial was completed in Uganda.

2003
The US and Royal Thai governments jointly initiated RV144, a phase III trial to evaluate a novel HIV vaccine strategy commonly referred to as "prime-boost."

2004
Both VaxGen candidates failed to confer protection against HIV in phase III trials.

2007
NIAID halted the phase II Step and Phambili studies due to safety concerns.

2009
The phase II HIV Vaccine Trials Network 505 study was initiated to evaluate a "prime-boost" vaccine regimen developed by the Vaccine Research Center (VRC).
  Results of the phase III Thai Trial (RV144) revealed that the vaccine combination demonstrated a modest preventive effect in humans. The trial, which enrolled more than 16,000 volunteers, was the first, and to date only, large clinical study to demonstrate efficacy for an investigational HIV vaccine.

2010
VRC scientists identified two potent antibodies that neutralize most strains of HIV in the laboratory (VRC01 and VRC02).
  The Pox Protein Public-Private Partnership (P5), an international collaborative team committed to building on the modest success of RV144, was formed.

2011
HVTN 505 was expanded to include protection from HIV as primary endpoint.

2012
Additional analyses of samples from RV144 provided insight into what types of immune responses may be needed for an effective vaccine.

2013
HVTN 505 immunizations were stopped due to lack of efficacy.

2015
The phase I/II HVTN 100 study, part of the P5 research endeavor, launched to test the safety of an experimental HIV vaccine regimen based on the RV144 findings, and also its ability to generate an immune response.

2016
NIAID launched the AMP Study to test whether intravenous infusions of the antibody VRC01 were safe, tolerable, and effective at preventing HIV infection. The trials were also designed to answer fundamental scientific questions for HIV prevention and vaccine research. In addition HVTN 702 was launched to test whether a new version of the RV144 HIV vaccine candidate safely prevented HIV infection among adults in South Africa.
  NIAID launched a clinical trial of a vaccine candidate, intended to prevent Zika virus infection, called the *NIAID Zika virus investigational DNA vaccine*.

2017
NIAID and partners launched Imbokodo or HVTN 705/HPX2008, a phase IIb proof-of-concept study evaluating the safety and efficacy of an experimental regimen based on a "mosaic" vaccine designed to induce immune responses against a wide variety of global HIV strains.

2019
As of 2019 the RV144 vaccine trial in Thailand was the only HIV vaccine to show efficacy against HIV infection to date.

2020
HIV Vaccine Research
HVTN 702
A trial of HVTN 702, started in 2016 in South Africa as an updated version of the RV144 HIV vaccine, was halted in February, 2020. The study sponsor made the call after interim results showed that the HVTN 702 vaccine was safe but did not prevent HIV. This disappointing outcome may have been attributable to differences between the HVTN 702 and RV144 study populations or to differences in the immune responses needed for protection against different global HIV subtypes.

Imbokodo (HPX2008/HVTN 705) and Mosaico (HPX3002/HVTN 706)
Another approach to an HIV vaccine is based on "mosaic" immunogens—vaccine components comprising elements from multiple HIV subtypes—that aim to induce immune responses against the wide variety of global HIV strains. Mosaic-based vaccine regimens are being evaluated in two late-stage clinical trials: Imbokodo (HPX2008/HVTN 705) and Mosaico (HPX3002/HVTN 706). A third approach, still in preclinical studies, involves placing HIV genes into an unrelated carrier virus, cytomegalovirus (CMV), to elicit a cell-based immune response. Efforts are underway to adapt this vaccine platform for testing in humans.

Broadly Neutralizing Antibodies (bNAbs)
Scientists also are exploring ways to harness the potential of broadly neutralizing antibodies (bNAbs) for long-acting HIV prevention tools and, ultimately,

> **BOX 27.1 Timeline for Human Immunodeficiency Virus Vaccine Research—cont'd**
>
> a vaccine. One gene transfer phase I trial began a few years ago in the United Kingdom to test an adeno-associated virus vector as a delivery vehicle for a gene encoding a bNAb.
>
> On May 14, 2020 an independent data and safety monitoring board (DSMB) found that the study data clearly indicated that long-acting injectable cabotegravir was highly effective at preventing HIV in the study population. Consequently, the DSMB recommended that NIAID stop the blinded phase of the trial, which was originally expected to continue until 2021, and share the results. NIAID accepted the recommendations, and HPTN 083 results are pending.
>
> *HPTN 084*
>
> The DSMB also reviewed data on May 14, 2020 from the phase III companion study of long-acting cabotegravir for HIV prevention in women in southern and eastern Africa, called HPTN 084. To date more than 3000 sexually active women in seven African countries have enrolled in the HPTN 084 study.

From History of HIV Vaccine Research, www.niaid.nih.gov. Accessed October 18, 2020; Mahomed S, Garrett N, Baxter C, Abdool Karim Q, Abdool Karim SS. Clinical trials of broadly neutralizing monoclonal antibodies for human immunodeficiency virus prevention: a review *J Infect Dis* 223(3):370–380, 2021.

Clinical Trials

RV144. RV144, also known as the *Thai Prime-Boost trial*, evaluated a poxvirus vector plus protein vaccine combination, which found evidence of modest protection. At the end of the trial, efficacy was 31.2% overall; efficacy at 12 months after immunization was higher.

Within 9 months, an international initiative was underway to analyze RV144 samples for correlates of risk. Correlates analysis identified one immune response (binding antibody to the V1/V2 region of the HIV envelope) associated with vaccine-induced protection. High levels of the immune substance immunoglobulin A (IgA) were associated with decreased protection.

Analysis of immune responses is ongoing. Scientists are seeking to improve on RV144; for example, is the binding antibody to V1/V2 responsible for protection or just a sign of it? What is the structure of the V1/V2 binding site?

Because the RV144 vaccine regimen did not induce neutralizing antibodies, researchers believe that antibody-mediated cellular cytotoxicity, in which nonneutralizing antibodies flag infected cells for destruction, played an important role. Work is underway to develop methods to maximize this activity with future vaccine candidates. Studies involving a replicating cytomegalovirus (CMV) vector have shown that effector T-cell responses could have the potential to clear HIV infections, and several vaccine candidates based on other replicating vectors are under evaluation in early clinical trials, with the CMV vector possibly entering human testing in the not-too-distant future.

VRC01. New technologies have contributed to the identification of many broadly neutralizing antibodies (bNAbs) capable of potently inhibiting multiple HIV isolates from all clades. There is now an intense focus on creating strategies capable of coaxing B cells into generating bNAbs using sequential immunizations with HIV antigens specifically designed for this purpose.

Researchers have also made progress in constructing HIV envelope proteins that more closely mimic the natural form—the three-prong trimer structure is unstable, making it difficult to preserve for creating vaccine antigens—and preliminary results in animal models suggest that this approach may induce antibodies with improved neutralization capacity.

In the past several years, researchers at the Vaccine Research Center, a section of NIAID, have discovered several different broadly neutralizing antibodies in specimens from patients living with HIV. These antibodies are rare and they have not been found until after a patient has been infected for at least several years. One of these antibodies is a bNAb called *VRC01*.

Most common antibodies bind to HIV by recognizing short pieces of protein, epitopes, but VRC01 binds to an entire region on the gp120 protein found on HIV's surface, the CD4-binding site. VRC01 is able to bind to the CD4 receptor and block HIV from attaching by "neutralizing" it.

Three early-phase safety studies of VRC01 have been conducted, with over 100 people receiving the antibody. The antibody is given to study participants intravenously. The strategy of using an IV infusion of antibodies is called *antibody-mediated prevention*, or *AMP*.

Early data show that the antibody seems safe and well tolerated by study participants. There have been few adverse reactions, and they were mild. The study has moved forward to phase IIb based on these results. Further research will focus on whether a bNAb can be protective in humans and on the required dose, if protection is demonstrated.

HVTN 100. In February, 2015 HVTN 100 was launched. This clinical trial evaluates the safety and immunogenicity of modified versions of the vaccines based on HIV-1 clade C, the prevalent virus in South Africa. In 2020, this study, a 12-month booster of subtype C pox-protein vaccines, restored immune responses and slowed response decay compared to the 6-month vaccination. Research studies continue in 2024.

Vaccine Expectations

Reasons for optimism about HIV vaccine development include the following:

1. Nonhuman primates vaccinated with products based on HIV or simian immunodeficiency virus have shown complete or partial protection against infection with the wild-type virus.
2. Successful vaccines have been developed against the feline immunodeficiency virus, also a retrovirus.
3. Almost all humans develop some form of immune response that is protective or able to control viral infection over a long period. Some individuals remain disease free for up to 25 years, frequently with undetectable viral load levels.
4. Vaccines that present epitopes to the immune system in a conformationally precise manner may induce the body to produce neutralizing antibodies and provide a high level of protection against HIV infection.
5. In the future, microbial and viral genome sequencing will become increasingly rapid and less expensive. One approach, known as *reverse vaccinology*, involves cloning and expressing all proteins that are predicted based on a complete genome to be secreted or surface associated, starting with the complete genome sequence. This approach allows for a small group of proteins from microorganisms (e.g., group B meningococcus, group B *Streptococcus*, and extraintestinal pathogenic *Escherichia coli*) to be candidates for multivalent subunit vaccines. To date, however, these organisms have eluded vaccine development.

Influenza

Influenza vaccines can provide moderate protection against virologically confirmed influenza, but such protection is greatly reduced or absent in some seasons. The efficacy of influenza vaccines may decline during years when the circulating viruses have drifted antigenically from those included in the vaccine.

WHO coordinates global influences and virus surveillance so that appropriate vaccine candidates can be identified by WHO and national authorities and vaccines can be reformulated each year. Vaccine viruses must be selected every year because genetic mutations arise continuously in influenza viruses, a process termed **antigenic drift** that results in the emergence of immunologically distinct variants. The process is repeated each year, which imposes severe time restrictions on all groups involved.

There are hundreds of influenza A strains that are mutating constantly and are hard to predict, whereas there are only two B strains. The trivalent vaccine protects against three different flu viruses: the two most common A strains (H1N1 and H3N2) and one B strain (either Massachusetts or Brisbane), whichever is predicted to affect citizens most strongly in a given year. A quadrivalent vaccine is a form that offers the same benefits as the trivalent vaccine, with the added bonus of covering both B strains, covering four strains total. Experts see this as beneficial because both B strains have been detected within the United States in the past 10 years.

Multiple approved 2024–2025 manufacturers will make the Influenza A (H1N1) 2024–2025 Monovalent vaccines using the established manufacturing processes for their seasonal influenza vaccines. The FDA approved these vaccines as a strain change to each manufacturer's seasonal influenza vaccine. There is considerable experience with seasonal influenza vaccine development and production, and influenza vaccines produced by this technology have a long and successful track record of safety and effectiveness in the United States. The Influenza A (H1N1) 2024–2025 Monovalent vaccines will undergo the usual testing and lot-release procedures that are in place for seasonal influenza vaccines.

Overall both the trivalent and quadrivalent types protect against the flu, and the CDC does not currently recommend one over the other. Eventually the quadrivalent vaccine will phase out the trivalent form. Right now the quadrivalent vaccine can cost almost double the trivalent form, and some insurance companies will not reimburse for the additional cost.

In a study of the safety and efficacy of intranasally administered live, attenuated influenza vaccine to children without a recent episode of wheezing illness or severe asthma, live, attenuated virus had significantly better efficacy than inactivated vaccine. Evidence for protection in adults aged 65 years or older is lacking. Studies consistently show the highest efficacy in young children (aged 6 months to 7 years). New vaccines with improved clinical efficacy and effectiveness are needed to further reduce influenza-related morbidity and mortality.

> **KEY CONCEPTS**
> **Vaccinations for International Travel**
> - International travelers frequently require vaccination against endemic diseases (e.g., hepatitis A) in a particular country. Healthcare professionals are now protected against hepatitis B through vaccines. Many adults receive the flu vaccine. Vaccines are also given to pets and livestock.
> - A vaccine stimulates active immunity and creates an immune memory so that exposure to the active disease microorganism will stimulate an already primed immune system to fight the disease.

INTERNATIONAL TRAVEL VACCINES

Vaccine-preventable diseases are an important consideration in the prevention of travel-related illnesses. Transmittable diseases are no longer only exotic diseases restricted by geography. For example measles and mumps epidemics have resulted in travel-related outbreaks in the United States.

The choice of vaccines for an individual traveler is based on risk of exposure to vaccine-preventable diseases on a traveler's itinerary. Specific risk and risk-taking behavior related to travel (e.g., type of accommodations, planned outdoor activities, use of insect repellent, and sexual behavior) need to be taken into consideration.

The Advisory Committee on Immunizations Practices provides comprehensive background and recommendations for administration of each kind of vaccine.

Epidemiology of Vaccine-Preventable Diseases

The worldwide epidemiology of travel-related diseases is constantly changing. Influenza is the most common vaccine-preventable disease and it is especially prevalent in environments in which there are mass gatherings or closely confined quarters (e.g., cruise ships). Other communicable diseases that present a high risk to nonimmune travelers are hepatitis A, symptomatic hepatitis B for long-stay travelers and expatriates, typhoid and paratyphoid among travelers to India, and yellow fever in travelers to Brazil. In contrast, the risk of cholera, Japanese encephalitis, meningococcal meningitis, polio, rabies, and varicella is considered low, even for travelers in highly endemic countries.

Travel-Only Vaccines and Chemoprophylaxis for Adults

Hepatitis A and typhoid vaccines are considerations for most travelers to developing countries. Other vaccines are dependent on risk areas in specific countries and specific risk activities (Table 27.2). Healthy travelers who are 65 years old or older should be current with pneumococcal vaccination with sequential doses of PPSV23.

Four categories of international travelers are more susceptible to acquiring transmittable diseases:
- Children
- Travelers with various chronic existing disorders (e.g., diabetes and liver disease)
- Immunocompromised and HIV-infected travelers
- Pregnant women

Immunocompromised and HIV-infected travelers represent up to 4% of travelers seen in some US travel clinics. Immunocompromised travelers have various conditions and medications that affect vaccinations. Health hazards at the destination that would potentially exacerbate the underlying conditions can be more severe for them than for immunocompetent travelers. Travelers with autoimmune diseases (e.g., systemic lupus erythematosus and rheumatoid arthritis) who are not being treated with immunosuppressive or immunomodulating drugs are not considered to be significantly immunocompromised.

It is important that travelers taking immunosuppressive drugs and most biological response-modifying drugs not receive live vaccines. Nonlive vaccines are safe but may have suboptimal efficacy in immunocompromised hosts. Unvaccinated travelers with severe immune compromise are discouraged from traveling to endemic areas for yellow fever even if they can enter the country without proof of yellow fever vaccination. In addition immunocompromised travelers may require additional nontravel vaccines compared with healthy travelers.

Travelers should receive routinely recommended vaccinations and specific travel immunizations based on destinations and activities. In addition malaria chemoprophylaxis is critical for those traveling to malaria-endemic areas. Malaria is found in more than 100 countries, mainly in tropical regions of the world, including large areas of Africa and Asia, Central and South America, Haiti, and the Dominican Republic.

TABLE 27.2 Available Vaccines for International Travelers.

Vaccine	High-Risk Travel Destinations	Recent Outbreaks or New Findings with Impact on Travelers
Cholera	Destinations with poor hygiene and sanitation practices where cholera is endemic, humanitarian aid work, some instances of visiting family and relatives	Haiti, Somalia, Yemen
Hepatitis A	Destinations with poor hygiene and sanitation practices, adventurous eating habits	Widespread
Hepatitis B	Adventure travel, medical tourism, or medical conditions that may require medical intervention	None
Influenza (+ avian influenza)	Mass gatherings, cruise ships, exposure to live poultry	Saudi Arabia, China, Vietnam, Thailand
Japanese encephalitis	Adventure travel in agricultural areas, open-air accommodations, rural homestays, some instances of visiting friends and relatives	Bali, China, Thailand
Measles, mumps, rubella	Mass gatherings, travel to one of many areas with current outbreaks, travel to areas with an antivaccine community (e.g., Amish communities)	South America (Venezuela, Brazil), Europe, Indonesia, Philippines
Meningococcal, quadrivalent ACYW-135	Mass gatherings; sub-Saharan Africa	Saudi Arabia
Polio virus	Endemic destinations with low vaccine coverage or disruption in healthcare infrastructure, humanitarian aid work	Afghanistan, Nigeria, Pakistan, Papua New Guinea, Somalia, Democratic Republic of Congo
Rabies	Remote areas with a high incidence of canine rabies; behaviors involving close contact with canines, wildlife, and bats	Indonesia (Bali), Malaysia, India, Thailand
Tetanus-diphtheria-pertussis (Tdap) or tetanus-diphtheria (Td)	Tetanus: participation in injury-prone activities, such as construction, cycling, and motorcycle riding. Diphtheria: humanitarian aid activities, destinations with low vaccine coverage	Diphtheria: Haiti, Venezuela, Bangladesh, Thailand, South Pacific, Vanuatu. Pertussis: Worldwide exposure
Tick-borne encephalitis	Unpasteurized dairy products, hiking, camping	Austria, Czech Republic, Finland, Germany, Latvia, Norway, Sweden, Switzerland
Typhoid	Destinations with poor hygiene or irregular destination travel requirement	Pakistan
Yellow fever	Destinations with known outbreaks or irregular destination travel requirement	Brazil, Angola, Democratic Republic of the Congo, Nigeria

From Freedman DO, Chen LH: Vaccines for international travel, *Mayo Clin Proc* 94(11):2314–2339, 2019.
* According to the CDC in 2024, measles cases are increasing globally, including in the United States. The majority of measles cases imported into the United States occur in unvaccinated U.S. residents who become infected during international travel. CDC recommends all travelers get fully vaccinated against measles before traveling to any international destination. Accessed September 28, 2024. https://wwwnc.cdc.gov/travel/.
** CDC Yellow Book (see Sec. 2, Ch. 5, Yellow Fever Vaccine & Malaria Prevention Information by Country). Accessed September 28, 2024.

CANCER VACCINES

Cancer treatment vaccines are designed to work by activating B cells and killer T cells and directing them to recognize and act against specific types of cancer. Cancer cells carry self and cancer-associated antigens. The cancer-associated antigens mark the cancer cells as abnormal (nonself) and can cause B cells and killer T cells to mount an attack against them.

Cancer vaccines belong to the class of substances known as *biological response modifiers*. There are two broad types of cancer vaccines:
- Preventive or prophylactic vaccines
- Therapeutic vaccines

Currently there are two FDA-approved preventive cancer vaccines and one therapeutic cancer vaccine.

Prophylactic Vaccines

Like traditional vaccines, preventive vaccines for cancer are based on antigens that are carried by infectious agents and that are relatively easy for the immune system to recognize as foreign antigens.

The FDA-approved preventive vaccines are Gardasil and Cervarix. These vaccines provide protection against two types of HPV, types 16 and 18, which cause approximately 70% of all cases of cervical cancer. These types can also cause some vaginal, vulvar, anal, penile, and oropharyngeal cancer. At least 17 other types of HPV are responsible for the remaining 30% of cervical cancer cases. More than 6 million people become infected with HPV every year in the United States, and almost 10,000 women are diagnosed with cervical cancer.

Gardasil

Gardasil was approved by the FDA in June, 2006. More than 30 countries had approved the vaccine before the FDA's approval. The vaccine can prevent cervical cancer and vaginal and vulvar precancers caused by HPV-16 and HPV-18. This vaccine also provides protection against two additional types of HPV for girls and women aged 9 to 26 years—types 6 and 11, which are responsible for about 90% of all cases of genital warts in males and females but do not cause cervical cancer. Because Gardasil targets four HPV types, it is called a *quadrivalent vaccine*. The quadrivalent vaccine is for use in patients not previously infected by one of the four covered HPV types.

Additional products in development include vaccines covering other high-risk HPV types for broader coverage, and also therapeutic vaccines designed to treat women who already have precancerous lesions or cancer.

Cervarix

Cervarix is a bivalent vaccine made from VLPs made with proteins from HPV types 16 and 18. It may provide partial protection against a few additional HPV types that can cause cancer. This vaccine is for girls and women aged 9 to 25 years.

Therapeutic vaccines

Therapeutic vaccines are a new form of vaccine. These vaccines are used to activate a patient's immune system to recognize and finally control an already established infectious pathogen. Therapeutic vaccines are different than those that are given for disease prevention such as measles, TB, and influenza vaccines. Therapeutic vaccines harness a patient's own immune system to fight an existing disease rather than immunizing for protection against future disease. In 2010 the US FDA approved the first therapeutic vaccine, Provenge, for prostate cancer.

> **KEY CONCEPTS**
> **Applications of Vaccines**
> - Cancer treatment vaccines are made using antigens from malignant cells or modified versions of them.
> - Pathogens or pathogen products adapted for biological warfare include smallpox, anthrax, plague, tularemia, brucellosis, Q fever, botulinum toxin, and staphylococcal enterotoxin B.
> - Vaccines emphasize public health safety (anthrax) or prevent the return of epidemic diseases.
> - Preventive AIDS vaccines are for HIV-negative individuals to prevent HIV infection. Therapeutic AIDS vaccines are for HIV-positive individuals to improve the immune system.
> - Anthrax vaccine is for emergency use in the event of an anthrax-based attack on the US population.
> - A therapeutic vaccine is directed at patients with acute myeloid leukemia (AML).
> - The threat of bioterrorism with smallpox has led to high-risk individuals already being vaccinated.

Cancer Treatment Vaccines

Cancer treatment vaccines are designed to treat cancers that have already developed. They are intended to delay or stop the growth of cancer, to cause shrinkage of tumors, to prevent cancer from coming back, or to eliminate cancer cells that have not been destroyed by other forms of treatment. Cancer vaccines might be designed to target tumor-associated antigens (TAAs), cancer germline antigens, virus-related antigens, or tumor-specific antigens (TSAs), which are also widely recognized as neoantigens.

Sipuleucel-T (Provenge) and Talimogene laherparepvec (T-VEC) are the two FDA-approved vaccines currently being utilized for advanced prostate cancer and advanced melanoma skin cancer, respectively. Researchers are testing vaccines for several types of cancers, including bladder cancer, brain tumor, breast cancer, cervical cancer, colorectal cancer, lung cancer, and many more. Although cancer vaccines as a single therapy are not sufficient to declare a complete victory over this deadly disease until now, it must be a comprehensive approach and existing treatments on the concept of cancer management.

Cancer treatment vaccines are made using antigens from malignant cells or modified versions of them. Antigens that have been used to date include proteins, carbohydrates, glycoproteins or glycopeptides, and gangliosides (carbohydrate–lipid). Other cancer vaccines may use weakened or killed cancer cells that carry a specific cancer-associated antigen or immune cells that are modified to express such an antigen. The source of these vaccine cells can be the patient (autologous) or another patient (allogeneic).

Developing a cancer vaccine is difficult because malignant cells have normal self-antigens and specific cancer-associated antigens. Cancer cells may undergo genetic changes that can lead to the loss of cancer-associated antigens. Additionally, malignant cells can produce chemical messages that suppress anticancer immune responses by killer T cells. The result is that even if the immune system recognizes a growing cancer as a threat, the malignant cells may escape a strong attack by the immune system.

It is much more difficult to develop a cancer treatment vaccine than a preventive vaccine. Understanding how cancer cells escape recognition and attack by the immune system is necessary in order to design cancer treatment vaccines. To be effective a cancer treatment vaccine must:

- Stimulate specific responses against the correct target, just as traditional vaccines do
- Be powerful enough to overcome the barriers that malignant cells use to protect themselves from attack by B cells and killer T cells

Clinical Trials

According to the National Cancer Institute–Molecular Analysis for Therapy Choice (NCI-MATCH) is a clinical trial that analyzes patients' tumors to determine whether they contain genetic abnormalities for which a targeted drug exists, an actionable mutation, and assigns treatment based on the abnormality. MATCH enrolled people with advanced solid tumors, lymphoma, or myeloma that progressed on standard treatment or people with a rare cancer for which there is no standard treatment. NCI-MATCH showed that people with advanced cancer may benefit from genomic sequencing to help plan their treatment.

As NCI-MATCH winds down in 2023, information learned from it is leading to new precision medicine trials, such as ComboMATCH, MyeloMATCHExit Disclaimer, and ImmunoMatch (iMATCH). Unlike NCI-MATCH, which tested single drugs, ComboMATCH will test combinations of drugs. MyeloMATCH will test treatments based on genetic changes in the cancer cells of people with acute myeloid leukemia (AML) and myelodysplastic syndromes (MDS). These cancers were not included in NCI-MATCH. The iMATCH trial will study how the immune status of a tumor affects the response to targeted treatments with immunotherapy.

Leukemia

According to the National Cancer Institute (www.cancer.gov), the mainstays of leukemia treatment for adults have been chemotherapy, radiation therapy, and stem cell transplantation.

CAR T-cell therapy is a type of treatment in which a patient's own immune cells are genetically modified to treat their cancer. Currently, one type of CAR T cell therapy is approved for the treatment of some children and young adults with B-cell precursor Acute lymphblastic leukemia. This CAR T cell therapy is now being explored for use in older adults with B-cell Acute lymphblastic leukemia. A second CAR T-cell therapy has also been approved for adults with B-cell precursor ALL that has not responded to treatment or has returned after previous treatment. CAR T-cell therapy is also being tested in adults with Chronic lymphocytic leukema. Researchers would like to know if using this type of immunotherapy early in the course of treatment would be more effective than waiting until the cancer returns.

New developments in leukemia in 2024 include FDA approved blinatumomab (Blincyto) for adults and children one month and older with CD19-positive Philadelphia chromosome-negative B-cell precursor acute lymphoblastic leukemia (Ph-negative BCP ALL). It is used as part of consolidation chemotherapy, which is given after cancer has disappeared following initial therapy.

Cancer Research UK, could be used to support advanced clinical studies in one or more of the following areas:
- AML
- Non–small cell lung cancer
- Other indications showing high levels of telomerase activity and susceptibility to immunotherapy
- In combination with checkpoint or immune pathway inhibitors
- In combination with additional antigens, including those arising from the exciting new field of tumor neoantigens

VACCINES IN BIODEFENSE

In regard to bioterrorism, the goal of the FDA is to foster the development of vaccines. Many products (e.g., FDA-regulated vaccines) could be affected by bioterrorism. Pathogens or pathogen products adapted for biological warfare include the following:
- Smallpox (variola)
- Anthrax (*Bacillus anthracis*)

Smallpox

Threats of bioterrorism with smallpox as a weapon have launched a high-profile discussion of the reintroduction of smallpox into the general US population. Individuals in high-risk occupations and positions have already begun to be vaccinated.

Category A Agents

Smallpox vaccination was stopped in 1972 after the disease was eradicated in the United States. Smallpox is classified as a Category A agent by the CDC. Other Category A agents include anthrax, plague, botulism, tularemia, and viral hemorrhagic fevers. These agents are believed to pose the greatest potential threat for an adverse public health effect and to have a moderate-to-high potential for large-scale dissemination.

Smallpox Vaccine

Smallpox vaccine, a preventive vaccine, is the only way to prevent smallpox. The vaccine is made from a live virus called *vaccinia*, which is another pox-type virus related to smallpox but unable to cause disease. A live virus vaccine (e.g., measles, mumps, rubella, chickenpox, and smallpox vaccines) is a vaccine that contains a living virus that can provide and produce immunity, usually without causing illness. For most people with a healthy immune system, live virus vaccines are safe and effective, but the live virus can be transmitted to other parts of the body or to other people from the unhealed vaccination site.

Vaccine administration. The smallpox vaccine is not injected, as are other types of vaccines. It is given using a bifurcated (two-pronged) needle that is dipped into the vaccine solution. The needle is used to prick the skin a number of times in a few seconds. It takes about 3 weeks for the site to heal, with a scar remaining. The first dose of vaccine offers protection from smallpox for 3 to 5 years, with decreasing immunity thereafter. A repeat vaccination offers longer immunity. Vaccination within 3 days of exposure completely prevents or significantly modifies smallpox in the vast majority of persons. Vaccination 4 to 7 days after exposure likely offers some protection from disease or may modify the severity of the disease.

Anthrax

Anthrax is an infectious disease caused by spores of the bacterium *Bacillus anthracis*. *B. anthracis* spores are highly resistant to inactivation; for example, they may be present in the soil for decades, occasionally infecting grazing animals that ingest the spores. Goats, sheep, and cattle are some animals that may become infected.

VACCINE SAFETY ISSUES

The safety of vaccines is a controversial public health issue because vaccines are in a unique niche in the marketplace. No vaccine is totally effective or 100% safe. The same components that make them effective may also cause serious adverse effects. It may not be possible to develop safer versions of vaccines without losing essential functions.

An FDA-approved vaccine must meet specific requirements, as follows:
1. Produce protective immunity with only minimal side effects
2. Be immunogenic enough to produce a strong and measurable immune response
3. Be stable during its shelf life, with potency remaining at a proper level

Inactivated vaccines are stored in powdered form and are reconstituted before administration. Live, attenuated vaccines require refrigeration.

The Center for Biologics Evaluation and Research (CBER) regulates vaccine products. Many of these are childhood vaccines that have contributed to a significant reduction of vaccine-preventable diseases. According to the CDC, vaccines have reduced preventable infectious diseases to an all-time low, and few people now experience the devastating effects of measles, pertussis, and other illnesses.

Vaccine development is an important focus of research related to AIDS, malaria, and other devastating diseases. Recently recommended vaccines include a new measles-mumps-rubella-varicella vaccine for 1-year-old children and a tetanus-diphtheria-pertussis (Tdap) vaccine for people aged 11 to 65 years.

Concerns About Vaccines

Vaccination requirements, even well-accepted laws on so-called classic childhood diseases (e.g., polio, measles, and pertussis), have been resisted in recent years based on philosophic, political, scientific, and ideologic issues. In the past 20 years, the number of recommended pediatric vaccines has increased dramatically, despite unproven theories alleging connections between vaccines and illnesses, including autism, diabetes, and multiple sclerosis. An estimated 1% to 3% of US children are excused by their parents from vaccine requirements, with rates as high as 15% to 20% in a few communities.

A vaccine for hepatitis E virus (HEV) has raised ethical concerns in Nepal. Testing of the recombinant protein (rHEV) vaccine in a civilian population led to concerns that residents might not have access to the vaccines after the clinical trials concluded. Hepatitis E is common (endemic) in Nepal.

Vaccine Side Effects and Adverse Events

Because vaccines contain live or killed laboratory-altered microorganisms and other constituents, unintended consequences can result. Although vaccines are designed to protect individuals from disease, side effects can occur, just as with any kind of medication. A possible side effect resulting from a vaccination is known as an *adverse event*. Most side effects from vaccination are mild, such as soreness, swelling, or redness at the injection site. Some vaccines are associated with fever, rash, and achiness. Serious side effects are rare but can include a seizure or life-threatening allergic reaction.

There is a range of possible vaccination side effects. Each year, due to chance alone, many babies will experience a medical event in close proximity to a vaccination. This does not mean, though, that the event is in fact related to the vaccination. The challenge is to determine when a medical event is directly related to a vaccination.

Side effects range from relatively few associated side effects, such as those associated with the vaccine for Hib, compared with vaccines known to have many potential side effects, such as the smallpox vaccine given to military personnel and others who might be first responders in the event of a bioterrorism attack.

Although no serious side effects are associated with Hib, side effects such as redness, warmth, or swelling at the injection site occur in up to 1 out of 4 children, and a fever of over 38°C (101°F) occurs in up to 1 out of 20 children. In comparison, the smallpox vaccine can produce mild to severe problems. These problems include a mild rash lasting 2 to 4 days, swelling and tenderness of lymph nodes lasting 2 to 4 weeks after the blister has healed, fever of over 37.8°C (100°F; about 70% of children, 17% of adults) or over 38.9°C (102°F; about 15% to 20% of children, under 2% of adults), and secondary blisters elsewhere on the body. For every 1 million people vaccinated for smallpox, between 14 and 52 could have a life-threatening reaction to the vaccine. Moderate to severe problems include serious eye infection or loss of vision due to spread of the vaccine virus to the eye; rash on the entire body (as many as 1 per 4000); severe rash on individuals with eczema (as many as 1 per 26,000); encephalitis (severe brain reaction), which can lead to permanent brain damage (as many as 1 per 83,000); severe infection beginning at the vaccination site (as many as 1 per 667,000, mostly in people with weakened immune systems); and death in 1 to 2 individuals per 1 million, mostly in people with weakened immune systems.

Monitoring of Adverse Events with Vaccines

In 1986 Congress enacted the National Childhood Vaccine Injury Act (NCVIA) to establish a no-fault compensation system for children who were harmed by adverse events after the administration of a vaccine if there was evidence that the vaccine actually caused the problem. In 2011 the US Supreme Court ruled that vaccine makers are immune from lawsuits, alleging that the design of a vaccine is defective. Many physicians and public health organizations support this ruling because they believe that it will ensure the availability and promote the use of childhood vaccines. Current vaccines are considered safer and more protective than early products.

Monitoring programs, such as the Vaccine Adverse Events Reporting System (VAERS) and the Clinical Immunization Safety Assessment Network, are systems to monitor and analyze reported adverse events and to determine whether they are likely related to vaccination. The goal of VAERS, according to the CDC, is "to detect possible signals of adverse events associated with vaccines." About 30,000 events are reported each year to VAERS. Between 10% and 15% of these reports describe serious medical events that result in hospitalization, life-threatening illness, disability, or death.

Rapid Cycle Analysis, another monitoring program, was launched in 2005. This program monitors real-time data to compare rates of adverse events in recently vaccinated people with rates among unvaccinated people. The system is used mainly to monitor new vaccines. Among the new vaccines being monitored in Rapid Cycle Analysis are the conjugated meningococcal vaccine, rotavirus vaccine, Tdap vaccine, and HPV vaccine.

CASE STUDY 27.1

A 25-year-old female medical student came to the emergency department because of a fever, cough, and shortness of breath. She noticed the shortness of breath after walking up one flight of stairs. She noticed increased fatigue with a dry cough.

The patient did not smoke, drink alcohol, or use illegal drugs. Eleven months earlier, she had traveled to Nairobi, Kenya, for a month-long volunteer assignment with a medical group. Since then, she had not traveled outside the United States. A tuberculin skin test performed before she went to Africa was negative. She received many vaccinations, including tetanus vaccine, before her international trip.

She was admitted to the hospital. A complete blood count and chest x-ray were ordered.

Laboratory and Radiology Results
The patient's complete blood count was essentially within reference ranges.

The chest x-ray showed a right pleural effusion and a possible infiltrate. A follow-up echocardiogram showed a pericardial effusion.

A cytologic examination of the pericardial fluid showed blood and no malignant cells. Gram staining showed red cells but no neutrophils or organisms, and a culture showed no growth of bacteria. A smear and culture were negative for acid-fast bacilli and mycobacteria. A repeat tuberculin skin test was performed during the hospitalization. There was no skin reaction. Smears and cultures of three specimens of sputum were negative for acid-fast bacilli and mycobacteria.

Questions
1. What are this patient's risk factors?
   a. Age
   b. Sex
   c. Global travel
   d. Contaminated vaccines
2. What can cause a negative TB skin test 5 months after traveling to Africa, even if TB is contracted?
   a. Technical problems (e.g., subcutaneous TB skin test)
   b. HIV infection
   c. Transient-specific anergy due to acute infection
   d. All of the above

See Appendix A for the answers to these questions.

Critical Thinking Group Discussion Questions
1. Is this patient at risk for developing an infectious disease?
2. Could this patient have tuberculosis even though the tuberculin skin test was nonreactive 5 months after returning from Africa and when repeated during this hospital admission?
3. What follow-up assay(s) could be ordered to assess the patient's ability to build antibodies in response to a tetanus vaccination?

REVIEW QUESTIONS

1. The Center for Biologics Evaluation and Research (CBER) regulates:
   a. Laboratory safety
   b. Vaccine products
   c. Personnel qualifications
   d. Research grants
2. Pathogens adapted for biological warfare include:
   a. Smallpox, *Bacillus anthracis*, chickenpox, viral hemorrhagic fevers
   b. Smallpox, *Bacillus anthracis*, Q fever
   c. *Bacillus anthracis*, tularemia, plague, *Staphylococcus*
   d. Epstein-Barr virus, *Bacillus anthracis*, tularemia, plague
3. Vaccines can be divided into _____ vaccines.
   a. Live, attenuated
   b. Nonreplicating
   c. Naked DNA
   d. Both a and b
4. To meet FDA requirements, a vaccine must:
   a. Produce protective immunity with only minimal side effects
   b. Be immunogenic enough to produce a strong and measurable immune response
   c. Be stable during its shelf life
   d. All of the above
5. The earliest host response to vaccination is a(n):
   a. Innate immune response
   b. Memory response
   c. Anamnestic response
   d. Both a and b
6. Preventive HIV vaccine is:
   a. Given to HIV-negative individuals
   b. For HIV-positive patients to improve their immune system and prevent progression to AIDS
7. Therapeutic HIV vaccine is:
   a. Given to HIV-negative individuals
   b. For HIV-positive patients to improve their immune system and prevent progression to AIDS
8. Anthrax vaccine:
   a. Offers protection against bioterrorism
   b. Offers protection against cervical cancer
   c. Is not available for preventing congenital infection
   d. Is a DNA-based vaccine
9. Influenza vaccine:
   a. Offers protection against bioterrorism
   b. Offers protection against cervical cancer
   c. Is not available for preventing congenital infection
   d. Is a required annual vaccination

Appendix A

Answers to Case Study Multiple-Choice Questions

CHAPTER 1: FOUNDATIONS OF INNATE AND ADAPTIVE IMMUNE SYSTEMS

Case Study 1.1
1. C
2. B

CHAPTER 2: SOLUBLE MEDIATORS OF THE IMMUNE SYSTEM

Case Study 2.1
1. B
2. A

CHAPTER 3: ANTIGENS AND ANTIBODIES

Case Study 3.1
1. B
2. D

CHAPTER 4: CELLULAR ACTIVITIES AND CLINICAL DISORDERS OF INNATE AND ADAPTIVE IMMUNITY

Case Study 4.1
1. D
2. C

Case Study 4.2
1. A
2. C

Case Study 4.3
1. D
2. D

CHAPTER 5: BASIC SAFETY IN THE IMMUNOLOGY-SEROLOGY LABORATORY

Case Study 5.1
1. D
2. C

CHAPTER 6: BASIC QUALITY CONTROL AND QUALITY ASSURANCE PRACTICES

Case Study 6.1
1. B
2. B

CHAPTER 7: BASIC SEROLOGIC LABORATORY: TECHNIQUES AND CLINICAL APPLICATIONS

Case Study 7.1
1. C
2. C

Case Study 7.2
1. D
2. A

CHAPTER 8: PRECIPITATION AND PARTICLE AGGLUTINATION METHODS

Case Study 8.1
1. D
2. D

CHAPTER 9: ELECTROPHORESIS TECHNIQUES AND CHROMATOGRAPHY

Case Study 9.1
1. B
2. B

CHAPTER 10: LABELING TECHNIQUES IN IMMUNOASSAY

Case Study 10.1
1. C
2. C

CHAPTER 11: FLOW CYTOMETRY

Case Study 11.1
1. A
2. D

CHAPTER 12: MOLECULAR LABORATORY TECHNIQUES

Case Study 12.1
1. A
2. D

CHAPTER 13: INFECTIOUS DISEASES: OVERVIEW AND TORCH DISEASES

Case Study 13.1
1. C
2. A

APPENDIX A Answers to Case Study Multiple-Choice Questions

Case Study 13.2
1. D
2. C

Case Study 13.3
1. B
2. A

Case Study 13.4
1. D
2. B

CHAPTER 14: STREPTOCOCCAL INFECTIONS

Case Study 14.1
1. B
2. D

CHAPTER 15: SYPHILIS

Case Study 15.1
1. D
2. B

CHAPTER 16: VECTOR-BORNE DISEASES

Case Study 16.1
1. A

Case Study 16.2
2. D

Case Study 16.3
1. A

Case Study 16.4
1. D

Case Study 16.5
1. C

CHAPTER 17: INFECTIOUS MONONUCLEOSIS

Case Study 17.1
1. D
2. D

CHAPTER 18: VIRAL HEPATITIS

Case Study 18.1
1. A
2. D

Case Study 18.2
1. B
2. A

Case Study 18.3
1. D
2. C

Case Study 18.4
1. C
2. C

CHAPTER 19: PRIMARY AND ACQUIRED IMMUNODEFICIENCY SYNDROMES

Case Study 19.1
1. A
2. C

Case Study 19.2
1. C
2. C

Case Study 19.3
1. B
2. D

CHAPTER 20: HYPERSENSITIVITY REACTIONS

Case Study 20.1
1. D

Case Study 20.2
1. B

Case Study 20.3
1. D

Case Study 20.4
1. A

Case Study 20.5
1. B

CHAPTER 21: PLASMA CELL NEOPLASMS AND OTHER DISEASES WITH PARAPROTEINS

Case Study 21.1
1. D
2. B

CHAPTER 22: TOLERANCE, AUTOIMMUNITY, AND AUTOIMMUNE DISORDERS

Case Study 22.1
1. D

Case Study 22.2
1. B

CHAPTER 23: SYSTEMIC LUPUS ERYTHEMATOSUS

Case Study 23.1
1. A
2. A

Case Study 23.2
1. D
2. D

CHAPTER 24: RHEUMATOID ARTHRITIS

Case Study 24.1
1. D
2. C

Case Study 24.2
1. C
2. D

CHAPTER 25: TRANSPLANTATION: HUMAN LEUKOCYTE ANTIGENS, SOLID ORGAN, TISSUES, AND HEMATOPOIETIC STEM CELLS

Case Study 25.1
1. D
2. A

CHAPTER 26: TUMOR IMMUNOLOGY AND APPLICATIONS OF MASSIVE PARALLEL SEQUENCING/NEXT-GENERATION SEQUENCING

Case Study 26.1
1. B
2. B

Case Study 26.2
1. C

CHAPTER 27: VACCINES: DEVELOPMENT AND APPLICATIONS

Case Study 27.1
1. C
2. D

APPENDIX B

Answers to Review Questions

CHAPTER 1: FOUNDATIONS OF INNATE AND ADAPTIVE IMMUNE SYSTEMS

1. b
2. b
3. c
4. a
5. a
6. a
7. d
8. b
9. b
10. d
11. b
12. c
13. d
14. b
15. a
16. b
17. b
18. a
19. a

CHAPTER 2: SOLUBLE MEDIATORS OF THE IMMUNE SYSTEM

1. c
2. d
3. a
4. a
5. b
6. c
7. a
8. b
9. a
10. b
11. a
12. b
13. a
14. c
15. a
16. a
17. a
18. d
19. b
20. c
21. a
22. a
23. a
24. d
25. d
26. a
27. d
28. d
29. d
30. d
31. b

CHAPTER 3: ANTIGENS AND ANTIBODIES

1. b
2. a
3. d
4. c
5. a
6. a
7. a
8. d
9. d
10. a
11. c
12. a
13. d
14. b
15. d
16. b
17. d
18. a
19. d
20. c
21. b
22. a
23. b
24. c
25. a
26. d
27. d
28. b
29. c
30. a
31. d
32. b
33. d
34. a
35. d
36. c
37. c
38. a
39. a
40. d
41. c
42. b

43. d
44. d
45. a
46. b
47. a
48. c
49. d
50. d
51. d
52. b
53. b
54. c
55. a

CHAPTER 4: CELLULAR ACTIVITIES AND CLINICAL DISORDERS OF INNATE AND ADAPTIVE IMMUNITY

1. b
2. d
3. c
4. a
5. b
6. a
7. a
8. a
9. a
10. a
11. b
12. c
13. c
14. d
15. a
16. c
17. b
18. b
19. d
20. b
21. d
22. a
23. a
24. b
25. c
26. a
27. d
28. d
29. b
30. d
31. a
32. b
33. d
34. d
35. b

CHAPTER 5: BASIC SAFETY IN THE IMMUNOLOGY-SEROLOGY LABORATORY

1. a
2. d
3. a
4. c
5. b
6. d
7. b
8. b
9. d
10. d

CHAPTER 6: BASIC QUALITY CONTROL AND QUALITY ASSURANCE PRACTICES

1. b
2. a
3. c
4. a
5. a
6. b
7. b
8. c
9. a
10. a
11. b
12. b
13. a
14. c
15. c
16. a
17. a
18. a
19. a
20. b

CHAPTER 7: BASIC SEROLOGIC LABORATORY: TECHNIQUES AND CLINICAL APPLICATIONS

1. d
2. c
3. d
4. c
5. c
6. d
7. d
8. c
9. a
10. b
11. b
12. d
13. a
14. a
15. a

CHAPTER 8: PRECIPITATION AND PARTICLE AGGLUTINATION METHODS

1. d
2. c
3. b
4. b
5. c
6. c
7. b
8. d
9. c
10. a
11. b

12. b
13. b
14. a
15. c
16. d
17. d
18. d
19. b
20. a
21. d
22. c
23. d
24. a
25. b
26. d
27. c
28. a
29. c
30. a
31. a
32. a
33. a
34. b
35. c
36. a
37. b
38. a
39. a
40. b
41. c

CHAPTER 9: ELECTROPHORESIS TECHNIQUES AND CHROMATOGRAPHY

1. c
2. c
3. b
4. d
5. b
6. a
7. b
8. c

CHAPTER 10: LABELING TECHNIQUES IN IMMUNOASSAY

1. d
2. a
3. b
4. d
5. a
6. b
7. b
8. c
9. a
10. c
11. b
12. a
13. a
14. a
15. a

CHAPTER 11: FLOW CYTOMETRY

1. a
2. c
3. b
4. d
5. d
6. d
7. a
8. b
9. a
10. a
11. a
12. c

CHAPTER 12: MOLECULAR LABORATORY TECHNIQUES

1. c
2. d
3. c
4. d
5. a
6. b
7. a
8. a
9. b
10. a
11. d
12. b
13. d
14. a
15. a
16. a
17. d

CHAPTER 13: INFECTIOUS DISEASES: OVERVIEW AND TORCH DISEASES

1. b
2. a
3. c
4. c
5. c
6. b
7. b
8. c
9. a
10. b
11. a
12. c
13. c
14. d
15. d
16. d
17. b
18. c
19. a
20. c
21. b
22. b
23. c

24. c
25. d
26. c
27. a

CHAPTER 14: STREPTOCOCCAL INFECTIONS

1. b
2. a
3. d
4. b
5. a
6. b
7. d
8. a
9. b
10. d
11. c
12. a
13. b
14. b
15. a
16. c
17. b
18. b
19. b
20. c

CHAPTER 15: SYPHILIS

1. b
2. d
3. a
4. c
5. c
6. d
7. a
8. b
9. b
10. a
11. a
12. b
13. d
14. b
15. b
16. b
17. b
18. c
19. c
20. d

CHAPTER 16: VECTOR-BORNE DISEASES

1. d
2. d
3. b
4. c
5. b
6. b
7. a
8. b
9. b
10. b
11. c
12. d
13. a
14. b
15. c
16. c
17. d
18. a
19. c
20. c
21. a
22. c
23. b
24. b
25. c
26. c
27. a
28. a
29. b
30. a
31. a

CHAPTER 17: INFECTIOUS MONONUCLEOSIS

1. d
2. b
3. b
4. c
5. d
6. d
7. d
8. d
9. a
10. c
11. c
12. d
13. c
14. c
15. c
16. a
17. b
18. a

CHAPTER 18: VIRAL HEPATITIS

1. b
2. a
3. c
4. d
5. d
6. a
7. c
8. b
9. a
10. d
11. b
12. c
13. a
14. d
15. b
16. a

17. d
18. c
19. b
20. d
21. b
22. d
23. d
24. a
25. b
26. d
27. b
28. a
29. b
30. b
31. a
32. b
33. d
34. c
35. b
36. a
37. a
38. a
39. c
40. c
41. a
42. b
43. b
44. b
45. d
46. a
47. b
48. c
49. a
50. a
51. a

CHAPTER 19: PRIMARY AND ACQUIRED IMMUNODEFICIENCY SYNDROMES

1. a
2. c
3. c
4. c
5. d
6. b
7. b
8. c
9. a
10. c
11. c
12. d
13. a
14. a
15. b
16. c
17. b
18. b
19. c
20. b
21. c
22. a
23. d
24. c
25. a
26. c
27. a
28. a
29. b
30. b
31. c
32. d
33. a
34. b

CHAPTER 20: HYPERSENSITIVITY REACTIONS

1. d
2. a
3. c
4. b
5. d
6. d
7. d
8. d
9. b
10. b
11. c
12. a
13. b
14. a
15. d
16. b
17. c
18. a
19. d
20. d
21. b
22. d
23. d
24. d
25. d
26. a
27. a
28. b
29. d

CHAPTER 21: PLASMA CELL NEOPLASMS AND OTHER DISEASES WITH PARAPROTEINS

1. c
2. d
3. b
4. d
5. c
6. d
7. c
8. b
9. d
10. d
11. a
12. b
13. b
14. d
15. b
16. b

CHAPTER 22: TOLERANCE, AUTOIMMUNITY, AND AUTOIMMUNE DISORDERS

1. c
2. d
3. a
4. c
5. b
6. d
7. c
8. d
9. d
10. a
11. c
12. d
13. b
14. c
15. d
16. d
17. a
18. b
19. c
20. d
21. a
22. a
23. d
24. b
25. c
26. c
27. d
28. c
29. c
30. b
31. d
32. b
33. c
34. b
35. b
36. a
37. b

CHAPTER 23: SYSTEMIC LUPUS ERYTHEMATOSUS

1. c
2. b
3. d
4. a
5. c
6. d
7. d
8. c
9. a
10. a
11. d
12. d
13. b
14. a
15. c
16. a
17. a
18. c
19. a
20. c
21. b
22. d
23. a
24. c
25. b

CHAPTER 24: RHEUMATOID ARTHRITIS

1. c
2. c
3. c
4. a
5. b
6. a
7. c
8. d
9. d
10. b
11. a
12. b
13. d
14. a
15. a
16. b

CHAPTER 25: TRANSPLANTATION: HUMAN LEUKOCYTE ANTIGENS, SOLID ORGAN, TISSUES, AND HEMATOPOIETIC STEM CELLS

1. a
2. c
3. c
4. c
5. b
6. a
7. c
8. c
9. b
10. d
11. d
12. b
13. a
14. a
15. c
16. b
17. b
18. d
19. b
20. c
21. d
22. a
23. d
24. c
25. d
26. a
27. d
28. a
29. c
30. a

CHAPTER 26: TUMOR IMMUNOLOGY AND APPLICATIONS OF MASSIVE PARALLEL SEQUENCING/NEXT-GENERATION SEQUENCING

1. d
2. b
3. d
4. a
5. c
6. b
7. d
8. b
9. b
10. c
11. a
12. d
13. a
14. d
15. a
16. b
17. a
18. d
19. c
20. a
21. b
22. d
23. d
24. c
25. a
26. a
27. d
28. b
29. d
30. c
31. a
32. a
33. c
34. d
35. a
36. d
37. b
38. d
39. a
40. c
41. b
42. d

CHAPTER 27: VACCINES: DEVELOPMENT AND APPLICATIONS

1. b
2. b
3. d
4. d
5. a
6. a
7. b
8. a
9. d

Appendix C

Origin and Immunoregulatory Activity of Cytokines

Cytokines	Origin	Prominent Biological Activities
Interleukins (ILs)		
IL-1 superfamily	IL-1α and IL-1β produced by activated macrophages, neutrophils, fibroblasts, and dendritic cells	Associated with innate immunity. Original members: IL-1α, IL-1β, and IL-1RA. IL-1α and IL-1β are proinflammatory cytokines involved in immune defense against infection. IL-1RA is a molecule that competes for receptor binding with IL-1α and IL-1β, blocking their role in immune activation. The principal function of IL-1 is mediating host inflammatory response to infections and other inflammatory stimuli. These cytokines increase the expression of adhesion factors on endothelial cells to enable transmigration of leukocytes to sites of infection and reset the hypothalamic thermoregulatory center, leading to increased body temperature (fever), which helps the immune system fight infection. IL-1 is also important in the regulation of hematopoiesis.
IL-2	Activated CD4 T cells, NK cells, and NKT cells	Associated with adaptive immunity. Has high capacity to induce activation of almost all clones of cytotoxic cells. Increases cytotoxic functions of T killer and NK cells; promotes production of perforins and IFN-γ by these cells. Activates monocytes-macrophages to synthesize and secrete TNF-α, IL-1β, IL-6, IL-8, G-CSF, and GM-CSF.
IL-3	Activated T cells, macrophages, eosinophils, mast cells, NK cells	Promotes expansion of early blood cells (hematopoiesis) that differentiate into all known mature cell types. Supports growth and differentiation of T cells from bone marrow through immune response.
IL-4	Th2 cells and mast cells	Associated with adaptive immunity. Induces differentiation of naïve helper T cells (Th0 cells) to Th2 cells. On activation by IL-4, Th2 cells subsequently produce additional IL-4. A cell that initially produces IL-4 and induces Th0 differentiation has not been identified. Early activation of resting B cells; upregulates MHC class II production (induces HLA-DR molecules on B cells, macrophages) and governs B-cell isotype switching to IgG1 and IgE. Key regulator in humoral and adaptive immunity.
IL-5	Th2 and mast cells	Associated with adaptive immunity. Principal function is to activate eosinophils and serve as a link between T-cell activation and eosinophilic inflammation. Stimulates growth and differentiation of eosinophils and activates mature eosinophils (IL-5 expressed on eosinophils). Growth and differentiation–inducing factor for activated T and B cells; induces class-specific B-cell differentiation (IgA production).
IL-6	Activated macrophages, T cells, osteoblasts, fibroblasts, endothelium, epithelia, and other	Functions in innate immunity and adaptive immunity; in the latter, stimulates growth of B cells that have differentiated into antibody producers. IL-1, TNF, and IL-6 appear to be major factors that induce the acute-phase response.
IL-7	Thymic stromal cells of red bone marrow, bone marrow, spleen, dendritic cells, keratinocytes, monocytes, macrophages	Stimulates proliferation of lymphoid progenitors; important for proliferation during certain stages of B-cell maturation and in T-cell and NK-cell survival, development, and homeostasis. IL-7 has recently been shown to have therapeutic potential and safety in several clinical trials designed to demonstrate T-cell restoration in immunodeficient patients.
IL-8	Macrophages and certain types of epithelial cells (e.g., endothelium)	Potent stimulator of neutrophils in chemotaxis. Activates "respiratory burst" and release of specific and azurophilic granular contents.
IL-9	Th2 and Th9 cells, mast cells, eosinophils	Promotes proliferation, survival, and activation of T cells, thymocytes, and mast cells. Supports proliferation of some T-cell lines and of bone marrow–derived mast cell progenitors; supports growth of erythroid blast-forming units. Inhibition of Th1 cells.
IL-10	Monocytes, Th2 cells, and B cells	Associated with adaptive immunity. Inhibits activated macrophages; displays potent abilities to suppress antigen-presenting capacity of APCs. Released by Tc cells to inhibit the actions of NK cells during immune response to viral infection. IL-10 is stimulatory toward certain T cells, mast cells, and B cells. It can downregulate the synthesis of other ILs.

APPENDIX C Origin and Immunoregulatory Activity of Cytokines

Cytokines	Origin	Prominent Biological Activities
IL-11	Stromal cells, synoviocytes, osteoblasts	Proliferation. Acts in a manner similar to IL-6 on hematopoietic progenitor cells. IL-11 has been shown to synergize with IL-3 to stimulate production of megakaryocyte and myeloid progenitors, and to increase the number of Ig-secreting B lymphocytes in vivo and in vitro.
IL-12	B cells, dendritic cells, macrophages	Although it shares functional properties of enhancing cytotoxic function of NK cells and activated T cells with IL-2, IL-12 appears to act through a distinct mechanism independent of IL-2. Biological actions of IL-12 include cytotoxicity, stimulating production of IFN-γ by NK and T cells, stimulating differentiation of naïve T cells into Th1 cells, and enhancing cytolytic functions of activated NK cells and CD8+ Tc cells.
IL-13	Activated T cells, NK cells, mast cells, basophils	Has many biological effects similar to IL-4 but appears to have less effect on T or B cells than IL-4. Major action of IL-13 on macrophages is to inhibit their activation and to antagonize IFN-γ. Important mediator of allergic inflammation and disease. Functions of IL-13 overlap considerably with those of IL-4, especially changes induced on hematopoietic cells, but these effects are probably less important given the more potent role of IL-4. IL-13 acts more prominently as a molecular bridge linking allergic inflammatory cells to nonimmune cells, altering physiologic function. It is associated primarily with induction of airway disease and also has antiinflammatory properties.
IL-14 (HMW-BCGF)	T cells and malignant B cells	Acts as BCGF in proliferation of normal and cancerous B cells. Hyperproduction of IL-14 enables progression of NHL-B; conversely, its antibodies slow down growth of NHL-B.
IL-15	Many cells	Biologically similar to IL-2; acts as synergist, particularly in LAK cell induction process; increases antitumoral activities of T killer and NK cells, and can be chemoattractant for T lymphocytes; endogenous IL-15 is a key condition for IFN-γ synthesis. IL-15 is produced in response to viral infection and other signals that trigger innate immunity; it is homologous to IL-2. The function of IL-15 is to promote proliferation of NK cells. Maintenance of memory cells does not appear to require persistence of the original antigen; instead, survival signals for memory lymphocytes are provided by cytokines such as IL-15.
IL-16	Monocytes, CD8+ lymphocytes, and B lymphocytes	Acts as a T-cell chemoattractant; increases mobility of CD8+ and CD4+ T cells and, with IL-2, promotes their activation. IL-16 is found in B lymphocytes. Recruits and activates many other cells expressing the CD4 molecule, including monocytes, eosinophils, and dendritic cells.
IL-17	CD4+ lymphocytes	Induces granulopoiesis through G-CSF; can reinforce antibody-dependent tumor cell destruction; participates in regulation of many cytokines (IL-1, IL-4, IL-6, IL-10, IL-12, and IFN-γ). Histamine and serotonin increase production of IL-17. IL-17 mimics many proinflammatory actions of TNF-α and TNF-β.
IL-18	Macrophages, keratocytes, osteoblasts	Produces enhanced Th2 responses. Acts as a synergist with IL-12 in some effects, especially induction of IFN-γ production and inhibition of angiogenesis; high IFN-γ production under integrated effect of IL-18 and IL-12 suppresses tumor growth. IL-18 stimulates production of IFN-γ by NK cells and T cells, synergistic with IL-12.
IL-19	Monocytes	LPS and GM-CSF stimulate synthesis of IL-19, which is then upregulated in monocytes. Biological function is similar to that of IL-10; regulates functions of macrophages and suppresses activities of Th1 and Th2.
IL-20	Activated keratinocytes and monocytes	Biological activities similar to those of IL-10 and can stimulate tumor growth. Regulates proliferation and differentiation of keratocytes during inflammation, particularly inflammation associated with the skin. Causes expansion of multipotential hematopoietic progenitor cells.
IL-21	Various lymphocytes	Regulates hematopoiesis and immune response and influences development of lymphocytes; similar to IL-2 and IL-15 in antitumor defense system; promotes high production of T lymphocytes, fast growth and maturation of NK cells, and fast growth of B lymphocytes. Has potent regulatory effects on immune cells, interacting with cell surface IL-21 receptors; expressed in bone marrow cells and various lymphocytes. Promotes plasma cell differentiation and Th17 differentiation.
IL-22	Activated T cells	Similar to IL-10 but does not prohibit production of proinflammatory cytokines through monocytes in response to LPS; somewhat similar to IFN-α, IFN-β, and IFN-γ.
IL-23	Macrophages, dendritic cells	Newly discovered cytokine that shares some in vivo functions with IL-12. Associated with IL-17 production. IL-23 is an important part of the inflammatory response against infection; as proinflammatory cytokine, it enhances T-cell priming and stimulates production of proinflammatory molecules (IL-1, IL-6, TNF-α, NOS-2, and chemokines), resulting in inflammation.

Continued

Cytokines	Origin	Prominent Biological Activities
IL-24	Activated monocytes-macrophages and Th2 cells	Appears to participate in cell survival and proliferation by inducing rapid activation of particular transcription factors called STAT1 and STAT3; predominantly released by and acts on nonhematopoietic (skin, lung, reproductive) tissues. Performs important roles in wound healing and cancer; cell death occurs in cancer cells and cell lines after exposure to IL-24.
IL-25	Th2 cells and mast cells	Biologically characterized as a member of the IL-17 cytokine family. Supports proliferation of cells in lymphoid lineage. Induces production of other cytokines (IL-4, IL-5, and IL-13) in multiple tissues, which stimulate the expansion of eosinophils. Important molecule in controlling immunity of the gut; implicated in chronic inflammation associated with the gastrointestinal tract; identified in chromosomal region associated with autoimmune diseases such as IBD, although no direct evidence suggests that IL-25 plays a role in IBD.
IL-26	T cells, many cells	Along with IL-19, IL-20, IL-22, and IL-24, IL-26 induces production of inflammatory cytokines, Th2 responses, and activation of epithelial cells. Induces rapid phosphorylation of transcription factors STAT1 and STAT3, which enhance IL-10 and IL-8 secretion and expression of CD54 molecule on surface of epithelial cells.
IL-27	Activated dendritic cells, macrophages, epithelial cells	Has important functions in regulating activity of B and T lymphocytes, including enhancement of Th1 differentiation responses and IL-10; inhibition of Th1, Th2, and Th17 responses.
IL-28	Dendritic cells, many cells	Plays role in immune defense against viruses (antiviral).
IL-29	Dendritic cells, many cells	Plays important role in host defenses against microbes; its gene is highly upregulated in cells infected with virus (antiviral).
IL-30 (also IL-27p28) New name of p28, a subunit of IL-27	Dendritic cells, many cells	Antiviral. IL-30, a member of the long-chain four-helix bundle cytokine family, and EBI3 form the IL-27 heterodimer, which is expressed by APCs. IL-27 triggers expansion of antigen-specific naïve CD4+ T cells and promotes polarization toward a Th1 phenotype with expression of IFN-γ. IL-27 acts in synergy with IL-12 and binds to WSX1.
IL-31	Produced preferentially by Th2 cells; receptor subunits expressed in activated monocytes and unstimulated epithelial cells	Believed to play a role in skin inflammation.
IL-32	T cells, NK cells, epithelial T and B cells, mast cells, eosinophils, and monocytes	Can induce cells of immune system to secrete TNF-α in addition to IL-1, IL-6, and IL-8. Induces expression of TNF-α and IL-8 in THP-1 monocytic cells. Expression of IL-32 is induced in human peripheral lymphocyte cells after mitogen stimulation, in human epithelial cells by IFN-γ, and in NK cells after exposure to an IL-12–IL-18 combination. Involved in activation-induced cell death. Expression of IL-32 is upregulated in T killer and NK cells after cell activation, and IL-32β is the predominant isoform in activated T cells. IL-32 is expressed specifically in T cells undergoing cell death; enforced expression of IL-32 induces apoptosis; downregulation rescues the cells from apoptosis.
IL-33	Helper T cells	Induces type 2 cytokine production from Th cells. Mediates biological effects by interacting with orphan IL-1 receptor, activating intracellular molecules in certain signaling pathways that drive production of type 2 cytokines (e.g., IL-4, IL-5, IL-13) from polarized Th2 cells. Constitutive expression of IL-33 is found in smooth muscle cells and bronchial epithelial cells. Expression in primary lung or dermal fibroblasts and keratinocytes is inducible by treatment with TNF-α and IL-1β; these two cytokines only induce low-level expression in dendritic cells and macrophages.
Interferons (IFNs)		
IFN-α	Plasmacytoid dendritic cells	Antiviral, increased MHC class I expression.
IFN-β	Th1 cells, fibroblasts, epithelial cells	Antiviral, increased MHC class I expression.
IFN-γ	Th1 cells, cytotoxic T cells, and NK cells	Associated with innate and adaptive immunity. Major macrophage activator; induces MHC class II molecules on many cells and can synergize with TNF; augments NK-cell activity; antagonist to IL-4.

APC, Antigen-presenting cell; *BCGF*, B-cell growth factor; *G-CSF*, granulocyte colony-stimulating factor; *GM-CSF*, granulocyte-macrophage colony-stimulating factor; *HMW-BCGF*, high-molecular-weight B-cell growth factor; *IBD*, inflammatory bowel disease; *IFN*, interferon; *IFN-β*, interferon beta; *IFN-γ*, interferon gamma; *Ig*, immunoglobulin; *IL-1RA*, interleukin-1 receptor antagonist; *LAK*, lymphokine-activated killer; *LPS*, lipopolysaccharides; *MHC*, major histocompatibility complex; *NHL-B*, B-cell non-Hodgkin lymphoma; *NK*, natural killer; *NKT*, natural killer T; *NOS-2*, nitric oxide synthase A2; *STAT1*, signal transducer and activator of transcription 1; *STAT3*, signal transducer and activator of transcription 3; *Tc*, cytotoxic T; *Th1*, type 1 helper T; *Th2*, type 2 helper T; *TNF*, tumor necrosis factor.

Immunoregulatory Activity of Other Cytokines

Factor	Target Cells	Prominent Biological Activities
Tumor Necrosis Factor (TNF)		
TNF-α (cachectin)	Activated macrophages, activated T cells, NK cells, and mast cells	Associated with innate immunity Local inflammation, endothelial activation
TNF-β (lymphotoxin)	T cells and B cells	Killing, endothelial activation
Tumor necrosis family	T cells and mast cells	–
CD40 ligand	–	B-cell activation, class switching
TNF Family		
CD27 ligand	T cells	Stimulates T-cell proliferation
CD30 ligand	T cells	Stimulates T- and B-cell proliferation
Chemokines		
Membrane cofactor protein (MCP-1)	Macrophages and others	Chemotactic for monocytes

MCP-1, Monocyte chemoattractant protein 1; *NK*, natural killer; *TNF*, tumor necrosis factor; *TNF-α*, tumor necrosis factor alpha; *TNF-β*, tumor necrosis factor beta.

Adapted from Abbas AK, Lichtman AH, Pillai S: Cytokines. In *Basic immunology,* ed 6, St. Louis, 2020, Elsevier; O'Shea JJ, Gadina M, Siegel RM: Cytokines and cytokine receptors. In Rich R, editor: ed 5, 2019, Table 9.1, 128–130; Ralston SH, editor: Clinical immunology. In Marshall SE, Johnston SI: *Davidson's principles and practice of medicine,* ed 23, 2018; Janeway C, Travers P: *Immunobiology,* ed 3, New York, 1997, Garland; and Abbas AK, Lichtman AH, Pober JS: *Cellular and molecular immunology,* ed 4, Philadelphia, 2000, Saunders.

Appendix D

Coronavirus Disease 2019 (COVID-19)

GUIDANCE FOR GENERAL LABORATORY SAFETY PRACTICES DURING THE COVID-19 PANDEMIC

General Guidance

This guidance is to address the general workflow safety concerns of laboratory personnel during the COVID-19 pandemic. All laboratories should perform site- and activity-specific risk assessments to determine the most appropriate safety measures to implement for particular circumstances. In addition, facilities should adhere to local policies and procedures as well as all applicable federal, state, and local regulations and public health guidelines.

Risk assessments should include the following considerations:
- Analyze the number of people that the laboratory space can realistically and safely accommodate while maintaining social distancing.
- Assess the flow of personnel traffic. Where possible, design one-way paths for staff to walk through the laboratory space.
- Assess procedures for cleaning and sanitizing commonly shared equipment and areas—for example, counters, benchtops, and desks—to ensure clean surfaces and equipment for all users.
- Review emergency communication and operational plans, including how to protect staff at higher risk for severe illness from COVID-19.

Every institution should have a COVID-19 health and safety plan to protect employees. This plan should be shared with all staff. Ideally, this plan would:
- Describe steps to help prevent the spread of COVID-19 if an employee is sick.
- Instruct sick employees to stay home and not return to work until the criteria to discontinue home isolation are met, in consultation with healthcare providers and state and local health departments.
- Provide information on whom employees should contact if they become sick.
- Implement flexible sick leave and supportive policies and practices. If sick leave is not offered to some or all employees, the institution should consider implementing emergency sick leave policies.
- Designate someone to be responsible for responding to employees' COVID-19 concerns. Employees should know who this person is and how to contact this person at all times.
- Provide employees with accurate information about COVID-19, how it spreads, and the risk of exposure.
- Reinforce training on proper handwashing practices and other routine infection control precautions to help prevent the spread of many diseases, including COVID-19.

Ensure that employees have access to personal protective equipment (PPE); disinfectant products that meet the US Environmental Protection Agency's (EPA's) criteria for use against SARS-CoV-2; and soap, clean running water, and drying materials for handwashing, or alcohol-based hand sanitizers that contain at least 60% ethanol or 70% isopropanol.

Social Distancing

To the extent possible, adhere to social distancing recommendations by adjusting staff schedules, adding additional shifts, or implementing nonoverlapping teams to minimize personnel contact. Identify laboratory tasks and activities that can be performed with reduced or no face-to-face interactions. Examples include limiting the number of laboratory meetings that occur and, when possible, using remote collaboration tools (such as video and phone conferencing), even for those who work in the same location or building.

To the extent possible, reconfigure workspaces and locations of shared equipment to reduce crowding. Create one-directional paths and workflows. Declutter workspaces and dispose of unnecessary items to help with reconfiguration. If reconfiguration is not possible, consider placing barriers (plexiglass, partition, plastic, etc.) between computer workstations, desks, or equipment that position staff six feet apart from each other.

Minimize personnel traffic and interactions by limiting visits from vendors and other external partners; engage with them virtually whenever possible.

Face Coverings

The Centers for Disease Control and Prevention (CDC) recommends wearing cloth face coverings in settings where social distancing measures are challenging to maintain, such as office spaces, computer workstations, and break rooms. Face coverings may prevent people who do not know they have the virus from transmitting it to others. These face coverings are not disposable face masks or respirators; they are not appropriate substitutes when risk assessments and work procedures recommend or require an employee to wear respiratory PPE.

In general, laboratory employees should wear a face covering in laboratory spaces that do not have requirements for respiratory PPE and where other social distancing measures are difficult to maintain. Any facial protection that is worn inside a laboratory area where personnel work with potentially infectious material should subsequently not be worn outside of that laboratory area. Site- and activity-specific risk assessments, as well as available resources, should determine where specific facial protection should be used.

Wash hands before putting on face coverings, and minimize the removal of face coverings. If a face covering becomes contaminated or dirty, follow the guidelines below to remove it and replace it with a clean face covering:
- Take off the face covering carefully.
- Untie the strings behind the head or stretch the ear loops.
- Handle only by the ear loops or ties.
- Fold outside corners together.
- Be careful not to touch eyes, nose, or mouth when removing a face covering, and place it in a sealed bag until it can be washed.
- Wash hands immediately after removing.

Face coverings should be washed frequently. Depending on the activity, each person may need to have multiple clean face coverings available to use at different times. Learn more about how to wash cloth face coverings.

Depending on the facility's design or configuration, additional physical barriers, such as a face shield, plexiglass, partition, or plastic barriers, may be needed to achieve social distancing goals.

Personal Hygiene and Disinfection

As more workers return to the laboratory, extra measures may be needed to ensure a clean and appropriate environment. Reevaluate current protocols for cleaning, use of PPE, and handwashing. High-touch locations and equipment with a high frequency of handling and contact present a higher probability of contamination in the work area and should be disinfected frequently. Increasing the number of available cleaning supplies and distributing them throughout the laboratory can encourage staff to more frequently clean surfaces and equipment.

Use visual reminders, such as posters displayed throughout the laboratory environment, common areas, and restrooms, to emphasize the importance of hand hygiene and to encourage frequent handwashing. Hands should be washed regularly with soap and water for at least 20 seconds. An alcohol-based hand sanitizer containing at least 60% ethanol or 70% isopropanol can be used when soap and water are not available. For more information, see the CDC's Hand Hygiene Recommendations.

Accessed June 1, 2020. www.cdc.gov.

APPENDIX E

Vaccines Licensed for Use in the United States by the Federal Drug Administration

Product Name	Trade Name
Adenovirus Type 4 and Type 7 Vaccine, Oral	No trade name
Anthrax Vaccine Adsorbed	Biothrax
BCG Live	BCG vaccine
BCG Live	TICE BCG
Cholera Vaccine Live Oral	Vaxchora
Dengue Tetravalent Vaccine, Live	DENGVAXIA
COVID-19 Vaccine, mRNA	Comirnaty
COVID-19 Vaccine, mRNA	SPIKEVAX
Diphtheria and Tetanus Toxoids Adsorbed	No trade name
Diphtheria and Tetanus Toxoids and Acellular Pertussis Vaccine Adsorbed	Infanrix
Diphtheria and Tetanus Toxoids and Acellular Pertussis Vaccine Adsorbed	DAPTACEL
Diphtheria and Tetanus Toxoids and Acellular Pertussis Vaccine Adsorbed, Hepatitis B (recombinant) and Inactivated Poliovirus Vaccine Combined	Pediarix
Diphtheria and Tetanus Toxoids and Acellular Pertussis Adsorbed and Inactivated Poliovirus Vaccine	KINRIX
Diphtheria and Tetanus Toxoids and Acellular Pertussis Adsorbed and Inactivated Poliovirus Vaccine	Quadracel
Diphtheria and Tetanus Toxoids and Acellular Pertussis Adsorbed, Inactivated Poliovirus, Haemophilus b Conjugate [Meningococcal Protein Conjugate] and Hepatitis B [Recombinant] Vaccine	VAXELIS
Diphtheria and Tetanus Toxoids and Acellular Pertussis Adsorbed, Inactivated Poliovirus and Haemophilus b Conjugate (Tetanus Toxoid Conjugate) Vaccine	Pentacel
Ebola Zaire Vaccine, Live	ERVEBO
Haemophilus b Conjugate Vaccine (Meningococcal Protein Conjugate)	PedvaxHIB
Haemophilus b Conjugate Vaccine (Tetanus Toxoid Conjugate)	ActHIB
Haemophilus b Conjugate Vaccine (Tetanus Toxoid Conjugate)	Hiberix
Hepatitis A Vaccine, Inactivated	Havrix
Hepatitis A Vaccine, Inactivated	VAQTA
Hepatitis A Inactivated and Hepatitis B (Recombinant) Vaccine	Twinrix
Hepatitis B Vaccine (Recombinant)	Recombivax HB
Hepatitis B Vaccine (Recombinant)	PREHEXBRIO
Hepatitis B Vaccine (Recombinant)	Engerix-B
Hepatitis B Vaccine (Recombinant), Adjuvanted	HEPLISAV-B
Human Papillomavirus Quadrivalent (Types 6, 11, 16, 18) Vaccine, Recombinant	Gardasil
Human Papillomavirus 9-valent Vaccine, Recombinant	Gardasil 9
Human Papillomavirus Bivalent (Types 16, 18) Vaccine, Recombinant	Cervarix
Influenza A (H1N1) 2009 Monovalent Vaccine	No trade name
Influenza A (H1N1) 2009 Monovalent Vaccine	No trade name
Influenza A (H1N1) 2009 Monovalent Vaccine	No trade name
Influenza A (H1N1) 2009 Monovalent Vaccine	No trade name
Influenza A (H1N1) 2009 Monovalent Vaccine	No trade name
Influenza Virus Vaccine, H5N1 (for National Stockpile)	No trade name
Influenza A (H5N1) Virus Monovalent Vaccine, Adjuvanted	No trade name
Influenza A (H5N1) Monovalent Vaccine, Adjuvanted	AUDENZ
Influenza Vaccine, Adjuvanted	Fluad Quadrivalent
Influenza Vaccine, Adjuvanted	FLUAD
Influenza Vaccine	Afluria Quadrivalent, Afluria Quadrivalent Southern Hemisphere

APPENDIX E   Vaccines Licensed for Use in the United States by the Federal Drug Administration

Product Name	Trade Name
Influenza Vaccine	Flucelvax Quadrivalent
Influenza Vaccine	Flulaval Quadrivalent
Influenza Virus Vaccine (Trivalent, Types A and B)	Afluria, Afluria Southern Hemisphere
Influenza Virus Vaccine (Trivalent, Types A and B)	FluLaval
Influenza Vaccine, Live, Intranasal (Trivalent, Types A and B)	FluMist
Influenza Virus Vaccine (Trivalent, Types A and B)	Fluarix
Influenza Virus Vaccine (Trivalent, Types A and B)	Fluarix
Influenza Virus Vaccine (Trivalent, Types A and B)	Fluvirin
Influenza Virus Vaccine (Trivalent, Types A and B)	Agriflu
Influenza Virus Vaccine (Trivalent, Types A and B)	Fluzone, Fluzone High-Dose and Fluzone Intradermal
Influenza Virus Vaccine (Trivalent, Types A and B)	Flucelvax
Influenza Vaccine (Trivalent)	Flublok
Influenza Vaccine (Quadrivalent)	Flublok Quadrivalent
Influenza Vaccine, Live, Intranasal (Quadrivalent, Types A and Types B)	FluMist Quadrivalent
Influenza Virus Vaccine (Quadrivalent, Types A and Types B)	Fluarix Quadrivalent
Influenza Virus Vaccine (Quadrivalent, Types A and Types B)	Fluzone Quadrivalent
Japanese Encephalitis Virus Vaccine, Inactivated, Adsorbed	Ixiaro
Measles, Mumps, and Rubella Virus Vaccine, Live	PRIORIX
Measles, Mumps, and Rubella Virus Vaccine, Live	M-M-R II
Measles, Mumps, Rubella and Varicella Virus Vaccine Live	ProQuad
Meningococcal (Groups A, C, Y, and W-135) Oligosaccharide Diphtheria CRM197 Conjugate Vaccine	Menveo
Meningococcal (Groups A, C, Y, and W-135) Polysaccharide Diphtheria Toxoid Conjugate Vaccine	Menactra
Meningococcal Group B Vaccine	BEXSERO
Meningococcal Group B Vaccine	TRUMENBA
Meningococcal Polysaccharide Vaccine, Groups A, C, Y, and W-135 Combined	Menomune-A/C/Y/W-135
Meningococcal (Groups A, C, Y, and W) Conjugate Vaccine	MenQuadfi
Plague Vaccine	No trade name
Pneumococcal Vaccine, Polyvalent	Pneumovax 23
Pneumococcal 13-valent Conjugate Vaccine (Diphtheria CRM197 Protein)	Prevnar 13
Pneumococcal 15-valent Conjugate Vaccine	VAXNEUVANCE
Pneumococcal 20-valent Conjugate Vaccine	Prevnar 20
Poliovirus Vaccine Inactivated (Human Diploid Cell)	Poliovax
Poliovirus Vaccine Inactivated (Monkey Kidney Cell)	IPOL
Rabies Vaccine	Imovax
Rabies Vaccine	RabAvert
Rabies Vaccine Adsorbed	No trade name
Rotavirus Vaccine, Live, Oral	ROTARIX
Rotavirus Vaccine, Live, Oral, Pentavalent	RotaTeq
Respiratory Syncytial Virus Vaccine	ABRYSVO
Respiratory Syncytial Virus Vaccine, Adjuvanted	AREXVY
Smallpox and Monkeypox Vaccine, Live, Non-Replicating	JYNNEOS
Smallpox (Vaccinia) Vaccine, Live	ACAM2000
Tetanus and Diphtheria Toxoids, Adsorbed	TDVAX
Tetanus and Diphtheria Toxoids Adsorbed for Adult Use	TENIVAC
Tetanus Toxoid Adsorbed	No trade name
Tetanus Toxoid, Reduced Diphtheria Toxoid and Acellular Pertussis Vaccine, Adsorbed	Adacel
Tetanus Toxoid, Reduced Diphtheria Toxoid and Acellular Pertussis Vaccine, Adsorbed	Boostrix
Tick-Borne Encephalitis Vaccine	TICOVAC
Typhoid Vaccine Live Oral Ty21a	Vivotif
Typhoid Vi Polysaccharide Vaccine	TYPHIM Vi
Varicella Virus Vaccine Live	Varivax
Yellow Fever Vaccine	YF-Vax
Zoster Vaccine, Live, (Oka/Merck)	Zostavax
Zoster Vaccine Recombinant, Adjuvanted	SHINGRIX

Accessed July 12, 2023 https://www.fda.gov/vaccines-blood-biologics/vaccines/vaccines-licensed-use-united-states. Note: Content current as of 06/01/2023

BIBLIOGRAPHY

PART I. BASIC IMMUNOLOGIC MECHANISMS

Chapter 1: Foundations of Innate and Adaptive Immune Systems

Abbas AK, Lichtman AH, Pillai S: *Basic immunology: functions and disorders of the immune system*, ed 6, Philadelphia, 2020, Elsevier.

Artis D, Spits H: The biology of innate lymphoid cells, *Nature* 517(1):293–301, 2015.

Lencer WI: von Andrian UH: Eliciting mucosal immunity, *N Engl J Med* 365(12):1151–1153, 2011.

Male D: Introduction to the immune system. In Male D, Peebles RS, Male V, editors: *Immunology*, ed 9, Elsevier, 2021, pp 1–13.

Maynard CL: The microbiota in immunity and inflammation. In Rich RR, editor: *Clinical Immunology*, ed 6, Elsevier, 2023, pp 281–294.

Rich RR, Cron RO: The human immune response. In Rich RR, editor: *Clinical Immunology*, ed 6, Elsevier, 2023, pp 1–17.

Sassone-Corsi M, Raffatellu M: No vacancy: how beneficial microbes cooperate with immunity to provide colonization resistance to pathogens, *J Immunol* 194(7):4081–4087, 2015.

Chapter 2: Soluble Mediators of the Immune System

Associated Regional and University Pathologists (ARUP) Laboratories: Complement deficiency testing algorithm, www.aruplab.org, last updated February, 2023. Accessed May 15, 2023.

Associated Regional and University Pathologists (ARUP) Laboratories: C1-INH deficiency testing algorithm, www.aruplab.org, last updated. Accessed May 15, 2023.

Atkinson JP, Liszewski MK, Java A, et al.: Complement and complement. In Rich RR, editor: *Clinical Immunology*, ed 6, Elsevier, 2023, pp 506–524.

Bean KV, Massey HD, Gupta G: Mediators of inflammation: complement. In McPherson RA, Pincus MR, editors: *Henry's clinical diagnosis and management by laboratory methods*, ed 24, St. Louis, 2022, Elsevier, pp 969–983.

Carroll MC: *Molecular and cellular mediators of inflammation*, American Association of Immunologists, Advanced Course in Immunology, Book 1, Boston, 2015.

Gabay C, Kushner I: Acute-phase proteins and other systemic responses to inflammation, *N Engl J Med* 340(6):448–454, 1999.

Human Gene Nomenclature Committee (HUGO): 2007, Available at www.genenames.org.

Larson RS, Springer TA: Structure and function of leukocyte integrins, *Immunol Rev* 18:181–217, 1990.

Male D: Mechanisms of innate immunity. In Male D, Peebles RS, Male V, editors: *Immunology*, ed 9, Elsevier, 2021, pp 46–60.

Mollah F, Tam S: Complement deficiency. In *StatPearls [Internet]*, Treasure Island (FL), 2023, StatPearls Publishing, PMID: 32491513.

Morgan BP: Complement. In Male D, Peebles RS, Male V, editors: *Immunology*, ed 9, Elsevier, 2021.

Murphy PM: Chemokines and chemokine receptors. In Rich RR, editor: *Clinical immunology*, ed 6, Elsevier, 2023, pp 215–227.

Shea JJ, Gadina M, Sciume G, et al.: Cytokines and cytokine receptors. In Rich RR, editor: *Clinical immunology*, ed 6, Elsevier, 2023, pp 186–214.

Pedrazzi AH: Acute phase proteins: clinical and laboratory diagnosis: a review, *Ann Pharm Fr* 56:108–114, 1998.

Prashant A, Vishwanath P, Kulkarni P, et al.: Comparative assessment of cytokines and other inflammatory markers for the early diagnosis of neonatal sepsis—a case control study, Schulz C, ed, *PLOS ONE* 8(7):e68426, 2013.

Roberts WL, Sedrick R, Moulton L, et al.: Evaluation of four automated high-sensitivity C-reactive protein methods: implications for clinical and epidemiological applications, *Clin Chem* 46:461–468, 2000.

Tham W, Schmidt CQ, Hauhart RE, et al.: *Plasmodium falciparum* uses a key functional site in complement receptor type-1 for invasion of human erythrocytes, *Blood* 118(6):1923–1933, 2011.

Chapter 3: Antigens and Antibodies

Abbas AK, Lichtman AH, Pillai S: *Cellular and molecular immunology*, ed 8, Philadelphia, 2015, Elsevier.

Abbas AK, Lichtman AH, Pillai S: *Basic immunology: functions and disorders of the immune system*, ed 6, Philadelphia, 2020, Elsevier.

Jeffries R, Vidarsson G, Rispens T: Antibodies. In Male D, Peebles RS, Male V, editors: *Immunology*, ed 9, Elsevier, 2021, pp 148–162.

Maynard CL: The microbiota in immunity and inflammation. In Rich RR, editor: *Clinical Immunology*, ed 6, Elsevier, 2023, pp 281–294.

Monos DS, Rajaliningam R: The major histocompatibility complex. In Rich RR, editor: *Clinical Immunology*, ed 6, Elsevier, 2023, pp 78–92.

Schroeder HW, Rich RR: Antigens and antigen presentation. In Rich RR, editor: *Clinical Immunology*, ed 6, Elsevier, 2023, pp 93–106.

Chapter 4: Cellular Activities and Clinical Disorders of Innate and Adaptive Immunity

Innate Immunity

Abbas AK, Lichtman AH, Pillai S: *Basic immunology: functions and disorders of the immune system*, ed 6, Philadelphia, 2020, Elsevier.

Aiuti A, Roncarolo MG: Ten years of gene therapy for primary immune deficiencies, *Hematology Am Soc Hematol Educ Program* 682–689, 2009.

Camous L, Roumenina L, Bigot S, et al.: Complement alternative pathway acts as a positive feedback amplification of neutrophil activation, *Blood* 117(4):1340–1349, 2011.

Faix J: Sepsis: new approaches to diagnosis and treatment, *Cl Lab News* 38:12–14, 2012.

Holland SM, Uzel G: Neutrophils and neutrophil disorders. In Rich RR, editor: *Clinical immunology*, ed 6, Elsevier, 2023, pp 491–505.

Klinke A, Nussbaum C, Kubala L, et al.: Myeloperoxidase attracts neutrophils by physical forces, *Blood* 117(5):1350–1358, 2011.

Kuhns D, Alvord WG, Heller T, et al.: Residual NADPH oxidase and survival in chronic granulomatous disease, *N Engl J Med* 363(27):2600–2610, 2010.

Maynard CL: The microbiota in immunity and inflammation. In Rich RR, editor: *Clinical immunology*, ed 6, Elsevier, 2023, pp 281–294.

McDonald DR: Innate immunity. In Rich RR, editor: *Clinical immunology*, ed 6, Elsevier, 2023, pp 39–54.

Meissner F, Seger RA, Moshous D, et al.: Inflammasome activation in NADPH oxidase defective mononuclear phagocytes from patients with chronic granulomatous disease, *Blood* 116(9):1570–1573, 2010.

Pillay J, den Braber I, Vrisekoop N, et al.: In vivo labeling with 2H2O reveals a human neutrophil lifespan of 5.4 days, *Blood* 116(4):625–627, 2010.

Priel DL, Kuhns DB: *Assessment of neutrophils in rich RR: Clinical immunology*, ed 6, Elsevier, 2023.

Turgeon ML: *Clinical hematology*, ed 6, Philadelphia, 2022, Lippincott Williams & Wilkins.

Yago T, Shao B, Miner JJ, et al.: E-selectin engages PSGL-1 and CD44 through a common signaling pathway to induce integrin αLβ2-mediated slow leukocyte rolling, *Blood* 116(3):485–494, 2010.

Zou J, Sweeney CL, Chou BK, et al.: Oxidase-deficient neutrophils from X-linked chronic granulomatous disease iPS cells: functional correction by zinc finger nuclease-mediated safe harbor targeting, *Blood* 117(21):5561–5572, 2011.

Adaptive Immunity

Abbas AK, Lichtman AH, Pillai S: *Basic immunology: functions and disorders of the immune system*, ed 6, Philadelphia, 2020, Elsevier.

Alanio C, Lemaitre F, Law HKW, et al.: Enumeration of human antigen-specific naïve CD8+ T cells reveals conserved precursor frequencies, *Blood* 115(19):3718–3725, 2010.

Artis D, Spits H: The biology of innate lymphoid cells, *Nature* 517(1):293–301, 2015.

Campbell DJ: Control of regulatory T cell migration, function, and homeostasis, *J Immunol* 195(6):2507–2511, 2015.

D'Acquisto F, Crompton T: CD3+CD4-CD8- (double negative) T cells: saviors or villains of the immune response? *Biochem Pharmacol* 82(4):333–340, 2011.

Desfrançois J, Moreau-Aubry A, Vignard V, et al.: Double positive CD4CD8 αβ T cells: a new tumor-reactive population in human melanomas, *PLOS ONE* 5:e8437, 2010.

Filipovich A, Zhang K, Snow AL, et al.: X-linked lymphoproliferative syndromes: brothers or distant cousins? *Blood* 116(18):3398–3408, 2010.

Gatto D, Brink R: B cell localization: regulation by EBI2 and its oxysterol ligand, *Trends Immunol* 34(7):336–341, 2013.

Horowitz B: *Innate immunity: gene regulation*, Boston, MA, 2015, American Association of Immunologists, AAI Advanced Course, Book 1.

Jenkins MK: *Anatomy of the immune response*, Boston, MA, 2015, American Association of Immunologists, AAI Advanced Course, Book 1.

Kagan JC: *Innate immunity: pattern recognition and anti-microbial mechanisms*, Boston, MA, 2015, American Association of Immunologists, AAI Advanced Course, Book 1, p AAI.

Haining WN: *T cell memory*, Boston, MA, 2015, American Association of Immunologists, AAI Advanced Course, Book 2.

Lee ST, Hogquist K: T-cell development. In Rich RR, editor: *Clinical immunology*, ed 6, Elsevier, 2023, pp 130–135.

Medina KL: *B cell development*, Boston, MA, 2015, American Association of Immunologists, AAI Advanced Course, Book 1.

Schroeder HW, Radbruch A, Berek C, cell development B: In Rich RR, editor: *Clinical immunology*, ed 6, Elsevier, 2023, pp 107–119.

Takata H, Naruto T, Takiguchi M: Functional heterogeneity of human effector CD8+ T cells, *Blood* 119(6):1390–1398, 2011.

Thaunat O, Morelon E, Defrance T: Am "B" valent: anti-CD20 antibodies unravel the dual role of B cells in immunopathogenesis, *Blood* 116(3):515–521, 2010.

Thrasher AJ: New insights into the biology of Wiskott-Aldrich syndrome (WAS), *Hematology Am Soc Hematol Educ Program* 132–138, 2010.

Tumanov A, Grivennikov SI, Kruglov AA, et al.: Cellular source and molecular form of TNF specify its distinct functions in organization of secondary lymphoid organs, *Blood* 116(17):3456–3464, 2010.

Turgeon ML: *Clinical hematology*, ed 6, Philadelphia, 2022, Lippincott Williams & Wilkins.

Yokoyama WM: *NK cells, their receptors and function in health and disease*, Boston, MA, 2015, American Association of Immunologists, AAI Advanced Course, Book 1.

Zhu J, Paul WE: CD4 T cells: fates, functions, and faults, *Blood* 112(5):1557–1569, 2008.

PART II. THE THEORY OF IMMUNOLOGIC AND SEROLOGIC PROCEDURES

Chapter 5: Basic Safety in the Immunology-Serology Laboratory

Centers for Disease Control and Prevention (CDC): Update: provisional public health service recommendations for chemoprophylaxis after occupational exposure to HIV, *MMWR Morb Mortal Wkly Rep* 45:468–472, 1995.

Centers for Disease Control and Prevention (CDC): Hand hygiene in healthcare settings: training, 2011. Available at http://www.cdc.gov/handhygiene/training.html.

Christopher JP: Laboratory safety management roles and responsibilities, *Med Lab Obs* 54(1):18–24, 2022.

Clinical Laboratory and Standards Institute (CLSI). *Clinical laboratory safety: approved guideline*, ed 3, Wayne, PA, 2012: GP17-A3. (Reaffirmed December 23, 2022).

ECRI: Special Report: Top 10 patient safety concerns, 2021. www.ecri.org. Accessed 2 February 2022.

Lybert L: *Deadly microbes lurking on healthcare surfaces*, Healthcare Surfaces Institute, webinar, 2022.

Miller LE: Recommended concentrations of bleach, *Lab Med* 21:116, 1990.

National Committee for Clinical Laboratory Standards: *Clinical laboratory waste management: approved guideline*, Villanova, PA, 1993, NCCLS Document GP5-A.

Occupational Safety and Health Administration: Occupational exposure to hazardous chemicals in laboratories: final rule, *Fed Regist* 55:3327–3335, 1990.

Occupational Safety and Health Administration: Occupational exposure to bloodborne pathogens: final rule, *Fed Regist* 56:64004–64182, 1991.

The Joint Commission (TJC). Laboratory service: 2023 national patient safety goals, www.jointcommission.org. Accessed December 6, 2022.

Turgeon ML: *Clinical laboratory science: concepts, procedures and clinical applications*, ed 9, St. Louis, 2022, Elsevier.

Van der Valk: SARS-CoV-2: The relevance and prevention of aerosol transmission, *J Occup Environ Med* 63(6):e395–e401, 2021.

Wyer LA: *Driving quality through a culture of safety*, San Diego, CA, 2017, 22nd Annual Management Sciences and Patient Safety Leadership Seminar, AACC Annual Meeting.

Chapter 6: Basic Quality Control and Quality Assurance Practices

Carraro P, Zago T, Plebani M: exploring the initial steps of the testing process: frequency and nature of preanalytic errors, *Clin Chem* 58(3):638–642, 2012.

Centers for Disease Control and Prevention (CDC): *Clinical Laboratory Improvement Amendments (CLIA): equivalent quality control procedures*, Brochure no. 4, Washington, DC, 2004, US Government.

Centers for Medicare & Medicaid Services, HHS: Medicare, Medicaid, and CLIA Programs: Laboratory requirements relating to quality systems and certain personnel qualifications: final rule, *Fed Regist* 68:3639–3714, 2003.

Clinical and Laboratory Standards Institute (CLSI): *Statistical quality control for quantitative measurement: principles and definitions: approved guideline*, ed 4, Wayne, PA, 2016:C24 reaffirmed document December 22, 2022.

Clinical and Laboratory Standards Institute (CLSI): *Defining, establishing, and verifying reference intervals in the clinical laboratory: approved guideline*, ed 3, Wayne, PA, 2010:EP28. reaffirmed document December 22, 2022.

Clinical and Laboratory Standards Institute (CLSI): *Using proficiency testing and alternative assessment to improve the clinical laboratory*, ed 3, Wayne, PA, 2016, QMS24. reaffirmed document December 22, 2022.

McPherson RA: Laboratory statistics. In *Henry's clinical diagnosis and management by laboratory methods*, ed 24, Philadelphia, 2022, Elsevier.

Miller WG: Quality control. In McPherson RA, Pincus M, editors: *Henry's clinical diagnosis and management by laboratory methods*, ed 24, Philadelphia, 2022, Elsevier.

Turgeon ML: *Clinical laboratory science: concepts, procedures and clinical applications*, ed 9, St. Louis, 2022, Elsevier.

Chapter 7: Basic Serologic Laboratory: Techniques and Clinical Applications

Bishop ML, Fody EP, Schoeff L: *Clinical chemistry principles, procedures, correlations*, ed 9, Burlington, MA, 2023, Jones & Bartlett.

Burtis CA, Bruns DB, editors: *Tietz fundamentals of clinical chemistry*, ed 7, St. Louis, 2015, Saunders.

McVoy LA, Lifshitz MS: Point-of-care testing and physician office laboratories. In *Henry's Clinical diagnosis and management by laboratory methods*, ed 24, Philadelphia, 2022, Elsevier, pp 81–88.

Turgeon ML: *Point-of-care testing. Clinical laboratory science: concepts, procedures and clinical applications*, ed 9, St. Louis, 2022, Elsevier, pp 218–220.

Chapter 8: Precipitation and Particle Agglutination Methods

Aoyagi K, Ashihara Y, Kasahara Y: Immunoassays and Immunochemistry. In *Henry's clinical diagnosis and management by laboratory methods*, ed 24, Philadelphia, 2022, Elsevier, pp 901–928.

Baines W, Noble P: Sensitivity limits of latex agglutination tests, *Am Clin Lab* 12:14–18, 1993.

Bishop ML, Fody EP, Schoeff L: *Clinical chemistry principles, procedures, correlations*, ed 9, Burlington, MA, 2023, Jones & Bartletts.

Kaplan LA, Pesce AJ: *Clinical chemistry: theory, analysis, correlation*, ed 5, St. Louis, 2009, Mosby.

Mahon CR, Lehman DC: *Textbook of diagnostic microbiology*, ed 7, St. Louis, 2022, Elsevier.

Chapter 9: Electrophoresis Techniques and Chromatography

Aoyagi K, Ashihara Y, Kasahara Y: Immunoassays and immunochemistry. In *Henry's clinical diagnosis and management by laboratory methods*, ed 24, Philadelphia, 2022, Elsevier, pp 901–928.

Bazydlo Landers JP: Electrophoresis. In Rifai N, Horvath AR, Wittwer CT, editors: *Tietz fundamentals of clinical chemistry and molecular diagnostics*, ed 8, Elsevier, 2019, pp 167–179.

Bishop ML, Fody EP, Schoeff L: *Clinical chemistry principles, procedures, correlations*, ed 9, Burlington, MA, 2023, Jones & Bartletts.

Hage DS: Chromatography and electrophoresis. In *Contemporary practice in clinical chemistry*, ed 4, Elsevier, 2019, pp 135–157.

Helena Laboratories Educational Presentations: Protein electrophoresis and IFE, immunofixation, and high res proteins, www.helena.com/educa_presentations.htm. Accessed August 2023.

Li SFY, Kricka LJ: Clinical analysis by microchip capillary electrophoresis, *Clin Chem* 52(42), 2006.

Chapter 10: Labeling Techniques in Immunoassay

Aoyagi K, Ashihara Y, Kasahara Y: Immunoassays and immunochemistry. In *Henry's clinical diagnosis and management by laboratory methods*, ed 24, Philadelphia, 2022, Elsevier, pp 901–928.

Gan SD, Patel KR: Enzyme immunoassay (EIA) and enzyme-linked immunosorbent assay (ELISA), *J Invest Dermatol* 133(9):e12, 2013.

Jandreski MA: Chemiluminescence technology in immunoassays, *Lab Med* 29(9):555–560, 1998.

Mark HFL: Fluorescent in situ hybridization as an adjunct to conventional cytogenetics, *Ann Clin Lab Sci* 24:153–163, 1994.

Wang Z, Hu J, Jin Y, Yao X, et al.: In situ amplified chemiluminescent detection of DNA and immunoassay of IgG using special-shaped gold nanoparticles as label, *Clin Chem* 52(10):1958–1961, 2006.

Chapter 11: Flow Cytometry

Abbas AK, Lichtman AH, Pillai S: Case 5 Human deficiency virus infection: acquired immunodeficiency syndrome. In *Basic immunology: functions and disorders of the immune system*, ed 6, Philadelphia, 2020, Elsevier, pp 308–311.

Aoyagi K, Ashihara Y, Kasahara Y: Immunoassays and Immunochemistry. In *Henry's clinical diagnosis and management by laboratory methods*, ed 24, Philadelphia, 2022, Elsevier, pp 901–928.

Bakke AC: The principles of flow cytometry, *Lab Med* 32(4):207–211, 2001.

Nunes-Santos CJ, Rosenweig SD, Fleisher TA: Flow cytometry. In Rich RR, editor: *Clinical immunology*, ed 6, Elsevier, 2023, pp 1185–1197.

Roshini SA, Barnidge DR, Lanza IR: Assessment of proteins of the immune system. In Rich RR, editor: *Clinical immunology*, ed 4, Elsevier, 2013, pp 1145–1159.

Turgeon ML: Applications of flow cytometry. In Turgeon ML, editor: *Clinical hematology: theory and procedures*, ed 6, Philadelphia, 2022, Lippincott Williams & Wilkins, pp 634–638.

Chapter 12: Molecular Laboratory Techniques

Bakker E: Is the DNA sequence the gold standard in genetic testing? Quality of molecular genetic tests assessed, *Clin Chem* 52(4):557–564, 2006.

Coleman WB, Tsongalis GJ: *Diagnostic molecular pathology: a guide to applied molecular testing*, St. Louis, MO, 2017, Elsevier.

Grada A, Weinbrecht K: Next-generation sequencing: methodology and application, *J Invest Dermatol* 133(8):1–4, 2013.

Heriot K: *Welcome to the beginning: molecular pathology for the community hospital pathologist and medical technologist*, Tampa, FL, 2014, ASCP Annual Meeting.

Miller JA: How should we assess PCR accuracy, *Clin Lab News* 48(5):24–25, 2022.

Palomaki GE, Eklund EE, Kloza EM: Lambert-Messerlian GMEt al: Assessment of a simplified cell-free DNA method for prenatal Down syndrome screening, *Clin Chem* 68(11):1449–1458, 2022.

Pratt GW, Platt M, Velez A, et al.: Utility of whole blood real-time PCR testing for the diagnosis of early Lyme disease, *Am J Clin Pathol* 158(3):327–330, 2022.

Rhea JM, Singh HV, Molinaro RJ: Next generation sequencing in the clinical molecular diagnosis of cancer: advantages and challenges to clinical laboratory implementation, *MLO Med Lab Obs* 43(12):8–10, 2011.

Rifai N, Horvath A, Wittwer C: *Tietz textbook of clinical chemistry and molecular diagnostics*, ed 8, Elsevier, 2019.

Sarker JS, Jones WD, Livasy CA: Microarray-based gene expression profiling for molecular classification of breast cancer and identification of new targets for therapy, *Lab Med* 41(6):364–372, 2010.

Strobl F: NAT in blood screening around the world, *Med Lab Obs* 43(4):12–21, 2011.

Tang Y, Procop GW, Persing DH: Molecular diagnostics of infectious diseases, *Clin Chem* 43(11):2021–2038, 1997.

Titus K: Growing pains put gene panels in a pinch, *CAP TODAY* 1:25–30, 2023.

Turgeon ML: *Clinical hematology: theory and procedures*, ed 6, Philadelphia, 2022, Lippincott, Williams & Wilkins.

PART III. IMMUNOLOGIC MANIFESTATIONS OF INFECTIOUS DISEASES

Chapter 13: Infectious Diseases: Overview and TORCH Diseases TORCH

Toxoplasmosis

Beaman MH, Luft BJ, Remington JS: Prophylaxis for toxoplasmosis in AIDS, *Ann Intern Med* 117(2):163–164, 1992.

Centers for Disease Control and Prevention (CDC). Toxoplasmosis, https://www.cdc.gov/parasites/toxoplasmosis/index.html Accessed August 29, 2023.

Goering RV, Dockrell HM, Zuckerman M, et al.: *MIM's medical microbiology and immunology*, ed 6, Congenital toxoplasmosis, Elsevier, 2019, pp 309–310.

Hill DE, Chirukandoth S, Dubey JP: Biology and epidemiology of *Toxoplasma gondii* in man and animals, *Anim Health Res Rev* 6(1):41–61, 2005.

Jones JL, Schulkin J, Maguire JH: Therapy for common parasitic diseases in pregnancy in the United States: a review and a survey of obstetrician/gynecologists' level of knowledge about these diseases, *Obstet Gynecol Surv* 60(6):386–393, 2005.

Kravetz JD, Federman DG: Toxoplasmosis in pregnancy, *Am J Med* 118(3):212–216, 2005.

Lopez A, Dietz VJ, Wilson M, et al.: Preventing congenital toxoplasmosis, *MMWR Recomm Rep* 49(RR-2):59–68, 2000.

Montoya JG: Laboratory diagnosis of *Toxoplasma gondii* infection and toxoplasmosis, *J Infect Dis* 185(Suppl 1):S73–S82, 2002.

Montoya JG, Kovacs JA, Remington JS: *Toxoplasma gondii*. In Mandell GL, Bennett JE, Dolin R, editors: *Principles and practice of infectious diseases*, ed 6, Philadelphia, 2005, Churchill Livingstone.

Montoya JG, Rosso F: Diagnosis and management of toxoplasmosis, *Clin Perinatol* 32(3):705–726, 2005.

Turgeon ML: *Clinical hematology*, ed 6, Philadelphia, 2022, Lippincott Williams & Wilkins.

Rubella

Centers for Disease Control and Prevention (CDC): Progress toward rubella and congenital rubella syndrome control and elimination—worldwide, 2012–2020, *MMWR Morb Mortal Wkly Rep* 71(6):196–201, 2022.

Goering RV, Dockrell HM, Zuckerman M, et al.: *MIM's medical microbiology and immunology*, ed 6, Congenital rubella, Elsevier, 2019, pp 307–308.

Goering RV, Dockrell HM, Zuckerman M, et al.: *MIM's medical microbiology and immunology*, ed 6, Measles virus infection, Elsevier, 2019, pp 360–362.

Hogan CA, Broadhurst MJ, Wang H, et al.: Viral infections, Rubella. In *Henry's clinical diagnosis and management by laboratory methods*, ed 24, Philadelphia, 2022, Elsevier, pp 1270–1271.

World Health Organization (WHO). Measles, mumps and rubella www.who.org. Accessed August 28, 2023.

Cytomegalovirus

Associated Regional and University Pathologists (ARUP) Laboratories: Cytomegalovirus—CMV https://arupconsult.com/content/cytomegalovirus. Accessed August 29, 2023.

Bowden R, Sayers M, Flournoy N, et al.: Cytomegalovirus immune globulin and seronegative blood products to prevent primary cytomegalovirus infection after marrow transplantation, *N Engl J Med* 314(16):1006–1010, 1986.

Brady MT: Cytomegalovirus infections: occupational risk for health professionals, *Am J Infect Control* 14(5):197–203, 1986.

Burny W, Liesnard C, Donner C, et al.: Epidemiology, pathogenesis and prevention of congenital cytomegalovirus infection, *Expert Rev Anti Infect Ther* 2(6):881–894, 2004.

Centers for Disease Control and Prevention (CDC): Cytomegalovirus (CMV) and congenital CMV infection, 2020. Available at http://www.cdc.gov/cmv/index.html.

Demmler GJ, Six HR, Hurst SM, et al.: Enzyme-linked immunosorbent assay for the detection of IgM-class antibodies to cytomegalovirus, *J Infect Dis* 153(6):1152–1155, 1986.

Goering RV, Dockrell HM, Zuckerman M, et al.: *MIM's medical microbiology and immunology* ed.6, Cytomegalovirus infection, Elsevier, 2019, pp 192–194.

Goering RV, Dockrell HM, Zuckerman M, et al.: *MIM's medical microbiology and immunology* ed.6, Congenital CMV, Elsevier, 2019, pp 308–309.

Josephson CD, Caliendo AM, Easley KA, et al.: Blood transfusion and breast milk transmission of cytomegalovirus in very low-birth-weight infants: a prospective cohort study, *JAMA Pediatr* 168(11):1054–1062, 2014.

Macé M, Sissoeff L, Rudent A, et al.: A serological testing algorithm for the diagnosis of primary CMV infection in pregnant women, *Prenat Diagn* 24(11):861–863, 2004.

Preiksaitis JK, Brennan DC, Fishman J, et al.: Canadian society of transplantation consensus workshop on cytomegalovirus management in solid organ transplantation: final report, *Am J Transplant* 5(3):218–227, 2005.

Ross SA, Boppana SB: Congenital cytomegalovirus infection: outcome and diagnosis, *Semin Pediatr Infect Dis* 16(1):44–49, 2005.

Rowshani AT, Bemelman FJ, van Leeuwen EM, et al.: Clinical and immunologic aspects of cytomegalovirus infection in solid organ transplant recipients, *Transplantation* 79(4):381–386, 2005.

Schrier RD, Nelson JA, Oldstone MB: Detection of human cytomegalovirus in peripheral blood lymphocytes in a natural infection, *Science* 230(4729):1048–1051, 1985.

Schuster V, Matz B, Wiegand H, et al.: Detection of human cytomegalovirus in urine by DNA-DNA and RNA-DNA hybridization, *J Infect Dis* 154(2):309–314, 1986.

Sia IG, Wilson JA, Espy MJ, et al.: Evaluation of the COBAS AMPLICOR CMV MONITOR test for detection of viral DNA in specimens taken from patients after liver transplantation, *J Clin Microbiol* 38(2):600–606, 2000.

Turgeon ML: *Clinical hematology*, ed 6, Philadelphia, 2022, Lippincott Williams & Wilkins.

Herpes Virus

Hall CB, Caserta MT, Schnabel KC, et al.: Transplacental human herpesvirus 6 (HHV-6) congenital infection caused by maternal chromosomally integrated virus, *J Infect Dis* 201(4):505–507, 2010.

General

Male D, Peebles Jr RS: Male V: Tuberculin type hypersensitivity. Table 26.3. In *Immunology*, ed 9, Elsevier, 2021.

Simmons CP, Farrar JJ, Chau NV, et al.: Dengue, *N Engl J Med* 366(15):1423–1432, 2012.

Chapter 14: Streptococcal Infections

Buchanan JT, Simpson AJ, Aziz RK, et al.: DNase expression allows the pathogen group A Streptococcus to escape killing in neutrophil extracellular traps, *Curr Biol* 16(4):396–400, 2006.

Centers for Disease Control and Prevention (CDC): *Streptococcus* laboratory, www.cdc.gov, Accessed August 28, 2023.

Filkins L, Hauser JR, Robinson-Dunn B, et al.: American Society for Microbiology provides 2020 guidelines for detection and identification of group B Streptococcus, *J Clin Microbiol* 59(1):e01230–20, 2020.

Tille PM, editor: Streptococcus, Enterococcus and similar organisms. In *Bailey and Scott's diagnostic microbiology*, ed 15, St. Louis, 2022, Elsevier, pp 269–286.

US Department of Health and Human Services, Centers for Disease Control and Prevention (CDC). Group A streptococcal (GAS) disease: strep throat: all you need to know. www.cdc.gov [Last reviewed: Jan 2022; Accessed: June 2022]

Chapter 15: Syphilis

Albert C: Getting testing right as case rates rise. *CAP, TODAY* 37(2):29–33, 2023, 1.

Associated Regional and University Pathologists (ARUP) Laboratories: Syphilis testing algorithm: traditional sequence algorithm and reverse sequence screening algorithm. http://www.aruplab.com. Last Updated October 2020, Accessed May 1, 2023.

Associated Regional and University Pathologists (ARUP) Laboratories: *Treponema pallidum* (VDRL), cerebrospinal fluid with reflex to titer. http://www.aruplab.com. Accessed August 13, 2023.

Centers for Disease Control and Prevention (CDC): Sexually transmitted diseases (STD)—syphilis, https://www.cdc.gov/std/syphilis/default.htm, Accessed August 13, 2023.

Centers for Disease Control and Prevention (CDC): Congenital syphilis—reported cases and rates of reported cases by year of birth, by state/territory and region in alphabetical order, United States, 2017–2021, Table 21. www.cdc.gov, Accessed August 13, 2023.

Centers for Disease Control and Prevention (CDC): Total syphilis—reported cases and rates of reported cases by state/territory and region in alphabetical order, United States, 2017–2021, Table 12. www.cdc.gov, Accessed August 13, 2023.

Centers for Disease Control and Prevention (CDC): Primary and secondary syphilis—reported cases and rates of reported cases by state/territory and region in alphabetical order, United States, 2017–2021 Table 14. www.cdc.gov, Accessed August 13, 2023.

Goering RV, Dockrell HM, Zuckerman M, et al.: MIM's Medical microbiology and immunology. In *Sexually transmitted infections*, ed 6, 2019, pp 241–245.

Leclerc G, Giroux M, Birry A, et al.: Study of fluorescent treponemal antibody test on cerebrospinal fluid using monospecific anti-immunoglobulin conjugates IgG, IgM, and IgA, *Br J Vener Dis* 54(5):303–308, 1978.

Miraglia C: Spirochetes. In Tille PM, editor: *Bailey and Scott's diagnostic microbiology*, ed 15, St. Louis, 2022, Elsevier, pp 586–592.

Chapter 16: Vector-Borne Diseases

Associated Regional and University Pathologists (ARUP) Laboratories: Toxoplasmosis serologic testing for pregnant individuals. http://www.aruplab.com. Last Updated November 2020, Accessed May, 2023.

Associated Regional and University Pathologists (ARUP) Laboratories: lyme disease-modified two-tiered testing algorithm http://www.aruplab.com. Last Updated May, 2023, Accessed June, 2023.

Centers for Disease Control and Prevention (CDC): Chikungunya virus, http://www.cdc.gov/chikungunya. Last Reviewed June 2, 2022. Accessed August 13, 2023.

Centers for Disease Control and Prevention (CDC): *Dengue*, 2023. Dengue cases reported to ArboNET by state or territory of residence—United States. http://www.cdc.gov/dengue. Last Reviewed February 9, 2023, Accessed August 13, 2023.

Centers for Disease Control and Prevention (CDC): *Locally acquired malaria cases identified in the United States*. CDC Health Alert Network, www.cdc.gov. Accessed June 26, 2023.

Centers for Disease Control and Prevention (CDC): *Average annual number of confirmed Lyme disease cases*, United States 1992-2022-http://www.cdc.gov. last reviewed: January 19, 2022, Accessed July 15, 2023.

Centers for Disease Control and Prevention (CDC): *Tick-borne relapsing fever (TBRF)*, 2023. http://www.cdc.gov/relapsing-fever. Last Reviewed: July 24, 2023, Accessed August 13, 2023.

Centers for Disease Control and Prevention (CDC): *Ticks*, 2023.: http://www.cdc.gov/ticks. last reviewed: October 21, 2021.

Centers for Disease Control and Prevention (CDC): *Average annual incidence of West Nile virus neuroinvasive disease reported to CDC by county*, 1999-2021, ArboNET, Arboviral Diseases Branch, CDC, www.cdc.gov. Accessed April 15, 2023.

Centers for Disease Control and Prevention (CDC): *West Nile virus*, 2023. www.cdc.gov. Last Reviewed: June 13, 2023, Accessed August 13, 2023.

Dimaio MA, Pereira IT, George TI, et al.: Performance of BinaxNOW for diagnosis of malaria in a U.S. hospital, *J Clin Microbiol* 50(9):2877–2880, 2012.

Goering RV, Dockrell HM, Zuckerman M, et al.: *MIM's medical microbiology and immunology, ed.6, Vector-borne infections Lyme disease*, 2019, pp 375–377.

Goering RV, Dockrell HM, Zuckerman M, et al.: *MIM's medical microbiology and immunology, ed 6, Infections of the skin, soft tissue, muscle and associated systems*, 2019, pp 340–343.

Gomes-Solecki M, Arnaboldi PM, Backenson PB, et al.: Protective immunity and new vaccines for Lyme disease, *Clin Infect Dis* 70(8):1768–1773, 2020.

Madison BM, De Jesus VR: *A review of diagnostic testing and automation for Lyme disease*, Clinical Laboratory News, 2023, pp 15–19, Sept/Oct 2023.

Mead P, Petersen J, Hinckley A: Updated CDC recommendation for serologic diagnosis of Lyme disease, *MMWR Morb Mortal Wkly Rep* 68:703, 2019. http://dx.doi.org/10.15585/mmwr.mm6832a4.

Miraglia C: Spirochetes. In *Bailey and Scott's diagnostic microbiology*, ed 15, St. Louis, 2022, Elsevier, pp 593–597.

Nikolic D: Spirochetes—lyme and lyme like diseases. In McPherson RA, Pincus MR, editors: *Henry's clinical diagnosis and management by laboratory methods*, ed 24, Philadelphia, 2022, Elsevier, pp 1237–1243.

Pantanowitz L, Ballesteros E, DeGirolami P: Laboratory diagnosis of babesiosis, *Lab Med* 32(4):184–186, 2001.

Paz BG, Adams L, Wong JM, et al.: Dengue vaccine: recommendations of the advisory committee on immunization practices, United States, *MMWR Morb Mortal Wkly Rep* 70(RR-6), 2021. www.cdc.gov. Accessed 30 August 2023.

Pratt GW, Platt M, Velez A, et al.: Utility of whole blood real-time PCR testing for the diagnosis of early Lyme disease, *Am J Clin Pathol* 158(3):327–330, 2022.

Ryff KR, Rivera A, Rodriguez DM, et al.: Epidemiologic trends of dengue in U.S. territories, 2020–2020, *MMWR Morb Mortal Wkly Rep* 72(4), 2023. www.cdc.gov. Accessed 30 August 2023.

Vannier E, Krause PJ: Human babesiosis, *N Engl J Med* 366(25):2397–2407, 2012.

Chapter 17: Infectious Mononucleosis

Bennett N: Laboratory-based investigations of IM and Epstein-Barr virus, *MLO Med Lab Obs* 39(1):10, 2007.

Greenough TC, Straubhaar JR, Kamga L, et al.: A gene expression signature that correlates with C8+ T cell expansion in acute EBV infection, *J Immunol* 195(9), 2015, 4185–4167.

Hogan CA, Broadhurst MJ, Wang H, et al.: Viral infections, infectious mononucleosis and related infections. In McPherson RA, Pincus MR, editors: *Henry's clinical diagnosis and management by laboratory methods*, ed 24, Philadelphia, 2022, Elsevier, pp 1270–1271.

Mori JA, Kurozumi H, Akagi K: Monoclonal proliferation of T cells containing Epstein-Barr virus in fatal mononucleosis, *N Engl J Med* 327(1):58, 1992.

Ortho Diagnostics: Monospot product brochures, Raritan, NJ, Ortho Diagnostics.

Papadopoulos EB, Ladanyi M, Emanuel D, et al.: Infusion of donor leukocytes to treat Epstein-Barr virus-associated lymphoproliferative disorders after allogeneic bone marrow transplantation, *N Engl J Med* 330(17):1185, 1994.

Robertson ES: Epstein-Barr virus, *N Engl J Med* 355(25):2708, 2006.

Sumaya CV: Serological testing for Epstein-Barr virus: development in interpretation, *J Infect Dis* 151(6):984, 1985.

Sumaya CV, Ench Y: Epstein-Barr virus infectious mononucleosis in children. I. Clinical and general laboratory findings, *Pediatrics* 75(6):1003, 1985.

Turgeon ML: *Clinical hematology: theory and procedures*, ed 6, Philadelphia, 2022, Lippincott Williams & Wilkins.

Chapter 18: Viral Hepatitis

Associated Regional and University Pathologists (ARUP) Laboratories: Viral hepatitis screening and diagnostic algorithm. http://www.aruplab.com. Accessed May 15, 2023.

Associated Regional and University Pathologists (ARUP) Laboratories: Chronic hepatitis B testing algorithm. http://www.aruplab.com. Accessed May 15, 2023.

Centers for Disease Control and Prevention (CDC): Number of reported cases of acute hepatitis B virus infection and estimated infections, United States, 2013-2020. https://www.cdc.gov/hepatitis/statistics. Accessed May 15, 2023.

Centers for Disease Control and Prevention (CDC): Number of reported cases of acute hepatitis C virus infection and estimated infections, United States, 2013-2020. https://www.cdc.gov/hepatitis/statistics. Accessed May 15, 2023.

Dammacco F, Tucci FA, Lauletta G, et al.: Pegylated interferon-α, ribavirin, and rituximab combined therapy of hepatitis C virus-related mixed cryoglobulinemia: a long-term study, *Blood* 116(3):343–353, 2010.

Dienstag JL: Hepatitis B virus infection, *N Engl J Med* 359(14):1486–1500, 2008.

Foran JM: Hepatitis C in the rituximab era, *Blood* 116(24):5081–5082, 2010.

Gibb DM, Goodall RL, Dunn DT, et al.: Mother-to-child transmission of hepatitis C virus, *Hosp Physician* 36:16, 2000.

Gudima S, Wu SY, Chiang CM, et al.: Origin of hepatitis delta virus mRNA, *J Virol* 74(16):7204–7210, 2000.

Hogan CA, Broadhurst MJ, Wang H, et al.: Viral infections, viral hepatitis pp.1279-1282. In *Henry's clinical diagnosis and management by laboratory methods*, ed 24, Philadelphia, 2022, Elsevier.

Jensen DM: A new era of hepatitis C therapy begins, *N Engl J Med* 364(13):1272–1273, 2011.

Kangxian J, Weifang L, Lian Z, Zhiying C: Epidemiological survey and follow-up of transfusion-transmitted virus after an outbreak of enterically transmitted infection, *J Viral Hepat* 7(4):309–312, 2000.

Klausner J, Baghdadi J: An update on diagnostics for hepatitis C, *MLO Med Lab Obs* 47(4):34–36, 2015.

National Institutes of Health (NIH): Hepatitis (viral), 2019. www.niddk.nih.gov/health-information/liver-disease/viral-hepatitis. Accessed July 15, 2023.

Ngo Y, Munteanu M, Messous D, et al.: A prospective analysis of the prognostic value of biomarkers (Fibro test) in patients with chronic hepatitis C, *Clin Chem* 52(10):1887–1896, 2006.

Rosen HR: Chronic hepatitis C infection, *N Engl J Med* 364(25):2429–2438, 2011.

Wang JT, Lee CZ, Kao JH, et al.: Incidence and clinical presentation of posttransfusion TT virus infection in prospectively followed transfusion recipients: emphasis on its relevance to hepatitis, *Transfusion* 40(5):596–599, 2000.

PART IV. IMMUNE DISORDERS

Chapter 19: Primary and Acquired Immunodeficiency Syndromes

Associated Regional and University Pathologists (ARUP) Laboratories: Algorithm—human immunodeficiency virus in adults and adolescent testing algorithm. http://www.aruplab.com. Accessed May 15, 2023.

Bio-Rad Laboratories: *GS HIV Combo Ab/Ab EIA*, product insert. www.bio-rad.com. Content current as of January 24, 2020. Accessed August 13, 2023.

Bousfiha AA, Jeddane L, Ailal F, et al.: Primary immunodeficiency diseases worldwide: more common than generally thought, *J Clin Immunol* 33(1):1–7, 2013.

Boztug K, Schmidt M, Schwarzer A, et al.: Stem-cell gene therapy for the Wiskott-Aldrich syndrome, *N Engl J Med* 363(20):1918–1927, 2010.

Cohen MS, Shaw GM, McMichael AJ, et al.: Acute HIV-1 infection, *N Engl J Med* 364(20):1943–1954, 2011.

Corey L, Gilbert PB, Tomaras GD, et al.: Immune correlates of vaccine protection against HIV-1 acquisition, *Sci Transl Med* 7(310):7–31, 2015.

Fauci AS, Marston HD: Ending the HIV–AIDS pandemic—follow the science, *N Engl J Med* 373(23):2197–2199, 2015.

Gallo RC, Montagnier L: AIDS in 1988, *Sci Am* 259:40–51, 1988.

Havlir D, Beyer C: The beginning of the end of AIDS? *N Engl J Med* 367(8):685–687, 2012.

Kapler R: CDC's HIV test algorithm matches protocol with latest technology, *MLO Med Lab Obs* 47(4):38–40, 2015.

Lallemant M, Chang S, Cohen R, et al.: Pediatric HIV—a neglected disease? *N Engl J Med* 365(7):581–583, 2011.

Malone B: 30 years of HIV/AIDS, *Clin Lab News* 37(1):3–4, 2011.

McCutchan FE: Understanding the genetic diversity of HIV-1, *AIDS* 14(Suppl 3):S31–S44, 2000.

Mills EJ, Bärnighausen T, Negin J: HIV and aging—preparing for the challenges ahead, *N Engl J Med* 366(14):1270–1273, 2012.

Moir S, Buckner CM, Ho J, et al.: B cells in early and chronic HIV infection: evidence for preservation of immune function associated with early initiation of antiretroviral therapy, *Blood* 116(25):5571–5579, 2010.

National Institutes of Health (NIH): Types of primary immune deficiency diseases. www.nih.gov. Accessed July 15, 2023.

National Institutes of Health (NIH): Possible clues found to why HIV vaccine showed modest protection, 2012. http://www.CDC.gov.

Schejbel L, Garred P: Primary immunodeficiency: complex genetics disorders? *Clin Chem* 53(2):159, 2007.

Schulman, Ronca & Bucuvalas, Inc: *Primary immune deficiency disease in America. 2002 The first national survey of patients and specialists—Primary Immunodeficiency Foundation*, MD, https://primaryimmune.org.

Scosyrev E: An overview of the human immunodeficiency virus featuring laboratory testing for drug resistance, *Clin Lab Sci* 19:231–248, 2006.

Turgeon ML, editor: *Clinical hematology: theory and procedures*, ed 6, Philadelphia, 2022, Lippincott Williams & Wilkins.

US Department of Health and Human Services: *Guidelines for the use of antiretroviral agents in HIV-1-infected adults and adolescents, what's new in the guidelines?* April 08, 2015. Available at https://www.nih.gov/news-events/news-releases.

US Department of Health and Human Services, Centers for Disease Control and Prevention (CDC): Revised surveillance case definition for HIV infection—United States, 2014, *MMWR Recomm Rep* 63(RR03):1–10, 2014.

US Food and Drug Administration (FDA): Approved HIV medicines (last reviewed March 23, 2023), https://fda.gov.

Wainberg MA, Zaharatos GJ, Brenner BG: Development of antiretroviral drug resistance, *N Engl J Med* 365(7):637–646, 2011.

Weber JN, Weiss RA: HIV infection: the cellular picture, *Sci Am* 259(4):100–109, 1988.

Wong-Stall F, Gallo RC: Human T-lymphotropic retroviruses, *Nature* 317:395–403, 1985.

Wong-Stall F, Haseltine WA: The molecular biology of the AIDS virus, *Sci Am* 259(4):52–63, 1988.

World Health Organization (WHO): HIV facts. www.WHO.org July, 2022. Accessed July 15, 2023.

Chapter 20: Hypersensitivity Reactions

Asthma & Allergy Foundation of American: *Latex allergy*. Available at https://aafa.org. Accessed September 29, 2024.

Bach J: The effect of infections on susceptibility to autoimmune and allergic diseases, *N Engl J Med* 347(12):911–920, 2002.

Choo-Kang LR: Specific IgE testing: objective laboratory evidence supports allergy diagnosis and treatment, *MLO Med Lab Obs* 38(1):10–14, 2006.

Choo-Kang LR: The progression of allergic disease, *MLO Med Lab Obs* 38(1):18, 2006.

Creticos PS, Schroeder JT, Hamilton RG: Immunotherapy with a ragweed–toll-like receptor 9 agonist vaccine for allergic rhinitis, *N Engl J Med* 355(14):1445–1454, 2006.

Kay AB: Allergy and allergic disease, *N Engl J Med* 344(2):109–113, 2001.

Kay AB: Natural killer T cells and asthma, *N Engl J Med* 354(11):1186–1188, 2006.

Kirchner DB: The spectrum of allergic disease in the chemical industry, *Int Arch Occup Environ Health* 75(Suppl):107–112, 2002.

Lundin P: *Evaluation of technical performance of four immunoassay systems for allergy testing: ImmunoCAP 1000, ImmunoCAP 250, Advia Centaur, and Immulite 2000*, Orlando, FL, 2005, AACC Annual Meeting (abstract).

National Institute of Allergy and Infectious Diseases (NIAID): Guidelines for clinicians and patients for diagnosis and management of food allergy in the United States. Available at https://www.niaid.nih.gov/diseases-conditions/guidelines-clinicians-and-patients-food-allergy.

Ollert M, Weissenbacher S, Rakoski J, et al.: Allergen-specific IgE measured by a continuous random-access immunoanalyzer: interassay comparison and agreement with skin testing, *Clin Chem* 51:1241–1249, 2005.

Quest Diagnostics: ImmunoCap: specific IgE blood test. 2012, http://www.questdiagnostics.com/home/physicians/testing-services/by-test-name/immunocap.

Tschopp CM, Spiegl N, Didichenko S, et al.: Granzyme B: a novel mediator of allergic inflammation: its induction and release in blood basophils and human asthma, *Blood* 108(7):2290–2298, 2006.

Chapter 21: Plasma Cell Neoplasms and Other Diseases with Paraproteins

Alaggio R, Amador C, Anagnostopoulos I, et al.: The 5th edition of the World Health Organization classification of haematolymphoid tumours: lymphoid neoplasms, *Leukemia* 36:1720–1748, 2022.

Associated Regional and University Pathologists (ARUP) Laboratories: Algorithm—plasma cell dyscrasia. http://www.aruplab.com. Accessed May 30, 2023.

Barlogie B, Tricot G, Anaissie E, et al.: Thalidomide and hematopoietic-cell transplantation for multiple myeloma, *N Engl J Med* 354(10):1021–1029, 2006.

Bladé J: Monoclonal gammopathy of undetermined significance, *N Engl J Med* 355(25):2765–2770, 2006.

Cohen AD, Comenzo RL: Systemic light-chain amyloidosis: advances in diagnosis, prognosis, and therapy, *Hematology Am Soc Hematol Educ Program* 287–294, 2010.

Grass S, Preuss KD, Wikowicz A, et al.: Hyperphosphorylated paratarg-7: a new molecularly defined risk factor for monoclonal gammopathy of undetermined significance of the IgM type and Waldenström macroglobulinemia, *Blood* 117(10):2918–2923, 2011.

Heher EC, Goes NB, Spitzer TR, et al.: Kidney disease associated with plasma cell dyscrasias, *Blood* 116(9):1397–1404, 2010.

Jakubikova J, Adamia S, Kost-Alimova M, et al.: Lenalidomide targets clonogenic side population in multiple myeloma: pathophysiologic and clinical implications, *Blood* 117(17):4409–4419, 2010.

Kyle A, Therneau TM, Rajkumar SV, et al.: Prevalence of monoclonal gammopathy of undetermined significance, *N Engl J Med* 354(13):1362–1369, 2006.

Kyle RA, Rajkumar SV: Multiple myeloma, *N Engl J Med* 351(18):1860–1871, 2004.

Leukemia: and Lymphoma Society Myeloma July 15, 2023. www.lymphoma.org/.

Moonen DH, Kohlhagen M, Dasari S, Willrich MA, et al.: Utilizing mass spectrophotometry to detect and isotype monoclonal proteins in urine: comparison to electrophoretic methods, *Clin Chem* 69(7):746–753, 2023.

Moreaux J, Hose D, Reme T, et al.: CD200 is a new prognostic factor in multiple myeloma, *Blood* 108(13):4194–4197, 2006.

Noonan K, Matsui W, Serafini P, et al.: A novel role of IL-17 producing lymphocytes in mediating lytic bone disease in multiple myeloma, *Blood* 116(18):3554–3563, 2010.

O'Keefe J, Robinson S, Ellerbrook, Spencer K: *An immunofixation tutorial, Helena Laboratories*, Texas, 2011, Beaumont.

Palumbo A, Anderson K: Multiple myeloma, *N Engl J Med* 364(11):1046–1058, 2011.

Prabhala RH, Neri P, Bae JE, et al.: Dysfunctional T regulatory cells in multiple myeloma, *Blood* 107(1):301–304, 2006.

Roccaro AM, Sacco A, Jia X, et al.: MicroRNA-dependent modulation of histone acetylation in Waldenström macroglobulinemia, *Blood* 116(9):1506–1514, 2010.

Treon Sp, Xu L, Yang G, et al.: *MYD88* L265P somatic mutation in Waldenström's macroglobulinemia, *N Engl J Med* 367(9):826–833, 2012.

Turgeon ML: *Clinical hematology: theory and procedures*, ed 6, Burlington, MA, 2024, Jones & Bartlett.

Usmani SZ, Sexton R, Hoering A, et al.: Second malignancies in total therapy 2 and 3 for newly diagnosed multiple myeloma: influence of thalidomide and lenalidomide during maintenance, *Blood* 120(8):1597–1600, 2012.

Waage A, Gimsing P, Fayers P, et al.: Melphalan and prednisone plus thalidomide or placebo in elderly patients with multiple myeloma, *Blood* 116(9):1405–1412, 2010.

Waxman A, Mink PJ, DeVesa SS, et al.: Racial disparities in incidence and outcome in multiple myeloma: a population-based study, *Blood* 116(25):5501–5506, 2010.

Chapter 22: Tolerance, Autoimmunity, and Autoimmune Disorders

Associated Regional and University Pathologists (ARUP) Laboratories: Algorithm celiac disease testing for symptomatic individuals. www.arup.org. Accessed August 1, 2023.

Associated Regional and University Pathologists (ARUP) Laboratories: Algorithm—Autoimmune liver disease testing. www.arup.org. Accessed August 1, 2023.

Bach JF: The effect of infections on susceptibility to autoimmune and allergic diseases, *N Engl J Med* 347(12):911–919, 2002.

Bakalar N: Crohn's disease and colitis are linked to mutant gene, *Dana Foundation Immunol News* 6:1–2, 2006.

Black A: Antiphospholipid syndrome: an overview, *Clin Lab Sci* 19(3):144–147, 2006.

Chang A, Toutellotte WW, Rudick R, et al.: Premyelinating oligodendrocytes in chronic lesions of multiple sclerosis, *N Engl J Med* 346(3):165–173, 2002.

Cho JH, Gregersen PK: Genomics and the multifactorial nature of human autoimmune disease, *N Engl J Med* 365(17):1612–1623, 2011.

Davidson A, Diamond B: Autoimmune disease, *N Engl J Med* 345(5):340–350, 2001.

Dyment DA, Ebers GC: An array of sunshine in multiple sclerosis, *N Engl J Med* 347(18):1445–1447, 2002.

Finkelberg D, Sahani D, Deshpande V, et al.: Autoimmune pancreatitis, *N Engl J Med* 355(25):2670–2676, 2006.

Foley KF, Kao P: Biomarkers for inflammatory bowel disease, *Clin Lab Sci* 20(2):84–88, 2007.

Frohman EM, Racke MK, Raine CS: Multiple sclerosis—the plaque and its pathogenesis, *N Engl J Med* 354(9):942–954, 2006.

Gosink J: Laboratory diagnostics for celiac disease, *MLO Med Lab Obs* 44(3):30–33, 2012.

Hafler D: *T cell tolerance and autoimmunity*, Boston, 2015, AAI Advanced Course in Immunology.

Hochberg EP, Gilman MD, Hasserjian RP: Case 17-2006: a 34-year-old man with cavitary lung lesions, *N Engl J Med* 354(23):2485–2493, 2006.

IMMCO Diagnostics: *Autoimmune gastritis and pernicious anemia*, Buffalo, NY, 2006, IMMCO Diagnostics. IMMCO Diagnostics: *Autoimmunity*, Buffalo, NY, 2006, IMMCO Diagnostics.

Johnson TP, Antiochos B, Rosen A: Mechanisms of autoimmunity. In Rich RR, editor: *Clinical immunology*, ed 6, Elsevier, 2023, pp 649–656.

Kahn AI, Susa J, Ansari Q: Systemic sclerosis (scleroderma), *Lab Med* 36(11):723–728, 2005.

Kappos L, Antel J, Comi G, et al.: Oral fingolimod (FTY 720) for relapsing multiple sclerosis, *N Engl J Med* 355(11):1124–1138, 2006.

Keren DF: Anti-ss DNA is not a useful diagnostic test, *College of American Pathologists*, 2001, Available at http://www.cap.org.

Krawitt EL: Autoimmune hepatitis, *N Engl J Med* 354(1):54–64, 2006.

Kuhle J, Pohl C, Mehling M, et al.: Lack of association between antimyelin antibodies and progression to multiple sclerosis, *N Engl J Med* 356(4):371–378, 2007.

Lechner K, Jäger U: How I treat autoimmune hemolytic anemias in adults, *Blood* 116(11):1831–1838, 2010.

Lyons PA, Rayner TF, Trivedi S, et al.: Genetically distinct subsets within ANCA-associated vasculitis, *N Eng J Med* 367(3):214–223, 2012.

Mackay IR: Autoimmune hepatitis: from the clinic to the diagnostic laboratory lab medicine, *Lab Med* 42(4):224–232, 2011.

Mannon PJ, Fuss IJ, Mayer L, et al.: Anti–interleukin-12 antibody for active Crohn's disease, *N Engl J Med* 351(20):2069–2078, 2004.

Mooney B: Diagnosing pediatric autoimmune diseases, *Adv Med Lab Prof* 4(1):13–14, 2002.

Mueller PW, Achenbach P, Lampasona V: Type 1 diabetes autoantibodies, *Clin Lab News* 36(1):8–10, 2010.

Mu Q, Zhang H, Luo XM: Is SLE influenced by microbes and diet? *Front Immunol* 6:608, 2015. www.frontiersin.org.

Nakamura RM, Barry M: Serologic markers in inflammatory bowel disease (IBD), *MLO Med Lab Obs* 33(1):8–15, 2001.

National MS Society: National MS Society information resource center, 2023. Available at http://www.nationalmssociety.org.

Newitt V: Sorting out celiac disease with serologic testing, *CAP TODAY* 37(4):138-xx, 2023. www.cap.org. Accessed 1 August 2023.

Nimmo M: Celiac disease: an update with emphasis on diagnostic considerations, *Lab Med* 36(6):366–369, 2005.

Noseworthy JH, Lucchinetti C, Rodriguez M, et al.: Multiple sclerosis, *N Engl J Med* 343(13):938–952, 2000.

Oksenberk J: Immune protein may play role in MS attacks and progression, *Science* 294(5547):1613, 2001.

Phelps RG, Jones V, Turner AN, et al.: The properties of HLA class II molecules divergently associated with Goodpasture's disease, *Intl Immunol* 12(8):1135–1143, 2000.

Podolsky DK: Inflammatory bowel disease, *N Engl J Med* 347(6):417–428, 2002.

Ramsery MK, Owens D: Wegener's granulomatosis: a review of the clinical implications, diagnosis and treatment, *Lab Med* 37(2):114–116, 2006.

Robert C, Kupper TS: Inflammatory skin disease, T cells, and immune surveillance, *N Engl J Med* 341(24):1817–1827, 1999.

Rosenbaum JT: The immune response—learning to leave well enough alone, *N Engl J Med* 373(24):2378–2379, 2015.

Rutgeerts P, Sandborn WJ, Feagan BG, et al.: Infliximab for induction and maintenance therapy for ulcerative colitis, *N Engl J Med* 353(23):2462–2473, 2005.

Saadeh RS, Ramos PA, Algeciras-Schimich, et al.: An update on laboratory-based diagnostic biomarkers for multiple sclerosis and beyond, *Clin Chem* 68(9):1134–1150, 2022.

Salama AD, Levy JB, Lightstone L, et al.: Goodpasture's disease, *Lancet* 358(9285):917–920, 2001.

Salama AD, Chaudhry AN, Ryan JJ, et al.: Goodpasture's disease, CD4+ T cells escape thymic deletion and are reactive with the autoantigen $\alpha 3(IV)NC1$, *J Am Soc Nephrol* 12(12):1908–1915, 2001.

Schulte-Pelkum J, Schulz-Knappe P: A multi-marker approach to diagnosing autoimmune disease, *MLO Med Lab Obs* 47(10):44–46, 2015.

Schwartz RS: Autoimmune folate deficiency and the rise and fall of "horror autotoxicus", *N Engl J Med* 352(19):1948–1950, 2005.

Sloand EM, Mainwaring L, Fuhrer M, et al.: Preferential suppression of trisomy 8 compared with normal hematopoietic cell growth by autologous lymphocytes in patients with trisomy 8 myelodysplastic syndrome, *Blood* 106(3):841–851, 2005.

Snyder MR, Murray JA: Celiac disease, *Clin Lab News* 36(1):8–10, 2010.

Tan FK: Autoantibodies against PDGF receptor in scleroderma, *N Engl J Med* 354(25):2709–2711, 2006.

Torassa U: Odd illnesses, strong clues: autoimmune woes target women, *San Francisco Chronicle* 69, 2001.

Turgeon ML: *Clinical hematology: theory and procedures*, ed 6, Philadelphia, 2022, Lippincott Williams & Wilkins.

Utiger RD: The pathogenesis of autoimmune thyroid disease, *N Engl J Med* 325(4):278–280, 1991.

Voulgarelis M, Dafni UG, Isenberg DA, et al.: Malignant lymphoma in primary Sjögren's syndrome, *Arthritis Rheum* 42(8):1765–1772, 1999.
Watanabe T, Tsuchida T, Kanda N, et al.: Anti–alpha-Fodrin antibodies in Sjögren syndrome and lupus erythematosus, *Arch Dermatol* 135(5):535–539, 1999.
Winter WE: Autoimmune disorders that influence carbohydrate metabolism, *Clin Lab News* 31(7):14–16, 2005.
Wright MZ, Dearing LD: The role of HLA testing in autoimmune disease, *Adv Med Lab Prof* 13:81–84, 2001.
Yorde L: Diagnosing thyroid disease, *Adv Med Lab Prof* 12(17), 2000.
Zeher M, Szodoray P, Gyimesi E, et al.: Correlation of increased susceptibility to apoptosis of CD4+ T cells with lymphocyte activation and activity of disease in patients with primary Sjögren's syndrome, *Arthritis Rheum* 42(8):1673–1681, 1999.
Zinkernagel RM: Maternal antibodies, childhood infections, and autoimmune diseases, *N Engl J Med* 345(18):1331–1335, 2001.

Chapter 23: Systemic Lupus Erythematosus

Aranow C, Diamond B, Mackay M: Systemic lupus erythematosus. In Rich RR, editor: *Clinical Immunology*, ed 6, Elsevier, 2023, pp 657–677.
Associated Regional and University Pathologists (ARUP) Laboratories: Antiphospholipid syndrome testing algorithm www.arup.org Last Updated August 2020, Accessed August 15, 2023.
Associated Regional and University Pathologists (ARUP) Laboratories: Antinuclear antibody disease testing patterns algorithm www.arup.org Last Updated December 2020, Accessed August 15, 2023.
Associated Regional and University Pathologists (ARUP) Laboratories: Antinuclear antibody disease testing—cytoplasmic patterns algorithm www.arup.org Last Updated August 2020, Accessed August 15, 2023.
Associated Regional and University Pathologists (ARUP) Laboratories: Antinuclear antibody disease testing—nuclear patterns algorithm www.arup.org Last Updated August 2020, Accessed August 15, 2023.
Bosch X: Systemic lupus erythematosus and the neutrophil, *N Engl J Med* 365(8):758–760, 2011.
Lupus Foundation of America: Understanding lupus. Available at http://www.lupus.org. Accessed August 1, 2023.
Lupus Research Alliance: What is lupus? http://www.lupusresearch.org. Accessed July 15, 2023.
Mills JA: Systemic lupus erythematosus, *N Engl J Med* 330(26):1871–1879, 1994.
Mu Q, Zhang H, Luo XM: Is SLE influenced by microbes and diet? *Front Immunol* 6:608, 2015. www.frontiersin.org.
Peebles CL: Antinuclear antibody profiles, *Clin Lab News* 31(1):10–12, 2005.
Rollins G: Antinuclear antibody testing dilemmas: does high throughput trump sensitivity? *Clin Lab News* 37(1):5–7, 2011.
Satoh M, Vázauez-Del Mercado M, Chan EK: Clinical interpretation of antinuclear antibody tests in systemic rheumatic diseases, *Mod Rheumatol* 19(3):219–228, 2009.
Sohn K, Khan WI: ANA testing from microscopy to multiplexing, *Clin Lab News* 40(6):1–6, 2014.
Tsokos GC: Systemic lupus erythematosus, *N Engl J Med* 365(22):2110–2121, 2011.
US Food and Drug Administration (FDA): *Approved Lupus Drugs*. Available at www.fda.gov.

Chapter 24: Rheumatoid Arthritis

Asthma & Allergy Foundation of American: Latex allergy. Available at https://aafa.org. Accessed September 29, 2024.
Barbour KE, Helmick CG, Boring M, et al.: Prevalence of doctor-diagnosed arthritis and arthritis-attributable activity limitation—United States, *MMWR Morb Mortal Wkly* 66(9):246–253, 2017.
Cope AP: Rheumatoid arthritis. In Rich RR, editor: *Clinical immunology*, ed 6, Elsevier, 2023, pp 678–692.
Fraenkel L, Bathon JM, England BR, et al.: 2021 American College of Rheumatology Guideline for the treatment of rheumatoid arthritis, *Arthritis Rheumatol* 73(7):1108–1123, 2021.
Genovese M, Becker J, Schiff M, et al.: Abatacept for rheumatoid arthritis refractory to tumor necrosis factor alpha inhibition, *N Engl J Med* 353(11):1114–1123, 2005.
Henderson WR: The role of leukotrienes, *Ann Intern Med* 121(9):684–696, 1994.
Jokar M, Jokar M: Prevalence of inflammatory rheumatic diseases in a rheumatologic outpatient clinic: analysis of 12626 cases, *Rheumatol Res* 3(1):21–27, 2018.
Mahajan TD, Mikuls TR: Recent advances in the treatment of rheumatoid arthritis, *Curr Opin Rheumatol* 30(3):231–237, 2018.
McInnes IB, Schett G: The pathogenesis of rheumatoid arthritis, *N Engl J Med* 365(23):2205–2219, 2011.
Roose JC, Oster AJ: A new approach to drug development, *N Engl J Med* 355(19):2046–2047, 2006.
Sangha O: Epidemiology of rheumatic diseases, *Rheumatology (Oxford)* 39(Suppl 2):3–12, 2000.
Scott DL, Kingsley GH: Tumor necrosis factor inhibitors for rheumatoid arthritis, *N Engl J Med* 355(7):704–712, 2006.
Sullivan E: Rheumatoid arthritis: test for anti-CCP antibodies joining RF test as key diagnostic tools, *Lab Med* 37:17–19, 2006.
Theis KA, Murphy LB, Guglielmo D, et al.: Prevalence of arthritis and arthritis-attributable activity limitation—United States, 2016–2018, *MMWR Morb Mortal Wkly Rep* 70:1401–1407, 2021. www.cdc.gov.
Turgeon ML: Synovial fluid. In Turgeon ML, editor: *Clinical hematology: theory and procedures*, ed 6, Burlington, MA, 2022, Jones & Bartlett.
Wong JB, Ramey DR, Singh G: Long-term morbidity, mortality, and economics of rheumatoid arthritis, *Arthritis Rheum* 44(12):2746–2749, 2001.

PART V. TRANSPLANTATION AND TUMOR IMMUNOLOGY

Chapter 25: Transplantation: Human Leukocyte Antigens, Solid Organ, Tissues, and Hematopoietic Stem Cells

Transplantation

Aiutii A, Roncarolo MG: Ten years of gene therapy for primary immune deficiencies, *Hematology Am Soc Hematol Educ Program* 682–689, 2009.
American Association of Blood Banks: *Standards for hematopoietic progenitor cell services*, ed 11, Bethesda, 2023, American Association of Blood Banks (newly rebranded to the Association for the Advancement of Blood & Biotherapies).
Baxter-Lowe LA, Busch MP: DNA microchimerism and organ transplant rejection, *Clin Chem* 52(3):559–560, 2006.
Baynes RD, Hamm C, Dansey R, et al.: Bone marrow and peripheral blood hematopoietic stem cell transplantation: focus on autografting, *Clin Chem* 46(Pt 2):1239–1251, 2000.
Bensinger W, Martin PJ, Storer B, et al.: Transplantation of bone marrow as compared with peripheral blood cells from HLA-identical relatives in patients with hematologic cancers, *N Engl J Med* 344(3):175–181, 2001.
Blaser B, Schwind NR, Karol S, et al.: Trans-presentation of donor-derived interleukin-15 is necessary for the rapid onset of acute graft-versus-host disease but not for graft-versus-tumor activity, *Blood* 108(7):2463–2469, 2006.
Blazer BR, Hill GR, Murphy WJ: Dissecting the biology of allogeneic HSCT to enhance the GvT effect whilst minimizing GvHD, *Na Rev Clin Oncol* 17(8):475–492, 2020.
Blume KG, Thomas ED: A review of autologous hematopoietic cell transplantation, *Biol Blood Marrow Transplant* 6(1):1–12, 2000.
Chabner BA, Longo DL, editors: *Cancer chemotherapy and biotherapy: principles and practice*, ed 3, Philadelphia, 2001, Lippincott Williams & Wilkins.
Copelan EA: Hematopoietic stem cell transplantation, *N Engl J Med* 354(17):1813–1826, 2006.
Cutler C, Antin JH: Peripheral blood stem cells for allogenic transplantation: a review, *Stem Cell* 19(2):108–117, 2001.
Dantal J, Soulillou JP: Immunosuppressive drugs and the risk of cancer after organ transplantation, *N Engl J Med* 353(13):1371–1372, 2005.
Debelak J, Shlomchik MJ, Snyder EL, et al.: Isolation and flow cytometric analysis of T-cell-depleted CD34+ PBPCs, *Transfusion* 40(12):1475–1481, 2000.

Delmonico FL, Burdick JF: Maximizing the success of transplantation with kidneys from older donors, *N Engl J Med* 354(11):411–412, 2006.

Fishbein TM: Intestinal transplantation, *N Engl J Med* 361(10):998–1008, 2009.

Focosi D, Petrini M: More on donor-derived T-cell leukemia after bone marrow transplantation, *N Engl J Med* 355(2):212–213, 2006.

Franks LM, Teich NM: *Introduction to the cellular and molecular biology of cancer*, ed 3, New York, 1999, Oxford University Press.

Gadi VK, Nelson JL, Boespflug ND, et al.: Soluble donor DNA concentrations in recipient serum correlate with pancreas-kidney rejection, *Clin Chem* 52(3):379–382, 2006.

Highfill SL, Rodriguez PC, Zhou Q, et al.: Bone marrow myeloid-derived suppressor cells (MDSCs) inhibit graft-versus-host disease (GVHD) via an arginase-1-dependent mechanism that is up-regulated by interleukin-13, *Blood* 116(25):5738–5747, 2010.

Ingelfinger JR: Risks and benefits to the living donor, *N Engl J Med* 353(5):447–449, 2005.

Keller M, Charya A, Andargie T, et al.: Laboratory considerations for successful xenotransplantation, *Clin Chem* 68(11):1368–1373, 2022.

LaHoz RM: The laboratory's role in solid organ transplantation-screening for infectious diseases in pre-transplant evaluations, *Clin Lab News* 42(9):17–22, 2016.

Laughlin MJ, Eapen M, Rubinstein P, et al.: Outcomes after transplantation of cord blood or bone marrow from unrelated donors in adults with leukemia, *N Engl J Med* 351(22):2265–2275, 2004.

Leisenrig WM, Martin PJ, Petersdorf EW: It's about time: a new prognostic tool for acute graft-versus-host disease, *Blood* 108(2):749–755, 2006.

Liu C, Chen BJ, Deoliveira D, et al.: Progenitor cell dose determines the pace and completeness of engraftment in a xenograft model for cord blood transplantation, *Blood* 116(25):5518–5527, 2010.

Lowsky R, Takahashi T, Liu YP, et al.: Protective conditioning for acute graft-versus-host disease, *N Engl J Med* 353(13):1321, 2005.

Mahdi BM: A glow of HLA typing in organ transplantation, *Clin Transl Med* 2(1):6, 2013.

Martin-Henao GA, Picón M, Amill B, et al.: Isolation of CD34+ progenitor cells from peripheral blood by use of an automated immunomagnetic selection system: factors affecting the results, *Transfusion* 40(1):35–43, 2000.

Moretta L, Locatelli F, Pende D, et al.: Killer Ig-like receptor-mediated control of natural killer cell alloreactivity in haploidentical hematopoietic stem cell transplantation, *Blood* 117(3):764–771, 2011.

Nakamae H, Storer B, Sandmaier BM, et al.: Cytopenias after day 28 in allogeneic hematopoietic cell transplantation: impact of recipient/donor factors, transplant conditions and myelotoxic drugs, *Haematologica* 96(12):1838–1844, 2011.

National Marrow Donor Program, 2023. Available at http://www.nmdp.org.

Nikolic B, Zhao G, Swenson K, et al.: A novel application of cyclosporin A in nonmyeloablative pretransplant host conditioning for allogeneic BMT, *Blood* 96(3):1166–1172, 2000.

Parolini O: In utero hematopoietic stem-cell transplantation—a match for mom, *N Engl J Med* 364(12):1174–1175, 2011.

Pellegrino B, Schmidt RJ: *Immunosuppression*, 2016. Available at www.emedicine.medscape.com.

Pham MX, Teuteberg JJ, Kfoury AG, et al.: Gene-expression profiling for rejection surveillance after cardiac transplantation, *N Engl J Med* 362(20):1890–1900, 2010.

Pietroni V, Toscano A, Citterio F: Donor-specific antibody in solid organ transplantation: where are we? *Int Trends Immun* 1(4):5–7, 2013.

Reya T: Illuminating immune privilege—a role for regulatory T cells in preventing rejection, *N Engl J Med* 365(10):956–957, 2011.

Rivière I, Dunbar CE, Sadelain M: Hematopoietic stem cell engineering at a crossroads, *Blood* 119(5):1107–1116, 2012.

Ross DW: *Introduction to oncogenes and molecular cancer medicine*, New York, 1998, Springer.

Rumpler MJ, McClosky C, Christopher L: *A new era in post-transplant monitoring*, Clinical Laboratory News, April, 2023, pp 14–17.

Serody JS, Sparks SD, Lin Y, et al.: Comparison of granulocyte colony-stimulating factor (G-CSF)–mobilized peripheral blood progenitor cells and G-CSF–stimulated bone marrow as a source of stem cells in HLA-matched sibling transplantation, *Biol Blood Marrow Transplant* 6(4A):434–440, 2000.

Socié G: Graft-versus-host disease: from the bench to the bedside? *N Engl J Med* 353(13):1396–1397, 2005.

Spitzer TR: Nonmyeloablative allogeneic stem cell transplant strategies and the role of mixed chimerism, *Oncologist* 5(3):215–223, 2000.

Spitzer TR, McAfee S, Sackstein R, et al.: Intentional induction of mixed chimerism and achievement of antitumor response after nonmyeloablative conditioning therapy and HLA-matched donor bone marrow transplantation for refractory hematologic malignancies, *Biol Blood Marrow Transplant* 6(3A):309–320, 2000.

Stevens CE, Carrier C, Carpenter C, et al.: HLA mismatch direction in cord blood transplantation: impact on outcome and implications for cord blood unit selection, *Blood* 118(14):3969–3978, 2011.

Storek J, Dawson MA, Storer B, et al.: Immune reconstitution after allogeneic marrow transplantation compared with blood stem cell transplantation, *Blood* 97(11):3380–3389, 2001.

Sykes M, Preffer F, McAfee S, et al.: Mixed lymphohaemopoietic chimerism and graft-versus-lymphoma effects after non-myeloablative therapy and HLA-mismatched bone marrow transplantation, *Lancet* 353(9166):1755–1759, 1999.

Titus K: Breast cancer biomarkers, classic and new, *CAP TODAY* 37(2):10–15, 2023, 1.

Ullmann AJ, Lipton JH, Vescle DH, et al.: Posaconazole or fluconazole for prophylaxis in severe graft-versus-host disease, *N Engl J Med* 356(4):335–346, 2007.

United Network for Organ Sharing: Data and Trends, 2023. Available at www.unos.org.

Upton H: Origin of drugs in current use: the cyclosporin story, 2001. Available at http://www.davidmoore.org.uk/Sec04_01.htm.

Venkataramanan R, Shaw LK, Sarkozi L, et al.: Clinical utility of monitoring tacrolimus concentrations in liver transplant patient, *J Clin Pharmacol* 41(5):542–551, 2001.

Vincent K, Roy DC, Perreault C: Next-generation leukemia immunotherapy, *Blood* 118(11):2951–2959, 2011.

Vincenti F, Rostaing L, Grinyo J: Belatacept and long-term outcomes in kidney transplantation, *N Engl J Med* 374(4):333–343, 2016.

Visigalli I, Delai S, Politi LS, et al.: Gene therapy augments the efficacy of hematopoietic cell transplantation and fully corrects mucopolysaccharidosis type I phenotype in the mouse model, *Blood* 116(24):5130–5139, 2010.

Wilde M: Rejection, retroviruses: major barriers to xenotransplantation, *Adv Med Lab Prof* 9:14–19, 1997.

Wils EJ, van der Holt B, Broers AEC, et al.: Insufficient recovery of thymopoiesis predicts for opportunistic infections in allogeneic hematopoietic stem cell transplant recipients, *Haematologica* 96(12):1846–1854, 2011.

Zambelli A, Poggi G, DaPrada G, et al.: Clinical toxicity of cryopreserved circulating progenitor cells infusion, *Anticancer Res* 18(6B):4705–4708, 1998.

Zhang C, Todorov I, Zhang Z, et al.: Donor CD4+ T and B cells in transplants induce chronic graft-versus-host disease with autoimmune manifestations, *Blood* 107(7):2993–3000, 2006.

Chapter 26: Tumor Immunology and Applications of Massive Parallel Sequencing/Next-Generation Sequencing

Alduaij W, Illidge TM: The future of anti-CD20 monoclonal antibodies: are we making progress? *Blood* 117(11):2993–3001, 2011.

Alexandrov LB, Nik-Zainal S, Wedge DC, et al.: Signatures of mutational processes in human cancer, *Nature* 500(7463):415–421, 2013.

American Association of Immunology (AAI): *AAI Advanced Course in Immunology, book 2*, 2015. Boston, MA.

Brugarolas J: Renal-cell carcinoma: molecular pathways and therapies, *N Engl J Med* 356(2):185–187, 2007.

Butterfield LH: Tumor immunology: harnessing the immune system to fight cancer. In Rosenblatt J, Podack E, Barber GN, editors: *Advances in immunology and immunotherapy*, New York, NY, 2013, Springer Science and Business Media.

Carr TH, McEwen R, Dogherty B, et al.: Defining actionable mutations for oncology therapeutic development, *Nat Rev Cancer* 16(5):319–329, 2016.

Choy, Peng W, Jiang P, Cheng S, et al.: Single molecule sequencing enables long cell-free DNA detection and direct methylation analysis for cancer patients, *Clin Chem* 68(9):1151–1163, 2022.

Christiani DC: Combating environmental causes of cancer, *N Eng J Med* 364(9), 2011, 791–791.

Corthay A: Does the immune system naturally protect against cancer? *Front Immunol* 5:197, 2014.

Dancey JE, Bedard PL, Oneto N, et al.: The genetic basis for cancer treatment decisions, *Cell* 148(3):409–420, 2012.

Diamandis EP: Oncopeptidomics: a useful approach for cancer diagnosis? *Clin Chem* 53(6):1004–1006, 2007.

Friend SH, Dryja TP, Weinberg RA: Oncogenes and tumor-suppressing genes, *N Engl J Med* 318(10):618–623, 1988.

Franks CE, Li J, Martinez M, et al.: Utility of commercially available quantitative hCG immunoassay as tumors markers in trophoblastic and non-trophoblastic disease, *Clin Chem* 69(6):606–614, 2023.

Gökmen-Polar Y, Badve S: Breast cancer prognostic markers: an overview of a changing menu, *MLO Med Lab Obs* 47(10):8, 2015.

Jelovac D, Armstrong DK: Recent progress in the diagnosis and treatment of ovarian cancer, *CA Cancer J Clin* 61(3):83–206, 2011.

Jeggo PA, Pear LH, Carr AM: DNA repair, genome stability and cancer: a historical perspective, *Nat Rev Cancer* 16(1):35–42, 2015.

Jordan CT, Guzman ML, Noble M: Cancer stem cells, *N Engl J Med* 356(12):1253–1260, 2006.

Joshi CJ, Ke W, Drangowska-Way A, et al.: What are housekeeping genes? *PLoS Comput Biol* 18(7):e1010295, 2022. https://doi.org/10.1371/journal.pcbi.1010295. PMID: 35830477; PMCID: PMC9312424.

Kerbel RS: Tumor angiogenesis, *N Engl J Med* 358(19):2039–2049, 2008.

Kiluk J, Carter WB: Markers of angiogenesis in breast cancer, *MLO Med Lab Obs* 38(10):12–16, 2006.

Krontiris TG: Molecular medicine: oncogenes, *N Engl J Med* 333(5):303–306, 1995.

Liu R, Wang X, Chen GY, et al.: The prognostic role of a gene signature from tumorigenic breast-cancer cells, *N Engl J Med* 356(3):217–226, 2007.

Loeb S: Germline sequence variants and prostate-specific antigen interpretation, *Clin Chem* 57(5):662–663, 2011.

Maris J: Defining why cancer develops in children, *N Engl J Med* 374(24):2373–2374, 2015.

McDermott U, Downing JR: Stratton MR: Genomics and the continuum of cancer care, *N Engl J Med* 364(4):340–350, 2011.

Mendelsohn J, Gray J, Howley P, et al.: *The molecular basis of cancer*, ed 4, Philadelphia, PA, 2015, Saunders.

Moonen DH, Kohlhagen M, Sadari S, et al.: Utilizing mass spectrophotometry detect and isotype monoclonal proteins in urine: comparison to electrophoretic methods, *Clin Chem* 69(7):746–753, 2023.

Mullin E: A bevy of biomarkers battle to replace PSA, *Clin Lab News* 42(2):16–18, 2016.

Rhea JM, Singh HV, Molinaro RJ: Next generation sequencing in the clinical molecular diagnosis of cancer: advantages and challenges to clinical laboratory implementation, *MLO Med Lab Obs* 43(1):8–10, 2011.

Roche: MabThera (Rituximab) Product monograph: Hertfordshire, England, 2004, Roche.

Schaapveld M, Aleman B, vanEggermond AM, et al.: Second cancer risk up to 40 years after treatment for Hodgkin's lymphoma, *N Engl J Med* 373(26):2499–2511, 2015.

Scott AM, Wolchok JD, Old LJ: Antibody therapy of cancer, *Nat Rev Cancer* 12(4):278–287, 2012.

Siegel R, Ward E, Miller KD, Wagle NS, Jemal A: Cancer statistics, *CA Cancer J Clin* 73(1):17–48, 2023.

Stratton MR, Campbell PJ, Futreal PA: The cancer genome, *Nature* 458(7239):719–724, 2009.

Cancer Genome Atlas Research Network, Linehan WM, Spellman PT, Ricketts CJ, et al.: Comprehensive molecular characterization of papillary renal-cell carcinoma, *New Engl J Med* 374(2):134–145, 2016.

Thorn SH, Negrin RS, Contag CH: Synergistic antitumor effects of immune cell–viral biotherapy, *Science* 311(5802):1780–1784, 2006.

Van Dyke T: p53 and tumor suppression, *N Engl J Med* 356(1):79–81, 2007.

Woeste S, Diagnosing prostate cancer: *Lab Med* 36(7):399–400, 2005.

Zhang J, Walsh MF, Wu G, et al.: Germline mutations in predisposition genes in pediatric cancer, *N Engl J Med* 374(24):2336–2346, 2015.

PART VI. VACCINES

Chapter 27: Vaccines: Development and Applications

AIDS Vaccine Advocacy Coalition: AIDS vaccine science for busy advocates - RV144: building on a breakthrough, 2016. Available at www.avac.org.

Associated Regional and University Pathologists (ARUP) Laboratories: Tetanus antibody, IgG, 2023. Available at http://www.aruplab.com.

Basu S: Hepatitis E vaccine, *N Engl J Med* 356(23):2421, 2007.

Centers for Disease Control and Prevention (CDC): Noninfluenza vaccination coverage among adults—United States, *MMWR Morb Mortal Wkly Rep* 63(5):95–102, 2014.

Centers for Disease Control and Prevention (CDC): Human papillomavirus vaccine. www.CDC.gov Accessed August 28, 2023.

Centers for Disease Control and Prevention (CDC): Smallpox, 2023. www.CDC.gov. Accessed 28 August 2023.

Centers for Disease Control and Prevention (CDC): Recommended adult immunization schedule—United States, www.CDC.gov Accessed August 28, 2023.

Charo RA: Politics, parents, and prophylaxis: mandating HPV vaccination in the United States, *N Engl J Med* 356(19):1905–1907, 2007.

Chaves S, Gargiullo P, Zhang JX, et al.: Loss of vaccine-induced immunity to varicella over time, *N Engl J Med* 356(11):1121–1128, 2007.

Dolin R: HIV vaccine trial results—an opening for further research, *N Engl J Med* 361(23):2279–2280, 2009.

Fred Hutch Research Center: How vaccines are developed. Accessed August 15, 2023 www.fredhutch.org.

Freedman DO, Chen LH: Vaccines for international travel, *Mayo Clin Proc* 94(11):2314–2339, 2019.

White Paper Gavi: *Malaria vaccine market shaping roadmap*, 2023. www.gavi.org.

Hoffmann P, Roumeguère T, van Velthoven R, et al.: Use of statins and outcome of BCG treatment for bladder cancer, *N Engl J Med* 355(25):2705–2707, 2006.

Johnston MI, Fauci AS: An HIV vaccine: evolving concepts, *N Engl J Med* 356(20):2073–2080, 2007.

Kesselheim A: Safety, supply, and suits—litigation and the vaccine industry, *N Engl J Med* 364(16):1485–1487, 2011.

Koff WC, Berkley SF: The renaissance in HIV vaccine development—future directions, *N Engl J Med* 363(5):e7, 2010.

Monath TP, Fowler E, Johnson CT, et al.: An inactivated cell-culture vaccine against yellow fever, *N Engl J Med* 364(14):1266–1326, 2011.

National Cancer Institute: Cancer vaccines, 2023. www.nci.org.

Osterholm MT, Kelley NS, Sommer A, et al.: Efficacy and effectiveness of influenza vaccines: a systematic review and meta-analysis, *Lancet* 12(1):36–44, 2012.

Pallansch MA, Sandhu HS: The eradication of polio: progress and challenges, *N Engl J Med* 355(24):2508–2511, 2006.

Poland GA, Jacobson RM: The age-old struggle against the antivaccinationists, *N Engl J Med* 364(2):97–100, 2011.

Relman DA: Microbial genomics and infectious diseases, *N Engl J Med* 365(4):347–357, 2011.

Rogers LS: Game changers: 5 Global Vaccine Innovations on the Horizon. Johns Hopkins Bloomberg School of Health, www.jhu.edu Accessed August 13, 2023.

Schmidt C, Schnierle BS: Chikungunya vaccine candidates: current landscape and future prospects, *Drug Des Devel Ther* 16(10):3663–3673, 2022.

US Food and Drug Administration (FDA): Vaccines licensed for use in the United States, 2023. www.FDA.gov. Accessed 15 August 2023.

US Food and Drug Administration (FDA): Anthrax, 2012. Available at http://www.fda.gov/BiologicsBloodVaccines/Vaccines/ucm061751.htm.

Verbeke R, Hogan MJ, Loré K, Pardi N: Innate immune mechanisms of mRNA vaccines, *Immunity* 55(11):1993–2005, 2022.

World Health Organization (WHO): Malaria. Available at https://www.who.int/news-room/fact-sheets/detail/malaria. Accessed November 29, 2019.

GLOSSARY

A

A Symbol for the nucleotide adenine.
ABL protooncogene 1 The gene that encodes for the enzyme tyrosine kinase. The enzyme is involved in various cellular processes, such as cell division, differentiation, and adhesion.
abruptio placentae The premature separation of a normally situated placenta.
accelerated rejection Transplant rejection that occurs 1 to 5 days after a second exposure to tissue antigens because of reactivation of T or B lymphocytes.
accuracy Degree of conformity of a measurement to a true value.
acquired Incurred because of external factors; not inherited.
acquired immunodeficiency disorders Abnormalities that are not genetic in origin but caused by another type of factor.
acquired immunity See adaptive immunity.
acquired immunodeficiency A defect in the normal immune response caused by external factors or an existing disease or condition; also called *secondary immunodeficiency*.
acquired immunodeficiency syndrome (AIDS) An immune disorder affecting T4 lymphocytes caused by the human immunodeficiency virus (HIV); previously called human T-lymphotropic retrovirus (HTLV) or lymphadenopathy-associated virus (LAV).
actinomycosis An infectious condition, usually of the mucosal surfaces (e.g., oral cavity) by *Actinomyces*, a bacterial genus.
actionable mutation A change in DNA that would be expected to predict a patient's response to treatment if detected in a patient's tumor.
activated partial thromboplastin time (aPTT) A coagulation procedure to detect factors active in the external mechanism (stage I) of blood coagulation.
activation unit The combination of complement components—C1, C4b, and C2b—that forms the enzyme C3 convertase whose substrate is C3.
active immunity The form of immunity produced by the body in response to stimulation by a disease-causing organism (naturally acquired active immunity) or by a vaccine (artificially acquired active immunity).
acute Referring to a condition of sudden and short duration.
acute cellular rejection The type of transplantation rejection that takes place from days to weeks after the procedure as a result of cellular mechanisms and antibody formation.
acute glomerulonephritis A sudden inflammation of the small, convoluted mass of capillaries of the kidney, primarily the capsule.
acute graft-versus-host disease (GVHD) See graft-versus-host disease.
acute phase The immediate time of reactivity to an infectious microorganism.
acute-phase antibody Immune protein produced during the initial or early stage of infection.
acute rejection Immediate response to a transplanted tissue or organ.
acute rheumatic fever Condition in which there is crossreactivity damage to cardiac tissue as the result of antibodies formed in response to group A streptococcal pharyngitis.
acute-phase proteins Group of glycoproteins associated with nonspecific inflammation of body tissues (also called *acute-phase reactants*).
acute-phase response Form of natural immunity in which the levels of soluble proteins and other cells increase rapidly in response to the presence of an infectious agent.
adaptive immunity The augmentation of body defense mechanisms in response to a specific stimulus, which can cause the elimination of microorganisms and recovery from disease. This response commonly leaves the host with a specific memory (acquired resistance), which enables the body to respond effectively if reinfection with the same microorganism occurs. Adaptive immunity is organized around T and B lymphocytes; also called *adaptive immune response*.
adaptive T regulatory 1 cells (TR1) CD4+ T lymphocytes induced from antigen-activated naïve T lymphocytes influenced by cellular regulators (e.g., interleukin-10 [IL-10]). These cells demonstrate suppressive actions.
adenocarcinoma A malignant new growth derived from glandular tissue or from recognizable glandular structures.
adenoma A tumor derived from glandular tissue.
adenopathy Swelling or enlargement of the lymph nodes.
adenosine A nucleoside found in RNA.
adjuvant Pertaining to a substance that enhances the effect of an antigen when the substance is given along with the antigen.
adrenal medulla The inner core of the small endocrine gland that rests on top of each kidney.
afferent lymphatic duct The vessel that carries transparent liquids (unfiltered lymph) and antigens into the lymph node.
affinity Propensity; the bond between a single antigenic determinant and an individual combining site.
agammaglobulinemia The absence of plasma gamma globulin, caused by a congenital or acquired condition; also called *common variable immunodeficiency*.
agglutination Process whereby particulate antigens aggregate (clump) to form a larger complex in the presence of a specific antibody.
agglutination inhibition reaction A type of agglutination reaction based on competition between antigen-coated particles and soluble patient antigens. The competition is for a limited number of antibody-combining sites. Failure to exhibit agglutination (clumping) is interpreted as a positive result.
agglutinin Former term for antibody.
agglutinogen Former term for antigen.
aggregation See agglutination.
AIDS (acquired immunodeficiency syndrome) An immunologic disease caused by the human immunodeficiency virus (HIV); see acquired immunodeficiency syndrome.
albumin A water-soluble protein found in blood (serum), egg whites, and other substances.
aliquot A representative portion of a larger sample or specimen.
allele An alternate form of one or more genes that occur(s) at the same locus on homologous chromosomes.
allergen A substance that causes an allergic response when it enters the body.
allergic rhinitis Inflammation of the mucous membranes of the nose caused by a hypersensitivity reaction to environmental substances, such as pollen or mold.
allergy An abnormal or altered and often harmful response of the immune system to foreign substances, or antigens; also called *atopy*.
allergy march Progression of allergic disease.
alloantibody Immunoglobulin produced in response to exposure to foreign antigens of the same species.
alloantigen An antigen found in another member of the host's species. This type of antigen is capable of eliciting an immune response in the host.
alloepitopes Specific HLA antigens in genetically different individuals.
allogenic (allogeneic) Genetically different individuals of the same species.
allograft A graft of tissue from a genetically different member of the same species (e.g., human kidney).
alloimmunization A recipient who is immunocompetent can mount an immune response to the donor antigens when exposed to foreign red blood cells, resulting in various clinical consequences depending on the type of blood cells and specific antigens involved. The antigens most commonly involved are classified in the following categories: (1) human leukocyte antigens [HLAs], class I, shared by platelets and leukocytes, and class II, present on some leukocytes; (2) granulocyte-specific antigens; (3) platelet-specific antigens (human platelet antigen [HPA]); and (4) red blood cell (RBC)–specific antigens.
allotype The protein of an allele that may be detectable as an antigen by another member of the same species.
alopecia Loss of hair; baldness.
alpha-fetoprotein (AFP) A major plasma protein produced by the yolk sac and the liver during fetal development. It is thought to be the fetal form of serum albumin.
alternate pathway The pathway of complement activation triggered by constituents (e.g., toxins) of microorganisms. This pathway does not involve an antigen-antibody reaction to become activated.
alveolar Pertaining to an alveolus or alveoli; the thin-walled chambers of the lungs are referred to as pulmonary alveoli.
amniocentesis The process of removing fluid from the amniotic sac for study (e.g., for biochemical analysis).
amplicon A DNA fragment produced by amplification of a specific DNA sequence.

amplification A process to produce multiple copies of a specific DNA sequence.
amyloidosis A condition of intercellular deposition of an abnormal protein with a waxy translucent appearance in various tissues.
anaerobic metabolism The major non–oxygen-associated, energy-yielding pathway connected with the breakdown of glucose (glycolysis) in body cells; also referred to as the *Embden-Meyerhof glycolytic pathway* or the *tricarboxylic acid (TCA) cycle*.
analyte The substance being assayed in an immunoassay.
anamnestic Pertaining to a memory response.
anamnestic antibody response An antibody memory response. This secondary type of response occurs on subsequent exposure to a previously encountered, recognized foreign antigen. It is characterized by the rapid production of IgG antibodies.
anamnestic response A memory response.
anaphylactic reaction A severe allergic reaction that can develop in IgA-deficient patients who have developed anti-IgA antibodies.
anaphylactic shock A severe allergic reaction.
anaphylactoid reaction A severe reaction to soluble constituents in donor plasma that produces edema.
anaphylatoxins Complement components C3a and C5a, which stimulate the release of their vasoactive amines by mast cells.
anaphylaxis An immediate (type I) hypersensitivity reaction characterized by local reactions such as urticaria (hives) and angioedema (redness and swelling), or by systemic reactions in the respiratory tract, cardiovascular system, gastrointestinal tract, and skin.
anaplasmosis A newer term for human granulocytic ehrlichiosis.
anaplastic tumor A tumor that is poorly differentiated by cell type but similar to embryonic or fetal tissue.
anergy A state of no immunologic response; absence of sensitivity to substances that would normally elicit an antigenic response.
aneuploidy A deviation from the normal number of chromosomes.
angioedema Redness and swelling.
angiogenesis Formation and differentiation of blood vessels.
anicteric Without icterus, or lacking a yellow discoloration of the skin and sclera.
anion A negatively charged particle in solution.
ankylosing spondylitis A rheumatologic disorder.
anneal The bonding or hybridization of two complementary nucleic acid strands to one another.
anomaly Marked deviation from normal.
anorexia nervosa An eating disorder that occurs primarily in adolescent females.
antenatal Before birth.
antibody (pl., antibodies) Specific glycoproteins (immunoglobulins) produced in response to an antigenic challenge. Antibodies can be found in blood plasma and body fluids (e.g., tears, saliva, milk). These serum globulins have a wide range of specificities for different antigens and can bind to and neutralize bacterial toxins or bind to the surfaces of bacteria, viruses, or parasites.
antibody affinity See affinity.
antibody screen A laboratory procedure for testing recipient serum for the presence of antibodies to human leukocyte antigen (HLA) on potential donor transplant cells.
antibody titer See titer.
antibody-dependent cell-mediated cytotoxicity reaction (ADCC) A cellular activity exhibited by K cells and phagocytic and nonphagocytic myelogenous-type leukocytes. The target cell in ADCC is coated with a low concentration of IgG antibody.
antibody-mediated immunity See humoral immunity.
antibody-producing B cells See B lymphocyte.
antibovine antibodies A protein formed in response to an antigen possessed by a cow.
anticardiolipin Anti–nuclear ribonucleoprotein (anti-nRNP) antibody associated with lupus erythematosus.
anticore window The period during which antigen cannot be detected in the circulating blood, such as in hepatitis B testing.
anti-DNase B (ADN-B) An antibody directed against anti-DNase B, a product secreted by group A streptococci.
antigen A foreign substance (immunogen) that can stimulate the production of antibodies (immune response).
antigen presentation The activity associated with conveying an altered antigenic molecule to T and B cells by macrophages. This process is necessary for most adaptive responses.
antigen switching A protective mechanism invoked by parasites that involves variable synthesis of surface antigens to evade an immune response by the host.
antigen-antibody precipitin arcs Arcs that form on a gel plate when a favorable antigen-to-antibody ratio exists (immunodiffusion).
antigenemia A foreign substance in the blood that can evoke an antibody response.
antigenic determinant See epitope.
antigenic drift Movement of a foreign substance, an antigen, in populations of people.
antigenicity Ability of an antigen to stimulate an immune response.
antigen-presenting cell (APC) Functionally defined cell capable of taking up antigens and presenting them to lymphocytes in a recognizable form.
anti-HBc Antibody to hepatitis B core antigen.
anti-HBe Antibody to hepatitis B capsid antigen.
anti-HBs Antibody to hepatitis B surface antigen.
anti–human globulin (AHG) reagent An enhancement medium to promote agglutination.
antilipoidal antibodies A protein substance formed against the biochemical class of lipids.
antimetabolite A substance that interferes with normal metabolic processes in cells.
antimitochondrial antibody (ANCA) Antibody produced against the mitochondria of a cell.
antimyelin antibody Antibody produced against the sheath (covering) of axons and other nervous tissues.
antineoplastic agent Substance with reactive properties against new cellular or tissue growth.
antineutrophil cytoplasmic antibody An autoantibody divided into antineutrophil cytoplasmic antibody (c-ANCA) or antibody producing a perinuclear staining of ethanol-fixed neutrophils (p-ANCA).
antinuclear antibody (ANA) Antibody produced in response to different components of the cellular nucleus in a variety of autoimmune disorders.
antinuclear factor A factor in serum that acts against the cellular nucleus.
antioncogene A tumor-suppressing gene that guards against unregulated cell growth.
antiparietal antibody Antibody against cells of the stomach. Parietal cells make and release a substance that the body needs to absorb vitamin B_{12}.
antiphospholipid antibodies A group of antibodies directed against plasma proteins that are uncovered by binding of these proteins to plasma membranes. Laboratory assays for antiphospholipid include lupus anticoagulant (LAC), anticardiolipin (ACL) antibodies, and anti-β2-glycoprotein I antibodies.
antiphospholipid syndrome A disorder in which the immune system mistakenly produces antibodies against certain normal proteins in the blood, antiphospholipid antibodies.
antiretroviral therapy Treatment against a retrovirus. Retroviruses contain a single, positive-strand RNA with the genetic information of the virus and a special enzyme called *reverse transcriptase* in their core.
$α_1$-antitrypsin An acute-phase protein.
antisera An antibody-containing test reagent.
antiserum (pl., antisera) A serum containing antibodies or immune serum.
antistreptolysin O antibody (ASO) An antibody produced against streptolysin O, a hemolysin produced by streptococci, particularly group A.
antitoxin An antibody that interlocks with and inactivates toxins produced by certain bacteria.
antitreponemal antibodies Predominantly immunoglobulin M (IgM) antibodies found in early or untreated early latent syphilis.
apheresis The process of removing a specific component of the blood, such as platelets or plasma, and returning the remaining components (red blood cells) to the donor.
aplastic anemia A deficiency of blood cells (e.g., erythrocytes) caused by the lack of cell production (hematopoiesis) in the bone marrow. This form of anemia may result from exposure to toxic chemicals or drugs such as chloramphenicol.
apoptosis Programmed or normal cell death.
arteriole Small blood vessel.
arteriosclerosis Loss of elasticity (hardening) in the walls of blood vessels (e.g., arteries).
arthralgia Pain in a joint.
arthritis Inflammation of a joint.
arthrocentesis Removal of fluid from a joint.
arthropathy Joint disease.
arthrospore An asexual body capable of developing into another organism found in the conidia of various fungi.

Arthus reaction A type III hypersensitivity reaction.
articular Related to a joint of the skeletal system.
ascites Abnormal accumulation of fluid in the spaces between tissues and organs of the abdominal cavity.
aseptic meningitis An inflammation of the covering of the brain (meninges) or spinal cord not caused by bacteria.
aseptic technique Handling of materials or specimens without the introduction of extraneous microorganisms.
aspergilloma A tumor-like growth caused by mold, *Aspergillus* (e.g., aseptic meningitis).
asthma Respiratory condition characterized by recurrent attacks of dyspnea (difficult or painful breathing) and wheezing; caused by spasmodic constriction of the bronchi (larger air passages to or within the lungs).
astrocyte A nerve cell characterized by fibrous or protoplasmic processes. Collectively, these cells are called *macroglia* or *astroglia*.
asymptomatic Exhibiting no symptoms of a disease or disorder.
ataxia Irregularity of muscular action or faulty muscular coordination.
ataxia-telangiectasia Abnormal dilation of blood vessels near the surface of the skin.
atherosclerotic Pertaining to arteriosclerosis.
atopic eczema Inflammation of the epidermis (skin) characterized by redness, itching, and weeping; caused by a hypersensitivity reaction.
atopy Immediate hypersensitivity reaction caused by the immunoglobulin E (IgE) antibody.
atrioventricular atrophy Wasting or lack of growth of tissues or organs.
autoantibody (autoagglutinin) An immunoglobulin produced against a self-antigen.
autoantigen An antigen belonging to the host that normally does not elicit an immune response.
autoclaving A method of destroying microorganisms by the use of heat and pressure.
autodiluter An instrument used to make various concentrations of liquids.
autograft Tissue that is moved from one part of a person's body to another part of the same person's body.
autoimmune Against one's immune system.
autoimmune disease An abnormal condition related to the reaction of building antibodies to self-antigens.
autoimmune disorder A disorder that results from the failure to recognize "immunologic" self-antigens and leads to destruction of body tissues.
autoimmune hemolytic anemia Destruction of erythrocytes by antibodies to self-antigens.
autoimmunity A condition in which the body's own antigenic structures stimulate an immune response and react with self-antigens in a manner similar to the destruction of foreign antigens. This process may cause autoimmune disease.
autologous A synonym for self or part of the same individual.
autonomic nervous system The branch of the nervous system that functions without conscious control.

autosomal dominant gene A genetic trait that expresses itself, if present; carried on 1 of the 22 pairs of (autosomal) chromosomes.
autosomal recessive gene A genetic trait carried on 1 of 22 pairs of chromosomes; expressed only if present in a homozygous state.
avascular necrosis Death of nonvascular cells or tissues.
avascularity Without blood or lymphatic vessels (e.g., cartilage or in a disease state).
avidity The strength with which a multivalent antibody binds to a multivalent antigen.

B

B cell See B lymphocyte.
B-cell growth factor 2 See interleukin-5.
B-cell–stimulating factor 1 See interleukin-4.
B-cell–stimulating factor 2 See interleukin-6.
B lymphocyte Lymphocyte subset type that secretes antibody, the humoral element of adaptive immunity; also called *B cell*.
babesiosis A potentially fatal tick-borne disease caused by a parasite that infects red blood cells.
bacteremia Infection of the blood caused by bacterial microorganisms.
bacteriostatic An agent that prevents the growth of bacteria.
bare lymphocyte syndrome Uncommon cause of severe combined immunodeficiency (SCID).
base pair A nucleotide (adenine, guanine, cytosine, thymidine, or uracil) and its complementary base on the opposite strand.
BCG (Bacille Calmette-Guérin) Tuberculosis vaccine also used to stimulate the immune system in patients with certain types of cancer.
Bence Jones (BJ) protein The abnormal protein commonly found in the urine of patients with multiple myeloma. It precipitates at 50°C (122°F), disappears at 100°C (212°F), and reappears on cooling to room temperature.
benign Nonmalignant or noncancerous.
beta hemolysis A clearing or disruption of red blood cells in agar because of the exotoxins produced by certain bacteria (e.g., group A beta streptococci).
beta pancreatic cells Insulin-producing cells of the pancreas.
bilirubin A breakdown product of erythrocyte catabolism. If increased levels of this substance accumulate in the circulation, they will be deposited in lipid-rich tissues, such as the brain, and manifested by the skin and sclera as jaundice (icterus).
biohazard A dangerous condition caused by an infectious microorganism.
biologic response modifiers Substances that boost, direct, or restore normal immune defenses.
biologics Refers to living substances.
biometrics Refers in biological studies to the collection, synthesis, analysis, and management of quantitative data on biological communities; also known as *biological statistics*.
biosafety policies Rules to ensure safety when a person is exposed to or working with disease-causing organisms.
blast transformation The conversion of a B lymphocyte into a plasma cell.

blotting Transfer or fixation of nucleic acids onto a solid matrix (e.g., nitrocellulose) so that the nucleic acids may be hybridized with a probe.
bond Physiochemical forces that hold atoms together to form molecules.
bone marrow The spongy material inside bones that contains hematopoietic (blood-forming) tissues.
bronchiectasis A chronic inflammatory condition of the airways (bronchi) caused by dilation and loss of elasticity of the vessel walls.
Bruton disorder See X-linked agammaglobulinemia.
Burkitt lymphoma An undifferentiated malignant neoplastic disorder of the lymphoid tissues.
bursa of Fabricius An outgrowth of the cloaca in birds that becomes the site of formation of lymphocytes with B-cell characteristics.

C

C The nucleotide cytosine.
C1 complex Interlocking enzyme system consisting of C1q, C1r, and C1s.
C3 The most abundant and important component of complement; produces a small (C3a) and large (C3b) peptide when activated.
C5 The complement component split by C3b into C5a and C5b.
C6789 The lytic complement sequence that is activated by C5b and terminates in lysing the cell membrane; called the *membrane attack complex (MAC)*.
cachexia Physical wasting away of the body (e.g., as in AIDS patients).
capillary electrophoresis A type of laboratory test method.
capillary zone electrophoresis Any electrophoresis method that separates components into bands or zones and stabilizes the reaction on a solid surface (e.g., gel or paper).
capsid A covering structure associated with a virus (e.g., hepatitis).
capture assay (capture enzyme immunoassay) A type of immunoassay that uses two antibodies. The first antibody binds the antigen to solid phase; the second antibody has an enzyme label and acts as an indicator.
carboxy-terminal region A section of an antibody molecule.
carcinoembryonic antigen (CEA) A detectable tumor marker.
carcinoma Another term for a malignant neoplasm of epithelial origin (cancer).
carcinoma in situ Cancer that has not spread beyond the origin tissue mass (organ) in which it is detected.
cardiolipid Antibody that is a subset of antiphospholipid antibodies; also referred to as *lupus anticoagulant antibody*. An antigen composed of cardiolipin, a lipid remnant of damaged cells, cholesterol, and lecithin is used to detect the nontreponemal reagin antibodies.
cardiolipin A type of antibody.
carditis Inflammation of the heart muscle.
carrier molecule A molecule that when coupled to a hapten makes the hapten capable of stimulating an immune response.

carrier state Asymptomatic condition of harboring an infectious organism. The term may also refer to a heterozygous individual or the carrier of a recessive gene who does not have symptoms of a disease.

caseous necrosis Soft, cheeselike tissue that forms as the result of tissue death.

catarrhal symptoms Term previously used to describe the manifestations of inflammation of the mucous membranes, particularly of the head or throat, with an accompanying discharge.

catecholamine A biologically active amine, such as epinephrine and norepinephrine, that has a marked effect on the nervous and cardiovascular systems, metabolic rate and temperature, and smooth muscle.

cation A positively charged particle in solution.

CD (cluster of differentiation) markers Molecules on the surface of lymphocytes that identify them to other immune system cells; also called *cell surface markers*.

CD34+ cells A cell surface marker, antigen, indicative of the most immature hematopoietic cell.

CD4 The protein receptor on the surface of a target cell to which the gp120 protein of the HIV viral envelope binds.

cDNA Complementary DNA, produced from mRNA using reverse transcriptase.

cell adhesion molecule (CAM) Protein located on the cell surface involved with binding with other cells or with the extracellular matrix in a process called cell adhesion.

cell flow cytometry A procedure that uses computerized equipment for the separation, classification, and quantitation of particles (e.g., blood cells or antibodies). The technique is based on passing a monocellular stream of particles through a beam of laser light. The particles are categorized by size and then analyzed. Monoclonal antibodies can be used for the determination of specific subsets of cells. Subsets of cells can be identified by clusters of differentiation (CD) surface membrane markers; also called *flow cell cytometry*.

cell surface marker The expression of antigens on the membrane of a cell; detectable by flow cell cytometry.

cell surface receptors Structures that mediate cell-to-cell binding (adhesion) of leukocytes.

cell-mediated immunity (also cellular immunity) The type of immunity dependent on the link between T cells and macrophages.

cellulitis Inflammation within solid tissues, usually loose tissues beneath the skin; manifested by redness, pain, swelling (edema), and interference with function.

central tolerance A condition that develops in the thymus during fetal development and eliminates cells that react with self-antigens.

centromere The constricted portion of a chromosome.

cerebrospinal fluid (CSF) The fluid formed by the choroid plexus in the ventricles of the brain; found within the subarachnoid space, central canal of the spinal cord, and four ventricles of the brain.

cerebrovascular accident (CVA) Stroke.

ceruloplasmin Substance often measured as copper in the blood.

cestode Tapeworm.

CH Constant region of the immunoglobulin heavy-chain gene locus.

chancre A lesion that begins as a papule and erodes into a red ulcer. It is the primary wound of syphilis; it occurs at the site of entry of the spirochete.

Chédiak-Higashi syndrome A rare inherited autosomal recessive trait characterized by the presence of large granules and inclusion bodies in the cytoplasm of leukocytes.

chemiluminescence Luminescence in which the light emission is caused by the products of a specific chemical reaction.

chemoattractant A chemical substance that is part of the process of attracting phagocytic cells to a site of injury in the body.

chemokines A large family of homologous cytokines.

chemotactic factor See interleukin-8.

chemotaxis Release of substances that attract phagocytic cells as the result of traumatic or microbial damage.

chimera Organisms whose bodies contain different cell populations of the same or different species, such as in the exchange of tissue between fraternal twins before birth so that each recognizes tissue antigens of the other and accepts them, or as the result of transplantation of donor cells such as bone marrow.

chimerism Different cell populations of the same or different species.

cholestasis Blockage or suppression of the flow of bile.

choreoathetosis A condition characterized by rapid, jerky, involuntary movements or slow, irregular, twisting, snakelike movements seen mostly in the upper extremities (e.g., hands, fingers).

chorioepithelioma A tumor arising from chorionic epithelium.

chorioretinitis Inflammation of the choroid (middle layer) and retina (innermost layer) of the eye.

chromaffin cell A deep-staining type of cell in adrenal tissue.

chromophore A chemical group that absorbs light at a specific frequency and consequently gives color to a molecule.

chromosomes Strands of DNA that carry all the genes, with 23 pairs of chromosomes in each human cell.

chronic Referring to a condition that persists for a long time.

chronic glomerulonephritis An inflammation of long duration of the small convoluted mass of capillaries of the kidney, primarily the capsule.

chronic graft-versus-host disease (GVHD) Ongoing rejection of a transplanted graft over a longer period.

chronic granulomatous disease (CGD) A long-lasting disease associated with a neutrophilic leukocyte disorder.

chronic rejection A negative reaction of a transplanted tissue or organ over a long period.

chronicity A condition of long duration.

chyle A milky bodily fluid consisting of lymph and emulsified fats, or free fatty acids (FFAs); from the Greek *chylos*, meaning juice.

circulating immune complex Antigen-antibody in the blood flow.

class I MHC (HLA) molecules Proteins coded for by genes at three loci (A, B, C) in the major histocompatibility complex (MHC). These molecules are expressed on all nucleated cells and are important to consider in tissue typing for transplantation.

class II MHC (HLA) molecules Proteins coded for by the DR, DP, and DQ loci of the major histocompatibility complex (MHC). These molecules are found on B lymphocytes, activated T lymphocytes, monocytes, macrophages, dendritic cells, and endothelium.

class switching Change in isotype of antibody produced after a B lymphocyte has encountered an antigen.

classic Ouchterlony gel diffusion A laboratory testing method for studying antigen-antibody reactions.

classic pathway A pathway of complement activation that is launched with an antigen-antibody interaction.

clinical manifestations Observable abnormalities.

clonal expansion Multiplication of a clone of identical cells.

clonal selection Activation and proliferation of a lymphocyte when an individual lymphocyte encounters an antigen that binds to its unique antigen receptor site.

clonality A group of genetically identical cells that are derived from the same cell.

clone A group of cells descended from the same single cell (daughter cells), all having identical phenotypes and growth characteristics as the original precursor cell.

cluster of differentiation (CD) A surface marker that identifies a particular cell line or stage of cellular differentiation with a defined structure; can be identified with a group or cluster of monoclonal antibodies (MAbs).

coagglutination (CoA) A variation of latex agglutination. Visible agglutination of the coated particles indicates an antigen-antibody reaction.

coalesce A fusion of components.

coefficient of variation A statistical quality control calculation of variation from the average (mean).

coinfection The existence of one infection with another because of multiple pathogenic organisms.

collagen A protein found in skin, tendons, bone, and cartilage.

collagen disease Disease of the skin, tendons, bone, or cartilage, such as systemic lupus erythematosus and rheumatoid arthritis.

collecting tubule A small duct that receives urine from several renal tubules.

colloid A gelatinous or mucoidlike substance.

colloidal charcoal An insoluble indicator used in testing for syphilis.

colony-stimulating factors (CSFs) Molecular substances that stimulate hematopoietic progenitor cells to form colonies.

colorimetric reaction Chemical reaction that results in a change in color.
combining site The portion of the Fab molecule that possesses specificity.
common immunocyte Any cell of the lymphoid series that can react with an antigen to produce an antibody or participate in cell-mediated reactions.
common thymocyte Lymphocytes arising in the thymus that precede mature thymocytes (e.g., OKT 10, OKT 6 surface antigen) in development.
competitive immunoassay (competitive enzyme immunoassay) A form of immunoassay in which unlabeled and labeled antigens compete for a limited number of binding sites on a reagent antibody.
complement A group of soluble blood proteins (enzymes) consisting of C1 to C9. It is present in the blood and can produce inflammatory effects and lysis of cells when activated.
complement cascade The sequential activation of plasma proteins that cause lysis of a cell.
complement fixation A traditional procedure that detects the presence of a specific antigen-antibody reaction by causing in vitro activation of complement. If complement is not fixed, lysis of the preantibody-coated reagent erythrocytes occurs.
complement receptor A part of the mediated innate immune system. Complement receptors are responsible for detecting pathogens by mechanisms not mediated by antibodies. Their activity can be triggered by specific antigens. Therefore complement (a group of proteins in the serum that help achieve phagocytosis and lysis of antigens) is also part of the humoral immune system.
complement-dependent cytotoxicity (CDC) Killing of cells as the result of attachment of antibody with activation of complement.
complete antibody Former term used for an IgM antibody.
concomitant Existing at the same time (a condition).
confidence limits Statistical standard deviations from a mean. Interval estimates are often desirable because the estimate of the mean varies from sample to sample.
congenital Pertaining to a condition present at birth.
congenital rubella syndrome See rubella syndrome.
conjugate vaccine A vaccine in which easily recognizable proteins are linked to the outer coat of the disease-causing organism to stimulate an immune response.
conjugated A term for combined.
conjugated antibody Paired or joined; a laboratory substrate prepared by joining two substances, such as fluorescein to an immunoglobulin molecule.
constant region The part of an antibody's structure that is the same in all antibodies of the same class.
control specimen A specimen such as serum with known assay values that is tested concurrently with patient specimens of unknown values.

convalescence The time of recovery from conditions such as illness, injury, or surgery; convalescent period.
convalescent phase The recovery period of a disease.
convalescent phase antibodies A protein (antibody) response to an infectious agent after the acute phase has receded.
convalescent sera See convalescent phase antibodies.
convertase An enzyme associated with the complement system.
Coombs test Traditional term for the anti–human globulin (AHG) test that can be performed as direct and indirect AHG procedures.
cooperativity Interaction of specific cellular elements (lymphocytes), cell products (immunoglobulins and cytokines), and nonlymphoid elements.
corpus luteum A yellow-colored mass of progesterone-secreting endocrine tissue.
cortical-hypothalamic-pituitary axis Interrelated association among the outer layer of the brain, the structure located at the base of the cerebrum, small endocrine gland, and the pituitary gland.
corticosteroid Any hormone produced by the outer layer of the gland located on top of each kidney.
cosmopolitan Referring to a wide distribution.
counterimmunoelectrophoresis (CIE) A procedure in which oppositely charged antigen and antibody are propelled toward each other by an electrical field. This allows detection of concentrations of antigens and antibodies 10 times smaller than the lowest concentrations measurable by immunodiffusion or double diffusion.
covalent (adv., covalently) Pertaining to a type of chemical bond.
cranial nerve neuritis Inflammation of any of the nerves attached to the brain that pass through the openings of the skull.
C-reactive protein (CRP) A nonspecific, acute-phase, reactant glycoprotein.
crossimmunity A phenomenon that occurs when an antibody reacts with an antigen structurally similar to the original antigen that induced antibody production.
crossreactivity A condition in which some of the determinants of an antigen are shared by similar antigenic determinants on the surface of apparently unrelated molecules, and a proportion of these antigens interact with the other kind of antigen.
cryoglobulin An abnormal protein that precipitates or forms a gel at 0°C (32°F) and redissolves at warm temperatures.
cryoglobulinemia Pertaining to a condition in which cold-reacting proteins (globulins) are found in the circulating blood.
cryptic plasmid A concealed or unrecognized extrachromosomal ring of DNA that replicates autonomously, especially in bacteria.
cryptogenic cirrhosis A condition of the liver with an obscure or a doubtful cause.
cutaneous Referring to the skin (epidermis).
cutaneous systemic infection An infection involving all of the skin.

cutaneous T-cell lymphoma Malignant neoplasm with epidermal manifestations that involves the T subset of lymphocytes.
cuvette A calibrated type of glass tube used for reading the color of a solution with a spectrophotometer.
cytochrome P450 One of a family of isozymes responsible for the biotransformation of several drugs. Drug metabolism via the cytochrome P450 system is an important determinant in the occurrence of several drug interactions that can produce drug toxicities, reduced pharmacologic effect, and adverse drug reactions.
cytogenetics The branch of genetics focusing on the study of chromosomes.
cytokine A polypeptide product of activated cells (lymphocytes or macrophages) that controls a variety of cellular responses and thereby regulates the immune system.
cytolysis Rupture of a cell membrane with release of the cellular cytoplasm.
cytomegalovirus (CMV) A herpes family virus that can cause congenital infections in the newborn and a clinical syndrome resembling infectious mononucleosis.
cytopathology The study of abnormal cells.
cytopenia Severe decrease in the number of hematologic cells.
cytotoxic Able to kill cells.
cytotoxic T cell Subset type of lymphocyte that can kill other cells infected by viruses, fungi, and some types of bacteria or cells transformed by malignancy.
cytotoxic T-cell responses A type of lymphocyte reaction that has a killing effect on a foreign cell.
cytotoxicity A condition in which macrophages can kill some targets (possibly tumor cells) without phagocytizing them.

D

Dane particle The intact, double-shelled, hepatitis B virus.
darkfield microscopy A specialized type of microscopic examination.
Davidsohn differential test The classic laboratory reference test for the diagnosis of infectious mononucleosis.
definitive host A host in which the parasite reaches maturity and, if possible, reproduces sexually.
delayed hypersensitivity An exaggerated immune response caused by chemicals released by sensitized T cells; usually peaks at 24 to 48 hours after reexposure to the antigen; also called a *type IV hypersensitivity reaction*.
delta agent An RNA virus that causes hepatitis but requires the coexistence of hepatitis B infection.
dementia An irreversible condition of organic loss of mental function.
denaturation The process of heating and separating two DNA strands.
denatured DNA Double-strand helix that separates into two single strands. Hydrogen bonds can break from heat, pH, nonphysiologic concentration of salts, organic solvents (e.g., alcohol), or detergents.

dendritic cells The weakly phagocytic Langerhans cell of the epidermis and similar non-phagocytic cells in the lymphoid follicles of the spleen and lymph nodes. These cells may be the main agent of T-cell stimulation, but their precise region has not yet been determined.
dengue fever A rapidly expanding RNA virus transmitted by an urban-adapted mosquito.
deoxynucleotide A single unit of DNA composed of three parts: a nitrogenous base, a deoxyribose sugar, and one phosphate group.
deoxyribonucleic acid See DNA.
dermatitis An inflammation of the skin.
dermatome An area of embryonic tissue that gives rise to skin.
dermatomyositis An inflammatory condition included in the collagen disorders in which the skin, subcutaneous tissues, and muscles are involved. Necrosis of the muscles is characteristic.
desensitization A treatment for allergies such as hay fever that involves stimulating the buildup of IgG antibodies to block the effects of IgE; also called *hyposensitization*.
dextran A product produced by fermenting sucrose (sugar); used as a blood volume substitute.
DH Diversity region of the immunoglobulin heavy-chain gene locus.
diagnosis Determination of the nature of a disorder or disease.
diapedesis Ameboid movement of cells such as monocytes and polymorphonuclear neutrophils to a site of inflammation in phagocytosis.
DiGeorge syndrome An immunodeficiency disease resulting from failure of the parathyroid and thymus glands to develop before birth.
diluent One of two parts of a solution; also called the *solvent*. The solute is added as the second part of a solution.
dilution Reducing the concentration of a chemical constituent in a solution.
dimer A chemical structure formed from two subunits.
direct agglutination Macroscopic clumping that can be observed because particulate reagents are used to indicate the presence of an antigen-antibody reaction; a general term.
direct antiglobulin test (DAT) A test performed to detect the coating of erythrocytes with antibodies.
direct fluorescent antibody (DFA) test A microscopic technique that conjugates antibody to detect an antigen-antibody reaction.
discoid lupus Term used to differentiate the benign dermatitis of cutaneous lupus from the cutaneous involvement of systemic lupus erythematosus (SLE).
disease A pathologic condition characterized by a specific and unique set of signs and symptoms.
disorder An abnormality of body function.
distal tubules Ducts in the kidney located farthest from the center of the structure.
DNA A molecule found in a cell's nucleus that carries the cell's genetic information (genome); the nucleic acid that forms the main structure of genes. The sugar of this nucleic acid is deoxyribose. DNA (deoxyribonucleic acid) is the primary genetic material of all cellular organisms and DNA viruses.
DNA amplification An ultrasensitive polymerase chain reaction (PCR) technique for the detection of HIV that amplifies minute amounts of viral nucleic acid in the DNA of lymphocytes.
DNA dot blot hybridization A rapid molecular biology technique used to detect the presence of a specific DNA in a specimen.
DNA ligase A chemical that can be used to link molecules.
DNA microarray technology A laboratory testing product of bonding or direct synthesis of numerous specific DNA probes on a stationary, often silicon-based support.
DNA sequencing Determining the order of nucleotides in a segment of DNA.
domain Basic unit of an antibody structure. Variations among the domains of different antibody molecules are responsible for differences in antigen binding and biological function.
donor-specific antibody (DSA) test A laboratory assay to monitor posttransplant development of clinically relevant antibodies directed against donor-specific HLA class I and class II mismatches.
dot blot Technique used to determine whether a particular nucleotide sequence is present in a patient's specimen.
double immunodiffusion method A simple, rather dated method used to detect extractable nuclear antigens (also known as *Ouchterlony immunodiffusion*, *agar gel immunodiffusion*, or *passive double immunodiffusion*).
double-negative lymphocytes Mature lymphocytes lacking CD4 and CD8 surface membrane markers. This phenotype of lymphocytes may have a pathogenic or an immunoregulatory role.
double-negative thymocytes A lymphocyte in the thymus that lacks CD4 and CD8 surface membrane markers.
double-positive thymocytes A lymphocyte in the thymus that expresses both CD4+ and CD8+ surface membrane markers at the second stage of thymocyte development.
downregulation Reduction in the number of receptors on the surface of target cells, making the cells less sensitive to a hormone or another agent.
downstream Toward the 3′ end of a nucleic acid molecule.
driver mutation A mutation in a gene that confers a selective growth advantage that in turn promotes cancer development.
dsDNA Double-strand DNA.
D^u An outdated term for a phenotype of the Rh blood group system; now referred to as *weak D*.
D^u rosette test An older procedure that uses D-positive indicator erythrocytes to form identifiable rosettes around individual D-positive fetal cells that may be in the maternal circulation.
dyscrasia A term formerly used to indicate an abnormal mixture of the "four humors"; now it is somewhat synonymous with a disease or pathologic condition.
dysgammaglobulinemia A disorder involving an abnormality in the structure, distribution, or frequency of serum gamma globulins.
dysplastic Pertaining to faulty or abnormal development of body tissue (dysplasia).
dyspnea Difficulty in breathing.
dysproteinemia An abnormality of the protein content of the blood.

E

early antigen (EA) Expressed by B lymphocytes infected with Epstein-Barr virus in infectious mononucleosis. EA consists of early antigen-diffuse (EA-D), which is found in the nucleus and cytoplasm of B cells, and early antigen-restricted (EA-R), which is usually found as a mass only in the cytoplasm.
early thymocyte Immature T cell in the thymus that precedes the common thymocyte in maturational development.
echinococcal Pertaining to a genus of tapeworm (*Echinococcus*).
ectopic pregnancy The gestation of a fertilized egg outside the uterus, most often in the fallopian tube.
eczema An inflammatory condition of the skin (epidermis) characterized by redness, weeping, and itching.
edema (edematous) Accumulation of fluid in the tissues that produces swelling.
EDTA Ethylenediaminetetraacetic acid, disodium salt; a common in vitro anticoagulant.
effector cells Active cells of the immune system responsible for destroying or controlling foreign antigens.
effector T cells See effector cells.
efferent lymphatic duct The tubule through which semitransparent fluid (lymph) and possibly antigens exit the lymph node.
efficacy Ability of a vaccine to produce the desired clinical effect at the optimal dosage and schedule.
ehrlichiosis See human ehrlichiosis.
EIA See enzyme immunoassay.
electromagnetic spectrum Form of radiation, including visible light, ranging from long to short wavelengths.
electrophoresis A method of separating macromolecules such as proteins on the basis of their net electrical charge and size (molecular weight). See also serum electrophoresis.
ELISA See enzyme-linked immunosorbent assay.
eluate The product obtained by purposely manipulating a red cell suspension to break an antigen-antibody complex, with the subsequent release of the antibody into the surrounding medium.
elution Removal of antibodies attached to antigen receptors on the red blood cell membrane.
embryogenesis The growth and development of a living organism. In human beings, this period is from the second to approximately the eighth week of gestation.
encephalopathy Any degenerative disease of the brain.
endemic Present at all times, such as the continual existence of a specific microorganism in a population of individuals or in a geographic location.
endocarditis An inflammation of the inner lining of the heart (endocardium).

endogenous Originating or produced within an organism, tissue, or cell.
endogenous pathway Antigens that are generated within a cell; for example viral proteins in any infected cell. In liver biochemistry, a route of lipoprotein metabolism.
endonuclease An enzyme that breaks down a nucleotide chain.
endoplasmic reticulum A component of a cell associated with protein production.
endosome A vesicle that has lost its coat.
endothelial cell The type of epithelial cell that lines body cavities such as the serous cavities, heart, and blood and lymphatic vessels.
endotoxemia A condition of having bacterial cell wall heat-stable toxins in the circulation. These toxins are pyrogenic and increase capillary permeability.
endotoxin A heat-stable toxin present in intact lipopolysaccharide complexes in the bacterial cell wall. If the toxin is produced outside of the cell, it is an endogenous endotoxin.
end-stage renal disease An irreversible pathologic condition of the kidneys.
engraftment The process in which hematopoietic cells migrate to the bone marrow, where they begin to produce new blood cells.
enterocolitis An inflammation of the small intestine and colon.
***env* gene** A structural gene of a retrovirus such as HIV that encodes for a polyprotein that contains numerous glycosylation sites. In HIV, the envelope proteins gp160, gp120, and gp41 are encoded.
envelope protein The outer structure of the HIV-1 virus.
enzyme immunoassay (EIA) A general term for quantitative testing of antigens and antibodies. The method uses color-changed products of an enzyme-substrate interaction or inhibition to measure the antigen-antibody reactions; also called *ELISA*.
enzyme-linked immunosorbent assay (ELISA) A quantitative method of laboratory analysis. Antigen or antibody can be measured using enzyme-labeled antibody or antigen bound to a solid support. A direct ELISA measures antigen using competition for antibody-binding sites between enzyme-labeled antigen and patient antigen. An indirect ELISA measures antibody concentrations using bound antigen to interact with specimen antibodies.
eosinophilia An increase in the numbers of certain blood cells, the eosinophils.
epidemic A situation in which a condition extremely exceeds the usual number of cases (e.g., infectious diseases).
epidemiologic Pertaining to epidemiology.
epidemiology The study of an infectious disease or conditions in many individuals in the same geographic location at the same time.
epilepsy A transient disturbance of nervous system function caused by abnormal electrical activity in the brain.
episomal Pertaining to a replicating form; see episomal DNA.
episomal DNA An accessory, extra chromosome-replicating genetic element.

epithelial cell Cell of a type of body tissue that forms the covering of external and internal surfaces or composes a body structure, such as glandular epithelium.
epitope A single antigenic determinant. It is functionally the portion of an antigen that combines with an antibody paratope, the part of the antibody molecule that makes contact with the antigenic determinant.
Epstein-Barr virus (EBV) A human DNA herpes virus found in association with leukocytes and B lymphocytes. It is the causative agent of infectious mononucleosis in Western countries and Burkitt lymphoma in Africa.
equivalence The relative concentration of antibody and antigen that produces the maximal binding of antibody to antigen.
erysipelas A febrile disease caused by group A streptococci. The disease is manifested by inflammation and redness of the skin and subcutaneous tissues, fever, vomiting, and/or headache.
erythema Redness of the skin caused by inflammation, infection, or injury.
erythema chronicum migrans (ECM) See erythema migrans (EM).
erythema migrans (EM) Characteristic red skin inflammation of *Borrelia* infection. Also referred to as *erythema chronicum migrans*.
erythematous Characterized by erythema (redness).
erythrocyte A red blood cell (RBC).
erythrocyte sedimentation rate (ESR) A nonspecific measurement reflecting inflammation; the rate at which red blood cells form a sediment in 1 hour.
erythrogenic toxin A substance producing redness.
erythropoiesis The process of producing red blood cells (RBCs).
estrogen A female sex hormone, such as estradiol, estriol, and estrone.
etiologic agent The substance, agent, or condition responsible for causing an abnormal condition.
etiology The study of the cause(s) of disease; also, the cause or origin of a disease.
exchange transfusion The replacement of an infant's coated erythrocytes with donor blood until the total blood volume is transferred.
excoriation Severe scratching leading to disruption of the integrity of the skin.
exocytosis Release of cellular substances contained in vesicles.
exogenous Pertaining to a source outside of a cell or system.
exogenous endotoxin A bacterial toxin in the bloodstream.
exogenous factors See exogenous.
exogenous insulin Insulin not produced by a person's own pancreas.
exogenous pathway The route of antigen introduction to the body (e.g., inhaled, ingested, or injected) that involves antigen-presenting cells (APCs).
exogenous reservoir A storage place outside of a system.
exome The protein-coding regions of the genome

exon The contiguous coding sequence that is expressed in the process of RNA splicing and the process of making mature mRNA.
exon polynucleotide Sequence coding for protein synthesis.
exotoxin A soluble poisonous substance produced by growth of microorganisms.
extra-articular Outside of a joint.
extracellular matrix Structures of great significance in embryogenesis, cellular growth and repair, and hemostasis.
extracutaneous Outside of the skin.
extramedullary hematopoiesis Production of erythrocytes outside the bone marrow, which can result in enlargement of the liver and spleen.
extrathecal synthesis Produced outside an enveloping sheath.
extravasation Forcing out of a vessel or channel (extravasating).
extravascular destruction The destruction of an erythrocyte through phagocytosis and digestion by macrophages of the mononuclear phagocyte system.
extravascular hemolysis The phagocytizing and catabolizing of erythrocytes by the mononuclear phagocyte system.
exudate A substance with a high content of protein and cellular debris, such as pus, that has escaped from blood vessels.

F

F(ab)2 Portion of an IgG molecule produced by pepsin digestion that contains two Fab fragments. Two light chains and portions of two heavy chains are joined by disulfide bonds in the hinge region; it has two antigen-combining sites.
Fab fragments Two of the three fragments formed if a typical monomeric IgG is digested with a proteolytic enzyme (e.g., papain). These fragments retain the ability to bind antigens (specific receptors on cells) and are called antigen-binding fragments.
factor H Major controlling factor of the alternate complement pathway. Factor H acts as a cofactor with factor I to break down complement component, C3b, which is formed during complement activation.
factor I A serine protease that cleaves the complement components, C3b and C4b, that are formed during complement activation. Separate cofactors are required for each of these reactions.
Fc portion (Fc fragment) The third fragment formed in addition to the two Fab fragments if a typical monomeric IgG is digested with a proteolytic enzyme (e.g., papain). This fragment is relatively homogeneous and sometimes crystallizable.
Fc receptor The portion of an antibody responsible for binding to antibody receptors on cells and the C1q component of complement.
Fd fragment The fragment consisting of a light chain and half of a heavy chain if the interchain disulfide bonds in the Fab fragment are disrupted.
febrile Hot or heat-producing.
febrile agglutinin Antibody demonstrated in microbial diseases that produce a high fever.
febrile disease A pathologic process in which an extremely high fever is a characteristic manifestation.

febrile purpura Discoloration of the skin associated with a high temperature or fever.
femur Bone of the leg that extends from the pelvic girdle to the knee (the thigh bone).
fibrin A mesh protein clot formed by the action of thrombin on fibrinogen.
fibroblast An immature fiber-producing cell of connective tissue capable of differentiating into a cartilage-forming cell (chondroblast), collagen-forming cell (collagenoblast), or bone-forming cell (osteoblast).
fimbriae Fringed or fingerlike structures.
FISH See fluorescent in situ hybridization.
flocculation tests (v., flocculate) Blood serum assays based on the clumping together of coated particles to form visible masses (aggregates) indicating an antigen-antibody reaction.
flow cytometry See cell flow cytometry.
fluorescence Property of some compounds that can absorb energy from an incident light source and convert that energy into light of a longer wavelength.
fluorescence polarization immunoassay (FPIA) A type of immunoassay based on the change in polarization of fluorescent light emitted from a labeled molecule when it is bound by antibody.
fluorescent antibody (FA) assay General term describing a procedure using fluorescent microscopy that uses the visual detection of fluorescent dyes coupled (conjugated) to antibodies that react with the antigen, when present.
fluorescent antibody A dye-antibody combination that emits light of another, longer wavelength.
fluorescent antinuclear antibody (FANA) test An assay that detects antibody to nuclear antigens using nucleated cells and a fluorescence-labeled antihuman immunoglobulin.
fluorescent in situ hybridization (FISH) A laboratory technique for demonstrating the presence of HIV-1 in lymphocytes in primary lymph nodes and in peripheral blood from HIV-infected patients.
fluorochrome dye or fluorochrome A stain for a specific component or other markers.
fluorophores Light-generating substances (e.g., fluorescent dye).
follicle-stimulating hormone (FSH) A protein that stimulates follicles in the ovary.
follicular Referring to follicles.
Forssman antibody A heterophil type of immunoglobulin that is stimulated by one antigen and reacts with an entirely unrelated surface antigen present on cells from a different mammalian species. It can be absorbed from human serum by guinea pig kidney cells.
Förster resonance energy transfer (FRET) A technique for studying molecular interactions inside living cells with improved spatial (angstrom) and temporal (nanosecond) resolution, distance range, sensitivity, and a broader range of biologic applications.
forward-angle light scatter The type of light scattered at an angle of less than 90 degrees that indicates overall cell size.
Franklin disease A dysproteinemia synonymous with gamma heavy-chain disease. This abnormality is characterized by the presence of monoclonal protein composed of the heavy-chain portion of the immunoglobulin molecule.
FTA-ABS test Fluorescent treponemal antibody absorption test, a confirmatory test for syphilis. This test detects antibodies to the bacterial spirochete *Treponema pallidum* using antihuman immunoglobulin and a fluorescent label (tag).
fulminant To occur suddenly with great intensity, such as lightning-like flashes of pain.
fulminant disease Sudden and severe onset of an abnormal condition.

G

G The nucleotide guanine.
gag gene A gene of a retrovirus such as HIV that encodes for the major core structural protein.
gag region (group-specific antigen) The genomic region encoding for core structural proteins.
gait disturbance Walking in an unusual or abnormal manner.
GALT See gut-associated lymphoid tissue.
gamma heavy-chain disease See Franklin disease.
gammopathy A disorder manifested by abnormality of gamma globulins.
gastroenteritis An inflammation of the lining of the stomach and intestine.
Gaucher disease A rare systemic enzymatic defect that permits the accumulation of cell debris normally cleared by macrophages and is characterized by undegraded lipid products accumulating in the macrophages.
Gaussian curve A frequency distribution curve represented by a deviation from the mean (average) of a test sample.
gel electrophoresis A method for separating proteins or DNA based on size and electrical charge. Specimens are placed into wells made in a gel and subjected to an electrical current.
gene A unit of genetic material that codes for hereditary traits.
gene cloning A method for producing quantities of a specific DNA sequence.
gene expression profiling A method that can, for example, distinguish between cells that are actively dividing or show how the cells react to a particular treatment. Microarray technology measures the relative activity of previously identified target genes.
genitalia The female and male reproductive organs and associated external structures such as the penis.
genome The complete DNA composition of an organism (hereditary factors).
genomics The study of an organism's entire genome.
genotype Actual alleles, coding for a specific trait, that are inherited.
germinal center The interior location of secondary follicles where B lymphocytes undergo blast transformation.
gestation The period of development and growth of the unborn in viviparous animals (e.g., human beings), from fertilization of the ovum to birth.
giant cell Macrophage-derived cell typically found at sites of chronic inflammation. A giant multinucleated cell is formed by the coalescing of cells into a solid mass, or granuloma; also called an epithelioid cell.
giardiasis A parasitic infection associated with the unicellular *Giardia* species.
glial cell The nonnervous or supportive tissue of the brain and spinal cord known to produce minute amounts of CD4 or an alternate receptor molecule, which allows it to be infected with HIV virus; also known as a neuroglial cell.
glomerulonephritis See acute glomerulonephritis or chronic glomerulonephritis.
glomerulus (pl., glomeruli) The small structure(s) in the malpighian body of the kidney composed of a cluster of capillary blood vessels enveloped in a thin wall.
glycolipid A molecule consisting of a carbohydrate plus a lipid.
glycoprotein A molecule consisting of a carbohydrate plus a protein.
goodness of fit The complementary matching of antigenic determinants and antigen-binding sites of corresponding antibodies that influences the strength of bonding between antigens and antibodies.
grading Strength of agglutination rated from negative (0) to 4+.
grafting The transfer of cells or organs from one individual to another or from one site to another in the same individual.
graft-versus-host disease (GVHD) An intense and often fatal immunologic reaction of engrafted cells against the host caused by the infusion of immunocompetent lymphocytes into individuals with impaired immunity; can be acute or chronic.
Gram-negative organisms Bacteria that appear red when stained with Gram stain and examined under the microscope.
grand mal seizure A major epileptic attack, with or without loss of consciousness.
granulocyte A type of leukocytic white blood cell.
granuloma A macrophage-derived lesion containing sequestered noxious agents such as foreign bodies, some types of bacteria, and others that cannot be eliminated.
granulomatous lesion A wound composed of a granuloma.
granulomatous reactions (gummas) A soft swelling characteristic of late-stage syphilis.
granzyme A/B Enzyme in granules.
Graves disease An autoimmune disorder of the thyroid gland.
Guillain-Barré syndrome A relatively rare disease of the nerves; also called *acute idiopathic polyneuritis*.
gumma Granulomatous reactions. A granuloma that may result from delayed hypersensitivity. It is the soft tumor of tissues characteristic of the tertiary stage of syphilis.
gut-associated lymphoid tissue (GALT) May play a role with bone marrow in the differentiation of stem cells into B lymphocytes; functions as the bursal equivalent in humans.

H

HAART Acronym for *highly active antiretroviral therapy*. This regimen consists of multiple drugs; it is conventional therapy for HIV infection and AIDS.

haplotype A single chromosome's set of genetic determinants.

hapten(s) Very small molecule(s) that can bind to a larger carrier molecule and behave as an antigen.

haptoglobin A protein produced by the liver.

harmonization To be in agreement; compatible interfacing.

HBeAg Antigen associated with the capsid of hepatitis B virus (HBV).

HbsAg Surface antigen of hepatitis B virus (HBV), the initially detectable evidence of hepatitis B infection.

hCG See human chorionic gonadotropic hormone.

heavy (H) chain One of the polypeptide units of an immunoglobulin molecule. Each monomer of an immunoglobulin consists of two heavy chains paired with two light chains.

Heidelberger curve The relationship between the quantity of antigen and measuring signal at a constant antibody concentration.

helminth A parasitic worm.

helper T (Th) cells CD4+ lymphocytes. Their function is to assist B lymphocytes in the recognition of foreign antigens.

helper-inducer T-cell subset A major phenotypic lymphocyte subset of T lymphocytes; also referred to as *T4 subset, helper T cells*.

hemagglutination A laboratory technique for the detection of antibodies that involves the agglutination of red blood cells.

hemagglutination assay A testing method that uses red blood cells to indicate clumping in an antigen-antibody reaction.

hemagglutination assays A laboratory method that uses red blood cells as an indicator (agglutination) of an antigen-antibody reaction.

hemagglutination inhibition technique (HAI) A laboratory technique for detecting antibodies that involves the blocking of agglutination of red blood cells.

hematology The study of blood.

hematopathology The study of diseases or disorders of the blood, bone marrow, lymph nodes, spleen, and hematolymphoid lesions.

hematopoiesis (hematopoietic tissues) Blood-producing structures of the body, such as the liver, spleen, and bone marrow.

hematopoietic cells Blood-producing cells.

hemodynamic shock A physiologic condition (e.g., decreased blood pressure) resulting from the rapid loss of 15% to 20% or more of the blood volume.

hemoflagellate A protozoan parasite found in the blood and body tissues.

hemoglobinuria The presence of hemoglobin from ruptured red blood cells in the urine.

hemolysin A substance such as streptolysin O and streptolysin S produced by most group A strains of streptococci that disrupts the membrane integrity of red blood cells, causing the release of hemoglobin.

hemolysis Rupturing of the cell membrane (e.g., erythrocyte), with subsequent release of cytoplasmic contents (hemoglobin).

hemolytic Pertaining to rupturing of circulating erythrocytes.

hemolytic anemia A condition manifested by a severe decrease in circulating erythrocytes, with associated findings caused by the rupturing of circulating erythrocytes.

hemolytic disease of the newborn (HDN) An immunologic incompatibility between mother and fetus that can produce severe or fatal consequences in the unborn or newborn; caused by destruction of erythrocytes and the accumulation of breakdown products; previously referred to as erythroblastosis fetalis.

hemolytic reaction See hemolytic.

hemolytic titration (CH50) assay A now obsolete assay used to measure complement-activating ability.

hemolyzed Pertaining to ruptured erythrocytes with the release of hemoglobin into the serum or plasma of a blood specimen.

hemolyzed specimens The condition of a whole blood specimen when red blood cells have been ruptured and free hemoglobin is released into the specimen.

hemoptysis Coughing and spitting up of blood as the result of bleeding from any part of the respiratory system.

hemostasis Process that causes bleeding to stop.

hemostatic Pertaining to cessation of bleeding.

Hepadnavirus A type of virus that infects the liver and causes hepatitis.

hepatitis Inflammation of the liver caused by a virus, other agents (e.g., drugs), or sexual contact.

hepatitis B core antigen (HBcAg) A structural nucleocapsid core protein.

hepatitis B virus (HBV) A DNA virus transmitted by the parenteral route or sexual contact.

hepatitis C virus (HCV) A virus transmitted by blood or sexual contact; can be an acute or chronic form.

hepatoma A tumor of the liver.

hepatomegaly Excessive enlargement of the liver.

hepatosplenomegaly An enlarged liver and spleen.

herd immunity Indirect protection from an infectious disease at a community level because the majority of a population has immunity to a specific microbe.

herpes virus Any of a large group of DNA viruses such as herpes simplex and varicella.

heterodimer A protein composed of two polypeptide chains differing in composition and in the order, number, and/or type of their amino acid residues.

heterogeneous Different; a mixed or dissimilar population such as different types of cells or different ethnic groups mixed together.

heterophile antigen An identical or closely related antigen in unrelated plants or animals. Antibodies produced to one heterophile antigen will crossreact with antibodies to the other.

heterosexual disease A pathologic condition transmitted between individuals of the opposite gender.

heterozygous Genetic state of having two dissimilar genes for the same trait.

highly active antiretroviral therapy (HAART) A type of therapy used in the treatment of AIDS.

hinge region The area of an antibody molecule between the Fc and Fab regions that allows the two regions to operate independently.

histamine An amine produced by the catabolism of histidine, which causes dilation of blood vessels.

histiocyte A large phagocytic interstitial cell of the mononuclear phagocyte system; a macrophage.

histocompatibility (HLA) antigen Cell surface protein antigen found on blood and body cells (e.g., leukocytes and platelets); readily provokes an immune response if transferred into a genetically different (allogenic) individual of the same species.

histone A simple protein found in combination with acidic substances such as nucleic acids.

histoplasmosis A severe respiratory infection caused by a fungus, *Histoplasma capsulatum*.

HIV Causative agent of acquired immunodeficiency syndrome (AIDS), also called *human immunodeficiency virus type 1 (HIV-1)*; formerly referred to as human T-lymphotropic virus (retrovirus) type III (HTLV-III) and lymphadenopathy-associated virus (LAV).

HLA allele A human leukocyte antigen allele named using a unique four-, six-, or eight-letter or digit name.

HLA genotype Actual inherited alleles for HLA antigens.

HLA match The pairing or matching of a transplant donor and recipient based on HLA antigens.

HLA phenotype HLA genes expressed as proteins on cells.

Hodgkin lymphoma A major form of malignant lymphoma; also called *Hodgkin disease*.

homogeneous Uniform; the same. All of the individual cells or organisms are the same.

homogeneous enzyme immunoassay An assay requiring no separation steps based on the principle of a decrease in enzyme activity when specific antigen-antibody combinations occur.

homologous The same.

homozygous In genetics, when the genes for a trait on homologous (paired) chromosomes are the same.

human B-cell lymphotropic virus (HBLV) A herpes virus that can interact with HIV in a way that might increase the severity of HIV infection.

human chorionic gonadotropin (hCG) A hormone secreted by placental tissue.

human ehrlichiosis A tick-borne illness in the same family as Rocky Mountain spotted fever.

human gonadotropic hormone (hCG) A glycoprotein hormone secreted by the trophoblast of a developing embryo in early pregnancy.

human herpes virus 6 (HHV-6) A herpes virus that can interact with HIV in a way that might increase the severity of HIV infection.

human immunodeficiency virus (HIV) See HIV.

human leukocyte antigen (HLA) Antigen on the cell surface that identifies the cells as

belonging to a specific body, rather than being foreign substances.
human T-lymphotropic virus type III (HTLV-III) See HIV.
humoral Pertaining to any fluid or semifluid in the body.
humoral and cellular immunity Forms of defense against disease associated with antibodies or antigens.
humoral immunity (humoral-mediated immunity) A form of body defense against foreign substances represented by antibodies and other soluble extracellular factors in the blood and lymphatic fluid.
Hutchinsonian triad The characteristic manifestation of congenital syphilis. The three major features are notched teeth, interstitial keratitis, and nerve deafness.
hyaluronidase An enzyme that breaks down hyaluronic acid found in connective tissue; also called *spreading factor*.
hybridization (hybridize) Interaction between two single-strand nucleic acid molecules to form a double-strand molecule.
hybridoma A cell line created in vitro by fusion of two different cell types. A hybridoma is usually formed from lymphocyte or plasma cells, one of which is a tumor cell.
hydatid cyst A parasitic infestation by a tapeworm of the genus *Echinococcus*.
hydatidiform mole An abnormal condition of degenerated chorionic villi in the uterus.
hydrophilic Water-loving.
hydrophobic Water-hating.
hygiene hypothesis A supposition or proposed explanation that states that a lack of early childhood exposure to infectious agents, symbiotic microorganisms (such as the gut flora or probiotics), and parasites increases a person's susceptibility to allergic diseases by suppressing the natural development of the immune system.
hyperacute rejection A type of transplant rejection that occurs rapidly (minutes to hours) after transplantation because of the presence of antibodies to blood group ABO or HLA antigens.
hypercalcemia A marked increase in ionized calcium in the circulating blood.
hypergammaglobulinemia An increased gamma globulin fraction of plasma protein.
hyperkeratosis A condition of increased growth of the upper layer of the skin (epidermis) or overgrowth of the cornea.
hyperplastic Abnormally increased cell growth.
hypersensitivity An unpleasant or damaging condition of the body tissues caused by antigenic stimulation. Hypersensitivity reactions include allergies such as hay fever.
hypervariable region A part of an antibody molecule that enables the antibody to single out one antigen to attack.
hyperviscosity An increase in the thickness (viscosity) of substances such as blood plasma.
hyperviscosity syndrome A collection of symptoms resulting from increased resistance (viscosity) of the flow of blood in the circulation.
hypervolemia An increase in total blood volume.
hypocomplementemia A decrease or deficiency of complement in the blood circulation.
hypogammaglobulinemia A decrease in the gamma globulin fraction of plasma protein.
hypoplastic Defective or incomplete development of a tissue or an organ.
hypothalamus The portion of the brain beneath the thalamus at the base of the cerebrum that forms the floor and part of the walls of the third ventricle.

I

icteric Pertaining to icterus.
icterus Synonym for jaundice, the yellow appearance of the skin and mucous membranes caused by accumulation of bilirubin (a product of red cell breakdown).
idiopathic Pertaining to a disorder or disease without an identifiable external cause, or self-originated.
idiopathic SLE (idiopathic systemic lupus erythematosus) A form of the autoimmune disorder lupus with no known cause.
idiotope An epitope in the variable region of an antibody.
idiotype The antigenic characteristic of the antibody-variable region.
IFA See immunofluorescent assay.
IF-blocking (intrinsic factor) antibodies A type of antibody associated with pernicious anemia.
IgA The second most abundant immunoglobulin in serum; the predominant form in tears, saliva, and colostrum.
IgD An immunoglobulin found in B-cell membranes; thought to play a role in B-cell response to antigens.
IgE The immunoglobulin responsible for allergic reactions.
IgG The most abundant immunoglobulin in serum; responsible for protection against viruses and bacteria.
IgM The largest immunoglobulin molecule and the first antibody produced in response to an antigen.
iliac node A small, rounded structure located in the lower 60% of the small intestines, from the jejunum to the ileocecal valve or in the inguinal region.
immature B cell The receptor cell that is finally programmed for insertion of specific IgM molecules into the plasma membrane.
immediate early antigen A marker for Epstein-Barr virus infection in infectious mononucleosis.
immediate hypersensitivity A subset of the body's antibody-mediated mechanisms.
immune adherence The ability of phagocytic cells to bind complement-coated particles, such as bacteria.
immune complex The noncovalent combination of an antigen with its specific antibody. An immune complex can be small and soluble or large and precipitating, depending on the nature and proportion of the antigen and antibody.
immune response The reaction of the immune system to foreign antigens in the body.
immune senescence Aging of the immune system, particularly its effect on changes in lymphocyte development and function, especially in older adults.
immune status The ability of a host (an individual) to recognize and respond to foreign (nonself) substances (e.g., antigens).
immune system The structures (e.g., bone marrow, thymus, lymph nodes), cells (e.g., macrophages, lymphocytes), and soluble constituents of the circulating blood (e.g., complement) that allow the host to recognize and respond to foreign (nonself) substances, such as antigens.
immunity The process of being protected against foreign antigens.
immunization A process of exposing the body to specific antigens to stimulate immunity.
immunoassay A laboratory procedure for analyzing immunoglobulins.
immunoblot See western blot.
ImmunoCAP A method used to detect *Aspergillus niger* IgE in serum.
immunochromatographic Pertaining to an analytic method used in immunology.
immunocompetent (immunocompetent cells) The ability to mount an immune response. A host is able to recognize a foreign antigen and produce specific antigen-directed antibodies. The term refers to lymphocytes that acquire thymus-dependent characteristics, which allow them to function in an immune response.
immunocompromised Pertaining to the condition that occurs when the immune system is unable to defend itself because of existing conditions.
immunodeficiency A dysfunction in body defense mechanisms that causes a failure to detect foreign antigens and produce antibodies against these foreign (nonself) substances.
immunodeficiency disease A condition in which a defect exists in the ability to detect antigens and/or produce antibodies against foreign antigens.
immunodeficiency syndrome A condition in which the immune system is not responding in an expected fashion.
immunodiffusion A laboratory method for the quantitative study of antibodies (e.g., radial immunodiffusion [RID]) or qualitative identification of antigens (e.g., Ouchterlony technique); also called *double diffusion*. This classic technique is used to detect the presence of antibodies and determine their specificity by visualizing lines of identity (precipitin lines).
immunoelectrophoresis (IEP) Two-step procedure involving the electrical separation of proteins, followed by the linear diffusion (immunofixation) of antibodies into the electrophoretic gel from a trough that extends through the length of the gel adjacent to the electrophoretic path. The reactions produce precipitin arcs at positions of equivalence.
immunofixation electrophoresis (IFE) A procedure in which specific antibodies help produce sensitive and specific qualitative visual identification of paraproteins by electrophoretic position.
immunofluorescence A laboratory technique that uses a microscope to study antibodies tagged with fluorophore (light-emitting dyes).
immunofluorescent assay (IFA) A laboratory method that uses a fluorescent substance in immunologic studies. For example, particular antigens can be identified microscopically in

tissues or cells by the binding of a fluorescent (light-emitting) antibody conjugate.
immunogen A large organic molecule that is a protein or large polysaccharide and rarely, if ever, a lipid.
immunoglobulin (immune globulin; Ig) Protein produced by the immune system (i.e., antibodies); a synonym for antibody. The term has replaced the term gamma globulin because not all antibodies have gamma electrophoretic mobility. Immunoglobulins are divided into five classes: IgM, IgG, IgD, IgA, and IgE. IgG is the most abundant.
immunohematology The study of antigen and antibody as related to blood transfusions and associated blood conditions.
immunohistochemistry The use of labeled antibodies to detect tumor markers in stained tissue specimens directly.
immunologic Related to antigens and antibodies.
immunologic dysfunction See immunodeficiency disease.
immunologic tolerance Self-tolerance or the failure to mount an immune response to an antigen.
immunology The study of molecules, cells, organs, and systems responsible for the recognition and disposal of nonself materials and how they work or can be manipulated. All aspects of body defense, such as antigens and antibodies, allergy, and hypersensitivity, are included.
immunomodulators Substances that influence regulation of the immune system.
immunoperoxidase A direct examination method for staining of cells taken from lesions in patients with human herpes virus.
immunophenotyping Procedure for identifying cells according to the presence of surface antigen expression.
immunoproliferation Overexpansion of cells or their products related to the immune system.
immunoproliferative Disorders of the immune system.
immunoprophylaxis Prevention of an immune response.
immunoregulation Control of the immune system.
immunoregulatory cells Specific cells that influence the operation of the immune system.
immunosorbent A laboratory method that uses the absorption of antibodies by insoluble preparations of antigens.
immunosorbent agglutination assay (ISAGA) An assay for the detection of IgM antibodies against *Toxoplasma gondii*.
immunosuppression Prevention of the recognition of antigen and/or production of antibody by repressing the normal adaptive immune response with drugs, chemicals, or other means. This process is commonly necessary before and after bone marrow or solid organ transplantation or to alter a severe hypersensitivity reaction.
immunosuppressive agent A drug, chemical, or other mechanism that prevents the immune system from recognizing and responding to nonself.
immunosurveillance A mechanism whereby the body rids itself of abnormal or transformed cells.

immunotherapy Desensitization or stimulation of a patient's own immune system to fight a tumor.
immunotoxin Antibodies conjugated to toxins to help destroy cancer cells.
impetigo A skin infection caused by streptococci that begins as a papule.
in situ In place, or existing within the tissue itself.
in situ hybridization The binding of a nucleic acid probe to target DNA located within intact cells.
in vitro Outside the body (e.g., in a test tube).
in vitro agglutination inhibition The blocking of the formation of clumps (agglutination) as the principle of a laboratory assay.
in vivo Inside the living organism.
inactivated toxins Toxins produced by bacteria and viruses that have been killed and are no longer capable of causing disease.
inactivated vaccine (killed vaccine) A vaccine made from a whole microorganism (bacteria or virus) whose biologic ability to grow or reproduce is ended.
inactivation Blocking the activity of a substance (e.g., complement).
incomplete antibody Formerly used term that refers to IgG-type antibodies.
indirect allorecognition pathways Presentation of processed donor HLA peptides bound to HLA class II molecules to CD4+ lymphocytes. The result is antibody formation directed against the donor graft.
indirect fluorescent assay (IFA) Procedure used to detect homogeneous antigen plus antigen with antiimmunoglobulins using fluorescent microscopy.
indirect hemagglutination technique Laboratory method that uses erythrocytes passively coated with substances such as extracts of bacterial cells, rickettsiae, pathogenic fungi, protozoa, purified polysaccharides, or proteins to detect antibody; also called *passive hemagglutination technique*.
indirect immunofluorescent assay A method to identify antigen by using two antibodies: one specific to the antigen and one that is an antihuman immunoglobulin with a fluorescent tag.
indolent Silent, inactive or slow growing.
induction A therapeutic phase during which cells are exposed to a variety of drugs or radiation so that they can be destroyed.
infarction Tissue death; an area of tissue, such as heart muscle, that undergoes necrosis (tissue breakdown) because of a lack of oxygen from the circulating blood. A condition of oxygen deprivation may be caused by narrowing of blood vessels (stenosis) or blockage of the blood circulation in the vessel (occlusion).
infection A pathogenic condition caused by microorganisms (e.g., viruses, bacteria, fungi) that produce injurious effects.
infectious material Body fluids or excretory products, or nonhuman substances contaminated with body fluids, that contain disease-causing microorganisms.
infectious mononucleosis A benign lymphoproliferative disorder.

infectious waste Contaminated discarded products that can cause infectious disease.
inflammation Tissue reaction to injury caused by physical or chemical agents, including microorganisms. Symptoms include redness, tenderness, pain, and swelling.
inflammatory response See inflammation.
inguinal adenopathy Enlarged lymph nodes in the region of the groin.
inhibition immunofluorescent assay A blocking test in which an antigen is first exposed to unlabeled antibody and then to labeled antibody, and is finally washed and examined.
innate immune response (innate immune system) Nonspecific immune system.
innate immunity Natural or inborn resistance to infection after microorganisms have penetrated the first line of resistance; innate immune system.
innate resistance Natural or inborn ability to resist infection.
integrin A transmembrane glycoprotein receptor that mediates attachment between a cell and the tissues surrounding it.
integrins Proteins that function mechanically, by attaching the cell cytoskeleton to the extracellular matrix (ECM).
interferons Cytokines produced by T lymphocytes and other cell lines that inhibit viral synthesis or act as immune regulators.
interferon-α (IFN-α) A protein that may be an immunosuppressive agent important in controlling the immune response in a negative manner; originally called leukocyte interferon.
interferon-β (IFN-β) Originally called fibroblast interferon or B-cell stimulatory factor-2; now reclassified as interleukin-6 (IL-6).
interleukin (IL) Cytokine or chemical messenger produced by leukocytes that affects the inflammatory process through an increase in soluble factors or cells.
interleukin-1 (IL-1) A cytokine whose most prominent biologic activity is activation of resting T cells; originally called lymphocyte-activating factor.
interleukin-2 (IL-2) A cytokine best known for its ability to initiate proliferation or clonal expansion of activated T cells. IL-2 also dramatically enhances the cytolytic activity of a population of natural (lymphokine-activated) killer cells against certain tumor cells; originally called T-cell growth factor.
interleukin-3 (IL-3) A cytokine that principally promotes the growth of early hematopoietic cell lines; originally called multicolony-stimulating factor (mCSF).
interleukin-4 (IL-4) A growth factor for the early activation of resting B cells that influences the synthesis of some immunoglobulins; originally called B-cell–stimulating factor-1.
interleukin-5 (IL-5) Shares many activities with IL-4 but is not active on early lymphoid cells; originally called T-cell–replacing factor or B-cell growth factor-2.
interleukin-6 (IL-6) A cytokine that induces secretion of immunoglobulin and is a major factor in induction of the acute-phase reaction; originally called interferon-β2 or B-cell–stimulating factor-2.

interleukin-7 (IL-7) A cytokine that stimulates early B-cell progenitor cells; originally called lymphopoietin-1.
interleukin-8 (IL-8) An inflammatory cytokine that is chemotactic for neutrophils and T cells; originally called monocyte-derived neutrophil chemotactic factor.
interleukin-9 (IL-9) A cytokine that is a potent lymphocyte growth factor.
interleukin-10 (IL-10) A cytokine that inhibits cytokine synthesis in various cells.
interleukin-11 (IL-11) A regulator of hematopoietic stroma that stimulates the production of megakaryocyte and myeloid progenitors; increases the number of immunoglobulin-secreting B lymphocytes.
interleukin-12 (IL-12) Enhances the activity of cytotoxic effector T cells; acts as a growth factor for natural (lymphokine-activated) killer cells and for activated T cells of the CD4+ and CD8+ subsets.
interleukin-13 (IL-13) Has many biological effects similar to those of IL-4; major action on macrophages is to inhibit their activation and antagonize interferon-γ (IFN-γ).
interleukin-14 (IL-14) Acts as a B-cell growth factor (BCGF).
interleukin-15 (IL-15) Biologically similar to IL-2. Endogenous IL-15 is a key condition for IFN-γ synthesis.
interleukin-16 (IL-16) Acts as a T-cell chemoattractant and participates in the regulation of many cytokines (e.g., IL-1, IL-4, IL-6, IL-10, IL-12, IFN-γ). Histamine and serotonin increase the production of IL-17. It mimics many of the proinflammatory actions of tumor necrosis factor-α (TNF-α) and TNF-β.
interleukin-17 (IL-17) Associated with allergic reactions.
interleukin-18 (IL-18) Acts as a synergist with IL-12 in some of their effects, especially in the induction of IFN-γ production and inhibition of angiogenesis. It stimulates the production of IFN-γ by natural killer cells and T cells and synergizes with IL-12 in this response.
interleukin-19 (IL-19) Has similar biological function to that of IL-10; regulates the functions of macrophages and suppresses the activities of helper T cells (Th1 and Th2).
interleukin-20 (IL-20) Plays an important role in skin inflammations.
interleukin-21 (IL-21) Regulates hematopoiesis and immune response and influences the development of lymphocytes; similar to the actions of IL-2 and IL-15 in regard to the antitumor defense system.
interleukin-22 (IL-22) Similar to IL-10 but does not prevent the production of proinflammatory cytokines through monocytes.
interleukin-23 (IL-23) Cytokine that shares some in vivo functions with IL-12, including the activation of STAT-4 (signal transducer and activator of transcription factor 4).
interleukin-25 (IL-25) A secreted bone marrow stroma-derived growth factor; also called *SF-20*.
internal defense system Defense mechanism in the body in which cells and soluble factors play essential roles.

interstitial pneumonitis An inflammation situated between or in the interspaces of the lung tissue.
intradermal Pertaining to forcing a liquid into a part of the body, as into the subcutaneous tissues, vascular tree, or organ.
intraerythrocytic Inside of a red blood cell.
intrahepatic cholestasis Failure of bile to flow in the liver.
intraleukocytic morulae Mulberry-shaped aggregates (balls) seen inside of white blood cells in ehrlichiosis.
intranasal spray application Treatment using a substance sprayed into the nostrils.
intraperitoneal fetal transfusion (IPT) Administration of blood to a fetus (unborn infant) via the abdominal cavity.
intrarenal obstruction Blockage within the kidney.
intrathecal Pertaining to something introduced into or occurring in the space under the arachnoid membrane of the brain or spinal cord.
intrathecal synthesis A process whereby something is introduced into or produced in the space under the arachnoid membrane of the brain or spinal cord.
intratubular precipitation Formation of a solid mass from soluble substances in the tubules of the kidney.
intrauterine Within the uterus.
intravascular coagulation Formation of a clot within a vessel (i.e., blood vessels of the circulatory system).
intravascular destruction An alternate pathway for erythrocyte breakdown, which normally accounts for less than 10% of red cell destruction.
intravascular hemolysis An alternate pathway of red cell destruction in which the cells are lysed in the vessels of the circulatory system.
intravascular thrombosis The formation of a clot in a blood vessel.
intravenous Pertaining to the administration of drugs or fluids directly into the veins.
intravenous urography Radiologic study of any part of the urinary tract by the administration of an opaque medium through a vein, which is rapidly excreted in the urine.
intrinsic coagulation mechanism Initial stage of blood coagulation that can be activated by antigen-antibody complexes.
intrinsic factor (IF) A glycoprotein synthesized and secreted by the parietal cells of the mucosa in the fundus region of the stomach in human beings. In a healthy state, the amounts of IF secreted by the stomach greatly exceed the quantities required to bind ingested cobalamin in its coenzyme forms.
intrinsic factor (IF) antibodies Antibodies to IF-factor.
intron A polynucleotide sequence that does not code for protein synthesis.
ischemic A decrease in the blood supply to a bodily organ, tissue, or part caused by constriction or obstruction of the blood vessels; causes death of cells not receiving oxygen.
islet cell An insulin-producing cell in the pancreas.

isoagglutinin An antibody type that reacts (agglutinates) with erythrocytes of other persons of the same species; also called *isohemagglutinin*.
isoelectric focusing Separation of molecules on the basis of their charge. Each molecule migrates to the point in the pH gradient at which it has no net charge.
isoimmune Possessing antibodies to antigens of the same system.
isotype Genetic variation in a family of proteins or peptides so that every member of the species will have each isotype of the family represented in its genome (e.g., immunoglobulin classes).
isotypic variant The heavy-chain constant region structure associated with the different classes and subclasses. Isotopic variants are present in all healthy members of a species.

J

jaundice A yellowish appearance of the skin, sclerae, and body excretions; see also icterus.
juvenile idiopathic arthritis A form of arthritis (joint inflammation) seen in young adults with no known cause.

K

Kahler disease An alternate term for multiple myeloma.
Kaposi sarcoma A rare, malignant, metastasizing disorder chiefly involving the skin. An increased incidence of this malignancy has been observed in patients with AIDS.
kappa (κ) chain One of two types of immunoglobulin light chains present in two-thirds of all immunoglobulin molecules.
keratinization Development of or conversion into keratin, an extremely tough scleroprotein found in structures such as hair and nails.
kernicterus Deposition of increased bilirubin, a red cell breakdown product, in lipid-rich nervous tissue such as the brain, which can produce mental retardation or death in the newborn. This condition can occur when circulating plasma bilirubin levels reach 20 mg/dL in a full-term infant and a lower level in a premature infant.
killer T cells Subset of lymphocytes that can kill cancer cells and cells infected with viruses, fungi, or certain bacteria; also referred to as *cytotoxic T cells* and *cytotoxic lymphocytes* (CTLs).
kinetochore A term for the centromere, the constricted area of the chromosome that demarcates the upper and lower arms of the structure.
kinetoplast An accessory structure/body found in many protozoa; also called *micronucleus*.
kinin A small, biologically active peptide.
kinin system A series of serum peptides sequentially activated to cause vasodilation and increased vascular permeability.
Kleihauer-Betke test A testing method based on the differences in solubility between adult and fetal hemoglobin. The test is performed on a maternal blood specimen for the detection of fetal-maternal hemorrhage.
Kupffer cell A phagocytic type of cell that lines the minute blood vessels (sinusoids) of the liver.

L

lag period The period between a stimulus (e.g., antigenic stimulation) and a reaction (e.g., immunoglobulin response).
lambda (λ) light chain One of two types of immunoglobulin light chains that are present in about one-third of all immunoglobulin molecules.
Langerhans cell A macrophage found in the skin.
large granular lymphocyte (LGL) Synonym for natural killer (NK) cell. About 75% of LGLs function as NK cells and appear to account fully for the NK activity in mixed cell populations.
laser Acronym for *light amplification by stimulated emission of radiation*; used in flow cell cytometry to identify cells.
latent Hidden or inactive.
latent infection Persistent infection characterized by periods of reactivation of the signs and symptoms of the disease.
latex agglutination A technique similar to hemagglutination except that smaller, antigen-coated latex particles are substituted for erythrocytes for the detection of antibodies. Antibodies can be absorbed into the latex particles by binding to the Fc region of antibodies, leaving the Fab region free to interact with antigens present in the patient specimen.
lattice formation The establishment of crosslinks between sensitized particles such as erythrocytes.
lattice hypothesis A theoretical step in the production of agglutination.
lecithin A waxy phospholipid.
lecithin pathway A pathway for activation of complement based on the attachment of mannose-binding protein to components of bacterial cell walls.
lesion A localized pathologic change in a bodily organ or tissue, such as a cut, abrasion, or sore.
leukocyte A white blood cell (WBC) that functions in antigen recognition and antibody formation.
leukocyte integrin A glycoprotein on the cell surface of white blood cells.
leukocytosis A marked increase in the total circulating white blood cell concentration.
leukopenia A marked decrease in the total circulating white blood cell concentration.
leukotriene Class of compounds that mediate the inflammatory functions of leukocytes. These substances are a collection of metabolites of arachidonic acid, with powerful pharmacologic effects.
ligand A linking or binding molecule.
ligase chain reaction (LCR) A means of increasing signal probes through the use of an enzyme called ligase, which joins two pairs of probes only after they have bound to a complementary target sequence.
light (L) chain A small chain in an immunoglobulin molecule that is bound to the larger chain by disulfide bonds. There are two types of light chains, kappa and lambda.
light-chain disease (LCD) A dysproteinemia of the monoclonal gammopathy type. In LCD, only kappa or lambda monoclonal light chains, or Bence Jones proteins, are produced.
linear epitope Amino acids that follow one another on a single chain that act as a key antigenic site; linear antigenic determinant.
lipemia Visibly cloudy blood serum.
lipemic Pertaining to lipemia.
lipopolysaccharide (LPS) The major component of some Gram-negative bacterial cell walls that protects them from phagocytosis but activates C3 directly. LPS can also act as a B-cell mitogen.
liposome A particle of fatlike substance held in suspension in tissues.
liposome-enhanced (liposome-enhanced testing) A variation of latex testing.
live, attenuated vaccine A vaccine whose biological activity has not been inactivated, but whose ability to cause disease has been weakened.
localized Confined to a specific area.
localized inflammatory response A tissue reaction confined to a specific area. This response is caused by physical or chemical agents, including microorganisms. The manifestations of the response include redness, tenderness, pain, and swelling.
long terminal redundancy (LTR) A structure that exists at each end of the proviral genome and plays an important role in the control of viral gene expression and the integration of the provirus into the DNA of the host.
lupus anticoagulants Antibodies against substances in the lining of cells. These substances prevent blood clotting in a test tube. They are called phospholipids. People with antibodies to phospholipids (PLs) may have an overly high risk of forming blood clots. Circulating anticoagulants are believed to be associated with the presence of false-positive serologic test results for syphilis.
lupus erythematosus An autoimmune disorder.
luteal phase A period of the menstrual cycle.
luteinizing hormone A hormone associated with ovulation.
Lyme borreliosis A multisystem illness that primarily involves the skin, nervous system, heart, and joints.
Lyme disease A mosquito-borne infectious disease.
lymphadenopathy Disease of the lymph nodes.
lymphoblast The most immature stage of the lymphocyte type of leukocyte.
lymphocyte A small white blood cell found in lymph nodes and circulating blood. Two major populations of lymphocytes are recognized, T and B cells.
lymphocyte recirculation Process that enables lymphocytes to come into contact with processed foreign antigens and disseminate antigen-sensitized memory cells throughout the lymphoid system.
lymphocyte-activating factor See interleukin-1.
lymphocytopenia A severe decrease in the total number of lymphocytes in the peripheral blood.
lymphocytosis A significant increase in the total number of lymphocytes in the peripheral blood.
lymphokine A soluble protein mediator released by sensitized lymphocytes on contact with an antigen. See soluble mediator.
lymphokine-activated killer (LAK) cells A population of natural killer (NK) cells with enhanced cytolytic activity resulting from the addition of IL-2.
lymphoma Solid malignant tumor of the lymph nodes and associated tissues or bone marrow.
lymphopoietin-1 See interleukin-7.
lymphoproliferative disorder A group of diseases characterized by the proliferation of lymphoid tissues and/or lymphocytes.
lymphosarcoma Malignant neoplastic disorders of the lymphoid tissues, excluding Hodgkin disease.
lyse (lysing) To break apart or dissolve.
lysis Irreversible leakage of cell contents that occurs after membrane damage.
lysozyme (muramidase) An enzyme secreted by macrophages that attacks the cell walls of some bacteria.
lytic Refers to lysis.

M

M protein See monoclonal protein.
macroglobulin A high-molecular-weight protein of the globulin type.
macroglobulinemia See Waldenström primary macroglobulinemia.
macromolecular complex The reaction between the protein being assayed and a specific antiserum.
macrophage A large mononuclear phagocytic cell of the tissues that exists as a wandering or fixed type; lines the capillaries and sinuses of organs such as the bone marrow, spleen, and lymph nodes. This cell phagocytizes, processes, and presents antigens to T cells and is also responsible for removing damaged tissue, cells, bacteria, and other substances from the host.
macrophage migration inhibitory factor (MIF) A lymphocyte product that is chemotactic for monocytes. Other similar factors stimulate monocyte and macrophage functions.
macular lesion A discolored unraised (flat) spot on the skin.
maculopapular A lesion with macular and papular characteristics.
maintenance of self-tolerance The continuing ability to recognize self-antigens.
major histocompatibility complex (MHC) A genetic region in human beings and other mammals responsible for signaling between lymphocytes and antigen-bearing cells. It is also the major determinant of transplant compatibility (or rejection).
malaise A general feeling of tiredness or discomfort.
malignant (malignancy) Cancerous.
malignant neoplasia (malignant neoplasm) A cancerous new growth.
manifestation The development of the signs and symptoms of a disease or disorder.
mannose-binding lectin A pattern recognition molecule of the innate immune system.
mannose-binding lectin pathway A complement activation pathway.
margination The process of white blood cells clinging to the lining of blood vessels.
mass spectrometry An analytic technique that identifies the chemical composition of a

specimen on the basis of the mass-to-charge ratio of charged particles.
mast cell A large tissue cell with basophilic granules containing vasoactive amines and heparin. When the cell is damaged, the granules release these inflammatory mediators, which increase vascular permeability and allow complement and phagocytic cells to enter damaged tissues from the circulating blood.
Material Data Sheet (MDS) (previously called *Material Safety Data Sheet* [MSDS]) A required informational sheet that describes various characteristics and cautions related to a product.
mature B cell A cell concerned with synthesis of circulating antibodies.
mean Statistical (arithmetic) average.
median A numerical value separating the halves of a sample; half the numbers in a series are above the median and half the numbers in the series are below the median.
mediastinum The tissues and organs such as the heart, trachea, esophagus, and lymph nodes that separate the sternum in the front (ventral side) from the vertebral column in the back (dorsal side) of the body.
medullary Refers to the middle of something; pertaining to a medulla, bone marrow, or spinal cord.
megakaryocyte A platelet cell.
megakaryocytic thrombocytopenic purpura A severe deficiency of cells (e.g., thrombocytes and platelets) related to blood clotting that causes large purple discolorations of the skin.
melanocyte A cell that produces melanin, the dark pigment normally found in structures such as the hair, eyes, and skin. It can also occur abnormally in certain tumors, called *melanomas*.
membrane attack complex (MAC) A unit created by action of the complement components (C7–C9) that punctures the wall of a cell and allows cytoplasm and organelles to flow out.
memory The immunologic response to an antigenic stimulus that usually leaves the immune system changed.
memory cells Long-lived T or B lymphocytes that have been stimulated by a specific antigen and recall prior antigen exposure.
meningoencephalitis An inflammation of the brain and its membranous covering (the meninges).
meningovascular A term that refers to the blood vessels of the covering of the brain and spinal cord (meninges).
meniscus The upside-down, half-moon shape of aqueous liquids in a glass vessel such as a pipette or flask.
mentation Mental activity.
mesothelium A type of epithelium, originally derived from the mesoderm lining the primitive embryonic body cavity, that becomes the serous membrane of body surfaces, such as the peritoneum (membrane viscera and lining of the abdominal cavity, except the kidneys), pleura (membrane covering the lungs), walls of the thoracic cavity (chest and diaphragm), and pericardium (sac enclosing the heart).
metastasis Spreading of malignant cells from the primary site of malignancy.

MHC See major histocompatibility complex.
microbial antigen A carbohydrate structure on a cell wall of a microorganism.
microbiology The study of microorganisms.
microbiota Microorganisms that inhabit the mammalian gut.
microencephaly Abnormally small brain.
microglia The phagocytic cells of the brain, thought to be derived from incoming blood monocytes.
microplate A compact plate of rigid or flexible plastic with multiple wells.
microspheres Tiny (microscopic) spheres that can carry vaccines or drugs and can pass easily through the body's tissues.
mitogen A substance that stimulates cell division (mitosis).
mixed-field agglutination An observation of some cells or particles clumping together whereas others do not clump.
mobility The ability of specific and nonspecific cells of the immune system to circulate.
mode The most frequent number in a group of numbers.
molecular mimicry Similarity between an infectious agent and a self-antigen that causes antibody formation in response to the infectious agent to crossreact with self.
molecule The smallest unit of a specific chemical substance that can exist alone.
monoclonal Genetically identical cells produced from the same original cell.
monoclonal antibody (MAb) Purified immunoglobulin produced by cells cloned from a single fusion-type hybridoma cell. Monoclonal antibodies are directed against antigens derived from a single cell line.
monoclonal antiserum (pl., antisera) Specific antibodies directed against antigens.
monoclonal gammopathy A dysproteinemia in which the level of a single type of immunoglobulin is increased. This immunoglobulin is secreted by a single clone of plasma cells.
monoclonal protein A protein characterized by a narrow peak or a localized band on electrophoresis, by a thickened bowed arc on immunoelectrophoresis, and by a localized band on immunofixation; also called *M protein* or *paraprotein*.
monocyte A type of leukocyte found in the peripheral blood.
monocyte-macrophage Related cell types.
monocytic Referring to monocyte(s).
monogenetic The theory that all living organisms are descended from a single cell or organism.
monokine A soluble protein mediator.
mononuclear cell A cell type that includes monocytes, promyelocytes, myelocytes, and blasts.
mononuclear phagocyte system (MPS) The body defense system composed of macrophages and a network of specialized cells of the spleen, thymus, and other lymphoid tissues; formerly called the reticuloendothelial system (RES).
monospecific Directed against one antigen site.
monovalent or monovalent receptor An antigen with only one antigenic determinant.
morbidity A condition of being diseased; the ratio of sick to healthy persons or the number of cases of a specific illness in a designated population.
morphologic The appearance of a structure.
mortality The rate of death or ratio of the number of deaths to living individuals in a designated population.
mucopurulent Refers to an exudate containing mucus and pus.
mucosal-associated lymphoid tissue (MALT) Lymphoid tissue found in the lining of the respiratory, gastrointestinal, and genitourinary tracts.
multimolecular lattice Crosslinkages of molecules.
multiple myeloma A malignant disorder of plasma cells, also known as *plasma cell myeloma* or *Kahler disease*.
multiple sclerosis (MS) An autoimmune disorder of the myelin sheath of nerve cell axons.
multipotential stem cell (MSC) Precursor cells in the bone marrow capable of differentiating into various blood cell (hematopoietic) types.
multivalent Having many charges.
murine hybridoma The fusion product of a malignant and normal cell that produces large quantities of monoclonal antibodies.
myalgia Pain or tenderness in the muscles.
myelin Covering of axons and other areas of the nervous system, such as the sheath of the spinal cord.
myelitis An inflammation of the spinal cord or bone marrow.
myeloablation Total destruction of bone marrow.
myeloma cell Plasma cells derived from malignant tumor strains.
myeloma clone A group of neoplastic cells that are descendants of a single neoplastic cell.
myeloma kidney disorders Abnormalities of the kidney associated with the neoplastic disorder multiple myeloma.
myelomatosis A term for multiple myeloma.
myeloperoxidase An important enzyme in the process of phagocytosis.
myelosuppressive An action to depress the growth of bone marrow cells.
myocarditis An inflammation of the cardiac muscle tissue.
myopericarditis Inflammation around the heart muscle.
myosin One of the two main contractile proteins found in muscles.

N

naked DNA vaccine A vaccine made up of deoxyribonucleic acid that is not encased or encapsulated.
nasopharyngeal carcinoma A malignancy involving the nose and throat.
natural immune system See innate immune response.
natural killer (NK) cells A population of effector lymphocytes that produce mediators as such interferon and IL-2; previously called null cells.
natural resistance Body resistance that is innate or inborn.
natural T regulatory (T_{reg}) cells A subclass of CD4+ T lymphocytes that plays a key role in

establishing tolerance to self-antigens, tumor cells, transplant antigens, and allergens.
necrosis The death of cells or a localized group of cells.
necrotic Dead.
necrotizing fasciitis Dying covering of muscles.
necrotizing vasculitis Inflammation of a vessel (e.g., blood vessel) that results in tissue destruction.
negative selection The process whereby T lymphocytes that are capable of responding to self-antigens are destroyed in the thymus gland.
neoantigens New antigens.
neonatal FC receptor A receptor involved in the transport of IgG from the maternal circulation across the placental barrier and the transfer of maternal IgG across the intestine in neonates.
neonatal lupus An autoimmune disorder in a newborn.
neonatal septicemia Systemic disease caused by pathogenic microorganisms or their toxins in the blood of an infant up to 4 weeks old.
neonate An infant up to 4 weeks old.
neoplasia (neoplastic) Referring to new abnormal tissue growth.
neoplasm Any new and abnormal tissue, such as a tumor.
nephelometry A laboratory assay method based on the measurement of the turbidity of particles in suspension. A nephelometer can be used for assays such as quantitating immunoglobulin concentrations in serum.
nephritis An inflammation of the kidney.
nephritogenic An agent or a microorganism capable of causing an inflammation of the kidney.
nephrolithiasis A disorder characterized by the formation of a kidney stone.
nephropathy Any inflammatory, degenerative, or sclerotic disease of the kidneys.
nephrosis A condition of the kidneys, particularly tubular degeneration, without the signs and symptoms of inflammation.
nephrotic syndrome A disorder of the kidneys characterized by a decreased concentration of albumin in the circulating blood, marked edema (swelling), increased protein levels in the urine (proteinuria), and increased susceptibility to infection.
nephrotoxic Refers to an agent, such as a specific toxin, that is destructive to kidney cells.
NETS Neutrophil extracellular traps.
neuralgia Acute pain radiating along the course of a nerve.
neurologic sequelae Morbid nervous system signs and symptoms that follow or are caused by a disease.
neurotoxic cytokine A substance able to destroy nervous tissue.
neutralization Procedure similar to complement fixation that can be used only when the antibody being measured is directed against a hemolysin (bacterial toxin capable of directly lysing red blood cells).
neutropenia A marked decrease in the neutrophil type of leukocytes.
neutrophil A granulocyte-containing type of leukocyte.
neutrophil chemotactic factor A preformed mediator whose function is to attract neutrophils to an inflammatory area.

neutrophil extracellular traps (NETs) The processed chromatin bound to granular and selected cytoplasmic proteins that can immobilize or kill invading microorganisms.
next-generation sequencing (NGS) A new form of molecular testing.
Niemann-Pick disease A qualitative disorder of monocytes-macrophages that is classified as a lipid storage disease.
noncompetitive assay or noncompetitive enzyme assay (immunoassay) An assay in which an excess of binding sites is present in order for all the specified analytes in the specimen to be bound and measured.
nonhistone (nonhistone proteins) In chromatin, those proteins that remain after the histones have been removed.
non-Hodgkin lymphoma (NHL) A condition of solid malignant tumors of the lymph nodes and associated tissues or bone marrow that is not of the Hodgkin's type.
nonintact Broken or disrupted, such as a cut in the skin.
nonmicrobial antigen A structure not related to microorganisms.
nonself Recognition of foreign material in body defenses; antigenically dissimilar from self.
nonsymptomatic An abnormal condition, such as an infectious disease, that does not manifest the signs and symptoms of the disorder.
nontreponemal antibodies (antibody assays) Antibodies that are not formed against *Treponema pallidum*. Serologic assays for syphilis that detect antibody to cardiolipin and are not specific to antitreponemal antibody are nontreponemal assays.
nontrophoblastic neoplasms A new growth that does not arise from abnormal trophoblast (embryonic) cells that grows inside the uterus after conception.
nonwaived assays Testing that requires qualified laboratory personnel for performance; does not include over-the-counter types of tests.
nonwaived testing A form of testing that requires compliance with governmental standards.
normal biota or normal flora Microorganisms that normally inhabit areas of the body such as the skin, mucous membranes, and intestinal tract; also called *normal biota*.
normal values See reference range.
normocytic normochromic anemia A deficiency of erythrocytes. However, the erythrocytes present in the circulation are of normal size and color.
Northern blot A molecular biology technique similar to the Southern blot, except that messenger RNA (mRNA) from the specimen is separated and blotted. If specific RNA is present, the radiolabel can be detected.
nosocomial transmission Pertaining to a hospital; a nosocomial infection is a hospital-acquired infection.
NSAID Nonsteroidal antiinflammatory drug.
nucleic acid probe A short strand of DNA or RNA of a known sequence used to identify a complementary nucleic acid strand in a patient sample.

nucleic acid sequence–based amplification (NASBA) A technique for amplifying RNA by first making a DNA copy and then making RNA transcripts from this template.
nucleocapsid Nucleic acid and surrounding protein coat of a virus.
nucleocapsid protein Coating around virus genetic material. Nonstructural nucleocapsid protein is a marker of HBV replication.
nucleotides DNA makeup of repeating bases (adenine-thymine, cytosine-uracil) that are linked together in a spiral helix.
null cell See natural killer cells.

O

occlusive Blocking.
Occupational Safety and Health Administration (OSHA) A government regulatory agency that helps ensure safe and healthful working conditions.
oligonucleotide probe A small portion of a single string of nucleotides used to detect the presence of a complementary nucleic acid sequence.
oligonucleotide Short nucleic acid polymers usually made up of 13 to 25 nucleotides.
oncofetal protein Gene product whose level is increased in malignant transformation.
oncogene A transforming gene of cellular origin found in retroviruses and associated with acute leukemias.
oncogenic Associated with tumor formation.
oncology The study of malignancy (diagnosis and treatment).
oncopeptidomics Protein profiling in cancer patients to determine the presence of new tumor markers or proteins that are consistent with cancer.
oocyst The encysted form of a fertilized gamete occurring in certain sporozoa; an immature ovum.
opportunistic infection A microbial disease that infects a debilitated host.
opsonin A chemical substance that binds to antigens and increases the rate and quality of action by phagocytes to destroy invading organisms.
opsonin effect The positive impact of the chemical substance, opsonin, on phagocytosis.
opsonization A process in which the complement component C3b is attached to a particle, which promotes the adherence of phagocytic cells because of the C3 receptors. Antibody, if present, augments this by binding to Fc receptors.
oropharynx The part of the throat between the soft palate and upper edge of the epiglottis.
osmosis The movement of water through a semipermeable membrane.
osmotic-cytolytic reaction or osmotic lysis Rupture of a cell caused by water intrusion that creates pressure on the cellular membrane.
osteoclast A giant multinucleated cell formed in the bone marrow of growing bones. This cell is associated with reabsorption and removal of unwanted tissue.
osteomyelitis An inflammation of bone or bone marrow.
osteonecrosis Accelerated destruction of bone tissue.

osteoporosis Increased porosity of bone that causes softening and thinning of the bone.
otitis media Inflammation of the middle ear.
Ouchterlony double diffusion A classic gel precipitation method in which antigen and antibody diffuse out from wells cut into the gel. The pattern indicates whether antigens are identical.
oxidative burst A state of increased oxygen consumption in phagocytic cells in which generated oxygen radicals kill engulfed (phagocytized) bacteria or parasites.

P

p24 A structural core antigen that is part of the human immunodeficiency virus (HIV).
p53 **gene or** *tp53* **gene** The gene that regulates the cell cycle.
PAMPs See pathogen-associated molecular patterns.
pancreatitis An inflammation of the pancreas.
papilloma Polyp of epithelial surfaces.
papule A small, solid, elevated lesion of the skin.
paracortical Around the cortex (outer portion) of an organ or gland.
paraprotein See monoclonal protein.
parenchymal Referring to the functional constituents of an organ as opposed to the framework (stroma).
parenteral Administered subcutaneously (beneath the skin), intramuscularly, or intravenously.
parotid gland The largest of the three salivary glands, located near the ear.
paroxysmal cold hemoglobinuria (PCH) A form of destruction of erythrocytes (red blood cells) caused by an IgG protein that reacts with the erythrocytes in colder parts of the body and subsequently causes complement components to bind to erythrocytes irreversibly. It is typically seen as an acute transient condition secondary to viral infection.
paroxysmal nocturnal hemoglobinuria (PNH) A disorder in which the patient's erythrocytes act as a complement activator. The activation of complement results in excessive lysis of the patient's erythrocytes.
passenger mutations Genetic mutations that do not impart a selective growth advantage.
passive hemagglutination technique (passive agglutination assay) See indirect hemagglutination technique.
passive immunity Temporary immune protection resulting from the transfer of antibodies from another individual who has actively formed antibodies; for example transfer from a mother to her unborn child. Also, it can be a transfer of lymphocytes from another individual known to be immune to a specific antigen.
passive immunodiffusion A precipitation reaction in a gel medium in which an antigen-antibody combination can result because of diffusion.
pathogen A disease-causing microorganism or agent.
pathogen-associated molecular patterns (PAMPs) Antigens on a few large groups of microorganisms.
pathogenesis The origin of disease.

pathogenic (pathogenicity) The disease-producing potential of a microorganism (pathogenicity).
pathologic Disease-causing.
pattern recognition receptors Receptors of the innate immune system that recognize pathogen-associated molecular patterns (PAMPs). Also called *pathogen recognition receptors*.
PCR Polymerase chain reaction.
peptide Short polymer of amino acid monomers linked by peptide bonds.
percutaneous (parenteral) Infused into a blood vessel.
perforation A hole or break in the wall or membrane of an organ or body structure.
periarteritis nodosa An inflammation of the layers of small and medium-sized arteries. This condition is manifested by a variety of systemic signs and symptoms, including febrile manifestations.
pericarditis An inflammation of the serous membrane lining of the sac surrounding the heart and origins of the great blood vessels.
perifollicular Around a follicle.
perinatal The period preceding, during, or after birth.
perineal region The external region between the vulva and anus in the female or between the scrotum and anus in the male.
peripheral blood stem cell (PBSC) A progenitor cell or the earliest form of an undifferentiated blood cell.
peripheral tolerance A process involving mature lymphocytes that occurs in the blood circulation.
peritonitis An inflammation of the serous membrane covering the intestines, abdominal organs (viscera), and abdominal cavity.
pernicious anemia An erythrocytic disorder associated with defective vitamin B_{12} uptake.
personal protective equipment (PPE) Clothing or accessories worn to protect against or reduce the risk of transmission of infectious agents.
pertussis Whooping cough.
petechiae Small, purple hemorrhagic spots on the skin or mucous membranes.
phagocyte Any cell capable of engulfing and destroying foreign particles, such as bacteria.
phagocytic Capable of engulfment.
phagocytosis A form of endocytosis. This important body defense mechanism is the process whereby specialized cells engulf and destroy foreign particles, such as microorganisms or damaged cells. Macrophages and segmented neutrophils (PMNs) are the most important phagocytic cells.
phagolysosome A vacuole (secondary lysosome) formed by the fusion of a phagosome and primary lysosome(s) in which microorganisms are killed and digested.
phagosome A membrane-bound vesicle in a phagocyte containing the engulfed material.
pharyngeal pouch An embryonic structure.
pharyngitis An inflammation of the throat.
pharynx The throat.
Phase I trials The earliest stage of drug approval testing.

Phase IV trials A latter stage of drug approval testing.
phenotype Visual expression of genetic makeup.
phlebotomy A procedure in which blood is drawn from a blood vessel.
photometrically A type of laboratory measuring system using light.
photomultiplier tube A vacuum tube that is an extremely sensitive detector of ultraviolet light.
photon A basic unit of radiation.
phototherapy A process that uses ultraviolet light to accelerate the breakdown of bilirubin that has abnormally accumulated in the skin.
phytohemagglutinin A specific substance, a lectin, that is derived from plants and has the ability to agglutinate erythrocytes.
picornavirus A single-strand RNA virus.
pipetting A method of measuring and transferring liquids via a calibrated tube.
plasma The straw-colored fluid component of blood in circulating or anticoagulated blood.
plasma cell A type of leukocyte, normally found in a low percentage in the bone marrow, that produces immunoglobulins.
plasma cell dyscrasias Abnormalities involving plasma cells.
plasma cell myeloma (plasma cell dyscrasia) See multiple myeloma.
plasmacytoid Resembling or similar to a plasma cell.
plasmacytoid lymphocyte A cell that resembles a plasma cell.
plasmin A proteolytic enzyme with the ability to dissolve formed fibrin clots.
plasminogen The inactive precursor to plasmin, which is converted to plasmin by the action of substances such as urokinase.
plasmodium A genus of parasitic protozoa (e.g., *Plasmodium vivax*).
platelet factor 3 An important blood coagulation factor associated with thrombocytes (platelets).
pleiotropy Many different actions of a single cytokine. It may affect the activities of more than one type of cell and have more than one type of effect on the same cell.
pleura The membrane covering the lungs, walls of the thoracic cavity (chest), and diaphragm.
pleuritis An inflammation of the serous membrane lining, the pleura.
pluripotent See multipotential stem cells.
PMN See polymorphonuclear leukocyte.
Pneumocystis jiroveci A protozoan that causes interstitial plasma cell pneumonia. This microorganism is commonly observed as an opportunistic pathogen in patients with AIDS; formerly called *Pneumocystis carinii*.
point-of-care testing (POCT) A term used to designate laboratory testing at or near the patient.
pol **gene** A gene of a retrovirus (e.g., HIV) that encodes for reverse transcriptase, endonuclease, and protease activities.
polyagglutinable RBCs Capable of reacting with many red blood cells.
polyarthritis Inflammation of several joints.
polyclonal antiserum (pl., antisera) Antibody directed against more than one antigen.

polyclonal gammopathy A dysproteinemia in which the products of a number of different cell types are demonstrated.
polyendocrinopathy A disease condition that involves several endocrine glands.
polymerase chain reaction (PCR) A molecular biology technique that uses amplification of low levels of specific DNA sequences in a sample to reach the threshold of detection. The reaction products are hybridized to a radiolabeled DNA segment complementary to a short sequence of the amplified DNA. After electrophoresis, the radiolabeled product of specific size is detected by autoradiography.
polymerization (polymerize) Coming together of many molecules.
polymorphonuclear leukocyte (PMN) A short-lived scavenger blood cell whose granules contain powerful bactericidal enzymes; also called *polymorphonuclear neutrophil leukocyte*.
polymyositis Inflammation of several muscles at the same time. This condition is manifested by a number of signs and symptoms, including pain, edema, deformity, and sleep disturbance.
polyneuropathy A disease involving several nerves.
polysaccharide Carbohydrates (e.g., starch, cellulose, or glycogen) in which many sugar molecules are bonded together.
polyserositis A condition of general inflammation of the serous membranes with effusion (escape of fluid). The inflammation is progressive and especially prevalent in the upper abdominal cavity.
polyspecific Refers to many antigen or antibody reactions.
positive selection The process of selecting immature T lymphocytes for survival on the basis of expression of high levels of CD3 cell surface markers and the ability to respond to self-MHC antigens.
posterior cervical In the back (dorsal surface); associated with the vertebral bone of the neck.
posterior pharynx Back of the throat.
postexposure prophylaxis A treatment protocol used after exposure to a potentially infectious microorganism.
postnatal After birth.
postoccipital lobe The back portion (lobe) of the cerebral hemisphere that is shaped like a three-sided pyramid.
postpartum After birth.
poststreptococcal glomerulonephritis An inflammation of a renal structure after an infection with streptococci.
postzone (postzone phenomenon) Excess of antigen resulting in no lattice formation in an agglutination reaction.
potency The strength of a substance.
prealbumin band The fraction of serum protein that migrates before albumin on electrophoresis.
preanalytic Before testing (preevaluation).
pre–B cell An early, rapidly dividing, mature B-cell precursor.
precipitating (precipitation) Formation of a solid mass (precipitate) from previously soluble components. An alternate definition is a process that occurs suddenly or unexpectedly.

precipitin A soluble particle that becomes insoluble particulate matter.
precipitin lines Observable lines of insoluble particulate matter.
precision The degree to which further measurements or analysis produce the same or very similar results; also called *reproducibility* or *repeatability*.
predictive value An expression of the probability that a given test result correlates with the presence or absence of disease. A positive predictive value is the ratio of patients with the disease who test positive to the entire population of individuals with a positive test result; a negative predictive value is the ratio of patients without the disease who test negative to the entire population of individuals with a negative test.
prenatal Before birth.
primary antibody response An immunologic (IgM antibody) response that occurs after a foreign antigen challenge.
primary biliary cirrhosis Cirrhosis (interstitial inflammation of an organ) of the liver caused by chronic retention of bile. The causative agent is unknown in the primary form of the disorder.
primary disorder An initial or a first condition.
primary follicle A cluster of B lymphocytes that have not yet been stimulated by antigen.
primary immune deficiency disorders (primary immunoglobulin deficiency disorder) A genetically determined disorder associated with certain diseases.
primary infection The first or original infection.
primary lymphoid tissue or organ The bone marrow and thymus gland are classified as primary or central lymphoid tissues.
primary response An initial antibody reaction to a foreign antigen.
prime To give an initial sensitization to antigen.
primer Short sequences of DNA, usually 20 to 30 nucleotides in length, used to hybridize specifically to a particular target DNA to help initiate replication of the DNA.
primitive stem cell The early form of uncommitted, multipotential blood cells that replicate themselves and generate more differentiated daughter cells.
probiotics Numerous microorganisms in the gut known to provide health benefits to the host when acquired in adequate amounts.
procainamide A drug that functions as a cardiac depressant; used in the treatment of cardiac arrhythmias.
procalcitonin (PCT) An indicator of sepsis.
prodromal period Earliest or initial sign or symptom of a developing disease or disorder. For example the prodromal period (prodrome) of an infectious disease manifested by rash would be the time between the earliest symptoms and the appearance of the rash or fever.
proficiency testing A comparison of in-house laboratory assay results with results from external laboratories; a valuable continuous improvement (quality assurance) tool.
progenitor cell Precursor (immature) blood cell.
prognosis A forecast of the probable outcome of a condition, disorder, or disease.

prognostic To predict an outcome.
progressive systemic sclerosis (PSS) A disorder of loss of tissue elasticity throughout the body that advances in severity over time.
properdin A normal protein of human plasma or serum.
prophylaxis A synonym for prevention.
prostaglandin A naturally occurring, unsaturated fatty acid that stimulates and suppresses the effects of many inflammatory processes and stimulates the contraction of uterine and other smooth muscle tissues; pharmacologically active derivative of arachidonic acid. Different prostaglandins are capable of modulating cell mobility and immune responses.
prostate-specific antigen (PSA) A cancer tumor marker for prostate cancer.
prostration A condition of extreme exhaustion (lack of strength or energy).
protease An enzyme that breaks down proteins and peptides.
protease inhibitors Substances that prevent or slow down the action of the enzyme protease.
protein A large molecule, composed of amino acids, that is a major constituent of cells.
proteinase An enzyme that can act on proteins.
proteinuria Protein (albumin) in the urine.
proteolysis (adj., proteolytic) The breaking apart of a protein molecule.
proteolytic enzyme A substance able to break apart a protein molecule.
proteomics Large-scale study of proteins, particularly their structures and functions.
prothrombin time (PT) A blood coagulation test that assesses the process of clotting, beginning with the formation of factor X.
protocol The steps usually followed in a situation such as laboratory testing or patient treatment.
protooncogene A regulatory gene that promotes cell division.
proviral genome A form of a virus that is integrated into the genome of a host cell.
proximal humerus The end portion of the upper bone of the arm nearest the center of the body (shoulder).
prozone phenomenon A possible cause of false-negative antigen-antibody reactions caused by an excessive amount of antibody.
pruritus Itching.
pseudoagglutination False clumping of cells or particles.
psychoneuroimmunology The relationship between the mind and body that combines research in basic science with psychological and psychosocial factors.
psychosocial factors Related to both psychological and social factors.
PT See prothrombin time.
purine Nitrogenous bases, adenine and guanine, incorporated into DNA or RNA, which represent a portion of the genetic code (genome).
purine analogues Antimetabolites that mimic the structure of metabolic purines (nucleotides; e.g., azathioprine).
purpura An extensive area of red or dark purple discoloration of the skin.

purulent Containing, discharging, or causing the production of pus.
pyelonephritis An inflammation of the kidney and pelvis region of the kidney, the funnel-shaped expansion of the upper end of the ureter into which the renal calices open.
pyoderma Any purulent (pus-producing) skin disease.
pyogen A microorganism causing fever.
pyogenic Producing pus.
pyrimidine Nitrogenous bases, cytosine and thymidine, in DNA, and cytosine and uracil in RNA, which form a portion of the genetic code (genome).
pyrogenic Inducing fever.
pyroglobulin An abnormal (IgM) globulin that precipitates on heating to 50°C to 60°C (122°F to 140°F) but does not redissolve on cooling or intensified heating, as do typical Bence Jones pyroglobulins.
pyroglobulinemia Presence in the blood of pyroglobulins.

Q

quality assurance (QA) Planned or systematic action necessary to provide confidence that a laboratory assay result will satisfy the given requirements for quality.
quality control (QC) A process used to ensure a certain level of quality in laboratory testing, including control of preanalytic, analytic, and postanalytic factors. The basic goal of quality control is to ensure that the results meet specific requirements and are dependable and satisfactory.
quantitation A process that measures the concentration of a substance.

R

radial immunodiffusion (RID) A quantitative variation of immunodiffusion. The diameter of the precipitin ring formed from evenly distributed antigen (or antibody) and its counterpart from the test sample diffuses into agar gel from a single well, resulting in a circular ring of precipitin around the sample well. The diameter of the precipitin ring is proportional to the concentration of specific antibody (or antigen) present in the test specimen. A comparison to a known standard allows for quantitation of the test specimen.
radioallergosorbent test (RAST) A procedure that detects the presence of IgE (and IgG) antibodies to allergens; a method used to measure antigen-specific IgE by means of a noncompetitive solid-phase immunoassay.
radioimmunoassay (RIA) An older and less frequently used laboratory technique using radioactive substances to evaluate immunoglobulins. Traditional RIA is done with specific antibodies in liquid solution. Solid-phase RIA uses antibody bound to a solid support (e.g., tube, glass beads).
radiolabeled A substance that is tagged with a radioactive element.
rapid plasma reagin (RPR) A laboratory screening test for syphilis.
RAST See radioallergosorbent test.
Raynaud phenomenon (Raynaud disease) A condition of episodic constriction of small arteries of the extremities (usually fingers or toes) induced by cold temperatures or emotional stress that would not affect a nonafflicted person. The signs and symptoms of the condition include two forms, a pale appearance and numb feeling followed by redness and tingling or a swollen, red, and painful condition. Heat relieves the condition if the stimulus was cold induced.
reactivated infection Another appearance of an infection.
reactive oxygen species (ROS) Chemically reactive molecules containing oxygen, such as H_2O_2.
reagent A chemical solution used in laboratory testing.
reagin An antibody-like protein that binds to a test antigen such as cardiolipin lecithin–coated cholesterol particles in the Venereal Disease Research Laboratory (VDRL) serologic method of testing for syphilis, a rapid plasma reagin (RPR) test; also a former term for IgE with a specificity for allergens.
reagin antibody Nontreponemal antibody produced by a patient infected with *Treponema pallidum* against components of their own or other mammalian cells.
real-time PCR A sensitive technique for measuring amplification of DNA by using fluorescent dyes or probes to take readings after each cycle instead of waiting until all the cycles have been completed.
re-anneal To reassemble or recombine two nucleic acid strands.
receptor A cell surface molecule that binds specifically to particular proteins or peptides in the fluid phase.
recessive The term used to describe a gene that is not expressed unless it is in the homozygous form.
recirculation Lymphocytes, mostly T cells, that pass from the circulating blood through the lymphatic system back to the circulating blood.
recognition unit The complement component that consists of the C1qrs complex. This unit must bind to at least two Fc regions to initiate the classic complement cascade.
recombinant DNA technology The technique whereby genetic material from one organism is inserted into a foreign cell or another organism to mass produce the protein encoded by the inserted genes; also called *recombinant genetic engineering*.
recombinant vector vaccine A vaccine that combines a vector, a harmless bacterium or virus, used to transport an antigen into the body to stimulate protective immunity and an antigen or immunogen from an organism other than the vector.
redundant Refers to different cytokines that have the same effect.
reference range or reference values Typical laboratory results for specific groups of patients, such as gender- or age-related average values. This term was previously referred to as normal values.
refractory anemia A form of anemia (decreased erythrocytes in the circulation) resistant to ordinary treatment.
regimen A schedule of treatment.
regional adenopathy Swelling or enlargement of the lymph nodes in a certain area or areas of the body.

reinfection A second or more incidence that manifests a prior infection.
relative lymphocytosis An increase of lymphocytes in the circulating blood in relation to the total number of leukocytes in the circulation.
reliability Dependability of results.
remission Withdrawal of symptoms of a disease or disorder; a temporary cure.
renal impairment Dysfunction of the kidneys.
renal insufficiency Inadequate functioning of the kidneys.
replicability The ability of specific and nonspecific cells of the immune system to produce daughter cells.
reproducibility The ability to obtain similar results when the same specimen is repeatedly tested.
respiratory burst The increase in oxygen consumption that occurs in a phagocytic cell as it begins to engulf a particle.
restriction endonuclease Bacterial enzyme that recognizes short sequences of DNA and cleaves the DNA near this restriction site. Each enzyme is named after the bacteria from which it has been isolated.
restriction endonuclease Enzymes that cleave DNA at specific recognition sites that are typically four to six base pairs long.
restriction fragment length polymorphism (RFLP) Variation in nucleotides in DNA that change where restriction enzymes cleave the DNA. Where mutations occur, different-sized segments of DNA are obtained, producing an altered electrophoretic pattern.
reticuloendothelial system (RES) See mononuclear phagocyte system (MPS).
retinal hemorrhage Extreme bleeding from the inner layer of the eye (retina) into the fluid-filled interior of the eye.
retinitis An inflammation of the inner layer (retina) of the eye.
retroauricular Behind the protruding portion of the external ear that surrounds the opening (auricle).
retrovirus A type of virus that carries a single, positive-strand RNA and uses a special enzyme, reverse transcriptase, to convert viral RNA into DNA.
reverse passive hemagglutination A laboratory method that uses erythrocytes as indicator cells to observe the absence of agglutination in the presence of antibodies. Carrier particles coated with antibody clump together because of a combination of antigen.
reverse transcriptase (RT) An enzyme found in the single, positive-strand RNA core of a retrovirus. This enzyme converts (copies) RNA to DNA.
Reye syndrome An acute and often fatal childhood disease that may follow a variety of common viral infections within several hours or days. The signs and symptoms of disease include persistent vomiting followed by delirium caused by edema of the brain, hypoglycemia, dysfunction of the liver, convulsions, and coma.
RFLPs (restriction fragment length polymorphisms) A variation in the DNA sequence of a genome that can be detected by a laboratory

technique known as gel electrophoresis. Analysis of RFLP variation is an important tool in genome mapping, localization of genetic disease genes, and determination of risk for a disease.

Rh factor A blood group antigen, named for the rhesus monkey, that was originally identified because an antibody agglutinated the erythrocytes of all rhesus monkeys and 85% of human beings. The antibody was later discovered to be the Landsteiner-Wiener antibody, which is different from the Rh antibody.

rheumatic disease A collection of rheumatoid disorders.

rheumatic fever A disease caused by the toxins produced by group A beta streptococci.

rheumatoid factor An IgM class antibody directed against IgG; detectable in patients with rheumatoid arthritis.

rhinitis Inflammation of the nose.

rhinorrhea Watery discharge from the nose.

RIA See radioimmunoassay.

ribonucleic acid (RNA) The nucleic acid containing the carbohydrate ribose.

***Rickettsia* (rickettsial)** A genus of nonmotile Gram-negative bacteria that causes infectious diseases (e.g., Rocky Mountain spotted fever, ehrlichiosis).

RIST Radioimmunosorbent test used to measure total IgE using a solid-phase immunoassay with anti-IgE.

rocket immunoelectrophoresis A classic method used to quantify antigens on the basis of the height of a rocket-shaped precipitin band obtained when radial immunodiffusion is combined with electrophoresis.

Rocky Mountain spotted fever (RMSF) A vector-borne infectious disease.

rouleaux (rouleaux formation) Pseudoagglutination or the false clumping of erythrocytes when the cells are suspended in their own serum. This phenomenon is caused by an abnormal protein in the serum, plasma expanders (e.g., dextran), or Wharton jelly, from cord blood samples. Rouleaux formation appears as rolls resembling stacks of coins on microscopic examination.

RPR (rapid plasma reagin) test A serologic test for venereal disease (syphilis).

rubella The RNA viral cause of German or 3-day measles.

rubella syndrome A term for a number of congenital anomalies such as mental retardation and cardiovascular defects caused by the rubella virus.

rubeola The single-strand RNA virus that cause measles.

S

S protein A control protein in the complement cascade that interferes with binding of the C5b67 complex to a cell membrane, thereby preventing lysis.

sandwich format immunoassay (sandwich format) An immunoassay method based on the ability of antibody to bind with more than one antigen.

sandwich hybridization A nucleic acid detection method using two probes, one of which is placed on a solid support (e.g., a membrane or microtiter plate) to capture the target DNA. A second labeled probe, which binds to a second site on the target DNA, is added to detect specific gene sequences.

sarcoma A malignant tumor of connective tissue origin.

scarlet fever An acute infectious disease caused by group A streptococcus. The rash and other signs and symptoms are caused by the erythema-producing toxin produced by the streptococci.

schistosomiasis An infectious disease caused by trematode worms.

sclerodactyly A chronic disorder characterized by progressive fibrosis of the fingers and toes.

scleroderma A progressive fibrosis beginning with the skin.

sebum The oily secretion of the sebaceous glands whose ducts open into the hair follicles.

second follicle A cluster of B lymphocytes that are proliferating in response to a specific antigen.

secondary immune response The second and subsequent response by the immune system to the same antigen encountered; the secondary response is shorter, faster, and wider than the primary response.

secondary immunoglobulin deficiency An acquired disorder associated with certain diseases.

secondary lymphoid tissue (secondary lymphoid organs) Secondary tissues include the lymph nodes, spleen, and Peyer patches in the intestine.

secretory component A protein in secretory IgA and IgM thought to protect against enzyme damage.

selectin One of three protein families that include immunoglobulin, integrin, and selectin and are associated in a network of cellular interactions in the immune system.

selectin A Sugar-binding lectin on the surface of cells.

self-limiting (self-limited) Confined; able to resolve over time.

senescence The process of growing old.

sensitivity The frequency of positive results obtained in testing a population of individuals who are positive for antibody.

sensitization Physical attachment of antibody molecules to antigens on the erythrocyte membrane.

sepsis Microbial infection throughout the systemic circulation.

septic arthritis An inflammation of the joints caused by the presence of pathogenic microorganisms.

septicemia The presence of pathogenic microorganisms in the blood.

sequela (pl., sequelae) A disease or condition occurring after or as a consequence of another condition or event.

serial dilution The stepwise decreasing strength (dilution) of a substance in solution.

seroconversion The development of a demonstrable antibody response to a disease or vaccine.

serodiagnostic test An assay of substances (Ag tab) in serum.

seroepidemiologic Pertaining to the evidence of antibodies to a disease in a defined population.

serogroups Groups of organisms that have related testing reactions.

serologic Pertaining to serology.

serologic testing An assay of constituents of serum.

serology The study of constituents of serum, the straw-colored fluid component of whole blood.

seronegative The lack of evidence of an antibody to a disease.

seronegative spondyloarthropathy Antibody-negative in a condition affecting the joints of the spine.

seropositive The presence of antibodies in a specimen.

seroprevalence The frequency of occurrence of a specific antibody in a specified population.

serositis An inflammation of the membrane consisting of mesothelium, a thin layer of connective tissue, manifested by lines enclosing the body cavities.

serotype A group of closely related microorganisms distinguished by a characteristic set of antigens.

serum Straw-colored fluid present in whole blood; seen after blood clots.

serum electrophoresis A technique for separating ionic molecules, principally proteins, into five fractions on a medium such as paper or cellulose acetate. The separation is based on the rate of migration, depending on size and ionic charge of the individual components in an electrical field. The components can be visualized by staining and quantitated using a densitometer.

serum sickness A type III hypersensitivity reaction occurring after a single large injection of serum from an animal of another species (passive immunization).

severe combined immunodeficiency disease (SCID) A life-threatening condition that results when a child is born without any major immune defenses.

sex-linked trait A genetic trait associated with the X chromosome.

sharps Objects that can cut.

sialic acid Found on red blood cell membranes; produces a negative surrounding charge.

sialoglycoprotein A sialic acid containing carbohydrate and a protein molecule.

sickle cell anemia An inherited form of anemia caused by genetically defective hemoglobin.

silent carrier A carrier of a disease who manifests no clinically obvious symptoms or signs.

single-base mutations A mutation that exchanges one DNA amino acid base for another (e.g., adenine to guanine).

single diffusion A precipitation reaction in which one of the reactants is incorporated in the gel and the other reactant diffuses out from the point of application.

single nucleotide polymorphism (SNP) The most common type of genetic variation among people.

single-strand conformational polymorphism assay A technique used to detect subtle differences in nucleotide sequences; typically used to compare sequences from two or more individuals to determine whether they are identical or if a mutation has occurred.

sinusitis An inflammation of the cavity in a bone, such as in the paranasal sinuses.
sinusoid A specialized capillary found in locations such as the bone marrow, spleen, and liver through which blood passes to reach the veins, allowing the lining macrophages to remove damaged or antibody-coated cells.
Sjögren syndrome An autoimmune disorder manifested by enlargement of the parotid glands; chronic polyarthritis; and dryness of the conjunctiva, throat, and mouth.
skin lesions Disruptions of the skin.
SLE See systemic lupus erythematosus.
smoldering multiple myeloma An out-of-sight or hidden form of plasma cell dyscrasia.
SNPs See specific nucleotide polymorphisms.
solid-phase assay A laboratory method in which one of the reactants is bound to the surface.
soluble Able to be dissolved in a liquid, or as if in a liquid, especially water.
soluble mediator A substance secreted by monocytes, lymphocytes, and neutrophils that provides the mechanism of cell-to-cell communication.
somnolence A condition of prolonged drowsiness or a state resembling a trance.
sor **gene** A gene of a retrovirus such as HIV. The product of the small, open-reading frame is a protein that induces antibody production in the natural course of infection.
Southern blot A molecular biology laboratory technique used in DNA analysis. DNA from a patient specimen is denatured and treated with enzymes to produce DNA fragments. The single-strand DNA fragments are then separated by electrophoresis. The fragments are further treated and radiolabeled. The resulting DNA with the radiolabel, if present, is then detected by autoradiography. Applications include studying the HIV sequence in peripheral blood cells and tissues such as lymph nodes, liver, and kidney.
specific nucleotide polymorphisms (SNPs) The most common type of genetic variation among human beings. Each SNP represents a difference in a single nucleotide. A SNP may replace a cytosine (C) with a thymine (T).
specific oligomer primers In PCR amplification, multiple nucleotide units (oligomers) are linked together for specific amplification of a fragment of a gene.
specificity Ability of a particular antibody to combine with one antigen instead of another; also the proportion of negative test results obtained in the population of individuals who actually lack the antibody in question.
spectrophotometry (adv., spectrophotometrically) A method for measuring the passage of colored light by reflection or transmission.
spirochete A type of bacteria with a twisted or spiral appearance when viewed microscopically.
spirochetemia The presence of spirochetes (e.g., in the disease syphilis) in the circulating blood.
spleen A large glandlike organ located in the upper left quadrant of the abdomen, under the ribs. The spleen is the body's largest reservoir of mononuclear phagocytic cells.
splenomegaly A disorder characterized by a greatly enlarged spleen.

spontaneous tumor antigen A unique antigen expressed by a tumor.
sporotrichosis An infection with or disease caused by a fungus.
sporotrichotic Pertaining to sporotrichosis.
SQUID See superconducting quantum interference device.
standard deviation (SD) The statistical calculation that demonstrates the distance (deviation) from a mean value in a group of measurements.
Standard Precautions Specific regulations and practices, such as wearing gloves, that conform to current state and federal requirements. These precautions assume that all specimens (e.g., blood) have the potential for transmitting disease; also called *Universal Blood and Body Fluid Precautions* (CDC), previously Uniform Precautions.
stasis Cessation of bleeding.
steric hindrance Mutual blocking of dissimilar antibodies with the same binding constant directed against antigenic determinants located in close proximity on a cell's surface.
stillborn (stillbirth) Dead at birth.
Stokes shift The difference in wavelength or frequency units between positions of the band maxima of the absorption and emission spectra.
strand displacement amplification A technique for amplifying DNA by using a DNA primer that is nicked by an endonuclease, allowing for displacement of the amplified strands.
streptococcal pharyngitis Sore throat caused by group A streptococcus.
Streptococcus pyogenes A species of streptococcus.
streptokinase An enzyme that dissolves clots by converting plasminogen to plasmin.
streptolysin O (SLO) A protein capable of lysing erythrocytes and leukocytes produced by some types of streptococci as they grow.
streptolysin S Associated with group A streptococcus.
stroma The connective, functionally supportive framework of a biologic cell, tissue, or organ.
structural protein Fibrous proteins (e.g., skin).
subclinical infection An early or mild form of a disease without visible signs.
substrate A substance on which another substance acts, such as an enzyme.
subunit vaccines Vaccines that use only a portion of a disease-causing virus.
superantigens A class of antigens that cause nonspecific activation of T cells, resulting in oligoclonal T-cell activation and massive cytokine production.
superconducting quantum interference device (SQUID) A very sensitive magnetometer used to measure extremely small magnetic fields, based on superconducting loops containing Josephson junctions.
superinfection An infection on top of another infection.
supernatant Fluid above the solid portion (e.g., cells in a centrifuged or sedimented specimen).
suppressor (cytotoxic) lymphocytes A major phenotypic lymphocyte subset of T lymphocytes; also referred to as T8 cells.
supraglottic larynx The area above the true vocal cords.

surface immunoglobulin (sIg) An immunoglobulin, at first cytoplasmic and later surface bound, that is the key feature of B cells whereby they recognize specific antigens.
surgical pathology The study of tissue or organs removed from the body.
surrogate testing Procedures performed in place of specific tests for an infectious agent such as non-A, non-B hepatitis.
susceptibility Having little resistance, such as resistance to infectious disease.
symptom An indication of a disorder or disease or a variation in normal body function.
symptomatic A deviation from usual function or appearance.
syncope Loss of balance.
syncytia Giant multinucleated groups or masses of cells.
syndrome A collection of symptoms that occur together.
synergistic The action of two or more agents that produces a much greater effect than the expected sum of the individual agents.
synovial fluid A viscous fluid in the joints.
synovitis Inflammation of the synovium.
synovium The soft tissue found between the articular capsule (joint capsule) and joint cavity of synovial joints. Also called *synovial membrane*.
systematic errors Errors in testing that occur on a repeated and regular basis.
systemic Throughout the body.
systemic circulation Blood circulation throughout the body.
systemic inflammatory response syndrome (SIRS) An inflammation that overwhelms the whole body.
systemic lupus erythematosus (SLE) An autoimmune disorder expressed as a group of multisymptom disorders that can affect almost every organ of the body.
systemic sclerosis Loss of tissue elasticity of vessels, such as blood vessels, throughout the whole body.

T

T cell See T lymphocyte.
T-cell receptor (TCR) A T-lymphocyte surface membrane marker.
T lymphocyte The cell responsible for the cellular immune response and involved in the regulation of antibody reactions; also called a *T cell*.
tabes dorsalis A slowly progressive degeneration of the nervous system caused by syphilis. In untreated patients, this condition may appear from 5 to 20 years after the initial infection with *Treponema pallidum*.
tachyarrhythmia Accelerated rhythm of the heartbeat.
tachycardia An abnormally fast heart rate.
tachypnea Accelerated breathing.
tart cell Cells that usually represent monocytes that have phagocytized another whole cell or nucleus, often a lymphocyte. When a blood preparation is microscopically examined for the presence of cells associated with systemic lupus erythematosus (SLE), tart cells may be seen. These cell formations can be mistaken for the classic lupus erythematosus (LE) cell connected with SLE.

TdT See terminal deoxynucleotidyl transferase.
telangiectasia A vascular lesion formed by the dilation of a group of capillaries and occasionally of terminal arteries.
teratocarcinoma A malignancy (see teratoma).
teratoma Malignant tumor derived from three germ layers.
terminal deoxynucleotidyl transferase (TdT) An intracellular DNA polymerase found mainly in cortical, and therefore young, thymocytes. These cells are lost from the thymus after corticosteroid treatment.
thermocycler A laboratory instrument used to amplify DNA and RNA specimens by the polymerase chain reaction (PCR). A thermocycler raises and lowers the temperature of the specimens in a holding block in discrete, preprogrammed steps, allowing for denaturation and reannealing of samples with various reagents.
thrombocytopenia A severe deficiency of circulating blood platelets (thrombocytes).
thrombocytopenia purpura Red discoloration of the skin due to patient deficiency of platelets.
thrombophlebitis An inflammation of a vein that develops before the formation of a thrombus (clot).
thrombosis Formation of a blood clot or thrombus.
thrombus A clot.
thymocyte An immature lymphocyte, found in the thymus gland, that undergoes differentiation to become a mature T cell.
thymoma A tumor derived from the epithelial or lymphoid elements of the thymus.
thymosin A humoral factor secreted by the thymus that promotes the growth of peripheral lymphoid tissue; also called thymic hormone.
thymus A primary or central lymphoid tissue responsible for processes of lymphocytes into the T type of cell. This ductless glandlike structure is located beneath the sternum (breastbone).
time-resolved fluoroimmunoassay The length of time measured of excitation by a pulse of light.
T-independent antigen Not dependent on T-cell recognition.
titer The concentration or strength of an antibody expressed as the highest dilution of the serum that produces agglutination (e.g., 1: 4, 1: 8).
Todd unit A unit that expresses antibody concentration in the testing for antistreptolysin antibodies.
tolerance Lack of immune response to self-antigens initiated during fetal development.
toll-like receptor (TLR) A class of proteins that are essential in the innate immune system.
TORCH A group of tests for infectious microorganisms. TORCH stands for *T*oxoplasma, other (viruses), *r*ubella, *c*ytomegalovirus (CMV), and *h*erpes.
toxic shock syndrome A serious and potentially fatal disorder caused by toxins produced by *Staphylococcus aureus*.
toxicology The study of drugs and related substances.
Toxoplasma gondii A protozoal microorganism that can be transmitted from an infected mother to an unborn infant. The disease can result in encephalomyelitis.
trans- A prefix meaning across, over, or through.
transaminase An enzyme (alanine transaminase [ALT], serum glutamic pyruvic transaminase [SGPT]) used in a surrogate test for non-A, non-B hepatitis.
transcriptase A polymerase that catalyzes the formation of RNA from a DNA template in the process of transcription. Reverse transcriptase (RNA-directed DNA polymerase) is an enzyme that generates complementary DNA (cDNA) from an RNA template.
transcription The process of generating a messenger RNA strand from DNA, used to code for proteins.
transcription-mediated amplification (TMA) A method of increasing target DNA through the use of two enzymes, an RNA polymerase and a reverse transcriptase, to synthesize new strands of DNA.
transferrin A plasma protein that transports iron through the blood to the liver.
transforming growth factor (TGF) The cytokine identified as the product of virally transformed cells (e.g., TGF-β). These molecules can induce phenotypic transformation in nonneoplastic cells.
translation The process whereby messenger RNA is used to make functional proteins.
transplacental The ability of a substance to move through the barrier of the placenta.
transplacental hemorrhage The entrance of fetal blood cells into the maternal circulation across the placenta.
transporter associated with antigen processing (TAP) The proteins responsible for the ATP-dependent transport of newly synthesized short peptides from the cytoplasm to the lumen of the endoplasmic reticulum for binding to class I HLA antigens.
Treponema pallidum **antibodies** Antibodies produced in response to a *Treponema pallidum* syphilis infection.
treponeme Spirochete of the genus *Treponema*.
trophoblast The outer layer of the blastocyst.
trophoblastic neoplasm A new growth involving trophoblastic tissue, such as a hydatiform mole.
tubular cell injury Damage to cells of the renal tubules.
tumor Proliferation of cells that produce a mass rather than a reaction or inflammatory condition.
tumor necrosis factor (TNF) A cytokine that can destroy tumor cells.
tumor suppressor gene(s) A gene that inhibits the growth of tumors.
tumor-associated antigen An antigen found on tumor cells that is not unique to those cells but that can be used to distinguish them from normal cells.
tumorigenesis Formation of tumors.
tumor-specific antigen (TSA) A tumor marker; an antigen that is only associated with a specific type of tissue.
turbid Cloudy.
turbidimetry See nephelometry.

U

ubiquitous Existing everywhere.
ulcerative lesion An open sore.
unilateral blindness The lack of vision in one eye.
Universal Blood and Body Fluid Precautions See Standard Precautions.
upregulation An increase in the number of receptors on the surface of target cells, making the cells more sensitive to a hormone or other agent.
urticaria Hives.

V

vaccination A method of stimulating the adaptive immune response and generating memory and acquired resistance without contracting disease; a form of artificial, active acquired immunity.
vaccine A suspension of killed or attenuated (inactivated) infectious agents administered to establish resistance to the disease.
variable lymphocyte A type of white blood cell that lacks the characteristics of a normal lymphocyte.
variable region The antigen-binding portion of an immunoglobulin molecule.
varicella-zoster virus (VZV) A virus that causes chickenpox.
varicosity A condition of having distended veins.
variolation Originally an Asian practice to cause a deliberate infection with smallpox. Dried smallpox scabs were blown into the nose of an individual who then contracted a mild form of the disease. Upon recovery the individual was immune to smallpox.
vasculitis An inflammation of a vessel such as a blood vessel.
vasculitis syndromes A group of symptoms that characterize inflammation of a blood vessel.
vasoamine Produced by mast cells, basophils, and platelets; vasoactive amines (e.g., histamine, 5-hydroxytryptamine) cause increased capillary permeability.
vasodilation Expansion of blood vessels.
vector (vector-borne) A bacterium or virus that does not cause disease in humans and is used in genetically engineered vaccines, or an organism, such as a mosquito or tick, that carries disease-causing microorganisms from one host to another.
Venereal Disease Research Laboratory (VDRL) A US Public Health Laboratory established in World War I for syphilis testing.
venereal route A sexually transmitted mode of infection.
viral capsid antigen (VCA) An antigen expressed by B lymphocytes infected with Epstein-Barr virus in infectious mononucleosis.
viral core protein Proteins found mainly in icosahedral DNA and RNA viruses.
viral load testing A quantitative measurement for HIV nucleic acid that is used principally to monitor the effects of antiretroviral therapy.
viremia A systemic (blood) infection caused by a virus.
virion A complete virus particle.
virulence The degree of pathogenicity or ability to cause disease of a microorganism.

W

Waldenström primary macroglobulinemia (WM) A neoplastic proliferation of the lymphocyte–plasma cell system; also called *Waldenström macroglobulinemia*.

Wasserman test The first diagnostic serologic test for syphilis; no longer in use.

West Nile virus A member of the Japanese encephalitis virus group of flaviviruses that cause febrile illness and encephalitis in human beings.

Wiskott-Aldrich syndrome A genetic disorder passed to males through the X chromosome; results in decreased production of specific antibodies and abnormal cellular immunity.

Western blot (WB) A molecular biology diagnostic technique similar to the northern blot and Southern blot procedures. WB is used to detect antibodies to specific epitopes of electrophoretically separated subspecies of antigens. WB is often used to confirm the specificity of antibodies detected by an ELISA screening procedure.

window period A period of undetectable evidence of infectious disease.

X

xenograft (xenotransplantation) A transplant (graft) between different species, such as pigs to humans.

X-linked agammaglobulinemia An inherited form of agammaglobulinemia, transmitted to males through the X chromosome, in which B cells fail to mature and to secrete immunoglobulins.

Z

zeta potential Difference in electrostatic potential between net charge at cell membrane and charge at surface of shear (net negative charge).

Zika virus A vector-borne virus.

zone electrophoresis See capillary zone electrophoresis.

zone of equivalence An area in which optimum precipitation occurs because the number of multivalent sites of antigen and antibody are approximately equal.

zoonosis (pl., zoonoses) Any infectious disease that can be transmitted (by a vector) from other animals, wild and domestic, to human beings or from human beings to animals (the latter is sometimes called *reverse zoonosis*).

zymosan A glucan with repeating glucose units connected by β-1,3-glycosidic linkages.

INDEX

A

A. *See* Adenine (A)
Abelson (ABL) kinase inhibitor, 473
ABL kinase inhibitor. *See* Abelson (ABL) kinase inhibitor
Abl proto-oncogene, 460
Abnormal nucleic acid, 471
Abruptio placentae, 345
Absolute lymphocyte count, determination of, 306b
ACA. *See* Acrodermatitis chronica atrophicans (ACA)
Accelerated rejection, 442. *See also* Grafts
Accessory cells. *See* Dendritic cells
Accrediting organizations, 108
Accuracy
    definition of, 109b, 110
    nonanalytic factors related to testing, 108–109
Acellular pertussis vaccines, 485–487
Acquired immunodeficiency syndrome (AIDS), 313–326
    analysis for measuring T cells in, 165
    case study of, 334b
    classification of, 318
    diagnostic evaluation and monitoring of, 322
        ARCHITECT HIV Ag/Ab Combo Assay, 326
        drug therapy, 327–328
        enzyme immunoassays (EIAs), 324
        fourth-generation testing, 326
        genome testing, 324
        HIV-1 antibody assays, 322–324
        HIV antigen tests, 324
        nucleic acid amplification testing (NAAT), 322–324
        OraQuick ADVANCE Rapid HIV-1/2 Antibody Test, 326, 327b
        pediatric testing, 326
        polymerase chain reaction, 324
        quantitative RNA assay, 326
        rapid testing, 326, 327b
        Western blot, 325–326, 325f
    encoding genes and antigens of, 316t
    epidemiology of, 316–317
        incidence, 306, 317t
        infectious patterns, 317–318
    etiology of, 313
        human T-lymphotropic retrovirus type III (HTLV-III), 313
        lymphadenopathy-associated virus (LAV), 313
        replication, 315–316, 316f
        viral characteristics of, 314–316
        viral genome components, 315t
        viral structure of, 314–315, 315f, 315t–316t
    HIV-1, 317–318
    HIV-2, 318
    immunologic manifestations of, 321
        cellular abnormalities, 321
        core antigen detection, 322, 322f
        HIV-1 antibodies, 322
        immune system alterations, 321
        serologic markers, 322
    mode of transmission, 318, 318b
    postexposure prophylaxis, 332–334
    preexposure prophylaxis, 332, 332b
    prevention of, 326
        vaccines, 326. *See also* Vaccines
        viral transmissions, reduction of, 326

Acquired immunodeficiency syndrome (Continued)
    proteins of serodiagnostic importance, 315t
    signs and symptoms of, 318–319, 319b
        cryptosporidiosis, 320
        disease progression, 321
        Kaposi sarcoma (KS), 320
        non-Hodgkin lymphoma, 320
        opportunistic infections, 319–320, 320f, 320t, 320b
    testing methods of, 322, 323t
    therapeutic monitoring, tests for, 326
        CD4+ T lymphocyte testing, 326, 327f
        viral load testing, 326
    treatments, antiretroviral therapy, 326–332
        drug resistance, 327, 329f, 330t–331t, 331–332
        entry inhibitors (ccr5 antagonist), 328
        fusion inhibitors, 328
        highly active antiretroviral therapy (HAART), 319–320
        integrase strand transfer inhibitors, 328
        investigational drugs, 331–332
        nonnucleoside reverse transcriptase inhibitors (NNRTIs), 328
        nucleoside reverse transcriptase inhibitors, 328
        protease inhibitors, 328
    treatments, postexposure prophylaxis (PEP), 332–334
    vaccines for, 491–493, 492b–493b
Acquired infection
    cytomegalovirus (CMV), 211–212. *See also* Cytomegalovirus (CMV)
    toxoplasmosis, 200–205. *See also* Toxoplasmosis
Acrodermatitis chronica atrophicans (ACA), 246
ACTH. *See* Adrenocorticotropic hormone (ACTH)
Actionable mutations, 459
Activation defects, T-cell, 309
Activator surfaces, 32
Active immunity, 24–25, 25t
Acute conditions, viral hepatitis, 274, 274t. *See also* Viral hepatitis
Acute, infectious mononucleosis, 268
Acute inflammation, 73, 73f
Acute-phase
    proteins, 41–45, 41b
        applications of, 42b
        catabolism, 42
        ceruloplasmin, 43
        clinically useful, 42t
        C-reactive protein (CRP), 42–43
        laboratory assessment methods for, 43–45
        overview of, 41–42, 42t, 42b
        synthesis of, 42
        α_1-antitrypsin, 43
    reactants, 41, 41b, 43
Acute rejection, 443
Acute respiratory distress coronavirus syndrome (ARDS), 197
Adaptive immune response, 374
    phases of, 80f
Adaptive (acquired) immunity, 6, 23
    cell-mediated, 25–26
    components of, 24b
    features of, 24t

Adaptive (acquired) immunity (Continued)
    humoral-mediated, 23
    vs. innate immunity, 19–26, 20t
    suppression of, 25
    types of, 24f
ADCC. *See* Antibody-dependent cell-mediated cytotoxicity (ADCC)
Adenine (A), 169
Adenocarcinomas, 455
Adenomas, 455
Adjuvants, 51, 485. *See also* Antigens (immunogens)
ADN-B. *See* Anti-DNase B (ADN-B)
Adrenal glands, 380
Adrenocorticotropic hormone (ACTH), as tumor markers, 469
ADVANCE Rapid HIV-1/2 Antibody Test, 326, 327b
AESOP syndrome, 363
Affinity, 58, 59f
Affymetrix arrays, 183
AFP. *See* Alpha-fetoprotein (AFP)
Agglutination, definition of, 129b
Agglutination inhibition, 131
Agglutination methods, 128–142.e2
    antibody influence on, 60–61
    case study of, 140b
    coagglutination, 131
    concepts, 130b
    direct bacterial agglutination, 132–133, 132b
    flocculation tests, 132
    hemagglutination, 133b, 134–138
        antibody type and, 134
        antigen-antibody ratio and, 134b, 135, 136t
        antigenic determinants, 135
        enhancing methods, 136
        graded reactions, 136, 136t, 137f–138f
        lattice formation, 135
        mechanisms of, 134–135
        microplate reactions of, 136–138
        particle charge and, 134
        pH of, 135
        sensitization, 134–135
        temperature and length of incubation, 135
    latex, 130–131, 133f–134f, 133t, 133b
    nephelometry, 138–140, 138b
        advantages and disadvantages of, 139
        assays performed by, 138b
        clinical application of, 139–140
        measuring methods of, 139
        optical system of, 139
        physical basis of, 139
        principle of, 138–139, 138b, 139f
    particle, 130, 132t
    pregnancy testing, 131
        agglutination inhibition, 131
        human chorionic gonadotropin, 131
    principles of, 129–130, 129f–130f, 130t
    procedural protocols, alternative, 131–132, 132b
AIDS. *See* Acquired immunodeficiency syndrome (AIDS)
Aliquot, 121
Alkaline phosphatase (ALP), 152, 154
Alleles
    human leukocyte antigen, 430–431, 430t. *See also* Human leukocyte antigens (HLAs)
    null, 430

Note: Page numbers followed by "b", "f" and "t" indicate boxes, figures, and tables respectively.

Allergens, 338
Allergy, 338
Allergy march, 341
Alloantibodies, 56
Alloantigens, 443
Alloepitopes, 432
Allogeneic transplantation, 440f, 439. *See also* Bone marrow transplantation
Allogenic antigens, 48. *See also* Antigens (immunogens)
Allografts, 25, 435t. *See also* Grafts
Alloimmunization, 345
Allophycocyanin (APC), 163
Allotype, 430
Allotype determinants, 56, 56t. *See also* Immunoglobulin (Ig) classes
ALP. *See* Alkaline phosphatase (ALP)
Alpha E integrin, 88
Alpha-fetoprotein (AFP), 467
Alpha helix, 169, 171f
ALPS. *See* Autoimmune lymphoproliferative syndrome (ALPS)
ALS. *See* Amyotrophic lateral sclerosis (ALS)
Amblyomma americanum, 241, 242t–243t. *See also* Ticks
American Rheumatism Association, 416–417, 417t
Amine precursor uptake and decarboxylational tumors, 455
Amphiregulin, 83
Amplicon, 170–171, 173b
Amplification products, analysis of, 175–183
Amyloidosis, 356
Amyotrophic lateral sclerosis (ALS), 386
Analytical specificity, 110
Anamnestic antibody response, 57. *See also* Antibodies
Anaphylactic reactions (type I), 339t, 339b, 340–343. *See also* Hypersensitivity reactions
  etiology of, 340, 340b
  immunologic activity of, 340–341
    anaphylactic reaction, 340
    anaphylactoid reaction, 340
    atopic reaction, 340–341
    hypersensitivity, immediate, 340, 341f
    stages of, 340
  laboratory evaluation of, 341
    chemiluminescent enzyme immunoassay, 343
    ImmunoCAP assays, 342–343, 342f, 343t
    intradermal testing, 343t
    skin patch testing, 342
    skin puncture test (SPT), 341
    skin testing protocols, 341–342
  mediators of, 341t
  signs and symptoms of, 341
    in children, 341
    generalized reaction, 341
    localized reaction, 341
  treatment for, 343
    desensitization, 343
    drug therapy, 343
Anaplasmosis, 241, 242t–243t, 250–251, 250b
Anergy, 87
Angioedema, 38
Anicteric, 275
Animal dander, hypersensitivity reactions to, 338
Ankylosing spondylitis, 420
Anneal process, 169
Anopheles mosquitoes, 254
Anthrax vaccine, 497. *See also* Vaccines
Anthropathology, 3
Antibiotics, 399
  bacteriostatic, 249
  for Lyme disease, 249–250

Antibodies, 47–66.e1
  case study of, 63b
  chemical composition of, 50b
  conjugated, 160–161
  definition of, 51
  functions of, 58, 58t
  general characteristics of, 51
  in graft rejection, 444
  half-life of, 25
  to histones, 405–406
  immunoglobulin (Ig) classes of, 51–53, 51b, 52t. *See also* Immunoglobulin (Ig) classes
    characteristics of, 52t
    IgA, 53
    IgD, 53
    IgE, 53
    IgG, 53, 54f
    IgM, 52
  interactions, antibody-antigen, 59–61. *See also* Antigens (immunogens)
    affinity, 58–59, 59f
    agglutination, influence on, 60–61
    avidity, 59, 59f
    cross-reactivity, 58
    detection of, 60, 60t
    electrostatic forces, 60
    goodness of fit, 60, 60f
    hydrogen bonds, 60
    hydrophobic bonds, 59–60
    immune complexes, 59
    molecular basis of, 59–61
    specificity, 58
    Van der Waals forces, 60
  isotypes (classes) of, 55f
  maternal, 25
  monoclonal (MAbs), 61–63
    characteristics of, 61b
    discovery of, 61
    production of, 61–62, 62f
    uses of, 62–63
  neutralizing, 61, 61b
  to nonhistone proteins, 406, 407t
  to nucleolar antigens, 406
  response types, 57b
  structure of, 53–56
    core of, 53
    diversity of, 53
    typical Ig molecule, 54–55, 54f
  synthesis of, 56–58, 56b
    clonal selection, 56–57
    primary antibody response, 57, 57f
    secondary (anamnestic) response, 57–58, 57f
  tumor immunology and, 462
Antibody-dependent cell-mediated cytotoxicity (ADCC), 443
Antibody detection
  capture enzyme immunoassay, 153
  competitive enzyme immunoassay, 153
  noncompetitive enzyme immunoassay, 153
Antibody testing, in serologic laboratory techniques, 121b, 122
Antibody titer, in serologic laboratory techniques, 121b, 122
Antibovine antibodies, 139
Anticardiolipin, 246
Anti-CD52 (alemtuzumab), 445
Anti-DNase B (ADN-B), 224
Antigen-antibody ratio, 134b, 135, 136t
Antigen-antibody reactions, 58b
Antigenic determinants, 25
Antigenic drift, 494
Antigen-presenting cells (APCs), 17, 87–88, 370
  cell-mediated immunity and, 25

Antigens (immunogens), 47–66.e1, 161–162. *See also* Antibodies
  adjuvants and, 51
  allogenic, 48
  antigen-presenting cells (APCs). *See* Antigen-presenting cells (APCs)
  case study of, 63b
  characteristics of, 48–50, 48b
    autoantigens, 50
    blood group, 50
    general, 48
    histocompatibility, 48–50, 49b
    human leukocyte antigen molecules, 49, 50f
    major histocompatibility complex regions (MHC), 49, 49f. *See also* Major histocompatibility complex (MHC)
  chemical composition of, 50b
  chemical nature of, 51
  distribution by age, examples of, 309t
  EIA/ELISAs for detection, 153
  haptens and, 51
  large polysaccharides as, 51
  lipids as, 51
  nucleic acids as, 51
  physical nature of, 51
    complexity, 51
    degradability, 51
    foreignness, 51
    molecular weight, 51
    structural stability, 51
  proteins as, 51
  T-cell-dependent and T-cell-independent, 89t
  triggers of, 338–339
    environmental substances, 338
    food allergies, 338–339, 339t
    infectious agents, 338
    latex allergies, 338
    self-antigens, 338
Antigen-specific immunosuppression, 445
Antiglobulin test, direct. *See* Direct antiglobulin test (DAT)
Antihuman globulin (AHG), 134
Anti-IL-2 receptor (CD25) antibody, 445t
Antilipoidal antibodies, 234
Antilymphocyte (antithymocyte) globulin (ATG), 445t, 446–447
Antineutrophil cytoplasmic antibodies (ANCAs), 403
Antinuclear antibodies (ANAs), 156, 372–373, 397, 405–406, 405t
Antinucleoprotein, rapid slide test for, 408
Antioncogenes, 461. *See also* Oncogenes
Antiphospholipid antibodies, 399, 400f
Antiphospholipid syndrome, 399
Antiretroviral therapy (ART), 317
  actions of mechanistic classes of, 328–331
  drug resistance, 327, 329f, 330t–331t, 331–332
  entry inhibitors (ccr5 antagonist), 328
  fusion inhibitors, 328
  highly active antiretroviral therapy (HAART), 319–320
Antistreptolysin O (ASO), 224
Antitreponemal antibodies, 233
α_1-Antitrypsin, 43
APC. *See* Allophycocyanin (APC)
APCs. *See* Antigen-presenting cells (APCs)
Apheresis, 439–440
ARCHITECT HIV Ag/Ab Combo Assay, 326
Arthralgia, 245
Arthritis
  classification of, 420t
  Lyme disease and, 245–246. *See also* Lyme disease
  oligoarthritis, 420t
  polyarthritis, 420t

Arthritis *(Continued)*
  psoriatic, 420t
  rheumatoid, 414–426. *See also* Rheumatoid arthritis (RA)
  systemic, 420t
Arthrocentesis, 417
Artificial passive immunity, 25
Aseptic meningitis, 246
Ashby technique, 4
Ashby, Winifred, 4
ASO. *See* Antistreptolysin O (ASO)
Aspergillosis, 194
Aspergillus spp., 194, 447
Association constant, 58
Assurance, quality. *See* Quality assurance and quality control
Asthma, 338
Asymptomatic hepatitis B virus (HBV) infections, 280–281. *See also* Viral hepatitis
Asymptomatic infections, 268
Ataxia-telangiectasia, hereditary (Louis Bar Syndrome), 312
ATG. *See* Antilymphocyte (antithymocyte) globulin (ATG)
Atopy, 338
Atrophic gastritis, 381
Autoantigens, 50, 340, 373. *See also* Antigens (immunogens)
Autoclaving, for decontamination, of waste materials, 104
Autograft, 435t. *See also* Grafts
Autoimmune diseases, 370, 372f, 373, 373b
  adaptive immune response, 374
  associated abnormalities of, 373t
  innate immune system, 373–374
  organ-nonspecific, comparison of, 374, 374f, 375t
  organ-specific and midspectrum, 374–389. *See also* Organ-specific and midspectrum diseases
    cardiovascular, 374–375
    collagen vascular disorders, 376
    endocrine gland disorders, 376–377
    exocrine gland disease, 380–381
    gastrointestinal disorders, 381–383
    hematologic disorders, 384–386, 385t
    immune markers, 383
    neuromuscular disorders, 386–389
    neuropathies, 389–390, 389t–390t
    pancreatic diseases, 377–380, 379f
    renal disorders, 390–391, 390b
    reproductive disorders, 380
    skeletal muscle disorders, 391
    skin disorders, 391–393, 391b
  organ-specific, comparison of, 374, 374f, 375t
  progression to, 371
Autoimmune disorders, in WAS, 313
Autoimmune enzyme immunoassay, 410
Autoimmune hematologic diseases, 384–386, 385t
  hemolytic anemia, 384–386, 385t
  idiopathic thrombocytopenic purpura, 386
  lymphoproliferative syndrome, 384
Autoimmune hemolytic anemia, 346
Autoimmune liver disease testing, 382f
Autoimmune lymphoproliferative syndrome (ALPS), 384
Autoimmune pancreatitis, 379–380
Autoimmunity, 369–395.e1
  factors influencing development of, 371–372
    exogenous factors, 371–372
    genetic factors, 371, 372f
    immunopathogenic mechanisms, 372, 372f, 373t
    patient age, 372
  major autoantibodies, 371b, 372–373

Automated procedures, 159–167.e1
  case study for, 166b–167b
  characteristics of, 159
  flow cell cytometry, 160–167
    acquired immunodeficiency syndrome analysis, 165
    basic lymphocyte screening panel, 166
    CD4 lymphocytes, 165–166
    clinical applications of, 163–167, 163b
    dot plots, 165f
    electromagnetic spectrum, 160, 160f
    flow process, 161, 161f
    fluorochromes and conjugated antibodies, 160–161
    fluorophores, 160
    HLA-B27 antigen, 166
    immunofluorescence in, 162–163
    laser technology, fundamentals of, 160, 160f
    Luminex flow cytometry system, 163, 164f
    lymphocyte subsets, 164, 165f
    monoclonal antibodies and, 161–162, 162f, 162t
    multicolor system, 163
    principles of, 160
    sample preparation for, 163
    tags and colors, 162b
    tandem dyes, 162–163
Automated testing, multiplex immunoassay, 410, 410f
Automatic dispensers, 120. *See also* Dispensers
Autosomal-dominant hyper-IgE syndrome (AD-HIES), 311
Avascularity, 437–438
Avidity, 59, 59f
  test, 204–205
Azathioprine, 446

B

Babesiosis, 241, 242t–243t, 252–253, 252b. *See also* Vector-borne diseases
  diagnostic evaluation, 253
  epidemiology of, 252–253
  etiology of, 252, 253f
  prevention of, 253
  signs and symptoms of, 253
  treatment for, 253
Bacillus Calmette-Guérin (BCG), 480
Bacteremia, 71
Bacterial agglutination, 132–133
  direct, 132–133, 132b
Bacterial diseases, 192–193
Bacteriostatic, 249
Bags, biohazard, for infectious waste, 104
BALT. *See* Bronchus-associated lymphoid tissue (BALT)
Bare lymphocyte syndrome, 308
Basic lymphocyte screening panel, 166
Basic mechanisms
  antigens and antibodies, 47–66.e1
  innate and adaptive immunity, 67–96.e1
  mediators, soluble, 28–46.e1
Basophils, 9–10, 9f
B-cell disorders, 303t
B-cell tolerance, 371
BD LSRII flow cytometer, 163
bDNA. *See* Branched DNA (bDNA)
Bead technology, in flow cytometry, 435
Bejel, 228–229. *See also* Syphilis
Bell palsy, 269
Benign, infectious mononucleosis, 268
Benign tumor, 455. *See also* Tumor immunology
BinaxNOW Malaria RDT, 123

Biodefense, vaccines in, 497. *See also* Vaccines
  anthrax, 497
  smallpox, 497
Biohazard, safety standards and, 103–104
Biohazard symbol, 104
Biological response modifiers (BRMs), 39
Biologics, 421
Biomarkers. *See also* Tumor immunology
  for rejection, 448
  surface membrane, 77–79, 78f
  for tumor, 462
    alpha-fetoprotein, 467
    bladder cancer, 470
    breast, ovarian, and cervical cancer, 469–470
    CA 15-3, 468
    CA 19-9, 468
    CA 27.29, 468
    CA 125, 467
    carcinoembryonic antigen, 468
    carcinofetal antigens, 467
    categories of, 465–467, 467f
    classic, 467–469
    enzyme, 469
    epidermal growth factor receptor (EGFR), 469–470
    HER2 (HER2/neu), 468–469
    hormone, 469
    human chorionic gonadotropin (hCG), 469
    human epididymis protein 4, 467
    lactic dehydrogenase (LDH), 469
    multiple-marker, 465, 466t
    neuron-specific enolase, 469
    nonneoplastic conditions, 462, 466t
    ovarian cancer, 469–470
    placental alkaline phosphatase (ALP), 469
    prostate-specific antigen, 468
    prostatic acid phosphatase, 468
    serum, 465, 466t
    spontaneous tumor antigens, 467
    thyroglobulin, 467–468
    tumor-associated antigens, 467
    tumor-specific antigens, 467
    variety of, 462–470, 463t–466t
Biomedical Advanced Research and Development Authority (BARDA), 111
Biometrics, 112–113, 112b
Biotechnology, 169
Bladder cancer, biomarkers for, 470
Blastomyces dermatitidis, 195
Blastomycosis, North American, 195
Blood, 19
Blood group antigens, 50
Blood transfusion, transmission of cytomegalovirus, 211
"Blueberry muffin" rash, 207f
B lymphocytes, 13–14, 77, 90–92
  activation of, 91–92
  B1 cells, 91
  B2 cells, 91
  cell surface markers, 90
  characteristics of, 80t, 89b
  development of, 90–92
  differentiation of, 90–92, 90t
  function of, 89b
  maturation stages, 12t
  MZ B cells, 91
  subsets of, 91
Body defenses, 20b, 21f
  early defense, 20
  first line of, 20, 22f–23f
  second line of, 20–22, 23b
  third line of, 22–26, 24f, 24t
  tumor immunology, 461–462, 461f. *See also* Tumor immunology

Bonding, of antigen, 59
  hydrogen bonds, 60
  hydrophobic bonds, 59–60
Bone marrow, 16
  B lymphopoiesis, 91
  in stem cell transplantation, 439
Bone marrow transplantation, 439, 440f. See also Transplantation
Bone matrix autograft, 437
Bone transplantation, 437. See also Transplantation
Booster vaccines, 24–25. See also Vaccines
Borrelia burgdorferi, 243
Borrelia mayonii, 241, 241
Borrelia miyamotoi infection, 241
Borreliosis. See Lyme disease
Bourbon virus, 241
Boylston, Zabdiel, 4
Branched DNA (bDNA), 174
BRCA1 mutation, 457–458
BRCA2 mutation, 457–458
Breast cancer
  biomarkers for, 469–470. See also Biomarkers
  molecular diagnosis of, 470
Breast carcinoma-associated antigen, 468
Breast milk
  maternal antibodies in, 25
  transmission of cytomegalovirus, 211
Brewster windows, 160
Bronchoalveolar lavage (BAL), 198
Bronchus-associated lymphoid tissue (BALT), 19
Bruton X-linked agammaglobulinemia (XLA), 309–310
Burkitt lymphoma, 267
Butterfly rash, 399–400, 401t, 402f. See also Systemic lupus erythematosus (SLE)
Bystander cells, 31

C

CA 15-3, 468
CA 19-9, 468
CA 27.29, 468
CA 125, 467
Cachectin, 72
Calcitonin, as tumor markers, 469
California encephalitis, 242t–243t
Cancer
  diagnostic testing, 470b
  genetics of, 459b
  immunoediting, 466, 467f
  incidence of, 456b
  in post-organ transplantation, 447
  process of, 459b
  stem cells, 455, 455f–456f
  treatment, 471b
  vaccines, 495–497
Cancer-predisposing genes, 459, 460t
Candida albicans, 193
Candida spp., 76, 193
CAP. See College of American Pathologists (CAP)
Capillary electrophoresis, 147, 147b
  microchip, 147
Capillary isoelectric focusing (CIEF), 147b
Capillary zone electrophoresis (CZE), 147b
Capsid, 275
Capture enzyme immunoassay, 153
Carcinoembryonic antigen (CEA), 468
Carcinofetal antigens, 467
Carcinogenesis, stages of, 459, 459b
Carcinoma in situ, 459

Carcinomas, 267, 455
  adenocarcinomas, 455
  nasopharyngeal, 267
  squamous cell, 455
  transitional cell, 455
Cardiolipin, 233
Cardiopulmonary characteristics, 402
Cardiovascular disorders, 374–375
Carditis, 374–375
Carrier state, of hepatitis B virus (HBV), 286–287. See also Viral hepatitis
Catecholamines, as tumor markers, 469
Category A agents, smallpox, 497
Cayenne tick, 252
CD. See Cluster of differentiation (CD)
CD4+ effector T lymphocytes, 82–84, 82f–84f
CD4 lymphocytes, 81–85, 81b
CD4+ T lymphocytes testing, 326, 327f
CD8+cytotoxic T lymphocytes, 84–85, 87f, 87b
CD8 lymphocytes, 81b
CD8+ T cells responses, induction, and effector phases of, 86f
CD34+ cells, 439
CEA. See Carcinoembryonic antigen (CEA)
Celiac disease, 383, 383b, 384f
Celiac disease testing, for asymptomatic individuals, 384f
Cell adhesion molecules (CAMs), 70
Cell-mediated immunity, 25–26
Cell-sorting, 162, 162f
Cell surface antigens, 90–92, 90t
Cell surface markers, B lymphocytes, 90
Cell surface receptors, 74
Cellular aspects, 403
Cellular component, 23. See also Natural immunity
Cellular interactions, 74b
Cellulitis, 223
Center for Biologics Evaluation and Research (CBER), 497
Centers for Disease Control and Prevention (CDC), 489
  safety standards of, 99
Central tolerance, 370
Centrifugation, 135t, 136
C-erbB-2 (HER2/neu) oncogene, 460
Ceruloplasmin, 43
Cervarix, 496
Cervical cancer, biomarkers, for tumor, 469–470. See also Biomarkers
Chains
  free light chains (FLCs), 360, 360t, 360b
  heavy-chain disease, 365
  light-chain disease, 365
Chédiak-Higashi syndrome, 75, 75b
Chemical carcinogens, 457
Chemiluminescence, 151t, 153b
  definition of, 153–154
  direct labels for, 154
  indirect labels for, 154
  specific clinical applications, 154
Chemiluminescence immunoassays, 235
Chemiluminescent enzyme immunoassay, anaphylactic reactions (type I), 343
Chemoattractant, 69
Chemokines, 17–19, 41, 69, 74
Chemotaxis, 68–69
Chemotherapeutic agents, 471–472, 472f
  cell cycle active
    phase nonspecific, 471
    phase specific, 471
  cytokines, 472
  interferon, 461
  non-cell cycle active, 471–472
Chemotherapy, 362–363

Chickenpox, 215. See also Varicella-zoster virus (VZV)
Chiggers, 242t–243t
Chikungunya disease, 258–259, 258b
  diagnostic evaluation, 258–259
  epidemiology of, 258
  etiology of, 258
  signs and symptoms, 258
  treatment and prevention, 259
Chikungunya vaccine, 490
Cholecystectomy, CRP levels after, 44f
Choristomas, 455
Chromatography
  definition, 147
  lateral/vertical flow immunoassays (immunochromatography), 147–149, 148f
  types, 147
Chronic conditions
  granulomatous disease (CGD), 75
  viral hepatitis, 274, 275t. See also Viral hepatitis
Chronic granulomatous diseases (CGDs), 75
Chronicity, 286–287
Chronic mucocutaneous candidiasis, 308–309
Chronic rejection, 443
Chyle, 118
Classic tumor markers, 467–469
Classification
  of acquired immunodeficiency syndrome (AIDS), 316
  of hypersensitivity reactions, 339t. See also Hypersensitivity reactions
    type I (anaphylactic reactions), 339b–340b, 340–343, 341f–342f, 341t, 343t. See also Anaphylactic reactions
    type II (cytotoxic reactions), 343–346, 343b, 344f, 345b. See also Cytotoxic reactions
    type III (immune complex reactions), 346–347, 346b, 347f, 347t. See also Immune complex reactions
    type IV (T cell-dependent reactions), 347–348, 347b, 348f. See also T cells
  of immunoglobulin (Ig), 56. See also Immunoglobulin (Ig) classes
  major histocompatibility complex (MHC)
    class I, 50f, 50t
    class II, 50f, 50t
CLIA '88. See Clinical Laboratory Improvement Amendments of 1988 (CLIA '88)
Clinical and Laboratory Standards Institute (CLSI), 101
Clinical Immunization Safety Assessment Network, 498
Clinical Laboratory Improvement Amendments of 1988 (CLIA '88), 108, 123, 159
Clinical manifestations, 206
Clinical sensitivity, 110
Clinical specificity, 110
Clonal selection, 19, 56–57
Cluster of differentiation (CD), 78, 78f
CMV. See Cytomegalovirus (CMV)
CN neuritis. See Cranial nerve (CN) neuritis
Coagglutination, 131
Coats, laboratory, as barrier protection, 101
Coccidioides immitis, 194
Coccidioidomycosis, 194–195
Coefficient of variation (CV), 110
Coinfections, 288
  hepatitis, 288. See also Viral hepatitis
Cold autoimmune hemolytic anemia, 346
Collagen vascular disorders, 376. See also Autoimmune diseases
College of American Pathologists (CAP), 108
Colony-stimulating factors (CSFs), 41

Colorado tick fever, 241
Colorectal cancer, DNA microarray technology in, 470
Colorimetric immunologic probe detection, 155
Combination drugs, multiclass, 328. See also Antiretroviral therapy
Combined cellular immune deficiency disorders, 312
Combining site, 58
Community-acquired hepatitis infections, 289. See also Viral hepatitis
Competitive enzyme immunoassay, 153
Competitive immunoassay, 154, 154f
Complement, 29b
   activation of, 29, 30f
      biological effects, 33–34, 33f, 33t, 33b
   assays, 37t
   components, 10
   deficiency, 34t–35t
      disorder, 38
      testing, 36f, 38
   definition of, 29
   enzyme activation and, 29
   fixation, 194
   inactivation of, 118
   levels, alterations in, 34–36, 34t–35t, 36b
      decreased levels, 34–36
      elevated levels, 34
   principal functions of, 29
   proteins, 22
Complementary-determining regions (CDRs), 54
Complement-mediated cytotoxicity, 433–434
Complement receptor 3 (CR3) deficiency, 75–76
Complement receptors, 29–30
Complete antibodies, 60–61
Complexity, of antigens, 51
Complex karyotype abnormalities, 356
Confidence limits, 109
Confirmatory laboratory evidence, Lyme disease, 247
Congenital cytomegalovirus (CMV), 212, 217f. See also Cytomegalovirus (CMV)
Congenital immunodeficiencies, lymphocyte subset for, 309t
Congenital rubella syndrome (CRS), 205, 207f, 207t
Congenital syphilis (CS), 232. See also Syphilis
Congenital toxoplasmosis, 201, 203b. See also Toxoplasmosis
Congenital transmission, 201
Conjugated antibodies, 155, 160–161
Conjugate vaccines, 487–488
Constant (C) region, 54
Containers, biohazard, for infectious waste, 104
Continuous field-flow-assisted dielectrophoresis (DEP), 471
Control, quality. See Quality assurance and quality control
Control specimen, 109b, 112
Convalescent sera, 233
Coombs reagent, 134
Corbett, Kizzmekia S., 4–5
Cord blood transplant, 439–440
Corneal grafts, 437–438. See also Grafts
Corneal transplants, 437. See also Transplantation
Coronavirus, 198–199
Corticosteroids, 445t
Corticosteroid therapy, 389
Corzyme test, 284
Costimulators, 51
Counterimmunoelectrophoresis, 130t
Countertop centrifuges, 136

COVID-19 pandemic, 195b, 196–199
   additional types of treatments, 199
   clinical complications, 197
   diagnostic laboratory evaluation, 196–197
      clinical chemistry laboratory, 197
      hematology and coagulation laboratory, 196
      immunology-serology laboratory, 196
   epidemiology of, 196
   etiology of, 196
   immunologic manifestations, 196
   living donor transplants, 435
   malaria and, 254
   molecular-based techniques, 197–198
   monocyte and macrophage activation in, 72
   pooled testing, 199
   prevention, 104–105
   qualitative chemiluminescent immunoassay, 199
   safety practices, 98
   serologic-based techniques, 198–199
   signs and symptoms, 196
   syphilis and, 233
   treatment and prevention, 199
      convalescent plasma, 199
      monoclonal antibodies, 199
   vaccinations, 105
   vaccine, 484–485, 484t, 486f
   vaccine innovations during, 479
Cranial nerve (CN) neuritis, 269
C-reactive proteins (CRPs), 41b, 42–43
   levels after cholecystectomy, 44f
Cross-reactivity, 58
CRPs. See C-reactive proteins (CRPs)
Cryoglobulins, 139–140
Cryococcosis, 194t, 195
Cryptococcus neoformans, 195
Cryptococcus spp, 447
Cryptosporidiosis, 320
Cryptosporidium parvum, 320
CS. See Congenital syphilis (CS)
CSFs. See Colony-stimulating factors (CSFs)
CTLA4-Ig (belatacept), 445t
Culex spp., 242t–243t
Culiseta melanura, 242t–243t
Curative therapy, risk factors of, 457–458
Cuvette, 139
CV. See Coefficient of variation (CV)
Cyclosporin A, 446
Cyclosporine, 445t, 446
Cytochrome P-450, 328, 457
Cytokines, 9, 68
   cell-mediated immunity and, 25
   chemotherapeutic agents, 472
   cytokine storm, 338
   as soluble mediators. See Soluble mediators
Cytokine storm, 40–41
Cytokine storm syndrome (CSS), 72–73, 197
Cytomegalovirus (CMV), 200, 210–214
   characteristics of, 210b
   epidemiology of, 210–211
   etiology of, 210
   immunologic characteristics of, 213b
   immunologic manifestations of, 212–213
      immune system alteration, 212–213
      serologic markers, 213
   laboratory evaluation of, 213, 214t
   signs and symptoms of, 211–212
      acquired infection, 211–212
      congenital infection, 212, 217f
   transmission, 211
      blood transfusion, 211
      breast milk, 211
      congenital infection, 211
      latent infection, 211

Cytometry, flow cell. See Flow cell cytometry
Cytotoxic reactions (type II), 89, 343–346, 343b, 344f, 345b. See also Hypersensitivity reactions
   antibody-dependent, complement-mediated, 344–346
   autoimmune hypersensitivity against solid tissue, 344, 344f
   complement-mediated, 344–346
   diagnostic evaluation of, 346
      direct antiglobulin tests (DAT), 346
      polyspecific antihuman globulin (AHG), 346
   prevention of, 346
   transfusion reactions, 345b
      delayed hemolytic reaction, 344–345
      hemolytic disease of the fetus and newborn (HDFN), 345–346
      immediate hemolytic reactions, 344
   treatment of, 347
Cytotoxic T-cell responses, 491
Cytotoxic T cells, 50, 80t

D

Da. See Daltons (Da)
Daltons (Da), 51
Dander, hypersensitivity reactions to, 338
Dane particles, 284
Darkfield microscopy, 233
DAT. See Direct antiglobulin test (DAT)
Decarboxylational tumors, amine precursor uptake and, 455
Decontamination
   of nondisposable equipment, 103
   SARS-CoV-2, guidance for, 104
   of spills, 103–104
   of waste materials, 104
   of work surfaces, 103
Deer tick, 244f
Defenses, body, 20b, 21f
   early defense, 20
   first line of, 20, 22f–23f
   second line of, 20–22, 23b
   third line of, 22–26, 24f, 24t
   tumor immunology, 461–462, 461f. See also Tumor immunology
Definitive host, 201
Degradability, of antigens, 51
Degranulation, of neutrophil, 70
Denaturation, of protein, 139
Dendritic cells (DCs), 11, 12t, 489
Dengue fever, 199, 242t–243t, 259–262
   characteristics of, 259b
   diagnostic evaluation of, 260, 261b
   epidemiology of, 259
   etiology of, 259
   nucleic acid amplification tests, 260–262
   signs and symptoms of, 259–260
   treatment and prevention, 262
   vaccine, 490–494
Deoxynucleotides (dNTPs), 179
Deoxyribonucleic acid (DNA), 169, 169b, 173f, 178
Dermacentor spp., 242t–243t
Dermacentor variabilis, 250
Determinants, antigenic, 48
Diabetes, in post-organ transplantation, 447
Diapedesis, 68, 72
Diet, cancer risk factors, 457
Differentiation, clusters of, 8, 8t
DiGeorge syndrome, 307
Diluent, 118–119
Diluter-dispensers, 120. See also Dispensers

Dilutions, in serologic laboratory techniques, 120–121, 120b
  dilution factor for, 120–121
  serial, 121, 121t, 122f
  single, 121
  specimens for, 120
Direct antiglobulin test (DAT), 346
Direct bacterial agglutination, 132–133, 132b
Direct immunofluorescent assay, 155, 155f
Discoid lupus, 397
Discoid rash, 398t
Disease manifestations, immunologic
  acquired immunodeficiency syndrome (AIDS), 313–326
  cytomegalovirus (CMV), 210–214
  infectious mononucleosis, 267–272.e2
  rubella and rubeola infections, 205–208
  streptococcal infections, 221–227.e1
  syphilis, 228–239.e2
  toxoplasmosis, 200–205
  vector-borne diseases, 240–266.e1
  viral hepatitis, 273–298
Disorders, immune
  hypersensitivity reactions, 337–352.e1
  systemic lupus erythematosus, 396–413.e3
Dispensers
  automatic, 120
  diluter, 120
Dispensers/syringes, automatic, 120
DNA microarray technology, 470, 470b
DNA vaccines, 482–484, 483f
Dog tick, 242t–243t
Donor-specific antibody tests, in flow cytometry, 435
Dot plots, flow cell cytometry, 165f
Double immunodiffusion, 129, 130f
Double-negative thymocytes, 79–80
Double-positive thymocytes, 80–81
Downregulation, 343
Driver mutation, 459
Drug-induced hemolysis, 385–386, 385t
Drug-induced immunosuppression, 472, 473t
Drug-induced lupus, 397, 398b
Drugs, hypersensitivity reactions to, 338
Dust phagocytes, 11
Dyscrasias, 92
  plasma cell, 354
Dysplastic, 312

E

EA. *See* Early antigen (EA)
Early antigen (EA), 213, 270
Eastern equine encephalitis, 242t–243t
EBNA. *See* Epstein-Barr nuclear antigen (EBNA)
EDTA. *See* Ethylenediaminetetraacetic acid (EDTA)
Effector T cells, 92
EGFR. *See* Epidermal growth factor receptor (EGFR)
Ehrlichia chaffeensis, 250
Ehrlichiosis, 241
  human, 250–251
  human monocytic, 242t–243t
Eight-color immunofluorescence, 163
Electrochemiluminescence, 151t
Electromagnetic spectrum, 160, 160f
Electronic devices, safety practices for, 103
Electrophoresis techniques, 143–149.e1, 130t, 143b, 144f, 144t
  capillary electrophoresis, 147, 147b
  case study for, 148b
  immunofixation electrophoresis, 144–147
    characteristics of, 146t
    clinical application of, 147

Electrophoresis techniques (Continued)
  definition of, 144–145
  follow-up laboratory testing with, 147
  interpretation of, 146–147, 146f
  principles for, 146
  procedure for, 145
  reference values, 144
  serum protein electrophoresis, 144
    clinical interpretation for, 144, 146f
    principles for, 144, 145f
    results for, 144
Electrostatic forces, 60
Elution, 134
Embryonic primary germ layers, 455f
Emergency Use Authorization (EUA), 110
Emission wavelength, 160
EMS. *See* Eosinophilia-myalgia syndrome (EMS)
Encephalitis
  California, 242t–243t
  St. Louis, 242t–243t
  West Nile, 242t–243t
Endocrine gland diseases. *See also* Organ-specific and midspectrum diseases
  thyroid disease, 376–377
    diagnostic evaluation of, 377, 377t–378t
    Graves' disease, 377, 378f
    immunologic manifestations of, 376–377, 376f
    lymphoid chronic thyroiditis, 376
Endogenous agents, 20–22
Endogenous pathway, 87–88
Endosomes, 88
Endotoxin, 11, 194
  exogenous, 225
Engerix-B hepatitis vaccine, 276–278
Engraftment, 432
Engulfment, 22
Entry inhibitors (ccr5 antagonist), 328. *See also* Antiretroviral therapy
Enveloped flavivirus, 288
Envelope protein, 315
Environmental factors, 397–399
Environmental Protection Agency (EPA), 103
Environmental substances, hypersensitivity reactions and, 338
Enzyme
  activation and, 29
  biomarkers, 469. *See also* Biomarkers
  as tumor markers, 469
Enzyme immunoassay (EIA), 38, 150b–151b, 173, 194, 321b, 324
  advantages and disadvantages of, 152b
  capture, 153
  competitive, 153
  enzymes for, 152t
  examples of, 153b
  modification of, 153
  noncompetitive, 153
Enzyme-linked immunosorbent assay (ELISA), 151, 151t, 235, 248
  advantages and disadvantages of, 152b
  for antigen detection, 153
  multiple and portable, 153
Eosinophilia-myalgia syndrome (EMS), 376
Eosinophils, 9, 9f
Epidemic proportion, 205
Epidemic typhus, 242t–243t
Epidermal growth factor receptor (EGFR), 469–470
Epitope, 48
Epstein-Barr nuclear antigen (EBNA), 270–271, 271t
Epstein-Barr virus (EBV), 213, 387
  characteristics of, 267b
  infectious mononucleosis associations, 267. *See also* Infectious mononucleosis
  serology of, 269–270, 270f, 270t

Equine encephalitis, Eastern and Western, 242t–243t
Equipment, preventive maintenance of, 109
Erythema migrans (EM) rash, 246, 246f
Erythrocytes, stabilized sheep, 132t
Erythrogenic toxin, 223
Ethylenediaminetetraacetic acid (EDTA), 163
Etiologic agent, 195
Excitation, 160
Exocrine gland disease, 380–381
Exogenous agents, 20–22
Exogenous endotoxin, 225
Exogenous factors, 371–372
Exogenous pathway, 87–88
Exome, 184
Exons, 430
Exposures, occupational, to viral hepatitis, 289. *See also* Viral hepatitis
Extracellular matrix (ECM), 74
Extracellular products, 222–223
Extravasation, 68
Exudate (pus), 68, 223

F

Facial barrier protection, 101
False-negative errors, 109b
False-positive errors, 109b
Farmer lung, 346
FAs. *See* Food allergies (FAs)
Fc portions, 59, 69. *See also* Antibodies
FDA. *See* Food and Drug Administration (FDA)
Febrile disease, murine typhus-like, 242t–243t
First-set rejection, 441, 443f
Flat chromatography, 147
Flavivirus, 260
Flavivirus, enveloped, 288
Flavivirus genus, 199
Fleas, in vector-borne diseases, 242t–243t
Flesh-eating bacteria. *See* Necrotizing fasciitis
Flocculation tests, 129, 129b, 132b
  in agglutination, 132
Floor-model centrifuges, 136
Flow cell cytometry, 160–167, 435. *See also* Automated procedures
  acquired immunodeficiency syndrome analysis, 165, 326, 327f
  basic lymphocyte screening panel, 166
  basics, 159b
  bead technology in, 435
  case study for, 166b–167b
  CD4 lymphocytes, 165–166
  clinical applications of, 163–167, 163b
  donor-specific antibody tests in, 435
  dot plots, 165f
  electromagnetic spectrum, 160, 160f
  flow process, 161, 161f
  fluorochromes and conjugated antibodies, 160–161
  fluorophores, 160
  HLA-B27 antigen, 166
  immunofluorescence in, 162–163
  laser technology, fundamentals of, 160, 160f
  Luminex flow cytometry system, 163, 164f
  lymphocyte subsets, 164, 165f
  molecular techniques in, 435
  monoclonal antibodies and, 161–162, 162f, 162t
  multicolor system, 163
  principles of, 160
  sample preparation for, 163
  tags and colors, 162b
  tandem dyes, 162–163
FlowMetrix system, 163
5-Fluorouracil, 471

Fluorescein, 155
Fluorescein isothiocyanate (FITC), 163
Fluorescence, 154b
Fluorescence in situ hybridization (FISH), 156b, 157–158, 179–180
Fluorescence polarization immunoassay, 156b, 157
Fluorescence-resonance energy transfer, 174
Fluorescent antibodies, 154b
Fluorescent antibody (FA) microscopy, 155
Fluorescent conjugates, 154b
Fluorescent dyes, 154
Fluorescent labeling, 154, 154b, 155f
Fluorescent treponemal antibody absorption (FTA-ABS), 236
Fluorochrome fluorescein isothiocyanate (FITC), 155
Fluorochromes, 160–161
Fluoroimmunoassay, 151t
  time-resolved, 157
Fluorophore quencher, 176–178
Fluorophore reporter, 176–178
Fluorophores, 154, 160
Flu vaccines. See Influenza vaccines
Follicular dendritic cells (FDCs), 11
Food allergies (FAs), 338–339, 339t
Food and Drug Administration (FDA)
  approvals, for hepatitis A virus (HAV) vaccines, 274, 277b–278b
  approved HIV medicines, 330t–331t
  FDA Regulatory Modernization Act of 1997, 331
  ImmunoCAP, 342–343
Foodborne toxoplasmosis, 201. See also Toxoplasmosis
Food intolerance, 338–339
Foods, hypersensitivity reactions to, 338
Foreignness, of antigens, 51
Förster resonance energy transfer (FRET), 162–163
Forward scatter light (FSC), 161
FOXP3 mRNA, 448–449
Free light chains (FLCs), 360
FTA-ABS. See Fluorescent treponemal antibody absorption (FTA-ABS)
Fulminant disease, 290
Fungal diseases, 193–195. See also Infectious disease immunologic manifestations
  aspergillosis, 194
  blastomycosis, North American, 195
  coccidioidomycosis, 194–195
  cryptococcosis, 195
  histoplasmosis, 194
  sporotrichosis, 195
  survival mechanisms, 193
  testing methods for, 194t
Fusion inhibitors, 328. See also Antiretroviral therapy

G

G. See Guanine (G)
G6PD. See Glucose-6-phosphate dehydrogenase (G6PD)
Gag region, 324
Gallbladder, radiographs of, 44f
GALT. See Gut-associated lymphoid tissue (GALT)
Gamma globulin, 51
Gammopathies
  malignant, 361b, 365
  monoclonal, 354–355
  monoclonal gammopathy of undetermined significance (MGUS), 365, 366t–367t
  polyclonal, 355
Gardasil, 495–496

Gas chromatography, 147
Gastrointestinal cancer-associated antigen, 468
Gaucher's disease, 76–77, 77f
Gaussian curve, 112, 112f
GBS. See Guillain-Barré syndrome (GBS)
GBS disease. See Group B streptococcal (GBS) disease
GBV-C. See GB virus type C (GBV-C)
Genes
  cancer-predisposing, 459, 460t
  tumor-suppressing, 461
Genetic factors, 371, 372f
Genetic predisposition, 397
Genome testing, 324
Genomic alterations, detection, 471
Genotypic assays, 331
Germ layers, embryonic primary, 455f
Germline-encoded receptors, 19
Gloves, selection and use of, 101, 102f
Glucocorticosteroids, 472
Glucose-6-phosphate dehydrogenase (G6PD), 152, 152t
Gluten, 383
Glycoproteins, 22
Goodness of fit, 60, 60f
Gowns, as barrier protection, 101
Graded agglutination reactions, 136, 136t
Graduated pipettes, 119f. See also Pipettes
Grafts
  allograft, 435t
  autograft, 435t
  graft-versus-host disease (GVHD), 449–451, 449t. See also Graft-versus-host disease (GVHD)
  heterograft, 435t
  homograft, 435t
  rejection of, 441–443, 441t, 441b, 442f
    accelerated, 443
    acute, 443
    chronic, 443
    first-set, 441, 443f
    hyperacute, 441–442
    second-set, 441, 443f
  syngraft, 435t
  types of, 437–439
    bone, 437
    cornea, 437–438
    heart, 438
    heart valves, 438
    hematopoietic or peripheral blood stem cells, 440f, 439, 440f
    intestine, 438
    kidney, 438
    liver, 438
    lung, 438–439
    pancreas, 439
    skin, 439
  xenograft, 435t
Graft-versus-host disease (GVHD), 449–451, 449b. See also Grafts; Transplantation
  acute, 449
  chronic, 449
  diagnostic evaluation of, 450
  drugs used for, 450b
  epidemiology of, 449
  etiology of, 449
  high-risk patients, 450
  immunologic manifestation of, 450
  intermediate-risk patients, 450–451
  low-risk patients, 451
  prevention of, 450–451
  radiation, on specific cellular components, 451
  requirements for, 449t
  signs and symptoms of, 449–450

Granulocytes
  basophils, 9–10, 9f
  eosinophils, 9, 9f
  neutrophils, 8–9, 8f
  radiation on, 451
  tissue basophils (mast cells), 9f, 10
Granulomatous reactions (gummas), 233
Granzyme A-B, 84
Grating-coupled surface plasmon resonance (GCSPR), 153
Graves' disease, 377, 378f
Group B streptococcal (GBS) disease, 225b. See also Streptococcal infections
  epidemiology of, 226
  etiology of, 226
  future directions in, 226
  laboratory data of, 226
  signs and symptoms of, 226
  Streptococcus agalactiae, 225b
GS HIV Combo Ag/Ab EIA, 326
Guanine (G), 169
Guillain-Barré syndrome (GBS), 269
Gummas (granulomatous reactions), 233
Gut-associated lymphoid tissue (GALT), 14, 19

H

HAART. See Highly active antiretroviral therapy (HAART)
Hand sanitizing, 101–103
Handwashing, 101–103
Haplotypes, 431
Haptens, 51
Harmonization, 159
HAV. See Viral hepatitis
Hay fever, hypersensitivity reactions and, 338
Hazard Communication Standard, 99
HBIG. See Hepatitis B immune globulin (HBIG)
HBV. See Viral hepatitis
HCV. See Viral hepatitis
HDV. See Viral hepatitis
HE4. See Human epididymis protein 4 (HE4)
Healthcare workers, vaccines for, 105
Heartland virus, 241
Heart transplant, 438. See also Transplantation
Heavy chains, of antibody molecule, 54
Heidelberger curve, 138
"HeLa" cells, 4, 5b
Helper T (Th) cells, 80t
  type 1, 82, 82f–83f
  type 2, 82–83, 83f–84f
  type 17, 83–84, 85f
Hemagglutination, 133b, 134–138. See also Agglutination methods
  antibody type and, 134
  antigen-antibody ratio and, 134b, 135, 136t
  antigenic determinants, 135
  assays, 118
  enhancing methods, 136
  graded reactions, 136, 136t, 137f–138f
  lattice formation, 135
  mechanisms of, 134–135
  microplate reactions of, 136–138
  particle charge and, 134
  pH of, 135
  sensitization, 134–135
  temperature and length of incubation, 135
Hematologic disorder, 398t
Hematopoiesis, 6, 7f
Hematopoietic stem cell (HSC), 436, 436b
  transplants, 439, 440f
Hematopoietic stimulators, 41
Hemoglobinuria, 225
Hemolysins, 222
Hemolytic anemia, 384–386

Hemolytic reactions, 344
Hemolyzed specimens, 109
Hepadnavirus, 278
Hepatitis B immune globulin (HBIG), 287
Hepatitis B virus vaccine, 485
Hepatitis vaccine, 277b–278b
Hepatitis, viral, 273–298
  case studies of, 293b–294b
  characteristics of, 274, 274t–275t, 275f
  definition of, 274
  forms of, 274, 275t
    acute, 275t
    chronic, 275t
    fulminant acute, 275t
    subclinical without jaundice, 275t
  general characteristics of, 274, 274t–275t
    differential diagnosis of, 274, 275f
    etiology of, 274
    incidence of, 274, 274t
    signs and symptoms of, 274, 275t
  hepatitis A virus (HAV), 274–278, 274b
    characteristics of, 274t
    diagnostic evaluations of, 276
    epidemiology of, 275
    etiology of, 275, 276f
    immunologic manifestations of, 276
    prevention of, 276–278, 277b–278b
    signs and symptoms of, 275–276
    treatments for, 276–278, 277b–278b
    vaccines for, 277b–278b
  hepatitis B virus (HBV), 275t, 278–287, 278b
    acute infection, 285–286
    antibodies, anti-HBe and anti-HBs, 285
    antigens, hepatitis B core (HBcAg), 284
    antigens, hepatitis B-related (HBeAg), 284
    antigens, hepatitis B surface (HBsAg), 281
    asymptomatic infections, 280–281
    carrier state of, 286–287
    chronic infection, 286
    coinfections with, hepatitis D virus, 288
    diagnostic evaluations of, 285
    epidemiology of, 278–280, 280f
    etiology of, 276f, 278, 279f
    hepatocellular necrosis and, 286
    laboratory assays of, 281–285, 281f–283f, 284t
    persistent infections, 280
    prevention of, 277b–278b, 287
    serologic patterns of, 286
    signs and symptoms of, 280–281
    treatment for, 287
    viral deoxyribonucleic acid (DNA), 285
  hepatitis C virus (HCV), 288–292, 288b
    acute infections, 291–292
    chronic infections, 291–292
    community-acquired infections, 289
    epidemiology of, 288–289, 289f
    etiology of, 288
    mother-to-infant transmissions, 289
    occupational exposure, 289
    parenteral exposure, 289
    polymerase chain reaction (PCR) amplification for, 290–291
    posttransfusion infections, 289
    prevention of, 292
    prognosis for, 289–290
    recombinant erythropoietin (EPO) for, 289
    sexual transmission of, 289
    signs and symptoms of, 290
    sporadic infections, 289
    testing algorithm for, 290f
    testing, traditional, 290–291, 290f, 291t
    transmission of, 289–290
    treatment for, 291

Hepatitis, viral (Continued)
  hepatitis D virus (HDV), 287–288
    chronic infections, 287
    coinfections, hepatitis B virus (HBV), 288
    diagnostic evaluations of, 288
    epidemiology of, 287–288
    etiology of, 287
    hepadnavirus and, 288
    immunologic manifestations of, 288
    signs and symptoms of, 288
    superinfections, 288
  hepatitis E virus (HEV), 292–293, 292b
    diagnostic evaluations of, 293
    epidemiology of, 292
    etiology of, 292
    immunologic manifestations of, 293
    prevention of, 293
    signs and symptoms of, 292–293
    treatments for, 293
    epidemiology of, 292
    etiology of, 292
    GB virus type C (GBV-C) and, 274
    prevention of, 293
    signs and symptoms of, 293
    transfusion-transmitted virus (TTV), 293–295, 293b
    epidemiology of, 293
    etiology of, 293
    signs and symptoms of, 293–295
Hepatocellular necrosis, 286
Hepatoma, 290
HER2 (HER2/neu), 468–469
Herceptin, 468
Herd immunity, 205–206, 481
Hereditary angioedema (HAE)
  epidemiology of, 38
  etiology of, 38
  laboratory assays, 36f, 38
  pathophysiology of, 38
  signs and symptoms, 38
Hereditary conditions, ataxia-telangiectasia, 312
Herpes simplex virus (HSV), 214–215, 214b
  congenital infection in, 215
  crossreacting antigen types of, 215
    type 1 (HSV-1), 215
    type 2 (HSV-2), 215
  laboratory diagnosis of, 215
  neonatal infection in, 215
Herpes viruses, 214–216, 214b
  cytomegalovirus (CMV), 210–214. See also Cytomegalovirus (CMV)
  Epstein-Barr virus, 214. See also Epstein-Barr virus (EBV)
  herpes simplex virus, 214–215. See also Herpes simplex virus (HSV)
  human herpes virus 6, 216
  varicella-zoster virus, 215–216
Herpes zoster (Shingles), vaccine for, 490–491
Heterogeneous immunoassays, 150, 150b
Heterograft, 435t. See also Grafts
Heterophile antibodies, 269
HEV. See Viral hepatitis
HGV. See Viral hepatitis
HHV-6. See Human herpesvirus 6 (HHV-6)
High complexity testing, 123
Highly active antiretroviral therapy (HAART), 319–320. See also Antiretroviral therapy
High-risk patients, in graft-versus-host disease, 450
Hinton, William Augustus, 3
Histidine-rich protein II (HRP-II) antigen, malaria, 256, 256f

Histocompatibility antigens, 48–50, 49b, 429–435, 430f. See also Antigens (immunogens)
  flow cytometry, 434–435
  human leukocyte antigen, 430–431, 430t–431t, 432f–434f
  major histocompatibility complex, 431, 431t
  potential transplant recipients and donor, evaluation of, 432–435, 433f–434f
Histones, antibodies to, 405–406
Histoplasma capsulatum, 194
Histoplasmosis, 194
HIV. See Human immunodeficiency virus (HIV)
HLA-B27 antigen, 163b, 166
HLAs. See Human leukocyte antigens (HLAs)
HME. See Human monocytic ehrlichiosis (HME)
Homogeneous immunoassays, 150b, 151
Homograft, 435t. See also Grafts
Hormonal influences, 399
Hormone, as tumor markers, 469
Horseradish peroxidase (HRP), 152, 154
Host, definitive, 201
Household chlorine bleach, for decontamination, 103
HSV. See Herpes simplex virus (HSV)
Human body louse, 242t–243t
Human chorionic gonadotropin (hCG), 131
Human cytomegalovirus (HCMV). See Cytomegalovirus (CMV)
Human ehrlichiosis, 250–251, 250b. See also Vector-borne diseases
  diagnostic evaluation of, 250–251, 251f
  epidemiology of, 250
  etiology of, 250
  signs and symptoms of, 250
  treatment and prevention of, 251
Human epididymis protein 4 (HE4), 467
Human Genome GeneChip set, 180–181
Human granulocytic ehrlichiosis, 242t–243t
Human herpes virus 6 (HHV-6), 214, 216b
Human immunodeficiency virus (HIV), 313b, 315f
  in adult testing algorithm, 325f
  alternative screening for, 324–326
  assays and characteristics, 323t
  characteristics, 315b
  enzyme immunoassay results, causes of false-positive and false-negative, 324t
  in infant testing, 326
  replication cycle, 329f
  stages of, 318b, 320t
  testing of, 123, 125f
  vaccines for, 491–493, 492b–493b. See also Vaccines
Human leukocyte antigens (HLAs), 48
  alleles, classification of, 430–431, 430t
    HLA-A, 16, 430t–431t
    HLA-B, 16, 430t–431t
    HLA-DRB1, 430t–431t
  impact of, 432, 432f
  major histocompatibility complex regions (MHC), 49f. See also Major histocompatibility complex (MHC)
  matching of, in stem cell transplantation, 441
  molecules, classes of, 431, 431t
  naming system, 430t
  role of, 431–432
  techniques, 433, 433f–434f
Human monocytic ehrlichiosis (HME), 242t–243t
Human papillomavirus vaccines, 487
Humoral and cellular immunity, 491
Humoral aspects, 403–404
Humoral component, 22
  adaptive immunity, 6

INDEX

Humoral-mediated immunity, 23, 25t
Hutchinson teeth, 232
HVTN 100, 493
Hyaluronan-mediated motility receptor (HMMR), 497
Hyaluronidase, 223
Hybridoma, 61
Hydrodynamic focusing, 161
Hydrophobic bonds, 59–60
Hygiene hypothesis, 398
Hyperacute rejection, 433, 441–442
Hypercalcemia, 356
Hypercholesterolemia, in post-organ transplantation, 447
Hyper-E syndrome (HIES), 311–312
Hypergammaglobulinemias, 354
Hyper-IgM. See Immune deficiency with elevated immunoglobulin M (Hyper-IgM)
Hyperimmunoglobulinemia E syndrome, 311
Hypersensitivity reactions, 337–352.e1
  antigens and reactions, types of, 338–339
    environmental substances, 338
    food allergies, 338–339, 339t
    infectious agents, 338
    latex allergies, 338
    self-antigens, 338
  case studies for, 350b–351b
  classification of, 339t
    type I (anaphylactic reactions), 339b–340b, 340–343, 341f–342f, 341t, 343t. See also Anaphylactic reactions
    type II (cytotoxic reactions), 343–346, 343b, 344f, 345b. See also Cytotoxic reactions
    type III (immune complex reactions), 346–347, 346b, 347f, 347t. See also Immune complex reactions
    type IV (T cell-dependent reactions), 347–348, 347b, 348f. See also T cells
  fundamentals of
    allergens, 338
    allergy, 338
    atopy, 338
    hypersensitivity, immediate and delayed, 338
    immunization, 338
    immunoglobulin E (IgE), 338
    major histocompatibility complex (MHC), 338
    sensitization, 338
  types of, 339–348, 339b, 341t
    comparison of, 348–351, 349f
Hypertension, in post-organ transplantation, 447
Hyperviscosity syndrome, 356
Hypocomplementemia, 36
  diseases associated with, 36b
Hypogammaglobulinemia of infancy, transient, 311

I

IBD. See Inflammatory bowel disease (IBD)
Icteric serum, 118
IDDM. See Insulin-dependent diabetes mellitus (IDDM)
Idiopathic disease, lupus, 397. See also Systemic lupus erythematosus
Idiopathic scleroderma, 376
Idiopathic thrombocytopenic purpura, 386
Idiotype determinants, 56. See also Immunoglobulin (Ig) classes
IF. See Intrinsic factor (IF)
IF-blocking antibodies, 382
IgE-mediated food allergy, diagnosis of, 340b
IgG antibody testing, 260–262
IgG index assay (CSF), 389–393
Illumina assays, 183
ILs. See Interleukins (ILs)
Immediate-early antigens, 213
Immediate hypersensitivity. See also Hypersensitivity reactions
  anaphylactic reactions (type I) and, 340, 341f
Immulite 2000, 154
Immune complex reactions, 339t. See also Hypersensitivity reactions
  antibody-antigen interactions, 59. See also Antibodies
  clinical manifestations of, 347
  disease associated with, 347t
    Arthus reaction, 346
    autoimmune disorders, 346, 346b
    Farmer lung, 346
    serum sickness, 346, 346b
  tests for, 347
  tissue injury, mechanism of, 346, 347f
  treatment for, 347
Immune deficiency with elevated immunoglobulin M (Hyper-IgM), 311
Immune disorders
  hypersensitivity reactions, 337–352.e1
  systemic lupus erythematosus, 396–413.e3
Immune markers, 383
  celiac disease, 383, 383b, 384f
  other gastrointestinal tract immunologic diseases, 383
Immune-mediated disease, 93–94, 93t
Immune precipitation methods in gel, 129, 129b
Immune response genes, 397
Immune senescence, 17
Immune system
  characteristics of, 6b
  importance in health and disease, 6t
  soluble mediators of. See Soluble mediators
Immunity, comparisons of, 5b, 19–26, 20t
  adaptive immunity, 6
  humoral-mediated, 23–25, 25t
  natural immunity, 20–22, 23b
Immunization. See also Vaccines
  for disease prevention, 104
Immunoassay
  antibody detection and, 153
    capture enzyme, 153
    competitive enzyme, 153
    noncompetitive enzyme, 153
  antigen detection and, 153
  chemiluminescence and, 153–154, 154f
  fluorescence polarization, 156b, 157
  formats, 150–151
  heterogeneous, 150, 150b
  homogeneous, 150b, 151
  immunofluorescence, 154–156, 154b, 155f
  labeling techniques, 150–158.e1
    alternative for, 156–158, 156b
    case study for, 157b
    types of labels, 151–153
  multiple and portable enzyme-linked immunosorbent assay, 153
  radioimmunoassay, 151
  solid-phase, 151–153
  types of, 151t
ImmunoCAP assays, anaphylactic reactions (type I), 342–343, 342f, 343t
Immunochromatography, 147–149
Immunocompetent
  cells, 372
  host, 24–25
Immunocompromised or debilitated patients, 195
Immunocompromised patients, 195
IMMUNO-COV antibody test, 61
Immunodiffusion, radial, 129–130, 130t, 132f
Immunofixation electrophoresis (IFE), 130t, 143b, 144–147
  characteristics of, 146t
  clinical application of, 147
  definition of, 144–145
  follow-up laboratory testing with, 147
  interpretation for, 146–147, 146f
  principles for, 146
  procedure for, 145
Immunofluorescence, 154–156, 154b, 155f
  direct immunofluorescent assay, 155, 155f
  eight-color, 163
  excitation in, 154
  excited-state lifetime, 155
  flow cell cytometry and, 162–163, 162b
    multicolor system, 163
    tandem dyes for, 162–163
  fluorescent emission in, 155
  indirect immunofluorescent assay, 156, 156b
  inhibition immunofluorescent assay, 155
Immunogens (antigens), 47–66.e1
  adjuvants and, 51
  allogenic, 48
  and antibodies, 47–66.e1. See also Antibodies
  antibody-antigen interactions, 58–59
  case study of, 63b
  characteristics of, 48–50, 48b
    autoantigens, 50
    blood group, 50
    general, 48
    histocompatibility, 48–50, 49b
    human leukocyte antigen molecules, 49, 50f
    major histocompatibility complex regions, 49, 49f. See also Major histocompatibility complex (MHC)
  chemical composition of, 50b
  chemical nature of, 51
  definition of, 48
  diagnostic evaluations of, serum protein electrophoresis procedures, 63b
  haptens and, 51
  large polysaccharides as, 51
  lipids as, 51
  nucleic acids as, 51
  physical nature of, 51
    complexity, 51
    degradability, 51
    foreignness, 51
    molecular weight, 51
    structural stability, 51
  proteins as, 51
Immunoglobulin (Ig) classes, 51–53, 51b. See also Antibodies
  characteristics of, 52t, 55–56, 55f
  IgA, 53, 56
  IgD, 53, 56
  IgE, 53, 56
  IgG, 53, 54f
  IgM, 52
Immunoglobulin E (IgE), 311
  hypersensitivity reactions and, 338
Immunoglobulins, 51
  functional characteristics, 52t
  levels in fetus, 53f
  variants of, 51b, 56t
    allotype determinants, 56
    idiotype determinants, 56
    isotype determinants, 56
Immunohistochemistry, 216
  in infectious diseases, 216
  polymer-based methods for, 217
  protocols for, 216–217
Immunologic consequences, 404

Immunologic disorders, 92–94, 92b, 398t
　antibody deficiency disorders, 309
　B-cell disorders, 309
　Bruton X-linked agammaglobulinemia, 309–310
　cellular immunodeficiency with immunoglobulin, 314t
　chronic mucocutaneous candidiasis, 308–309
　combined cellular immune deficiency disorders, 312
　common variable immune deficiency, 303
　DiGeorge syndrome, 307
　hereditary ataxia-telangiectasia, 312
　hyper-E syndrome (HIES), 311–312
　hyperimmunoglobulinemia E syndrome, 311
　immunodeficiency with elevated immunoglobulin M (Hyper-IgM), 311
　immunoglobulin subclass deficiencies, 311
　Nezelof syndrome, 314t
　partial combined immune deficiency disorders, 312–313
　primary immune deficiency disorders, 302, 302b
　secondary immune deficiency disorders, 313, 314b
　severe combined immune deficiency, 307–308, 307t
　T-cell activation defects, 309
　T-cell immune deficiency disorders, 302, 303t, 306
　transient hypogammaglobulinemia of infancy, 311
　Wiskott-Aldrich syndrome (WAS), 312–313
　X-linked lymphoproliferative disease (XLP) syndromes 1 and 2, 312
Immunologic manifestations, 376–377, 376f, 388, 388b
　acquired immunodeficiency syndrome (AIDS), 321
　cytomegalovirus (CMV), 210–214
　infectious mononucleosis, 267–272.e2
　rubella and rubeola infections, 205–208
　streptococcal infections, 221–227.e1
　syphilis, 228–239.e2
　toxoplasmosis, 200–205
　vector-borne diseases, 240–266.e1
　viral hepatitis, 274t
Immunologic organs, development of, 14f
Immunologic thrombocytopenic purpura (ITP), 386
Immunologic tolerance, 370–371, 370t
Immunology
　body defense
　　first line of, 20, 22f–23f
　　second line of, 20–22, 23b
　　third line of, 22–26, 24f, 24t
　case study for, 25b–26b
　definition of, 5–6
　diversity in, 3
　history of, 3
　immunity, comparisons of
　　adaptive immunity, 6
　　humoral-mediated, 23–25, 25t
　　natural immunity, 20–22, 23b
　milestones in, 3, 3t
　pioneer women in, 4–5
Immunology and serology concepts
　basic mechanisms
　　antigens and antibodies, 47–66.e1
　　innate and adaptive immunity, 67–96.e1
　　mediators, soluble, 28–46.e1
　immune disorders
　　autoimmune diseases, 373, 373b
　　hypersensitivity reactions, 337–352.e1
　　rheumatoid arthritis (RA), 414–426
　　systemic lupus erythematosus, 396–413.e3

Immunology and serology concepts (Continued)
　infectious disease immunologic manifestations
　　acquired immunodeficiency syndrome (AIDS), 321
　　cytomegalovirus (CMV), 210–214
　　infectious mononucleosis, 267–272.e2
　　rubella and rubeola infections, 205–208
　　streptococcal infections, 221–227.e1
　　syphilis, 228–239.e2
　　toxoplasmosis, 200–205
　　vector-borne diseases, 240–266.e1
　　viral hepatitis, 273–298
　procedural theory and techniques
　　agglutination methods, 128–142.e2
　　automated procedures, 159–167.e1
　　electrophoresis techniques, 143–149.e1, 144t
　　immunoassay labeling techniques, 150–158.e1
　　molecular laboratory techniques, 168–188
　　quality assurance and quality control, 107–116.e1
Immunology-serology laboratory, safety in, 97–106.e1
　case study of, 105b
　COVID-19 prevention, 104–105
　decontamination
　　of nondisposable equipment, 103
　　SARS-CoV-2, guidance for, 104
　　of spills, 103–104
　　of waste materials, 104
　　of work surfaces, 103
　disposal of infectious laboratory waste in, 104
　electronic devices, 103
　hand sanitizing and handwashing, 101–103, 103b
　nail care, 103
　patient safety in, 100
　prevention of transmission of infectious diseases in, 100–101
　protective techniques for infection control in, 101
　risk and risk management, 98–99
　safety manual, 99–100
　safety standards and agencies in, 99
　safe work practices for infection control in, 101
　shoes, 103
Immunopathogenic mechanisms, 372, 372f, 373t
Immunoperoxidase staining, 216b
Immunophenotyping, 78, 161–162, 163b
　for cancer diagnosis, 163b, 164
Immunoregulation, 382
Immunoregulatory cells, 92
Immunosuppression, 19, 444–445, 444b, 445t. See also Solid organ transplantation
　antigen-specific, 445
　drug-induced, 472, 473t
　in human solid organ transplantation, 444b
　new approaches in, 447
　protocols, 447
　types of, 445t
　　antilymphocyte (antithymocyte) globulin (ATG), 446–447
　　azathioprine, 446
　　corticosteroids, 446
　　cyclosporine (cyclosporin A), 446
　　monoclonal antibodies, 447
　　mycophenolate mofetil (MMF, RS-61443), 446
　　nulojix, 447
　　sirolimus, 446
　　tacrolimus (FK-506), 446
Immunosurveillance, 462

Impetigo, 223, 223f
Inactivated vaccines, 482
Inactivation, of complement, 118
Incomplete antibodies, 60–61
Indirect immunofluorescent assay, 156, 156b
Indirect immunofluorescent technique, 408f, 408f, 406–408, 407f–409f
Indirect immunofluorescent tests, 406, 407f–408f
Infection control, 100b
Infections. See Infectious disease immunologic manifestations
Infectious agents, 338
Infectious disease immunologic manifestations
　acquired immunodeficiency syndrome (AIDS), 321
　cytomegalovirus (CMV), 210–214
　infectious mononucleosis, 267–272.e2
　rubella and rubeola infections, 205–208
　streptococcal infections, 221–227.e1
　syphilis, 228–239.e2
　toxoplasmosis, 200–205
　vector-borne diseases, 240–266.e1
　viral hepatitis, 273–298
Infectious diseases, 189–220.e3
　alternate immunology laboratory techniques for, 216–219, 216b
　bacterial diseases, 192–193
　characteristics of, 191–192
　COVID-19 (SARS-COV-2 virus), 196–199
　dengue fever, 199
　development of, 192
　fungal diseases, 193–195
　immunohistochemistry of, 216–219
　laboratory testing of, 192, 437
　molecular testing approaches for, 217–219
　mycoplasmal diseases, 195
　parasitic diseases, 193
　in post-organ transplantation, 447
　rickettsial diseases, 195
　TORCH test panel, 200, 200t
　viral diseases, 195
Infectious laboratory waste, disposal of, 104
Infectious mononucleosis, 267–272.e2
　case study of, 271b
　diagnostic evaluations of, 269, 269t, 269b
　　leukopenia, 269
　　morphologic features, 269
　epidemiology of, 268
　　cytomegalovirus (CMV) associations, 268. See also Cytomegalovirus (CMV)
　etiology of, 267–268
　　Epstein-Barr virus (EBV) associations, 267
　immunologic manifestations of, 269–272
　　early antigen (EA), 270
　　Epstein-Barr nuclear antigen (EBNA), 270–271, 271t
　　Epstein-Barr virus (EBV) serology, 269–270, 270f, 270t
　　viral capsid antigen (VCA), 270
　pathophysiology of, 268, 268b
　screening test for, 113t–114t
　signs and symptoms of, 268–269
　transmission of infection, 268, 268b
Infectious mononucleosis postperfusion syndrome, 268
Inflammation, 72b
　acute, 73, 73f
　definition of, 9
Inflammatory bowel disease (IBD), 382–383
Inflammatory polyneuropathies, 386
Influenza SARS-CoV-2 (Flu SC2), 198
Influenza vaccines, 485, 493–494. See also Vaccines
Inform HER2 Dual ISH test, 469

Inhibition immunofluorescent assay, 155
Innate and adaptive immunity, 67–96.e1
   acute inflammation, 73, 73f
   blood and tissue cells, 8
   blood cells, origin and development, 6–8
   case studies of, 93b
   cells of, 6, 6b
   cell surface receptors, 74
   comparative features of, 40t
   comparisons of, 19–26, 20t, 22f–23f
   cytokines of, 39t
   cytokine storm syndromes, 72–73
   dendritic cells, 11, 12t
   extracellular matrix (ECM), 74
   features of, 24t
   leukocyte adhesion defect (LAD), 75, 77
   leukocyte integrin disease states, 77
   lymphoid cells, 16–19, 16f
   monocytes-macrophages, 71–72, 71b, 76t
      antigen presentation, 72
      biologically-active molecules, secretion, 72
      Gaucher's disease, 76–77, 77f
      immune response induction, 72
      Niemann-Pick disease, 77
      phagocytosis and, 71–72, 72b
      qualitative disorders of, 76
      signs and symptoms of, 76
   neutrophil disorders, 74–76
      abnormal neutrophil function, 75
      Chédiak-Higashi syndrome, 75
      chronic granulomatous diseases (CGDs), 75
      complement receptor 3 (CR3) deficiency, 75–76
      innate (congenital) neutrophil abnormalities, 75–76, 75b
      myeloperoxidase deficiency, 76
      noninfectious neutrophil-mediated inflammatory diseases, 74–75, 74b
      specific granule deficiency, 76
   neutrophil extracellular traps (NETs), 71
   phagocytosis, process of, 68–71, 69f
      adhesion, 69–70
      bacteremia and, 71
      cell adhesion molecules (CAMs) and, 70
      chemoattractant substances and, 69
      chemotaxis, 68–69
      degranulation and, 70
      digestion, 70–71
      engulfment, 70, 70f
      ligands and, 69
      margination and, 69
      subsequent phagocytic activity, 71
   polymorphonuclear neutrophils (PMNs), 68
   principal mechanisms of, 7f
   sepsis, 73–74
   systemic inflammatory response syndrome (SIRS), 73–74
Innate immune response, 489
Innate immune system, 373–374
Innate lymphoid cells, 88
Innate resistance, 22–23
Insect stings, hypersensitivity reactions to, 338
In situ synthesized arrays, 180
Institute of Medicine recommendations, 206
Instrumentation, characteristics of, 159
Insulin-dependent diabetes mellitus (IDDM), 373b, 378–379
Integrase inhibitors, Antiretroviral therapy, 330t–331t
Interactions, antibody-antigen, 59–61. See also Antibodies
   affinity, 58–59, 59f
   agglutination, influence on, 60–61
   avidity, 59, 59f
   cross-reactivity, 58

Interactions, antibody-antigen (Continued)
   detection of, 60, 60t
   electrostatic forces, 60
   goodness of fit, 60, 60f
   hydrogen bonds, 60
   hydrophobic bonds, 59–60
   immune complexes, 59
   molecular basis of, 59–61
   specificity, 58
   Van der Waals forces, 60
Interferon-gamma (IFN-γ), 192
Interferons (IFNs), 40
   chemotherapeutic agents, 461
   functions of
      IFN-α, 287
      peginterferon-alpha, 287
   natural immunity and, 22, 23b
Interleukin 1 (IL-1), 192
Interleukins (ILs), 25, 40
   cell-mediated immunity and, 25
   IL-24, 459
Intermediate-risk patients, in graft-*versus*-host disease, 450–451
International Agency for Research on Cancer (IARC), 457
International Cancer Genome Consortium and the Cancer Genome Atlas, 473–474
International Organization for Standardization (ISO), 108
International Pancreas Transplant Registry (IPTR), 439
Intestine transplantation, 438. See also Transplantation
Intolerance, food, 338–339
Intradermal (ID) injection, 490
Intradermal testing, anaphylactic reactions (type I), 343t
Intraerythrocytic organisms, 253
Intraleukocytic morulae, for anaplasmosis, 250
Intramuscular (IM) injection, 490
Intranasal spray application, 490
Intrinsic factor (IF), definition of, 381
Investigational drugs, antiretroviral, 331–332. See also Antiretroviral therapy
In vitro agglutination inhibition, 131
IPTR. See International Pancreas Transplant Registry (IPTR)
I. scapularis, 242t–243t
ISO. See International Organization for Standardization (ISO)
Isoelectric focusing, 147
Isolated intestinal transplant, 438
Isolated islet cell transplantation, 439
Isotachophoresis, 147b
Isotype determinants, 56. See also Immunoglobulin (Ig) classes
Ixodes spp., 242t–243t. See also Ticks

J

Job syndrome, 311

K

Kaposi sarcoma (KS), 320
Kappa (κ) monoclonal light chains, 354–355
Karikó, Katalin, 5
Karyotype abnormalities, complex, 356
Kidney transplantation, 438. See also Transplantation

L

Labeling, accuracy and, 108–109
Labeling techniques, in immunoassay, 150–158.e1

Labeling techniques, in immunoassay (Continued)
   alternative, 156–158, 156b
      fluorescence polarization immunoassay, 156b, 157
      magnetic labeling technology, 156, 157f
      signal amplification technology, 156
      time-resolved fluoroimmunoassay, 157
   case study for, 157b
   chemiluminescence, 153–154, 154f
   fluorescence in situ hybridization, 154b, 157–158
   immunoassay formats, 150–151
   immunofluorescence, 154–156, 154b, 155f
   types of labels, 151–153, 151t
Laboratory immunology and serology concepts basic mechanisms
   antigens and antibodies, 47–66.e1
   innate and adaptive immunity, 67–96.e1
   mediators, soluble, 28–46.e1
immune disorders
   autoimmune diseases, 373, 373b
   rheumatoid arthritis (RA), 414–426
   systemic lupus erythematosus, 396–413.e3
infectious disease immunologic manifestations
   acquired immunodeficiency syndrome (AIDS), 321
   cytomegalovirus (CMV), 210–214
   infectious mononucleosis, 267–272.e2
   rubella and rubeola infections, 205–208
procedural theory and techniques
   agglutination methods, 128–142.e2
   automated procedures, 159–167.e1
   electrophoresis techniques, 143–149.e1, 144t
   immunoassay labeling techniques, 150–158.e1
   molecular laboratory techniques, 168–188
   quality assurance and quality control, 107–116.e1
   streptococcal infections, 221–227.e1
   syphilis, 228–239.e2
   toxoplasmosis, 200–205
   vector-borne diseases, 240–266.e1
   viral hepatitis, 273–298
Laboratory policies, established, accuracy and, 108
Laboratory procedure manual, accuracy and, 108, 108b
Laboratory techniques, serologic, 117–127.e1, 118b
   blood specimen preparation in, 118–122
   case study of, 124b
   dilutions in, 120–121, 120b
      dilution factor for, 120–121
      serial, 121, 121t, 122f
      single, 121
      specimens for, 120
   inactivation of complement in, 118
   pipettes for, 118–120, 119f
      automatic dispensers/syringes, 120
      diluter-dispensers, 120
      micropipettors, 119–120, 119f
   pipetting techniques for, 118–120
      automatic, 120
      manual, 119b
   procedures manual of, 118
   types of specimens tested in, 118
Lactic dehydrogenase (LDH), 469
LADA. See Latent autoimmune diabetes in adults (LADA)
Lambda (λ) monoclonal light chains, 354–355
Lancefield, Rebecca Craighill, 4
Lancefield Streptococcus classifications, 222t

Laser, 160
 technology, fundamentals of, 160
Latent autoimmune diabetes in adults (LADA), 377–378
Latent infection, of cytomegalovirus, 211
Latent syphilis, 231–232
Late-onset lupus, 402
Lateral or vertical flow immunoassays, 202b
Lateral/vertical flow immunoassays, 147–149, 148f
Late (tertiary) syphilis, 232–233
Latex
 agglutination, 130–131, 133f–134f, 133t, 133b. See also Agglutination methods
 particles, 132t
Lattice hypothesis, 135
LAV. See Lymphadenopathy-associated virus (LAV)
LCD. See Light-chain disease (LCD)
LDH. See Lactic dehydrogenase (LDH)
Leading-edge vaccines, 479–481
 malaria, 479–480
 Shigella, 480
 tuberculosis, 480–481
LED. See Light-emitting diode (LED)
L'Esperance, Elise, 4
Leukapheresis, 439–440
Leukemia, vaccine for, 496–497
Leukocyte adhesion defect (LAD), 75, 77
Leukocyte adhesion deficiency, 76b
Leukocyte integrins, 74, 76b
 disease states involving, 77
Leukocytes, 6
 polymorphonuclear (PMN), 26f, 222
Leukopenia, 269
Leukotrienes, 93, 419
Lewis, Julian H., 3
Lice, in vector-borne diseases, 242t–243t
Ligands, 69
Light chain
 kappa (κ), 354–355
 lambda (λ), 354–355
 monoclonal, 354–355
Light-chain disease (LCD), 365
Light chains, of antibody molecule, 54–55
Light-emitting diode (LED), for nephelometry, 139
Limits of detection (LOD), 111
Lipids, 51
Liposome assay, 38
Liposome-enhanced latex agglutination, 131, 134f
Liquid biopsy tests, 462
Liquid chromatography, 147
Listeria spp, 447
Live, attenuated vaccines, 482
Liver transplant, 438
Living donor transplants, 437
Load tests, viral, 326
Lone star tick, 242t–243t
Long terminal redundancies (LTRs), 314
Louse-borne relapsing fever, 242t–243t
Lower respiratory tract disease (LRTD), 479–480
Low-risk patients, in graft-*versus*-host disease, 451
Luminex flow cytometry system, 163, 164f
Lung transplantation, 438–439. See also Transplantation
Lupoid hepatitis, 382
Lupus. See Systemic lupus erythematosus (SLE)
Lupus anticoagulants, 197, 404
Lupus erythematosus microbiota, 397–398

Lyme disease (Lyme borreliosis), 241, 243–250. See also Vector-borne diseases
 antibiotics for, 249–250
 antibody detection of, 247–249
 arthritis in, 245–246
 cardiac manifestations of, 246
 cerebrospinal fluid analyses, 249
 characteristics of, 243b
 confirmatory laboratory evidence, 247
 cutaneous manifestations of, 246, 246f
 diagnostic evaluation of, 247–249, 249t
 enzyme-linked immunosorbent assay for, 248
 epidemiology of, 244, 245f
 etiology of, 243, 244f
 immunologic manifestations of, 246–247
 neurologic manifestations of, 246
 polymerase chain reaction, 248–249
 pregnancy in, 246
 presumptive laboratory evidence, 247
 prevention of, 249–250
 signs and symptoms of, 244–247, 245t
 stages of, 244
 treatment for, 249–250
 Western blot analysis for, 248, 249f
Lymphadenopathy, 402
Lymphadenopathy-associated virus (LAV), 313
Lymph nodes, 17–19
 internal structure of, 18f
 structure of, 18f
Lymphocyte recirculation, 19
Lymphocytes, 13–16, 13f
 characteristics of, 79b, 80t
 circulation of, 19
 development, 13–14, 13b, 14f–15f
 distribution of, 18t
 dysfunction, 92b
 facts about, 77b
 functions of, 79b
 natural killer (NK) cells, 15–16, 88–89, 88b
 plasma cells, 14–15, 15f
 radiation on, 451
 recirculations of, 19
 suppressor cytotoxic, 92
 T-regulatory, 88–89, 88b
 viral responses by, 87b
Lymphocytes and plasma cells
 B lymphocytes, 90–92
  activation of, 91–92
  development of, 90–92
  differentiation of, 90–92, 90t
  subsets of, 91
 case studies of, 93b
 immunologic disorders, 92–94, 92b
  antibody deficiency disorders, 309
  B-cell disorders, 309
  Bruton X-linked agammaglobulinemia (XLA), 309–310
  combined cellular immune deficiency disorders, 312
  common variable immune deficiency, 303
  DiGeorge syndrome, 307
  hereditary ataxia-telangiectasia, 312
  hyper-E syndrome (HIES), 311–312
  hyperimmunoglobulinemia E syndrome, 311
  immunodeficiency with elevated immunoglobulin M (Hyper-IgM), 311
  immunoglobulin subclass deficiencies, 311
  partial combined immune deficiency disorders, 312–313
  primary immune deficiency disorders, 302, 302b
  secondary immune deficiency disorders, 313, 314b
  selective immunoglobulin A deficiency, 311

Lymphocytes and plasma cells (Continued)
  severe combined immune deficiency, 307–308, 307t
  T-cell activation defects, 309
  T-cell immune deficiency disorders, 302, 303t, 306
  transient hypogammaglobulinemia of infancy, 311
  Wiskott-Aldrich syndrome (WAS), 313
  X-linked lymphoproliferative disease (XLP) syndromes 1 and 2, 312
 innate lymphoid cells, 88
 lymphocyte subset alterations, 92
  aging changes, 92
 plasma cell biology, 92
 surface membrane markers, 77–79, 78f
 T lymphocyte development, 79–88, 80t
  antigen-presenting cells (APCs), 87–88
  antigen processing, 87–88
  antigen recognition, 86–87
  CD4+ effector T lymphocytes, 82–84, 82f–84f
  CD4 lymphocytes, 81–85, 81b
  CD8+cytotoxic T lymphocytes, 84–85, 87f, 87b
  double-negative thymocytes, 79–80
  double-positive thymocytes, 80–81
  early cellular differentiation and development, 79–81
  later differentiation and development, 81
  T cell activation, 87
  T-independent antigen triggering, 87
Lymphocyte subsets, 164, 165f
Lymphoid cells, innate, 16–19, 16f–18f
Lymphoid chronic thyroiditis, 376
Lymphoid markers, 77–79
Lymphokine-activated killer cells, 462
Lymphoproliferative syndrome, 384
Lymphotoxin, 17
Lysozymes, 70, 71b

M

MAC. See Membrane attack complex (MAC)
Macroglobulinemia, Waldenström's primary, 363–365
 cardiopulmonary abnormalities and, 364
 cutaneous manifestations of, 364
 diagnostic evaluation of, 364–365
 epidemiology of, 363
 etiology of, 363
 hematologic abnormalities of, 363–364
 hematologic assessment of, 364
 immunologic assessment of, 364–365
 immunologic manifestations of, 364
 neuropsychiatric problems and, 364
 ocular manifestations of, 364
 renal dysfunction and, 364
 signs and symptoms of, 363–364
 skeletal features of, 363
 treatment of, 365
Macromolecular complex, formation of, 138
Macrophage activation syndrome (MAS), 72
Macrophages, 10–11, 11f, 71, 71b, 462
 vs. neutrophils, 12t
 primary functions of, 72b
Magnetic labeling technology, 156, 156b, 157f
Major histocompatibility complex (MHC), 370. See also Antigens (immunogens)
 cell-mediated immunity and, 25
 class I, 50f, 50t
 class II, 50f, 50t
 definition of, 48
 human leukocyte antigen (HLA) system and, 49. See also Human leukocyte antigens (HLAs)

Major histocompatibility complex (MHC) (Continued)
    hypersensitivity reactions and, 338. See also Hypersensitivity reactions
    regions of, 49, 49f
Malaria, 253–258
    characteristics of Plasmodium species, 254, 255f
    COVID-19 pandemic and, 254
    diagnostic laboratory evaluation, 256–258
        histidine-rich protein II (HRP-II) antigen, 256, 256f
        microscopic examination, 256, 256f
        molecular testing, 256–258
        rapid device testing (RDT), 256, 257f
    disease phase in humans, 254
    epidemiology of, 254
    etiology of, 253–254
    global distribution and statistics, 254
    lifecycle, 480f
    risk of, 254
    signs and symptoms, 255–256
    testing, 123, 125f
    treatment and prevention, 258
    vaccines, 479–480
Malar rash, 398t
Malignant tumor, 455–456. See also Tumor immunology
Manifestations, immunologic
    acquired immunodeficiency syndrome (AIDS), 313–326
    cytomegalovirus (CMV), 210–214
    infectious mononucleosis, 267–272.e2
    rubella and rubeola infections, 205–208
    streptococcal infections, 221–227.e1
    syphilis, 228–239.e2
    toxoplasmosis, 200–205
    vector-borne diseases, 240–266.e1
    viral hepatitis, 273–298
Marginal zone B cells, 91
Margination, 69
Markers, 165
    surface membrane, 77–79, 78f
Massively parallel sequencing, 178, 183–186, 183t, 184f, 185b
Massive parallel sequencing, 470
Mast cells, 10
Maternal antibodies, 25
Mature red blood cells, radiation on, 451
MCV. See Mutated and citrullinated vimentin (MCV)
Mean, statistical, 112
Measles (rubeola infections), 208–210
    antibody testing of, 210t
    case study of, 218b
    definition of, 208
    epidemiology of, 208
    laboratory testing of, 209–210
    prevention of, 208–209
Mechanisms
    antigens and antibodies, 47–66.e1
    innate and adaptive immunity, 67–96.e1
    mediators, soluble, 28–46.e1
Median, statistical, 112
Mediators, soluble, 28–46.e1
    acute-phase proteins, 41–45, 41b
        applications of, 42b
        catabolism, 42
        ceruloplasmin, 43
        clinically useful, 42t
        C-reactive protein (CRP), 42–43
        laboratory assessment methods for, 43–45
        overview of, 41–42, 42t, 42b
        synthesis of, 42
        α_1-antitrypsin, 43
    biological response modifiers, 39

Mediators, soluble (Continued)
    case study, 43b
    complement system, 29–30
        activation of, 29, 30f, 31t
        biological functions, 33–34, 33f, 33t, 33b
        complement levels, alterations in, 34–36, 34t–35t, 36b
        enzyme activation and, 29
        membrane attack complex, 31–32, 32f
        proteolytic complement cascade, 31
        recognition stage, 31
    cytokines, 39–40, 39t
    diagnostic evaluation of, 36–38, 36f, 37t
        enzyme immunoassay, 38
        hemolytic method, 38
        liposome assay, 38
    hematopoietic stimulators, 41
        chemokines, 41
        colony-stimulating factors (CSFs), 41
        stem cell factor (c-kit Ligand), 41
        transforming growth factors (TGFs), 41
    interferons (IFNs), 40
    interleukins (ILs), 40
    mannose-binding lectin pathway, 33
    pathways, alternative, 32–33
    pathways, classic, 30–32
        membrane attack complex, 31–32
        proteolytic complement cascade, 31
        recognition stage, 31
    pathways, mannose-binding lectin, 33
    tumor necrosis factor (TNF), 41
Mediterranean spotted fever, 242t–243t
Membrane attack complex (MAC), 31–32, 32f
Membranoproliferative glomerulonephritis, 390
Memory cells, 79
Meningeal syphilis, 232
Meningitis, aseptic, 246
Meningococcal protein conjugate, 487
Meningococcal vaccines, 487
Meningovascular syphilis, 232
6-Mercaptopurine, 444b, 446, 473t
Metals, hypersensitivity reactions to, 338
Method theory and techniques
    agglutination methods, 128–142.e2
    automated procedures, 159–167.e1
    electrophoresis techniques, 143–149.e1, 144t
    immunoassay labeling techniques, 150–158.e1
    molecular laboratory techniques, 168–188
    quality assurance and quality control, 107–116.e1
MGUS. See Monoclonal gammopathy of undetermined significance (MGUS)
MHC. See Major histocompatibility complex (MHC)
Microarrays, 180–183, 180b, 181f
Microbial antigens, 118
Microbial carcinogens, 457, 458t
Microbiome, 19–20
Microbiota, 19–20
Microchip capillary electrophoresis, 147
Microcirculation, 69
β_2-Microglobulin, multiple myeloma and, 356
Micropipettors, 119–120, 119f. See also Pipettes
Microplate agglutination reactions, 136–138
Microscopy, fluorescent antibody (FA), 155
Midspectrum diseases, organ-specific and, 374–389. See also Autoimmune diseases
    autoimmune hematologic disorders, 384–386, 385t
    cardiovascular disorders, 374–375
    collagen vascular disorders, 376
    comparison of, 374f
    endocrine gland disorders, 376–377
    exocrine gland disease, 380–381
    gastrointestinal disorders, 381–383

Midspectrum diseases, organ-specific and (Continued)
    neuromuscular disorders, 386–389
    neuropathies, 389–390, 389t–390t
    pancreatic diseases, 377–380, 379f
    renal disorders, 390–391, 390b
    reproductive disorders, 380
    skeletal muscle disorders, 391
    skin disorders, 391–393, 391b
Milestones, immunology, 3, 3t
Mites, in vector-borne diseases, 242t–243t
MM. See Multiple myeloma (MM)
MOB-5, 459. See also Interleukins (ILs)
Moderately complex tests, 123
Mode, statistical, 112
Mold, hypersensitivity reactions to, 338
Molecular laboratory techniques, 168–188, 186b
    for amplicons, 170–171, 173b
    amplification methods, 171–175, 171b
        branched deoxyribonucleic acid, 174
        general characteristics of, 170b
        nucleic acid sequence–based amplification (NASBA), 174
        polymerase chain reaction and, 171–173, 174f, 176f
        probe amplification methods, 175
        serial invasive signal amplification, 175
        strand displacement amplification, 175
        target amplification methods, 171, 175
        transcription-mediated amplification (TMA), 174, 177f
    amplification products, 175–183
        DNA methylation analysis, 183
        electrophoresis-based techniques, 176, 177t
        fluorescence in situ hybridization (FISH), 179–180
        hybridization assays, 179, 179b
        illumina assays, 183
        microarrays, 180–183, 180b, 181f
        pyrosequencing, 179
        Sanger (chain termination) sequencing, 178–179, 178f
        self-assembled arrays, 181–183
        spotted arrays, glass, 180–181, 182f
        SYBR green dye–based assays, 176–179
        TaqMan assays, 176–179
    case study, 186b
    massively parallel sequencing/next-generation sequencing technology, 183–186, 183t, 184f, 185b
    for nucleic acids
        characteristics of, 169–170, 170f–173b
        comparison of, 169
        deoxyribonucleic acid (DNA) as, 169, 173f
        mutations and polymorphisms, 169–170
        ribonucleic acid as, 169–170, 173f
    polymerase chain reaction techniques in, 171–173, 173f
    modified polymerase chain reaction in, 173
    nucleic acid probes and, 173
    nucleic acid sequence–based amplification in, 174
    oligonucleotides and, 171
    reverse transcriptase polymerase chain reaction in, 176
    thermocycler and, 175
    transcription-mediated amplification in, 174, 177f
Molecular patterns, pathogen-associated. See Pathogen-associated molecular patterns (PAMPs)
Molecular weight, of antigens, 51

Monoclonal antibodies (MAbs), 16, 61–63, 447.
　　See also Antibodies
　characteristics of, 61b
　direct immunofluorescent assay and, 155
　discovery of, 61
　for flow cell cytometry, 161–162, 162f, 162t
　production of, 61–62, 62f
　therapy, 472–475, 472f, 473t–474t
　uses of, 62–63
Monoclonal gammopathies. See also
　　Gammopathies, 17, 145, 354–355
Monoclonal gammopathy of undetermined
　　significance (MGUS), 365, 366t–367t
Monoclonal light chain, 354–355
Monoclonal protein, 354. See also M
　　(monoclonal) protein
Monocyte-macrophage disorders, 76b
　Gaucher's disease, 76–77, 77f
　Niemann-Pick disease, 77
　qualitative disorders of, 76
　signs and symptoms of, 76
Monocyte-macrophage host defense functions,
　　71–72, 71b, 76t
　antigen presentation, 72
　biologically-active molecules, secretion, 72
　immune response induction, 72
　phagocytosis and, 71–72, 72b
Monocytes, 10–11, 10f
Mononuclear phagocyte system, 10, 12f
Mononucleosis, infectious, 267–272.e2
　case study of, 271b
　diagnostic evaluations of, 269, 269t, 269b
　　leukopenia, 269
　　morphologic features, 269
　epidemiology of, 268
　　cytomegalovirus (CMV) associations, 268.
　　　See also Cytomegalovirus (CMV)
　etiology of, 267–268
　　Epstein-Barr virus (EBV) associations, 267
　immunologic manifestations of, 269–272
　　early antigen (EA), 270
　　Epstein-Barr nuclear antigen (EBNA),
　　　270–271, 271t
　　Epstein-Barr virus (EBV) serology,
　　　269–270, 270f, 270t
　　viral capsid antigen (VCA), 270
　pathophysiology of, 268, 268b
　signs and symptoms of, 268–269
　transmission of infection, 268, 268b
Morbidity, 228–229
Morphologic features, 269
Mosquitoes, in vector-borne diseases, 242t–243t
Mosquito vector diseases, 253
　chikungunya disease. See Chikungunya
　　disease
　dengue fever. See Dengue fever
　malaria. See Malaria
　West Nile virus. See West Nile virus (WNV)
Mother-to-infant hepatitis transmission, 289. See
　　also Viral hepatitis
M protein, 146, 354
M (monoclonal) protein (MAbs), 354
MS. See Multiple sclerosis (MS)
MSAs. See Myositis-specific autoantibodies (MSAs)
MUC-2 gene, 468
Mucor spp, 447
Mucosal immune system, 23f
Multiple and portable enzyme-linked
　　immunosorbent assay, 153
Multiple-marker, for tumor, 465, 466t
Multiple myeloma (MM), 146, 355–363
　Bence Jones protein in, 359–360, 365b–366b
　definition of, 355
　diagnostic evaluation of, 358
　epidemiology of, 355–356, 356t

Multiple myeloma (MM) (Continued)
　etiology of, 355
　free light chains for, 360, 360t, 360b
　hematologic assessments for, 358, 359f
　hematologic features of, 356–357
　immunologic manifestations of, 358
　immunologic testing for, 360–361, 360t, 361f,
　　361b
　infectious diseases in, 358
　interleukin-6 (IL-6) and, 356
　molecular testing for, 358–359, 359t
　neurologic features of, 358
　pathophysiology of, 356
　prognosis for, 361–362, 362t
　renal disorders of, 357–358
　skeletal abnormalities of, 356, 357f
　staging system for, 361
　treatment of, 362–363
Multiple sclerosis (MS), 387–389, 388b
　albumin quotient, 388
　categorization of, 387–388
　clinical laboratory evaluations, 388
　detection of oligoclonal banding, 388
　diagnostic methods, overview of, 387–388
　epidemiology, 387
　etiology, 387
　glucose in CSF and serum, 388
　leukocyte cell counts, 388
　overview of diagnostic methods, 388
　pathophysiology, 387
　radiological examination, 388
　ruling in, 388
　ruling out, 388
　significance of oligoclonal bands, 388–389
　signs and symptoms, 387
　total protein in CSF, 388
　treatment, 389
Murine typhus, 242t–243t
Musculoskeletal features, 402
Mutated and citrullinated vimentin (MCV), 419
Mutation, 459
MW. See Molecular weight (MW)
Myasthenia gravis, 386–387, 386b
Mycobacterium spp, 447
Mycobacterium tuberculosis, 192–193
　etiology of, 192
　pathophysiology of, 192–193
Mycophenolate mofetil (MMF, RS-61443), 445t,
　　446
Mycoplasmal diseases, 195
Myelitis, 269
Myeloma, multiple, 355–363
　Bence Jones protein in, 359–360, 365b–366b
　definition of, 355
　diagnostic evaluation of, 358
　epidemiology of, 355–356, 356t
　etiology of, 355
　free light chains for, 360, 360t, 360b
　hematologic assessments for, 358, 359f
　hematologic features of, 356–357
　immunologic manifestations of, 358
　immunologic testing for, 360–361, 360t, 361f,
　　361b
　infectious diseases in, 358
　interleukin-6 (IL-6) and, 356
　molecular testing for, 358–359, 359t
　neurologic features of, 358
　pathophysiology of, 356
　prognosis for, 361–362, 362t
　renal disorders of, 357–358
　skeletal abnormalities of, 356, 357f
　staging system for, 361
　treatment of, 362–363
Myeloperoxidase deficiency, 76
Myositis-specific autoantibodies (MSAs), 391b

N

NA. See Nuclear antigen (NA)
NAAT. See Nucleic acid amplification tests
　　(NAAT)
NADPH oxidase. See Nicotinamide-adenine
　　dinucleotide phosphate (NADPH) oxidase
Nail care, safety practices for, 103
Naïve lymphocytes, 79
Nanoparticles, 485
Nasopharyngeal carcinoma, 267
National Childhood Vaccine Injury Act
　　(NCVIA), 498
National Healthcare Safety Network (NHSN), 99
National Institute of Allergy and Infectious
　　Diseases (NIAID), 338
National Organ Transplant Act, 436
Natural immunity, 20–22, 23b
Natural killer (NK) cells, 15–16, 88–89, 462
　characteristics of, 80t, 88b
　functions of, 88b
Natural Treg cells, 88
Necrosis, 286
　hepatocellular, 291–292
Necrotizing fasciitis, 221
Needlestick injuries, 289
Negative predictive value (NPV), 111
Negative selection, 19, 370
Neisseria gonorrhoeae, direct fluorescent
　　antibody test for, 154
Neonatal Fc receptor (FcRn), 53
Neonatal lupus, 397
Neonatal septicemia, 221
Neonatal varicella infection, 215. See also
　　Varicella-zoster virus
Neoplasms, 455
　thymus, 267
Nephelometry. See also Automated procedures
　for agglutination, 130t, 138–140, 138b
　advantages and disadvantages of, 139
　assays performed by, 138b
　clinical application of, 139–140
　measuring methods of, 139
　optical system of, 139
　physical basis of, 139
　principle of, 138–139, 138b, 139f
Neuroendocrine tumors, 455
Neurologic disorder, 398t
Neuromuscular disorders, 386–389
Neuron-specific enolase, as tumor markers, 469
Neuropathies, 389–390, 389t–390t
Neuropsychiatric features, 402
Neurosyphilis, 232–233. See also Syphilis
Neutralizing antibodies (NAbs), 61, 61b, 198
Neutrophil disorders, 74–76
　abnormal neutrophil function, 75
　Chédiak-Higashi syndrome, 75
　chronic granulomatous diseases (CGDs), 75
　complement receptor 3 (CR3) deficiency,
　　75–76
　innate (congenital) neutrophil abnormalities,
　　75–76, 75b
　myeloperoxidase deficiency, 76
　noninfectious neutrophil-mediated inflamma-
　　tory diseases, 74–75, 74b
　specific granule deficiency, 76
Neutrophil extracellular traps (NETs), 71, 403
Neutrophils, 8–9, 8f
　antimicrobial systems of, 71b
　defense activities, 68b
　degranulation of, 70
　function and types of granules in, 68t
　vs. macrophages, 12t
Next-generation sequencing (NGS), 470
Next-generation sequencing technology, 178,
　　183–186, 183t, 184f, 185b

Nezelof syndrome, 314t
NGS. *See* Next-generation sequencing (NGS)
NHSN. *See* National Healthcare Safety Network (NHSN)
NIAID. *See* National Institute of Allergy and Infectious Diseases (NIAID)
Nicotinamide-adenine dinucleotide phosphate oxidase (NADPH) oxidase, 70–71
Niemann-Pick disease, 77
NK cells. *See* Natural killer (NK) cells
NNRTIs. *See* Non-nucleoside reverse transcriptase inhibitors (NNRTIs)
Nocardia spp, 447
Noncoding substitutions, 430
Noncompetitive enzyme immunoassay, 153
Nonerosive arthritis, 398t
Non-Hodgkin lymphoma, 320
Noninfectious neutrophil-mediated inflammatory diseases, 74–75, 74b
Non-instrument-based testing, 123–127
   human immunodeficiency virus testing in, 123, 125f
   malaria testing in, 123
   pregnancy testing in, 123–127
Nonlymphoid markers, 77–79
Nonnucleoside reverse transcriptase inhibitors (NNRTIs), 328. *See also* Antiretroviral therapy
Nonpermissive cells, 457
Nonreplicating mRNA, 484
Nonspecific soluble factors, 25
Nontreponemal antibodies, 233
Nontreponemal methods, 233–234
North American blastomycosis, 195
Nosocomial infections, 169
Nosocomial transmission, 101
Nuclear antigen (NA), 271
Nucleic acid amplification tests (NAATs), 260–262, 322–324
   crossreactive flaviviruses, 260
   IgG antibody testing, 260–262
   serologic tests, 260
Nucleic acid probe, 173
Nucleic acids, characteristics of, 169–170, 170f–173f
Nucleic acid vaccines, 482–484
Nucleocapsid proteins, 278
Nucleoside reverse transcriptase inhibitors (NRTIs), 328
Nucleotides, 169, 170f
Null alleles, 430. *See also* Alleles
Nulojix, 447

O

Oat cell carcinomas, hormone markers for, 469
Occlusive bandages, 101
Occupational exposures, to viral hepatitis, 289. *See also* Viral hepatitis
Occupational Safety and Health Administration (OSHA), safety standards of, 99
Ocrelizumab (Ocrevus), 389
Oligoarthritis, 420t
Oligoclonal bands, significance of, 388–389, 389b
Oligonucleotides, 171
Oncofetal proteins, 467
Oncogenes. *See also* Tumor immunology
   activation mechanism of, 460–461, 460t
   classes of, 460
   overexpression of, 460
   role of, 460–461, 460t
   viral, 461, 461b
Oncogenic viruses, 461b
Onesimus, 4

Opportunistic infections, 319–320, 320f, 320t, 320b
Opsonization, 69
Oral ulcers, 398t
Organ-nonspecific autoimmune diseases, comparison of, 374, 374f, 375t
Organ-nonspecific, comparison of, 374f
Organochlorine substances, 457
Organ-specific and midspectrum diseases, 374–389. *See also* Autoimmune diseases
   autoimmune hematologic disorders, 384–386, 385t
   cardiovascular disorders, 374–375
   collagen vascular disorders, 376
   comparison of, 374, 374f, 374b, 375t
   endocrine gland disorders, thyroid disease, 376–377
   exocrine gland disease, 380–381
   gastrointestinal disorders, 381–383
   immune markers, 383
   neuromuscular disorders, 386–389
   neuropathies, 389–390, 389t–390t
   pancreatic diseases, 377–380, 379f
   renal disorders, 390–391, 390b
      associated with anti-glomerular basement membrane antibody, 390, 390f
      associated with circulating immune complexes, 390
      membranoproliferative glomerulonephritis, 390
      tubulointerstitial nephritis, 391
   reproductive disorders, 380
   skeletal muscle disorders, 391
      inflammatory myopathy, 391, 391b
   skin disorders, 391–393, 391b
Organ transplantation, 427–453.e1. *See also* Transplantation
   biomarkers, for rejection, 448
   case study of, 451b–452b
   current directions in, 451–452
   FOXP3 mRNA in, 448–449
   general facts about, 435–436
   graft rejection in, 441–443, 441t, 441b, 442f
      accelerated, 443
      acute, 443
      chronic, 443
      first-set, 441, 443f
      hyperacute, 441–442
      second-set, 441, 443f
   graft-*versus*-host disease (GVHD), 449–451, 449b
      diagnostic evaluation of, 450
      drugs used for, 450b
      epidemiology of, 449
      etiology of, 449
      high-risk patients, 450
      immunologic manifestation of, 450
      intermediate-risk patients, 450–451
      low-risk patients, 451
      prevention of, 450–451
      radiation, on specific cellular components, 451
      requirements for, 449t
      signs and symptoms of, 449–450
   hematopoietic stem cells in, 436, 436b
   histocompatibility antigens, 429–435, 430f
      flow cytometry, 434–435
      human leukocyte antigen, 429–435, 430f, 430t–431t, 432f–434f
      major histocompatibility complex, 431, 431t
      potential transplant recipients and donor, evaluation of, 432–435, 433f–434f
   mechanisms of rejection in, 443–447
      antibody effects, 444

Organ transplantation *(Continued)*
   general characteristics, 443–444
   immunosuppression, 444–445, 444b, 445t
   immunosuppressive protocols, 447
   representative immunosuppressant drugs, pharmacologic activity of, 447
   T cells, 446
   post-organ transplantation, complications of, 447
      cancer, 447
      diabetes, 447
      hypercholesterolemia, 447
      hypertension, 447
      infectious diseases, 447
      osteoporosis, 447
   post-stem cell transplantation, 448
   posttransplant immune status, longitudinal assessment of, 453.e1f, 453.e1t
   pretransplant screening, 436–437, 437t
   stem cells sources
      bone marrow, 439
      engraftment, 440
      HLA matching, 441
      peripheral blood stem cells, 439–440
      umbilical cord blood, 440
   types of, 437–439
      bone, 437
      cornea, 437–438
      heart, 438
      heart valves, 438
      hematopoietic or peripheral blood stem cells, 440f, 439, 440f
      intestine, 438
      kidney, 438
      liver, 438
      lung, 438–439
      pancreas, 439
      skin, 439
   xenotransplantation and, 448, 448b
OSHA. *See* Occupational Safety and Health Administration (OSHA)
Osmotic cytolytic reaction, 31–32
Osmotic lysis, 223
OSOM Card Pregnancy Test, 123
Osteoclasts, 356
Osteoporosis, in post-organ transplantation, 447
Ostwald pipettes, 119f
Ouchterlony double-diffusion technique, 129, 131f
Ouchterlony gel diffusion, 129
Ovarian cancer biomarkers, 469–470. *See also* Biomarkers

P

p53 protein, 460
PA. *See* Pernicious anemia (PA)
PAHO. *See* Pan American Health Organization (PAHO)
PAMPs. *See* Pathogen-associated molecular patterns (PAMPs)
Pan American Health Organization (PAHO), 205
Pancreas transplantation, 439. *See also* Transplantation
Pancreatic disorders, 377–380, 379f
   adrenal glands, 380
   autoimmune pancreatitis, 379–380
   insulin-dependent diabetes mellitus, 373b, 378–379
   latent autoimmune diabetes, in adults, 379
   parathyroid gland, 380
   pituitary gland, 380
   polyglandular syndromes, 380
Paper chromatography, 147

Papillomas, 455
Paraprotein, 354
Parasite-specific pLDH, 256
Parasitic diseases, 193
Parathyroid gland, 380
Parenchymatous syphilis, 233. See also Syphilis
Paroxysmal cold hemoglobinuria, 385
Partial combined immune deficiency disorders, 312–313
Particle agglutination assays, 130, 132t
Passenger mutations, 459
Passive agglutination assays, 118
Passive immunity, 25, 25t
Pasteur, Louis, 3
Pathogen-associated molecular patterns (PAMPs), 22
  definition of, 22
  pattern recognition receptors (PRRs), 22
  phagocytosis receptors and, 22
  toll-like receptors (TLRs) and, 22
Pathogen recognition receptors, 489
Pathogens, 481
  Aspergillus spp., 194
  Blastomyces dermatitidis, 195
  Candida spp., 193
  Coccidioides immitis, 194
  Cryptococcus neoformans, 195
  Flavivirus genus, 199
  Histoplasma capsulatum, 194
  Sporothrix schenckii, 195
  Toxoplasma gondii, 200, 202f
  Treponema spp
    Treponema carateum, 228–229, 229t
    Treponema pallidum, 229t
    Treponema pallidum (variant), 229t
    Treponema pertenue, 229t
Patient age and sex, 372
Patient identification, accuracy and, 108–109
Pattern recognition receptors (PRRs), 22
PBSCs. See Peripheral blood stem cells (PBSCs)
PE. See Phycoerythrin (PE)
PEG. See Polyethylene glycol (PEG)
Penicillins, 249–250
PEP. See Postexposure prophylaxis (PEP)
PerCP. See Peridinin chlorophyll protein (PerCP)
Percutaneous (parenteral) inoculation, of blood, 100
Performance indicators, 112b
Pericarditis, 398t
Peridinin chlorophyll protein (PerCP), 163
Peripheral blood stem cells (PBSCs), 439
  in stem cell transplantation, 439–440
Peripheral blood stem cell transplant, 440f, 440f, 439, 440f
Peripheral tolerance, 370
Pernicious anemia (PA), 381–382, 382t
Personal protective equipment (PPE), 101
Pertussis, 481
Phagocyte system, mononuclear, 10, 12f
Phagocytic cells, 11
Phagocytosis, 9, 192–193
  process of, 68–71, 69f
    adhesion, 69–70
    bacteremia and, 71
    cell adhesion molecules (CAMs) and, 70
    chemoattractant substances and, 69
    chemotaxis, 68–69
    degranulation and, 70
    digestion, 70–71
    engulfment, 70, 70f
    ligands and, 69
    margination and, 69
    subsequent phagocytic activity, 71
Phagocytosis receptors, 22
Phase I trials, 331

Phase IV trials, 331
Phenotypic assays, 331
Photon, 159b, 160
Photosensitivity, 398t
Phycoerythrin (PE), 163
Pinta, 228–229. See also Syphilis
Pipettes, 118–120, 119f
  graduated, 119f
  micropipettors, 119–120, 119f
  serologic, 119f
PIs. See Protease inhibitors (PIs)
Piston-type automatic micropipette, 119f
Pituitary gland, 380
Placental alkaline phosphatase (ALP), as tumor markers, 469
Plaque-reduction neutralization tests (PRNT), 198
Plasma cell dyscrasias, 354
Plasma cell neoplasms, 353–368.e1
  with associated paraneoplastic syndrome, 363
    AESOP syndrome, 363
    POEMS syndrome, 363
    TEMPI syndrome, 363
  multiple myeloma, 355–363
    Bence Jones protein in, 359–360, 365b–366b
    definition of, 355
    diagnostic evaluation of, 358
    epidemiology of, 355–356, 356t
    etiology of, 355
    free light chains for, 360, 360t, 360b
    hematologic assessments for, 358, 359f
    hematologic features of, 356–357
    immunologic manifestations of, 358
    immunologic testing for, 360–361, 360t, 361f, 361b
    infectious diseases in, 358
    interleukin-6 (IL-6) and, 356
    molecular testing for, 358–359, 359f
    neurologic features of, 358
    pathophysiology of, 356
    prognosis for, 361–362, 362t
    renal disorders of, 357–358
    skeletal abnormalities of, 356, 357f
    staging system for, 361
    treatment of, 362–363
  Waldenström's primary macroglobulinemia, 363–365
    cardiopulmonary abnormalities and, 364
    cutaneous manifestations of, 364
    diagnostic evaluation of, 364–365
    epidemiology of, 363
    etiology of, 363
    hematologic abnormalities of, 363–364
    hematologic assessment of, 364
    immunologic assessment of, 364–365
    immunologic manifestations of, 364
    neuropsychiatric problems and, 364
    ocular manifestations of, 364
    renal dysfunction and, 364
    signs and symptoms of, 363–364
    skeletal features of, 363
    treatment of, 365
Plasma cells, 13–15, 15f, 77, 92b
  biology of, 92
  dyscrasias, 354
Plasmodium, 253
Plasmodium falciparum (malaria), 253–254
Plasmodium knowlesi, 254
Plasmodium malariae, 254
Plasmodium ovale, 254
Plasmodium species, 254, 255f
Plasmodium vivax, 254
Platelets, HLA-matched, 48
Platelets, radiation on, 451

Pleuritis, 398t
Pneumococcal vaccines, 487
Pneumocystis jiroveci (*P. carinii*), 320f, 447
PNEUMOVAX 23, 90
POCT. See Point-of-care testing (POCT)
POEMS syndrome, 363
Point-of-care testing (POCT), 122–127
  characteristics of, 122b
  testing categories of, 123
    quality control for, 123
    staff competency for, 123
    waived, 123
Pollens, hypersensitivity reactions to, 338
Polyarthritis, 420t
Polyclonal gammopathies, 355
Polyclonal protein, 355
Polyethylene glycol (PEG), 61
Polyglandular syndromes, 380
Polymerase chain reaction, 170–173
  weakness of, techniques for, 173b
Polymorphonuclear leukocytes (PMN), 26f, 222
Polymorphonuclear neutrophils (PMNs), 68
Polyps, 455
Polysaccharide and conjugate vaccines
  meningococcal protein conjugate, 487
  meningococcal vaccines, 487
Polysaccharides, 487
Polysaccharide vaccines, 90, 487
Positive antinuclear antibody, 398t
Positive predictive value (PPV), 111
Positive selection, 19, 79b, 80, 370
Postanalytical errors, 109b
Postexposure prophylaxis (PEP), 332–334
Post-organ transplantation, complications of, 447
Post-stem cell transplantation, complications of, 448
Poststreptococcal glomerulonephritis, 221
Posttransfusion hepatitis infections, 289. See also Viral hepatitis
Posttransplantation lymphoproliferative disorder (PTLD), 268
Posttransplant immune status, longitudinal assessment of, 453.e1f, 453.e1t
Postzone phenomenon, in hemagglutination, 135, 136t
Povitzky, Olga Raissa, 4–5
Powassan disease, 241
PPE. See Personal protective equipment (PPE)
Prealbumin band, 388
Preanalytical errors, 109b, 123
Precipitation, 128–142.e2
  assays, 129–130, 130t
  definition of, 129b
  principles of, 129–130
Precipitins, 130b
Precision, 109b, 110
Predictive value (PV), 111
Preexposure prophylaxis, 332, 332b
Pregnancy
  Lyme disease and, 246. See also Lyme disease (Lyme borreliosis)
  risk of cytomegalovirus, 211
  testing of, 123–127
Pregnancy testing, agglutination methods, 131
  agglutination inhibition, 131
  human chorionic gonadotropin, 131
Presumptive laboratory evidence, Lyme disease, 247
Prevnar 13, 90
Primary antibody response, 57, 57f. See also Antibodies
Primary cellular immunodeficiencies, examples of, 314t
Primary cytomegalovirus (CMV) infections, 212. See also Cytomegalovirus (CMV)

Primary immune deficiency disorders (PIDs), 302, 302b, 314t
　absolute lymphocyte count, 306b
　autoimmune inflammatory conditions, 304, 304t, 305f
　B-cell disorders, 302, 303t, 304f
　Bruton X-linked agammaglobulinemia (XLA), 309–310
　categories of, 303b
　characteristics, 304
　chronic mucocutaneous candidiasis (CMC), 309t, 308–309, 309t, 310b
　common variable immunodeficiency, 310–311
　DiGeorge syndrome, 307
　　etiology, 307
　　immunologic manifestations, 307
　　signs and symptoms, 307
　features, 302, 302f
　hereditary ataxia-telangiectasia, 312
　hyper-E syndrome, 311–312
　immunodeficiency with elevated immunoglobulin M, 311
　incidence, 303
　laboratory evaluation, 304–306, 306f
　origin and effects of, 302b
　selective immunoglobulin A deficiency, 311
　severe combined immune deficiency (SCID), 307–308, 307t
　T-cell disorders, 302, 303t, 306
　transient hypogammaglobulinemia, infancy, 311
　treatment for, 311–312
　Wiskott-Aldrich syndrome, 312–313
　X-linked lymphoproliferative disease (XLP) syndromes 1 and 2, 312
Primary immune deficiency syndromes, 299–336.e1
Primary lymphoid organs, 16–17, 16b
　bone marrow, 16
　thymus, 16–17, 17f
Primary syphilis, 230, 230f, 232f
Primers, 171
Probe amplification, 171
Probiotics, 20
Procalcitonin (PCT), 43
Procedural theory and techniques
　agglutination methods, 128–142.e2
　automated procedures, 159–167.e1
　electrophoresis techniques, 143–149.e1, 144t
　immunoassay labeling techniques, 150–158.e1
　molecular laboratory techniques, 168–188
　quality assurance and quality control, 107–116.e1
Prodromal, 292
Prodromal period, 215
Proficiency testing (PT), 109b, 111–112
Prognostic indicator, 269–270
Progressive systemic sclerosis (scleroderma), 376
Properdin, 32
Prophylactic vaccines, 495–496
Prostate-specific antigen (PSA), 468
Prostatic acid phosphatase, as tumor markers, 468
Protease, 315
Protease inhibitors (PIs), 328, 330t–331t
Proteinases, 29
Protein-based subunit vaccine, 485
Protein-conjugated vaccines, 90
Proteins, 144
　acute phase, 22
　as antigens, 51
　complement, 22
Proteolytic complement cascade, 31
Proteomics, 448
Proteomic technology, 470

Proto-oncogenes, 460. See also Oncogenes
Provider-performed microscopy tests, 123
Proviral genome, 315
Prozone phenomenon, 134b, 135, 136t
PRRs. See Pattern recognition receptors (PRRs)
PSA. See Prostate-specific antigen (PSA)
Pseudoagglutination, 136. See also Hemagglutination
Psoriatic arthritis, 420t. See also Arthritis
Psychotic disorders, 269
PTLD. See Posttransplantation lymphoproliferative disorder (PTLD)
Pulmonary alveolar macrophages, 11
Purine, 169, 170f
Purine analogs, 472
Purulent, 223
Pyoderma, 224
Pyrimidine, 169, 170f

Q

Q fever, 242t–243t
Qualified personnel, 108
Quality assurance and quality control, 107–116.e1
　accrediting organizations for, 108
　case study of, 115b
　errors related to phase of testing in, 109, 109b
　monitoring quality for, 111–112
　　control specimens in, 112
　　proficiency testing in, 111–112
　nonanalytical factors related to testing accuracy in, 108–109
　quality descriptors, 109
　　coefficient of variation of, 110
　　limits of detection, 111
　　positive and negative predictive values related to SARS-CoV-2, 111
　　predictive values of, 111
　　sensitivity and specificity of, 110
　reference range statistics for, 112, 112f
　testing outcomes of, 112–113
　validating new procedures of, 113–115, 113t–114t
　test kits in, parallel testing of, 113–115
Quality methods, 108b
Quality metrics, 109b
Quality regulators, 108b

R

R21/Matrix-M vaccine, 479
RA. See Rheumatoid arthritis (RA)
Radial immunodiffusion (RID), 129–130, 130t, 132f
Radiation
　carcinogenesis, 457
　exposure, 457
　graft-versus-host disease and, 451
Radioimmunoassay, 151, 151t
RANTES gene, 321
Rapamycin, 445t
Rapid device testing (RDT), malaria, 256, 257f
Rapid diagnostic tests (RDTs), for malaria, 123
Rapid plasma reagin (RPR) tests, 132, 233–234
Rapid testing, 122–127
　non-instrument-based, 123–127
　　human immunodeficiency virus testing in, 123, 125f
　　malaria testing in, 123
　　pregnancy testing in, 123–127
　　quality control standards for, 123
　　testing categories of, 123
　　　quality control for, 123
　　　staff competency for, 123
　　　waived, 123

Ras proto-oncogene, 460
Rat flea, 242t–243t
Raynaud's phenomenon, 401
Reactants, acute phase, 22
Reactions, hypersensitivity, 337–352.e1
　antigens and reactions, types of, 338–339
　　environmental substances, 338
　　food allergies, 338–339, 339t
　　infectious agents, 338
　　latex allergies, 338
　　self-antigens, 338
　case studies for, 350b–351b
　classification of, 339t
　　type I (anaphylactic reactions), 339b–340b, 340–343, 341f–342f, 341t, 343t
　　type II (cytotoxic reactions), 343–346, 343b, 344f, 345b
　　type III (immune complex reactions), 346–347, 346b, 347f, 347t
　　type IV (T cell-dependent reactions), 347–348, 347b, 348f
　fundamentals of
　　allergens, 338
　　allergy, 338
　　atopy, 338
　　hypersensitivity, immediate and delayed, 338
　　immunization, 338
　　immunoglobulin E (IgE), 338
　　major histocompatibility complex (MHC), 338
　　sensitization, 338
　type I (anaphylactic reactions), 339b–340b, 340–343, 341f–342f, 341t, 343t. See also Anaphylactic reactions
　type II (cytotoxic reactions), 343–346, 343b, 344f, 345b. See also Cytotoxic reactions
　type III (immune complex reactions), 346–347, 346b, 347f, 347t. See also Immune complex reactions
　type IV (T cell-dependent reactions), 347–348, 347b, 348f. See also T cells
　types of, 339–348, 341t
　　comparison of, 348–351, 349f
Reactivated cytomegalovirus (CMV) infections, 212. See also Cytomegalovirus (CMV)
Reactive oxygen species (ROS), 70–71
Reagin antibodies, 233
Receptor for hyaluronan-mediated motility (RHAMM), 497
Receptors
　pattern recognition (PRRs), 22
　phagocytosis, 22
　toll-like (TLRs), 22
Recirculation, lymphocyte, 19
Recombinant protein vaccine, 485–487
Recombinant vaccines, 287. See also Vaccines
Recombinant vector vaccines, 488
Red blood cell agglutination reactions, 137f
Reduced nicotinamide-adenine dinucleotide phosphate oxidase, 70–71
Reference range statistics, 112, 112f
Reference values, for electrophoresis, 144
Regulatory T (T_{reg}) cells, 371
Renal disorders, 390–391, 390b, 398t
Replicating and nonreplicating viral vector-based vaccines, 488
Replication, 169, 173f
Respiratory burst, 70–71
Respiratory syncytial virus (RSV), 479
　vaccines, 479–480
Respiratory virus panels, 217–219
Resting lymphocytes, 13
Retrovirus, 315
Reverse grouping, 140b

Reverse-screening algorithm protocols, 236–238
Reverse transcriptase (RT), 176, 328
Reverse-transcriptase polymerase chain reaction (RT-PCR), 197
Reye syndrome, 269
Rheumatic diseases, 415
Rheumatic fever, 223–224
Rheumatoid arthritis (RA), 414–426
  arthritis-attributable activity limitation, 414
  associated disorders, 420b
  case study of, 424b, 425t
  characteristics of, 415b, 416, 416f
  classification for, 416–417, 417t
  complications of, 415–416
  definition of, 416
  diagnostic evaluation of, 419
    agglutination tests, 419
    anti-keratin antibodies (AKA), 419
    antinuclear antibodies (ANA), 420
    anti-perinuclear factor (APF), 419
    comparisons of, 425t
    complement levels, 420
    cryoglobulins, 420
    cyclic citrullinated peptide (CCP) antibodies, 419–420
    enzyme-linked immunosorbent assays (ELISAs), 419
    immune complexes, 419
    immunoturbidimetric assays, 419
    lateral flow immunoassay (LFIA), 419
    rheumatoid factor (RF), 419
  epidemiology of, 415–416
  etiology of, 415, 415f
    articular and extraarticular manifestations, 415
  extraarticular manifestations of, 416b
  inflammation in, 414, 415f
  joints, anatomy and physiology of, 417–418
  juvenile idiopathic arthritis (JIA) and, 420–421
    antinuclear antibodies (ANAs) and, 421
    definition of, 420
    epidemiology of, 420
    etiology of, 420
    human intracisternal A-type particles (HIAPs) and, 420
    immune complexes and, 419–420
    immunologic manifestations of, 420–421
    rheumatoid factors (RFs) of, 420
    signs and symptoms of, 420
    subgroups of, 420t
  manifestations of
    extraarticular, 416b
    leukotriene responses, 419
  National Health Interview Survey (NHIS) on, 414
  pathogenesis of, 418–419, 418f
  polyarthritis and, 416
  serology of, 419b
  signs and symptoms of, 416–417, 416f, 416b
  treatment for, 421–424, 421b
    classes of drugs, 421, 422t–423t
    corticosteroids, 421
    cyclooxygenase enzyme (COX)-1/2 blockers, 421
    disease-modifying antirheumatic drugs, 421–424
    glucocorticoids, 421
    goals of, 421
    nonsteroidal antiinflammatory drugs (NSAIDs), 421
Rheumatoid factor (RF), 417
Rhinitis, 338
Rhipicephalus sanguineus, 242t–243t. See also Ticks

Ribonucleic acid (RNA), 169–170, 169b, 173f
Rickettsial diseases, 195
Rickettsial infection, 250
Rickettsia parkeri, 241
Risk, definition of, 98
RMSF. See Rocky Mountain spotted fever (RMSF)
RNA vaccines, 484
Rocky Mountain spotted fever (RMSF), 241, 242t–243t, 252, 252b
  diagnostic evaluation of, 252
  epidemiology of, 252
  etiology of, 252
  signs and symptoms of, 252
  treatment and prevention of, 252
ROS. See Reactive oxygen species (ROS)
Rouleaux, 358
Rouleaux formation, 136
RPR tests. See Rapid plasma reagin (RPR) tests
RT. See Reverse transcriptase (RT)
RTS, S/AS01 vaccine, 479
Rubella infections, 205–208
  case study of, 218b
  characteristics of, 205b
  diagnostic evaluations of, 208, 209t
    indirect immunofluorescence assays (IFAs), 209t
    TORCH antibodies, 209t
  epidemiology of, 205–206
    epidemic, 205
    stillbirths and, 205
  etiology of, 205
  healthcare personnel, 206
  immunologic manifestations of, 208
    acquired rubella infection, 208
    congenital rubella syndrome, 208, 212f
  laboratory testing for, 207b
  natural history of, 212f
  pregnant women, 206
  signs and symptoms of, 206–207
    acquired rubella infection, 206–207, 207f
    clinical manifestations, 206
    congenital rubella infection, 207, 207t, 208f
Rubeola infections (measles), 208–210
  antibody testing of, 210t
  case study of, 219b
  definition of, 208
  epidemiology of, 208
  laboratory testing of, 209–210, 210t
  prevention of, 208–209
RV144, 493

S

Sabin-Feldman dye test, 205
Safety data sheets, 99
Safety, in immunology-serology laboratory, 97–106.e1
  case study of, 105b
  COVID-19 prevention, 104–105
  decontamination
    of nondisposable equipment, 103
    SARS-CoV-2, guidance for, 104
    of spills, 103–104
    of waste materials, 104
    of work surfaces, 103
  disposal of infectious laboratory waste in, 104
  electronic devices, 103
  hand sanitizing and handwashing, 101–103, 103b
  nail care, 103
  patient safety in, 100
  prevention of transmission of infectious diseases in, 100–101
  protective techniques for infection control in, 101

Safety, in immunology-serology laboratory (Continued)
  risk and risk management, 98–99
  safety manual, 99–100
  safety standards and agencies in, 99
  safe work practices for infection control in, 101
  shoes, 103
Safety issues, 99b
Salmonella typhi (Vi) vaccine, 487
Sandwich immunoassay, 154, 154f
Sanger (chain termination) sequencing, 178–179
Sarcomas, 455
SARS-CoV-2
  decontamination, guidance for, 104
  positive and negative predictive values related to, 111
  sensitivity and specificity related to, 110–111
Scarlet fever, 223–224
SCID. See Severe combined immune deficiency (SCID)
Scleroderma, 376, 416. See also Collagen vascular disorders
Scrub typhus, 242t–243t
SD. See Standard deviation (SD)
Secondary (anamnestic) antibody response, 57–58, 57f. See also Antibodies
Secondary immune deficiency disorders, 313, 314b
Secondary lymphoid organs, 17–19, 17t
Secondary syphilis, 230–231, 230f, 232f
Second colloid antigen, 377
Second-set rejection, 441, 443f. See also Grafts
Secretory component, 53
Secretory IgA, 53
Selectin, 74
Selective immunoglobulin A deficiency, 311
Self
  antigens, 338. See also Antigens (immunogens)
  self-renewal, of stem cells, 456, 456f
Self-amplifying mRNA vaccines, 484
Self-assembled arrays, 180
Sepsis, 73–74
Septic shock, 41
Sequelae, 276
Serial dilutions, 120b, 121, 122f. See also Dilutions
  preparation of, 121t
  principle of, 122
Serodiagnostic tests, 194
Serogroups, 222
Serologic laboratory techniques, basic, 117–127.e1, 118b
  blood specimen preparation in, 118–122
  case study of, 124b
  dilutions in, 120–121, 120b
    dilution factor for, 120–121
    serial, 121, 121t, 122f
    single, 121
    specimens for, 120
  inactivation of complement in, 118
  pipettes for, 118–120, 119f
    automatic dispensers/syringes, 120
    diluter-dispensers, 120
    micropipettors, 119–120, 119f
  pipetting techniques for, 118–120
    automatic, 120
    manual, 119b
  procedures manual of, 118
  types of specimens tested in, 118
Serologic pipettes, 119f. See also Pipettes
Serologic tests, 260

Serology and immunology concepts
    acquired immunodeficiency syndrome (AIDS), 313–326
        cytomegalovirus (CMV), 210–214
        infectious mononucleosis, 267–272.e2
        rubella and rubeola infections, 205–208
        streptococcal infections, 221–227.e1
        syphilis, 228–239.e2
        toxoplasmosis, 200–205
        vector-borne diseases, 240–266.e1
        viral hepatitis, 273–298
    basic mechanisms
        antigens and antibodies, 47–66.e1
        innate and adaptive immunity, 67–96.e1
        mediators, soluble, 28–46.e1
    immune disorders
        autoimmune diseases, 373, 373b
        hypersensitivity reactions, 337–352.e1
        rheumatoid arthritis (RA), 414–426
        systemic lupus erythematosus, 396–413.e3
    procedural theory and techniques
        agglutination methods, 128–142.e2
        automated procedures, 159–167.e1
        electrophoresis techniques, 143–149.e1, 144t
        immunoassay labeling techniques, 150–158.e1
        molecular laboratory techniques, 168–188
        quality assurance and quality control, 107–116.e1
Serology, technical errors in, 109b
Seropositivity, 214–215
Seroprevalence, 201
Serositis, 402
Serum
    protein electrophoresis procedures, 144
        clinical interpretation for, 144, 146f
        principles of, 144, 145f
        results for, 144
    as tumor markers, 462b, 466t
Severe combined immune deficiency (SCID), 307–308, 307t
Sexually transmitted infections (STIs), 229
Sexual transmission, of hepatitis, 289. See also Viral hepatitis
Sheath, 161
Shigella vaccines, 480
Shigellosis, 480
Shingles, 215. See also Varicella-zoster virus vaccine for, 490–491
Shoes, safety practices for, 103
Side scatter light (SSC), 161
Signal amplification technology, 156, 156b, 171
Signatures, mutational, 458
Silent substitutions, 430
Single dilutions, 121
Single nucleotide polymorphisms (SNPs), 169–170, 320
Sipuleucel-T (Provenge), 496
Sirolimus, 446
SIRS. See Systemic inflammatory response syndrome (SIRS)
Six-color flow cytometry, 163b
Sjögren's syndrome, 380–381, 381t
Skeletal muscle disorders, 391
Skin allografts, 439
Skin-associated lymphoid tissue, 19
Skin disorders, 391–393, 391b
Skin patch testing, anaphylactic reactions (type I), 342
Skin puncture test (SPT), 341
SLE. See Systemic lupus erythematosus (SLE)
SLO. See Streptolysin
Smallpox, vaccine for, 497
Smoking, as cancer risk factors, 457

Smoldering multiple myeloma, 356
SNPs. See Single nucleotide polymorphisms (SNPs)
Sodium hypochlorite solutions, for decontamination, 103
Solid organ transplantation, 427–453.e1, 437. See also Transplantation
    biomarkers, for rejection, 448
    case study of, 451b–452b
    current directions in, 451–452
    FOXP3 mRNA in, 448–449
    general facts about, 435–436
    graft rejection in, 441–443, 441t, 441b, 442f
        accelerated, 443
        acute, 443
        chronic, 443
        first-set, 441, 443f
        hyperacute, 441–442
        second-set, 441, 443f
    graft-*versus*-host disease (GVHD), 449–451, 449b
        diagnostic evaluation of, 450
        drugs used for, 450b
        epidemiology of, 449
        etiology of, 449
        high-risk patients, 450
        immunologic manifestation of, 450
        intermediate-risk patients, 450–451
        low-risk patients, 451
        prevention of, 450–451
        radiation, on specific cellular components, 451
        requirements for, 449t
        signs and symptoms of, 449–450
    hematopoietic stem cells in, 436, 436b
    histocompatibility antigens, 429–435, 430f
        flow cytometry, 434–435
        human leukocyte antigen, 429–435, 430f, 430t–431t, 432f–434f
        major histocompatibility complex, 431, 431t
        potential transplant recipients and donor, evaluation of, 432–435, 433f–434f
    immunosuppression in, 444b
    mechanisms of rejection in, 443–447
        antibody effects, 444
        general characteristics, 443–444
        immunosuppression, 444–445, 444b, 445t
        immunosuppressive protocols, 447
        representative immunosuppressant drugs, pharmacologic activity of, 447
        T cells, 446
    post-organ transplantation, complications of, 447
        cancer, 447
        diabetes, 447
        hypercholesterolemia, 447
        hypertension, 447
        infectious diseases, 447
        osteoporosis, 447
    post-stem cell transplantation, 448
    posttransplant immune status, longitudinal assessment of, 453.e1f, 453.e1t
    pretransplant screening, 436–437, 437t
    stem cells sources
        bone marrow, 439
        engraftment, 440
        HLA matching, 441
        peripheral blood stem cells, 439–440
        umbilical cord blood, 440
    types of, 437–439
        bone, 437
        cornea, 437–438
        heart, 438
        heart valves, 438

Solid organ transplantation (Continued)
        hematopoietic or peripheral blood stem cells, 440f, 439, 440f
        intestine, 438
        kidney, 438
        liver, 438
        lung, 438–439
        pancreas, 439
        skin, 439
    xenotransplantation and, 448, 448b
Solid-phase enzyme-linked immunosorbent assay, 151b, 152, 434
Solid-phase immunoassay, 151–153
    principle of, 152f
Soluble mediators, 28–46.e1
    acute-phase proteins, 41–45, 41b
        applications of, 42b
        catabolism, 42
        ceruloplasmin, 43
        clinically useful, 42t
        C-reactive protein (CRP), 42–43
        laboratory assessment methods for, 43–45
        overview of, 41–42, 42t, 42b
        synthesis of, 42
        α_1-antitrypsin, 43
    biological response modifiers, 39
    case study, 43b
    complement system, 29–30
        activation of, 29, 30f, 31t
        biological functions, 33–34, 33f, 33t, 33b
        complement levels, alterations in, 34–36, 34t–35t, 36b
        enzyme activation and, 29
        membrane attack complex, 31–32, 32f
        proteolytic complement cascade, 31
        recognition stage, 31
    cytokines, 39–40, 39t
    diagnostic evaluation of, 36–38, 36f, 37t
        enzyme immunoassay, 38
        hemolytic method, 38
        liposome assay, 38
    hematopoietic stimulators, 41
        chemokines, 41
        colony-stimulating factors (CSFs), 41
        stem cell factor (c-kit Ligand), 41
        transforming growth factors (TGFs), 41
    interferons (IFNs), 40
    interleukins (ILs), 40
    mannose-binding lectin pathway, 33
    pathways, alternative, 32–33
    pathways, classic, 30–32
    tumor necrosis factor (TNF), 41
Somatic mutations
    identification of, 470–471
    in tumor immunology, 458–459
Southern tick-associated rash illness (STARI), 241
Specific granule deficiency, 76
Specificity, 58
Specific oligomer primers, 324
Specimen, procurement of, 108–109
S phase-active drugs, 471
Spills, decontamination of, 103–104
Spirochaeta pallida, 228. See also *Treponema* spp
Spirochetes, 230
    direct observation of, 233
Splenomegaly, 269
Spontaneous tumor antigens, 467
Sporadic hepatitis infections, 292. See also Viral hepatitis
Sporadic/isolated errors, 109
Sporothrix schenckii, 195
Sporotrichosis, 195
SPT. See Skin puncture test (SPT)
Squamous cell carcinomas, 455
Squirrel flea and louse, 242t–243t

Stabilized sheep erythrocytes, 132t
Staff competency, in point-of-care testing, 123
Stages and staging. *See also* Classification
   of carcinogenesis, 459, 459b
   syphilis, 231t
      latent, 231t
      primary, 231t, 232f
      secondary, 231t, 232f
      secondary, relapse of, 231t
      tertiary (late), 231t
Standard deviation (SD), 110
Standard Precautions, 101
Stellate macrophages, 11
Stem cell factor (c-kit Ligand), 41
Stem cells. *See also* Transplantation
   cancer, 455, 455f–456f
Stem cell transplantation, 436
   diseases treatable by, 436b
   sources of, 439–441
      bone marrow, 439
      engraftment in, 440
      HLA matching in, 441
      peripheral blood stem cells, 439–440
      umbilical cord blood, 440
Steric hindrance, 135
Stillbirths, 205
STIs. *See* Sexually transmitted infections (STIs)
St. Louis encephalitis, 242t–243t
Stokes shift, 155, 160
Streptococcal infections, 221–227.e1
   case study of, 226b
   diagnostic evaluation of, 224–225
   epidemiology of, 223
   etiology of
      extracellular products, 222–223
      Lancefield Streptococcus classifications, 222t
      morphologic characteristics, 222, 222f
      necrotizing fasciitis, 221
      poststreptococcal glomerulonephritis, 221
   group B streptococcal (GBS) disease, 225b
      epidemiology of, 226
      etiology of, 226
      future directions in, 226
      laboratory data of, 226
      signs and symptoms of, 226
      Streptococcus agalactiae, 225b
   immunologic manifestations of, 224
      anti-DNase B (ADN-B), 224
      antistreptolysin O, 224
   signs and symptoms of, 223–224
      cellulitis, 223
      complications of, 224
      erysipelas, 223
      impetigo, 223, 223f
      scarlet fever, 223–224
      upper respiratory infection, 223
   streptococcal toxic shock syndrome (STSS), 225–226
      definition of, 225
      epidemiology of, 225
      etiology of, 225
      immunologic mechanisms of, 225
      laboratory data of, 225
      signs and symptoms, 225
      treatment for, 225
   Streptococcus pyogenes, complications of, 224
Streptococcal toxic shock syndrome (STSS), 225–226. *See also* Streptococcal infections
   definition of, 225
   epidemiology of, 225
   etiology of, 225
   immunologic mechanisms of, 225
   laboratory data of, 225
   signs and symptoms, 225
   treatment for, 225

Streptococcosis, 223
Streptococcus spp
   Streptococcus agalactiae, 225b
   Streptococcus pyogenes, 221, 222f
Streptokinase, 223
Streptolysin
   O (SLO), 224
   S, 223
Strongyloides spp, 447
Structural proteins, 314
Structural stability, of antigens, 51
STSS. *See* Streptococcal toxic shock syndrome (STSS)
Subclass deficiencies, immunoglobulin, 311
Subcutaneous (SC) injection, 490
Substances, environmental, 338
Substitutions, 430
Subunit vaccines, 485–488
Superinfections, hepatitis D virus (HDV), 288. *See also* Viral hepatitis
Suppressor
   cytotoxic lymphocytes, 92
   genes, 460
Surface-based infection, risk reduction of, 103
Surface immunoglobulin (sIg), 74, 89b
Surface membrane markers, 77–79, 78f
Survival mechanisms, of fungi, Fungal diseases, 193
Survivin, 459
SYBR Green, 178
Syndromes
   acquired immunodeficiency (AIDS), 313–326. *See also* Acquired immunodeficiency syndrome (AIDS)
   antiphospholipid, 399
   autoimmune lymphoproliferative, 384
   Chédiak-Higashi, 75, 75b
   congenital rubella, 205, 207f
   DiGeorge, 307
   eosinophilia-myalgia, 376
   Felty, 419
   Guillain-Barré (GBS), 269
   hyperimmunoglobulinemia E, 311
   Nezelof, 314t
   Reye, 269
   Sjögren's, 380–381, 381t
   streptococcal toxic shock (STSS), 225–226
   Wiskott-Aldrich (WAS), 312–313
Syngraft, 435t. *See also* Grafts
Synonymous nucleotide substitutions, 430
Synovitis, 416
Synovium, 416
Syphilis, 228–239.e2, 229b
   case study of, 238b
   congenital, 232
   diagnostic evaluation of, 233
      algorithm protocols, 234f
      chemiluminescence immunoassays, 235
      darkfield microscopy, 233
      fluorescent treponemal antibody absorption (FTA-ABS), 236
      nontreponemal methods, 233–234
      positive test data, 236t
      rapid plasma reagin, 233–234
      spirochetes, direct observation of, 233
      tests for, 235t
      traditional vs. reverse-screening algorithm protocols, 236–238, 237t–238t
      treponemal methods, 234–236
      Treponema pallidum antibody, 235
      Venereal Disease Research Laboratory Test, 234
   epidemiology of, 229–230
   etiology of, 228–229, 229f, 229t
      bejel, 228–229

Syphilis *(Continued)*
      pinta, 228–229
      Treponema carateum, 228–229, 229t
      Treponema pallidum, 229t
      Treponema pallidum (variant), 229t
      Treponema pertenue, 229t
      treponemes, 229
      yaws, 228–229
   immunologic manifestations of, 233
      antitreponemal antibodies, 233
      granulomatous reactions (gummas), 233
      nontreponemal antibodies, 233
      reagin antibodies, 233
      Treponema pallidum antibodies, 233
   laboratory characteristics, 233b
   late (tertiary), 232–233
   latent, 231–232
   neurosyphilis, 232–233
   primary, 230, 230f, 232f
   secondary, 230–231, 230f, 232f
   signs and symptoms, 230, 231t
   stages of, 231t
Syringes, 120
Systematic errors, 109
Systemic arthritis, 420t. *See also* Arthritis
Systemic inflammatory response syndrome (SIRS), 73–74
Systemic lupus erythematosus (SLE), 396–413. e3, 397b, 398t
   case studies of, 411b–412b
   clinical and serologic features of, 398b
   definition of, 397
   diagnostic evaluation of, 404–410
      antinuclear antibody visible method, 408f, 406, 407f–408f
      antinucleoprotein, rapid slide test for, 408
      autoimmune enzyme immunoassay, 410
      automated testing, multiplex immunoassay, 410, 410f
      hematologic, 404
      hemostatic findings, 404
      histologic changes, 404
      laboratory evaluation, 406–408
      serologic findings, 404–406, 406t–407t
   different forms of, 397
      discoid lupus, 397
      drug-induced lupus, 397, 398b
      neonatal lupus, 397
      systemic (SLE), 397
   epidemiology of, 399
   etiology, 397–399
      antibiotics, 399
      environmental factors, 397
      genetic predisposition, 397
      hormonal influences, 399, 400f
      vitamins, 399
   immunologic characteristics of, 402b
   immunologic manifestations of, 403
      antineutrophil cytoplasmic antibodies (ANCAs), 403
      antinuclear antibodies (ANAs), 420
      antiphospholipid antibodies, 399, 400f
      antiphospholipid syndrome, 399
      cellular aspects, 403
      humoral aspects, 403–404
      immunologic consequences, 404
      neutrophil extracellular traps (NETs), 403
   laboratory testing, 404b
   signs and symptoms of, 399–404, 401f, 401t
      butterfly rash, 399–400
      cardiopulmonary characteristics, 402
      cutaneous features, 399, 402f
      gastrointestinal manifestations, 402
      infection, 399
      late-onset lupus, 402

Systemic lupus erythematosus (Continued)
  lymphadenopathy, 402
  musculoskeletal features, 402
  neuropsychiatric features, 402
  Raynaud's phenomenon, 401
  renal characteristics, 402
  serositis, 402
  treatments for, 411–412
System, immune. See Immune system

T

T. See Thymine (T)
TAAs. See Tumor-associated antigens (TAAs)
Tachyzoites, 205
Tacrolimus (FK-506), 444b, 446
Talimogene laherparepvec (T-VEC), 496
Tandem dyes, for flow cytometry, 162–163
TaqMan method, 176–178
Target amplification, 171
Target enrichment strategies, 184–185, 184f, 185b
T-cell-dependent antigens, 89t
T-cell-independent antigens, 89t
T-cell receptor (TCR), 54, 79, 432
  peptide-MHC by, recognition of, 87f
T-cell receptor excision circles (TREC), 305
T cells
  antigen recognition by, 86–87
  in graft rejection, 444
  immune deficiency disorders, 302, 303t, 306
  reactions, T cell-dependent, 339t, 348. See also Hypersensitivity reactions
    characteristics of, 348, 348f
    latex sensitivity, 348
    test for, 348
    treatment for, 348
  tolerance, 371
Techniques and theory
  agglutination methods, 128–142.e2
  automated procedures, 159–167.e1
  electrophoresis techniques, 143–149.e1, 144t
  immunoassay labeling techniques, 150–158.e1
  molecular laboratory techniques, 168–188
  quality assurance and quality control, 107–116.e1
Telomerase, 470
TEMPI syndrome, 363
Teratomas, 455
Terminal redundancies, long (LTRs), 314
Testing methods, accuracy and, 109
Test requisitioning, accuracy and, 108
Tetracyclines, 249
Tg. See Thyroglobulin (Tg)
TGFs. See Transforming growth factors (TGFs)
Thai Prime-Boost trial, 493
Theories and techniques
  agglutination methods, 128–142.e2
  automated procedures, 159–167.e1
  electrophoresis techniques, 143–149.e1, 144t
  immunoassay labeling techniques, 150–158.e1
  molecular laboratory techniques, 168–188
  quality assurance and quality control, 107–116.e1
Therapeutic vaccines, 496
Thermocycler, 175
6-Thioguanine, 471, 473t
Thoracic duct, 19
364D rickettsiosis, 243
Thymine (T), 169
Thymocytes
  double-negative, 79–80
  double-positive, 80–81
Thymopoiesis, 440

Thymus, 16–17
  development of, 14f, 17f
Thyroglobulin (Tg), 50, 467–468
Thyroid disease, 376–377. See also Organ-specific and midspectrum diseases
  diagnostic evaluation of, 377, 377t–378t
  Graves' disease, 377, 378f
  immunologic manifestations of, 376–377, 376f
  lymphoid chronic thyroiditis, 376
Thyroid membrane receptors, 377
Thyroid microsomes, 377
Thyronine, 377
Tickborne, airborne vector, 242t–243t
Tickborne relapsing fever (TBRF), 241, 242t–243t
Ticks, in vector-borne diseases, 242t–243t
Time-resolved fluoroimmunoassay, 157
T-independent antigen triggering, 87
Tissue and eye bank, 437
Tissue basophils. See Mast cells
Tissue specimens, storage of, 163
Titers, 275
T lymphocytes, 13–14, 77, 79–88, 80t
  antigen and, 338
  CD4+ effector, 82–84, 82f–84f
  CD8+cytotoxic, 84–85, 87f, 87b
  cell-mediated immunity and, 25
  development
    antigen-presenting cells (APCs), 87–88
    antigen processing, 87–88
    antigen recognition, 86–87
    CD4 lymphocytes, 81–85, 81b
    double-negative thymocytes, 79–80
    double-positive thymocytes, 80–81
    early cellular differentiation and development, 79–81
    later differentiation and development, 81
    T cell activation, 87
    T-independent antigen triggering, 87
  maturation stages, 12t
  subsets, 81
  tumor immunology and, 461–462. See also Tumor immunology
TNF. See Tumor necrosis factor (TNF)
Tolerance, 369–395.e1
  B-cell, 371
  central, 370
  immunologic, 370–371, 370t
  layers of, 370t
  maintenance of, 370–371
  peripheral, 370
  T-cell, 371
Toll-like receptors (TLRs), 22, 489
TORCH test panel, 200, 200t
Toxic shock syndrome, streptococcal (STSS), 225–226
  definition of, 225
  epidemiology of, 225
  etiology of, 225
  immunologic mechanisms of, 225
  laboratory data of, 225
  signs and symptoms, 225
  treatment for, 225
Toxoid vaccines, 487–488
Toxoplasma gondii, 200, 202f. See also Toxoplasmosis
Toxoplasma spp, 447
Toxoplasmic meningoencephalitis, 203f
Toxoplasmosis, 200–205
  case study of, 218b
  characteristics of, 200b
  diagnostic evaluation of, 203–205, 206f
    avidity test, 204–205
    cell culture, 205
    histologic diagnosis, 205

Toxoplasmosis (Continued)
  IgM antibodies, 204
  indirect fluorescent antibody test, 205
  polymerase chain reactions (PCRs), 205
  Sabin-Feldman dye test, 205
  serologic tests, 204–205, 204t, 206f
  tachyzoites, 205
epidemiology of, 200–201, 202f
  definitive host, 201
  seroprevalence, 201
  Toxoplasma gondii life cycle, 202f
  transmission, congenital, 201
  transmission, foodborne, 201
  transmission, transplacental, 201, 203b
  transmission, zoonotic, 201
etiology of, 200
immunologic manifestations of, 203
laboratory testing for, 203b
signs and symptoms of, 201–203
  acquired infection, 201
  congenital infection, 201–203
Tp53 gene, 460
TPPA. See Treponema pallidum particle agglutination (TPPA)
Transcriptase, 324
Transcription, 169
Transforming growth factors (TGFs), 41
Transfusion reactions, types of, 345b
Transfusion-transmitted virus (TTV), 293–295, 293b. See also Viral hepatitis
  epidemiology of, 293
  etiology of, 293
  signs and symptoms of, 293–295
Transient hypogammaglobulinemia, of infancy, 311
Transitional cell carcinomas, 455
Translation, 169
Transmission of infection, 268, 268b
Transplacental transmission, 201, 203b
Transplantation
  complications of, 447–448
  general facts about, 435–436
  solid organ, 427–453.e1
    biomarkers in, for rejection, 448
    case study of, 451b–452b
    current directions in, 451–452
    FOXP3 mRNA in, 448–449
    graft rejection in, 441–443, 441t, 441b, 442f
    graft-versus-host disease in, 449–451, 449t
    histocompatibility antigens in, 429–435, 430f
    post-organ transplantation, 447
    post-stem cell transplantation, 448
    xenotransplantation, 448, 448b
  stem cells for, sources of, 439–441
  terminology in, 435, 435t
  tissue and organ, 435–436
  types of, 437–439
T-regulatory lymphocytes, 88–89, 88b
Trench fever, 242t–243t
Treponemal methods, 234–236
Treponema pallidum antibodies, 235
Treponema pallidum particle agglutination (TPPA), 236
Treponema spp
  Treponema carateum, 229t
  Treponema pallidum, 229t
  Treponema pallidum (variant), 229t
  Treponema pertenue, 229t
Treponemes, 229
Triggers, antigen, 338–339
  environmental substances, 338
  food allergies, 338–339, 339t
  infectious agents, 338
  latex allergies, 338
  self-antigens, 338

Triiodothyronine, 377
Tris(2,2'-bipyridyl)-ruthenium, 154
Tropism tests, 332
TSAs. *See* Tumor-specific antigens (TSAs)
TTV. *See* Transfusion-transmitted virus (TTV)
Tuberculin skin test (TST), 192
Tuberculin type hypersensitivity, 192, 193f
Tuberculosis (TB)
    blood test, 193
    skin test, 193
    vaccine, 480–481
Tubulointerstitial nephritis, 391
Tularemia, 243
Tumor
    definition of, 455
    types of, 455–456, 455b
        benign, 455
        malignant, 455–456, 456f
Tumor-associated antigens (TAAs), 467
Tumorigenesis, 181
Tumor immunology, 454–476.e1
    body defenses, 461–462, 461f
        antibodies, 462
        macrophages, 462
        natural killer cells, 462
        T lymphocytes, 461–462
    cancer diagnostic testing, 470–471
        continuous field flow-assisted dielectrophoresis, 471
        genomic alterations, detection, 471
        improved management of cancer treatment, 471
        massive parallel sequencing/next-generation sequencing, 470
        somatic mutation identification, 470–471
    cancer-predisposing genes, 459, 460t
    cancer stem cells, 455, 456f
    case study of, 460t, 474b
    causative factors in, 457–458, 457t–458t
        disease associations, 457–458, 458t
        environmental, 457, 457t
        host, 457–458
        microbial carcinogens, 457, 458t
    DNA microarray technology, 470
    epidemiology of, 457
        adults, 457
        children, 457
        risk factors, 457
    oncogenes
        activation mechanism, 460–461, 460t
        classes of, 460
        overexpression of, 460
        role of, 460–461, 460t
        tumor-suppressing genes, 461
        viral, 461, 461b
    p53 protein, 460
    proto-oncogenes, 460
    somatic mutations in, 458–459
    stages of carcinogenesis, 459, 459b
    treatment modalities, 471–475
        chemotherapeutic agents, 471–472, 472f
        drug-induced immunosuppression, 472, 473t
        monoclonal antibody therapy, 472–475, 472f, 473t–474t
    tumor markers, 462, 462b
        alpha-fetoprotein, 467
        bladder cancer, 470
        breast, ovarian, and cervical cancer, 469–470
        CA 15-3, 468
        CA 19-9, 468
        CA 27.29, 468
        CA 125, 467
        carcinoembryonic antigen, 468
        carcinofetal antigens, 467
        categories of, 465–467, 467f

Tumor immunology *(Continued)*
        classic, 467–469
        enzyme, 469
        HER2 (HER2/neu), 468–469
        hormone, 469
        human chorionic gonadotropin (hCG), 469
        human epididymis protein 4, 467
        lactic dehydrogenase (LDH), 469
        multiple-marker, 465, 466t
        neuron-specific enolase, 469
        placental alkaline phosphatase (ALP), 469
        prostate-specific antigen, 468
        prostatic acid phosphatase, 468
        serum, 465, 466t
        spontaneous tumor antigens, 467
        thyroglobulin, 467–468
        tumor-associated antigens, 467
        tumor-specific antigens, 467
        variety of, 462–470, 463t–466t
    tumor types, 455–456
        benign, 455
        malignant, 455–456, 456f
Tumor-infiltrating lymphocytes, 461–462
Tumor necrosis factor (TNF), 17, 41, 462
Tumor necrosis factor-alpha (TNF-α), 225
Tumor necrosis factor gamma (TNF-α), 192
Tumor-specific antigens (TSAs), 467
Tumor-suppressing genes, 461
Turbidometry, 130t
Turbid serum, 118
Twinrix hepatitis vaccine, 276–278
Type 1 helper T (Th1) Cells, 82
    development of, 82f
    functions of, 83f
Type 2 helper T (Th2) Cells, 82–83
    development of, 83f
    functions of, 84f
Type 17 helper T (Th17) Cells, 83–84
    development of, 85f
    functions of, 85f
Types, of hypersensitivity reactions, 339t. *See also* Hypersensitivity reactions
    type I (anaphylactic reactions), 339b–340b, 340–343, 341f–342f, 341t, 343t. *See also* Anaphylactic reactions
    type II (cytotoxic reactions), 343–346, 343b, 344f, 345b. *See also* Cytotoxic reactions
    type III (immune complex reactions), 346–347, 346b, 347f, 347t. *See also* Immune complex reactions
    type IV (T cell-dependent reactions), 347–348, 347b, 348f. *See also* T cells
Typhus
    epidemic, 242t–243t
    murine, 242t–243t
    scrub, 242t–243t
Tyramide signal amplification (TSA), 156

U

U. *See* Uracil (U)
Umbilical cord blood, in stem cell transplantation, 440
    issue related to, 440
Upper respiratory infection, streptococcal, 223. *See also* Streptococcal infections
Uracil (U), 169
Urticaria, 341

V

Vaccination
    goal of, 481
    host response to, 489
    rates of, 489

Vaccine Adverse Events Reporting System (VAERS), 498
Vaccines, 477–499.e1
    adjuvants and, 485
    administration, sites of, 490
    in biodefense, 497
        anthrax, 497
        smallpox, 497
    booster, 24–25
    cancer, 495–497
    concerns about, 497
    COVID-19 vaccine, 484–485, 484t, 486f
        development for, 488
    definition of, 481
    development model, 488–489
    DNA, 482–484, 483f
    for healthcare providers, 105
    history of, 481
    inactivated, 482
    international travel vaccines, 494, 495t
    live, attenuated, 482
    monitoring of adverse events with, 498–499
    nucleic acid, 482–484
    polysaccharide, 90
    polysaccharide and conjugate
        meningococcal protein conjugate, 487
        meningococcal vaccines, 487
        pneumococcal vaccines, 487
        Salmonella typhi (Vi) vaccine, 487
        toxoid vaccines, 487–488
    protein-conjugated, 90
    recombinant protein, 485–487
    replicating and nonreplicating viral vector, 488
    representative, 490
        for Chikungunya, 490
        for dengue fever, 490–494
        for herpes zoster, 490–491
        for HIV-AIDS, 491–493, 492b–493b. *See also* Acquired immunodeficiency syndrome (AIDS)
        for influenza, 493–494
    RNA, 484
    safety issues in, 497–499
    side effects and adverse events, 497–498
    subunit vaccines and carriers, 485–488
    types of, 481–488
    for viral hepatitis, 276
        hepatitis A virus (HAV), 276, 277b–278b
        hepatitis B virus (HBV), 277b–278b
    virus-like particle (VLP) vaccines, 485
Valvular heart disease, 223
Van der Waals forces, 60
Variable (V) region, 54
Variants, immunoglobulin (Ig), 51b, 56t. *See also* Immunoglobulin (Ig) classes
    allotype determinants, 56
    idiotype determinants, 56
    isotype determinants, 56
Variation, coefficient. *See* Coefficient of variation (CV)
Varicella-zoster virus (VZV), 215–216, 215b
    epidemiology of, 215
    etiology of, 215
    laboratory diagnosis of, 215–216
    prevention of, 216
    shingles and, 215
    signs and symptoms of, 215
        complications of, 215
        neonatal varicella infection, 215
        zoster infection, 215
    vaccine for, 216
Variolation, 481
Vasculitic syndromes, 375, 375b
Vasculitis, 375, 375b

INDEX

Vasodilation, 341
VCA. See Viral capsid antigen (VCA)
VDRL. See Venereal Disease Research Laboratory (VDRL) Test
Vector-borne diseases, 240–266.e1
  babesiosis, 242t–243t, 252–253
    diagnostic evaluation, 253
    epidemiology of, 252–253
    etiology of, 252, 253f
    prevention of, 253
    signs and symptoms of, 253
    treatment for, 253
  case study for, 263b–264b
  Chikungunya disease, 258–259, 258b
    diagnostic evaluation, 258–259
    epidemiology of, 258
    etiology of, 258
    signs and symptoms, 258
    treatment and prevention, 259
  dengue fever, 199, 242t–243t, 259–262
    characteristics of, 259b
    diagnostic evaluation of, 260, 261b
    epidemiology of, 259
    etiology of, 259
    nucleic acid amplification tests, 260–262
    signs and symptoms of, 259–260
    treatment and prevention of, 262
  examples of, 242t–243t
  human ehrlichiosis, 250–251, 250b
    diagnostic evaluation of, 250–251, 251f
    epidemiology of, 250
    etiology of, 250
    signs and symptoms of, 250
    treatment and prevention of, 251
  Lyme disease, 243–250
    antibiotics for, 249–250
    antibody detection of, 249
    arthritis in, 245–246
    cerebrospinal fluid analyses, 249
    characteristics of, 243b
    cutaneous manifestations of, 246, 246f
    diagnostic evaluation of, 247–249, 249t
    enzyme-linked immunosorbent assay for, 248
    epidemiology of, 244, 245f
    etiology of, 243, 244f
    immunologic manifestations of, 246–247
    neurologic manifestations of, 246
    polymerase chain reaction, 248–249
    pregnancy in, 246
    prevention of, 249–250
    signs and symptoms of, 244–247, 245t
    stages of, 244
    treatment for, 249–250
    Western blot analysis for, 248, 249f
  malaria, 253–258
    characteristics of *Plasmodium* species, 254, 255f
    COVID-19 pandemic and, 254
    diagnostic laboratory evaluation, 256–258, 256f–257f
    disease phase in humans, 254
    epidemiology of, 254
    etiology of, 253–254
    global distribution and statistics, 254
    risk of, 254
    signs and symptoms, 255–256
    treatment and prevention, 258
  Rocky Mountain spotted fever, 252, 252b
    diagnostic evaluation of, 252
    epidemiology of, 252
    etiology of, 252
    signs and symptoms of, 252
    treatment and prevention of, 252

Vector-borne diseases *(Continued)*
  West Nile virus, 262–265, 262b
    diagnostic evaluation of, 263
    epidemiology of, 262, 262–263, 262f
    etiology of, 262
    signs and symptoms of, 263
    treatment and prevention of, 263–265
Venereal Disease Research Laboratory (VDRL) Test, 132, 234
Vertical flow immunoassays, 197
Viral capsid antigen (VCA), 267, 270
Viral core protein, 315
Viral diseases, 195
  cellular replication and, 195
  cytomegalovirus (CMV), 210–214
  dengue fever, 199
  hepatitis, 273–298. See also Viral hepatitis
    general characteristics of, 274, 274t
    hepatitis A virus (HAV), 274t
    hepatitis B virus (HBV), 274t
    hepatitis C virus (HCV), 274t
  herpes viruses, 214–216
    cytomegalovirus, 214. See also Cytomegalovirus (CMV)
    Epstein-Barr virus, 214. See also Epstein-Barr virus (EBV)
    herpes simplex virus, 214–215
    human herpes virus 6, 214
    varicella-zoster virus, 215–216
  mutation and, 195
  zoonoses and, 195
Viral hepatitis, 273–298
  case studies of, 293b–294b
  characteristics of, 274, 274t–275t, 275f
  definition of, 274
  forms of, 274, 275t
    acute, 275t
    chronic, 275t
    fulminant acute, 275t
    subclinical without jaundice, 275t
  general characteristics of, 274, 274t–275t
    differential diagnosis of, 274, 275f
    etiology of, 274
    incidence of, 274, 274t
    signs and symptoms of, 274, 275t
  hepatitis A virus (HAV), 274–278, 274b
    characteristics of, 274t
    diagnostic evaluations of, 276
    epidemiology of, 275
    etiology of, 275, 276f
    immunologic manifestations of, 276
    prevention of, 276–278, 277b–278b
    signs and symptoms of, 275–276
    treatments for, 276–278, 277b–278b
    vaccines for, 277b–278b
  hepatitis B virus (HBV), 275t, 278–287, 278b
    acute infection, 285–286
    antibodies, anti-HBe and anti-HBs, 285
    antigens, hepatitis B core (HBcAg), 284
    antigens, hepatitis B-related (HBeAg), 284
    antigens, hepatitis B surface (HBsAg), 281
    asymptomatic infections, 280–281
    carrier state of, 286–287
    chronic infection, 286
    coinfections with, hepatitis D virus, 288
    diagnostic evaluations of, 285
    epidemiology of, 278–280, 280f
    etiology of, 276f, 278, 279f
    hepatocellular necrosis and, 286
    laboratory assays of, 281–285, 281f–283f, 284t
    persistent infections, 280
    prevention of, 277b–278b, 287
    serologic patterns of, 286
    signs and symptoms of, 280–281

Viral hepatitis *(Continued)*
    treatment for, 287
    viral deoxyribonucleic acid (DNA), 285
  hepatitis C virus (HCV), 288–292, 288b
    acute infections, 291–292
    chronic infections, 291–292
    community-acquired infections, 289
    epidemiology of, 288–289, 289f
    etiology of, 288
    mother-to-infant transmissions, 289
    occupational exposure, 289
    parenteral exposure, 289
    polymerase chain reaction (PCR) amplification for, 290–291
    posttransfusion infections, 289
    prevention of, 292
    prognosis for, 289–290
    recombinant erythropoietin (EPO) for, 289
    sexual transmission of, 289
    signs and symptoms of, 290
    sporadic infections, 289
    testing algorithm for, 290f
    testing, traditional, 290–291, 290f, 291t
    transmission of, 289–290
    treatment for, 291
  hepatitis D virus (HDV), 287–288
    chronic infections, 287
    coinfections, hepatitis B virus (HBV), 288
    diagnostic evaluations of, 288
    epidemiology of, 287–288
    etiology of, 287
    hepadnavirus and, 288
    immunologic manifestations of, 288
    signs and symptoms of, 288
    superinfections, 288
  hepatitis E virus (HEV), 292–293, 292b
    diagnostic evaluations of, 293
    epidemiology of, 292
    etiology of, 292
    immunologic manifestations of, 293
    prevention of, 293
    signs and symptoms of, 292–293
    treatments for, 293
  epidemiology of, 292
  etiology of, 292
  GB virus type C (GBV-C) and, 274
  prevention of, 293
  signs and symptoms of, 293
  transfusion-transmitted virus (TTV), 293–295, 293b
    epidemiology of, 293
    etiology of, 293
    signs and symptoms of, 293–295
Viral load testing, 326
Viral oncogenes, 461, 461b. See also Oncogenes
Viremia, 275
Virgin (naïve) lymphocytes, 13
Virions, 286
Virus-like particle (VLP) vaccines, 485
Vitamin B_{12} (cobalamin) transport, 381, 382t
Vitamins, 399
Volumetric pipettes, 119f
VRC01, 493
VZV. See Varicella-zoster virus (VZV)

W

Waived testing, 123
Waldenström's primary macroglobulinemia (WM), 363–365
  cardiopulmonary abnormalities and, 364
  cutaneous manifestations of, 364
  diagnostic evaluation of, 364–365
  epidemiology of, 363
  etiology of, 363

Waldenström's primary macroglobulinemia (WM) *(Continued)*
   hematologic abnormalities of, 363–364
   hematologic assessment of, 364
   immunologic assessment of, 364–365
   immunologic manifestations of, 364
   neuropsychiatric problems and, 364
   ocular manifestations of, 364
   renal dysfunction and, 364
   signs and symptoms of, 363–364
   skeletal features of, 363
   treatment of, 365
Warm autoimmune hemolytic anemia, 346
WAS. *See* Wiskott-Aldrich syndrome (WAS)
Waste, containers for, 104
Waste, infectious
   disposal of, 104
   final decontamination of, 104
Western blot analysis, for Lyme disease, 248, 249f
Western equine encephalitis, 242t–243t
West Nile encephalitis, 242t–243t
West Nile fever, 242t–243t
West Nile virus (WNV), 241, 262–265, 262b
   diagnostic evaluation of, 263
   epidemiology of, 262, 262–263, 262f
   etiology of, 262
   signs and symptoms of, 263
   treatment and prevention of, 263–265

WHO. *See* World Health Organization (WHO)
Wiskott-Aldrich syndrome (WAS), 312–313
   malignancies in, 313
WM. *See* Waldenström's primary macroglobulinemia (WM)
WNV. *See* West Nile virus (WNV)
Wood tick, 242t–243t
Work surfaces, decontamination of, 103
World Health Organization (WHO)
   classification for dengue severity, 259–260
   congenital syphilis elimination strategies, 232
   geographic data, of dengue fever, 199
   incidence data, 316
      of acquired immunodeficiency syndrome (AIDS), 306
      of viral hepatitis, 274
   influenza vaccines and, 494
   of viral hepatitis, 274

X

X-CGD. *See* X-linked diseases
Xenogenic valve replacement, 438
Xenograft, 435t. *See also* Grafts
Xenopsylla cheopis, 242t–243t
Xenotransplantation, 448, 448b
   milestones in, 448b
X-linked chronic granulomatous disease (X-CGD), 75
X-linked diseases
   agammaglobulinemia, Bruton, 309–310
   chronic granulomatous disease (X-CGD), 75
X-linked lymphoproliferative disease (XLP) syndromes 1 and 2, 312

Y

Yaws, 228–229. *See also* Syphilis

Z

Zeta potential, 60, 133b, 135f
   of hemagglutination, 134
   techniques to reduce, 135t
Zone of equivalence, 129
Zoonoses, 195
Zoonotic toxoplasmosis, 201. *See also* Toxoplasmosis
Zoster infection, 215. *See also* Varicella-zoster virus (VZV)
Zymosan, 32